Blood and
Bone Marrow
PATHOLOGY

Commissioning Editor: Michael J Houston
Project Development Manager: Sheila Black
Project Manager: Camilla Rockwood
Designer: Sarah Russell
Illustration Manager: Mick Ruddy
Illustrator: Robin Dean

Blood and Bone Marrow PATHOLOGY

Edited by

Sunitha N. Wickramasinghe

ScD PhD MB BS FRCP FRCPath FIBiol

Emeritus Professor of Hematology, University of London
Visiting Professor of Hematology, University of Oxford
Formerly Head of the Department of Hematology
St Mary's Hospital Medical School
Imperial College of Science, Technology and Medicine
London, UK

Jeffrey McCullough MD

Professor of Laboratory Medicine and Pathology
Variety Children's Association Chair in Molecular and Cellular Therapy
Director, Biomedical Engineering Institute
University of Minnesota
Minneapolis, Minnesota, USA

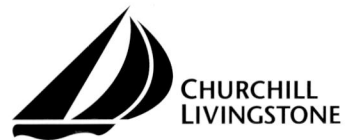

CHURCHILL
LIVINGSTONE

CHURCHILL LIVINGSTONE
An imprint of Elsevier Science Limited

First published 2003
Reprinted 2003

ISBN 0 443 06436 9

British Library Cataloguing in Publication Data
A catalogue record for this book is available from the British Library

Library of Congress Cataloging in Publication Data
A catalog record for this book is available from the Library of Congress

Note
Medical knowledge is constantly changing. As new information
becomes available, changes in treatment, procedures, equipment and
the use of drugs become necessary. The editors and the publishers
have taken care to ensure that the information given in this text is
accurate and up to date. However, readers are strongly advised to
confirm that the information, especially with regard to drug usage,
complies with the latest legislation and standards of practice.

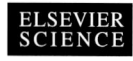 your source for books,
journals and multimedia
in the health sciences
www.elsevierhealth.com

The
publisher's
policy is to use
**paper manufactured
from sustainable forests**

Colour Separation and Typesetting by RDC Tech Group
Printed in China

Contents

Preface   vii

List of contributors   ix

SECTION 1
Normal blood and bone marrow cells

1   Normal blood cells   3
    S.N. Wickramasinghe

2   Normal bone marrow cells:
    development, cytology and
    ultrastructure   23
    S.N. Wickramasinghe

3   Normal bone marrow: histology,
    histochemistry and
    immunohistochemistry   53
    R. Bartl, B. Frisch

4   Regulation of hematopoiesis   71
    C. Verfaillie

SECTION 2
Pathology of the marrow

5   General considerations   89
    S.N. Wickramasinghe, B.J. Bain

SECTION 3
Disorders affecting erythroid cells

6   Investigation and classification
    of anemia   131
    S.N. Wickramasinghe

7   Abnormalities of the red cell
    membrane   141
    J. Delaunay

8   Erythroenzyme disorders   149
    D.M. Layton, D.R. Roper

9   Abnormalities of the structure
    and synthesis of hemoglobin   159
    S.L. Thein

10 Acquired hemolytic anemias   185
    J.G. Kelton, H. Chan, N. Heddle,
    S. Whittaker

11 Iron deficiency anemia, anemia of
    chronic disorder and iron overload   203
    M.J. Pippard

12 Macrocytic anemia   229
    S.N. Wickramasinghe

13 Aplastic anemia   249
    E.C. Gordon-Smith

14 Pure red cell aplasia and
    sideroblastic anemias   265
    S.N. Wickramasinghe

15 Congenital dyserythropoietic anemias   273
    S.N. Wickramasinghe

16 Polycythemia (the erythrocytoses)   283
    M. Messinezy, J.D. van der Walt,
    T.C. Pearson

SECTION 4
Disorders affecting leukocyte lineages

17 Abnormalities in leucocyte
    morphology and number   299
    S.N. Wickramasinghe

18 Disorders of phagocyte function   321
    J.R. Brown, A.J. Thrasher

19 Myelodysplastic disorders   331
    T.J. Hamblin, B.S. Wilkins

20 Acute leukemias   351
    D.M. Swirsky, S.J. Richards, P.A.S. Evans

21 The chronic lymphoid and myeloid leukemias and systemic mastocytosis   381
D.M. Clark, B.J. Bain

22 Lymphoma   405
B.S. Wilkins, D. Oscier

23 Abnormalities in immunoglobulin synthesising cells   437
F. Davies, K. Anderson

Abnormalities of hemostasis

24 Hemostasis: principles of investigation   473
D.H. Bevan

25 Disorders affecting megakarocytes and platelets: inherited conditions   493
J.G. White

26 Acquired disorders affecting megakaryocytes and platelets   525
D. Provan, A.C. Newland

27 Inherited disorders of coagulation   557
C.A. Lee

28 Acquired bleeding disorders   577
D.J. Perry

29 Natural anticoagulants and thrombophilia   599
M.A. Laffan

Immunohematology

30 Blood groups on red cells, platelets and neutrophils   615
G. Daniels, A. Hadley

31 Transfusion medicine for pathologists   637
J. McCullough

32 Histocompatibility: HLA and other systems   665
P.E. Posch, R.J. Hartzman, C.K. Hurley

Index   709

Preface

The science and practice of hematology continues to advance at an impressive pace. This book provides a concise and up-to-date account of the anatomy, physiology and pathology of the blood and bone marrow. The appearances of blood and marrow smears and of histological sections of bone marrow in disease are extensively illustrated in color. To complement these discussions of hematopathology, chapters on the HLA system and transfusion medicine are included. The contributors, all experts in their field, have written in their own style with their own preference regarding the balance between biochemistry, pathophysiology, cytology, histopathology and clinical aspects. The book does not deal with the treatment of hematological disorders in any detail; usually only principles underlying treatment are provided. As in other multi-author books there is inevitably some overlap between the contributions of various authors and the editors have not attempted to eliminate all such overlap. We are grateful to the contributors, all busy scientists or clinicians, for taking time to provide excellent chapters for this book. We hope that *Blood and Bone Marrow Pathology* will serve as a useful reference text for both histopathologists and hematologists.

Sunitha N Wickramasinghe   2002
Jeffrey McCullough

Contributors

Kenneth C Anderson MD PhD
Professor of Medicine, Harvard Medical School
Director, Jerome Lipper Multiple Myeloma Center
Dana-Farber Cancer Institute
Boston, MA
USA

Barbara J Bain FRACP FRCPath
Reader in Hematology
Department of Hematology
St Mary's Hospital
London, UK

Reiner Bartl
Osteologische Ambulanz
Klinikum Großshadern
Medizinische Klinik und Poliklinik III
Klinikum der Universität
München
Germany

David Huw Bevan FRCP FRCPath
Senior Lecturer and Honorary Consultant in
  Hematology
Department of Hematology
St George's Hospital Medical School
London, UK

Joanne R Brown PhD
Post-doctoral Research Fellow
Immunobiology Unit
The Institute of Child Health
Great Ormond Street Hospital
London, UK

Howard H W Chan MBChB FRCPC
Clinical Fellow, Transfusion Medicine
McMaster University
Hamilton
Ontario, Canada

David M Clark MD MRCP (UK) FRCPath
Consultant Cellular Pathologist
Pathlinks Department of Pathology
Grantham and District Hospital
Lincolnshire, UK

Geoff Daniels PhD MRCPath
Senior Research Fellow
Bristol Institute for Transfusion Sciences
Bristol, UK

Faith E Davies MB BCh MRCP MD
Department of Health Clinician Scientist
Academic Department of Hematology and
  Oncology
University of Leeds
Leeds, UK

Jean Delaunay MD PhD
Professor of Genetics
Service d'Hématologie, d'Immunologie et de
  Cytogénétique
Hôpital de Bicêtre
Faculté de Médecine
Paris
France

Paul A S Evans PhD FIBMS
Chief Biomedical Scientist
Hematological Malignancy Diagnostic Service
Institute of Pathology
Leeds, UK

Bertha Frisch MD
Professor of Hematology
Department of Pathology
Ichilov Hospital
Tel-Aviv
Israel

E C Gordon-Smith
MA MSc FRCPATH FRCP FRCP (E) FMedsci
Professor of Hematology
Department of Hematology
St George's Hospital Medical School
London, UK

Andrew G Hadley BSc DPhil
National Stem Cell Services Manager
National Blood Service
Bristol, UK

T J Hamblin MB ChB DM FRCP FRCPath FMedSci
Professor of Immunohematology
Department of Hematology
The Royal Bournemouth Hospital
Bournemouth, UK

Robert J Hartzman MD
Director, CW Bill Young/Department of Defense
Marrow Donor Recruitment and Research Program
Naval Medical Research Center
Kensington, MD
USA

Nancy Heddle MSc ART
Associate Professor
Department of Medicine
McMaster University
Ontario
Canada

Carolyn K Hurley PhD
Professor of Oncology
Department of Oncology
Georgetown University Medical Center
Washington, DC
USA

John G Kelton MD FRCPC
Professor
Departments of Medicine and Pathology and Molecular Medicine
McMaster University Medical Centre
Hamilton, Ontario
Canada

Michael Laffan DM FRCP FRCPath
Senior Lecturer In Hematology
Department of Hematology
Imperial College
London, UK

D Mark Layton MB BS FRCP FRCPCH
Consultant and Honorary Reader
Department of Hematology
Hammersmith Hospital
Imperial College of Science, Technology and Medicine
London, UK

Christine Lee MA MD DSc(Med) FRCP FRCPath
Director & Consultant Hematologist
Hemophilia Centre & Hemostasis Unit
London, UK

Jeffrey McCullough MD
Department of Laboratory Medicine and Pathology
University of Minnesota
Minneapolis, MN
USA

Maria Messinezy FRCP FRCPath
Formerly Clinical Assistant
Hematology Department
Guy's King's & St Thomas' School of Medicine
London, UK

A C Newland MA FRCP FRCPath
Professor of Hematology
Department of Hematology
The Royal London Hospital
London, UK

David Oscier MA FRCP FRCPath
Honorary Clinical Senior Lecturer, Southampton University
Consultant Hematologist
Department of Hematology
Royal Bournemouth Hospital
Bournemouth, UK

Thomas C Pearson MD FRCPath
Professor of Hematology
Hematology Department
Guy's King's & St Thomas' School of Medicine
London, UK

David J Perry MD PhD FRCP FRCPath
Senior Lecturer
Hemophilia Centre & Hemostasis Unit
Royal Free Hospital
London, UK

Martin J Pippard BSc MB ChB FRCP FRCPath
Professor of Hematology
Department of Molecular & Cellular Pathology
Ninewells Hospital and Medical School
Dundee, UK

Phillip E Posch PhD
Instructor
Department of Microbiology and Immunology
Georgetown University Medical Center
Washington, DC
USA

Drew Provan MD FRCP FRCPath
Senior Lecturer in Hematology
Department of Hematology
Barts and the London School of Medicine and Dentistry
London, UK

Stephen J Richards PhD MRCPath
Consultant Clinical Scientist
Department of Hematology
Hematological Malignancy Diagnostic Service
Leeds General Infirmary
Leeds, UK

David Roper
Diagnostic Laboratory
Hammersmith Hospital
London, UK

David M Swirsky FRCP, MRCPath
Consultant Hematologist
Hematological Malignancy Diagnostic Service
Leeds General Infirmary
Leeds, UK

Swee Lay Thein MB BS, FRCP, FRCPath, DSc
Professor of Molecular Hematology
Department of Hematological Medicine
Guy's, King's & St Thomas' School of Medicine
London, UK

Adrian Thrasher PhD MBBS MRCP(Vh) MRCPCH
Reader in Pediatric Immunology
Molecular Immunology Unit
Institute of Child Health
London, UK

Jon D Van Der Walt MB BCh FRCPath
Senior Lecturer and Honorary Consultant in
Histopathology
Department of Histopathology
St Thomas' Hospital
London, UK

Catherine Verfaillie MD
Professor of Medicine and Director
Stem Cell Institute
University of Minnesota
Minneapolis, MN
USA

James G White MD
Regents Professor
Laboratory Medicine and Pathology, and Pediatrics
University of Minnesota School of Medicine
Minneapolis, MN
USA

Susan Whittaker BSc BA MSc
Research Fellow
Transfusion Medical Trials Centre
Hamilton
Ontario
Canada

Sunitha N Wickramasinghe ScD PhD MB BS FRCP FRCPath
FIBiol
Emeritus Professor of Hematology, University of London
Visiting Professor of Hematology, University of Oxford
Formerly Head of the Department of Hematology
St Mary's Hospital Medical School
Imperial College of Science, Technology and Medicine
London, UK

Bridget S Wilkins MB BCh DM PhD FRCPath
Consultant/Honorary Senior Lecturer in Pathology
Department of Histopathology
Royal Victoria Infirmary
Newcastle upon Tyne, UK

Normal blood and bone marrow cells and hematopoiesis

Normal blood cells 3

Normal bone marrow cells: Development, cytology and ultrastructure 23

Normal bone marrow: histology, histochemistry and immunohistochemistry 53

Regulation of hematopoiesis 71

Normal blood cells 1

SN Wickramasinghe

Erythrocytes

Morphology

Red cell parameters

Red cell life span

Functions of red cells

Reticulocytes

Granulocytes (polymorphonuclear leukocytes)

Neutrophil granulocytes
Morphology and composition
Number and life span
Functions of neutrophils

Eosinophil granulocytes
Morphology and composition
Number and life span
Functions

Basophil granulocytes

Monocytes

Lymphocytes

Platelets
Morphology and composition
Number and life span

Functions

Alterations in the blood in pregnancy

Blood consists of a pale-yellow, coagulable fluid called plasma in which various types of blood cells are suspended. The cells comprise the erythrocytes, granulocytes, monocytes, lymphocytes and platelets. Blood also contains very small numbers of circulating hemopoietic stem cells and progenitor cells, mast cell progenitors, megakaryocytes and megakaryocyte bare nuclei.

Erythrocytes

Morphology

Erythrocytes are highly differentiated cells that have no nuclei or cytoplasmic organelles. Normal erythrocytes are circular biconcave discs with a mean diameter of 7.2 µm (range 6.7–7.7 µm) in dried fixed smears and about 7.5 µm in the living state. They are eosinophilic and

consequently appear red with a central area of pallor in smears stained by a Romanowsky stain (Fig. 1.1).

Red cell parameters[1]

The three basic parameters which can be measured in relation to the red cell population are: (1) the concentration of hemoglobin per unit volume of blood after lysis of the red cells (hemoglobin concentration); (2) the number of red cells per unit volume of blood (red cell count); and (3) the hematocrit. The hemoglobin concentration is usually determined spectrophotometrically, after conversion to cyanmethemoglobin. The red cell count was previously determined visually using counting chambers but modern automated blood-counting machines determine this parameter more precisely using electrical impedance or light-scattering techniques. The hematocrit (packed cell volume – PCV) was originally determined after centrifugation of the blood in tubes of

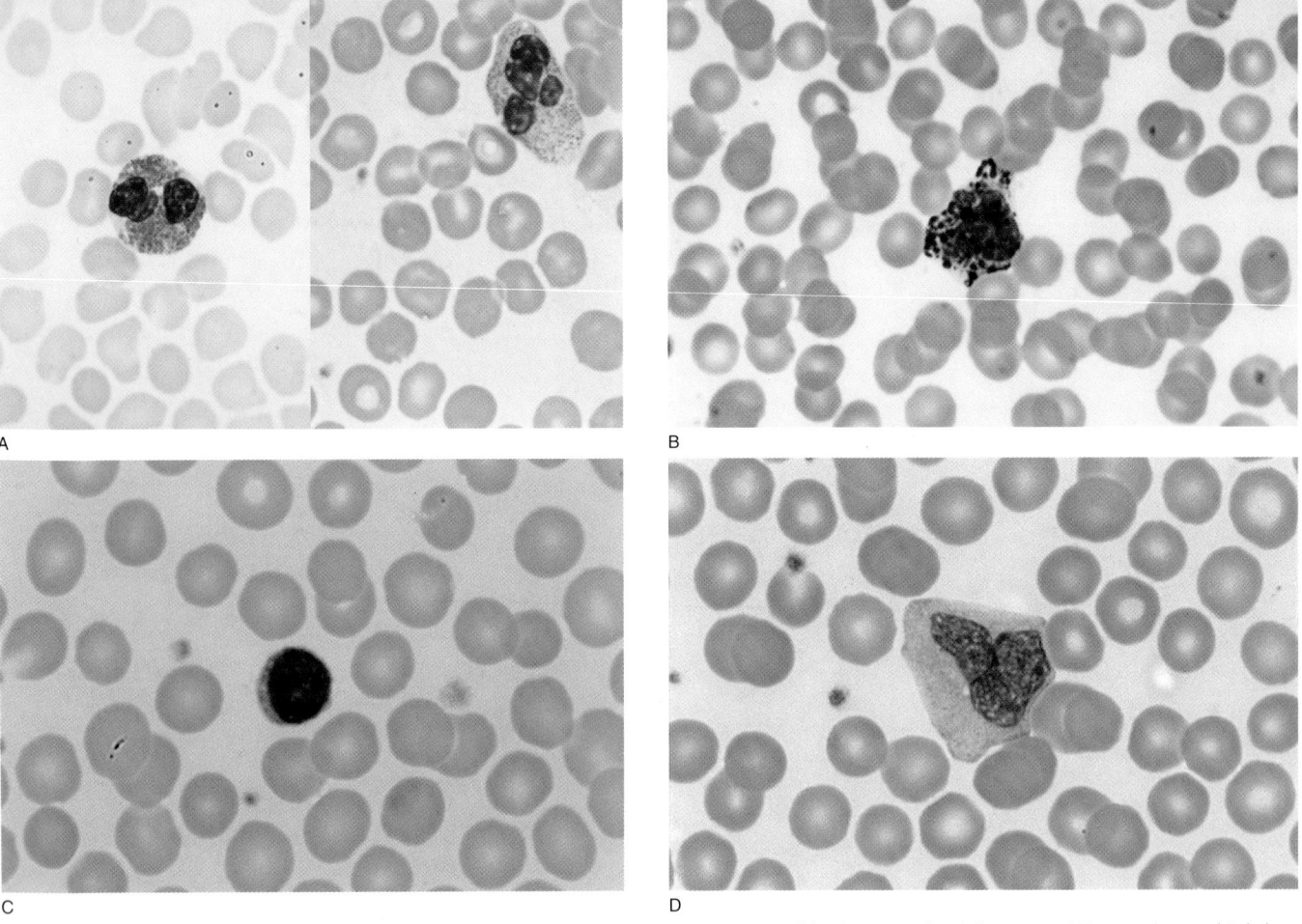

A

B

C

D

Fig. 1.1 (A–D) Cells from peripheral blood smears of normal individuals. May–Grünwald–Giemsa stain. (A) Neutrophil granulocyte (right) and eosinophil granulocyte (left). (B) Basophil granulocyte. (C) Small lymphocyte. (D) Monocyte. Red cells and platelets are seen in all the photomicrographs. (C) and (D) are at a slightly higher magnification than (A) and (B).

standard specification under a fixed centrifugal force and for a fixed time. It was defined as the length of the column of resulting packed red cells expressed as a fraction or percentage of the length of the column of cells plus plasma. The value obtained for the PCV includes the volume of some plasma trapped between the red cells. From the values obtained for the hemoglobin concentration, red cell count and PCV, it is possible to calculate the mean cell volume (MCV), mean cell hemoglobin (MCH) and mean cell hemoglobin concentration (MCHC) as shown in Table 1.1. Automatic blood-counting machines determine the MCV using electrical impedance or light-scattering techniques and calculate the PCV from the measured MCV and red cell count. The normal values for various red cell parameters at different ages are given in Tables 1.2 and 1.3. Between the age of 2 years and the onset of puberty there is a gradual rise in the hemoglobin concentration in both sexes. In the next few years there is a further rise in males but not females with the result that the mean hemoglobin value is higher in adult males than in adult females. In healthy infants aged 4 months and over, and in healthy young children, the average MCV is lower than in healthy adults.[4,6,9] Whereas the lower limit for the MCV in unselected healthy adults is 82 fl, the corresponding figure for children between 1 and 7 years

(who show no biochemical evidence of iron deficiency) is about 70 fl. The MCV increases progressively with age both in children and, to a much lesser extent, in adults.

Red cell life span[10–12]

As red cells do not contain ribosomes, they cannot synthesize new protein to replace essential molecules (e.g. enzymes, structural proteins) which become denatured in the course of time. Red cells therefore have a limited life span of 110–120 days, at the end of which they are ingested and degraded by the macrophages of the marrow, spleen, liver and other organs. A variety of changes affect red cells as they age within the circulation. These include a progressive decrease in MCV and in surface area, a progressive increase in density and osmotic fragility, a decrease in deformability, a decreased ability to reduce methemoglobin and a decrease in the rate of glycolysis. Recent studies suggest that the critical change which causes a red cell to be destroyed at the end of its life span could be the formation of denatured/oxidized hemoglobin (hemichromes) which induces clustering of the integral membrane protein, band 3. This clustering generates an epitope on the red cell surface that binds autologous IgG and the antibody-coated aged erythrocytes are recognized and phagocytosed by macrophages.[13] A second mechanism that may be involved in the recognition of aged red cells by macrophages is the exposure of phosphatidylserine on the outer surface of their cell membrane.[14]

Functions of red cells[15–17]

Normal function of the erythrocyte requires a normal red cell membrane, and normal enzyme systems providing

Table 1.1 Calculation of red cell indices

MCV (in fl)	$= PCV^a \div RBC$ per liter $\times 10^{15}$
MCH (in pg)	$= Hb^b \div RBC$ per liter $\times 10^{13}$
MCHC (in g/dl)	$= Hb^b \div PCV^a$

Hb, hemoglobin; MCH, mean corpuscular hemoglobin; MCHC, mean corpuscular hemoglobin concentration; MCV, mean corpuscular volume; PCV, packed cell volume; RBC, red blood cells.
[a] Expressed as a fraction.
[b] In g/dl.

Table 1.2 95% reference limits for some hematologic parameters in healthy Caucasian adults[a] determined in the UK using a Coulter Counter Model S Plus III or IV[2]

	Men		Women
Hb (g/dl)	13.4–16.7 ($n = 100$)		11.9–14.7 ($n = 100$)
Red cell count (10^{12}/l)	4.4–5.7 ($n = 100$)		3.9–5.0 ($n = 100$)
PCV	0.40–0.51[b] ($n = 100$)		0.36–0.45[b] ($n = 100$)
MCV		82.5–99 fl[b] ($n = 200$)	
MCH		27–32.8 pg ($n = 200$)	
MCHC		32–34 g/dl ($n = 200$)	
Platelet count (10^9/l)	168–411 ($n = 148$)		188–445 ($n = 225$)

Hb, hemoglobin; MCH, mean corpuscular hemoglobin; MCHC, mean corpuscular hemoglobin concentration; MCV, mean corpuscular volume; PCV, packed cell volume.
[a] Aged 18–60 years.
[b] 3% correction for plasma trapping.

Table 1.3 Age-dependent changes in the mean values (and 95% reference limits) for red cell parameters in normal individuals

Age	n	Hemoglobin (Hb)(g/dl)	Red blood cell count (RBC) ($\times 10^{12}$/l)	Mean corpuscular volume (MCV) (fl)	Reference and other details
Cord blood	59	17.1(13.5–20.7)	4.6(3.6–5.6)	113(101–125)	a
1 day	59	19.4(15.1–23.7)	5.3(4.2–6.4)	110(99–121)	a
1 month*	240	13.9(10.7–17.1)	4.3(3.3–5.3)	101(91–112)	b
2 months*	241	11.2(9.4–13.0)	3.7(3.1–4.3)	95(84–106)	b
4 months*	52	12.2(10.3–14.1)	4.3(3.5–5.1)	87(76–97)	b
6 months*	52	12.6(11.1–14.1)	4.7(3.9–5.5)	76(68–85)	b
12 months	56*	12.7(11.3–14.1)	4.7(4.1–5.3)	78(71–84)	b
	51	11.1(7.7–14.5)	4.8(3.8–5.8)	73(58–88)	a
	163	10.1(7.5–12.7)	4.7(3.5–5.5)	72(58–86)	c
10–17 months*	59			77(70–84)	d
3 years	103	12.4(10.1–14.7)	4.7(3.9–5.5)	78(68–88)	a
	128	11.0(8.6–13.4)	4.5(3.5–5.5)	78(64–92)	c
18 months–4 years*	26			80(74–86)	d
5 years	97	12.7(10.7–14.7)	4.7(3.7–5.6)	80(72–88)	a
	24	11.8(9.2–14.4)	4.4(3.7–5.1)	83(69–97)	c
4–7 years*	42			81(76–86)	d
7 years	103	12.9(9.2–16.6)	4.8(3.8–5.8)	79(61–97)	a
7–8 years	151	12.5(10.3–14.7)	4.6(4.0–5.2)	81(72–89)	e
10 years	111	13.2(10.8–15.6)	4.8(3.9–5.7)	81(68–94)	a
14 years	45	13.6(10.7–16.5)	4.9(3.9–5.9)	81(66–96)	a
20 years male	–	15.9(13.7–18.3)	5.3(4.6–6.2)	89(78–99)	f
20 years female	–	13.8(11.7–15.8)	4.6(4.0–5.4)	89(76–99)	f
60 years male	–	15.9(13.8–18.4)	5.0(4.3–5.9)	93(82–103)	f
60 years female	–	13.9(11.8–15.9)	4.6(3.9–5.3)	90(77–100)	f

* Data in which cases with iron deficiency were excluded.
a = Healthy and sick American whites; used microhematocrit and counting chambers.[3]
b = Healthy full-term infants from Finland; continuous iron supplementation; normal transferrin saturation and serum ferritin level; used Coulter counter model S.[4]
c = Healthy Jamaican blacks; cohort study; HbS and β-thalassemia excluded; used Coulter ZBI 6.[5]
d = Healthy Caucasian, Asian and black children in America; Hb > 11.0 g/dl, transferrin saturation ≥ 20%, normal serum ferritin; hemoglobinopathy and β-thalassemia trait excluded; used Coulter counter model S.[6]
e = Healthy individuals; mostly American blacks; used Coulter counter model S.[7]
f = Reference intervals derived form 1744 healthy Americans (ethnic origin not stated) aged 16–89 years using Hemac 630 laser cell counter.[8]

energy and protecting against oxidant damage. The erythrocyte membrane is composed of a lipid bilayer (containing integral proteins) and is bound to a sub-membranous cytoskeletal network of protein molecules including spectrin, actin and the proteins constituting bands 4.1a and 4.1b[18] (Chapter 7). This cytoskeletal network is responsible for maintaining the biconcave shape of a normal red cell. The membrane also contains ATP-dependent cation pumps that continuously pump Na^+ out of and K^+ into the red cell, against concentration gradients, thereby counteracting a continuous passive diffusion of ions across the membrane in the opposite direction. Mature erythrocytes derive their energy from glycolysis by the Embden–Meyerhof pathway (Chapter 8). They can also metabolize glucose through the pentose phosphate pathway, which generates the reduction potential of the cell and protects the membrane, the hemoglobin and erythrocyte enzymes from oxidant damage (Chapter 8). Both a normal cell membrane and normal energy production are required to enable the biconcave red cells to repeatedly and reversibly deform during numerous transits through the microcirculation.

The prime function of the red cell is to combine with oxygen in the lungs and to transport and release this oxygen for utilization by tissues. The red cells also combine with CO_2 produced in tissues and release this in the lungs.

The function of oxygen transport resides in the hemoglobin molecule which is ideally structured for this purpose. Most of the hemoglobin (Hb) of an adult is HbA which is a tetramer consisting of two α-globin chains and two β-globin chains. Each of these globin chains is associated with a heme molecule which is inserted deeply within a pocket which excludes water but allows O_2 to enter and interact with the iron atom at the center of the heme molecule. In the deoxygenated state, the iron atom is in the ferrous state (Fe^{++}) and has a 'spare' electron. In the oxygenated state there is a weak ionic link between the oxygen molecule and the iron atom as a result of the 'sharing' of the 'spare' electron, but the iron remains in the ferrous state. This reaction between the oxygen molecule and the iron atom of the heme ring is reversible and the oxygen is readily released at the low oxygen concentrations found in tissues. The importance of excluding water from the heme pocket is that the water could oxidize the iron atom to the ferric state by accepting the spare electron. Hemoglobin in which the iron atoms are in the ferric state is called methemoglobin and does not combine with oxygen.

The ability of red cells to combine with and release oxygen is illustrated in the oxygen dissociation curve shown in Figure 1.2. The shape of the oxygen dissociation curve of HbA is sigmoid and this is a function of the interaction of the four monomers which make up its tetrameric structure; the shape of the oxygen dissociation curve of the monomer, myoglobin, is hyperbolic. The

advantage of the sigmoid curve over the hyperbolic curve is that much more oxygen is released from the hemoprotein at the low P_{O_2} values obtained in tissues (35–40 mmHg) with the former than with the latter. The percentage saturation of hemoglobin at this P_{O_2} is about 70%. The biochemical basis of the interaction between the four heme groups of the globin chains of the hemoglobin molecule (heme–heme interaction), which determines the sigmoid shape, appears to be related to conformational changes resulting from the combination of oxygen with heme and is dependent on movement at the α_1–β_2 contact. The changes are such that the combination of O_2 with one heme moiety facilitates combination with the other heme moieties. The capacity of hemoglobin to combine with O_2 at a given P_{O_2} is referred to as its oxygen affinity and is expressed as the P_{O_2} required to cause 50% saturation (P_{50}). A decrease in pH leads to a shift of the oxygen dissociation curve to the right and a decrease in oxygen affinity. This effect, which is known as the Bohr effect, facilitates the release of oxygen at the low pH of tissues. A shift of the oxygen dissociation curve to the right also results from the combination of hemoglobin with 2,3-diphosphoglycerate that is produced as a result of the metabolism of glucose via the Rapoport–Luebering shunt of the Embden–Meyerhof pathway (Chapter 8).

The CO_2 produced in the tissues enters the blood. Most of this CO_2 enters the red cells and is converted there to carbonic acid by the enzyme carbonic anhydrase. The hydrogen ions released from the dissociation of this weak acid combine with the hemoglobin, and are largely responsible for the Bohr effect referred to above. A small proportion of the CO_2 entering red cells combines with hemoglobin to form carbaminohemoglobin. When the blood circulates through the lungs, where the P_{CO_2} is lower than that in the blood, the CO_2 is released from the red cells into the alveolar air. The release of CO_2 from red cells results in a reversal of the Bohr effect (i.e. a shift of the oxygen dissociation curve to the left) and the uptake of considerable amounts of O_2. The oxygen saturation and P_{O_2} of arterial blood is greater than 95% and 100 mmHg respectively.

The biconcave shape of normal erythrocytes facilitates the diffusion of gases in and out of the cytoplasm and also imparts adequate flexibility and deformability to enable these cells to repeatedly traverse the microcirculation.

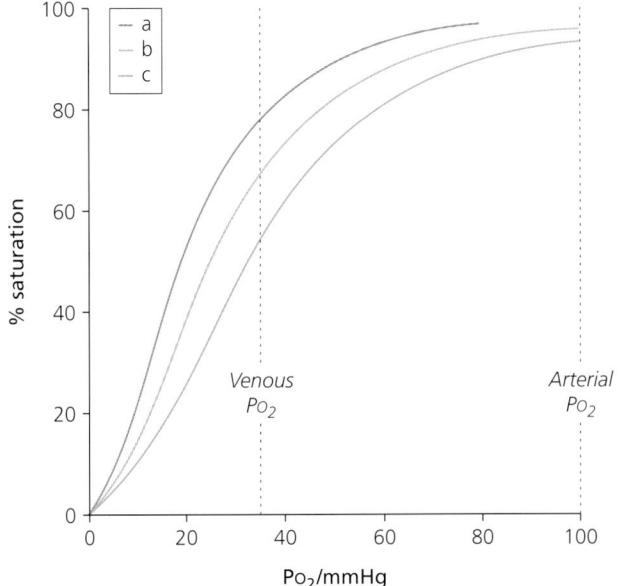

Fig. 1.2 Oxygen dissociation curve of normal adult blood and the effect of varying the pH. P_{O_2} and P_{CO_2} = partial pressure of O_2 and CO_2 respectively. a = pH 7.6 (P_{CO_2} 25 mmHg); b = pH 7.4 (P_{CO_2} 40 mmHg); c = pH 7.2 (P_{CO_2} 61 mmHg).

Reticulocytes

These are the immediate precursors of the red cells. They are rounded anucleate cells that are about 20% larger in volume than mature red cells and appear faintly polychromatic when stained by a Romanowsky method. When stained supravitally with new methylene blue or brilliant cresyl blue, the diffuse basophilic material responsible for the polychromasia (i.e. ribosomal RNA) appears as a basophilic reticulum (Fig. 1.3). Electron-

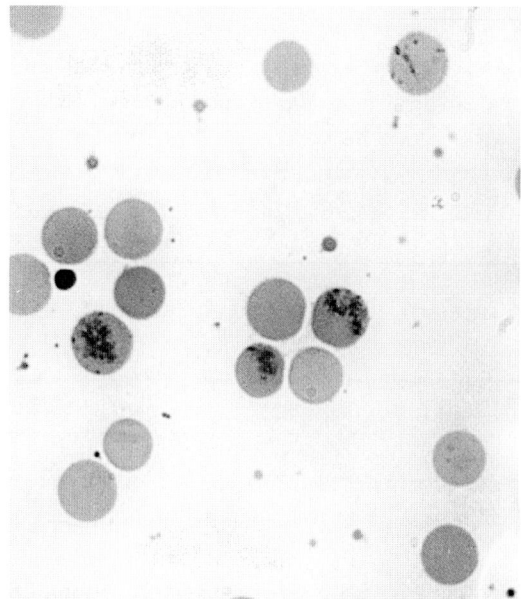

Fig. 1.3 Blood smear containing four reticulocytes, one of which is more mature and contains much less basophilic reticulum than the others. The blood was stained supravitally with brilliant cresyl blue at 37°C for 20 min prior to the preparation of the smear. × 940.

microscope studies[19] have shown that reticulocytes are rounded cells with a tortuous surface and that in addition to ribosomes they contain mitochondria and autophagic vaculoes (Fig. 1.4). Circulating reticulocytes mature into red cells over a period of 1–2 days during which there is a progressive degradation of ribosomes and mitochondria and the acquisition of the biconcave shape. Reticulocytes actively synthesize hemoglobin and non-hemoglobin proteins. They contain enzymes of the Embden–Meyerhof pathway and the pentose phosphate shunt and, unlike the mature red cells, can also derive energy aerobically via the Krebs cycle that operates in the mitochondria and oxidizes pyruvate to CO_2 and water. Supravitally stained preparations were traditionally used and are still frequently used to assess reticulocyte numbers by microscopy with an eyepiece micrometer disc to facilitate counting. In one study of normal adults, reticulocytes counted in this way comprised 0.8–2.6% of the total circulating erythrocyte plus reticulocyte population in males and 1.0–3.7% in females.[20] Although several laboratories still express reticulocyte counts as a percentage, it is more useful to express them as the total number per liter of blood, that is as an absolute reticulocyte count. The latter is directly proportional both to the rate of effective erythropoiesis and the average maturation time of blood reticulocytes.[21] In normal adults the absolute reticulocyte count determined by microscopy was

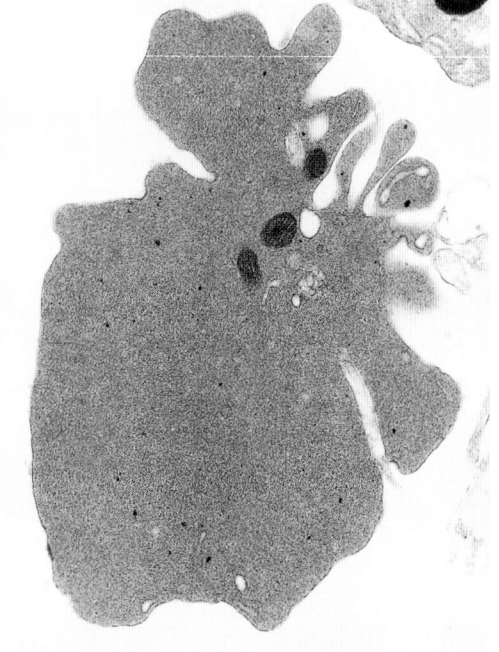
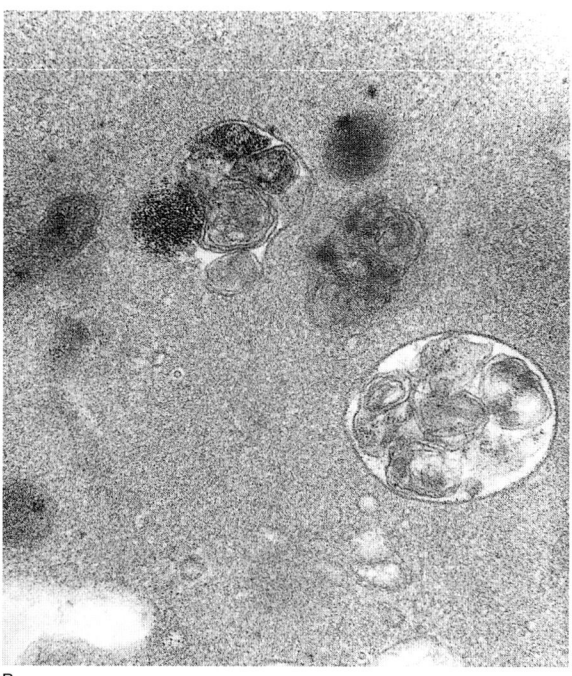

A   B

Fig. 1.4 (A, B) Electron micrographs of two normal reticulocytes. Uranyl acetate and lead citrate. (A) The reticulocyte profile has an irregular outline and contains three mitochondria. × 14 400. (B) Higher power view of part of another reticulocyte showing three autophagic vacuoles. These vacuoles contain structures which may represent mitochondria in the process of degradation. × 19 200.

$18–158 \times 10^9/l.^{22}$ It is now possible to count reticulocytes after staining their RNA with fluorescent reagents such as acridine orange, thioflavin-T, thiazol orange or auramine O, using automated machines employing flow cytometry. Results obtained by flow cytometric methods are more accurate and reproducible than by the traditional method. In one study employing the new techniques, the reference range for adults was $20–70 \times 10^9/l.^{23}$ Another study involving larger numbers of subjects gave slightly higher values and showed that the percentage and absolute reticulocyte counts were significantly higher in men than in women (97.5th percentile: 95.6×10^9 in males and 88×10^9 in females aged 20–29 years).[24]

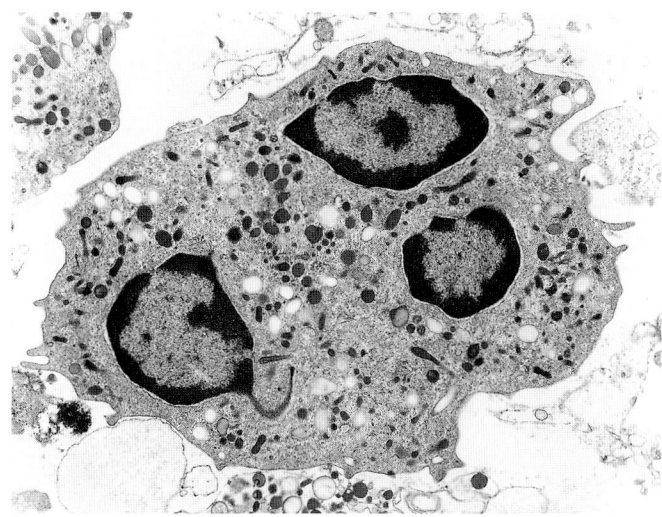

Fig. 1.5 Electron micrograph of a neutrophil granulocyte. The three nuclear segments contain a large quantity of condensed chromatin at their periphery. The cytoplasmic granules vary considerably in size, shape and electron-density. Uranyl acetate and lead citrate. × 5500.

Granulocytes (polymorphonuclear leukocytes)

These cells contain characteristic cytoplasmic granules and a segmented nucleus. The latter consists of two or more nuclear masses (nuclear segments) joined together by fine strands of nuclear chromatin.

The nuclear masses contain moderate quantities of condensed chromatin. The granulocytes are subdivided into neutrophil, eosinophil and basophil granulocytes according to the staining reactions of the granules.

Neutrophil granulocytes

Morphology and composition

Neutrophil granulocytes have a mean volume of 500 fl and, in dried fixed smears, have a diameter of 9–15 µm. Their cytoplasm is slightly acidophilic and contains many very fine granules that stain with neutral dyes; the granules stain a faint purple color with Romanowsky stains (see Fig. 1.1A). The nucleus usually contains two to five nuclear segments; the average values for the proportions of cells with two, three, four and five or more segments are 32, 46, 19 and 3% respectively. In the female, 1–17% of cells contain a drumstick-like appendage attached by a fine strand of chromatin to one of the nuclear masses; these appendages correspond to Barr bodies (inactivated X-chromosomes). Neutrophils possess a variety of surface receptors including those for C3 and IgG-Fc and the CXC chemokine receptors.

Neutrophil granules show a considerable heterogeneity with respect to their ultrastructure[19] (Fig. 1.5) and composition; granule membrane proteins may be incorporated into the cell membrane and soluble granule proteins are exocytosed. Some granules are electron-dense

and ellipsoidal; they are referred to as primary granules and are formed at the promyelocyte stage. Others are less electron-dense and are very pleomorphic; they are termed specific granules and are formed at the myelocyte (secondary granules) and the metamyelocyte (tertiary granules) stages. The primary granules are 0.5–1.0 µm in their long axis and contain myeloperoxidase, lysozyme (muramidase), defensins, bacterial permeability inducer, acid phosphatase, β-glucuronidase, α-mannosidase, elastase, cathepsins B, D and G, and proteinase 3. The specific granules vary considerably in size being frequently quite small (0.2–0.5 µm long) and the granule membrane contains NADPH oxidase (cytochrome b$_{558}$), vitronectin and laminin receptors and CR3. The granule proteins include lysozyme, transcobalamin I (a vitamin B_{12} binding protein), collagenase, $β_2$ microglobulin, lactoferrin or lactoferrin and gelatinase, SGP28 (specific granule protein of 28 kDa),[25] hCAP-18 (human cationic antimicrobial protein) and NGAL (a matrix protein). A third type of granule contains gelatinase but little or no lactoferrin (gelatinase granules) and neutrophils also contain secretory vesicles.[26] The secretory vesicles are involved in adhesion of neutrophils to the endothelium, the gelatinase granules in migration through basement membrane and the primary and specific granules mainly in phagocytosis, killing and digestion of microorganisms.[27] The alkaline phosphatase activity of neutrophils is present within membrane-bound intracytoplasmic vesicles called phosphosomes. In addition to the various organelles mentioned above, the cytoplasm contains a centrosome, a poorly developed Golgi apparatus (Fig. 1.6), microtubules

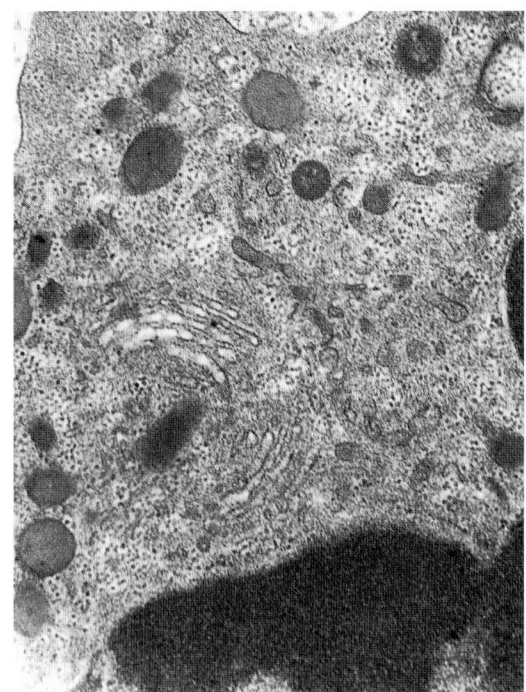

Fig. 1.6 Electron micrograph of part of a neutrophil granulocyte showing the flattened saccules of the Golgi apparatus. The numerous electron-dense particles scattered within the cytosol consist of glycogen. Uranyl acetate and lead citrate. × 33 400.

multivesicular bodies suggesting that only the latter are true lysosomes.[28]

Number and life span

In the blood, the neutrophil granulocytes are distributed between a circulating granulocyte pool (CGP) and a marginated granulocyte pool (MGP).[29] The latter, which is in a rapid equilibrium with the CGP, consists of cells that are loosely associated with the endothelial cells of small venules. The CGP accounts for 16–99% (mean 44%) of the total blood granulocyte pool in healthy subjects. Exercise and adrenaline cause a rapid shift of cells from the MGP to the CGP and bacterial endotoxin causes a shift from the CGP to the MGP. The concentrations of neutrophil granulocytes in the peripheral venous blood of healthy Caucasians of different ages and sexes are given in Tables 1.4 and 1.5. Healthy blacks have lower neutrophil counts than Caucasians (Table 1.4); Chinese and Indians have similar counts to those in Europeans.[32] Considerably lower total white cell and neutrophil counts have been reported from East Africa than those shown in Table 1.4 for American blacks, and West Indian and African blacks living in England. However, the former studies have not allowed for the skewed distribution of leukocyte numbers in calculating reference ranges, and thus have exaggerated the difference between the black and Caucasian populations.[35] Despite this, total white cell and neutrophil counts are probably genuinely lower in Africans living in African countries, particularly if taking an African diet, than in Africans living in Western countries.[36] Neutrophil granulocytes leave the circulation in an exponential fashion with a $T_{1/2}$ of 2.6–11.8 h (mean 7.2 h)[29] and appear in normal

and microfilaments, a few small mitochondria, a few ribosomes, a little endoplasmic reticulum, occasional multivesicular bodies and numerous glycogen particles (Fig. 1.6). As primary granules contain a variety of acid hydrolases, they have been considered the lysosomes of the neutrophil. However, studies of ultrathin cryosections by immuno-electron microscopy have shown that the lysosome-associated membrane proteins are not demonstrable in primary granules but are found in vesicles and

Table 1.4 95% reference limits for the concentration of circulating leukocytes in the peripheral venous blood of healthy adults

	Caucasians[a]			Blacks	
	Male (n = 100)		Female (n = 100)	Female (West Indian plus African)[a] (n = 158)	Male plus female (American)[b] (n = 226)
White blood cell count (WBC) (10^9/l)	3.5–9.5[c]		4.1–10.9[c]	3.1–8.7[d]	3.6–10.2
Neutrophil count (10^9/l)	1.6–6.0[c]		2.0–7.3[c]	1.1–6.1[d]	1.3–7.4
Lymphocyte count (10^9/l)		1.2–3.5		1.0–3.6	1.45–3.75
Monocyte count (10^9/l)		0.2–0.8		0.14–0.77	0.21–1.05
Eosinophil count (10^9/l)		0.02–0.59		0.01–0.82	0.03–0.72
Basophil count (10^9/l)		0–0.15		0–0.08	0–0.16

[a] Based on total WBCs determined on a Coulter S Plus and 500-cell manual differential counts.
[b] Based on total WBCs determined on a Coulter counter A or F and 200-cell manual differential counts. Only 22 cases were female.[30]
[c] Men have WBC and neutrophil counts significantly lower than women (P < 0.001).[31]
[d] Black women[32] and men have WBC and neutrophil counts significantly lower than Caucasian women (P < 0.001) and men.

Table 1.5 Age-related ranges for the concentration of circulating white blood cells ($\times 10^9$/l) in normal individuals. (Adapted from Dittmer[33] and Bain[34])

Age	White blood cell count (WBC)	Neutrophils[a]	Eosinophils	Basophils	Lymphocytes	Monocytes
Cord blood	5.0–23.0[b]	1.7–19.0	0.05–2.0	0–0.64	1.0–11.0	0.1–3.7
12 h	13.0–38.0	6.0–28.0	0.02–0.95	0–0.50	2.0–11.0	0.4–3.6
24 h	9.4–34.0	4.8–21.0	0.05–1.00	0–0.30	2.0–11.5	0.2–3.1
7–8 days	9.0–18.4	1.8–8.0	0.16–0.94	0–0.25	3.0–9.0	0.03–0.98
2 months	5.1–18.0	0.7–9.0	0.07–0.84	0.02–0.20	3.0–16.0	0.13–1.8
5–6 months	5.9–17.5	1.0–8.5	0.01–1.0	0.02–0.20	3.2–13.5	0.10–1.3
1 year	5.6–17.5	1.5–8.5	0.05–0.70	0.02–0.20	2.5–10.5	0.05–1.28
2 years	5.6–17.0	1.5–8.5	0.04–1.19	0.02–0.20	2.2–9.5	0.05–1.28
4 years	4.9–15.5	1.5–8.5	0.02–1.40	0.03–0.20	1.7–8.0	0.15–1.28
6 years	4.4–14.5	1.5–8.9	0.08–1.10	0.02–0.20	1.5–7.0	0.15–1.28
9–10 years	3.9–13.5	1.5–8.0	0.06–1.03	0.01–0.54	1.4–6.5	0.15–1.28
13–14 years	3.9–13.0	1.4–8.0	0.04–0.76	0.01–0.43	1.2–5.8	0.15–1.28
18 years	4.5–12.5	1.8–7.7	0–0.45	0–0.20	1.0–5.0	0–0.8

[a] Includes a small percentage of myelocytes during the first few days after birth.
[b] Includes 0.03–5.4 $\times 10^9$/l of erythroblasts.

secretions (saliva, secretions of the respiratory and gastrointestinal tracts and urine) and in various tissues. They probably survive outside the blood for up to 30 h.

Functions of neutrophils[37]

These cells are highly motile. They move towards, phagocytose and degrade various types of particulate material such as bacteria and damaged tissue cells. Neutrophils are attracted to sites of infection or inflammation as a result of chemotactic gradients generated around such sites. The chemotactic factors include activated complement components (C3a, C5a, C567), membrane phospholipids and other factors released from tissue cells, lymphokines released from activated lymphocytes, products of mononuclear phagocytes (e.g. tumor necrosis factor, IL-8), platelet-derived factors (platelet factor 4, the β-thromboglobulin neutrophil-activating peptide 2 (NAP-2), platelet-derived growth factor) and products of certain bacteria. IL-8, platelet factor 4 and NAP-2 bind to CXC chemokine receptors on the surface of neutrophils and activate these cells. Activated neutrophils adhere to endothelial cells via adhesion molecules on their cell membrane (Chapter 18). The arrival of neutrophils at sites of inflammation is probably facilitated by an increased permeability of adjoining blood vessels caused by activated complement components such as C3a and C5a.

The first stage in the phagocytosis of a particle such as a bacterium is the adherence of the neutrophil to the particle. The adherence is mediated through specific receptors on the neutrophil cell membrane: these include Fc (IgG$_1$, IgG$_3$) and C3 receptors. Both the adherence and the subsequent ingestion of such particles are enhanced by their interaction with opsonizing factors such as C3 generated via the classical or alternative complement activation pathway, antibody and mannose-binding lectin (Chapter 18). Following adhesion, pseudopodia form around the particle and progressively encircle it, probably via a zipper-like mechanism dependent on the interaction between receptors on the cell membrane and opsonizing factors present all over the particle. Both the movement of neutrophils towards a particle and the act of phagocytosis may be dependent on the activity of intracytoplasmic microfilaments composed of actin. The act of phagocytosis is associated with a burst of oxygen consumption (respiratory burst) and the production of hydrogen peroxide.

The ingestion of a particle is followed by the fusion of both primary and specific granules with the membrane of the phagosome and the discharge of granule contents into the phagocytic vacuole. Neutrophils contain considerable quantities of glycogen that can be converted to glucose. They obtain much of their energy by breaking down glucose anaerobically via the Embden–Meyerhof pathway but can oxidize some glucose aerobically through the Krebs cycle. The killing of certain bacteria (e.g. *Staphylococcus aureus, Escherichia coli, Salmonella typhimurium, Klebsiella pneumoniae, Proteus vulgaris*) is oxygen dependent and the killing of others (e.g. *Pseudomonas aeruginosa, Staphylococcus epidermidis, 'viridans'* streptococci, various anaerobes) oxygen independent. The mechanisms responsible for the killing of bacteria are complex.

NADPH serves as the electron donor in the biochemical processes leading to the reduction of O_2 to O_2^- and oxygen-dependent killing; the bactericidal agents derived from O_2^- include hydrogen peroxide, hydroxyl radicals, hypochlorite ions (generated from halides by hydrogen peroxide in the presence of the enzyme myeloperoxidase) and chloramines. The generation of O_2^- requires the membrane-associated enzyme known as the respiratory burst oxidase, the components of which only assemble when the neutrophil is activated by various stimuli, including the phagocytosis of opsonized bacteria. These components are cytochrome b_{558} (the electron transferring oxidase), two phosphoproteins (p47-phox and p67-phox) and two GTP-binding proteins (Rac 2 and Rap 1a) (also see Chapter 18).

The substances mediating oxygen-independent killing include defensins (three small peptides) and bactericidal permeability increasing protein that damage and make leaky the membranes of microorganisms, lysozyme and lactoferrin. At the acid pH of the phagocytic vacuole, lysozyme (muramidase) hydrolyses peptidoglycans in bacterial cell walls and consequently allows the osmotic swelling and lysis of certain bacteria. Lactoferrin is bacteriostatic as it binds iron at a low pH and thus deprives bacteria of this growth factor.

Eosinophil granulocytes[38–40]

Morphology and composition

Eosinophil granulocytes have a diameter of 12–17 µm in fixed smears. Their cytoplasm is packed with large rounded granules which stain reddish-orange with Romanowsky stains (see Fig. 1.1A). The proportions of cells with one, two, three and four nuclear segments are 6, 68, 22 and 4%, respectively. Eosinophils possess surface receptors for IgG-Fc (Fc$_\gamma$RI, Fc$_\gamma$RIII), IgE, IgM, C4, C3b and C3d[39,41] and the CC chemokine receptor 3.

The electron microscope reveals two types of eosinophil granules: a few rounded homogeneously electron-dense granules and many rounded, elongated or oval crystalloid-containing granules[19] (Fig. 1.7) (also see Chapter 2). Both homogeneous and crystalloid-containing granules contain an arginine- and zinc-rich basic protein, a peroxidase (distinct from neutrophil peroxidase) and acid phosphatase. Eosinophil granules also contain phospholipase B and D, histaminase, ribonuclease, β-glucuronidase, cathepsin and collagenase but not lysozyme. The eosinophil ribonucleases include eosinophil-derived neurotoxin (Rnase 2) and eosinophil cationic protein (Rnase 3). The Charcot–Leyden crystal protein, which has lysophospholipase activity and carbohydrate-binding properties, is found both in the cytosol and in some of the eosinophil granules.[42]

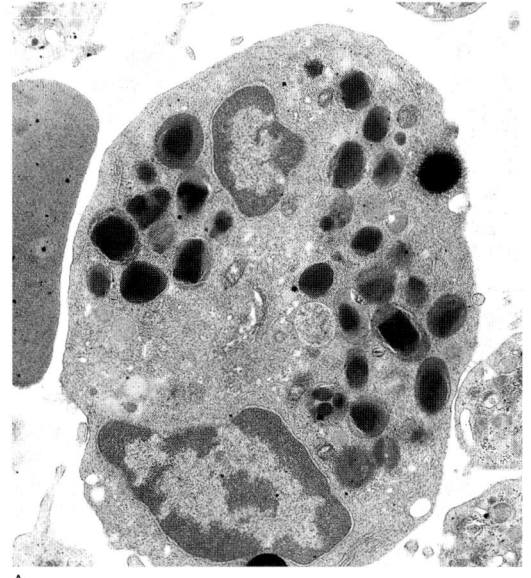
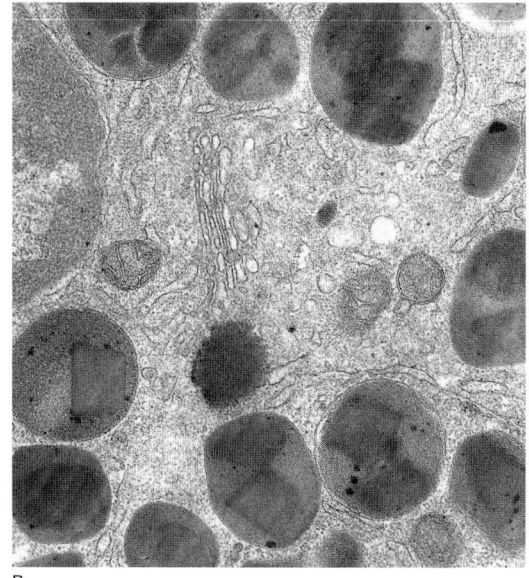

A   B

Fig. 1.7 (A, B) Electron micrographs of normal eosinophil granulocytes. Uranyl acetate and lead citrate. (A) The two nuclear segments contain a large quantity of condensed chromatin at their periphery. One homogeneous granule and several crystalloid-containing granules are present in the cytoplasm. There is a small Golgi apparatus at the center of the cell (this apparatus is usually somewhat better developed in eosinophils than in neutrophils). × 10 000. (B) Higher power view of part of another eosinophil granulocyte showing the Golgi apparatus and strands of rough endoplasmic reticulum. × 24 600.

Number and life span

The 95% confidence limits for the eosinophil count in normal adult venous blood is given in Table 1.4. Contrary to earlier reports, eosinophil counts in healthy black people and people from the Indian subcontinent are the same as in Caucasians.[32] Eosinophil granulocytes leave the circulation in a random manner with a $T_{1/2}$ of about 4.5–8 h; they probably survive in the tissues for 8–12 days.

Functions[43,44]

Eosinophils share several functions with neutrophils: both cell types are motile, respond to specific chemotactic agents and phagocytose and kill similar types of micro-organisms. Eosinophils tend to be somewhat slower at ingesting and killing bacteria than neutrophils but appear to be metabolically more active than these cells. Eosinophils, but not neutrophils, function as the effector cell (killer cell) in antibody-dependent damage to metazoal parasites. Eosinophils bind to IgG- and C3-coated helminths via their corresponding surface receptors and discharge their granule contents around the parasite. The killing of the parasite is caused by the eosinophilic cationic proteins and the major basic protein, which generate defects and pores in the cuticle and cell membrane, as well as eosinophil peroxidase, which exerts its effect through the production of H_2O_2 and hypochlorous acid. It has been suggested recently that the two eosinophil ribonucleases, Rnase 2 and Rnase 3, may be involved in hitherto unrecognized innate and specific defense against viruses.[45] Eosinophils also have a role in regulating immediate-type hypersensitivity reactions. In these reactions chemical mediators of anaphylaxis such as histamine and leukotrienes C_4 (LTC_4) and B_4 as well as the small peptides known as eosinophil chemotactic factor of anaphylaxis (ECF-A) are released from mast cells and basophils as a result of the interaction between specific antigen and IgE on the surface of these cells. Eosinophils are attracted to the site of the activated mast cells or basophils by mast cell- and basophil-derived ECF-A, platelet-activating factor (PAF) and leukotriene B_4 (LTB_4) and by several other chemoattractants (chemokines) produced at sites of allergic inflammation; some of the chemokines are also activators of eosinophils. The most potent eosinophil chemokines are eotaxin (produced by macrophages, eosinophils and some other tissue cells), RANTES, the 5 lipoxygenase product 5-oxo-6, 8, 11, 14-eicosatetraenoic acid[46] and monocyte chemoattractant protein (MCP). Eotaxin is a ligand of the CC chemokine receptor 3 (CCR3) that is expressed on eosinophils, basophils and T_H2 lymphocytes. C5a, monocyte-derived LTB$_4$ and PAF, and some lymphokines are also involved in attracting eosinophils. The attracted eosinophils then release prostaglandin E_2 (PGE_2) which inhibits further release of basophil- and mast-cell-derived mediators. Eosinophils also release specific enzymes that inactivate these mediators, including histaminase and phospholipase B and D which break down histamine and PAF, respectively. Eosinophil-derived arylsulphatase inactivates various chemotactic peptides and LTC_4. Eosinophils may enhance hypersensitivity reactions by their phospholipase-A_2-dependent synthesis and release of LTC_4 and PAF, and also via the release of eosinophil-derived major basic protein, peroxidase and cationic proteins that activate basophils and mast cells and cause histamine release.

Basophil granulocytes[47]

In Romanowsky-stained blood smears, basophil granulocytes have an average diameter of about 12 μm and display large rounded purplish-black cytoplasmic granules (see Fig. 1.1B). Some of these granules lie over the nucleus. The nucleus usually has two segments. The granules stain metachromatically (i.e. reddish-violet) with toluidine blue or methylene blue. Basophils stain strongly by the periodic acid-schiff (PAS) reaction (due to the presence of glycogen aggregates) and do not stain for acid or alkaline phosphatase. Basophil granules undergo varying degrees of extraction during processing for electron microscopy and characteristically show a particulate substructure with each particle measuring about 20 nm in diameter[48] (Fig 1.8). Basophils possess at their cell surface high-affinity receptors for IgE (Fc$_γ$RI) and receptors for IgG, C and histamine, and CC chemokine receptors.

Basophil granules contain histamine (which is synthesized by the cell), sulphated mucopolysaccharides (predominantly chondroitin sulphate), peroxidase, low levels of chymase (a serine protease) and negligible amounts of tryptase. The mucopolysaccharides account for the metachromatic staining of the granules. Basophils also contain Charcot–Leyden crystal protein[42] and possibly PAF (which causes platelets to aggregate and release their contents) and eosinophil chemotactic factor of anaphylaxis (ECF-A). Both basophils and mast cells play a key role in immediate-type hypersensitivity reactions. When IgE-coated basophils react with specific antigen, they degranulate, release histamine and ECF-A and generate and release LTC_4. The release of histamine and other substances from basophils (and mast cells) is mediated via the transport of vesicles between the secretory granules and plasma membrane (piecemeal

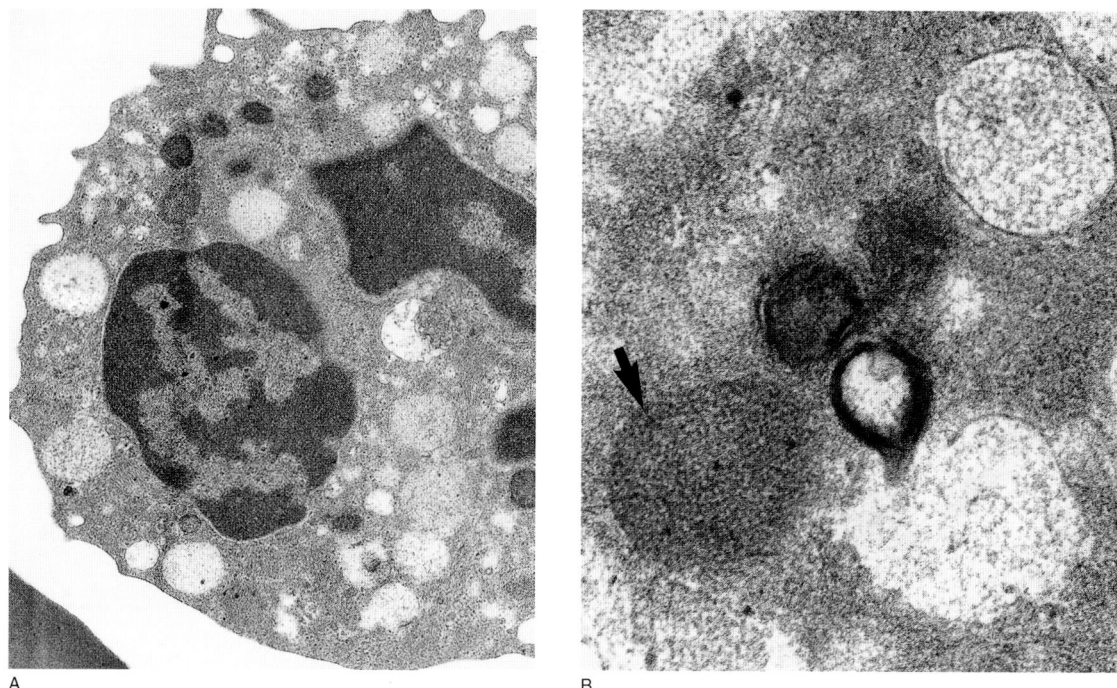

A   B

Fig. 1.8 (A, B) Ultrastructure of basophil granulocytes from normal peripheral blood. Uranyl acetate and lead citrate. (A) There are several large distinctive granules within the cytoplasm. Most of the granules have been partially or completely extracted during the processing for electron microscopy. × 18 300. (B) Higher power view of part of another basophil granulocyte showing a well-preserved cytoplasmic granule (arrowed) and two virtually completely extracted granules. The unextracted granule shows a characteristic particulate substructure. × 36 500.

degranulation).[49] The released histamine causes contraction of bronchial and gastrointestinal smooth muscle, inhibition of cytotoxic T-cell activity and lymphokine release, chemotactic attraction of other granulocytes, upregulation of C3b receptors on eosinophils and release of lysosomal enzymes from neutrophils. The response of eosinophils to basophil degranulation is discussed on page 13. The accumulation of basophils at sites of hypersensitivity reactions is mediated by chemokines such as MCP and eotaxin and the preferential recruitment of these cells may depend on the pattern of usage of the CC chemokine receptors.[50] Apart from participating in immediate-type hypersensitivity reactions, basophils may also be involved in the histamine-mediated killing of intestinal parasites.

Basophils represent the most infrequent type of leukocyte in the blood (see Tables 1.4 and 1.5).

Monocytes[51] (see Figs 1.1D and 1.9)

These are the largest leukocytes in peripheral blood. In stained smears, they vary considerably in diameter (15–30 μm) and in morphology. The nucleus is large and eccentric and may be rounded, kidney- or horseshoe-shaped or lobulated. The nuclear chromatin has a skein-like or lacy appearance. The cytoplasm is plentiful, stains grayish-blue and contains few to many fine azurophilic granules. One or more intracytoplasmic vacuoles may be present. Cytochemical studies with the light microscope have shown the presence of many hydrolytic enzymes, including acid phosphatase, NaF-resistant esterase, galactosidases and lysozyme. Monocytes also contain defensins, myeloperoxidase, collagenase, elastase and coagulation system proteins (tissue factor, factors V, VII, IX, X and XIII, plasminogen activator) and have membrane receptors for IgG-Fc and C3. In addition, they have two CC chemokine receptors, CCR2 and CCR5, that bind various CC chemokines such as monocyte chemo-attractant protein-1 (MCP-1), MCP-2, MCP-3, RANTES, macrophage inflammatory protein-1α (MIP-1α) and MIP-1β.

Under the electron microscope, monocyte granules are seen to vary considerably in size and shape and to be more or less homogeneously electron-dense. Some of these granules contain acid phosphatase and peroxidase. The peroxidase-positive granules are characteristically smaller than those of neutrophils. In thin sections, monocytes display finger-like projections of their cell membrane. Their cytoplasm contains appreciable amounts of rough endoplasmic reticulum, moderate numbers of dispersed ribosomes, a well-developed Golgi apparatus,

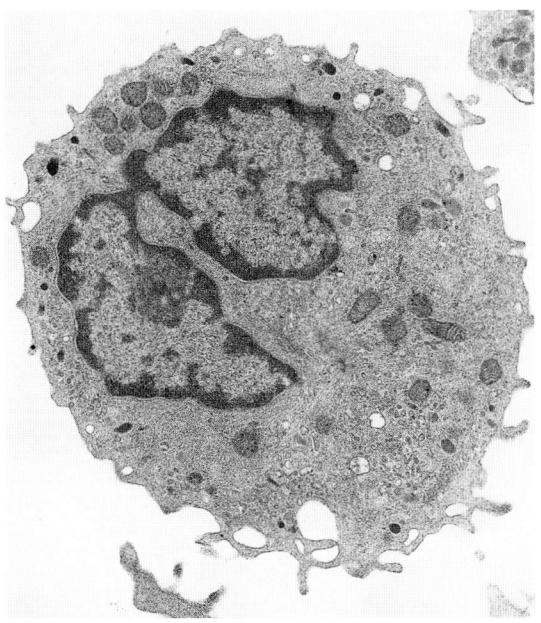 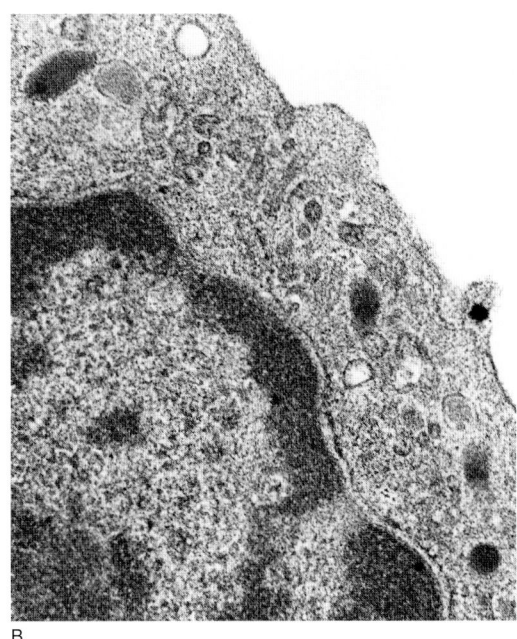

A   B

Fig. 1.9 (A, B) Electron micrograph of a monocyte from normal peripheral blood. Uranyl acetate and lead citrate. (A) The cytoplasm contains numerous mitochondria, several small pleomorphic electron-dense granules and short strands of rough endoplasmic reticulum. The nucleus has an irregular outline. It contains moderate quantities of condensed chromatin and a prominent nucleolus. × 11 300. (B) Higher power view of part of the cell shown in (A). The electron-dense granules are clearly seen as are a large number of small vesicular structures. These vesicles are typically found around the Golgi apparatus. × 25 200.

several mitochondria and bundles of microfibrils. The nucleus has moderate quantities of heterochromatin and although nucleoli are not usually detectable by light microscopy, they are frequently seen by electron microscopy.

Blood monocytes are distributed, as are neutrophils (see p. 10), between a circulating and a marginated pool; there are, on average, 3.6 times more marginated than circulating cells. The concentration of circulating monocytes in the peripheral venous blood of healthy adults is given in Table 1.4. Monocytes leave the circulation in an exponential manner, with an average $T_{1/2}$ of 71 h. They transform into macrophages in various tissues and may survive in this form for several months.

Monocytes are actively motile cells that respond to chemotactic stimuli (e.g. MCP-1, RANTES, MIP-1α and MIP-1β), phagocytose particulate material and kill microorganisms in a manner similar to that described for neutrophil granulocytes (p. 11). Monocytes and monocyte-derived macrophages are particularly conspicuous at sites of chronic inflammation. Macrophages play important roles in various aspects of the immune response. These include the processing and presentation of antigen on class II major histocompatibility complex (MHC) molecules (Ia molecules) in a form recognizable by helper T-lymphocytes, and the degradation of excess antigen. The macrophages of the liver, spleen and bone marrow

destroy senescent red cells and those in the marrow produce several cytokines regulating various aspects of hemopoiesis. The cytokines produced include G-CSF, M-CSF, GM-CSF, erythropoietin, thymosin B_4, IL-1, IL-6, IL-8, tumor necrosis factor (TNF), fibroblast growth factor and platelet-derived growth factor.

Lymphocytes

Lymphocytes have an average volume of approximately 180 fl[52] and in stained smears have a diameter which varies from about 7 to 12 μm. Most of the lymphocytes in normal blood are small (see Fig. 1.1C). In Romanowsky-stained smears, they have scanty bluish cytoplasm; the nucleus is round or slightly indented and there is considerable condensation of nuclear chromatin. The cytoplasm, which sometimes merely consists of a narrow rim around the nucleus, may contain a few azurophilic granules. Ultrastructural studies reveal that small lymphocytes contain a few scattered monoribosomes, an inactive Golgi apparatus, a few mitochondria, a few lysosomal granules and a small nucleolus (Fig. 1.10). About 10% of lymphocytes are large lymphocytes. These are about 12–16 μm in diameter and contain more cyto-plasm and less condensed chromatin than small lym-phocytes. In normal blood an occasional large

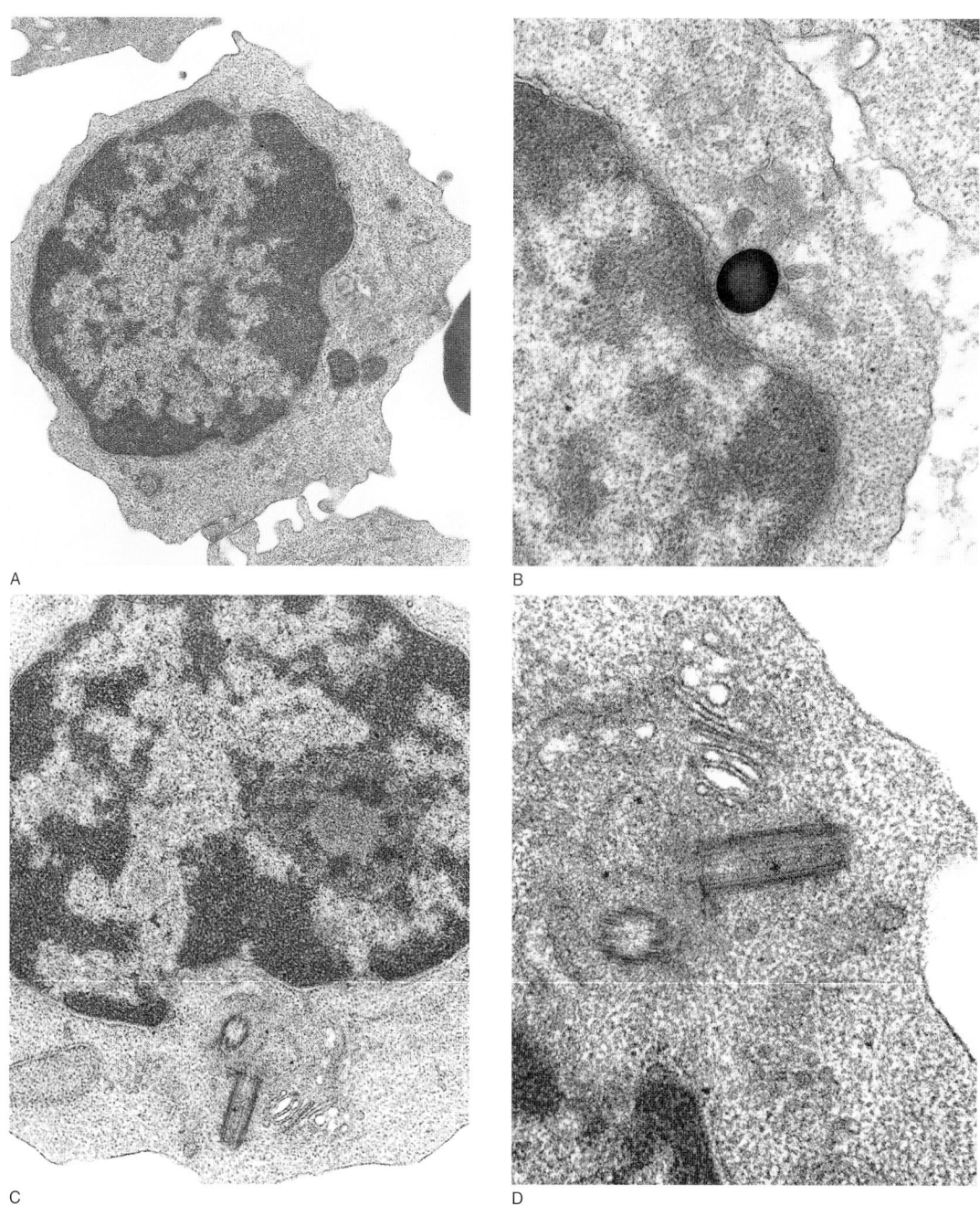

Fig. 1.10 (A–D) Various ultrastructural appearances of lymphocytes from the peripheral blood of a normal adult. Uranyl acetate and lead citrate. (A) Typical lymphocyte with a high nucleus: cytoplasm ratio, a rounded nuclear outline and large quantities of nuclear-membrane-associated condensed chromatin. The cytoplasm lacks granules but has a few mitochondria and a few moderately long strands of rough endoplasmic reticulum. × 14 200. (B) Part of a lymphocyte showing a large electron-dense intracytoplasmic inclusion (Goll body) of uncertain nature. The cytoplasm contains numerous monoribosomes and there is a cluster of small membrane-bound granule-like structures adjacent to the Goll body. × 34 700. (C) Small lymphocyte with a nucleus containing a nucleolus as well as large quantities of condensed chromatin. There is a slight indentation of the nucleus adjacent to two centrioles and the Golgi apparatus. × 22 000. (D) Higher-power view of the centrioles and the Golgi apparatus shown in (C) × 44 000.

lymphocyte has voluminous cytoplasm and several coarse azurophilic granules (large granular lymphocytes). The large granular lymphocytes include natural killer cells (see below).

The concentration of lymphocytes in the blood is age dependent: normal values are given in Tables 1.4 and 1.5. Lymphocytes recirculate: they leave the blood through the endothelial cells of the postcapillary venules of lymphoid organs and eventually find their way back into lymphatic channels and re-enter the blood via the thoracic duct. The life span of lymphocytes varies considerably. The average life span in humans appears to be about 4 years but some cells survive for over 10 years.

Although most mature lymphocytes are morphologically similar to one another they can be divided into two major functionally distinct groups, designated B-lymphocytes (B-cells) and T-lymphocytes (T-cells). Some characteristics of these two types of cell, including their various functions, are summarized in Table 1.6. On the basis of the nature of the two disulfide-linked chains of the T-cell receptor (TcR), T-cells are divided into $\alpha\beta$ T-cells (with $\alpha\beta$TcR or TcR-2) and $\gamma\delta$ T-cells (with $\gamma\delta$TcR or TcR-1); most T-cells are $\alpha\beta$ T-cells. Two functionally different groups of $\alpha\beta$ T-cells exist, termed helper cells or T_H cells and suppressor/cytotoxic cells or T_C cells. T_H cells are CD4-positive, recognize antigen and release lymphokines involved in promoting the functions of B-cells and the maturation of other kinds of T-cells including T_C cells. Using antibodies, it is possible to distinguish between T_H cells that provide helper functions

for B-cells and those that activate CD8+ suppressor T-cells. T_H cells are also subdivided into T_H1 cells that produce the inflammatory cytokines IFN-γ and IL-2, T_H2 cells that produce cytokines such as IL-4 and IL-5 that affect growth and differentiation of B-cells, and T_H0 cells that are not restricted to producing a particular group of cytokines. T_C cells are CD8-positive, inhibit the functions of other lymphocytes and also have cytotoxic capability against malignant or virus-infected cells. They recognize peptides presented with class I MHC molecules and when activated by antigen acquire azurophilic cytoplasmic granules containing acid hydrolases and other substances that mediate target cell lysis. Lymphocytes that are neither B-cells nor T-cells also exist. For example, K (killer) cells, which have Fc receptors but not the other surface receptors of B-cells, lyse antibody-coated cells, and NK (natural killer) cells (large granular lymphocytes) which lack antigen-specific receptors, play a role in the body's defense against viruses and certain tumors.

T_H-lymphocytes regulate normal hemopoiesis including eosinophil granulocytopoiesis and erythropoiesis.[53] Furthermore, abnormalities in T-cell subpopulations

Table 1.6 Some characteristics of T- and B-lymphocytes

		T-lymphocyte	B-lymphocyte
Identifying characteristics		T-cell receptor complex (CD3) Form rosettes with sheep red blood cells Surface antigens CD2, CD5, CD6	Surface membrane immunoglobulin (SmIg) Receptors for complement components C3b, C3d, C4 Receptors for Fc end of immunoglobulin molecule in immune complex or in aggregated immunoglobulin (FcR) Surface antigens CD19, CD20, CD22 Receptors for Epstein–Barr virus (some cells only)
Origin		Derived from a lymphoid stem cell initially detectable in fetal liver and subsequently in bone marrow; develop under the influence of thymic epithelium	Derived from a lymphoid stem cell initially detectable in fetal liver and subsequently in bone marrow
Relative distribution	Peripheral blood	70%	20–30%
	Bone marrow	70%	15%
	Lymp node	75% Paracortical distribution; medullary sinuses	25% Follicles; medullary cords
	Lymph	75%	25%
	Spleen	50% Periarteriolar lymph sheath	50% Follicles; marginal zone between T zone and red pulp; cords of red pulp
Function		Cellular immunity (e.g. against viruses, fungi, low-grade intracellular pathogens such as mycobacteria) Graft rejection Tumor rejection Delayed hypersensitivity Interaction with B-cells in production of antibodies against certain antigens Suppression of B-cell function Production of eosinophilia	Maturation into plasma cells for the production of antibodies (immunoglobulin)

seem to play a role in the pathogenesis of the cytopenias in some cases of aplastic anemia, pure red cell aplasia associated with chronic lymphocytic leukemia and chronic idiopathic neutropenia (Chapters 13 and 17).

Platelets

Morphology and composition[54]

Platelets are small fragments of megakaryocyte cytoplasm with an average volume of 7–8 fl. When seen in Romanowsky-stained blood smears, most platelets have a diameter of 2–3 μm. They may be found lying singly but show a tendency to form small clumps. Platelets have an irregular outline, stain light blue and contain a number of small azurophilic granules that are usually concentrated at the center. Newly formed platelets are larger than more mature ones.

Electron microscope studies have revealed that non-activated (resting) platelets are shaped like biconvex discs, have a more-or-less smooth but convoluted surface and contain mitochondria, granules, two systems of cytoplasmic membranes (a surface-connected canalicular system and a dense tubular system), microfilaments, microtubules and many glycogen molecules that are often found in clumps (Fig. 1.11) (also see Chapter 25). The discoid shape is actively maintained by a cytoskeleton consisting of many short contractile microfilmanets composed of actomyosin and an equatorial bundle of

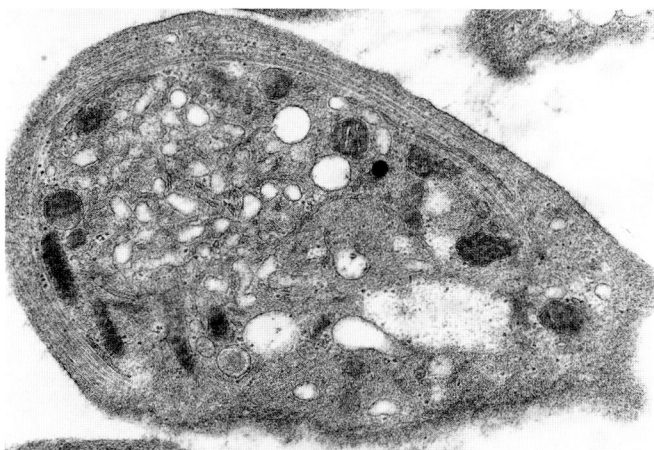

Fig. 1.11 Electron micrograph of a platelet sectioned in the equatorial plane showing the circumferential band of microtubules. Many electron-lucent vesicles belonging to the surface-connected canalicular system, a few mitochondria and some platelet granules (including one dense body) can be seen. The dense tubular system is present between the vesicles of the surface-connected canalicular system, but is only just visible at the present magnification. Uranyl acetate and lead citrate. × 20 000.

microtubules composed of tubulin. The microfilaments are situated between various organelles and may be attached to specific proteins at the inner surface of the cell membrane. In addition to maintaining cell shape, the microfilaments are probably involved in clot retraction. The equatorial bundle of microtubules is situated in an organelle-free sol-gel zone just beneath the cell membrane and appears to be connected to this membrane by filaments. When platelets change shape during activation, the microtubules break their connections with the cell membrane and contract inwards; the platelet granules also become concentrated at the center of the cell. The cell membrane of the resting platelet is extensively invaginated to form a surface-connected open canalicular system. This canalicular system provides a large surface area through which various substances, including the contents of platelet granules, can be released to the exterior via multiple openings in the cell membrane. It is thought that the contraction of the microfilaments during platelet activation brings the platelet granules close to special areas of this canalicular system which are capable of fusing with granules. The contraction of microtubules may also play a role in this process. The platelet also contains a specialized form of endoplasmic reticulum known as the dense tubular system, elements of which are found adjacent to the bundle of microtubules and in between the invaginations of the open canalicular system. This system is the main site of synthesis of thromboxane A_2 which plays an important role in the reactions leading to the release of the contents of platelet granules. In addition, the dense tubular system contains a high concentration of calcium ions when compared with that elsewhere in the cytoplasm and may regulate the activity of several calcium-dependent reversible cytoplasmic processes such as the activation of actomyosin, depolymerization of microtubules and glycogenolysis.

On the basis of the ultrastructural appearances and ultrastructural cytochemistry of the granules, and of studies of patients with a selective lack of one type of granule, the platelet granules can be divided into four types, namely dense bodies, α granules, lysosomal granules and peroxisomes (Table 1.7).[19] The characteristics of these granule types are summarized below and discussed in more detail in Chapter 25. Dense bodies (δ granules) are very electron-dense, usually show a bull's eye appearance because of the presence of an electron-lucent zone between the central electron-dense material and the limiting membrane and contain the storage pool of ADP and ATP which is concerned with secondary platelet aggregation. They also contain calcium and adrenaline as well as 5HT (which causes both vasoconstriction and platelet aggregation). The α granules (the

Table 1.7 Characteristics of various types of platelet granules[54,55]

Granule	Contents	Appearance
Dense bodies (δ granules)	Serotonin, calcium, storage pool of ATP and ADP, pyrophosphate	Very dense, may have 'bull's eye' appearance
α granules[a]	β thromboglobulin, platelet factor 4, platelet-derived growth factor, fibrinogen, fibronectin, factor-VIII-related antigen (vWF), thrombospondin	Less electron-dense than dense bodies
Lysosomal granules[a] (λ granules)	Acid phosphatase, cathepsin, β-glucuronidase, β-galactosidase, arylsulphatase	Less electron-dense than dense bodies
Peroxisomes	Catalase	Smaller than α and λ granules

[a] Distinguished from each other by ultrastructural cytochemisty.

most frequent type of platelet granule) and lysosomal (λ) granules are slightly larger than dense granules, and are moderately electron-dense. The α- and λ-granules can be distinguished only on the basis of their ultrastructural cytochemistry; for example, λ granules but not α granules contain acid phosphatase. The peroxisomes are smaller than α and λ granules. Substances present in α granules (Table 1.7) include platelet factor 4 which has heparin-neutralizing activity and may thus potentiate the action of thrombin, and the platelet mitogenic factors that stimulate growth of endothelial and smooth muscle cells and of skin fibroblasts.

Number and life span

The normal range for the platelet count in peripheral blood is about $160–450 \times 10^9/l$ (see Table 1.2); slightly lower values are seen during the first 3 months of life. Small cyclical variations in the platelet count may be seen in some individuals of both sexes, with a periodicity of 21–35 days; in premenopausal women the fall usually occurs during the 2 weeks preceding menstruation. The platelet counts of women are slightly higher than those of men.[56,57] There are also slight racial variations in the normal platelet count. For example, values lower than those quoted above have been reported in Australians of Mediterranean descent.[58] In addition, Nigerians have lower platelet counts than Caucasians,[59] as have Africans and West Indians living in the UK.[60]

The life span of normal platelets is 8–10 days.

Functions[61]

Large quantities of energy are used during various platelet functions. This energy is mainly derived from the metabolism of glucose by the glycolytic pathway and tricarboxylic acid cycle. The energy is held as ATP within a metabolic pool that is distinct from the storage pool of adenine nucleotides situated in the dense bodies.

Platelets play an essential role in the hemostatic mechanism. When endothelial cells of vessel walls are damaged and shed, platelets adhere to subendothelial connective tissue (basement membrane and non-collagen microfibrils) via von Willebrand factor (vWF) attached to a specific receptor on the platelet membrane, glycoprotein Ib-IX. This adhesion requires calcium ions. Platelets may also adhere to collagen via other specific membrane receptors (see Chapter 26). Adhesion is followed within seconds by the transformation of the platelet from its original discoid shape to a spiny sphere (a potentially reversible process) and within a few minutes by the release of the contents of some platelet granules (the release reaction). Initially, the contents of the dense bodies are released; with stronger stimulation, some α granules are also discharged. The ADP released from the dense bodies, and possibly also traces of thrombin generated by the activation of the clotting cascade, cause an interaction of other platelets with the adherent platelets and with each other (secondary platelet aggregation) with further release of ADP from the aggregating platelets. Aggregation induced by ADP (and by adrenaline and collagen) is preceded by an alteration of the cell membrane leading to calcium-dependent binding of fibrinogen to specific platelet receptors on membrane glycoprotein IIb–IIIa;[62] the fibrinogen molecules link adjacent platelets. To a lesser extent, aggregation may also be mediated by binding of vWF and vitronectin to glycoprotein IIb–IIIa. In addition, platelet- and endothelial-cell-derived thrombospondin stabilize aggregation after binding to receptors on glycoprotein IV. The process of secondary aggregation continues until a platelet plug occludes the damaged vessel. The release reaction may be mediated through thromboxane A_2 synthesized in the platelet from arachidonic acid released from membrane phospholipids (the conversion of arachidonic acid to thromboxane A_2

requires the enzymes cyclo-oxygenase and thromboxane synthetase). The formation of a fibrin clot around the platelet plug is initiated by the activation of factor VII by tissue factor exposed on various cells (Chapter 24). The exposure of certain membrane phospholipids (platelet factor 3) in aggregated platelets plays a role in the formation of this fibrin clot. These platelet phospholipids participate in: (1) the formation of factor Xa through a reaction involving factors IXa, VIII, X and calcium; and (2) in the reaction between factors II, V, Xa and calcium.

In addition to their primary role in hemostasis, platelets have several other functions. They participate in the generation of the inflammatory response by releasing factors that increase vascular permeability and attract granulocytes. The α granules of the platelet contain mitogenic factors that may promote the regeneration of damaged/detached endothelial cells. These mitogenic factors also stimulate fibroblast proliferation and may therefore promote the healing of wounds. Furthermore, platelets remove the pharmacologically active substance 5HT from their microenvironment by taking it up and concentrating it in the dense granules; they thus serve as 'detoxifying' cells. Platelets also have a limited capacity for phagocytosis. Finally, platelets play a role in pathological processes such as thrombosis and the rejection of transplants and have also been implicated in the pathogenesis of atherosclerosis.

Platelet function may be tested *in vivo* or *in vitro*. The bleeding time is the most useful *in vivo* measure of platelet function and may be determined according to the method of Ivy or Duke. The Ivy test, which is performed on the forearm, is more sensitive in detecting an abnormality than the Duke test, which is performed on the ear lobe. In the Ivy test, a sphygmomanometer cuff is applied and inflated to a pressure of 40 mm to raise the venous pressure. A set number of punctures of defined depth are made in the skin with a lancet and the time till bleeding stops is measured.[63] In a variation of the Ivy test an incision through a template is used rather than a puncture.[64] The bleeding time is predominantly a measure of platelet number and function though some prolongation is caused by severe defects of coagulation factors, including overdose of oral anticoagulants. If platelet numbers are known to be normal, then a prolonged bleeding time usually indicates an intrinsic platelet defect (e.g. an inherited or an aspirin-induced defect) or an extrinsic defect (e.g. inhibition by uremic toxins, or failure to interact with an abnormal surface due to a lack of high-molecular-weight vWF). The Hess test is also an *in vivo* test of platelet function, but is not very useful because a positive result is often consequent on increased capillary fragility rather than a platelet defect.

Platelet functions that may be investigated *in vitro* include adhesion, aggregation, clot retraction and contribution to the intrinsic coagulation pathway (also see Chapter 24). Adhesion can best be tested by passing whole blood through rabbit aorta stripped of its endothelium and quantitating the number of adherent platelets.[65] Both adhesion and aggregation are tested by passing blood through a glass bead column and determining the percentage of retained platelets; this test is difficult to standardize. Recently, automated equipment has been developed to test these linked functions using whole blood (Chapter 24). Aggregation is most readily tested by the use of an aggregometer which measures optical density of platelet-rich plasma; as aggregation is induced (e.g. by ADP, adrenaline [epinephrine], collagen or the antibiotic ristocetin) the optical density falls; if platelets disaggregate the optical density rises again. It is also possible to measure adenosine triphosphate (ATP) release during platelet aggregation. Clot retraction is assessed by measuring the volume of serum expressed by whole blood that is allowed to clot in a glass tube at 37°C for 1 h; a high hematocrit may interfere with clot retraction. The contribution of the platelet to the intrinsic pathway of blood coagulation may be tested by the prothrombin consumption test (which shows defective conversion of prothrombin to thrombin when there is a deficiency of platelet number or function) or the platelet factor 3 availability test or the thromboplastin generation test (which test for the ability of the platelet to accelerate the intrinsic pathway of coagulation).

Alterations in the blood in pregnancy

In most women, the hemoglobin level begins to fall at about the sixth to eight week of a normal pregnancy, reaches its lowest level at about the thirty-second week and increases slightly thereafter. The extent of fall varies markedly from woman to woman but hemoglobin levels less than 10 g/dl are probably abnormal. The average fall is about 1.5–2 g/dl. This physiologic 'anemia' occurs despite an average increase in the red cell mass of about 300 ml and results from an average increase in the plasma volume of about a liter.[66] The reticulocyte percentage is increased, plateauing at about 6% between 25 and 35 weeks. The mean corpuscular volume and MCH rise during pregnancy in the absence of any deficiency of vitamin B_{12} or folic acid. Serum iron falls. Transferrin synthesis increases due to a direct hormonal effect (similar changes are seen in subjects taking oral contraceptives); the transferrin concentration and total iron-binding capacity increase. The serum vitamin B_{12} level falls steadily throughout pregnancy reaching its lowest level at term; this is a physiological change and is not indicative of deficiency. About 10% of normal women have serum vitamin B_{12} levels below 100 ng/l during the last trimester. There is a return to non-pregnant levels by 6 weeks postpartum.[67] Red cell and serum folate levels also fall[67] and 20–30% of women have subnormal red cell folate levels at term. Physiologic needs for iron and folic acid are increased, and in subjects with reduced stores and/or poor intake (Chapters 11 and 12) deficiency may occur. The hemoglobin F level increases slightly. The percentage of F-cells is increased at mid-term but returns to non-pregnant levels by term. The erythrocyte sedimentation rate (ESR) rises early in pregnancy and is highest in the third trimester. The white-cell count increases, due to an increase of neutrophils and monocytes. Total white blood cell counts (WBCs) of $10-15 \times 10^9/l$ are common during pregnancy, and postpartum levels may reach $20-40 \times 10^9/l$. Metamyelocytes and myelocytes are seen in the blood in about a quarter of subjects and promyelocytes may also be present. 'Toxic' granulation and Döhle bodies[68] (see Chapter 17) are common and are a physiologic change. The neutrophil alkaline phosphatase rises early in pregnancy and remains elevated; a further rise occurs during labor, with a return to non-pregnant levels by 6 weeks postpartum. The bactericidal capacity of neutrophils is increased and in 40–60% of subjects in the second and third trimester, an increased proportion of neutrophils are positive in the nitro-blue tetrazolium reduction test. Lymphocyte and eosinophil counts are decreased. The basophil count may rise. Consistent changes in the platelet count have not been reported, but some fall may occur.[69,70] Throughout pregnancy, factors VII, VIIIC, VIIIR:Ag, X, fibrinogen and α_1 antitrypsin increase markedly. Factors II and V increase early in pregnancy but decrease steadily thereafter.[63] Pregnancy is also associated with some increase in factor IX, a slight fall in antithrombin IIIC and antithrombin Ag and from 11–15 weeks onwards a marked decrease in fibrinolytic activity. Fibrin degradation products increase after 21–25 weeks in about 40% of subjects.

Fetal cells, for example fetal red cells and fetal lymphocytes,[71] enter the maternal circulation during pregnancy as well as at delivery. This phenomenon is common enough to be regarded as physiologic, although it may have adverse effects when the mother becomes sensitized to fetal antigens (see Chapters 10 and 30).

REFERENCES

1. Lewis SM, Bain BJ, Bates I 2001 Dacie & Lewis Practical haematology, 9th edn. Churchill Livingstone, Edinburgh
2. Bain BJ 1989 Blood cells. A practical guide. Gower Medical Publishing, London
3. Guest GM, Brown EW 1957 Erythrocytes and hemoglobin of the blood in infancy and childhood. III. American Journal of Diseases of Childhood 93: 486
4. Saarinen UM, Siimes MA 1978 Developmental changes in red blood cell counts and indices of infants after exclusion of iron deficiency by laboratory criteria and continuous iron supplementation. Journal of Pediatrics 92: 412–416
5. Serjeant GR, Grandison Y, Mason K et al 1980 Haematological indices in normal negro children: a Jamaican cohort from birth to five years. Clinical and Laboratory Haematology 2: 169–178
6. Koerper MA, Mentzer WC, Brecher G, Dallman PR 1976 Developmental change in red blood cell volume: implication in screening infants and children for iron deficiency and thalassemia trait. Journal of Pediatrics 89: 580–583
7. Schmaier BA, Maurer HM, Johnston CL et al 1974 Electronically determined red cell indices in a predominantly black urban population of children 4 to 8 years of age. Journal of Pediatrics 84: 559–561.
8. Giorno R, Clifford JH, Beverly S, Rossing RG 1980 Hematology reference values. Analysis of different statistical technics and variations with age and sex. American Journal of Clinical Pathology 74: 765–770
9. Hows J, Hussein S, Hoffbrand AV, Wickramasinghe SN 1977 Red cell indices and serum ferritin levels in children. Journal of Clinical Pathology 30: 181–183
10. Mollison PL, Veal N 1955 The use of the isotope ^{51}Cr as a label for red cells. British Journal of Haematology 1: 62–74
11. Donohue DM, Motulsky AG, Giblett ER et al 1955 The use of chromium as a red cell tag. British Journal of Haematology 1: 249–263
12. Mollison PL, Engelfriet CP, Contreras M 1997 Blood transfusion in clinical medicine, 10th edn. Blackwell Science, Oxford
13. Rettig MP, Low PS, Gimm JA et al 1999 Evaluation of biochemical changes during *in vivo* erythrocyte senescence in the dog. Blood 93: 376–384
14. Boas FE, Forman L, Beutler E 1998 Phosphatidylserine exposure and red cell viability in red cell aging and in hemolytic anemia. Proceedings of the National Academy of Sciences USA 95: 3077–3081
15. Grimes AJ 1980 Human red cell metabolism. Blackwell Scientific Publications, Oxford
16. Harris JW, Kellermeyer RW 1970 The red cell. Production, metabolism, destruction: normal and abnormal. Harvard University Press, Cambridge, MA.
17. Barcroft J 1928 The respiratory function of the blood. Cambridge University Press, Cambridge
18. Marchesi VT 1983 The red cell membrane skeleton: recent progress. Blood 61: 1–11
19. Bessis M 1973 Living blood cells and their ultrastructure. Springer, Berlin
20. Deiss A, Kurth D 1970 Circulating reticulocytes in normal adults as determined by the new methylene blue method. American Journal of Clinical Pathology 53: 481–484
21. Hillman RS, Finch CA 1969 The misused reticulocyte. British Journal of Haematology 17: 313–315
22. Wintrobe MM, Lee GR, Boggs DR et al 1981 Clinical hematology, 8th edn. Lea and Febiger, Philadelphia, 1885
23. Bowen D, Bentley N, Hoy T, Cavill I 1991 Comparison of a modified thiazole orange technique with a fully automated analyzer for reticulocyte counting. Journal of Clinical Pathology 44: 130–133
24. Tarallo P, Humbert J-C, Mahassen P et al 1994 Reticulocytes: biological variations and reference limits. European Journal of Haematology 53: 11–15
25. Kjeldsen L, Cowland JB, Johnsen AH, Borregaard N 1996 SGP28, a novel matrix glycoprotein in specific granules of human neutrophils with similarity to a human testis-specific gene product and a rodent sperm-coating glycoprotein. FEBS Letters 380: 246–250
26. Kjeldsen L, Sengelov H, Borregaard N 1999 Subcellular fractionation of human neutrophils on Percoll density gradients. Journal of Immunological Methods 232: 131–143
27. Borregaard N 1997 Development of neutrophil granule diversity. Annals of the New York Academy of Sciences 832: 62–68
28. Bainton DF 1999 Distinct granule populations in human neutrophils and lysosomal organelles identified by immuno-electron microscopy. Journal of Immunological Methods 232: 153–168
29. Cartwright GE, Athens JW, Wintrobe MM 1964 The kinetics of granulopoiesis in normal man. Blood 24: 780–803

30. Orfanakis NG, Ostlund RE, Bishop CR, Athens JW 1970 Normal blood leukocyte concentration values. American Journal of Clinical Pathology 53: 647–651

31. Bain BJ, England JM 1975 Normal haematological values: sex difference in neutrophil count. British Medical Journal 1: 306–309

32. Bain B, Seed M, Godsland I 1984 Normal values for peripheral blood white cell counts in women of four different ethnic origins. Journal of Clinical Pathology 376: 188–193

33. Dittmer DS 1961 Blood and other body fluids. Federation of American Societies for Experimental Biology, Washington, 125

34. Bain BJ 2001 Blood cells: a practical guide, 3rd edn. Blackwell Science, Oxford

35. Shaper AG, Lewis P 1971 Genetic neutropenia in people of African origin. Lancet ii: 1021–1023

36. Ezeilo GC 1972 Non-genetic neutropenia in Africans. Lancet ii: 1003–1004

37. Soothill JF, Segal AW 1983 Phagocyte function and its defects. In: Hardisty RM, Weatherall DJ (eds), Blood and its disorders, 2nd edn. Blackwell Scientific Publications, Oxford, 629

38. Beeson PB, Bass DA 1977 The eosinophil. Saunders, Philadelphia

39. Tachimoto H, Bochner BS 2000 The surface phenotype of human eosinophils. Chemical Immunology 76: 45–62

40. Dvorak AM, Weller PF 2000 Ultrastructural analysis of human eosinophils. Chemical Immunology 76: 1–28

41. Anwar AR, Kay AB 1977 Membrane receptors for IgG and complement (C4, C3b and C3d) on human eosinophils and neutrophils and their relation to eosinophilia. Journal of Immunology 119: 976–982

42. Calafat J, Janssen H, Knol EF et al 1997 Ultrastructural localization of Charcot–Leyden crystal protein in human eosinophils and basophils. European Journal of Haematology 58: 56–66

43. Kay AB 1976 Functions of the eosinophil leucocyte. British Journal of Haematology 33: 313–318

44. Butterworth AE, David JR 1981 Eosinophil function. New England Journal of Medicine 304: 154–156

45. Rosenberg HF, Domachowske JB 1999 Eosinophils, ribonucleases and host defense: solving the puzzle. Immunologic Research 20: 261–274

46. Powell WS, Ahmed S, Gravel S, Rokach J 2001 Eotaxin and RANTES enhance 5-oxo-6, 8, 11, 14-eicosatetraenoic acid-induced eosinophil chemotaxis. Journal of Allergy and Clinical Immunology 107: 272–278

47. Dvorak AM, Dvorak HF 1979 The basophil. Its morphology, biochemistry, motility, release reactions, recovery, and role in the inflammatory responses of IgE-mediated and cell-mediated origin. Archives of Pathology and Laboratory Medicine 103: 551–557

48. Zucker-Franklin D 1980 Ultrastructural evidence for the common origin of human mast cells and basophils. Blood 56: 534–540

49. Dvorak AM 1998 Histamine content and secretion in basophils and mast cells. Progress in Histochemistry and Cytochemistry 33: 169–320

50. Heinemann A, Hartnell A, Stubbs VE et al 2000 Basophil responses to chemokines are regulated by both sequential and cooperative receptor signaling. Journal of Immunology 165: 7224–7233

51. van Furth R, Raeburn JA, van Zwet TL 1979 Characteristics of human mononuclear phagocytes. Blood 54: 485–500

52. Chapman EH, Kurec AS, Davey FR 1981 Cell volumes of normal and malignant mononuclear cells. Journal of Clinical Pathology 34: 1083–1090

53. Goodman JW, Goodman DR 1983 Involvement of cells of the immune system in regulation of erythropoiesis. In: Dunn CDR (ed), Current concepts in erythropoiesis. Wiley, Chichester, 59–79

54. White JG 1987 Platelet structural physiology: The ultrastructure of adhesion, secretion and aggregation in arterial thrombosis. In: Thrombosis and platelets in myocardial ischemia. Cardiovascular Clinics 18: 13–33

55. Berndt MC, Castaldi PA, Gordon S et al 1983 Morphological and biochemical confirmation of gray platelet syndrome in two siblings. Australian and New Zealand Journal of Medicine 13: 387–390

56. Stevens RF, Alexander MK 1977 A sex difference in the platelet count. British Journal of Haematology 37: 295–300

57. Bain BJ 1985 Platelet count and platelet size in males and females. Scandinavian Journal of Haematology 35: 77–79

58. von Behrens WE 1975 Mediterranean macrothrombocytopenia. Blood 46: 199–208

59. Essien EM, Usanga EA, Ayeni O 1973 The normal platelet count and platelet factor 3 availability in some Nigerian population groups. Scandinavian Journal of Haematology 10: 378–383

60. Bain BJ, Seed M 1986 Platelet count and platelet size in healthy Africans and West Indians. Clinical and Laboratory Haematology 8: 43–48

61. Packham MA 1983 Platelet function inhibitors. Thrombosis and Haemostasis 50: 610–619

62. Agam G, Livne A 1983 Passive participation of fixed platelets in aggregation facilitated by covalently bound fibrinogen. Blood 61: 186–191

63. Bain B, Forster T 1980 A sex difference in the bleeding time. Thrombosis and Haemostasis 43: 131–132

64. Mielke CH Jr, Kaneshiro MM, Maher IA et al 1969 The standardized normal Ivy bleeding time and its prolongation by aspirin. Blood 34: 204–215

65. Tschopp TB, Weiss HJ, Baumgartner HR 1974 Decreased adhesion of platelets to subendothelium in von Willebrand's disease. Journal of Laboratory and Clinical Medicine 83: 296–300

66. Chesley LC 1972 Plasma and red cell volumes during pregnancy. American Journal of Obstetrics and Gynecology 112: 440–450

67. Chanarin I 1990 The megaloblastic anaemias, 3rd edn. Blackwell Scientific Publications, Oxford.

68. Abernathy MR 1966 Dohle bodies associated with uncomplicated pregnancy. Blood 27: 380–385

69. Sejeny SA, Eastham RD, Baker SR 1975 Platelet counts during normal pregnancy. Journal of Clinical Pathology 28: 812–813

70. Stirling Y, Woolf L, North WRS et al 1984 Haemostasis in normal pregnancy. Thrombosis and Haemostasis 52: 176–183

71. Schroder J, de la Chapelle A 1972 Fetal lymphocytes in the maternal blood. Blood 39: 153–162

Normal bone marrow cells: development, cytology and ultrastructure

2

SN Wickramasinghe

Hemopoietic cells

Development of hemopoiesis

Postnatal changes in the distribution of red marrow

General characteristics of hemopoiesis
Hemopoietic stem cells and progenitor cells

Erythropoiesis
Light microscope cytology of erythroblasts
Cytochemistry
Ultrastructure
Regulation of erythropoiesis

Neutrophil granulocytopoiesis and monocytopoiesis
Neutrophil granulocytopoiesis
Monocytopoiesis: mononuclear phagocyte system

Eosinophil granulocytopoiesis
Light microscope cytology
Cytochemistry
Ultrastructure

Basophil granulocytopoiesis

Megakaryocytopoiesis
Light microscope cytology
Ultrastructure

Lymphopoiesis

Plasma cells
Ultrastructure

Stromal cells

Cells of marrow sinusoids

Bone marrow macrophages (phagocytic reticular cells)
Ultrastructure

Non-phagocytic reticular cells

Mast cells

Osteoblasts and osteoclasts

Cellularity and marrow differential count

There are two categories of cell in the bone marrow, namely, the hemopoietic cells (and the mature blood cells derived from them) and the stromal cells. Some types of stromal cell are derived from the hemopoietic stem cells.

Hemopoietic cells

Development of hemopoiesis

Erythropoiesis begins within the blood islands of the yolk sac on the 14th to 19th day of development of the human embryo and persists there until the end of the 12th week of gestation.[1-3] Yolk sac erythropoiesis occurs intravascularly and is megaloblastic in type. It is associated with the synthesis of three embryonic hemoglobins, Gower I ($\zeta_2\varepsilon_2$), Gower II ($\alpha_2\varepsilon_2$) and Portland I ($\zeta_2\gamma_2$) and results in the production of cells which usually remain nucleated throughout their life span (Fig. 2.1). In the 6th and 7th weeks of gestation, the blood islands also contain a few megakaryocytes. Erythropoietic foci appear in the fetal liver in the 6th week of gestation and the liver becomes the main site of erythropoiesis from the 3rd to the 6th month when erythroblasts account for about 50% of the nucleated cells of the liver.[2,4] The erythroblasts are found extravascularly within the liver parenchyma (Fig. 2.2) and are initially megaloblastic in type but subsequently become macronormoblastic. Fetal hepatic erythropoiesis is associated with the synthesis of fetal hemoglobin (HbF; $\alpha_2\gamma_2$) and results in the production of anucleate, macrocytic red cells. The liver continues to produce red cells in decreasing numbers after the 6th month of gestation until the end of the 1st postnatal week.

Occasional foci of erythropoietic cells can be seen in the vascular connective tissue of certain marrow cavities between 2.5 and 4 months of gestation;[3] after the 6th month the marrow is the major site of fetal hemopoiesis. The myeloid/erythroid (M/E) ratio in this tissue is about 1:4 after $6\frac{1}{2}$ months of gestation.[5] Erythropoiesis in fetal bone marrow occurs extravascularly, is macronormoblastic in type and results in the production of macrocytic red cells containing HbF and HbA ($\alpha_2\ \beta_2$): the mean cell volume (MCV) in the cord blood of full-term babies ranges between 90 and 118 fl. Erythropoieisis in fetal bone marrow appears to be regulated by erythropoietin produced extrarenally, probably in the liver. Small foci of erythroblasts, a few granulocytopoietic cells and occasional megakaryocytes occur in many embryonic and fetal tissues and organs but their contribution to total hemopoietic activity is probably small. Tissues containing such foci include the lymph nodes, spleen and kidneys.

Postnatal changes in the distribution of red marrow[6,7]

At birth all the marrow cavities contain red marrow consisting mainly of hemopoietic cells. By the age of 1 year, virtually all of the hemopoietic cells in the terminal phalanges are replaced by fat cells. After the first 4 years an increasing number of fat cells appear amongst the hemopoietic cells of other marrow cavities. Between the ages of 10 and 14 years, the hemopoietic cells in the middle of the shafts of the long bones become virtually completely replaced by fat cells. Subsequently, these zones of non-hemopoietic yellow marrow spread both proximally and distally. Distal spread is more rapid than

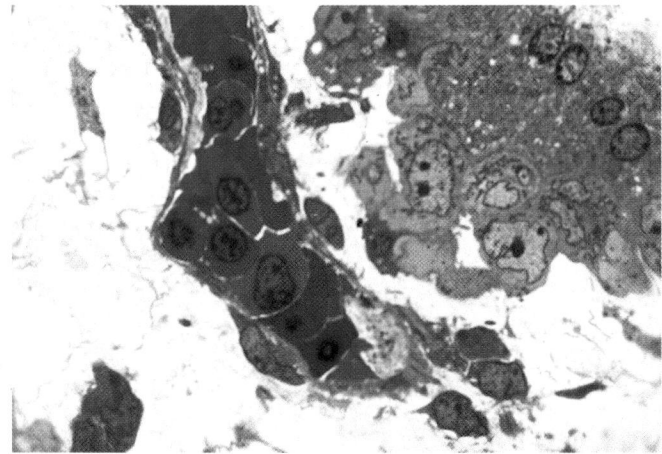

Fig. 2.1 Semithin section of a plastic-embedded chorionic villus biopsy taken at 7 weeks of gestation showing a blood vessel containing nucleated embryonic red cells. Toluidine blue.

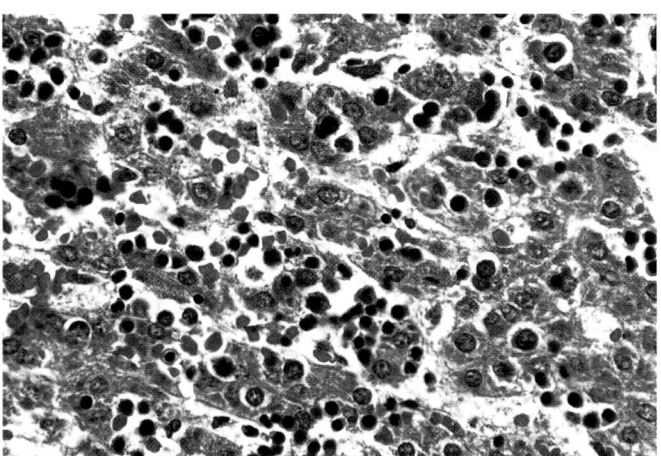

Fig. 2.2 Histologic appearances of normal fetal liver during the middle trimester of pregnancy. About 40% of the area of the section consists of erythropoietic cells which are present singly or in clusters between the plates of liver cells. Hematoxylin–eosin.

proximal spread and by about the 25th year the only regions of the long bones that contain red, hemopoietic marrow are the proximal quarters of the shafts of the femora and humeri. Other sites of hemopoiesis in an adult are the skull, ribs, clavicles, scapulae, sternum, vertebrae and pelvis.

General characteristics of hemopoiesis

During intrauterine life and in the growing child, there is a progressive increase with time in the total number of hemopoietic and blood cells. By contrast, in normal adults, the total number of such cells remains more or less constant. All the hemopoietic systems of normal adults are examples of steady-state cell renewal systems in which a relatively constant rate of loss of mature cells (erythrocytes, granulocytes, monocytes and platelets) is balanced fairly precisely by the production of new cells.

The formation of blood cells of all types involves two processes: (1) the progressive development of biochemical, functional and structural characteristics specific for a given cell type (i.e. cytodifferentiation); and (2) cell proliferation. The latter serves to amplify the number of mature cells produced from a cell that has become committed to any particular blood cell production line.

Hemopoietic stem cells and progenitor cells

The hemopoietic cells can be divided into two categories: (1) the early precursors that cannot be recognized morphologically with certainty but that can be studied by functional tests (described as the 'morphologically unrecognized precursors'); and (2) the morphologically recognizable precursors. The morphologically unrecognized precursors consist of two categories: (1) hemopoietic stem cells that have both the ability to develop into various types of blood cell and an extensive capacity to maintain their own numbers by cell proliferation; and (2) hemopoietic progenitor cells that are committed to one or more hemopoietic differentiation pathways but that do not have a substantial capacity for self-renewal.

The most primitive hemopoietic stem cells are pluripotent and generate both multipotent myeloid stem cells, whose progeny develop into erythrocytes, granulocytes, monocytes, platelets, osteoclasts and mast cells, and lymphoid stem cells that give rise to all types of lymphocyte.[8-10] Thus, cytogenetic studies have not only shown that the Philadelphia (Ph) chromosome is present

in the granulocytic, erythroid and megakaryocytic lineages of most patients with chronic granulocytic leukemia (CGL), but also that this chromosome is present in the lymphoblasts of some patients with lymphoblastic leukemia whose disease later evolves into CGL and in those of some patients with CGL whose disease has evolved into a lymphoblastic crisis. Further evidence for the existence of a pluripotent stem cell in humans comes from the demonstration that in one case of sideroblastic anemia with glucose-6-phosphate-dehydrogenase (G6PD) mosaicism, a single G6PD isoenzyme was present in myeloid cells as well as in T- and B-lymphocytes[11] and from studies of xenogeneic transplant models in immuno-incompetent animals[12] (also see Chapter 4). As is evident from Chapter 4, several investigators now restrict the term hemopoietic stem cell to what has been termed the pluripotent hemopoietic stem cell in the present chapter. The multipotent myeloid stem cells and the lymphopotent stem cells referred to above are then considered to be early committed progenitor cells.

Initially, the multipotent myeloid stem cell was defined by its ability to form within the spleen macroscopically visible colonies composed of a mixture of cell types when injected into lethally irradiated mice; this stem cell is therefore frequently referred to as the 'colony-forming unit in spleen' or CFU-S. Subsequently, cells that are closely related to these stem cells became assayable in semi-solid culture media in which they give rise to colonies containing cells of all four myeloid lineages, that is granulocyte–erythrocyte–macrophage–megakaryocyte (GEMM) colonies. The morphology of the myeloid stem cell may resemble that of medium-sized lymphocytes (transitional lymphocytes).

In healthy adults most of the myeloid stem cells are in a quiescent state (i.e. in the G_0 phase) or in a prolonged G_1 phase. However, when there is an increased need for hemopoiesis, these normally quiescent stem cells become triggered into active proliferation. Unlike the myeloid stem cells, a high proportion of the more mature hemopoietic progenitor cells are engaged in cell proliferation. The hemopoietic progenitor cells are interposed between the stem cells and the earliest morphologically recognizable precursor cells and undergo progressive restriction in their differentiation potential until they eventually become unipotent.

The complex mechanisms involved in the regulation of hemopoietic stem cells and progenitor cells are described in Chapter 4. Growth-promoting cytokines such as granulocyte–macrophage colony stimulating factor (GM-CSF) and granulocyte colony stimulating factor (G-CSF) not only influence hemopoiesis but also enhance some functions of the mature cells.

Erythropoiesis[8]

There are several generations of hemopoietic progenitor cells that are committed to erythropoiesis. These have been defined and studied operationally in terms of the characteristics of the erythroid colonies they generate in appropriate semi-solid media. The most immature of such cells are referred to as the erythroid burst-forming units (BFU-E) and the most mature as the erythroid colony-forming units (CFU-E). The CFU-E develop into proerythroblasts which are the earliest morphologically recognizable red cell precursors in the marrow. The proerythroblasts then progress through several morphologically-defined cytologic classes. These are, in order of increasing maturity, the basophilic erythroblasts, the early polychromatic erythroblasts, the late poly-chromatic erythroblasts and the marrow and blood reticulocytes. Cell division occurs in the proerythroblasts, basophilic erythroblasts and early polychromatic erythroblasts but not in more mature cells. By contrast, the results of cytodifferentiation can be seen in all classes of morphologically recognizable precursors, both proliferating and non-proliferating. There are, on average, four cell divisions in the morphologically-recognizable precursor pool so that one proerythroblast may give rise to 2^4 or 16 red cells. In normal adults, the time taken for a proerythroblast to mature into marrow reticulocytes and for these reticulocytes to enter the circulation is about 7 days; of this, about 2.5 days is spent in the marrow reticulocyte pool. The time taken for blood reticulocytes to mature into erythrocytes is 1–2 days. In normal individuals erythrocytes circulate for 110–120 days before they are removed and broken down by cells of the mononuclear phagocyte system.

Both in normal subjects and in various pathologic states, the erythroblasts are organized into erythroblastic islands composed of one or more central macrophages surrounded by one or two layers of erythroblasts (Figs 2.3 and 2.4). Studies in experimental animals indicate that erythropoietic islands are necessary functional units for active erythropoiesis.[13] Surface receptors on central macrophages are involved in macrophage–erythroblast interactions and one such receptor, Emp, is required for terminal erythroid differentiation and enucleation.[14] The central macrophages produce both stimulatory and inhibitory cytokines.

Some of the erythropoietic cells do not develop successfully into erythrocytes but are recognized as being abnormal and phagocytosed by the bone marrow macrophages. This loss of potential erythrocytes is referred to as ineffective erythropoiesis. The extent of ineffective erythropoiesis is small in normal marrow but is substantial in certain diseases.

Light microscope cytology of erythroblasts

In this chapter, the term *erythroblast* is used to describe any nucleated red cell precursor, normal or pathologic; the term *normoblast* is applied only to nucleated red cells that resemble those seen in normal bone marrow. The various classes of normal erythroblast are termed, in increasing order of maturity, pronormoblasts, basophilic

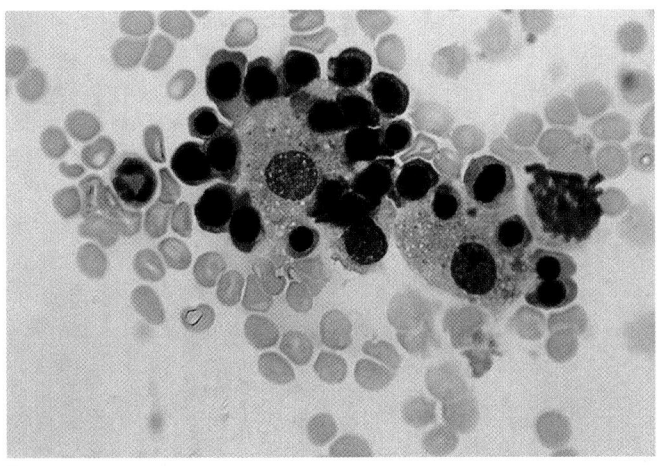

A

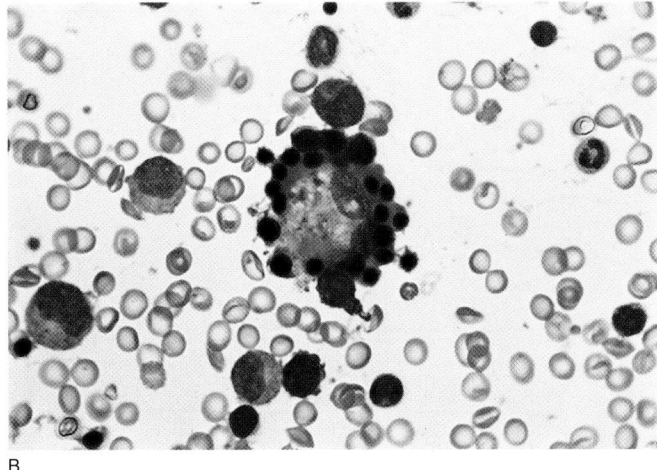

B

Fig. 2.3 (A,B) Erythroblastic islands from a normal subject (A) and a patient with iron deficiency anemia (B). (A) The island consists of several early and late polychromatic erythroblasts that are closely associated with a macrophage. A second macrophage lying near the erythroblastic island is partially surrounded by erythroblasts. The nucleus of each macrophage has a pale-staining lace-like chromatin structure. (B) The central macrophage is attached to a pronormoblast and several early and late polychromatic erythroblasts. May–Grünwald–Giemsa stain.

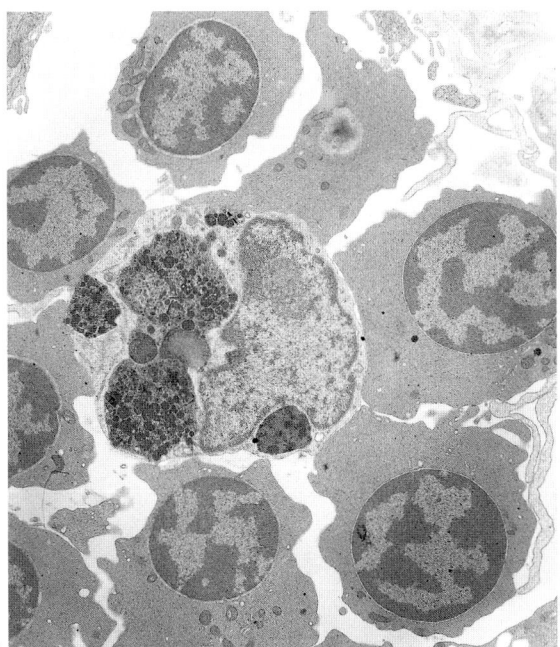

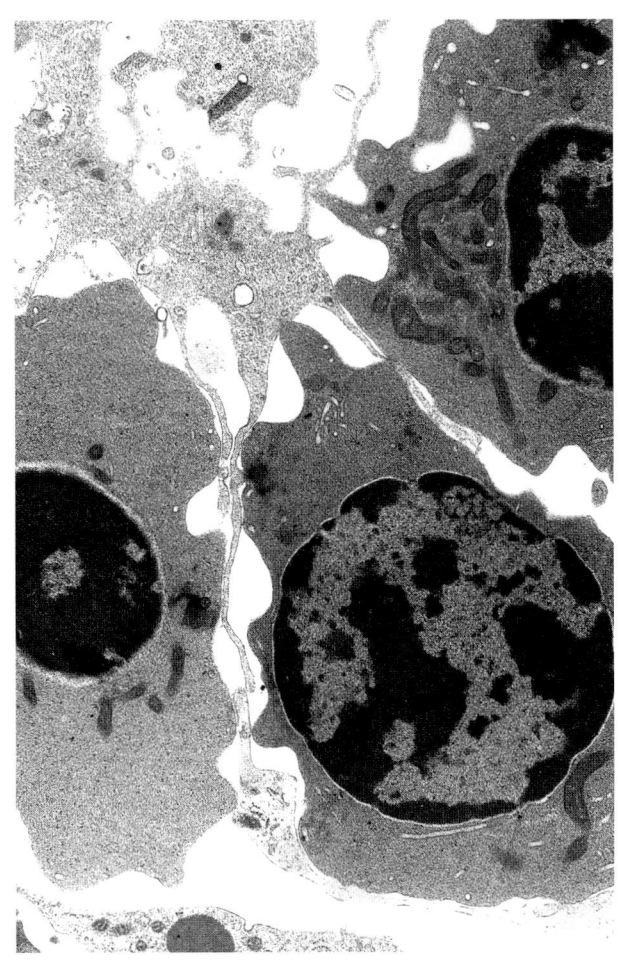

Fig. 2.4 (A,B) Electron micrographs of two erythroblastic islands from normal bone marrow. (A) The central macrophage, which contains large intracytoplasmic inclusions, is surrounded by a layer of erythroblasts. Thin processes of macrophage cytoplasm can be seen between and around the three erythroblasts on the right. (B) A higher power view of part of another island showing thin processes of macrophage cytoplasm partially surrounding three erythroblasts. Uranyl acetate and lead citrate.

normoblasts, early polychromatic normoblasts, late polychromatic normoblasts, marrow reticulocytes and blood reticulocytes.

In Romanowsky-stained marrow smears, the pronormoblast (Fig. 2.5A) appears as a large cell with a diameter of 12–20 μm. It has a large rounded nucleus that is surrounded by a small amount of deep-blue cytoplasm; the intensity of cytoplasmic basophilia is greater than that shown by myeloblasts. The cytoplasm may show a pale area adjacent to the nucleus (corresponding to the Golgi apparatus) and frequently displays small blebs at the periphery. The nuclear chromatin has a finely granular or finely reticular appearance and there are prominent nucleoli. Cells belonging to successive cytologic classes show a progressive decrease in average cell and nuclear diameter and a progressive increase in the volume of cytoplasm relative to that of the nucleus. The cytoplasm of the basophilic normoblast (Fig. 2.5B) is even more blue-staining than that of the pronormoblast. Its nuclear chromatin has a coarsely granular appearance and there are no nucleoli. The early polychromatic normoblast (Figs 2.5C, D) has polychromatic cytoplasm and a nucleus containing small or moderately large clumps of con-

densed chromatin. The late polychromatic normoblasts (Fig. 2.5E) have a diameter of 8–10 μm, a faintly polychromatic cytoplasm and a small eccentric nucleus with a diameter less than about 6.5 μm and containing large clumps of condensed chromatin. Eventually the nucleus becomes pyknotic and is extruded. The morphology of the resulting marrow reticulocytes is similar to that of circulating reticulocytes as described in Chapter 1.

Cytochemistry

Normal erythroblasts are periodic acid-Schiff (PAS)-, Sudan black- and peroxidase-negative. Occasional erythroblasts contain a few alpha-naphthol AS-D chloroacetate esterase-positive granules. Cells in all classes of erythroblast frequently contain coarse acid-phosphatase-positive paranuclear granules. When normal marrow smears are stained by Perls' acid ferrocyanide method, one to five very small blue–black granules are seen in 20–90% of the polychromatic erythroblasts, randomly distributed in the cytoplasm. These iron-containing granules are termed siderotic granules and erythroblasts containing such granules are termed sideroblasts.

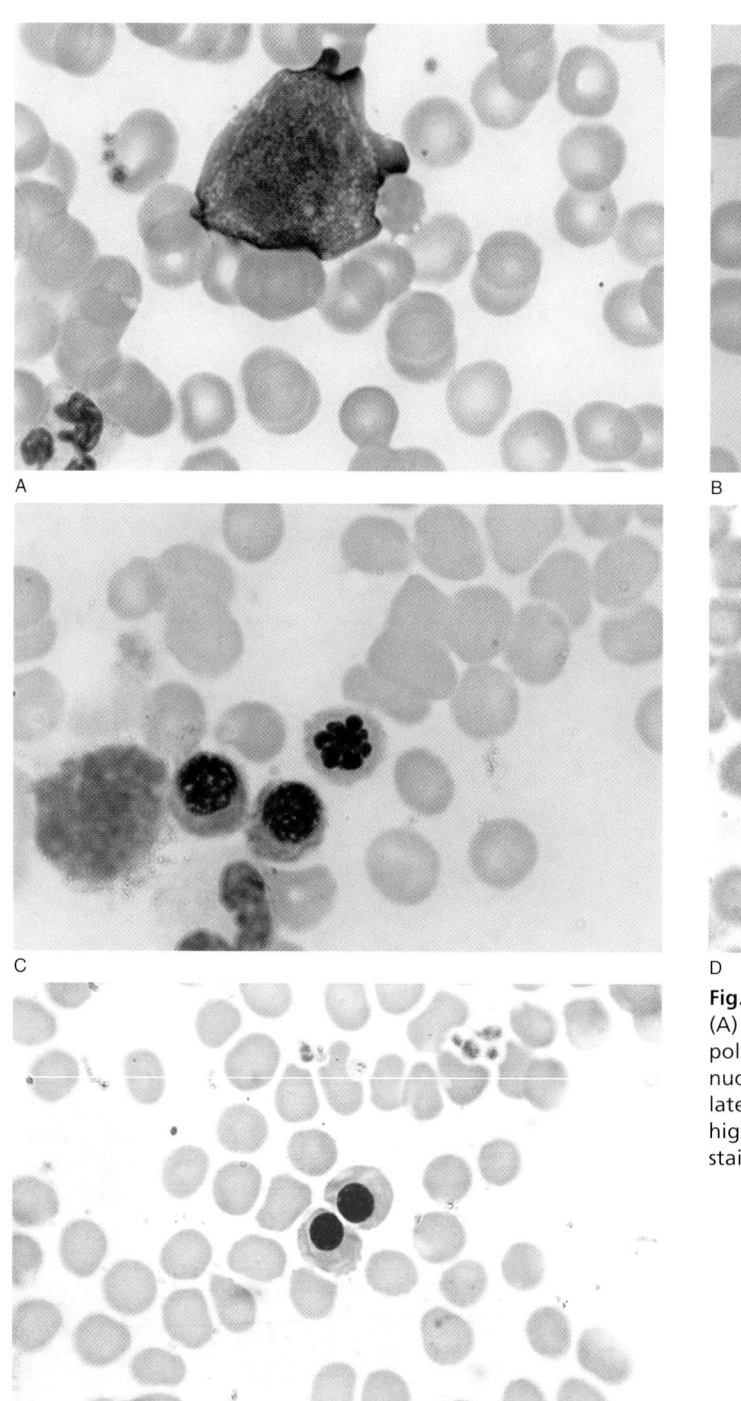

A

B

C

D

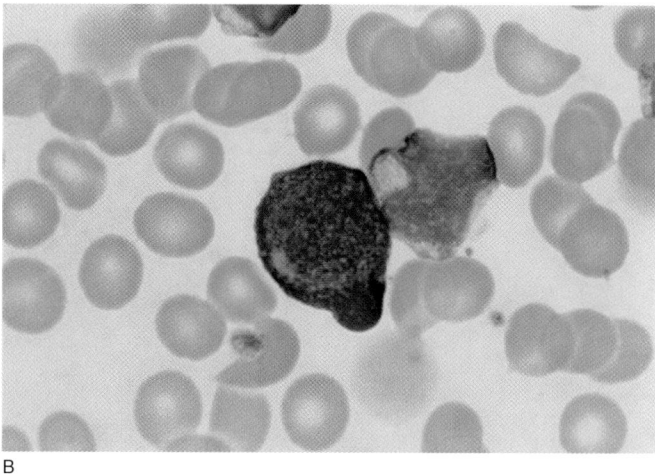

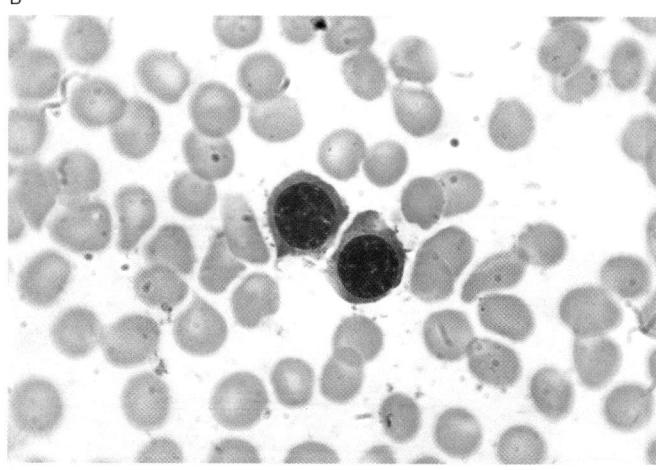

Fig. 2.5 Erythroblasts from a smear of normal bone marrow. (A) Pronormoblast. (B) Basophilic normoblast. (C) Three early polychromatic normoblasts, including one with a karyorrhectic nucleus (rare). (D) Two early polychromatic normoblasts. (E) Two late polychromatic normoblasts. (A), (B) and (C) are at a slightly higher magnification than (D) and (E). May–Grünwald–Giemsa stain.

E

Ultrastructure

Electron microscope studies[15] show that all erythroblasts contain characteristic surface invaginations (Fig. 2.6) which develop into small intracytoplasmic vesicles (rhopheocytotic vesicles); the function of these vesicles is uncertain. The walls of rhopheocytotic vesicles are made up of a single membrane whose inner surface is coated with an amorphous material; the vesicles sometimes contain ferritin molecules. Pronormoblasts possess cytoplasm of low electron-density and nuclei in which the chromatin is predominantly in the form of euchromatin (expanded chromatin) with little nuclear-membrane-associated heterochromatin (condensed chromatin) (Fig. 2.7A). They have a fairly well-developed Golgi apparatus adjacent to a moderately deep indentation of the nucleus,

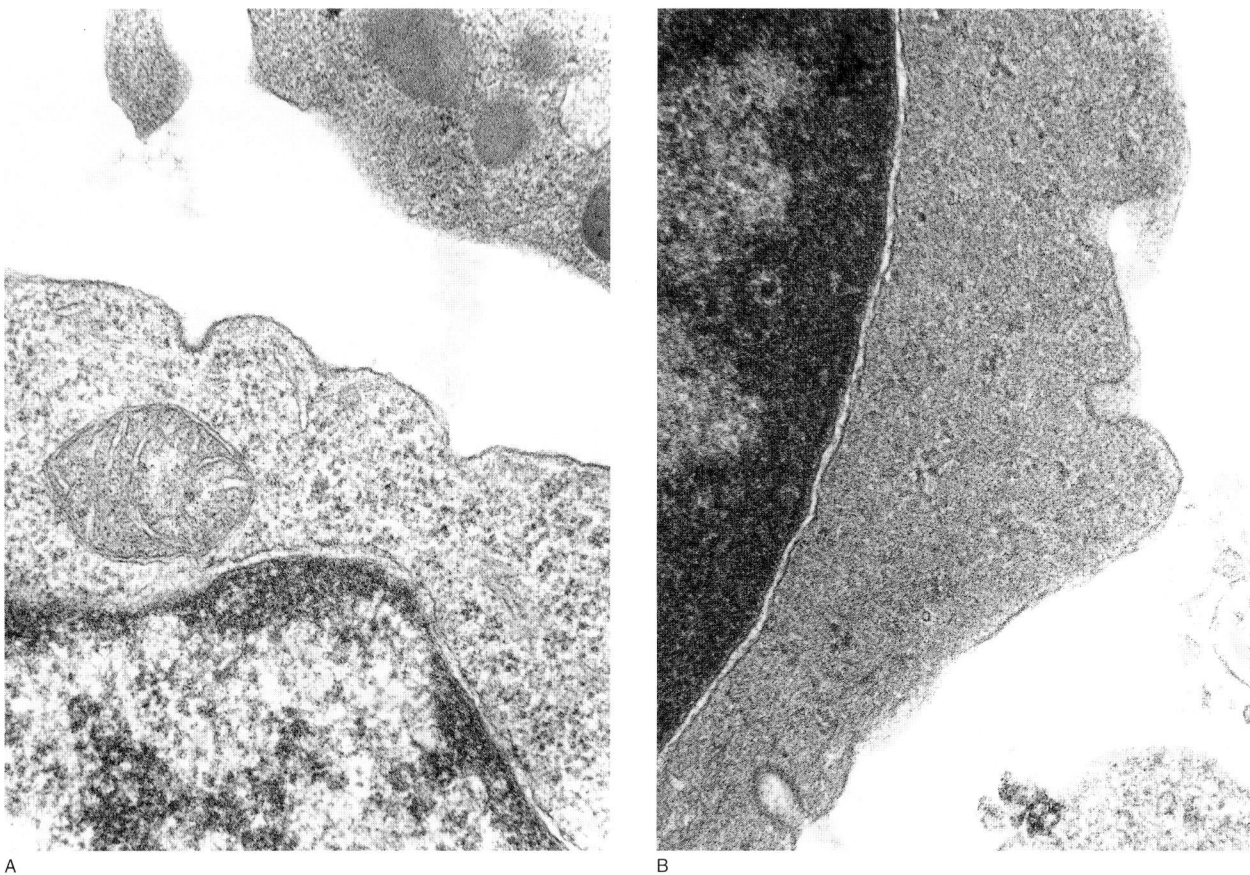

A   B

Fig. 2.6 (A,B) Electron micrographs of two normal erythroblasts showing characteristic surface invaginations (formation of rhopheocytotic vesicles). (A) Basophilic normoblast ($\times$ 45 800). (B) Late polychromatic normoblast ($\times$ 54 200). Clusters of polyribosomes and a mitochondrion are seen in the basophilic normoblast. Uranyl acetate and lead citrate.

numerous polyribosomes, several mitochondria, some strands of endoplasmic reticulum, some scattered ferritin molecules and a few pleomorphic electron-dense acid-phosphatase-positive lysosomal granules usually grouped near the Golgi saccules. The maturation of pronormoblasts into late polychromatic normoblasts (Figs 2.7B,C) is accompanied by: (1) a progressive increase in the amount of heterochromatin both in the nucleoplasm and adjacent to the nuclear membrane; (2) a progressive decrease in the number of ribosomes; (3) a progressive increase in the electron-density of the cytoplasm due to the accumulation of hemoglobin; (4) a decrease in the number and size of the mitochondria; and (5) a tendency of intra-cytoplasmic ferritin molecules to aggregate into siderosomes. A Golgi apparatus persists in polychromatic erythroblasts (Fig. 2.8). The extruded nucleus of the late polychromatic erythroblast is surrounded by a very thin rim of cytoplasm and is enclosed within a cytoplasmic membrane. It is rapidly phagocytosed by adjacent macrophages. The entry of newly formed reticulocytes into the marrow sinusoids occurs through temporary and rather narrow transendothelial channels (Fig. 2.7D).

Regulation of erythropoiesis

The various elements involved in the regulation of hemopoiesis, including erythropoiesis, are discussed in detail in Chapter 4. A key factor determining the rate of red cell production is the hormone erythropoietin (a glycoprotein). Receptors for eythropoietin are expressed on erythroid cells and the binding of erythropoietin to its receptor results in the activation of an incompletely characterized intracellular signaling pathway. An important effect of erythropoietin is to maintain the viability and proliferation of erythroid progenitor cells, by preventing programed cell death. It is probably by this mechanism that erythropoietin stimulates the rate of conversion of CFU-E to pronormoblasts. Erythropoietin also stimulates terminal differentiation and decreases the time taken for the maturation of a pronormoblast to a marrow reticulocyte and the release of the latter into the circulation. The plasma level of erythropoietin is inversely related to the capacity of the blood to deliver oxygen to the kidneys and other tissues. Thus, in most anemic states there is an increased level of erythropoietin in the

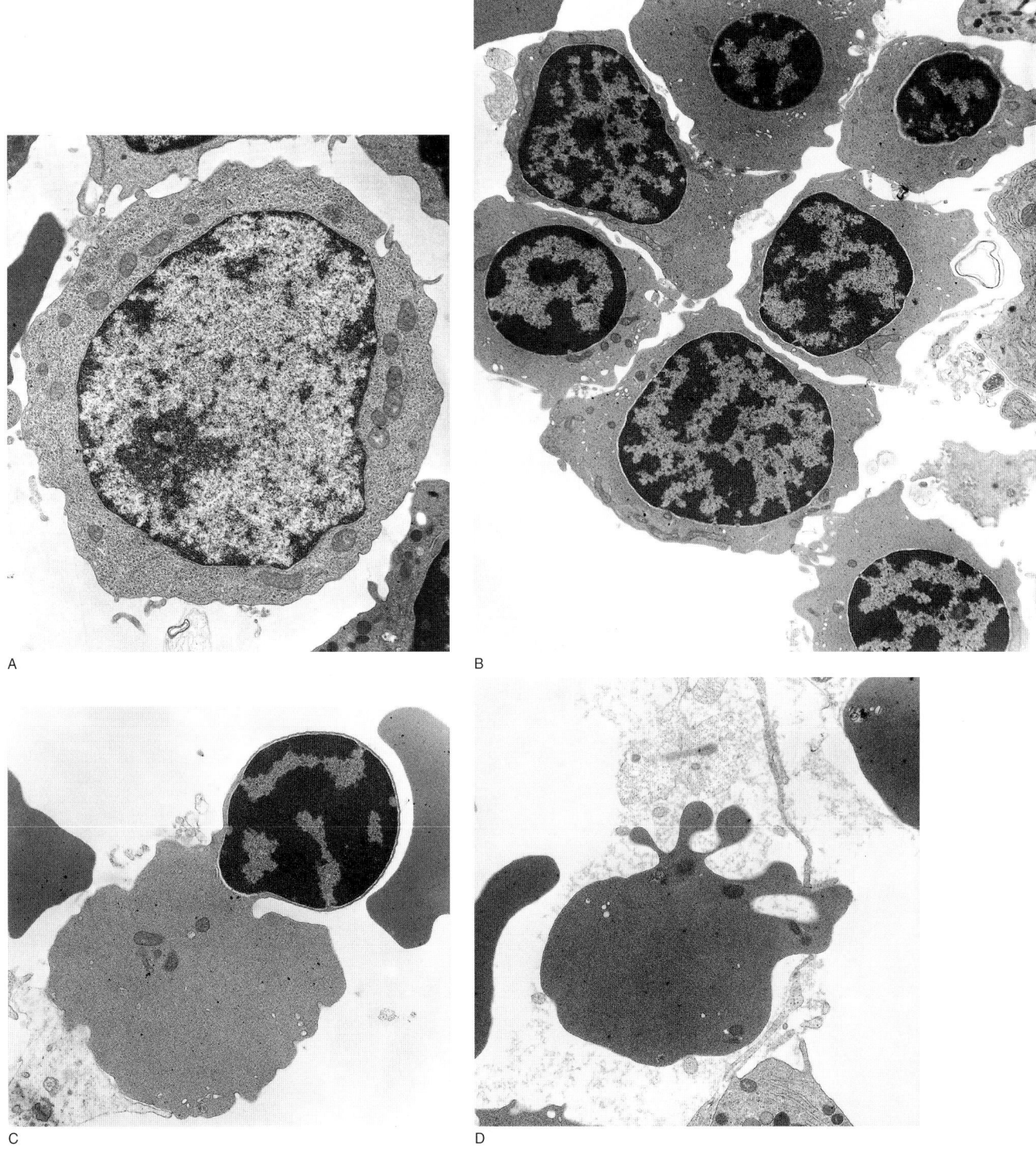

A

B

C

D

Fig. 2.7 (A–D) Electron micrographs of erythroblasts from normal bone marrow. (A) Pronormoblast. (B) Group of early and late polychromatic normoblasts. (C) Late polychromatic normoblast immediately prior to extruding its nucleus. (D) Reticulocyte in the process of entering a marrow sinusoid. Most of the cell has passed through the endothelial cell of the sinusoidal wall. Uranyl acetate and lead citrate. (A) × 7700, (B) × 7100, (C) × 7800, (D) × 7700.

plasma, which in turn causes an enhancement of the rate of erythropoiesis. The kidneys are the organs mainly concerned with erythropoietin production in adults and the hormone is produced by peritubular cells. Bone marrow macrophages may also produce erythropoietin.

The secretions of various endocrine glands influence erythropoiesis and patients with hypofunction of the thyroid, testes, adrenal glands or anterior lobe of the pituitary gland develop a mild to moderate anemia. Thyroxine, androgens and growth hormone stimulate

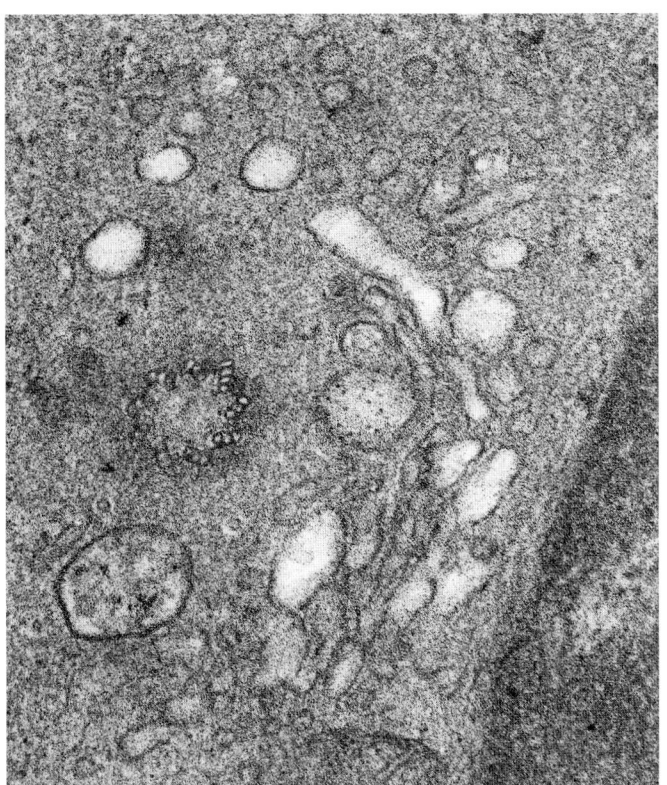

Fig. 2.8 Electron micrograph of part of a polychromatic erythroblast from normal marrow showing a centriole lying adjacent to sacs of a relatively poorly developed Golgi apparatus. Uranyl acetate and lead citrate. × 86 300.

erythropoiesis partly by an effect on the kidneys which results in an increased production of erythropoietin. Thyroxine also stimulates erythropoiesis by modulating β-adrenergic receptor activity in CFU-E and androgens directly stimulate the proliferation of multipotent hemopoietic stem cells and CFU-E. Corticosteriods enhance erythropoiesis both by a stimulation of erythropoietin production and by a direct effect on the bone marrow. There is some evidence that estrogens may inhibit erythropoiesis; the sex difference in the hemoglobin levels of adults appears to be largely due to the higher androgen levels in males.

Neutrophil granulocytopoiesis and monocytopoiesis

There are several generations of hemopoietic progenitor cells concerned with the production of neutrophil granulocytes and macrophages. These have been defined on the basis of their ability to form colonies of granulocytes, macrophages or both when grown *in vitro* in semi-solid media containing appropriate colony-stimulating factors or *in vivo* within diffusion chambers implanted

intraperitoneally in mice. Cells giving rise to granulocyte or macrophage colonies *in vitro* are described as granulocyte–macrophage colony-forming units (CFU-GM). The multipotent myeloid stem cell generates a bipotent granulocyte–macrophage progenitor cell and the latter develops into progenitor cells that are irreversibly committed to mature either into neutrophils (CFU-G) or into macrophages (CFU-M). The earliest morphologically recognizable precursors in the neutrophil and monocyte–macrophage series are the myeloblasts and monoblasts respectively.

Neutrophil granulocytopoiesis[8]

The morphologically recognizable cells of the neutrophil series are, in order of increasing maturity, the myeloblasts, neutrophil promyelocytes, neutrophil myelocytes, neutrophil metamyelocytes, juvenile neutrophils and the marrow neutrophil granulocytes. Cell division occurs up to and including the myelocyte stage; more mature cells are non-dividing. Cytodifferentiation occurs both in the proliferating and non-proliferating cells. The time taken for a myeloblast to mature into a marrow granulocyte and for the latter to enter the circulation is 10–12 days; about half of this time is spent in the proliferating cell pool. In normal individuals the blood neutrophils leave the circulation with an average $T_{1/2}$ of 7.2 h.

Light microscope cytology of neutrophil precursors

In Romanowsky-stained marrow smears, myeloblasts have a diameter of 10–20 μm, a large rounded or oval nucleus with finely dispersed chromatin, two to five nucleoli and a relatively small quantity of agranular, moderately deep-blue cytoplasm (Fig. 2.9A). The neutrophil promyelocyte is larger than the myeloblast and is characterized by the presence of a few to several purplish-red (azurophilic) granules (primary granules), a somewhat coarser nuclear chromatin pattern and prominent nucleoli (Figs. 2.9B,C). The neutrophil myelocyte has a greater volume of cytoplasm relative to that of the nucleus when compared with the promyelocyte and usually has an eccentric nucleus. The cytoplasm is initially slightly basophilic but eventually becomes predominantly acidophilic. It contains many fine, light-pink (neutrophilic) granules (specific granules) in addition to some azurophilic ones. The nucleus is rounded, oval, flattened on one side or slightly indented (see Figs. 2.9C,D), contains coarsely granular chromatin and usually lacks a distinct nucleolus. The neutrophil metamyelocyte has a C-shaped nucleus which displays a

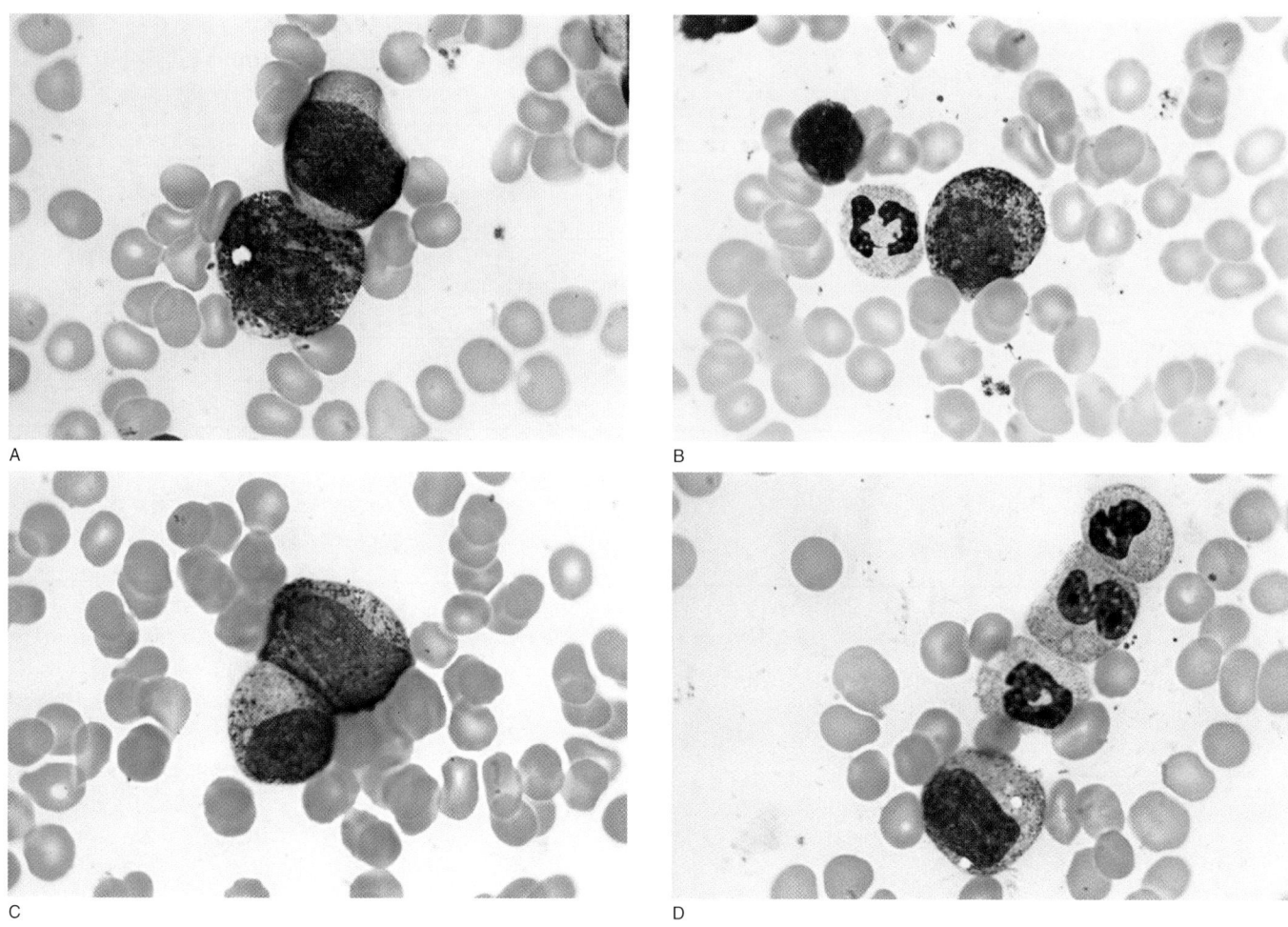

A

B

C

D

Fig. 2.9 (A–D) Granulocytopoietic cells from a smear of normal bone marrow. (A) Myeloblast and eosinophil myelocyte. (B) Neutrophil promyelocyte and neutrophil granulocyte. (C) Neutrophil promyelocyte and neutrophil myelocyte. (D) Neutrophil myelocyte and three band neutrophils. May–Grünwald–Giemsa stain.

greater degree of condensation of nuclear chromatin than the myelocyte nucleus. Its cytoplasm stains pale pink and contains numerous neutrophilic granules but few or no azurophilic granules. The 'band' or juvenile neutrophil (also called a 'stab form') has a U-shaped or long, relatively-narrow band-like nucleus which shows no further condensation of the chromatin. The nucleus is frequently twisted into various configurations and may show one or more partial constrictions along its length (Fig. 2.9D). The neutrophil granulocyte differs from the 'band' neutrophil in having a segmented nucleus in which two to five nuclear masses are strung together by fine stands of chromatin; the nuclear masses contain large clumps of condensed chromatin (Fig. 2.9B, also see Figs 1.1A and 1.5).

Cytochemistry[16–19]

Myeloblasts are peroxidase-negative and, usually, alpha-naphthol AS-D chloroacetate-esterase-negative. They do not stain with Sudan black or show a few small stained granules near the nucleus. They are diffusely stained pale red–purple by the PAS reaction and there may sometimes also be a fine granular positivity. Neutrophil promyelocytes and more mature cells show granular cytoplasmic staining with the PAS reagent and Sudan black and with reactions for peroxidase and alpha-naphthol AS-D chloroacetate esterase activity. The intensity of PAS staining and, to a lesser extent, Sudan black staining increases in cell classes of increasing maturity. Alpha-naphthyl acetate esterase activity is present in promyelocytes and myelocytes but not granulocytes. Promyelocytes and more mature cells are acid-phosphatase-positive with the more immature cells showing stronger positivity than the more mature ones. Segmented neutrophil granulocytes show weak to strong staining for alkaline phosphatase activity and a few metamyelocytes stain weakly. Immunocytochemical investigations have demonstrated lysozyme and elastase in promyelocytes and more mature cells and lactoferrin in myelocytes, metamyelocytes and granulocytes.

Ultrastructure and granule composition

Electron microscope studies[15,20–22] reveal that the myeloblast nucleus contains one or more well-developed nucleoli and has only a small amount of peripheral condensed chromatin. The cytoplasm is rich in ribosomes and has a few strands of endoplasmic reticulum and a small Golgi apparatus. Neutrophil promyelocytes contain large quantities of rough endoplasmic reticulum (RER), many polyribosomes, a highly-developed Golgi apparatus, several large mitochondria and relatively little condensed chromatin. In successive cytologic classes of increasing maturity, there is a reduction in the quantity of RER, ribosomes and mitochondria, a diminution of the Golgi apparatus (after the myelocyte stage) and an increase in the amount of condensed chromatin. In addition, a large number of glycogen particles appear at the metamyelocyte and granulocyte stages.

The primary (azurophilic) granules that develop at the promyelocyte stage are ellipsoidal, very electron-dense, about 0.5–1.0 μm in their long axis, and contain peroxidase, acid phosphatase, lysozyme, elastase, α_1 antitrypsin and sulphated mucosubstances. Some primary granules have a core with a linear periodic substructure. There are at least two subpopulations of specific granules, the secondary and tertiary granules, that are synthesized *de novo* at the myelocyte (Figs 2.10 and 2.11) and metamyelocyte stages, respectively. The secondary granules are larger, more spherical and less electron-dense than primary granules, and undergo a variable degree of extraction during processing. They contain lysozyme and transcobalamin I and are peroxidase-negative; they are peroxidase-positive only if a high concentration of diaminobenzidine is used at alkaline pH when staining for this enzyme. They are also acid-phosphatase-negative. The tertiary granules are small (0.2–0.5 μm in their long axis), rounded, elongated or dumb-bell-shaped, peroxidase-negative and acid-phosphatase-negative; their electron-density is between that of the primary and secondary granules. Some of the secondary and tertiary granules contain lactoferrin or lactoferrin and gelatinase. A subpopulation of tertiary granules (termed gelatinase granules) contains gelatinase but little or no lactoferrin.[23] (Some investigators reserve the term tertiary granules for the gelatinase granules and use the term specific granule for all other granules excluding primary granules.) Human cationic antimicrobial protein (hCAP-18) is synthesized in myelocytes and metamyelocytes and is found with lactoferrin in specific granules.[24] The primary granules formed at the promyelocyte stage remain in the

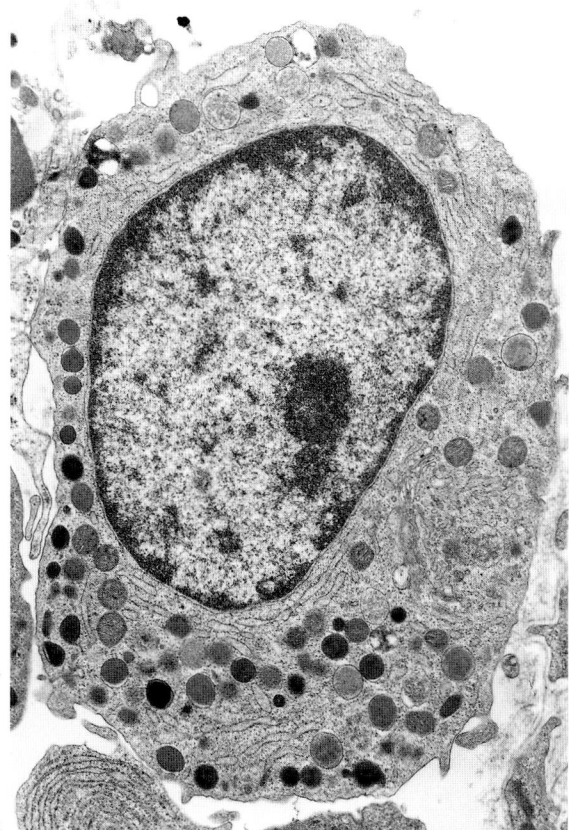

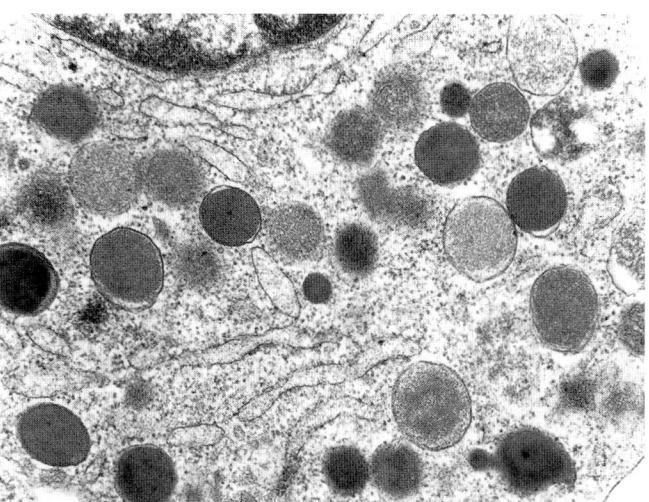

Fig. 2.10 (A) Electron micrograph of a neutrophil myelocyte from normal bone marrow. The nucleus is rounded, contains a nucleolus and shows a small amount of nuclear-membrane-associated heterochromatin (condensed chromatin). The cytoplasm contains two morphologically distinct types of granules and many strands of rough endoplasmic reticulum. Uranyl acetate and lead citrate. × 11 100. (B) The lower part of the cell in (A) at higher magnification, showing the different appearances of the two types of granules: the very electron-dense granules are known as primary granules (and are formed at the promyelocyte stage) and the less electron-dense granules are known as secondary granules (and are formed at the myelocyte stage). Uranyl acetate and lead citrate. × 26 000.

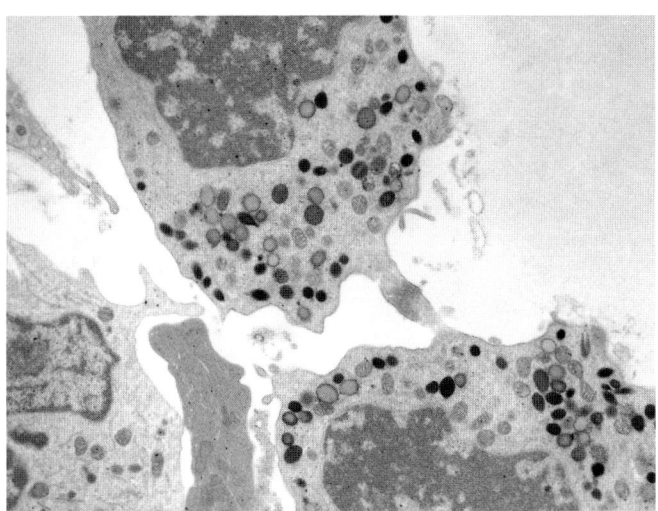

Fig. 2.11 A neutrophil myelocyte from normal bone marrow at a late stage of cell division. The two daughter cells contain telophase nuclei and are joined together by an intercellular spindle bridge. Their cytoplasm contains a mixture of primary and secondary granules. Uranyl acetate and lead citrate. × 8400

more mature cells, including granulocytes, but lose their azurophilic property and are therefore not seen by light microscopy in metamyelocytes and more mature cells. The cytoplasm of neutrophil granulocytes contains small membrane-bound vesicles with alkaline phosphatase activity, called phosphosomes. There are also secretory vesicles, formed by endocytosis in band cells and neutrophils representing a store of mobilizable surface-membrane-bound receptors.[25] The diversity in the composition of neutrophil granules is based on the synthesis of individual granule proteins at different times during granulocytopoiesis, which in turn appears to be based on transcriptional control of mRNAs for individual granule proteins.[26]

Monocytopoiesis: mononuclear phagocyte system[27]

The morphologically recognizable precursors of the blood monocytes are, in order of increasing maturity, the monoblasts, promonocytes and marrow monocytes; only the first two of these cell types undergo division. The blood monocytes leave the circulation with an average $T_{1/2}$ of 71 h and transform into tissue macrophages. In the normal steady state there is a constant loss of tissue macrophages (e.g. by shedding of alveolar macrophages), which is balanced by the formation of new macrophages from blood monocytes and to a small extent from the division of some existing macrophages. The system of cells concerned with macrophage production is called the mononuclear phagocyte system. At sites of inflammation,

macrophages may transform into epithelioid cells or develop into multinucleate giant cells.

Light microscope cytology of monocyte precursors

Monoblasts are agranular cells with basophilic cytoplasm and resemble myeloblasts except for the tendency of their nuclei to be cleft or slightly lobulated. When compared with monoblasts, promonocytes are larger, have a lower nucleus-to-cytoplasm ratio and contain less-basophilic cytoplasm. They have a rounded, oval or clearly lobulated nucleus which consists predominantly of euchromatin and one or more prominent nucleoli may be visible. A small number of azurophilic granules are present in their cytoplasm. Marrow monocytes and blood monocytes have less cytoplasmic basophilia, a lower nucleus-to-cytoplasm ratio (< 1) and a greater number of azurophilic granules than promonocytes. Their cytoplasm is pale gray–blue with a ground-glass appearance and sometimes contains vacuoles. They have an eccentric oval, kidney-shaped, horse-shoe-shaped or lobulated nucleus with skein-like or lacy chromatin.

Cytochemistry[16,19,28]

Monocytes stain positively for alpha-naphthyl acetate esterase (non-specific esterase) and alpha-naphthyl butyrate esterase but are alpha-naphthol AS-D chloroacetate-esterase-negative. Whereas in the granulocytes series both the alpha-naphthyl acetate and butyrate esterase activities are fluoride-insensitive, in monocytes and macrophages these activities are inhibited by fluoride. Other cytochemical characteristics of monocytes are some granular PAS- and Sudan black-positivity, slight granular peroxidase-positivity, strong staining for acid phosphatase and absence of alkaline phosphatase activity. Monocytes contain lysozyme. Similar proportions of promonocytes, marrow monocytes and blood monocytes have IgG-Fc, IgE-Fc and C3b receptors.

Ultrastructure[15,20]

The electron microscope shows that the cytoplasm of promonocytes contains many ribosomes, some RER, bundles of fibrils, a well-developed Golgi apparatus, several mitochondria and a few characteristic granules of two types. The immature granules consist of a central zone of flocculent electron-dense material and a peripheral clear zone. The mature granules are smaller than the immature ones, show considerable variation in size and shape and are homogeneously electron-dense. The promonocyte nucleus contains only small amounts of nuclear-membrane-associated condensed chromatin and has one or more nucleoli. The maturation of promonocytes to marrow monocytes and blood monocytes is associated with an increase in the number of cytoplasmic granules, a progressive decrease in the number of ribosomes, strands of endoplasmic reticulum and cytoplasmic fibrils, and some increase in the amount of condensed chromatin. In addition, mostly mature granules are present in marrow monocytes and only mature granules (i.e. granules without a peripheral clear zone) in blood monocytes. The cell membranes of promonocytes and monocytes show characteristic ruffles which appear as finger-like surface projections in thin sections.

Peroxidase-positivity is found in all the promonocyte granules and some of the monocyte granules and acid phosphatase activity in some of the large round granules, especially in promonocytes.

Eosinophil granulocytopoiesis

There is a progenitor cell committed to eosinophil granulocytopoiesis which can be detected by its ability to form colonies consisting of eosinophil granulocytes when grown in a semi-solid medium containing various hemopoietic growth factors including IL-3, GM-CSF and IL-5. This progenitor cell is described as the eosinophil colony-forming unit or CFU-Eo. The earliest morphologically recognizable eosinophil precursor is the eosinophil promyelocyte. The other more mature cells of the eosinophil series are the eosinophil myelocytes, eosinophil metamyelocytes, eosinophil band cells and marrow eosinophil granulocytes. The CFU-Eo, eosinophil promyelocytes and eosinophil myelocytes undergo cell division; the metamyelocytes, band cells and granulocytes are non-dividing cells.

Light microscope cytology

In Romanowsky-stained smears, the eosinophil promyelocyte has a large rounded nucleus with a finely-granular chromatin pattern and nucleoli. It has a moderate quantity of basophilic cytoplasm containing coarse granules, some of which are reddish-orange and others bluish in color. The eosinophil myelocytes have a coarsely-granular chromatin pattern and polychromatic cytoplasm containing several typical eosinophil granules and few or no blue-staining granules (see Fig. 2.9A). The eosinophil metamyelocytes have a C-shaped nucleus, moderate quantities of condensed chromatin, a faintly polychromatic or acidophilic cytoplasm and several eosinophilic granules. The band or juvenile eosinophils

are similar to eosinophil metamyelocytes except that they have a U-shaped or long band-like nucleus. The morphology of the eosinophil granulocyte is described in Chapter 1.

Cytochemistry[16]

Eosinophil granules do not stain by the PAS reaction, but PAS-positive material is found between the granules. In all cells of the eosinophil series, the periphery of the granules is strongly Sudan-black-positive and the core stains weakly or does not stain. In addition, the granules are peroxidase- and acid-phosphatase-positive, essentially alpha-naphthol AS-D chloroacetate-esterase-negative and contain lysozyme. The peroxidase present in human eosinophil granules is biochemically and immunochemically distinct from the myeloperoxidase present in granules of the neutrophil series. Other constituents of eosinophil granules are eosinophil cationic proteins, an arginine- and zinc-rich major basic protein, histaminase and aryl sulphatase.

Ultrastructure

Two types of eosinophil granules termed primary and secondary can be recognized under the electron microscope.[15,29] Primary granules are large, homogeneous and electron-dense. Secondary granules contain a crystalloid inclusion, composed largely of polymerized major basic protein, at their center. Secondary granules are derived from the maturation of primary granules. Eosinophil promyelocytes contain several homogeneous granules and the more mature promyelocytes also contain an occasional crystalloid-containing granule. In eosinophil myelocytes, several granules of both types are present (Fig. 2.12) and in the metamyelocytes and granulocytes crystalloid-containing granules predominate (Fig. 2.13) (also see Chapter 1). The primary granules of eosinophil promyelocytes are larger and more rounded than those of neutrophil promyelocytes.

Basophil granulocytopoiesis

The basophil granulocyte is derived from the multipotent myeloid stem cell via a committed progenitor cell designated the basophil colony-forming unit (CFU-Baso). This progenitor cell may be closely related to the mast cell progenitor.[31] The morphologically recognizable precursors of basophil granulocytes are rounded in shape and may be subdivided into basophil promyelocytes and myelocytes, which have round or oval nuclei, and basophil metamyelocytes, which have C-shaped,

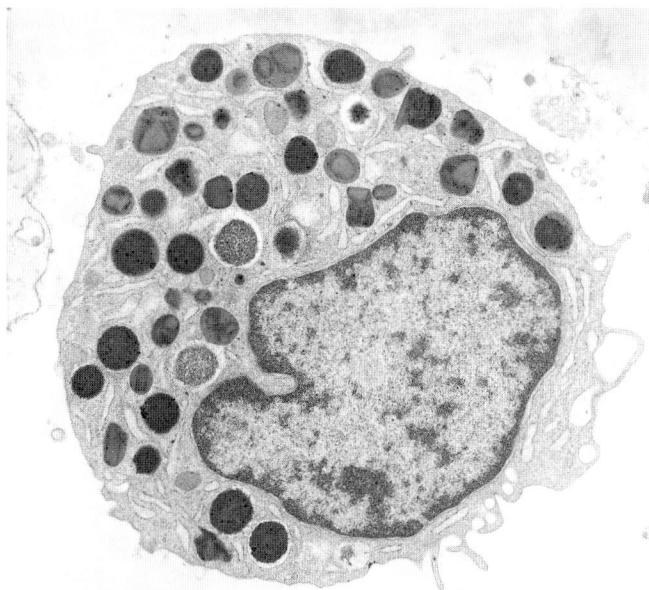

Fig. 2.12 Electron micrograph of an early eosinophil myelocyte from normal bone marrow. The nucleus shows a slight to moderate amount of condensed chromatin. The majority of the cytoplasmic granules consist of very electron-dense primary granules but there are also a few crystalloid-containing secondary granules. Two of the cytoplasmic granules contain granular material of a relatively low electron-density and display a clear halo at their periphery; these probably represent immature primary granules. The cytoplasm contains many dilated sacs of rough endoplasmic reticulum. Uranyl acetate and lead citrate. × 8500.

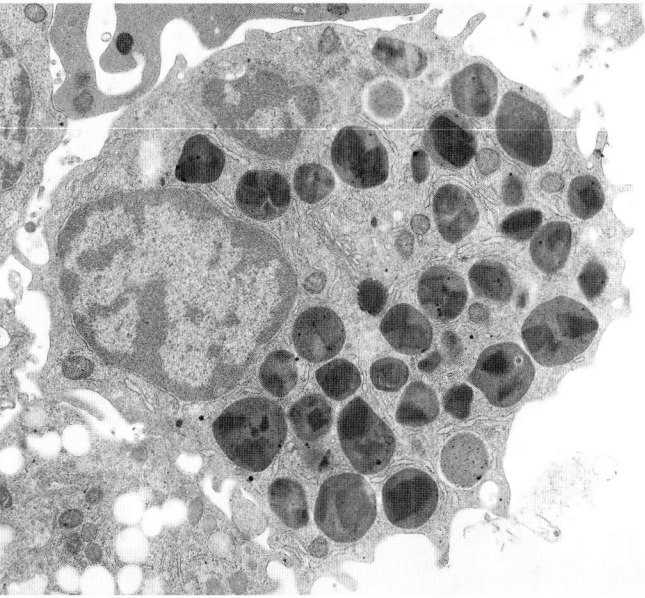

Fig. 2.13 Electron micrograph of an eosinophil granulocyte in normal bone marrow. Most of the granules are crystalloid-containing secondary granules. Uranyl acetate and lead citrate. × 9500.

unsegmented nuclei. Characteristically, in Romanowsky-stained smears all these cell types have large round deeply basophilic cytoplasmic granules that often overlie and obscure the nucleus. However, the granules are water-soluble and so their contents may be extracted during fixation and staining.

With basic dyes such as toluidine blue or methylene blue, the more mature basophil granules stain metachromatically (i.e. a reddish-violet). Basophil granules are PAS-negative (with PAS-positive deposits between the granules), Sudan black- and peroxidase-positive (most strongly in promyelocytes and myelocytes), acid-phosphatase-positive and essentially alpha-naphthol AS-D chloroacetate-esterase-negative.[16,30]

The ultrastructure of the granules in basophil promyelocytes and myelocytes is similar to that of the granules of mature basophil granulocytes (see Chapter 1) except that the intragranular particles are finer.[31]

Megakaryocytopoiesis[32]

The progenitor cells committed to megakaryocytopoiesis are called the megakaryocyte colony-forming units (CFU-Meg). The latter are derived from the multipotent myeloid stem cells and develop into the earliest morphologically recognizable member of the megakaryocyte series, the megakaryoblast. The CFU-Meg is defined operationally in terms of its ability to form a small colony of megakaryocytes when grown in suitable semi-solid medium in the presence of megakaryocyte colony-stimulating factors (e.g. mitogen-stimulated spleen cell supernatants or the conditioned medium from a myelomonocytic leukemia cell line, WEHI-3, or a mixture of hemopoietic growth factors including IL-3, IL-11, GM-CSF and thrombopoietin). The megakaryocytes in these colonies show more or less normal maturation and shed platelets.[33] The CFU-Meg are a diploid cell population in which DNA synthesis and nuclear division (karyokinesis) is followed by cell division (cytokinesis).

There are four types of megakaryocytes in Romanowsky-stained marrow smears. These are, in increasing order of maturity, megakaryoblasts (group I megakaryocytes), promegakaryocytes (group II megakaryocytes), granular megakaryocytes (group III megakaryocytes) and 'bare nuclei'. DNA synthesis occurs in 44% of megakaryoblasts, 18% of promegakaryocytes and in only 2% of granular megakaryocytes.[34] This DNA synthesis is not associated with cytokinesis and cycles of DNA synthesis result in the production of mononucleate polyploid cells. The DNA content of a megakaryoblast ranges from 4 to 32c and that of a promegakaryocyte or granular megakaryocyte from 8 to 64c; cells with higher DNA content are larger than those with lower content (1c = the haploid DNA content, i.e. the DNA content of a spermatozoon). The time taken for a megakaryoblast to mature into a platelet-producing granular megakaryocyte may be about 6 days.

Although the majority of the megakaryocytes are found in the marrow parenchyma, some whole cells enter the circulation via the marrow sinusoids. Most of the circulating megakaryocytes are trapped in the lungs and some of pulmonary megakaryocytes appear to produce platelets.

Light microscope cytology

Megakaryoblasts and megakaryocytes are larger than other immature hemopoietic cells and are therefore relatively easily identified. In marrow smears, most cells with a diameter > 20 μm belong to the megakaryocyte series.[35] The megakaryoblasts are 20–30 μm in diameter and have a single large oval, kidney-shaped or lobed nucleus with several nucleoli, a very high nucleus to cytoplasm ratio and a deeply-basophilic agranular cytoplasm. Promegakaryocytes are usually larger than megakaryoblasts and have a lower nucleus to cytoplasm ratio and a less basophilic cytoplasm. The overlapping nuclear lobes of a promegakaryocyte are arranged in a C-shaped formation, the concavity of which sometimes contains a group of azurophilic cytoplasmic granules. The granular megakaryocytes (Fig. 2.14) are up to 70 μm in diameter and possess abundant pale-staining cytoplasm and numerous azurophilic cytoplasmic granules. The nucleus has coarsely granular chromatin and multiple lobes which extend through much of the cell. Prior to the formation of platelets by the fragmentation of cytoplasmic processes, the nuclear lobes become fairly tightly packed together. Following completion of platelet formation, a 'bare' nucleus remains.

Ultrastructure

Electron microscope studies[15,36,37] show that the nucleus of the megakaryoblast is lobulated and contains only small quantities of condensed chromatin and several prominent nucleoli. The cytoplasm is relatively scanty and contains a well-developed Golgi apparatus within a deep indentation of the nucleus. It also contains many polyribosomes, scattered RER, several mitochondria, a few microtubules, a few membrane-lined vesicles representing the beginning of the demarcation membrane system and both a few lysosomal vesicles containing acid phosphatase and aryl sulphatase and a few immature α granules situated near the Golgi apparatus. The demarcation membrane system (DMS) consists of a system of cytoplasmic vesicles which arise as invaginations of the surface membrane; the cavities of these vesicles are continuous with the exterior. During maturation of a megakaryoblast into promegakaryocytes and granular megakaryocytes, there is a progressive increase in the amount of nuclear-membrane-associated condensed chromatin, in the number of α granules and in the development of the DMS and a decrease in the number of ribosomes, RER and mitochondria. Granular megakaryocytes (Fig. 2.15) have considerably more cytoplasm and a larger, more lobulated and segmented nucleus than a megakaryoblast. Three zones can often be seen in the cytoplasm: a narrow outer zone just internal to the cell membrane, a wide intermediate zone and a narrow perinuclear zone. Hardly any organelles are present in the outer zone. Many ovoid electron-dense α granules, numerous vesicles and saccules belonging to the DMS (which demarcate future platelet zones) and some lysosomal vesicles are found in the intermediate zone, together with microtubules, ribosomes, RER and

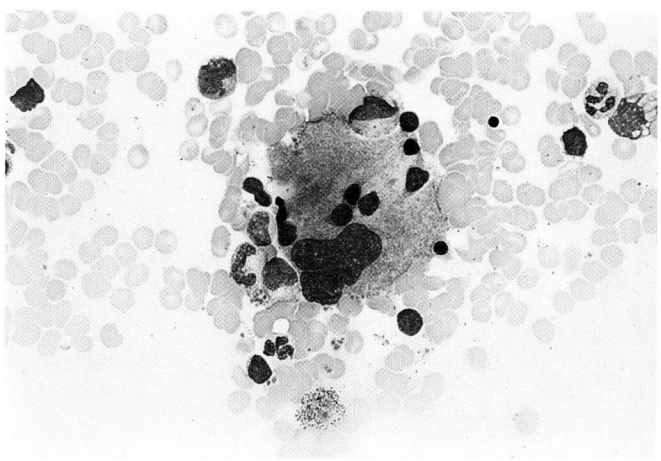
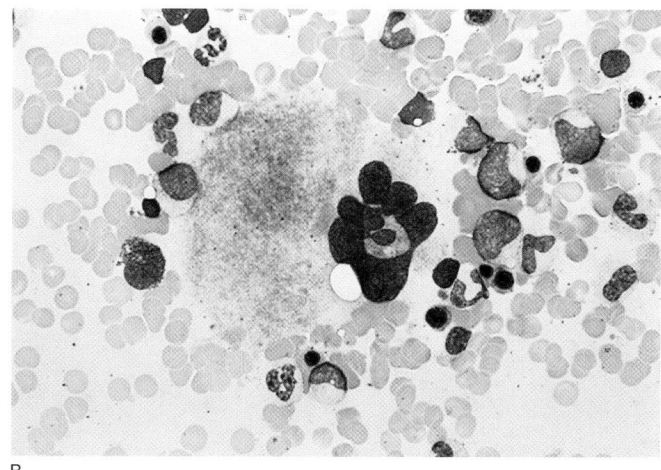

A   B

Fig. 2.14 (A, B) Two granular megakaryocytes from a smear of normal bone marrow. The megakaryocyte in (A) contains a granulocyte within its cytoplasm (emperipolesis). May–Grünwald–Giemsa stain.

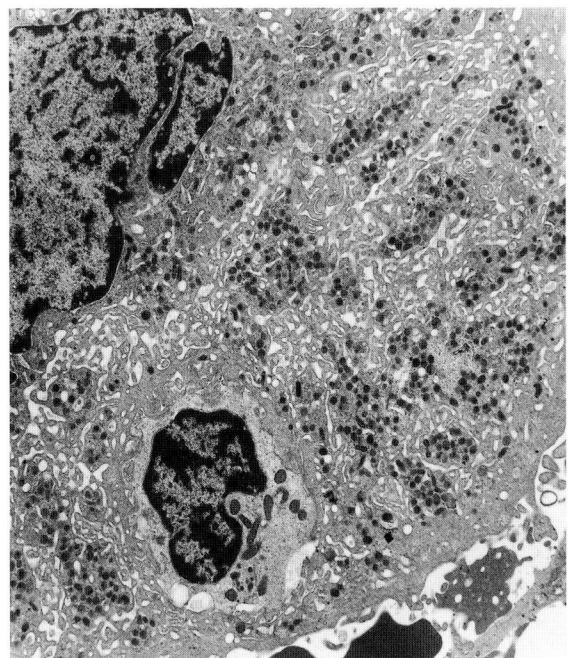

Fig. 2.15 Electron micrograph of part of a granular megakaryocyte. The extensive demarcation membrane system and numerous cytoplasmic granules can be seen in the wide intermediate zone of the cytoplasm. The cytoplasm also contains a normal-looking lymphocyte which may have been traveling through the megakaryocyte (emperipolesis). Uranyl acetate and lead citrate. × 5300.

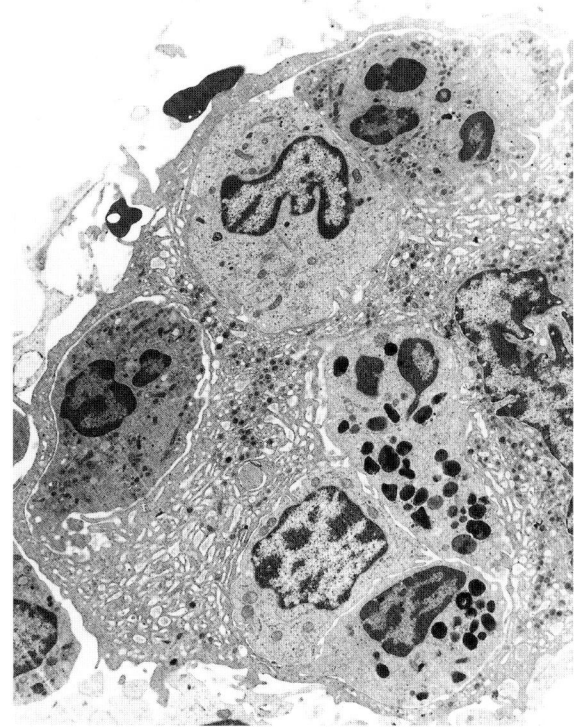

Fig. 2.16 Electron micrograph of a megakaryocyte which is apparently showing an unusual degree of emperipolesis. Although sections of six other cells (including two eosinophil granulocytes, two neutrophil granulocytes and a monocyte) are seen within the megakaryocyte profile, it is possible that at least some of these cells are not completely within the megakaryocyte but merely protruding into it. Uranyl acetate and lead citrate. × 6800.

mitochondria. The perinuclear zone contains the Golgi apparatus, ribosomes, RER and mitochondria. During platelet release, the granular megakaryocytes protrude cytoplasmic processes[38] close to or directly into the marrow sinusoids, pieces of cytoplasm break away from these processes and subsequently fragment into platelets. The DMS appears to provide extra membrane for the formation of the cytoplasmic processes and to be involved in the fragmentation of these processes. The almost bare nucleus that remains after the release of platelets is surrounded by a narrow rim of cytoplasm containing a few granules and other organelles.

Ultrastructural cytochemical studies have demonstrated a platelet peroxidase (PPO), distinct from myeloperoxidase, in the endoplasmic reticulum and perinuclear space (but not in the Golgi apparatus) of megakaryoblasts, megakaryocytes[39] and a few small rounded marrow cells identified as promegakaryoblasts.[40] PPO is also present in the dense bodies and dense tubular system of platelets.

Emperipolesis[41,42]

This term describes the presence and movement of one cell inside the cytoplasm of another; the 'engulfed' cell can subsequently leave the 'engulfing' cell and appears to be morphologically unaltered as a result of the interaction. If a sufficiently large number of megakaryocytes are examined, some are regularly found to display the phenomenon of emperipolesis both in normal marrow and in a wide range of clinical conditions. The cell types that may be found within megakaryocytes include neutrophil and eosinophil granulocytes and their precursors, and lymphocytes, erythroblasts and red cells. Megakaryocytic emperipolesis may be seen in marrow smears as well as in histologic sections of marrow, including thin sections used for electron microscopy; sometimes one megakaryocyte may contain several cells 'inside' it (Figs 2.15 and 2.16). Megakaryocytic emperipolesis is of uncertain significance but may represent a transmegakaryocytic route for the entry of blood cells into the circulation; it has been suggested that some of the intramegakaryocytic cells may enter the circulation via the processes of megakaryocytic cytoplasm which protrude into adjacent marrow sinusoids. Emperipolesis is not confined to megakaryocytes. It has been described also in various non-hemopoietic cells and in malignant cells, including blast cells from patients in the acute phase of chronic granulocytic leukemia.

Lymphopoiesis[43-45]

Lymphopotent stem cells exist in fetal and postnatal hemopoietic tissues and a substantial degree of lymphopoiesis occurs in these. The lymphopotent stem cells generate both B-cell and T-cell progenitors and give rise to all types of lymphocyte. Much of the lymphopoiesis that occurs in normal bone marrow appears to be independent of antigenic stimulation and serves to supply the body with partially differentiated cells, some of which mature into B-lymphocytes in the marrow or T-lymphocytes in the thymus. The newly-formed mature B- and T-cells enter the circulation and then migrate to peripheral lymphoid tissues (spleen, lymph nodes, Peyer's patches, Waldeyer's ring). The development of bone marrow-derived precursor cells into T-lymphocytes is dependent on an interaction of the precursor cells with the surface molecules or secretory products of the epithelial elements of the thymus. In the case of birds, the development of the precursor cells into B-lymphocytes requires the bursa of Fabricius, an epithelial structure in the avian hind-gut. The bursa-equivalent in mammals is thought to be the marrow stromal cells. Newly formed B-cells that enter peripheral lymphoid tissues may undergo antigen-dependent proliferation and further maturation. Some B-cells undergo antigen-dependent development into plasma cells in the marrow itself. Specific antigens (short peptide fragments of degraded antigen presented on specific antigen-presenting cells) also stimulate T-lymphocytes present in peripheral lymphoid tissues to undergo maturation and proliferation. There is a high rate of cell death during antigen-independent lymphopoiesis in both the marrow and the thymus that serves to delete clones of B- and T-cells recognizing self-antigens. Over 99% of T-cells bearing the T-cell receptor generated in the thymus undergo apoptosis within this organ. The main features of the maturation of a lymphoid stem cell into an antibody-secreting plasma cell are shown in Table 2.1; the maturation of pre-B cells and immature B-cells is antigen-independent. Some antigen-activated B-cells develop into memory B-cells rather than plasma cells, allowing rapid antibody production in a secondary immune response. The stages in the development of lymphoid stem cells into mature peripheral blood T-cells are shown in Table 2.2. During T-lymphopoiesis, the maturation of thymic lymphoblasts and stage I and II thymocytes is antigen-independent.

Early lineage-specific markers expressed on lymphoid progenitors include CD-10 and CD-38. CD-19 is expressed on B-lymphoid progenitors and CD-7 on early T-lymphoid progenitors (prothymocytes) and natural killer (NK)-cell progenitors. Some other surface markers appearing during lymphopoiesis are shown in Tables 2.1 and 2.2. The cytokines influencing lymphocyte progenitor cells and precursors include IL-2, IL-4, IL-5, IL-6 and IL-11 for the B-lineage and IL-2, IL-3, IL-4 and IL-10 for the T-lineage.

Table 2.1 Scheme of B-lymphocyte differentiation[43]

Cell type	Immunoglobulin gene rearrangement and secretion status	TdT	Surface antigens (monoclonal antibodies)						
			CD10 (CALLA)	CD9 (BA2)	CD24 (BA1)	CD20 (B1), CD19	CD21 (B2)	FcR	C3R
Lymphoid stem cell	–	+	–	+	+/–	–	–		
Early pre B-cell	μ gene rearranged	+	+	+	+/–	+	–		
Pre B-cell	μ gene expressed; κ gene rearrangement followed by λ gene rearrangement	+	+	+	+/–	+	–		
Immature B-cell	(1) Cμ SmIgM	–	+/–	+	+	+	–		
	(2) SmIgM	–	–	–	+	+	+		
	(3) SmIgM SmIgD	–	–	–	+	+	+	+	+/–
Mature B-cell	(1) SmIgM SmIgD SmIgA or IgG	–	–	–	+	+	+	+	+/–
	(2) SmIgA or IgG	–	–	–	+	+	–	+	+/–
Immunoblast		–	–		–		–		
Plasma cell	CIg	–	–	–	–	–	–		+/–

Ig, immunoglobulin; μ, heavy chain of IgM; Cμ, cytoplasmic μ chain; κ, λ, light chains of immunoglobulin. FcR, receptor for Fc segment of Ig molecule; C3R, receptor for the third component of complement; CALLA, common ALL antigen, BA1, BA2, B1, B2, monoclonal antibodies against B-cells or their precursors; TdT, terminal deoxynucleotidyl transferase; SmIg, surface membrane immunoglobulin; CIg, cytoplasmic immunoglobulin.

The distribution of lymphoid cells and plasma cells in the marrow is described in Chapter 3. The light and electron microscope features of these cells are similar to those of the same cells in peripheral lymphoid tissue. A description of bone marrow plasma cells is given below.

Table 2.2 Maturation of T-lymphocytes[44,45]

Cell	Site		TdT	CD2, SRC receptor	CD5 (pan-T, pan-thymocyte)	CD3 (pan-mature T)	CD4	CD8
Thymic lymphoblast (prothymocyte)	Thymic subcapsular cortex		+	–	–	–	–	–
Stage I or early thymocyte	Thymic cortex		+	+/–	+	–	–	–
Stage II or common thymocyte[a]	Thymic cortex		+/–	+/–	+	–/+	+	+
Stage III or mature thymocyte	Thymic medulla	T_H	–	+	+	+	+	–
		T_C	–	+	+	+	–	+
Mature T-cell	Peripheral blood, lymph nodes	T_H	–	+	+	+	+	–
		T_C	–	+	+	+	–	+

TdT, terminal deoxynucleotidyl transfase; SRC, sheep red blood cells; CD3 = T-cell receptor (TcR) complex.
[a] T-cell receptor rearrangements occur in the more mature cells; TcR-1 cells develop before TcR-2 cells.

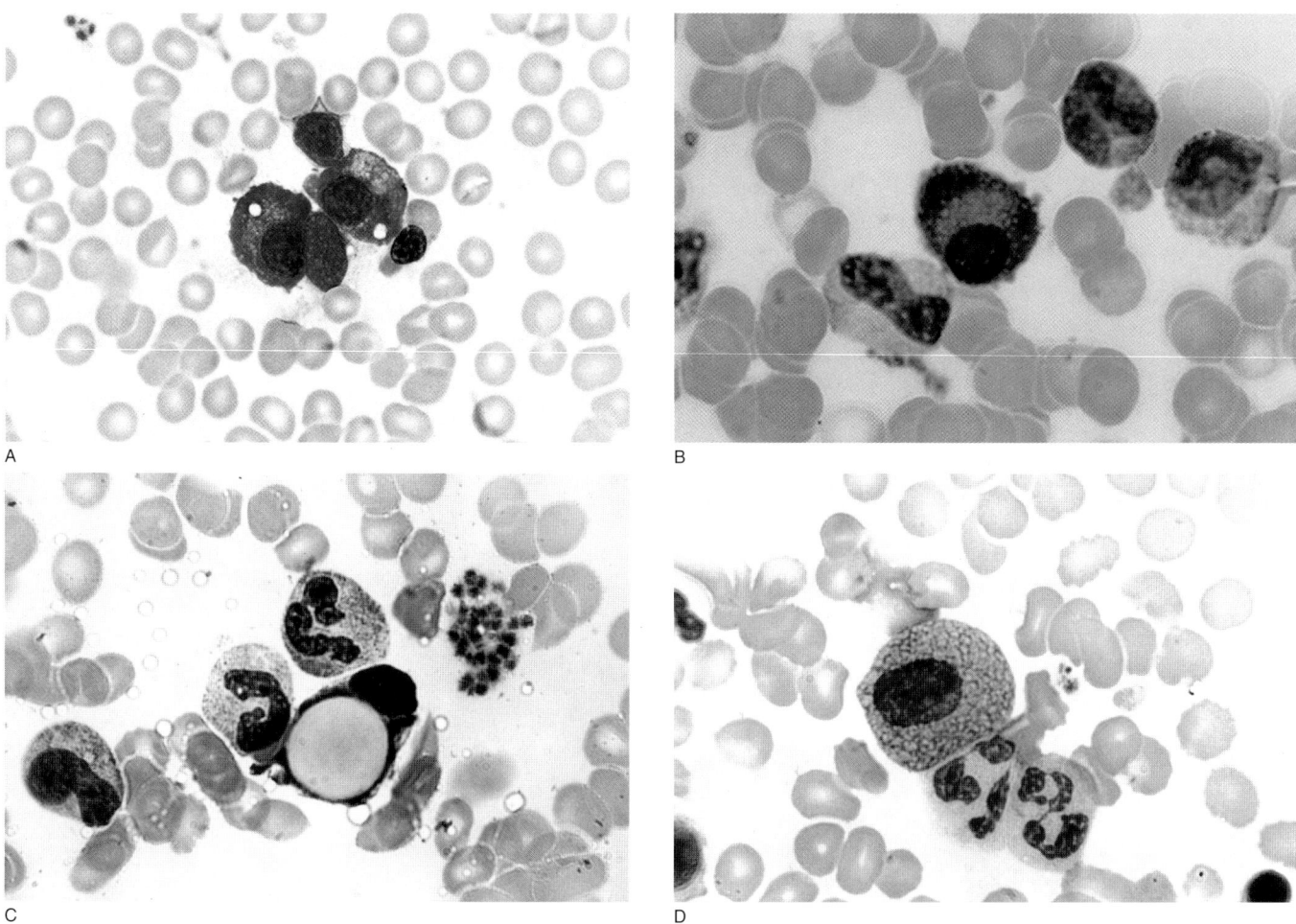

A

B

C

D

Fig. 2.17 (A–D) Different appearances of plasma cells from smears of normal bone marrow. (A) Cluster of five cells in which the two largest are plasma cells. Each of the two plasma cells contains a large intracytoplasmic vacuole and displays a large paler-staining crescentic zone immediately adjacent to the nucleus. This zone corresponds to the position of the Golgi apparatus. (B) Plasma cell with a pinkish cytoplasmic tinge and a prominent crescentic Golgi zone. (C) Plasma cell containing a single Russell body. (D) Plasma cell with a 'reticulated' cytoplasm. May–Grünwald–Giemsa stain.

Plasma cells

The mature plasma cells seen in Romanowsky-stained smears of normal bone marrow may vary markedly in their morphology. The majority are 14–20 μm in diameter and have deep-blue cytoplasm with a paler paranuclear zone corresponding to the site of the Golgi apparatus; the cytoplasm may have one or more vacuoles (Fig. 2.17A,B). The nucleus is eccentric and small relative to the volume of the cytoplasm and contains moderate amounts of condensed chromatin (Figs 2.17 and 2.18). The characteristic cartwheel appearance of the nucleus is only seen in histologic sections, not in smears. A small proportion of normal plasma cells show various additional cytologic features and have then been given different names. Some plasma cells contain Russell bodies (Fig. 2.17C) which are very large, rounded, acidophilic, PAS-positive cytoplasmic inclusions; there is usually only one Russell body per cell. Mott cells (grape cells, or morular cells) are plasma cells containing several smaller, slightly basophilic, rounded inclusions. Some plasma cells have a reticulated appearance due to the presence of many pleomorphic inclusions (Fig. 2.17D) and others are described as 'flaming cells' as they are eosinophilic at their periphery (occasionally, the entire cytoplasm may take on an eosinophilic hue). Rarely, a plasma cell may contain azurophilic rods with a crystalline ultrastructure. These resemble Auer rods found in acute myeloid leukemia, but unlike Auer rods are PAS-, Sudan black- and peroxidase-negative. Plasma cells show strong acid phosphatase positivity, especially around the nucleus and over the Golgi zone, and are alpha-naphthol chloroacetate-esterase-negative.

Ultrastructure

When examined with the electron microscope, the cytoplasm of the mature plasma cell is seen to be packed with flattened sacs of RER (Figs 2.19 and 2.20A,B) which are frequently aligned parallel to each other, in a concentric arrangement or in whorls; the sacs contain an amorphous material composed mostly of immunoglobulin. The cytoplasm also contains a well-developed Golgi zone (Fig. 2.20A), some rounded acid-phosphatase-positive primary lysosomes (which vary considerably

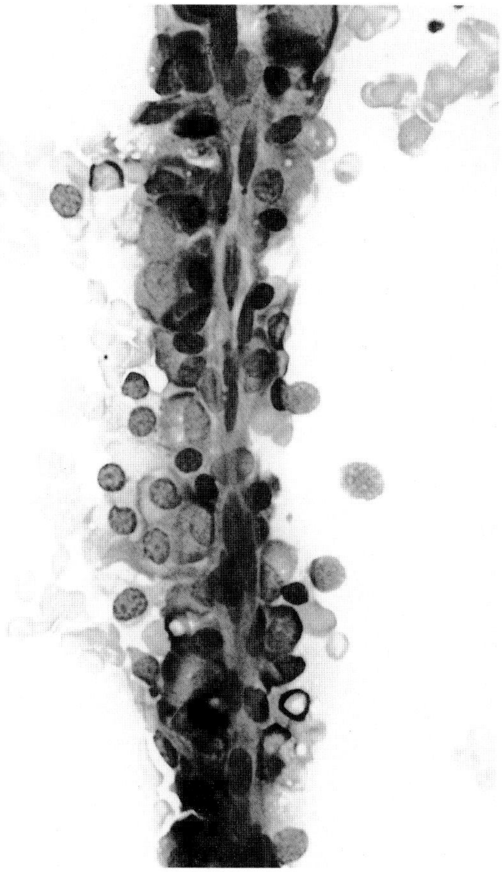

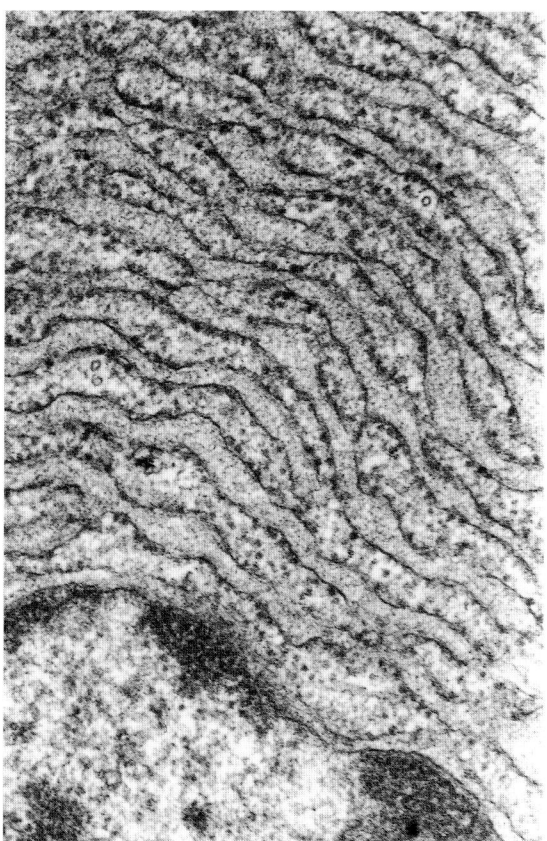

Fig. 2.19 Electron micrograph of part of a plasma cell from a normal bone marrow. There are several sacs of rough endoplasmic reticulum arranged more or less parallel to each other. The sacs contain a finely granular material (presumably antibody) and have ribosomes attached to their outer surfaces. Uranyl acetate and lead citrate. × 116 000.

Fig. 2.18 A capillary from a smear of normal bone marrow showing plasma cells arranged along it. May–Grünwald–Giemsa stain.

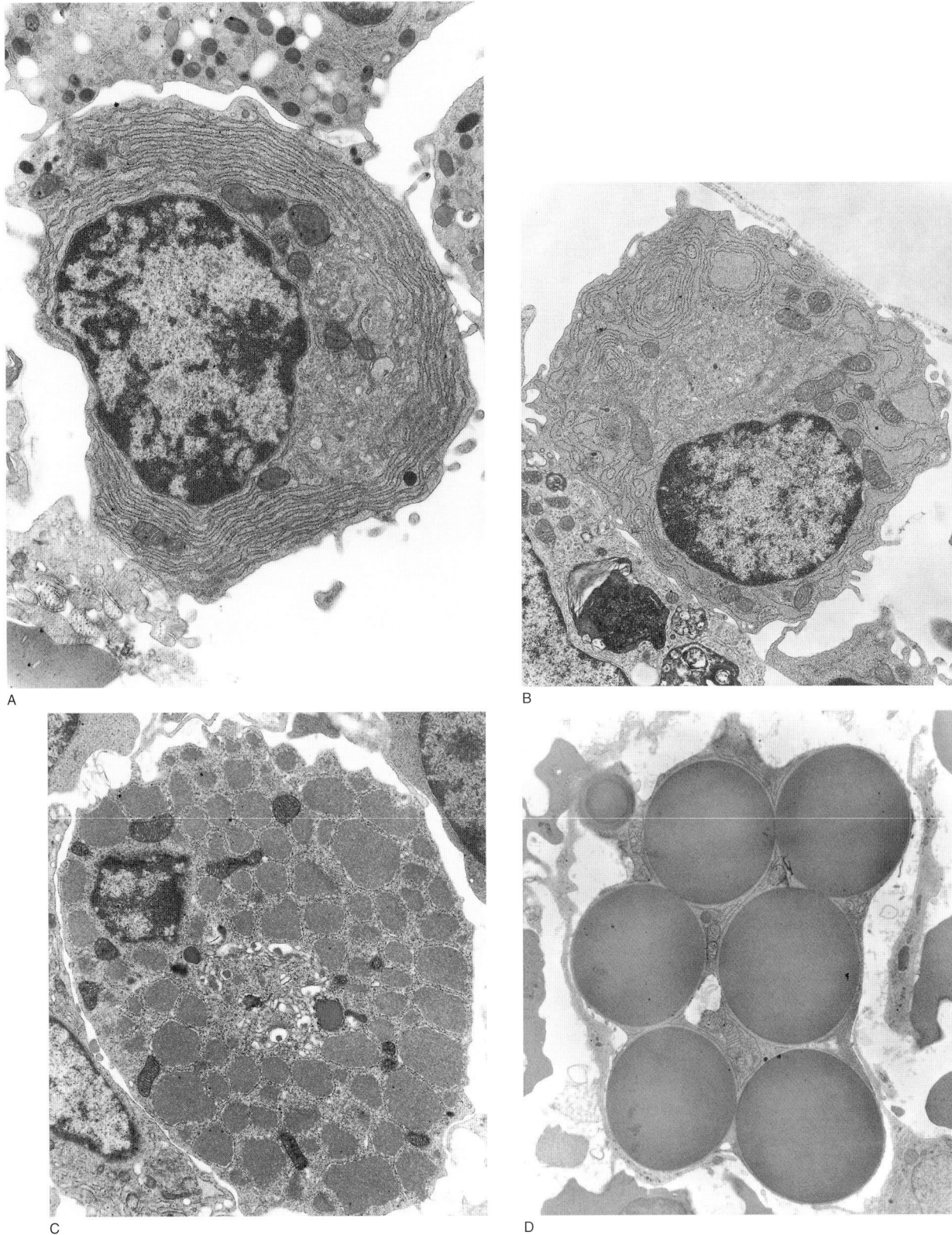

Fig. 2.20 (A–D) Various appearances of the ultrastructure of plasma cells from normal bone marrow. (A) The cytoplasm is packed with rough endoplasmic reticulum aligned more or less parallel to each other. There is a large paranuclear Golgi zone, which is devoid of endoplasmic reticulum. (B) The endoplasmic reticulum is arranged in concentric whorls and parts of it are distended to varying extents with relatively electron-lucent material. (C, D) Rounded intracytoplasmic inclusions consisting of sacs of endoplasmic reticulum distended with electron-dense material. Uranyl acetate and lead citrate. (A) × 10 700; (B) × 7700; (C) × 7200; (D) × 5800.

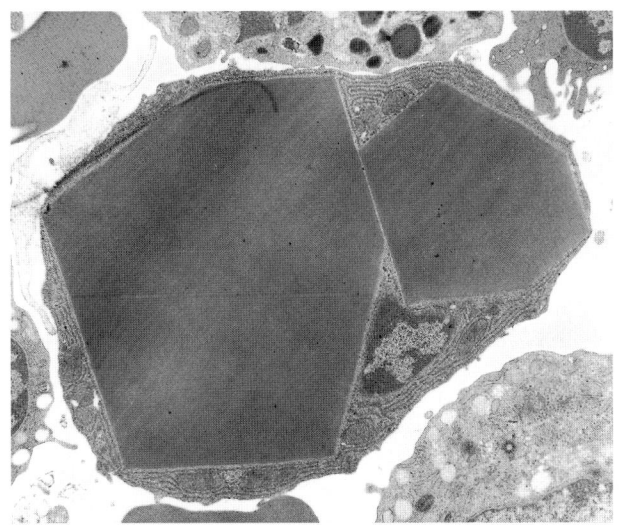

Fig. 2.21 Plasma cell with polygonal crystalline inclusions lined by rough endoplasmic reticulum. Uranyl acetate and lead citrate. From Wickramasinghe,[46] with permission.

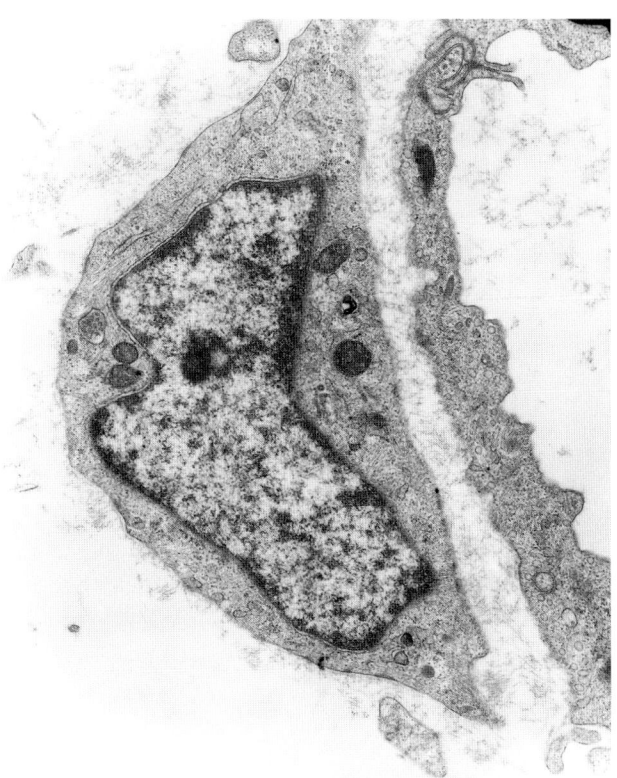

Fig. 2.22 Ultrastructure of a trilaminar region of the wall of a sinusoid in normal bone marrow showing an inner layer of two interdigitating endothelial cells, an outer adventitial cell and some intercellular matrix between these layers. From Wickramasinghe,[48] with permission.

in size and are located near the Golgi complex) and moderate numbers of mitochondria. Russell bodies and the inclusions within Mott cells and 'reticulated cells' consist of masses of homogeneous electron-dense material which are usually lined by RER (Fig. 2.20B–D); these inclusions result from the condensation of immunoglobulin within distended cisternae of the RER. Very occasional plasma cells have rhomboidal or needle-like crystalline inclusions (Fig. 2.21). The nuclei of plasma cells contain a variable quantity of condensed chromatin (which is generally, but not always, proportional to the degree of cytoplasmic maturity) and frequently contain a well-developed nucleolus.

Stromal cells

Several types of stromal cell (endothelial cells, macrophages, non-phagocytic reticular cells including myofibroblasts, and osteoblasts) are involved in the regulation of hemopoiesis through the expression of adhesive ligands, the synthesis of extracellular matrix and the production of cytokines.

Cells of marrow sinusoids

The thin walls of marrow sinusoids are composed of an inner complete layer of flattened endothelial cells, little or no associated basement membrane material, and an outer incomplete layer of adventitial cells (Fig. 2.22). Thus some areas of the sinusoidal wall are only composed of

thin endothelial cells. Endothelial cells overlap and may interdigitate extensively. They have numerous small pinocytotic vesicles along their luminal and abluminal surfaces and some cells have more electron-dense cytoplasm than others. The adventitial cells protrude long cytoplasmic processes; some of these lie on the external surface of the sinusoid and others are found between surrounding hemopoietic cells. Some adventitial cells have very electron-lucent cytoplasm.

Bone marrow macrophages (phagocytic reticular cells)

These cells, which are derived from monocytes, are 20–30 μm in diameter, irregular in shape, and have voluminous cytoplasm with long cytoplasmic processes at their periphery (see Figs. 2.3 and 2.4). In Romanowsky-stained normal marrow smears, the cytoplasm appears pale blue and contains azurophilic granules, vacuoles, lipid droplets and, often, phagocytosed material, including extruded erythroblast nuclei and, occasionally, whole granulocytes. The nucleus of the macrophage is large, round or oval, and has a pale-staining lace-like chromatin structure and one or more large nucleoli. Macrophages are relatively fragile and their cytoplasm is frequently ruptured during the preparation of smears.

When stained by the Perls' acid ferrocyanide method, the macrophages of iron-replete individuals contain blue or blue-black granules. Macrophages are PAS-positive, strongly alpha-naphthyl acetate-esterase- and acid-phosphatase-positive, and alpha-naphthol AS-D chloroacetate-esterase-negative. Most are Sudan black- and alkaline-phosphatase-negative.

Ultrastructure

Electron microscope studies reveal that some macrophages occur within erythroblastic islands, plasma cell islands and lymphoid nodules, and that others lie adjacent to marrow sinusoids and actually form part of the incomplete adventitial layer of the sinusoidal wall. The long thin cytoplasmic processes of bone marrow macrophages not only extend for considerable distances between erythropoietic and other marrow cells but also may protrude through endothelial cells into the sinusoidal lumen (Fig. 2.23). The intrasinusoidal cytoplasmic processes[47,48] appear to recognize and phagocytose senescent erythrocytes, abnormal or damaged cells (e.g. heat-damaged red cells, sickled red cells, red cells containing malarial parasites) and circulating particulate or colloidal material.

The eccentric nucleus of a macrophage often has an irregular outline and shows relatively little peripheral chromatin condensation (Fig. 2.24). The cytoplasm contains many strands of RER, moderate numbers of mitochondria, scattered ferritin molecules, a moderately well-developed Golgi apparatus, centrioles and several primary lysosomes. There are also a number of membrane-bound electron-dense intracytoplasmic inclusions which vary markedly in size, shape and ultrastructure, are sometimes up to 7 μm in diameter, contain both lipid

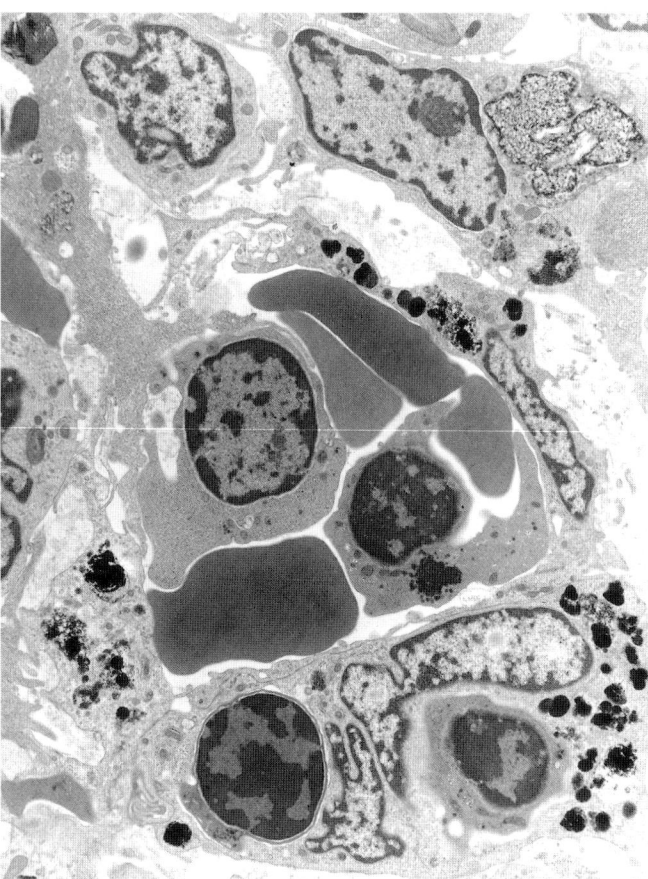

Fig. 2.23 Process of macrophage cytoplasm protruding through an endothelial cell into the lumen of a bone marrow sinusoid in a patient with homozygous β-thalassemia. The sinusoid contains erythrocytes and two erythroblasts, one of which contains large quantities of precipitated α-globin chains. Both the endothelial cell and the larger adventitial cell contain iron-laden secondary lysosomes. The adventitial cell also contains a phagocytosed erythroblast nucleus and a phagocytosed erythroblast. Uranyl acetate and lead citrate. × 6400. From Wickramasinghe,[48] with permission.

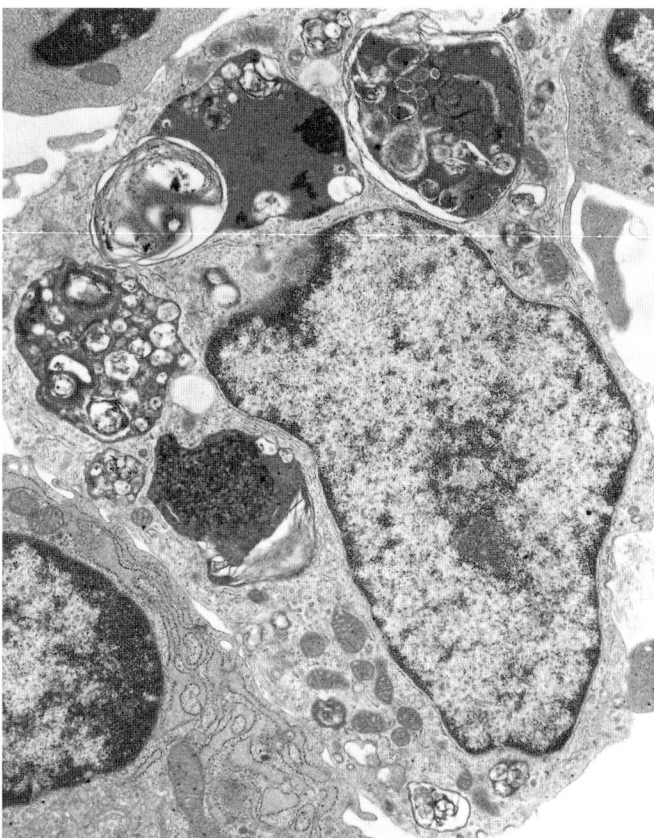

Fig. 2.24 Electron micrograph of a macrophage from normal bone marrow. The nucleus has a central nucleolus and the cytoplasm has several large pleomorphic inclusions. Uranyl acetate and lead citrate. × 9700.

(e.g. myelin figures) and large numbers of ferritin and hemosiderin molecules, and probably represent phagocytosed cells at an advanced stage of degradation. The phagosomes of normal macrophages sometimes contain clearly recognizable extruded erythroblast nuclei, red cells, neutrophils or eosinophils (Fig. 2.25A). A very occasional mature macrophage may be found in mitosis (Fig. 2.25B).[48]

Non-phagocytic reticular cells

In stained marrow smears, these are irregular in outline or are fibroblast-like (i.e. spindle-shaped) and resemble macrophages except that they do not contain large intracytoplasmic inclusions (Fig. 2.26). Electron microscopy reveals either no secondary lysosomes or only an occasional secondary lysosome (Fig. 2.27). Some of the

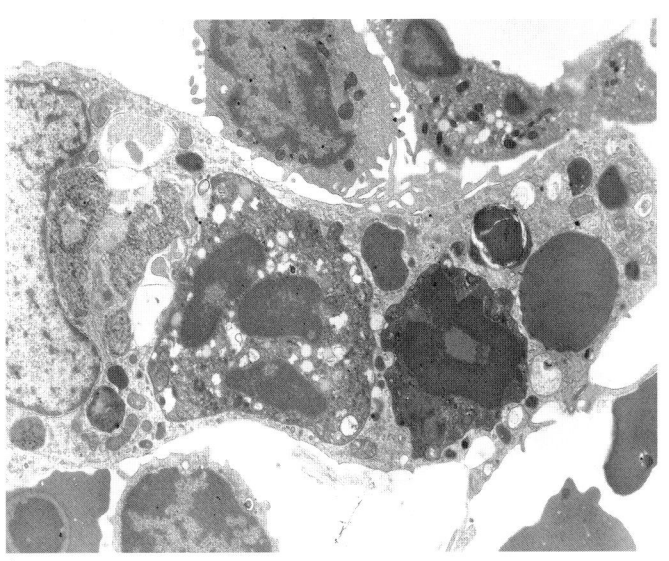

A

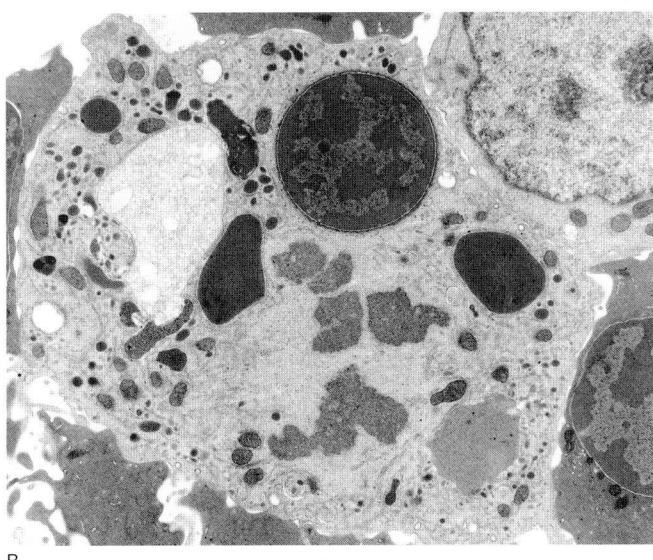

B

Fig. 2.25 (A) Electron micrograph of a macrophage from normal bone marrow. The cytoplasm contains two phagocytosed granulocytes. Uranyl acetate and lead citrate. × 9500. (B) Electron micrograph of a macrophage from normal bone marrow undergoing mitosis. The cytoplasm contains a phagocytosed extruded erythroblast nucleus and phagocytosed red cell material. Uranyl acetate and lead citrate. × 9700. From Wickramasinghe,[48] with permission.

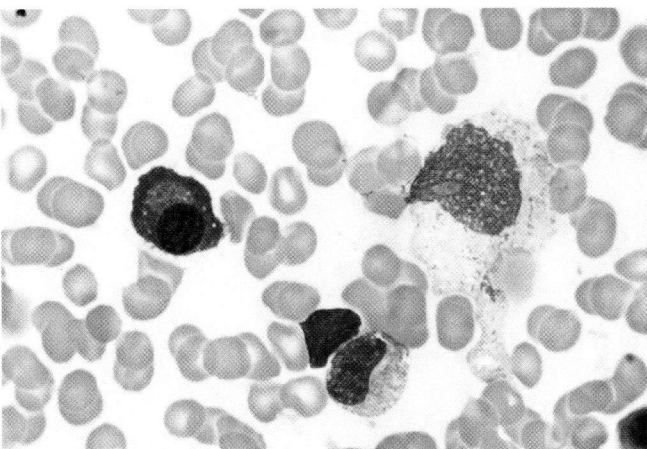

Fig. 2.26 Non-phagocytic reticular cell in a smear of normal bone marrow. The nucleus has pale-staining lace-like chromatin and a large nucleolus. The cytoplasm is voluminous and granular but does not contain large inclusions. The other cells in the photomicrograph are a plasma cell, a lymphocyte and a neutrophil myelocyte. May–Grünwald–Giemsa stain.

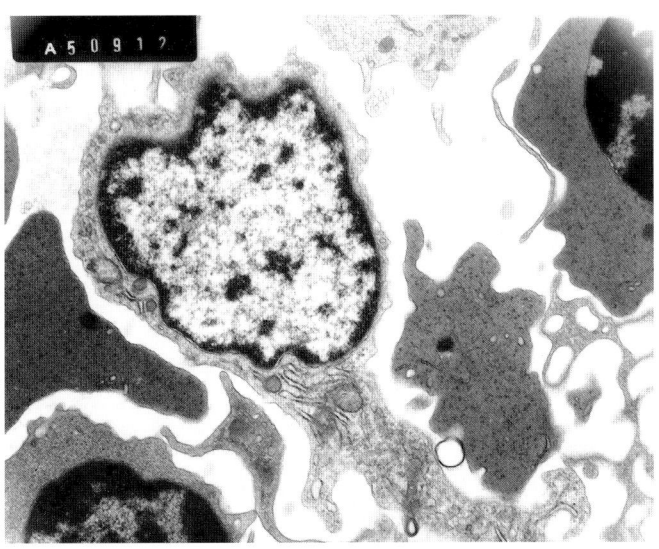

Fig. 2.27 Electron micrograph of spindle-shaped non-phagocytic reticular cell from normal bone marrow. The cytoplasm lacks secondary lysosomes.

spindle-shaped non-phagocytic reticular cells are probably not derived from the hemopoietic stem cell but from the cell capable of generating fibroblast colonies *in vitro.*

Mast cells

Tissue mast cells are derived from CFU-S and the latter develop within the marrow into progenitors of mast cells.[49] The most mature mast cell progenitors enter the peripheral blood,[50,51] circulate and migrate into tissues where they proliferate and mature into mast cells. There are some data suggesting that both the basophil granulocyte and the mast cell might share a common bipotent progenitor cell.[31,51]

Mast cells vary considerably in size (long axis of 5–25 µm in smears) and can be distinguished from basophils by their generally larger size, tendency to have an elongated or ovoid shape, and the fact that the coarse, purplish-black to red-purple granules (Romanowsky stain) that pack the cytoplasm are less water-extractable and seldom overlie the nucleus (Fig. 2.28). The nucleus of the mast cell is small, round or oval, contains less condensed chromatin than that of a basophil and stains more or less uniformly. It is centrally or, occasionally, eccentrically placed. Mast cells are less strongly PAS-positive than basophils. Unlike basophil granulocytes, mast cells may undergo mitosis.

Mast cell granules are rich in heparin and chondroitin sulphates and stain metachromatically with toluidine blue. They contain large amounts of three serine proteinases, namely tryptase, chymase and cathepsin G as well as stem cell factor,[52] a cytokine involved in the regulation of mast cell growth and functions. Mast cells also contain histamine, carboxypeptidase, other hydrolytic enzymes (e.g. acid and alkaline phosphatase and alpha-naphthol AS-D chloroacetate esterase) and high affinity surface receptors for IgE but, unlike basophil granulocytes, they also contain 5-hydroxytryptamine (serotonin) and do not contain peroxidase. As in the case of basophils, when activated by antigen and IgE, the histamine and other constituents of mast cell granules are released by a process termed piecemeal degranulation (see Chapter 1). Stimulated mast cells also release products of arachidonic acid oxidation such as leukotriene C_4 (LTC$_4$) and prostaglandin D_2 (PGD$_2$) as well as the cytokines tumor necrosis factor α(TNF-α) and IL-4.

The mast cell granules vary markedly in their ultrastructure. They may be dense and amorphous or may contain both dense amorphous regions as well as less dense crystalline regions appearing at high magnification as scrolls or whorls of lamellae, a lattice, or parallel lamellae (Fig. 2.29). Tryptase is found preferentially in the crystalline regions and chymase and cathepsin G in the amorphous regions.[53] The cytoplasm of a mast cell contains some mitochondria, a few strands of endoplasmic reticulum, some fibrils and occasional lipid droplets but does not contain glycogen deposits. Unstimulated mast cells differ from basophils in having long thin cytoplasmic processes projecting from their surface. Cells with characteristics between those of basophils and mast cells have been described.[31]

Apart from being involved in immediate-type hypersensitivity reactions, mast cells (and basophils) appear to participate in IgE-dependent host defense against parasites. Mast cells accumulate at sites of resolving inflammation and may modulate inflammatory responses by releasing heparin (which prevents further fibrin deposition) and proteases (which may inhibit coagulation and promote fibrinolysis). By virtue of their heparin content, mast cells may also be involved in triglyceride metabolism.

Osteoblasts and osteoclasts

Groups of osteoblasts and individual osteoclasts can be seen in Romanowsky-stained normal marrow smears. Osteoblasts (Fig. 2.30) appear oval or elongated and are 20–50 µm in diameter. They have a single small eccentric nucleus with small quantities of condensed chromatin and one to three nucleoli. The cytoplasm is abundant and blue-staining and frequently has somewhat indistinct margins. Although these cells superficially resemble plasma cells, they are larger and their Golgi zone is not

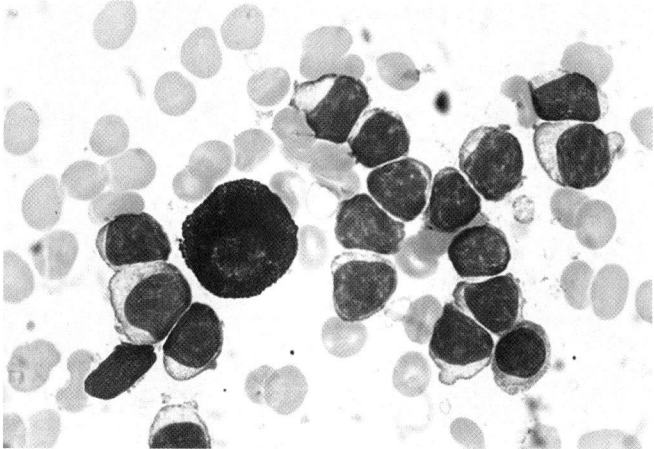

Fig. 2.28 Normal-looking mast cell from the bone marrow smear of a case of Waldenström's macroglobulinemia. The cytoplasm is packed with coarse granules only a few of which overlie the nucleus. May–Grünwald–Giemsa stain.

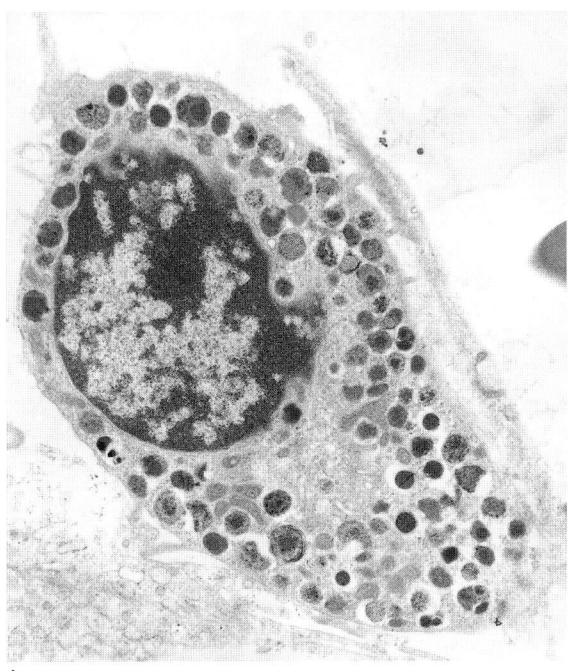

A

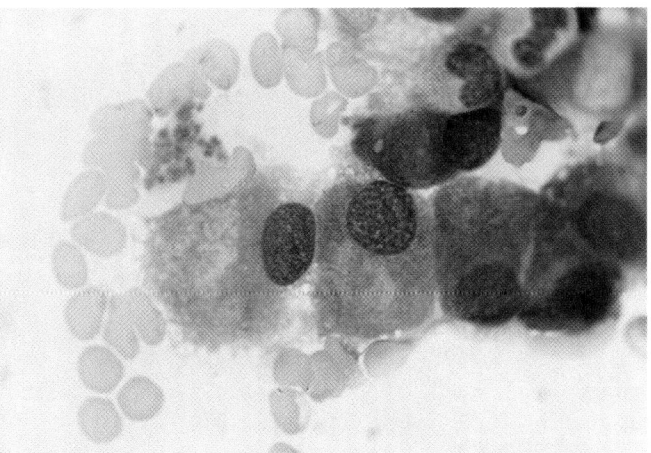

Fig. 2.30 A group of osteoblasts from a smear of normal bone marrow. The cytoplasm of each cell contains a large pale-staining area (occupied by the Golgi apparatus). As is the case in three of the cells in the photomicrograph, the Golgi zone is usually situated at some distance from the nucleus. May–Grünwald–Giemsa stain.

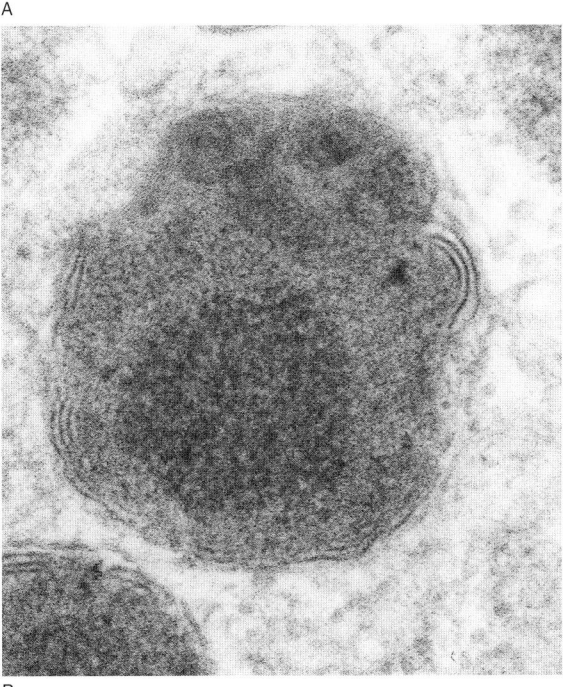

B

Fig. 2.29 (A) Electron micrograph of a mast cell in normal bone marrow. The cytoplasmic granules vary considerably in their ultrastructure. There are long thin cytoplasmic projections at the cell surface. Uranyl acetate and lead citrate. × 8500. (B) A single granule from the cell in (A), at high magnification, showing central condensations and peripheral lamellae. × 103 700.

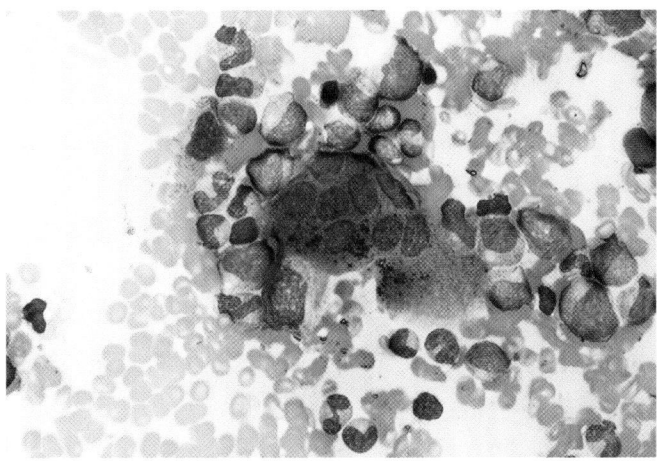

Fig. 2.31 A multinucleate osteoclast from a smear of normal bone marrow. May–Grünwald–Giemsa stain.

Osteoclasts (Fig. 2.31) are giant multinucleate cells with abundant pale-staining cytoplasm containing many fine azurophilic granules. The individual nuclei within a single cell are small, round or oval, uniform in size, and have a single prominent nucleolus. There is usually no overlap between adjacent nuclei within the same cell. Osteoclasts must be distinguished from the other polyploid giant cells in the marrow, the megakaryocytes. Unlike osteoclasts, the latter (when normal) have a single large segmented and lobulated nucleus. Osteoclasts are strongly acid-phosphatase-positive. Recent data clearly indicate that osteoclasts are derived from the multipotent myeloid stem cell, but the relationship of the osteoclast progenitor cell to the CFU-GM or CFU-M remains unclear.

immediately adjacent to the nucleus. Furthermore, the nucleus of an osteoblast does not show the heavily-stained coarse clumps of condensed chromatin that are characteristically seen in plasma cells. Osteoblasts are alkaline-phosphatase-positive.

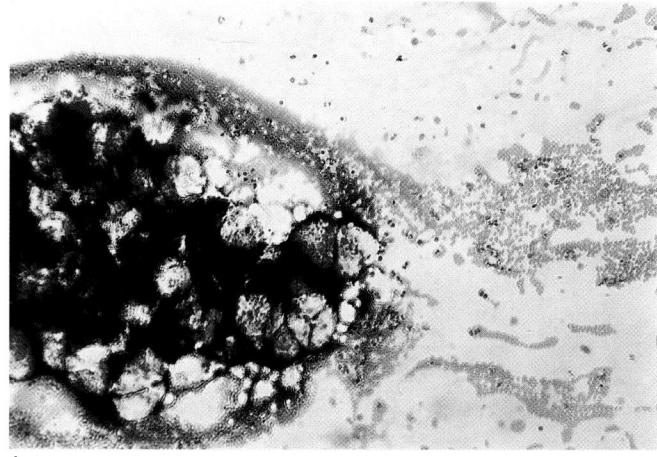

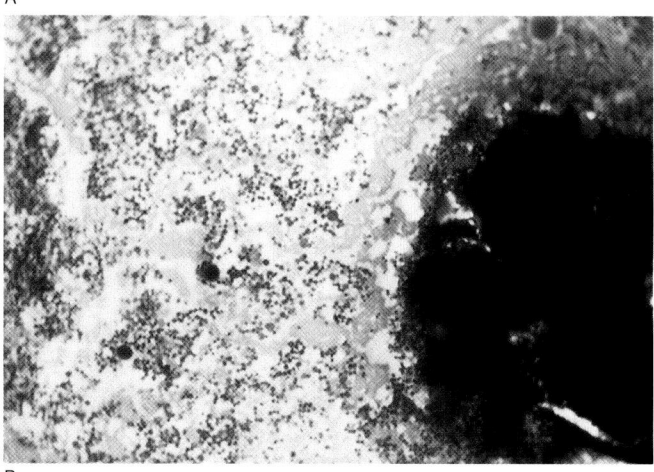

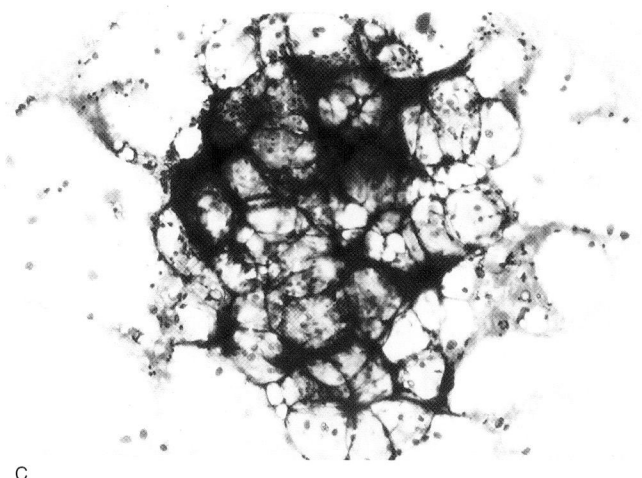

Fig. 2.32 (A–C) Different degrees of cellularity of marrow fragments in bone marrow smears from three different individuals. (A) Normocellular fragments in which a little over half the volume of the fragment consists of hemopoietic cells (normal adult). (B) Hypercellular fragment showing virtually complete replacement of fat cells by hemopoietic cells (congenital dyserythropoietic anemia, type I). (C) Hypocellular fragment in which under 25% of the volume of the fragment consists of hemopoietic cells (aplastic anemia). May–Grünwald–Giemsa stain.

Cellularity and marrow differential count

The bone marrow contains a mixture of fat cells and hemopoietic cells in various proportions. The proportion of hemopoietic cells relative to fat cells (i.e. the cellularity of the marrow) can be roughly assessed by examining several marrow fragments in stained marrow smears (Fig. 2.32). However, cellularity is more accurately assessed from histologic sections of aspirated marrow fragments or, preferably, of specimens obtained by trephine biopsy of bone (see Chapter 3). In histologic studies, cellularity is expressed as the percentage of the area of a microscopic field of marrow tissue which is occupied by hemopoietic cells. Studies of histologic sections of marrow fragments aspirated from the tibia, iliac crest and sternum of normal infants and children have shown 100% cellularity at birth, the appearance of fat cells as early as 2 weeks after birth (85% cellularity), and a cellularity of 35–80% (mean, 50%) in iliac crest and sternal aspirations from children between the ages of 18 months and 11 years.[54] In trephine biopsies from normal

adults, marrow cellularity varies between 30 and 70%. Samples from adults with a cellularity of 25% or less are therefore described as hypocellular and those with a cellularity of 75% or more as hypercellular. However, in subjects aged 70 years or more, the cellularity of the marrow may normally be less than 25%, particularly in the sternum but also in the iliac crest (also see Chapter 3).[55]

The percentage distribution of various cell types in smears of bone marrow from normal adults is given in Table 2.3.[56] In one study of 10 normal adults, in which differential counts were performed on very large numbers of nucleated cells in marrow smears, there were 99.9–266.9 (average, 183) megakaryocytes per 10^6 nucleated marrow cells.[57] When differential counts are performed on only 200–250 nucleated marrow cells, the proportion of megakaryocytes encountered varies between 0 and 6.1%.[58] However, careful quantitative histologic studies of trephine biopsies of normal marrow have given higher figures, with average values of about 650 megakaryocytes per 10^6 nucleated marrow cells presumably because megakaryocytes tend to be firmly fixed within marrow fragments and do not readily separate and spread in conventional smears.

There are marked changes in the cellular composition of the marrow during the first 3 months of life. The percentage of erythroblasts falls progressively from 40% (range, 18.5–65%) on the first day to 8% (range, 0–20.5%) between the 8th and 10th days and remains low for a period of about 3 weeks. It then gradually increases again

Table 2.3 Differential counts on smears of bone marrow aspirated from healthy adults. Means, 95% confidence limits and observed ranges form 28 cases aged between 20 and 29 years and observed ranges for 63 cases aged between 20 and 93 years.[56] 2000 cells were studied in each case

| Cell type | Percentages | | | |
	Mean (20–29 years)	95% confidence limits (20–29 years)	Observed range (20–29 years)	Observed range (20–93 years)
Myeloblasts	1.21	0.75–1.67	0.75–1.80	0.75–1.90
Promyelocytes	2.49	0.99–3.99	1.00–3.75	
Myelocytes				
Neutrophil	17.36	11.54–23.18	12.25–22.65	12.00–24.35
Eosinophil	1.37	0–2.85	0.25–3.45	0.25–3.45
Basophil	0.08	0–0.21	0.00–0.25	0.00–0.25
Metamyelocytes				
Neutrophil	16.29	11.40–22.44	11.45–23.60	8.75–27.35
Eosinophil	0.63	0.07–1.19	0.25–1.30	0.15–1.70
Juvenile neutrophils				
(Stab form)	8.70	3.58–13.82	4.85–13.95	2.60–13.95
Polymorphs				
Neutrophil	13.42	4.32–22.52	8.70–28.95	6.40–28.95
Eosinophil	0.93	0.21–1.65	0.45–1.55	0.25–2.35
Basophil	0.20	0–0.48	0.05–0.50	0.05–0.65
Monocytes	1.04	0.36–1.72	0.65–2.10	0.50–2.95
Plasma cells	0.46	0–0.96	0.10–0.95	0.10–2.00
Lymphocytes	14.60	6.66–22.54	9.35–25.05	6.85–25.05
Basophilic erythropoietic cells	0.92	0.40–1.44	0.50–1.60	0.50–1.60
Early polychromatic erythroblasts	6.76	2.56–10.96	3.30–12.20	1.80–12.20
Late polychromatic erythroblasts	11.58	6.16–1.70	7.85–19.55	6.15–19.90
Reticulum cells	0.24	0–0.54	0.50–0.65	0.05–0.80

Table 2.4 Changes in the cellular composition of the marrow during infancy and childhood

	0–24 hours[59] (n = 19)	2 months–1 year[60] (n = 16)	2–20 years[60] (n = 92)	20–29 years[56] (n = 28)
Neutrophil series				
Mean	46.4	54.4	60.6	60.1
Range	20–73		45–77	
Lymphocytes				
Mean	12.1	25.1	16.0	14.6
Range	2–22.5		12–28	9.3–25.0
Erythroblasts				
Mean	40	19.8	23.1	19.3
Range	18.5–65		12.7–19.3	
Myeloid/erythroid ratio				
Mean	1.16	3.5	2.9	3.1
Range			1.2–5.2	2.0–8.3[54]

to reach a value of 16% (range, 6.5–31.5%) in the 3-month-old infant.[59] These changes appear to be secondary to an increase of arterial oxygen saturation to adult levels within 3 h of birth resulting in a suppression of erythropoietin production. Erythropoietin production increases again when the infant is 6–13 weeks old. The proportion of granulocytes and their precursors increases during the first 2 weeks after birth and then decreases to stabilize at about 50% after the 2nd month (Table 2.4); a slight increase is seen after the age of 4 years.[56,59–61] The proportion of lymphocytes is relatively low in the neonate, increases markedly during the first 7–10 days and

Table 2.5 Changes in the prevalence of lymphocytes in the bone marrow during infancy and childhood[59,60,62,63]

Age	Total number of cases	Percentage of lymphocytes	
		Mean	Range or ±2 standard deviations
0–48 h	24	12.3	4.0–22.0
7–10 days	28	32.7	7.5–62.0
1 month	23	46.9	12.0–73.0
3 months	12	47.0	31.0–81.0
6 months	22	47.5	±15.7
12 months	18	47.1	±22.6
1.5 years	19	43.5	±17.1
4–4.5 years	9	19.1	12.0–27.0
2–20 years	89	15.9	5.0–36.0

Table 2.6 The prevalence of plasma cells in normal bone marrow.[64] 5000 nucleated marrow cells were assessed in each case

Age	Total number of cases	Percentage of plasma cells	
		Mean	Range
New born	6	0.016	0–0.04
0.5–6 months	6	0.024	0–0.06
6–12 months	5	0.068	0.02–0.16
1–2 years	7	0.118	0–0.30
2–4 years	6	0.184	0.08–0.50
4–6 years	5	0.228	0.12–0.28
6–12 years	6	0.350	0.20–0.62
12–15 years	6	0.386	0.28–0.56
21–29 years	5	0.384	0.26–0.48

remains high throughout the first year. Adult values are reached by the age of 4 years (Table 2.5).[59,60,62,63] Plasma cells are rarely seen in the marrow at birth but increase progressively to reach adult values by the age of about 12 years (Table 2.6).[64]

REFERENCES

1. Bloom W, Bartelmez GW 1940 Hemopoiesis in young human embryos. American Journal of Anatomy 67: 21–44
2. Gilmour JR 1941 Normal haemopoiesis in intrauterine and neonatal life. Journal of Pathology and Bacteriology 52: 25–55
3. Kelemen E, Calvo W, Fliedner TM 1979 Atlas of human hemopoietic development. Springer-Verlag, Berlin
4. Emura I, Sekiya M, Ohnishi Y 1983 Two types of immature erythrocytic series in the human liver. Archivum Histologicum Japonicum 46: 631–643
5. Kalpaktsoglou PK, Emery JL 1965 Human bone marrow during the last three months of intrauterine life. A histological study. Acta Haematologica (Basel) 34: 228–238
6. Piney A 1922 The anatomy of the bone marrow with special reference to the distribution of the red marrow. British Medical Journal ii: 792–795
7. Custer RP, Ahlfeldt FE 1932 Studies on the structure and function of bone marrow. II Variations in cellularity in various bones with advancing years of life and their relative response to stimuli. Journal of Laboratory and Clinical Medicine 17: 960–962
8. Wickramasinghe SN 1975 Human bone marrow. Blackwell Scientific Publications, Oxford
9. Gordon MY 1993 Human haemopoietic stem cell assays. Blood Reviews 7: 190–197
10. Ogawa M 1994 Hematopoiesis. Journal of Allergy and Clinical Immunology 94: 645–650
11. Prchal JT, Throckmorton DW, Carroll AJ et al 1978 A common progenitor for human myeloid and lymphoid cells. Nature 274: 590–591
12. McCune JM, Namikawa R, Kaneshima H et al 1988 The SCID-hu mouse: murine model for the analysis of human hematolymphoid differentiation and function. Science 24: 1632–1639
13. Giuliani AL, Wiener E, Lee MJ et al 2001 Changes in murine bone marrow macrophages and erythroid burst-forming cells following the intravenous injection of liposome-encapsulated dichloromethylene diphosphonate (Cl₂MDP). European Journal of Haematology 66: 1–9
14. Hanspal M, Smockova Y, Uong Q 1998 Molecular identification and functional characterisation of a novel protein that mediates the attachment of erythroblasts to macrophages. Blood 92: 2940–2950
15. Bessis M 1973 Living blood cells and their ultrastructure. Springer-Verlag, Berlin
16. Hayhoe FGJ, Quaglino D 1988 Haematological cytochemistry, 2nd edn. Churchill Livingstone, Edinburgh
17. Rheingold JJ, Wislocki GB 1948 Histochemical methods applied to hematology. Blood 3: 641–655
18. Gibb RP, Stowell RE 1949 Glycogen in human blood cells. Blood 4: 569–579
19. Rozenszajn L, Leibovich M, Shoham D, Epstein J 1968 The esterase activity in megaloblasts, leukaemic and normal haemopoietic cells. British Journal of Haematology 14: 605–610
20. Scott RE, Horn RG 1970 Ultrastructural aspects of neutrophil granulocyte development in humans. Laboratory Investigation 23: 202–215
21. Bainton DF, Ullyot JL, Farquhar MG 1971 The development of neutrophilic polymorphonuclear leukocytes in human bone marrow. Origin and content of azurophil and specific granules. Journal of Experimental Medicine 134: 907–934
22. Cawley JC, Hayhoe FGJ 1973 Ultrastructure of haemic cells. A cytological atlas of normal and leukaemic blood and bone marrow. Saunders, London
23. Kjeldsen L, Sengelov H, Borregaard N 1999 Subcellular fractionation of human neutrophils on Percoll density gradients. Journal of Immunological Methods 232: 131–143
24. Sorensen O, Arnljots K, Cowland JB et al 1997 The human antibacterial cathelicidin, hCAP-18, is synthesized in myelocytes and metamyelocytes and localized to specific granules in neutrophils. Blood 90: 2796–2803
25. Borregaard N, Lollike K, Kjeldsen L et al 1993 Human neutrophil granules and secretory vesicles. European Journal of Haematology 51: 187–198
26. Cowland JB, Borregaard N 1999 The individual regulation of granule protein mRNA levels during neutrophil maturation explains the heterogeneity of neutrophil granules. Journal of Leukocyte Biology 66: 989–995
27. Furth R van (ed) 1980 Mononuclear phagocytes. Functional aspects, part II. Martinus Nijhoff, The Hague
28. Leder LD 1967 The origin of blood monocytes and macrophages. Blut 16: 86–98
29. Scott RE, Horn RG 1970 Fine structural features of eosinophil granulocyte development in human bone marrow. Journal of Ultrastructural Research 33: 16–28
30. Parwaresch MR 1976 The human blood basophil. Springer-Verlag, Berlin
31. Zucker-Franklin D 1980 Ultrastructural evidence for the common origin of human mast cells and basophils. Blood 56: 534–540
32. Williams N, Levine RF 1982 The origin, development and regulation of megakaryocytes. British Journal of Haematology 52: 173–180
33. Vainchenker W, Bouguet J, Guichard J, Breton-Gorius J 1979 Megakaryocyte colony formation from human bone marrow precursors. Blood 54: 940–945
34. Queisser U, Queisser W, Spiertz B 1971 Polyploidization of megakaryocytes in normal humans, in patients with idiopathic

thrombocytopenia and with pernicious anaemia. British Journal of Haematology 20: 489–501

35. Levine RF, Hazzard KC, Lamberg JD 1982 The significance of megakaryocyte size. Blood 60: 1122–1131
36. Jean G, Lambertenghi-Deliliers G, Ranzi T, Poirier-Basseti M 1971 The human bone marrow megakaryocyte. An ultrastructural study. Haematologia 5: 253–264
37. Breton-Gorius J, Reyes F 1976 Ultrastructure of human bone marrow cell maturation. International Review of Cytology 46: 251–321
38. Radley JM, Haller CJ 1982 The demarcation membrane system of the megakaryocyte: a misnomer? Blood 60: 213–219
39. Breton-Gorius J 1980 The value of cytochemical peroxidase reactions at the ultrastructural level in haematology. Histochemical Journal 12: 127–137
40. Breton-Gorius J, Gourdin MF, Reyes F 1981 Ultrastructure of the leukemic cell. In: Catovsky D (ed), Methods in hematology. The leukemic cell. Churchill Livingstone, Edinburgh, 87–128
41. Larsen TE 1970 Emperipolesis of granular leukocytes within megakaryocytes in human hemopoietic bone marrow. American Journal of Clinical Pathology 53: 485–489
42. Rozman C, Vives-Corrons JL 1981 On the alleged diagnostic significance of megakaryocytic 'phagocytosis' (emperipolesis). British Journal of Haematology 48: 510
43. Cooper MD 1987 Current concepts. B lymphocytes: Normal development and function. New England Journal of Medicine 317: 1452–1456
44. Lobach DF, Haynes BF 1987 Ontogeny of the human thymus during fetal development. Journal of Clinical Immunology 7: 81–97
45. Strominger JL 1989 Developmental biology of T cell receptors. Science 244: 943–950
46. Wickramasinghe SN 1997 Bone marrow. In: Sternberg SS (ed) Histology for pathologists, 2nd edn. Lippincott-Raven, Philadelphia, 737
47. Marton PF 1975 Ultrastructural study of erythrophagocytosis in the rat bone marrow. I. Red cell engulfment by reticulum cells. Scandinavian Journal of Haematology (suppl) 23: 1–26
48. Wickramasinghe SN 1991 Observations on the ultrastructure of sinusoids and reticular cells in human bone marrow. Clinical and Laboratory Haematology 13: 263–278
49. Kirshenbaum AS, Kessler SW, Goff JP, Metcalfe DD 1991 Demonstration of the origin of human mast cells from CD34+ bone marrow progenitor cells. Journal of Immunology 146: 1410–1415

50. Zucker-Franklin D, Grusky G, Hirayama N, Schnipper E 1981 The presence of mast cell precursors in rat peripheral blood. Blood 58: 544–551
51. Denburg JA, Richardson M, Telizyn S, Bienenstock J 1983 Basophil/mast cell precursors in human peripheral blood. Blood 61: 775–780
52. dePaulis A, Minopoli G, Arbustini E et al 1999 Stem cell factor is localized in, released from, and cleaved by human mast cells. Journal of Immunology 163: 2799–2808
53. Whitaker-Menezes D, Schechter NM, Murphy GF 1995 Serine proteinases are regionally segregated within mast cell granules. Laboratory Investigation 72: 34–41
54. Sturgeon P 1951 Volumetric and microscopic pattern of bone marrow in normal infants and children. III. Histologic pattern. Pediatrics 7: 774–781
55. Harstock RJ, Smith EB, Petty CS 1965 Normal variations with ageing of the amount of hematopoietic tissue in bone marrow from the anterior iliac crest. A study made from 177 cases of sudden death examined by necropsy. American Journal of Clinical Pathology 43: 326–331
56. Jacobsen KM 1941 Untersuchungen über das Knockenmarkspunktat bei normalen Individuen verschiedener Altersklassen. Acta Medica Scandinavica 106: 417–446
57. Dameshek W, Miller EB 1946 The megakaryocytes in idiopathic thrombocytopenic purpura, a form of hypersplenism. Blood 1: 27
58. Pizzolato P 1948 Sternal marrow megakaryocytes in health and disease. American Journal of Clinical Pathology 18: 891
59. Gairdner D, Marks J, Roscoe JD 1952 Blood formation in infancy. Part I. The normal bone marrow. Archives of Diseases in Childhood 27: 128–133
60. Glaser K, Limarzi LR, Poncher HG 1950 Cellular composition of the bone marrow in normal infants and children. Pediatrics 6: 789–824
61. Young RH, Osgood EE 1935 Sternal marrow aspirated during life. Cytology in health and in disease. Archives of Internal Medicine 55: 186–203
62. Diwany M 1940 Sternal marrow puncture in children. Archives of Diseases in Childhood 15: 159–170
63. Rosse C, Kraemer MJ, Dillon TL et al 1977 Bone marrow cell populations of normal infants: the predominance of lymphocytes. Journal of Laboratory and Clinical Medicine 89: 1225–1240
64. Steiner ML, Pearson HA 1966 Bone marrow plasmacyte values in childhood. Journal of Pediatrics 68: 562–568

Normal bone marrow: histology, histochemistry and immunohistochemistry

R Bartl   B Frisch

3

Normal bone marrow – organization, structure and function

Marrow cellularity

Age-related changes

Topography and bone marrow architecture

Hematopoietic microenvironment

Bone marrow stroma: cells, fibers and extracellular matrix
Extracellular matrix
Fibers
Nerves
Blood vessels

Hematopoiesis
Erythropoiesis
Myelopoiesis – granulocytes
Mast cells
Magekaryocytes and thrombopoiesis

Monocytes, macrophages and iron-containing reticular cells
Macrophages (histiocytes, reticular cells)
Lymphocytes
Plasma cells
Evaluation of normal bone marrow sections
Artifacts and pitfalls

Methods

Plastic embedding
Fixation for plastic
Composition of the fixative
Glucose phosphate buffer pH 7.4
Reagents
Dehydration

Embedding and staining
Methyl methacrylate embedding mixture
Procedure for coating glass slides
Gelatin solution
Removal of methacrylate from the sections
Methanol ammonia solution
Giemsa stain – for cytologic details
Phosphate buffer pH 6.7, 0.066 mol/l
Phosphate buffer pH 6.6, 0.066 mol/l
Giemsa pH 6.7 (prepare fresh before use)
Giemsa solution pH 6.6
Toluidine blue stain

Paraffin embedding and immunohistology
Fixation

Rapid processing
For plastic embedding
For paraffin embedding

Normal bone marrow – organization, structure and function

The term 'bone marrow' refers to the tissue occupying the cavities under the cortex within the honeycomb of trabecular bone (Figs 3.1A,B). Normal marrow is either red, consisting of the hematopoietic tissue, or yellow, composed mainly of fat cells (adipose tissue). In children most bones contain hematopoietic marrow, almost to the exclusion of fat cells. In the adult, red marrow is found in the skull, sternum, scapulae, vertebrae, ribs, pelvic bones and the proximal ends of the long bones (e.g. femora and humeri). The hematopoietic marrow produces the mature blood cells, which have a finite life span and must be

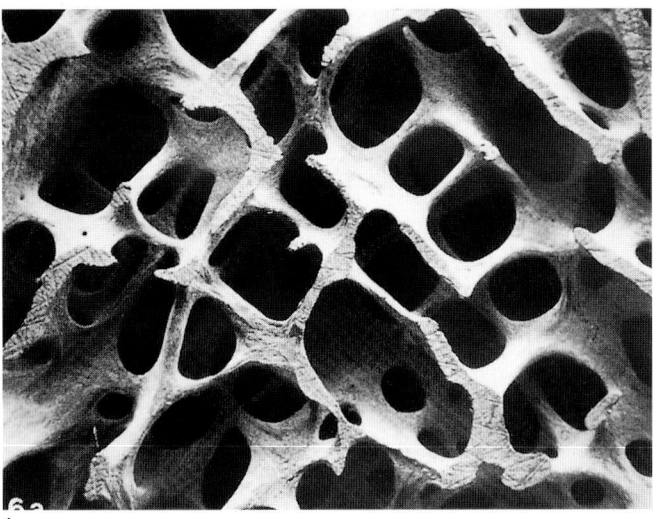

A

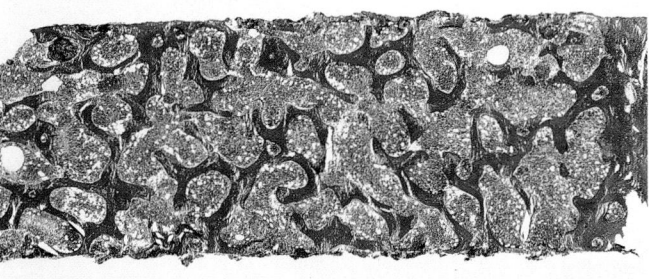

B

Fig. 3.1 (A) Scanning electron microscope view of representative cancellous bone structure of iliac crest. Reproduced from: Whitehouse WJ (1977) Cancellous bone in the anterior part of the iliac crest. Calcif. Tissue Res 26: 67–76, with permission. (B) Bone marrow biopsy section (BMBS) showing trabecular bone structure of normal adult. Plastic-embedded, Gomori.

constantly replaced. The weight of the total bone marrow is 1600–3700 g, about 1000 g of which is red marrow. If and when a greater hematopoietic capacity is required, expansion into, for example, the shafts of the long bones may occur. The red marrow can also expand or contract by means of an increase or decrease in the proportion of adipose tissue present, as well as by changes in the microcirculation. Under special circumstances other bones and organs, (liver, spleen, lymph nodes) also support hematopoiesis. Stem cells (and early hematopoietic progenitor cells) circulate in the peripheral blood and 'home' to the bone marrow. Proliferation of normal bone marrow cell populations can be assessed by use of the antibodies Ki67 and PCNA (proliferating cell nuclear antigen).[1–4]

A continuous supply of precursor cells is provided by the pluripotent stem cell compartment which is capable of self-renewal, and also has the ability to differentiate into progenitor cells committed to erythro-, granulo-, mono-, lympho- and megakaryopoiesis. The bone marrow supports lymphopoiesis and maturation of plasma cells. Stem and progenitor cells are not recognizable as such by the usual morphologic (including histochemical and immunohistologic) techniques, and are therefore not visualized on sections of biopsies. The bone marrow is composed of: (1) the parenchyme: the precursors and all maturation stages of the red cells, white cells, megakaryocytes, and (2) the stroma: fat cells, histiocytes/

Table 3.1 Histomorphometry of normal bone and bone marrow[1]

Variables	Mean value (SD)	Dimension
Hematopoietic tissue	40 (9)	Vol%
Fatty tissue	28 (8)	
Trabecular bone	26 (5)	
Osteoid	0.3 (0.2)	
Sinusoids	4.5 (2.1)	
H/F index[2]	1.4	
G/E index[3]	2.8	
Lymphocytes (diffuse)	20 (12)	/mm²
Mast cells	2 (1)	
Megakaryocytes	8 (4)	
Macrophages (containing iron)	16 (10)	
Plasma cells	21 (18)	
Lymphoid nodules	2	%
Arteries	3 (4)	/100 mm²
Arterioles	26 (18)	
Capillaries	101 (61)	
Sinusoids	1700 (825)	
Osteoblastic index (OB)[4]	5 (5)	%
Osteoclastic index (OC)[5]	4 (3)	/100 mm

[1] These values are derived from 158 biopsies of normal healthy individuals.
[2] H/F index = hematopoietic tissue (vol%)/fatty tissue (vol%).
[3] G/E index = granulopoietic cells (n)/erythropoietic cells (n).
[4] OB = percentage of trabecular circumference covered by cuboidal osteoblasts.
[5] OC = number of osteoclasts per 100 mm trabecular circumference.

macrophages (reticulum cells), fibroblasts, blood vessels and intercellular matrix. Plasma cells, mast cells and lymphocytes complete the picture (Table 3.1). However, it must be borne in mind that bone and its cells are also an integral component of connective tissue and must be included in any histologic evaluation of bone marrow.

A short list of antibodies for confirmation of cellular identities is given in Table 3.2.

Marrow cellularity

This term includes both hematopoietic and adipose tissue and it indicates the relative amounts of these two components.[5-7] *Normocellular* (Fig. 3.2A) indicates about equal proportions or somewhat more hematopoiesis than fat cells. *Hypocellular* (Fig. 3.2B and 3.3A) indicates a reduction in hematopoiesis and a corresponding increase

Table 3.2 Immunohistology: short list of antibodies for normal bone marrow

Antibody	Cell	Source	Mono or polyclonal
Myeloperoxidase	Granulocytes	Dako	P
Glycophorin	Erythroid cells	Dako	M
Factor VIII Rag	Megakaryocytes	Dako	P
CD34 (Qbend 10)	Stroma endothelium	Oxoid	M
CD68	Mononuclear phagocytes (MPs), some granulocytes	Dako	M
CD20	B-lymphocytes	Dako	M
Ig, kappa, lambda	Plasma cells	Dako	P
CD45	T, B, some MPs	Dako	M
CD4	T-helper cells	Biomen	M
CD8	T cytotoxic cells	Dako	M
KI 67	Proliferating cells	Novocast	M

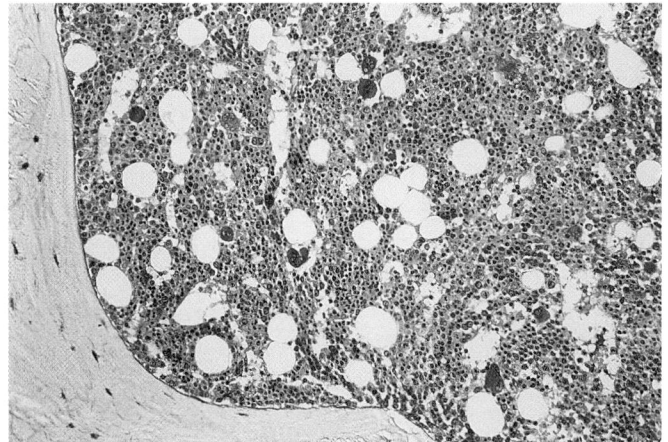

A

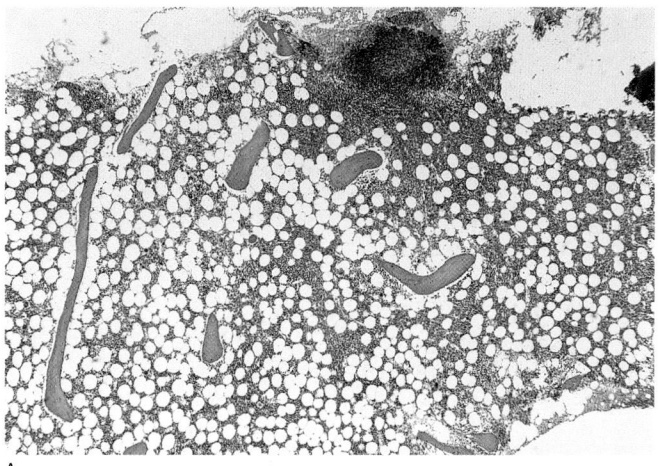

A

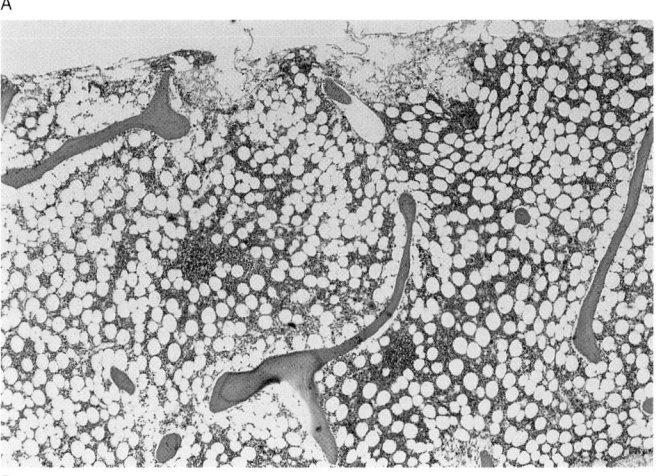

B

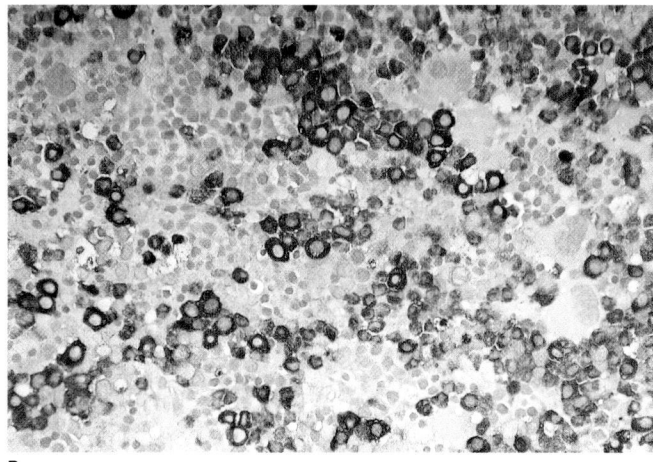

B

Fig. 3.2 (A) BMBS showing a bone trabeculum and normocellular bone marrow. Plastic-embedded, Giemsa. (B) BMBS showing hypocellular bone marrow. Note reduction in trabecular bone, increase in fat cells, decrease in hematopoiesis and lymphocytic aggregates. Paraffin-embedded, H&E.

Fig. 3.3 (A) BMBS showing osteopenia and hypocellularity. Note lymphocytic nodule with germinal center – top, middle. Paraffin-embedded, H&E. (B) BMBS showing variable marrow cellularity. Paraffin-embedded, H&E.

in fat cells, particularly in the subcortical marrow spaces. Moreover, variable marrow cellularity (hypocellular intertrabecular spaces alternating with hyper or normo-

cellular ones) may also be found (Fig. 3.3B). *Hypercellular* is used when the fat is decreased (Fig. 3.4A). An almost aplastic bone marrow is shown for comparison (Fig. 3.4B).

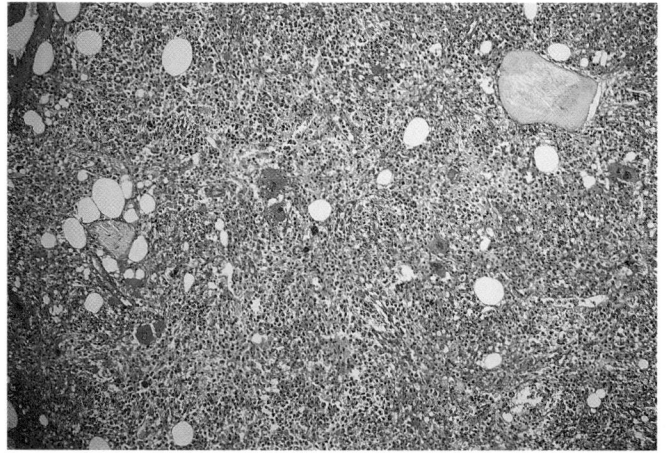

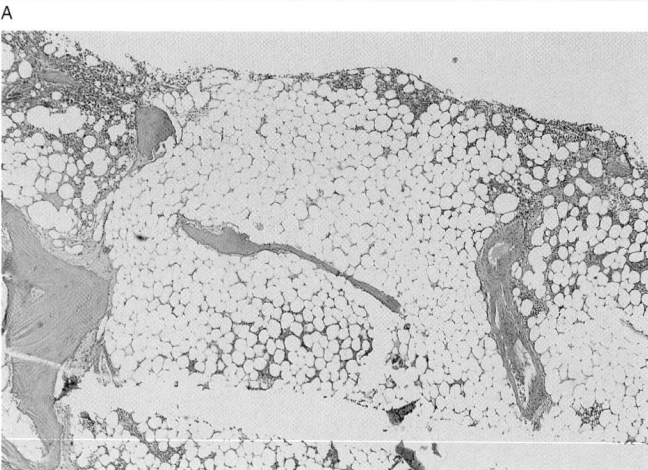

Fig. 3.4 (A) BMBS showing hypercellular marrow. Note few residual fat cells. Plastic-embedded, Giemsa. (B) BMBS showing almost aplastic marrow for comparison. Paraffin-embedded, H&E.

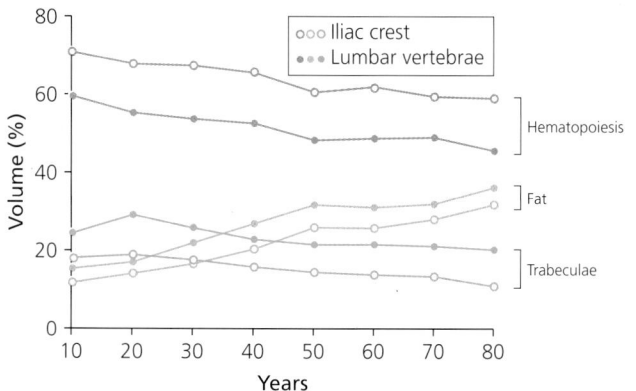

Fig. 3.5 Quantitative estimation of hematopoiesis, fat and trabecular bone in bone biopsies of 158 individuals without evidence of disease. Note steady decline in hematopoiesis and trabecular bone with increasing age.

Age-related changes

With advancing age, there is a reduction in the amount of trabecular bone and of hematopoiesis, accompanied by an increase in fat cells, particularly, but not only, in the subcortical regions (Fig. 3.5). In addition, other cells normally present in the bone marrow, such as lymphocytes, plasma and mast cells, may increase in the bone marrow of older people.[8–10] Stromal changes are also found, such as alterations in walls of blood vessels, especially sclerosis.

Topography and bone marrow architecture

The hematopoietic tissue is localized in the extravascular compartment, erythropoietic islands and megakaryocytes are associated with the marrow sinusoids in the central regions of the marrow cavities, early myeloid precursors lie close to the endosteal surfaces and to the arterioles, while the more mature forms of the granulocytic series are also found in the central intertrabecular areas (Fig. 3.6). There are, however, normally considerable variations, especially in hyper- and hypoplastic conditions and when osseous changes are present. Nevertheless, deviations from the marrow architecture, changes in the composition of the cell populations and alterations in the stromal compartment are all indicators of functional disturbances, especially in proliferation, maturation, and cellular composition of the bone marrow. It should also be remembered that bone and bone marrow are functionally closely linked and interdependent, so that alterations in one invariably induce changes in the other. Consequently, cortical and trabecular bone and their cells (osteoblasts, endosteal lining cells, osteocytes and osteoclasts) should always be examined together with the bone marrow (Table 3.1, Fig. 3.6).

Hematopoietic microenvironment

The constituents of the normal bone marrow are closely packed within a hard bony 'container'. The stromal elements form an extensive, closely woven network in which the hematopoietic precursors are embedded, attached in various ways and to different components by the adhesive proteins and by other cells, such as the central macrophages in the erythroid islands. The integrins are transmembrane glycoproteins that mediate cell-to-cell and cell matrix interactions. Hematopoietic precursors receive their nutrients, vitamins, hormones, regulatory factors, cytokines and modulators through the extracellular matrix. Indeed, the correct processing of signals from the extracellular matrix (ECM) contributes to the regulation of the cell cycle, cellular differentiation and apoptosis. All cells of a particular organism have the same genetic information, but there are striking differences in morphology and function of different types, for example a leukocyte and a liver cell. Remove a cell from its normal microenvironment and it loses many of its distinguishing characteristics. Thus the ECM is an essential factor in normal cell survival and activity, and in tissue integrity.

Bone marrow stroma: cells, fibers and extracellular matrix

The stroma provides the framework 'scaffolding' for hematopoiesis. The stroma consists of reticular cells, fat cells, fibroblasts and their fibrils and the extensive network of blood vessels, including the sinusoids.[11-15] Fat cells occupy about a third of the marrow volume in the iliac crest biopsy (Table 3.1, Fig. 3.2A). They serve a supporting, filling and metabolic function as shown, for example by their ability to participate in steroid aromatization. There are close associations between the mesenchymal elements – the endothelium, the advential cells, fibroblasts and osteoblasts, and the endosteal lining cells as well as reticular cells and macrophages. Osteoblasts, for example, produce growth factors for myeloid cells (Chapter 4), which may contribute to their paratrabecular localization. Fibroblasts, elongated cells with elongated nuclei, may be indistinguishable from the so-called reticular cells. Fibroblasts produce the reticular fibers of which there are few in the normal bone marrow, mainly in association with blood vessels and endosteum; smooth muscle actin and vimentin may occasionally be useful in demonstration of connective tissue elements (Fig. 3.7).

Extracellular matrix

This consists of a variety of components – mainly proteins – produced by the stromal cells. These include cell adhesion molecules (CAMs), collagen, fibronectin, vitronectin, proteoglycans as well as the growth and other factors involved in the highly complex regulatory mechanisms controlling the production of the formed elements of the blood (see Chapter 4).

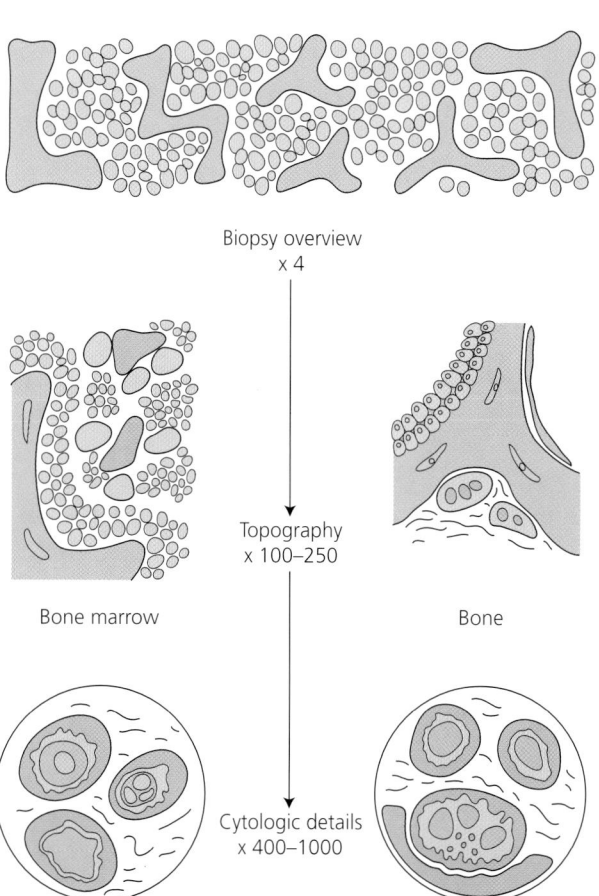

Fig. 3.6 Microscopic evaluation of bone marrow biopsy: overview – cortical and trabecular bone and cellularity; topography and cytologic detail; note magnifications – these are used throughout this text.

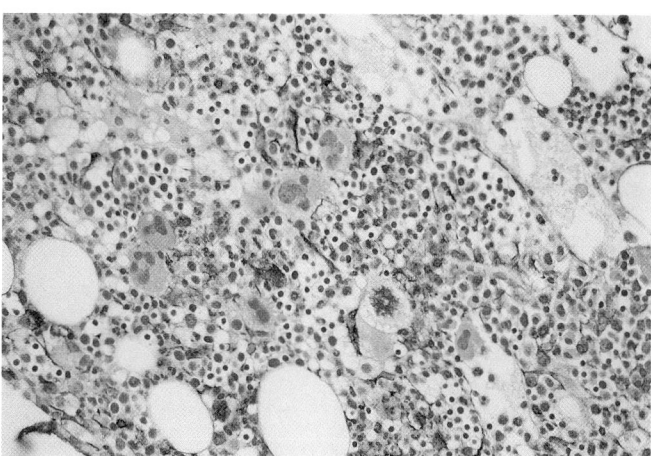

Fig. 3.7 BMBS. Note connective tissue elements stained brown. Paraffin-embedded, vimentin.

Fibers

The normal bone marrow contains only thin reticular fibers near bone and blood vessels, best visualized by the Gomori stain for reticulin or similar stains and by polarized light (Fig. 3.8). Fibrosis in the marrow may involve reticulin fibers only, or also collagen (i.e. bundles of reticulin). All these components of the bone marrow stroma constitute the microenvironment which provides the niches for the stem cells and the inductive influences which direct them to one or other line of differentiation, support their maturation and facilitate their egress from the extravascular compartment into the systemic circulation.[16,17]

Nerves

Nerves are rarely found in biopsy sections, but occasionally may be seen next to blood vessels in the periosteum.

Blood vessels

The medullary arteries enter via the cortical bone and branch within the marrow and the trabeculae. The smaller branches divide into arterioles, and then into capillaries which frequently have a cuff of plasma cells around them, and flow into the sinusoids whose walls consist of a single layer of endothelial cells, an incomplete outer covering of adventitia and, when large, a very loose network of reticulin fibers (Figs. 3.9–3.11). The sinusoids in turn drain into the periosteal veins. The endothelial cells of postcapillary, or postsinusoidal venules may be plump, with vesicular nuclei and distinct nucleoli. The endothelium forms the interface between the intra- and the extravascular compartments, through which the

blood cells enter the circulation. The sinus endothelial cells possibly contribute to regulation of entry of mature cells into the circulation. The hematopoietic progenitor

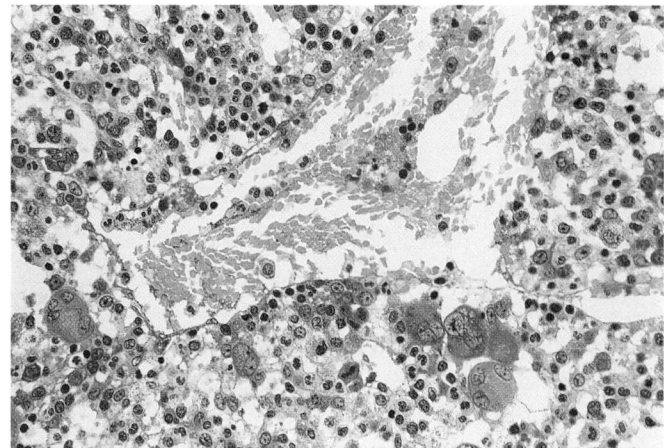

Fig. 3.9 BMBS. Note large sinus and megakaryocytes lower right. Plastic-embedded, Giemsa.

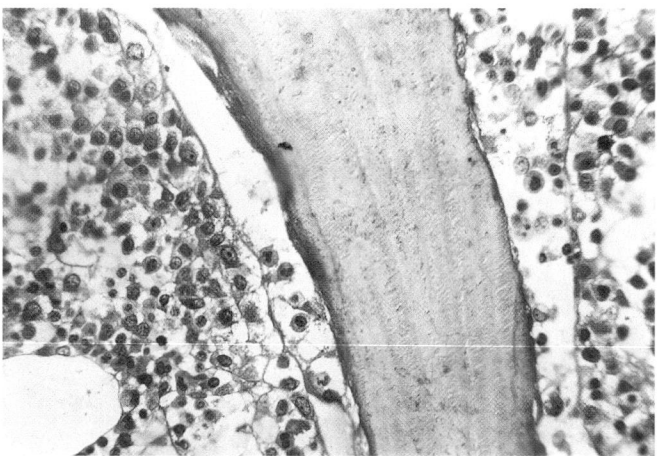

Fig. 3.10 BMBS. Note paratrabecular sinus and myeloid precursors, left. Plastic-embedded, Giemsa.

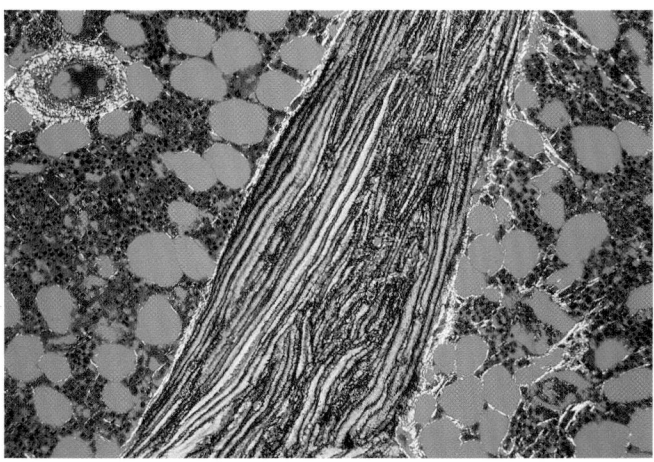

Fig. 3.8 BMBS viewed in polarized light. Note paratrabecular and perivascular reticulin fibers, Plastic-embedded, Gomori.

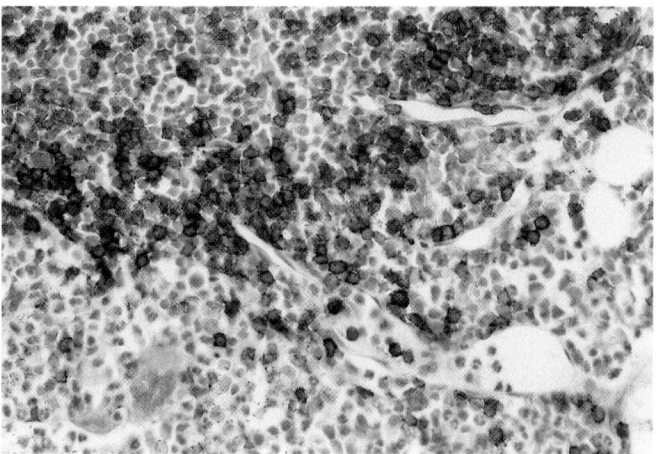

Fig. 3.11 BMBS. Note myeloid precursors adjacent to blood vessels. Paraffin-embedded, myeloperoxidase.

cell antigen CD34 is also present in vascular endothelial cells. Thus a bone marrow biopsy (BMB) illustrates the normal range of blood vessels and may therefore supply additional information in diseases which affect them, such as arteriosclerosis, arteritis and amyloidosis. Physiologically, parts of the sinusoidal channels are collapsed at any one time and the expansion and contraction of the vascular system within the rigid bony cage contribute (together with quantitative changes in fat cells) to the extreme fluctuations in the production of blood cells of which the marrow is capable. When the need arises, an increase of up to 10-fold its usual hematopoietic capacity is possible. It should be remembered that the parenchyme of the bone marrow is at all times composed of a rapidly evolving, highly mobile population so that a section of a biopsy is comparable to a still of a motion picture. This helps to account for the great variety seen in biopsy sections, which is nevertheless within the 'normal' range. Moreover, many processes in the bone marrow are highly efficient and fast and leave few traces, as witness the disposal of normoblast nuclei and the transendothelial passage of reticulocytes and granulocytes which is so rarely observed in contrast to megakaryocytes.

Hematopoiesis

This is the process of production of the formed elements of the blood; there are cords, islands or clusters of precursor cells between the sinusoids, through whose endothelial cells the erythrocytes, leukocytes and platelelets enter the blood stream. The normal cell populations in the peripheral blood are maintained by the hematopoietic tissues in the bone marrow. Stem cells, the earliest cells capable of hematopoiesis, possess the capacity for self-renewal and the potential for multilineage differentiation. The pluripotent stem cell compartment gives rise to the stem cells for both myeloid and lymphoid cell lines, which in turn produce progenitor cells of progressively restricted potential. In addition to erythrocytes, granulocytes, lymphocytes, megakaryocytes and platelets, the stem cells give rise to mast cells, macrophages and osteoclasts, but not to the bone marrow fibroblasts and osteoblasts, whose origin is in the mesenchyme.[18–24]

Erythropoiesis

The nucleated precursors of the red cells are found in small and large 'islands' consisting of immature and mature erythroblasts (Fig. 3.12A,B). These are easily identified, and may be stained by antibodies to glycophorin and hemoglobin. A macrophage (reticular cell) with long cytoplasmic processes, and containing hemosiderin and

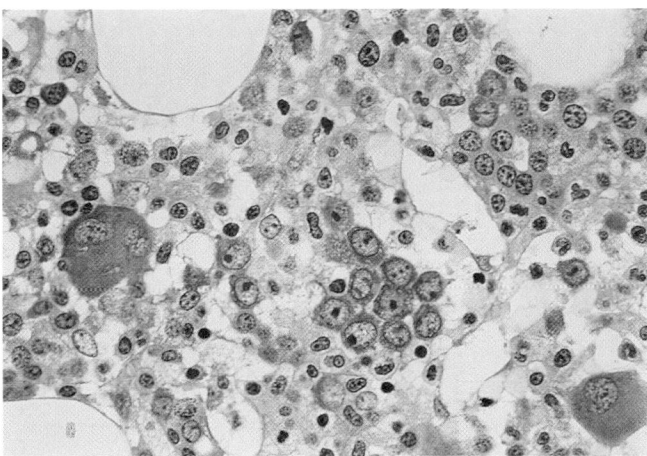

A

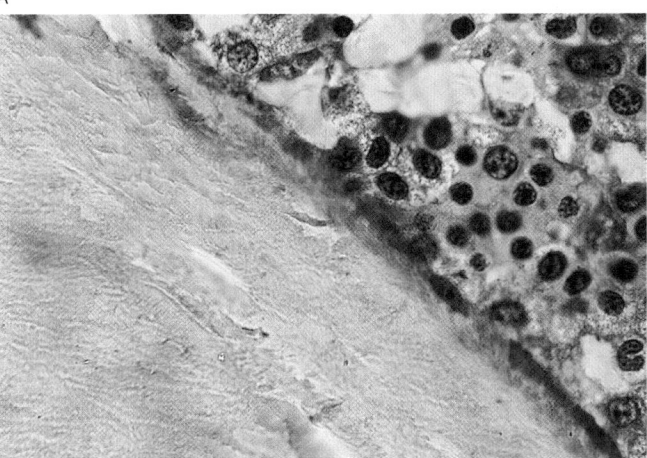

B

Fig. 3.12 (A) BMBS showing erythroid precursors. Note large erythroblasts (lower left of center) intertrabecular area. Plastic-embedded, Giemsa. (B) BMBS showing erythroid precursors next to the bone indicating disorganization of marrow architecture. Plastic-embedded, Giemsa.

possibly some cellular or nuclear debris, is usually found in the middle or the vicinity of such 'islands'. Using the proliferation antigen Ki67, the highest proliferative activity in normal bone marrow was found in the erythroid cells.[25] The macrophage appears to play a supporting role in normal red cell production (Fig. 3.12). It takes approximately 5 days from erythroblasts to reticulocytes, though this process may be accelerated in acute conditions. The myeloid:erythroid ratio is 1.5:1 to 3:1 in BMB. When one considers the astronomical numbers of erythrocytes produced per unit time (millions per mm^3 per second) it is astonishing that extruded nuclei and macrophages containing them are so rarely observed in normal BMB. This strongly indicates that the engulfment and/or lysis of normoblast nuclei must be remarkably efficient and fast. In contrast, cellular debris reminiscent of granulocytic nuclei may be found within macrophage cytoplasm much more frequently.

Myelopoiesis – granulocytes

The granulocytic series consists of neutrophils, eosinophils, basophils and mast cells. Myeloblast, promyelocyte, myelocyte, metamyelocyte, band and segmented forms are all identifiable in sections of the bone marrow.[26–29] The paratrabecular[30] and the periarteriolar regions constitute the granulocytic 'generation zones', but precursors are also scattered throughout the rest of the marrow (Fig. 3.13A,B). Neutrophilic (punctuate, brownish) granules and eosinophilic (slightly larger and yellowish-red) granules are readily distinguished, even in early myelocyte development. Basophils (having partially water-soluble granules) are recognized infrequently though mature basophils are occasionally seen. They have fewer, larger and darker red granules.

Under normal circumstances, granulopoiesis is very effective, so that practically all the cells produced reach the circulation. Mature granulocytes migrate through the endothelium into the sinusoids. Myeloid cells are positive for CD13, CD15 and CD33 and myeloperoxidase, myeloblasts may express CD34. Myeloperoxidase appears at the promyelocyte stage and is present in the azurophilic granules.

Mast cells

Mast cells lie adjacent to the endothelial cells of sinusoids, at the endosteal surface of the trabecular bone (Fig. 3.14), in the periosteum, in the walls of small arteries, scattered in the bone marrow, and frequently at the edges of and within lymphoid aggregates or nodules. Mast cells produce numerous factors that influence proliferation, differentiation and function of practically all components of bone marrow, as well as bone cells (Table 3.3). Mast cells are characterized by oval to round nuclei and cytoplasm densely packed with bright red granules in Giemsa-stained sections of undecalcified BMBs, and of paraffin-embedded biopsies. Mast cells may be round, oval or spindle shaped, with abundant cytoplasm, or thin and elongated resembling fibroblasts, in which case they are best identified in sections stained by toluidine blue and under high magnification as only few granules may

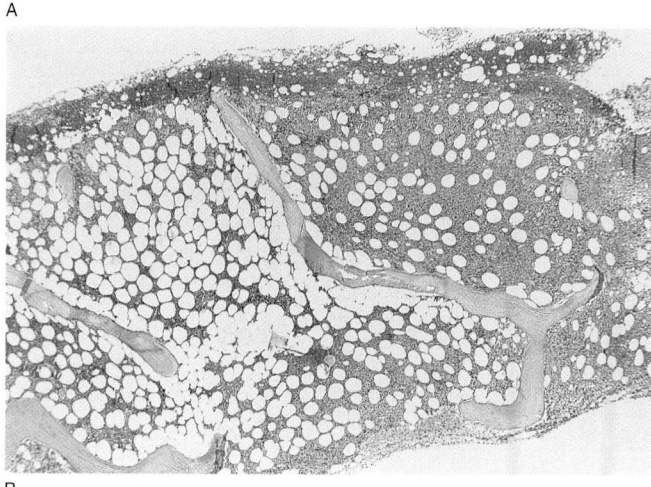

A

B

Fig. 3.13 (A) BMBS showing myeloperoxidase-positive cells at the trabecular surface. Paraffin-embedded, myeloperoxidase. (B) BMBS showing myeloid precursors dispersed in the marrow. Paraffin-embedded, myeloperoxidase.

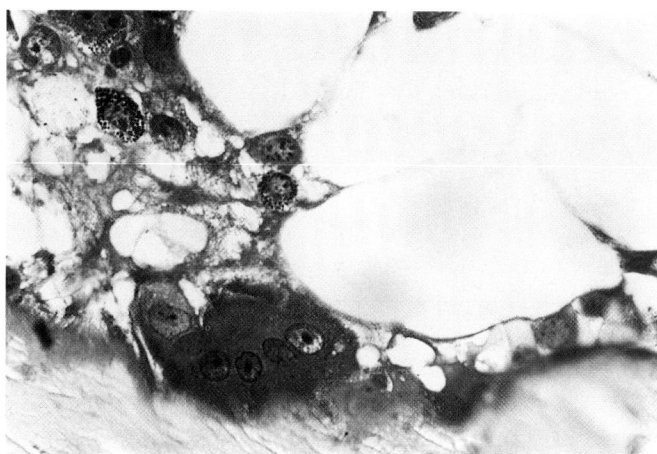

Fig. 3.14 BMBS. Note mast cells upper right, and osteoclast on trabecular surface, lower right of center. Plastic-embedded, Giemsa.

Table 3.3 Responses to mast cell factors

Leukocyte	Fibroblast	Microvascular
Adherance	Proliferation	Augmented vascular
Chemotaxis	Collagen production	permeability
Phagocytosis	Substrate responses	Leukocyte adherance
IgE production	Protein degradation	Constriction
Mast cell	Coagulation	Dilation
proliferation	activation	
Eosinophil		
activation		

be present. Small accumulations of mast cells and histiocytes, sometimes in association with endothelial cells (previously designated fibro-histiocytic lesions) may also be found in the bone marrow; their significance is unknown. They may be increased in infections, or occur as reactions to drugs. Mast cells may also be stained by antibodies to IgE.

Megakaryocytes and thrombopoiesis

These are the largest cells normally present in the bone marrow.[31–33] They range from 12 to 150 μm and show considerable variation in shape as well as size and nuclear configuration (Fig. 3.15A–C). The smaller ones may be difficult to identify so that enzymic or marker techniques are required, such as Factor VIII related antigen (Fig. 3.15A). Three stages are recognized:

1. The megakaryoblast, 15–20 μm, with an oval or kidney-shaped nucleus and basophilic cytoplasm. These measurements are approximate and related to the method of preparation (i.e. paraffin or plastic embedding, and plane of section).
2. The pro-megakaryocyte, 20–80 μm, cytoplasm less basophilic, but with a zone of developing granules, especially perinuclear.
3. Mature megakaryocytes, with eosinophilic cytoplasm, and with variable granularity.

The nucleus is coarsely cerebriform and often multilobed. DNA synthesis proceeds as polyploidization goes through 8, 16, 32 or $64n$, while lobulation may continue after that: 95% of platelet-shedding megakaryocytes are $16-32n$. Differentiation of the cytoplasm commences after DNA synthesis has ceased (in most cases) and three cytoplasmic zones are distinguished in the mature megakaryocyte: perinuclear, intermediate and marginal. The first contains the synthetic apparatus, the second the developing demarcation membranes and the third, which is found only in non-platelet-releasing megakaryocytes, contains filaments. In cases of extreme demand, large megakaryocyte fragments are released into the circulating blood – megaplatelets or megathrombocytes. Emperipolesis – the presence of other intact cells (erythroblasts, granulocytes) within megakaryocyte cytoplasm – may be found in megakaryocytes of any size, and such cells are not apparently phagocytosed.

Topographically, megakaryocytes are dispersed singly in the intertrabecular spaces and typically they abut on or project into the sinusoids, so that the platelets are shed directly into their lumina (see Fig. 3.9). Whole megakaryocytes or portions of their cytoplasm may also enter the sinuses and fragment in the vascular system; occasional denuded megakaryocyte nuclei are also found in normal bone marrows. There is a close association between megakaryocytes and fibroblasts whose proliferation is stimulated by PDGF (platelet-derived growth factor) and

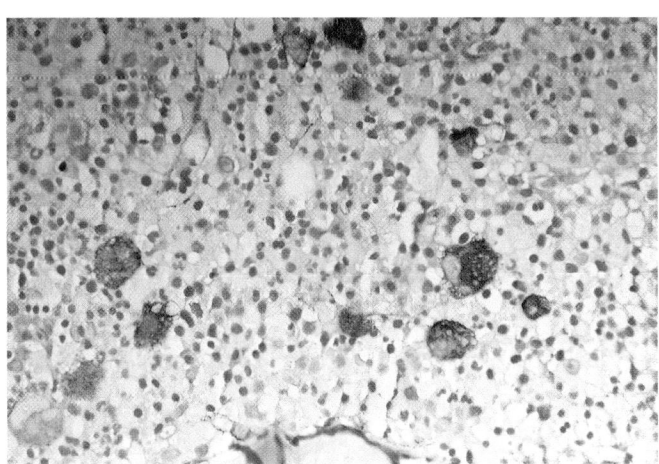

A

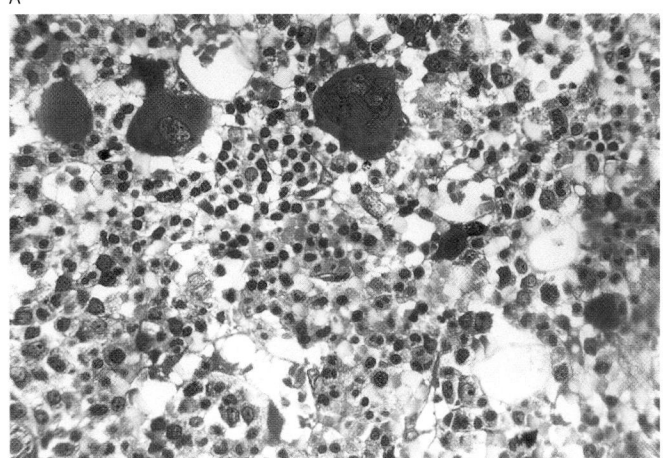

B

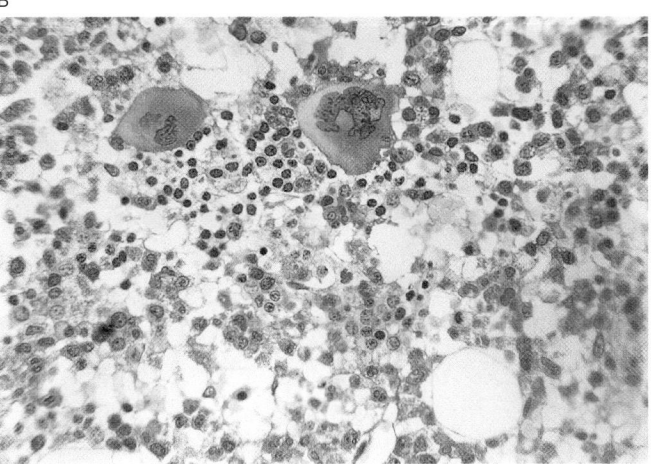

C

Fig. 3.15 (A) BMBS. Note large and small megakaryocytes. Paraffin-embedded, FVIII-related antigen. (B) BMBS. Note megakaryocytes, erythroblasts and myeloid cells, and lymphocytes near the megakaryocytes. Plastic-embedded, H&E. (C) BMBS. Same as (B) for comparison. Plastic-embedded, Giemsa.

by TGF β1 (transforming growth factor β1) both secreted by megakaryocytes. Small clusters of lymphocytes may also be found near megakaryocytes (Fig. 3.15B,C).

Monocytes, macrophages and iron-containing reticular cells

Monocytes (though produced in the bone marrow) are not often recognized, even in optimal histological sections, as they are easily confused with granulocytic precursors. Although they are larger, like the latter they have oval to kidney-shaped vesicular nuclei and abundant eosinophilic cytoplasm with no or variable granulation.[34] They are not fixed, but are mobile cells, even within the bone marrow. They are recognized in greater quantities by immunohistochemistry than in conventionally stained sections (Fig. 3.16).

Macrophages (histiocytes, reticular cells)

Macrophages appear to be a heterogeneous population and there are several views as to their origin, which may be from the fixed reticular cells or their derivatives, from the granulocyte–monocyte precursors, or from mature monocytes.[35,36] Macrophages may be very large, with nuclei resembling those of histiocytes, and their abundant cytoplasm may contain granules, vacuoles, lipid, cellular and nuclear debris (Fig. 3.17). They are stained by CD68 (Fig. 3.16). Typical bone marrow macrophages (reticular cells) may contain hemosiderin and/or cellular debris (Fig. 3.17). These cells form part of the reticulo-endothelial

system (RES) or the mononuclear phagocyte system, responsible for the breakdown of senescent red cells and the storage of iron. There are about 16 iron-containing macrophages per mm^2 of bone marrow. Iron stains on bone marrow sections demonstrate normal storage, overload and depletion. Iron stores in bone marrow sections may be graded: none; small particles in a few reticular cells; more numerous particles in more cells; and large particles as well as deposition on osteoid seams. Up to 50% of erythroid precursors may contain cytoplasmic iron, but unevenly distributed, not in the form of 'ring' sideroblasts. There is generally a good correlation between serum ferritin levels, iron absorption, and marrow stores, except in cases of sideroblastic anemia, hemosiderosis, some cases of neoplasia, infections and hepatic diseases. Lipo-macrophages and foam cells, sea blue histiocytes and pseudo-Gaucher cells, as well as Gaucher cells, as seen in the storage diseases, are also thought to develop out of reticular or adventitial cells (or even endothelial cells). Tissue histiocytes (cells which take up vital dyes and are capable of phagocytosis) are derived partly by recruitment of monocytes and partly by mitotic division of local histiocytes. Tissue histiocytes have oval or kidney-shaped vesicular nuclei, with variable amounts of cytoplasm and inclusions. Histiocytes in different situations may have different properties.

Some subgroups of histiocytes are recognized. Littoral cells are the sinus histiocytes which line the venous sinuses of the bone marrow (and other organs); they are spindle shaped with cytoplasmic processes. Epithelioid histiocytes have nuclei similar to those of histiocytes, and abundant eosinophilic and granular cytoplasm. Giant cells are thought to be derived from the histiocyte–monocyte series by endomitosis and/or by fusion or coalescence.

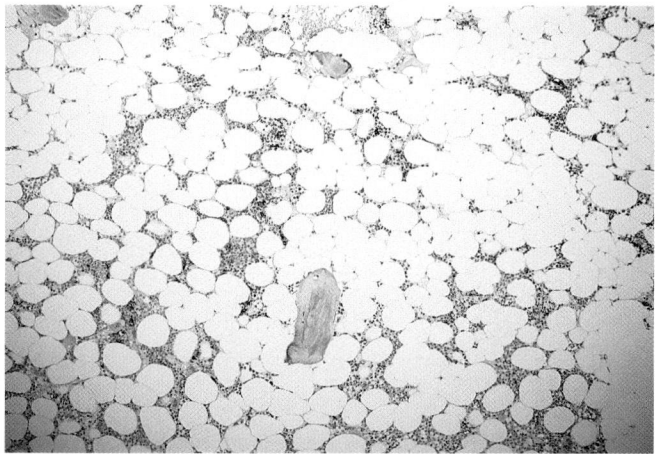

Fig. 3.16 BMBS. CD68 for monocytes/macrophages, which are dispersed throughout the marrow. Paraffin-embedded Giemsa.

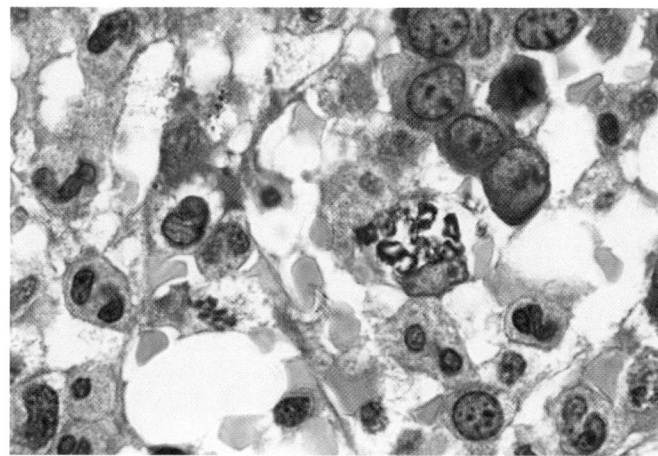

Fig. 3.17 BMBS. Note macrophage, center left, with cellular debris. Plastic-embedded, Giemsa.

Lymphocytes

Lymphoid cells are part of the normal marrow population and may constitute up to 15–20% of the nucleated cells.[37–41] In new-born babies up to 50% of the nucleated cells may be lymphocytes. Regulation of the migration, localization and function of lymphocytes is also partly controlled by cellular adhesion molecules (CAM), broadly divided into three groups – immunoglobulins, integrins and selectins. Integrin-associated proteins in particular have been shown to participate in regulation of motile activity in B-cell lines.[42] On immunohistology, most lymphocytes are T-cells, very few B-lymphocytes are present, reflecting the proportions in the peripheral blood: T-cells 65–75%, B-cells 10–15%, natural killer (NK) cells 10–20%. It should also be noted that bone marrows of children without any hematologic disorder have higher numbers of B-cell precursors and B-cells, which may resemble leukemic blasts. This must be taken into account when checking for minimal residual disease. Lymphocytes are dispersed among the hematopoietic and fat cells, or aggregated to form lymphoid nodules whose incidence increases with age and such nodules are found in 1% to over 40% of BMB with the higher incidence in the older age groups (Figs 3.2B and 3.3A). The nodules or aggregates especially when small, are more readily observed in sections stained for reticulin fibers, as they contain more fibers than their surroundings. Capillaries, reticular cells, a few plasma cells and mast cells are usually also associated with these lymphoid nodules. On immunohistology, the aggregates or nodules consist of a heterogeneous population of T- and B-cells, mainly T-cells. They are stained by LCA, and markers for B-cells such as CD20, and for T-cells such as CD3, 4, 8 (Figs 3.18, 3.19 and 3.20). Four types of lymphoid accumulations have been described: (1) nodules with germinal centers; (2) sharply demarcated nodules; (3) nodules with irregular borders; and (4) small aggregates of lymphoid cells (Figs 3.2B, 3.3A, 3.18–3.21). When multiple nodules are found in a section, immunohistology may be required to rule out or to confirm involvement by a neoplastic lymphoproliferative disorder. Immunohistology is required for identification of B- and T-cells in the bone marrow. The number of T-cells may increase considerably in reactive conditions. Normally, lymphoid cell aggregates are found mainly in the intertrabecular and perivascular regions. Aggregates may be found anywhere in the sections, intertrabecular and perivascular aggregates are common in reactive conditions and older age groups, while paratrabecular aggregates are more characteristic of a neoplastic infiltration. Recognition of the type and classification of lymphoid aggregates is likely to be greatly influenced in

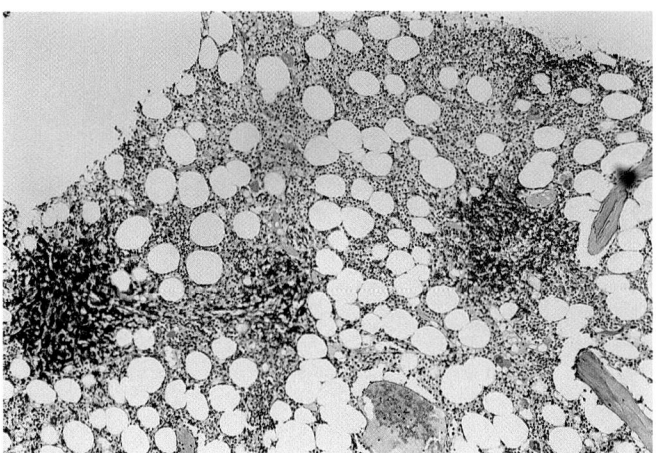

Fig. 3.18 BMBS. Note lymphocytic aggregates and interstitial lymphocytes. Paraffin-embedded, LCA (Leukocyte common antigen).

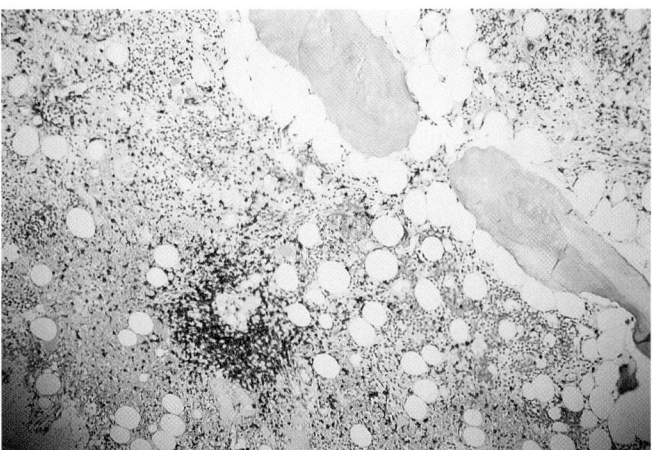

Fig. 3.19 BMBS. Note positive small aggregate and interstitial lymphocytes. Paraffin-embedded, Pan T-cell antigen.

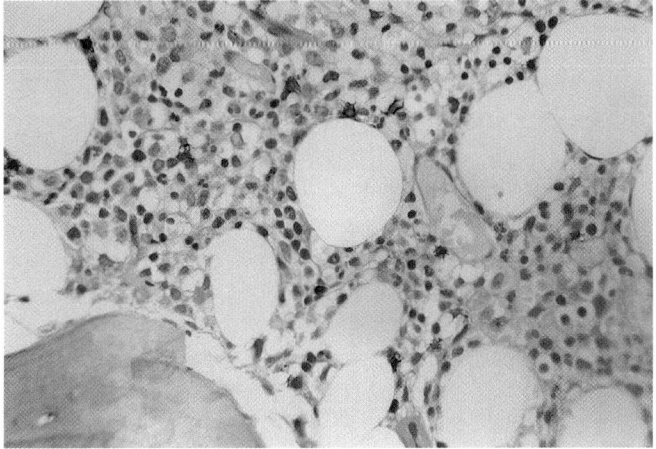

Fig. 3.20 BMBS. Note few positive cells in normal bone marrow. Paraffin-embedded, B-cell antigen (CD20).

the not too distant future by characterization of gene expression. Molecular classification based on gene expression will supplement existing criteria for identifi-

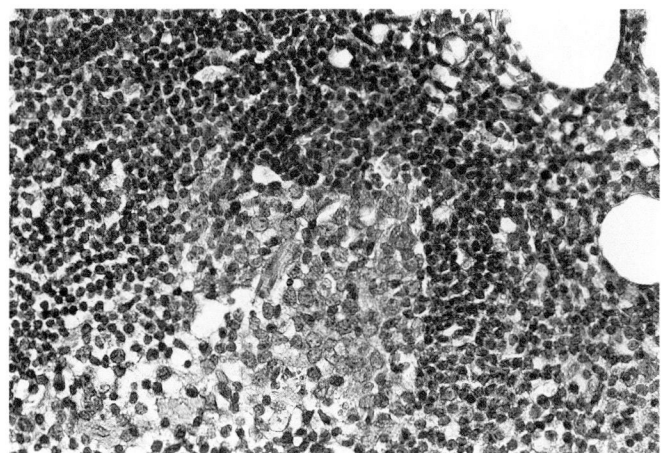

Fig. 3.21 BMBS. High magnification of nodule with germinal center. Paraffin-embedded, H&E.

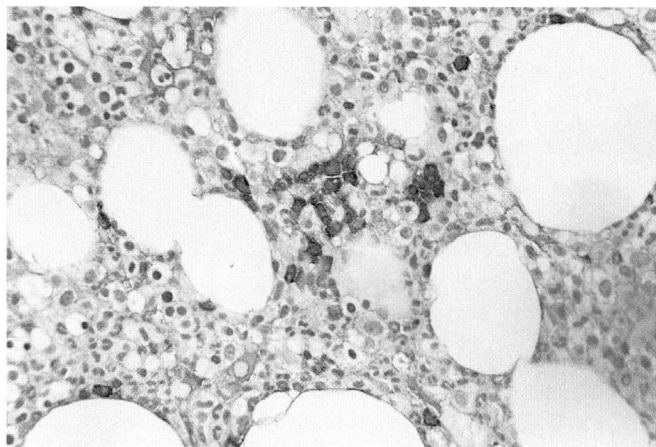

Fig. 3.22 BMBS. Note small cluster and interstitial plasma cells. Paraffin-embedded, Kappa.

ation and subtyping of lymphoproliferative disorders and other hematologic neoplasias.[43,44]

Plasma cells

These represent the final developmental stage, that is the effector cells of the B-cell lineage. They constitute about 1–4% of the nucleated cells of the adult marrow. Plasma cells are equally distributed throughout the red marrow with no significant differences between various skeletal sites (i.e. iliac crests, sternum and vertebrae), while they are almost absent from the yellow marrow. Altogether, there are more than 100 million plasma cells in the red marrow, producing more than 90% of the serum immunoglobulins. They react with CD138.[45]

When B-lymphocytes differentiate to plasma cells, large amounts of rough endoplasmic reticulum (RER) are synthesized, assembled and occupy the cytoplasm, often dilated by accumulation of immunoglobulins. Plasma cells and their immediate precursors have a very low proliferative activity, as indicated by the labeling index with tritiated thymidine.

There are normally two types of bone marrow plasma cells:

The reticular plasma cells ('Marschalko')

This is the predominant plasma cell (80%) in normal marrow and reactive plasmacytosis. It is oval, has an eccentric nucleus, perinuclear 'hof' and basophilic cytoplasm. In sections, plasma cell nuclei have a 'spoke-wheel' pattern; nucleoli are rare. Plasma cells exhibit acid phosphatase, β glucuronidase and non-specific esterase activity. Plasma cells are normally found in close

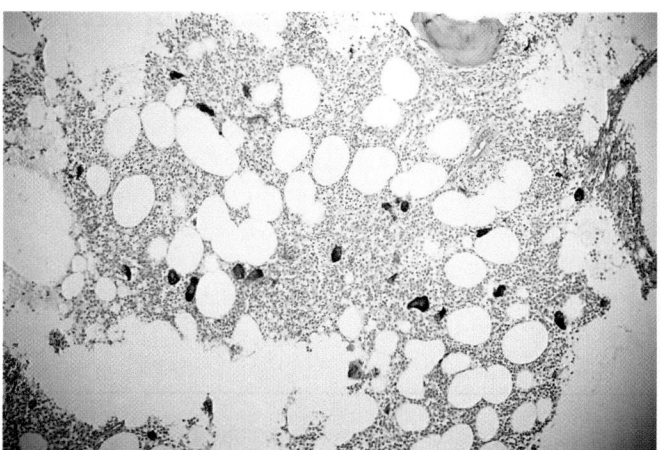

Fig. 3.23 BMBS. Note fewer positive cells than with kappa. Paraffin-embedded, Lambda.

apposition to capillaries and small blood vessels as well as singly and in clusters of two or three within the bone marrow. Demonstration of light chain restriction (i.e. reactivity with either Kappa or Lambda antibodies) is a useful indicator of possible monoclonality when most of the plasma cells present stain with either kappa or lambda. Normally, some stain with each – usually more kappa than lambda (Figs 3.22 and 3.23).[46]

The 'lymphoplasmacytoid' plasma cells

These derive directly from IgM-bearing B1 lymphocytes and produce low-affinity IgM. They are smaller, have a less eccentric nucleus, a narrower rim of cytoplasm and a poorly defined Golgi zone; they often appear in viral infections and may be found in peripheral blood as well as dispersed in the bone marrow.

Evaluation of normal bone marrow sections

It is clear from the process of hematopoiesis described above that a highly characteristic feature of normal bone marrow morphology is its heterogenous cell population and its typical architectural pattern. These two aspects should be carefully assessed to begin with, because any deviation will immediately indicate a possible perturbation of normal function and which additional investigations should be initiated. Therefore, a systematic evaluation, as shown in Table 3.4, should always be carried out.[47]

Artifacts and pitfalls

Displaced pieces of epidermis, skeletal muscle, periosteal tissue, cartilage and blood clots may be found in the sections. Variability in cellularity such as hypo- and hyperplastic areas may be misleading if the biopsy is small and therefore insufficiently representative.

It should also be remembered that evaluation of immunohistology should always be carried out with appropriate controls, and the possibility of cross-reactivity should also be considered in unusual cases or results.[47]

Methods

Plastic embedding

Fixation for plastic

Put the specimen into the fixative (Schaffer's solution) and leave for 4–16 h depending on biopsy width and amount of bone and time of receipt of the biopsy. Biopsies received in the afternoon may have to be left in fixative longer (overnight).

Composition of the fixative

Methanol absolute G.R. (Merck)–96 ml
Glucose phosphate buffer–4 ml
Formol neutralized G.R.–50 ml

Formol is neutralized by the addition of CaCo–c.50 g/l. The fixative can be kept in the refrigerator at 4°C.

Glucose phosphate buffer pH 7.4

Na_2HPO_4, $2H_2O$–48.0 g
KH_2PO_4–8.7 g

Table 3.4 Diagnostic evaluation of bone marrow biopsy sections: normal bone marrow

Overview of the biopsy section
Cortical bone and trabeculae
Fatty tissue
Cellularity

Examination of trabecular bone
Trabecular structure
Osteoid
Osteoblasts and osteocytes
Osteoclasts

Examination of hemopoiesis
Erythropoiesis
Megakaryopoiesis
Granulopoiesis
Topography of the cell lines

Examination of bone marrow stroma
Vasculature
Macrophage
Plasma cells
Lymphocytes and lymphoid nodules
Mast cells
Fibers
Iron content

Glucose. $1H_2O$ (mol.wt. 198-17)–154.0 g
Aqua dest. Ad–5000 ml

Sterilize by filtration through a bacterial funnel. The buffer can be kept for 3–4 weeks in the refrigerator at 4°C. The bottled, sterile and unopened buffer can be kept for longer (±5 months).

Reagents

Formaldehyde solution GR35% – Merck no. 4003
Methanol GR – Merck no. 6009
Na_2HPO_4, $2H_2O$ (di-sodium hydrogen phosphate 2-hydrate GR) – Merck no. 6580
KH_2PO_4 (potassium dihydrogen phosphate GR) – Merck no. 4873
D(+)Glucose (–monohydrate) – Merck no. 8342

Dehydration

Transfer specimen (biopsy) from fixative directly to absolute methanol (100%), change the methanol after 0.5, 1 and 2 h; dehydrate in the absolute methanol 4–6 h altogether, depending on the size of the biopsy. The vial should be tightly closed during dehydration. Dehydration times may also vary, and longer times (up to 12 h) do not cause any apparent damage or alteration in the appearance of the stains subsequently applied.

Embedding and staining

The biopsy is transferred directly from 100% methanol to the fluid methyl methacrylate in a glass vial with just enough methacrylate to cover the specimen, left for 0.5 h, the methacrylate is poured off and the vial filled with fresh methacrylate. The vial is tightly closed and placed in a water bath (or in a dish with water) in an incubator overnight at ±45°C. In the morning the vial is placed in the freezer for about 0.5 h, then the glass vial is smashed and the hardened block trimmed. Sections are cut at 2 or 3 μm, floated on hot (>70°C) water to stretch them, picked up on gelatin-coated glass slides, blotted dry with some pressure, and left for ±30 min in the incubator at ±45°C. The sections are now ready for staining, and any of the stains routinely used in histopathology can be applied after the removal of the methacrylate; for example Giemsa, hematoxylin and eosin, toluidine blue for calcified bone and osteoid; fiber stains for reticulin and collagen; periodic acid-Schiff (PAS) for glycoproteins; Perls' stain for iron, or the Prussian blue stain (potassium ferrocyanide).

Methyl methacrylate embedding mixture

Methacrylate 500 ml
Benzoyl peroxide 17.5 g
Plastoid N 125 ml

This mixture can be kept in a tightly stoppered bottle in the refrigerator for up to a month.

The exact times required for optimal staining are usually determined by each laboratory individually, but it should be borne in mind that, generally speaking, thin sections require longer staining times; the procedures are the same as those given for paraffin sections in any text on histopathologic techniques, Giemsa and toluidine blue are given below as examples.

Procedure for coating glass slides

Clean glass slides are dipped into the gelatin solution, drained and dried for a few minutes at room temperature or in an incubator at 37–46°C, and used to pick up the sections from the water bath.

Gelatin solution

Dissolve 6.75 g gelatin in 1500 ml distilled water at 60°C; cool to 50°C and add 58 ml 4% potassium chromium (III) sulfate solution; add several crystals of thymol and four drops of Plastoid N. The gelatin solution is stable at room temperature for about 10–14 days, and longer when kept in the refrigerator; gelatinized slides can be kept for 2 days or longer if put into boxes and kept in the refrigerator.

Removal of the methacrylate from the sections

Sections mounted on the glass slides are used. The slides are placed into benzene (Benzol).

Benzene I – 20 min
Benzene II – 20 min
Then into absolute methanol – 2 min
96% methanol – 2 min
80% methanol – 2 min
Methanol ammonia solution – 10 min
Aqua dest. – 10 min

The sections are now ready for staining.

Methanol ammonia solution

70% methanol – 100 ml
Ammonia 25% – 10 ml
Benzol (benzene) GR – Merck no. 1783
Methanol GR – Merck no. 6009
Ammonia solution GR (mon 25%) – Merck no. 5432

Giemsa stain – for cytologic details

Remove the methacrylate and put the slides into distilled water for 10 min. Drain and put into Giemsa solution pH 6.7 at 50°C for 45 min; then into Giemsa solution pH 6.6 at 40°C for 25 min. Dip in distilled water and dry the slides immediately by gentle blotting with filter paper, dip into xylol, cover with a mounting medium (Entallan) and cover glass; as mentioned above, these staining times are approximate.

Phosphate buffer pH 6.7, 0.066 mol/l

0.066 mol/l disodium hydrogen phosphate (Na_2HPO_4):43.4 ml
0.066 mol/l potassium dihydrogen phosphate (KH_2PO_4):56.6 ml

Phosphate buffer pH 6.6, 0.066 mol/l

0.066 mol/l disodium hydrogen phosphate (Na_2HPO_4):36 ml
0.066 mol/l potassium dihydrogen phosphate (KH_2PO_4):64 ml

Giemsa pH 6.7 (prepare fresh before use)

Distilled water: 49 ml
Phosphate buffer pH 6.6: 1 ml
Giemsa solution: 2 ml

Giemsa solution pH 6.6

Distilled water: 49 ml
Phosphate buffer pH 6.7: 1 ml
Giemsa solution: 2 ml

The times for staining are calculated for 3 µm section thickness; thinner sections need more time.

Toluidine blue stain

This is used for rapid diagnostic evaluation, as well as for calcified bone and osteoid. Dissolve the methylmethacrylate as described above. Then stain in toluidine blue 0.1% in distilled water, at *c*.50°C for 5–20 min, dip in water, blot gently, dry in air for 1–5 min, dip in xylol, cover with mounting medium and cover glass.

Paraffin embedding and immunohistology

Fixation

The biopsies are fixed in 10% neutral buffered formalin for 4–6 h or overnight, depending on the size (width) of the biopsy. The biopsies are then placed in the decalcification liquid (De Cal Rapid N° HS 105 National Diagnostics, Atlanta, GA, USA) for 0.5–1.0 h, depending on the width of the biopsy and the estimated amount of bone present.

The biopsies are rinsed in distilled water for 30 min and transferred to 70% methanol. The specimens can then be processed automatically in a tissue processor as any other piece of tissue for histopathologic examination. Sections for immunohistology are picked up on polylysine-coated slides, dried overnight in the incubator at 37°C and used the next day after removal of the paraffin. Antigen retrieval and antigen–antibody reactions are carried out according to the manufacturer's instructions or data-sheets. Bone-biopsy sections must be checked against tissues known to react with the antibody being used, to avoid errors in interpretation. In many cases, kits are available which contain detailed instructions, and it is advisable to follow these carefully.

Rapid processing

For plastic embedding

For plastic embedding the following times are used: a 4–6 h fixation, 4–6 h dehydration (two 0.5–1 h changes) infiltration (two changes) polymerization 12–14 h (overnight), cut, mount and dry 0.5–1 h, stain by Giemsa or H&E (hematoxylin and eosin) and cover 0.5–1 h, total time 24–26 h.

The plastic blocks are cut in a standard histopathology microtome such as the Leica (Jung Reichert) 2055, with manual and/or automatic sectioning which is carried out with a heavy-duty tungsten tipped knife. The sections are floated on hot water (>70°C), which straightens them; they are then picked up on glass slides from the hot water, covered with filter paper and pressure briefly applied by means of a roller to flatten and attach them to the slides.

For paraffin embedding

For paraffin embedding only about 16–24 h are required when short decalcification times are used (0.5–1.5 h) depending on the width of the biopsy and the amount of bone present: fixation 3–4 h, decalcification 0.5–1.5 h, rinse in distilled water 30 min, transfer to 70% methanol and process in an automatic tissue processor such as a Tissue-Tek (VIP300, Miles, UK), followed by cutting, mounting and staining by routine histopathologic methods.

This method is also used for immunohistology, but longer periods are required for drying the sections on the polylysine-coated slides, to prevent their detachment later during processing.

The methods for plastic embedding and immunohistology is given in Table 3.5. Additional methods and details are given in the following references:

Blythe D, Hand NM, Jackson P et al 1997 Use of methyl methacrylate resin for embedding bone marrow trephine biopsy sections. Journal of Clinical Pathology 50: 45–49
Frisch B, Bartl R 1999 Histology and immunohistology in paraffin and plastic. Biopsy interpretation of bone and bone marrow. Arnold, London and Oxford University Press, NY
Kreft A, Büsche G, Bernhards J, Georgh A 1997 Immunophenotype of hairy-cell leukaemia after cold polymerization of methyl-methacrylate embeddings from 50 diagnostic bone marrow biopsies. Histopathology 30: 145–151

Table 3.5 Method for plastic embedding and immunohistology

Time	Procedure
8–18 h (over night) (for biopsies of 1–2 mm diameter shorter times can be used)	**Fixation** 45 ml tetrahydrofuran 45 ml ethanol 96% 10 ml ethylenglycol
3 h overall, 3 changes	**Dehydration** Tetrahydrofuran 100%
3 h overall, 2 changes, under vacuum	**Infiltration** 84% methylmethacrylate 14% dibutylphthalate } A 1% polyethylenglycol 600 0.7% benzoylperoxide, dried
16–18 h (overnight)	**Polymerization** 15 ml A and 50 μl dimethyltoluidine in a waterbath in the refrigerator at 4°C, each biopsy in a small glass vial

Reagents: Merck & Sigma

REFERENCES

1. Duda SH, Laniado M, Schick F et al 1995 Normal bone marrow in the sacrum of young adults: differences between the sexes seen on chemical-shift MR imaging. American Journal of Roentgenology 164(4): 935–940
2. Budke H, Orazi A, Neiman RS et al 1994 Assessment of cell proliferation in paraffin sections of normal bone marrow by the monoclonal antibodies Ki-67 and PCNA. Modern Pathology 7(8): 860–866
3. Pellegrini W, Facchetti F, Marocolo D et al 1995 Assessment of cell proliferation in normal and pathological bone marrow biopsies: a study using double sequential immunophenotyping on paraffin sections. Histopathology 27(5): 397–405.
4. Ahr A, Scharl A, Muller M et al 1999 Cross-reactive staining of normal bone marrow cells by monoclonal antibody 2E11. International Journal of Cancer 84(5): 502–505
5. Babyn PS, Ransom M, McCarville ME et al 1998 Normal bone marrow: signal characteristics and fatty conversion. Magnetic Resonance Imaging Clinics of North America 6(3): 473–495
6. Vande-Berg BC, Malghem J, Lecouvet FE Maldague B 1998 Magnetic resonance imaging of normal bone marrow. European Radiology 8(8): 1327–1334
7. Shin SS, Sheibani K, Kezirian J et al 1992 Immunoarchitecture of normal human bone marrow: a study of frozen and fixed tissue sections. Human Pathology 23(6): 686–694
8. Rozman C, Feliu E, Berga L et al 1989 Age-related variations of fat tissue fraction in normal human bone marrow depend both on size and number of adipocytes: a stereological study. Experimental Hematology 17(1): 34–37
9. Baur A, Stabler A, Bartl R et al 1997 MRI gadolinium enhancement of bone marrow: age-related changes in normals and in diffuse neoplastic infiltration. Skeletal Radiology 26(7): 414–418
10. Taccone A, Oddone M, Dell'Acqua AD et al 1995 MRI 'road-map' of normal age-related bone marrow. II. Thorax, pelvis and extremities. Pediatric Radiology 25(8): 596–606
11. Schmitt-Graff A, Skalli O, Gabbiani G 1989 Alpha-smooth muscle actin is expressed in a subset of bone marrow stromal cells in normal and pathological conditions. Virchows Archive B-Cell Pathology including Molecular Pathology 57(5): 291–302
12. Schmitz B, Thiele J, Kaufmann R et al 1995 Megakaryocytes and fibroblasts – interactions as determined in normal human bone marrow specimens. Leukemia Research 19(9): 629–637
13. Siebertz B, Stocker G, Drzeniek Z et al 1999 Expression of glypican-4 in haematopoietic-progenitor and bone marrow-stromal cells. Biochemical Journal 344(3): 937–943
14. Soini Y, Kamel D, Apaja-Sarkkinen M et al 1993 Tenascin

immunoreactivity in normal and pathological bone marrow. Journal of Clinical Pathology 46(3): 218–221
15. Tao M, Li B, Nayini J et al 2000 SCF, IL-lbeta, IL-lra and GM-CSF in the bone marrow and serum of normal individuals and of AML and CML patients. Cytokine 12(6): 699–707
16. Beckman EN, Brown AW, Jr Normal reticulin level in iliac bone marrow. Archives of Pathology and Laboratory Medicine 114(12): 1241–1243
17. Apaja-Sarkkinen M, Autio-Harmainen H, Alavaikko M et al 1986 Immunohistochemical study of basement membrane proteins and type III procollagen in myelofibrosis. British Journal of Haematology 63(3): 571–580
18. Reuss-Borst MA, Buhring HJ, Klein G, Muller CA et al 1992 Adhesion molecules on CD34+ hematopoietic cells in normal human bone marrow and leukemia. Annals of Hematology 65(4): 169–174
19. Kastan MB, Radin AI, Kuerbitz SJ et al 1991 Levels of p53 protein increase with maturation in human hematopoietic cells. Cancer Research 51(16): 4279–4286
20. Loyson SA, Rademakers LH, Joling P et al 1997 Immunohistochemical analysis of decalcified paraffin-embedded human bone marrow biopsies with emphasis on MHC class I and CD34 expression. Histopathology 31(5): 412–419
21. Majka M, Ratajczak J, Machalinski B et al 2000 Expression, regulation and function of AC133, a putative cell surface marker of primitive human haematopoietic cells. Folia Histochemica et Cytobiologica 38(2): 53–63
22. Cohen PR, Rapini RP, Farhood AI et al 1993 Expression of the human hematopoietic progenitor cell antigen CD34 in vascular and spindle cell tumors. Journal of Cutaneous Pathology 20(1): 15–20
23. Servida F, Soligo D, Lambertenghi Deliliers G 2000 Functional differences between dendritic cells derived from CD34+ bone marrow and peripheral blood stem cells. Haematologica 85(4): 352–355
24. Toba K, Koike T, Watanabe K et al 2000 Cell kinetic study of normal human bone marrow hematopoiesis and acute leukemia using 7AAD/PY. European Journal of Haematology 64(1): 10–21
25. Thiele J, Meuter RB, Titius RB et al 1993 Proliferating cell nuclear antigen expression by erythroid precursors in normal bone marrow, in reactive lesions and in polycythaemia rubra vera. Histopathology 22(5): 429–435
26. Kurrascyh RH, Rutherford AV, Rick ME et al 1989 Characterization of a monoclonal antibody, OVBI, which binds to a unique determinant in human ovarian carcinomas and myeloid cells. Journal of Histochemistry and Cytochemistry 37(1): 57–67
27. Miranda RN, Briggs RC, Shults K et al 1999 Immunocytochemical analysis of MNDA in tissue sections and sorted normal bone marrow cells documents expression only in maturing normal and neoplastic myelomonocytic cells and a subset of normal and neoplastic B lymphocytes. Human Pathology 30(9): 1040–1049
28. Moore S, McDiarmid LA, Hughes TP 2000 Stem cell factor and chronic myeloid leukemia CD34+ cells. Leukemia and Lymphoma 38(3–4): 211–220
29. Tsuruta T, Tani K, Hoshika A Asano S et al 1999 Myeloperoxidase gene expression and regulation by myeloid cell growth factors in normal and leukemic cells. Leukemia and Lymphoma 32(3–4): 257–267
30. Taichman RS, Emerson SG 1994 Human osteoblasts support hematopoiesis through the production of granulocyte colony-stimulating factor. Journal of Experimental Medicine 179(5): 1677–1682
31. Calapso P, Vitarelli E, Crisafulli C, Tuccari G et al Tuccari G 1992 Immunocytochemical detection of megakaryocytes by endothelial markers: a comparative study. Pathologica 84(1090): 215–223
32. Beckstead JH, Stenberg PE, McEver RP et al 1986 Immunohistochemical localization of membrane and alpha-granule proteins in human megakaryocytes: application to plastic-embedded bone marrow biopsy specimens. Blood 67(2): 285–293
33. Thiele J, Wagner S, Dienemann D et al 1990 Megakaryocyte precursors (promegakaryoblasts and megakaryoblasts) in the normal human bone marrow. An immunohistochemical and morphometric study on routinely processed trephine biopsies. Analytical and Quantitative Cytology and Histology 12(4): 285–289
34. Wilkins BS, Jones DB 1992 Cell-stroma interactions in monocytopoiesis. FEMS Microbiology Immunology 5(5–6): 347–353
35. Thiele J, Braeckel C, Wagner S et al 1992 Macrophages in normal human bone marrow and in chronic myeloproliferative disorders: an immunohistochemical and morphometric study by a new monoclonal antibody (PG-ML) on trephine biopsies. Virchows Archive A-Pathological Anatomy and Histopathology 421(1): 33–39

36. Titius BR, Thiele J, Schaefer H et al 1994 Ki-SI and proliferating cell nuclear antigen expression of bone marrow macrophages. Immunohistochemical and morphometric study including reactive (inflammatory) myelitis, secondary aplastic anemia, AIDS, myelodysplastic syndromes and primary (idiopathic osteomyelofibrosis. Acta Haematologica 91(3): 144–149

37. Horny HP, Engst U, Walz RS Kailserling E. 1989 *In situ* immunophenotyping of lymphocytes in human bone marrow: an immunohistochemical study. British Journal of Haematology 71(3): 313–321

38. O'Donnell LR, Alder SL, Balis UJ et al 1995 Immunohistochemical reference ranges for B lymphocytes in bone marrow biopsy paraffin sections. American Journal of Clinical Pathology 104(5): 517–523

39. Orazi A, Cotton J, Cattoretti G et al 1994 Terminal deoxynucleotidyl transferase staining in acute leukemia and normal bone marrow in routinely processed paraffin sections. American Journal of Clinical Pathology 102(5): 640–645

40. Caldwell CW, Poje E, Helikson MA et al 1991 B-cell precursors in normal pediatric bone marrow. American Journal of Clinical Pathology 95(6): 816–823

41. Ciudad J, Orfao A, Vidrieles B et al 1998 Immunophenotypic analysis of CD19+ precursors in normal human adult bone marrow: implications for minimal residual disease detection. Haematologica 83–12, 1069–1075

42. Yoshida H, Tomiyama Y, Ishikawa J et al 2000 Integrin-associated protein/CD47 regulates motile activity in human B-cell lines through CDC42. Blood 96(1):

43. Alizadeh A, Eisen M, Dabis R et al 2000 Distinct types of diffuse large B-cell lymphoma identified by gene expression profiling. Nature 403(6769): 503–511

44. Dworzak MN, Fritsch G, Fleischer C et al 1998 Comparative phenotype mapping of normal vs. malignant pediatric B-lymphopoiesis unveils leukemia-associated aberrations. Experimental Hematology 26(4): 305–313

45. Chilosi M, Adami F, Lestani M et al 1999 CD138/syndecan-1: a useful immunohistochemical marker of normal and neoplastic plasma cells on routine trephine bone marrow biopsies. Modern Pathology 12(12): 1107–1116

46. Lenormand P, Crocker J 1987 Distribution of IgAl and IgA@ subclassed in bormal bone marrow trephines and in trephines infiltrated by IgA producing multiple myeloma. Journal of Clinical Pathology 40(2): 200–205

47. Frisch B, Bartl R 1999 Histology and immunohistology in paraffin and plastic. Biopsy interpretation of bone and bone marrow. Arnold, London and Oxford University Press, NY.

Regulation of hematopoiesis

C Verfaillie

4

Introduction

Hematopoietic stem and progenitor cells

Phenotyic characterization

Functional characterization

Factors that govern hematopoiesis

'Stromal' cells
Myofibroblasts
Endothelial cells
Osteoblasts
Mesenchymal stem cells

Cytokines

Adhesion receptors and extracellular matrix components
β1-integrins and hematopoiesis
Sialomucins and hematopoietic progenitors
Proteoglycans

Other signal molecules
Notch
Wnt/Frizzled

The hematopoietic process

Conclusions

Introduction

Hematopoiesis, or the process of myelopoiesis and lymphopoiesis, occurs in close proximity with a permissive microenvironment. In adult life, the hematopoietic microenvironment is provided in the bone marrow. Earlier in ontogeny, hematopoiesis takes place in the aorto-gonads-mesonephros (AGM) region,[1–3] yolk sac[4,5] and fetal liver.[6,7] The marrow microenvironment contains both hematopoietic and 'stromal' cells.[8,9] These stromal cells are of mesenchymal (endothelial cells, fibroblasts, myocytes, adipocytes and osteoblasts) and non-mesenchymal (macrophage) origin. Stromal cells produce and deposit a complex extracellular matrix (ECM), and produce and concentrate locally hematopoietic cytokines that induce or inhibit progenitor proliferation and differentiation.[10,11] Hematopoietic cells interact through specific cell-surface receptors with either immobilized or secreted cytokines, with adhesive ligands present on stromal cells or ECM components, and ligands presented by other hematopoietic cells. The combined effect of these cell–cytokine, cell–cell and cell–ECM interactions underlies the normal hematopoietic process.

Hematopoietic stem and progenitor cells

The minimal definition of an hematopoietic stem cell (HSC) is as a cell capable of prolonged self-renewal as well as generation of myeloid and lymphoid progeny.

Phenotypic characterization

Primitive human progenitors that can initiate long-term cultures or can repopulate immunodeficient animals are CD34+, AC133+, lineage−, CD38−, HLA-DR^{low} and Thy$_1$^{low}.[12–15] Committed progenitors also express CD34 antigens, but acquire lineage-specific markers. Expression of CD38 and HLA-DR is associated with loss of 'stemness'. Acquisition of CD33 and CD38 is seen on committed myeloid progenitors,[16] and appearance of CD10 and CD38 signals lymphoid commitment.[17] Expression of CD7 is seen for T-lymphoid and natural killer (NK) progenitors[18,19] and CD19 for B-lymphoid progenitors.[20]

Although Lin−CD34+CD38− cells are enriched in primitive progenitors, they are still heterogeneous and contain cells at different stages of differentiation. Stem cells can also be selected based on functional parameters: stem cells are quiescent, and therefore are spared from cell cycle-specific cytotoxic agents such as 5-fluorouracil.[21,22]

In addition, stem cells express functional multidrug resistance p-glycoprotein,[23] which extrudes toxins as well as certain dyes from the cell. This allows selection of stem cells based on negative staining for Rhodamine or Hoechst 33342.[24] In addition, Rhodamine staining may, at least in mice, reflect mitochondrial activation.[25] Addition of these markers to cell-surface markers further enriches for HSC.

There is also mounting evidence that some HSC may be CD34.[26,27] Both in mouse and man, cells that express low levels of CD34 antigen have the ability to repopulate the hematopoietic system following transplantation. In mouse, there is evidence that expression of CD34 antigens varies with the 'activation' state of the progenitors. Sato *et al* showed that the repopulating stem cell is found in the CD34+ fraction of marrow in prenatal life and in young mice, whereas repopulating cells do not express CD34 in older mice.[28] Following stimulation with cytokines *in vivo*, or following transplantation, repopulating cells re-express CD34 for a limited period after which they again downregulate CD34 antigen expression. Furthermore, there is evidence that Hoechst-33342-negative cells contain a large proportion of CD34− cells that may have repopulating ability.[29,30] As the function of CD34 is unknown, it is unclear what the functional repercussion of the reversible gain and loss of expression of this antigen is.

Functional characterization

HSC are cells that can undergo self-renewing cell divisions, as well as generate progeny capable of differentiating in the myeloid and lymphoid direction. HSC are thus cells capable of repopulating a myeloablated host. Although the expanded number of cell-surface markers and functional markers associated with 'stem cells' may identify more primitive progenitors within the CD34+ population, less than 5–10% of such cells are HSC. One depends therefore on functional assays to enumerate HSC, including *in vitro* culture assays or *in vivo* xenogeneic repopulating assays.

Colony-forming-unit (CFU)- granulocyte-macrophage (GM), burst-forming-unit (BFU)-E, CFU-Mix assays enumerate committed hematopoietic progenitors (HPC), but not HSC. A second progenitor measured in semi-solid methylcellulose assay is the high proliferative potential colony-forming cell or HPP-CFC.[31] The HPP-CFC gives rise to visually detectable large myeloid cell colonies in methylcellulose cultures that can be replated. Therefore, in contrast to BFU-E, CFU-GM and CFU-Mix, the HPP-CFC measures a more primitive progenitor as HPP-CFC can sustain myelopoiesis. However, this assay does not allow determination of lymphoid differentiation and self-renewal of cells with myeloid and lymphoid differentiation potential.

Long-term cultures in which cells are cocultured with hematopoietic supportive stromal feeders[32] with or without exogenous cytokines enumerate a more primitive progenitor capable of sustaining hematopoiesis for 5–8 weeks *in vitro,* also termed long-term-culture initiating cell (LTC-IC).[33] Some investigators have extended these cultures to 20 weeks.[34] Such extended LTC-IC (E-LTC-IC) assays reflect a more primitive progenitor than LTC-IC capable of generating secondary colony-forming cells for 5–8 weeks. The LTC-IC, and the E-LTC-IC, fulfill the HSC criterion of being able to initiate and sustain myelopoiesis, but not the two other criteria, self-renewal and long-term lymphopoiesis.

In vitro assays that can assess lymphoid differentiation of human primitive progenitors have only recently been developed. A number of groups have now also established culture systems that allow NK, B-lymphoid and dendritic cell differentiation from immature human CD34+Lin- cells.[35] When these assays are combined with thymic organ cultures to induce T-cell differentiation,[36,37] multilineage lymphoid differentiation of a given cell can be demonstrated *in vitro.* As is true for the LTC-IC assay, none of the lymphoid differentiation assays can evaluate myelopoiesis or self-renewal of HSC.

To address the multilineage differentiation potential, a number of groups have developed 'switch' cultures, in which the ability of single cells to give rise to both myeloid and lymphoid long-term-culture initiating cells can be tested. Whitlock and Witte were the first to describe an *in vitro* system that allows detection of cells with both myeloid and B-lymphoid differentiation potential.[38] Since then several groups have developed culture systems for human and murine progenitors that can measure at the single-cell level whether a cell has the ability to differentiate into myeloid and lymphoid progenitors.[39,40] However, these assays still do not allow measurement of self-renewal of stem cells, nor of 'engraftment' ability of stem cells.

In animals, identification of HSC is done by transplanting cells in syngeneic lethally irradiated animals[41–44] and transferring engrafted bone marrow (BM) cells to a secondary recipient. Detection of multilineage hematopoiesis in such secondary recipients demonstrates that the initial cell population contained HSC. The recent development of xenogeneic transplant models in immuno-incompetent animals (immunodeficient mice such as severe combined immunodeficient [SCID] mice,[45] non-obese diabetic [NOD]-SCID mice[14] and beige-nude-SCID [BNX] mice[46] or preimmune fetal lambs)[47] has provided us with *in vivo* models that allow not only demonstration of multilineage differentiation but also self-renewal and repopulating ability, two other characteristics of HSC. As human HSC have to repopulate a xenogeneic microenvironment which may support homing, growth and differentiation of human HSC less well than a human microenvironment it remains to be proven that these assays enumerate all human HSC. Finally, testing of the effect of certain manipulations on stem cells can also be done in large non-human primate.[48,49] Most investigators agree that results seen in the non-human primate transplant model may most closely reflect what can be expected in humans.

Factors that govern hematopoiesis

Hematopoietic cells with an immature morphology can be found lining the subendosteal region in close proximity with osteoblasts as well as surrounding small blood vessels.[50] More differentiated progenitors and precursors of the myeloid, erythroid and lymphoid lineage are located throughout the marrow. However, the distribution is not random. For instance, erythroid progenitors and precursors can be found associated with macrophages,[51] megakaryocytes are concentrated around endothelial cells[52,53] and myeloid as well as B-lymphoid progenitors are associated with myofibroblast cells.[19,54,55] This apparent association of lineage-specific progenitors and their more differentiated precursors in islands suggests that lineage-specific differentiation may depend on specialized progenitor – stromal cell interactions. This has led to the concept of 'stem cell/progenitor niches' (Fig. 4.1).[56,57] Such niches would consist of specialized stromal cells that produce ECM components and hematopoietic-supportive cytokines that are conducive for the commitment and/or differentiation of progenitor cells at a specific stage of differentiation.

'Stromal' cells

A number of investigators have cloned murine or human stromal cell lines from hematopoietic-supportive organs, including AGM region,[58,59] yolk sac,[5,60,61] fetal liver[55,62] and adult marrow.[63–65] These cell lines are from mesenchymal origin and have characteristics of fibroblasts, myoblasts, endothelial cells and osteoblasts. Independent of their lineage, some but not all stromal cell lines support multipotent stem cell populations, while they support poorly more committed progenitors.[55,62–64] Other

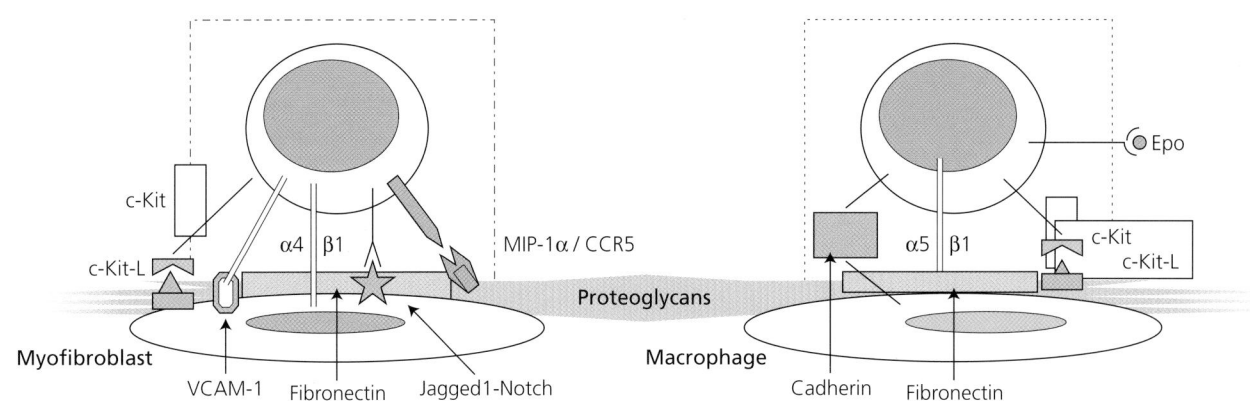

Fig. 4.1 Putative "niche" that harbors either stem cells or committed progenitors, such as erythroblasts. Such a niche would consist of a specialized 'stromal' cell, which produces locally extracellular matrix components, cytokines and other ligands important for the survival, self-renewal, or differentiation and proliferation of a progenitor cell at a certain stage of differentiation.

A putative 'stem cell niche' would be built around a myofibroblast cell or endosteal cell, which locally secretes proteoglycans and fibronectin. Myofibroblasts/endosteal cells would express adhesive receptors such as VCAM and cell-surface-expressed cytokines such as c-Kit ligand. Hematopoietic stem cells are equipped with integrins that allow them to adhere to VCAM and fibronectin. Aside from retaining cells within the stem cell niche, integrins may also regulate cell survival and proliferation. Hematopoetic progenitors express c-Kit which allows them to interact with c-Kit-ligand. Proteoglycans concentrate, protect and present cytokines to cells, including chemokines. For instance, stroma-specific proteoglycans can present MIP-1α or SDF-1α that interacts with the CCR-5 receptor and CXCR-4 receptor on stem cells. Finally, stromal cells within the stem cell niche may present ligands for the Notch receptor such as Jagged-1 or DLK, which may help stem cells decide whether to proliferate or differentiate.

Other niches that harbor more committed progenitors such as erythroblasts may also exist. An 'erythroblast niche' would be built around a macrophage. Macrophages would produce fibronectin to which erythroblasts can adhere through the α5β1 integrin. This interaction is important not only for retaining erythroblasts in the erythroblast niche but also to regulate their differentiation. Erythroblasts would also interact with c-Kit ligand either in soluble form or as a cell-surface-expressed isoform. In addition, cell–cell interactions between cadherins present on macrophages and erythroblasts direct the differentiation process of erythroblasts to mature erythroid elements.

cell lines support myelopoiesis or B-cell development but not more immature, multilineage progenitors.[55,62] The availability of these cell lines provides a powerful tool to begin characterizing factors required for self-renewal or lineage commitment of stem cells, or factors necessary for the proliferation or differentiation of lineage-committed progenitors.

Myofibroblasts

Numerous investigators have cloned murine marrow or fetal liver fibroblast-like cell lines.[62–70] Different cell lines appear to have differing abilities to support HSC, committed myeloid and/or lymphoid progenitors, or do not support hematopoiesis at all. The type of cytokines and ECM components secreted by the cell lines has been extensively studied.

However, the type and quantity of cytokines produced by the different cloned fibroblast-like feeders does not correlate with the ability of certain feeders to support primitive progenitors or committed myeloid or lymphoid progenitors. This has led several groups to initiate molecular studies aimed at identifying novel or known genes, expressed in feeders that can or cannot support hematopoietic stem cells or committed progenitors. These efforts have already shown that a murine delta-(dlk) like

protein[71] and the human Jagged-1 protein[72] are found almost exclusively in feeders that support immature progenitors. As both may serve as a ligand for Notch receptors on hematopoietic cells,[73] they may serve to prevent commitment or differentiation and contribute to the ability of these feeders to support immature progenitors. It is also of interest to note that fibroblast-like feeders derived from non-hematopoietic organs express the same types of cytokines as hematopoietic organ-derived fibroblasts[64] but do not support hematopoiesis. Gupta *et al* have shown that this may in part be related to differences in the type of glycosaminoglycans produced by feeders from hematopoietic and non-hematopoietic organs.[74,75] Such differences may change the presentation or local concentration of cytokines and affect the support of hematopoiesis. Finally, as adhesive interactions *per se* may influence the growth and differentiation of progenitors,[10] differences in adhesive ligands on the fibroblasts themselves or in the cell ECM may be important determinants of their hematopoietic-supportive capacity.

Endothelial cells

In vivo, endothelial cells line the sinusoids of the bone marrow cavity. As in other tissues, entry in and exit from the marrow will require that progenitors and mature blood cells pass through the endothelial barrier of the sinusoids. Cells with an immature phenotype as well as megakaryocytes are found surrounding small blood vessels.[50,51] Microvascular endothelium may thus not only act as a gatekeeper, controlling the trafficking and homing of hematopoietic progenitors, but also provide cellular contacts and cytokines for the support of steady-state hematopoiesis. That endothelium–stem cell interactions may play an important role in hematopoiesis is illustrated by the fact that hematopoiesis is also found in association with endothelial cells lining the AGM region[58,59] as well as the 'blood islands' in the yolk sac.[5,60,61]

Bone marrow microvascular endothelial cells (BMEC) have been generated.[53,76,77] Migration of progenitors through marrow microvascular endothelium is required for the homing and engraftment of stem cells in the marrow microenvironment.[78,79] A number of very elegant studies have started to unravel the mechanisms underlying HSC homing and engraftment through endothelium *in vitro* and *in vivo* and have shown a role for selectins, integrins and chemokines in the process.[76,80,81] Aside from the obvious role of endothelium in regulating homing and engraftment of HSC, there is also mounting evidence that endothelium is one of the cell types in the marrow microenvironment that govern HSC and progenitor growth and differentiation.[53] Endothelial cells produce ECM and express adhesive ligands that modulate progenitor growth. In addition, BMEC produce large amounts of stem cell factor (SCF), IL-6, granulocyte–macrophage colony-stimulating factor (GM-CSF), IL-1α, IL 11 and granulocyte colony stimulating factor (G-CSF). BMEC support long-term proliferation of hematopoietic progenitor cells.[53]

Osteoblasts

Primitive progenitors can be found in close proximity with the endosteal lining of the marrow cavity.[50] Emerson and colleagues have shown that human CD34+ cells adhere tightly to osteoblast feeders, even though the nature of the receptor–ligand pairs in this interaction are not yet known.[82] Like other mesenchymal cells, osteoblasts produce cytokines, such as G-CSF, GM-CSF and IL-6, known to support hematopoiesis. When human CD34+ cells are cocultured with osteoblast feeders, primitive LTC-IC can be maintained/expanded to the same or greater extent than when cocultured with mixed marrow stromal feeders. Thus, these studies suggest an important role for the osteoblast component of the marrow microenvironment in hematopoiesis.

Mesenchymal stem cells

A cell that has recently gained a lot of attention, the mesenchymal stem cell (MSC) may be the precursor for the cells listed above. MSC were first identified by Fridenshtein[83] who demonstrated that when BM is plated in fetal-calf-serum containing medium, colonies consisting of adherent fibroblast-like cells develop that differentiate into bone and adipocytes. Since then several investigators have shown that these cells can also differentiate into chondrocytes, adipocytes, and at least in rodents, skeletal myocytes.[84–86] MSC can be purified based on their ability to adhere to plastic or with monoclonal antibodies (SH2 and SH4, or Stro 1).[84,86] There is now also evidence that this cell population may be capable of differentiating into smooth muscle cells and endothelium. Furthermore, treatment with IL-1α transforms MSC into cells that support hematopoiesis. As MSC may be able to home to and engraft[87,88] and can be culture expanded extensively (10^4–10^8-fold in 4–8 weeks)[86,89] studies are ongoing to test whether coinfusion of MSC and HSC may improve hematopoiesis after transplantation.

Cytokines

Over the last two decades, a large number of growth-promoting and inhibitory cytokines and their receptors have been identified. Stem and progenitor cells are thought to express most cytokine receptors. What dictates whether cells respond to some but not all cytokines is not known. It is also not completely understood why stem and progenitor cells undergo self-renewing cell divisions vs differentiation. Cytokine receptors belong to three groups, as is detailed elsewhere.[90,91] Tyrosine kinase receptors, such as c-kit, the receptor for steel factor or stem cell factor (SCF),[92] and the fetal liver tyrosine kinase receptor-3 (FLT3-R).[93] Both play an important role in the stimulation of primitive stem and progenitor cells. The second family is the cytokine receptor family, which lacks endogenous tyrosine kinase activity but recruits and activates non-receptor tyrosine kinases such as Jak/Stat and Ras/MAPK.[90,91] Ligands for these receptors include interleukin (IL)-3[90] and thrombopoietin (TEPO),[94] both of which are active on primitive progenitors. Of note, IL-3 may be detrimental to the pluripotentiality of murine progenitors, and when added in too high a concentration to human progenitors induces terminal differentiation and loss of primitive HPC.[95,96] The third family consists of the gp130 family, which includes receptors for IL-6,[97] IL-11,[98] oncostatin-M[99] and leukemia inhibitory factor (LIF).[100] As for the cytokine-receptor family, these receptors do not have intrinsic tyrosine kinase activity.

All these cytokines interact with a receptor complex, which contains the gp130 signal molecule.[101] Lack of expression of the IL-6 receptor can be circumvented by the addition of a soluble form of the IL-6 receptor to the cultures.[102] No such soluble receptor has been identified for the other cytokines signaling through gp130.

Aside from growth-promoting cytokines a number of growth-inhibitor cytokines, such as transforming growth factor (TGF)-β,[103,104] tumor necrosis factor (TNF)-α[105] and the interferons[106] have been characterized. What the normal physiologic role is *in vivo* of the growth-inhibitory cytokines is not fully understood.

Chemokines also affect hematopoiesis. Chemokines are 70–100 amino acid long polypeptides, containing four cysteine residues.[107] The family has diverged into two groups: the C-X-C or α chemokines in which the first two of the four cysteine residues are separated by an additional amino acid and the C-C or β chemokines in which the first two cysteine residues are adjacent to each other. Originally, they were considered as inducible mediators of inflammation, but in recent years, several chemokines have been identified that are expressed constitutively and function in the physiologic traffic and homing of stem and progenitor cells[108] as well as in the regulation of progenitor and stem cell proliferation and survival. Like TGF-β, addition of macrophage inflammatory protein (MIP)-1α to cultures prevents cells from cycling[69,70,87,88] and MIP-1α has therefore been tested in clinical trials as a chemoprotectant for HSC. The chemokine, stroma-derived factor-1 (SDF-1), and its receptor, CXCR-4,[109] have been implicated in the homing and mobilization of human CD34+ cells (Fig. 4.1). The chemokine SDF-1α, which binds to the CXCR-4 receptor, is the major chemoattractant for stem and progenitor cells in the BM.[110,111] This can be measured *in vitro*, where migration of normal progenitor cells through endothelium or fibronectin-coated transwells is significantly enhanced when SDF-1α is present in the compartment opposite to the cell compartment.[78,80,112] Furthermore, SDF-1α is responsible for homing of stem and progenitor cells to the BM microenvironment when human CD34+ cells are transplanted into NOD-SCID mice,[79] by affecting the function of a number of adhesion receptors, including β1- and β2-integrins.[79,112,113] (Other studies have shown that SDF-1a also affects progenitor and stem cell survival.)

As the concentration of cytokines found in stromal cultures is well below what is commonly added to *ex vivo* stroma-free cultures[64,114,115] it is thought that the combination of several different growth factors in small concentrations may induce progenitor proliferation and differentiation. Because growth factors can be bound and concentrated by ECM components, such as glycosaminoglycans,[74,116,117] it is likely that the local concentration of cytokines is actually significantly higher that the concentration found in culture supernatants. There is also evidence that interaction with these ECM components may present cytokines in a biologically more active form to progenitors.[118,119] Stromal cells also produce membrane-bound cytokines that may be significantly more active than in their soluble form.[120] Finally, adhesive interactions between HPC and stromal cells or ECM components may serve a permissive role in that they modulate responsiveness of HPC to the small concentrations of cytokines available.[121–125]

Adhesion receptors and extracellular matrix components

HSC and progenitors adhere to several ECM components, including fibronectin, heparan-sulfate and thrombospondin, among others. These adhesive events may affect growth and differentiation of HPC either directly or indirectly by changing the response of progenitors to cytokines. Several excellent reviews have been published that address the role of ECM components in hematopoiesis.[10,126–130] We review the interactions between CD34+ cells and fibronectin/vascular cell adhesion model (VCAM)-1 via β1-integrins, proteoglycans and the role of sialomucins in hematopoiesis as they represent examples of the complexity of interactions in the bone marrow microenvironment.

β1-integrins and hematopoiesis

Stem cells, progenitors and precursors bind to fibronectin[131,132] and VCAM[133] through β1-integrins. As is true for other cell types, adhesion via integrins is important to localize progenitors in the marrow microenvironment, and a number of studies have shown an important role for integrin–fibronectin or VCAM interactions for 'homing' and engraftment of progenitors.

β1-integrin-mediated interactions between progenitors and fibronectin or other stromal components may also directly influence their survival, proliferation and differentiation. For instance, coculture of CD34+ cells with fibronectin or engagement of β1-integrins on CD34+ cells with blocking monoclonal antibodies under physiologic cytokine conditions (picogram concentrations of cytokines as found in LTC) inhibits colony-forming cell (CFC) proliferation,[124,125,134,135] whereas proliferation of primitive progenitors in response to cytokines is increased in the presence of fibronectin.[123,136–138] In addition, engagement of integrins on progenitors cultured without cytokines provides an anti-apoptotic signal.[121,122] The functional state of β1-integrins on progenitors is influenced by other environmental signals. For instance, serum and cytokine starvation decreases the ability of CD34[+] cells to adhere to fibronectin.[136–139] Addition of supraphysiologic concentrations of cytokines (nanogram concentrations of for instance IL3 or SCF) to serum-starved cells significantly upregulates adhesion of CD34[+] cells to levels above that seen under steady-state conditions. As integrins, like all adhesion receptors, do not have intrinsic kinase activity, activation of signal pathways requires recruitment of non-receptor kinases.[140–142] Integrins activate the focal adhesion kinase[141] or the related kinase, Pyk-2[143,144] which serve to bind and activate a number of Src-homology domain (SH)2- and SH3-containing adaptor proteins,[145–148] and activate the Pl3-kinase pathway and the Ras/mitogen activated protein kinase (MAPK) pathway,[149,150] both of which mediate growth and survival regulatory signals (Fig. 4.1). Which signal pathways are involved in inhibiting or enhancing growth of progenitors in response to combined integrin and cytokine signaling is currently being studied by a number of investigators. Likewise, the signal pathways involved in the anti-apoptotic effects of integrins on hematopoietic progenitors is just starting to be determined.

Once progenitors differentiate, the expression pattern and functional status of α5β1 and α4β1 integrins change. For instance, CFU-E adhere significantly better to fibronectin than more differentiated pre-proerythroblasts.[151–153] Differentiation into erythroblasts and normoblasts is accompanied with a complete loss of adhesion to fibronectin and a concomitant loss of expression of the α5β1 integrin receptor at the reticulocyte stage. Differentiation of CFU-E to erythroblasts and erythrocytes requires interaction with fibronectin. Similar observations have been made for B-lymphocyte maturation. Upon differentiation, B-cell precursors and mature B-cells lose their capacity to adhere to fibroblasts, which is due to a decreased α5β1 and α4β1 integrin expression.[154–156] Generation of B-cells in stroma-dependent cultures requires close interaction between the immature progenitors and the stromal layer, as survival and proliferation of B-cell precursors depends on α4β1/VCAM and possibly fibronectin interactions.

Sialomucins and hematopoietic progenitors

A second group of receptors on CD34[+] cells that are important regulators of progenitor proliferation, apoptosis and differentiation, is the sialomucin family of receptors. The role of this family of receptors in hematopoiesis has only recently been established. The ligands for the receptors are not all known. Sialomucins play a role in the localization and homing of progenitors and stem cells in the microenvironment, and have important effects on proliferation and survival of progenitor and stem cells.

CD34

The CD34 antigen was the first sialomucin to be described on progenitors, and is also expressed on the majority of stem cells.[26,157] Some studies have provided evidence that CD34 may play a role in progenitor adhesion. However, the exact role of CD34 in stem and progenitor cell interaction with the BM is still unclear.[158] The subpopulation of murine and human stem cells that does not express CD34 antigens on the cell surface is capable of engrafting,[159,160] suggesting that CD34 may not be required for homing and engraftment of stem and progenitor cells to the BM. Whether engagement of CD34 affects progenitor and stem cell growth and/or survival is not known. There is, however, evidence that CD34 may play a role in differentiation. Enforced expression of CD34[161] prevents terminal differentiation of cell-lines. Consistent with this finding, CD34[+] mice showed a significantly decreased number of progenitors in the yolk sac or fetal livers, possibly related to premature terminal differentiation.[162]

CD43

CD43 is a transmembrane sialomucin expressed on the majority of progenitor cells, including myeloid and lymphoid committed and primitive progenitors.[163,164] Its role in adhesion of progenitor cells to stroma is unknown. However, engagement of CD43 directly affects progenitor survival.[163,165] Whether similar effects occur at the stem cell level is not yet known.

CD164

CD164 is expressed both on CD34[+] progenitor cells and on BM stromal cells.[166] Three different epitopes of CD164 have been described, with class-I and -II being expressed on hematopoietic cells at different stages of differentiation.[167] For instance, lymphocytes express class-I epitopes whereas endothelium in high-endothelium venules are class-II positive, suggesting reciprocal homing functions in this tissue.[168,169] The ontogeny-, differentiation- and tissue-specific expression pattern of the different isoforms of this receptor may provide a certain degree of specificity in homing of HPC, although *in vivo* studies will be needed to clarify this.[168,169] Engagement of CD164 on CD34[+] cells prevents recruitment of quiescent progenitor cells into cycle when stimulated with a cocktail of cytokines and induces apoptosis of a fraction of CD34[+]CD38[−] cells.[166] Engagement of P-selectin via antibodies or with immobilized or soluble ligand for P-selectin glycoprotein ligand (PSGL)-1 has marked growth-inhibitory effect of HPC, implicating P-selectin in regulation of HPC cell cycle.[170] Likewise, engagement of CD43 inhibits CD34[+] cell growth and induces death of committed but not primitive progenitors.[163,165] What effects CD164 have on HSC proliferation is not yet known and will require transplantation of stem cells cultured with or without mucin-receptor simulation *in vivo*.

Like integrins, mucin cytoplasmic tails lack tyrosine kinase activity, so interactions through other signaling and adaptor proteins are required.[171,172] The nature of downstream signaling from mucins in progenitors is still unclear, even though there is evidence that mucins interact with the cytoskeleton through the actin-binding proteins ezrin and moesin and that stimulation of mucin receptors induces activation of protein tyrosine kinases, the phospholipase C/phosphoinositides and G proteins signaling pathways.[164]

Proteoglycans

As in most tissues, the marrow microenvironment is rich in proteoglycans. These include heparan, dermatan and chondroitin sulfate proteoglycans and hyaluronic acid.[118,173] Proteoglycans consist of a core protein to which one or more glycosaminoglycans (GAGs) are attached. GAGs are long, negatively charged, unbranched polysaccharide chains composed of repeating sulfated disaccharide units.[174] The type of sugar residues, the type of linkage between these residues and the number and location of sulfate groups are important for the interaction of GAGs with ECM components, cells and growth factors and provide specificity.

Heparan-sulfate GAGs secreted by hematopoietic supportive stromal cell lines play an important role in the maintenance and expansion of LTC-IC.[74,75,175] Characteristics associated with the hematopoietic supportive nature of heparan-sulfate GAGs include a high degree of sulfation, localization of the sulfate groups (6-O rather than N-sulfation) and length of the GAG-chains. Marrow-specific haparan sulfate GAGs allow adhesion of CD34[+] cells.[175] The receptors on human hematopoietic progenitors responsible for their interaction with marrow-derived heparan sulfate GAGs have not yet been identified. In addition, marrow-specific heparan sulfate

GAGs can concentrate a number of hematopoietic growth factors, including IL3,[117] IL7,[176] GM-CSF,[116] basic-fibroblast growth factor (b-FGF)[119,175] and chemokines such as MIP-1α,[75] MIP-1β[177] and platelet factor (PF)4.[178] The ability of marrow-specific heparan-sulfate GAGs to selectively colocalize certain growth factors and progenitors at a specific stage of differentiation may be crucial for the regulation of proliferation and differentiation. Heparan-sulfate GAGs can therefore be seen as the orchestrators of the putative progenitor or stem cell niche.

Several studies have also suggested a role for chondroitin-sulfate GAGs in the hematopoietic process. When β-D-xyloside, an agent that uncouples chondroitin sulfate glycosaminoglycan synthesis from proteoglycan synthesis, is added to LTC, a significant increase in chondroitin/ dermatan sulfate GAGs is seen in stromal supernatants.[118] Hematopoiesis in β-D-xyloside-treated LTC is significantly increased, suggesting a role for chondroitin sulfate in hematopoiesis.

Other signal molecules

Aside from classical adhesion receptors that allow interaction with adhesive ligands on ECM or stromal cells, several other receptors, including Notch[179] and Wnt,[180,181] are present on HPC and stem cells. As during development,[182–186] it is thought that signaling through these pathways may affect proliferation and differentiation of HSC and progenitors.

Notch

Differentiation into multiple cell types from a population of initially equivalent cells is a fundamental process in the development of all multicellular organisms.[182–184] Studies initially in *Drosophila* and later in mammalian cells have shown that intercellular signaling through the Notch/LIN-12 transmembrane receptors is imperative for normal growth and differentiation during the development of all species. Binding of the Notch receptor to its ligand causes proteolysis of the Notch receptor. As a result, the receptor's intracellular domain enters the nucleus where it functions as a transcriptional coactivator. If and how growth factors control these genetic circuits, and the manner in which these signals then lead to expression of a particular cell identity, is far from clear. Given the wide variety of cell types influenced by Notch, signals relayed through Notch activation may not be instructive, but signaling via Notch may influence the ability of the cell to respond to other microenvironmental signals which then alters cell fate.

Notch-1 and Notch-2 are expressed on human CD34+ cells.[179] Forced expression of the activated intracellular domain of Notch-1 and Notch-2 in the murine cell line, 32D, prevented growth arrest and differentiation to granulocytes when the cells were cultured with G-CSF or GM-CSF respectively.[73] Overexpression of the activated form of Notch in murine HSC causes lymphoid leukemia.[187]

The human homolog of one of the Notch ligands, Jagged-1, is expressed in human-marrow-derived stromal cells that support growth of primitive human hematopoietic progenitors *in vitro*.[188] Culture experiments show that Jagged-1 affects growth of primary hematopoietic cells *in vitro*. Jagged-1 expressed in a Jagged-1-negative stromal cell line or on the surface of beads, increases the production of immature HPP-CFC and LTC-IC, and to a lesser extent of more mature CFC present in either adult human marrow or in the mouse embryo AGM region.[72,188,189] Thus, Jagged-1 may well be a novel candidate regulator of stem cell growth. Recent studies have also shown that other ligands for Notch, Delta-1, Delta-4 and delta like (dlk) affect as regulators of primitive hematopoietic progenitors.[71,190]

Wnt/Frizzled

Yet another receptor–ligand pair that has recently been recognized as important in cell fate decision making, especially in cells of mesodermal origin, is the Wnt family of secreted glycoproteins[185,186] that bind transmembrane receptors from the Frizzled family.[191] Wnt sequences, patterns of expression and activities are highly conserved in evolution. Wnt binds to cell-surface-expressed Frizzled receptors. This causes complex formation between cytoplasmic beta-catenin[192] and the lymphoid enhancing binding/T-cell transcription factor (LEF/TCF) family of transcription factors. As a result of this complex formation, beta-catenin–LEF/TCF translocates to the nucleus,[193] LEF/TCF function is activated and induces transcription of a number of genes, including homeobox genes.

Transcripts for Wnt-5a have been found in human CD34+ and for Wnt-5a and Wnt-10b in murine AA4+/Sca+/c-Kit+ cells. Wnt-1, Wnt-5a, Wnt-2b and Wnt-10b have been cloned from human fetal bone stromal cells.[180,181,194] Recent *in vitro* studies have suggested that signaling via Wnt may affect the cell fate decision-making process in hematopoiesis. Presence of either Wnt-5a, Wnt-2b or Wnt-10b in stromal feeders used to culture CD34+ cells increased the number of CFU-MIX by 8–10-fold, CFU-GM by 1.5–2.4 fold and BFU-E by 8–10-fold. The frequency of CD34+ cells in Wnt-expressing stromal cultures was higher than in cultures in which Wnt was not expressed. Likewise, culture of murine progenitors in medium conditioned by Wnt-1, Wnt-5a or Wnt-10b expressing stromal cell lines stimulated a 7-fold, 8-fold, and 11-fold expansion in cell number, respectively. Although little is known about the function of Wnt in hematopoiesis, these initial studies would suggest that Wnts may stimulate the survival/proliferation of hematopoietic progenitors and may comprise a novel class of hematopoietic cell regulators.

The hematopoietic process

Hematopoiesis is a highly regulated process in which the majority of hematopoietic stem cells remains quiescent. Per definition, hematopoietic stem cells can undergo self-renewing cell divisions. Upon division, they can also generate more mature myeloid and lymphoid lineage-committed hematopoietic progenitor cells. Compared with hematopoietic stem cells, committed progeny has more limited proliferative capacity. They undergo further multiplications before they terminally differentiate into mature blood elements, which egress in the blood or secondary hematopoietic organs.

The marrow microenvironment is a complex organ that provides factors that support hematopoietic stem and progenitor survival and proliferation. Whether external factors are also responsible for induction of cell commitment and differentiation is the subject of intense debate. One school of thought is that the decision of a hematopoietic stem cell to self-renew or commit to multipotent progenitors as well as the decision of a multipotent progenitor to differentiate along a given pathway is 'stochastic'.[195,196] In this model, commitment and differentiation is dictated by factors intrinsic to the stem or progenitor cell but not by the external environment. The microenvironment then simply provides signals for stem and progenitor cell survival and proliferation, but not signals that affect commitment or differentiation decisions. This model is based on results from studies showing that the nature of lineage-specific progenitors generated by isolated primitive progenitor is not influenced by the type of cytokine used to stimulate the cells.[197–199] The observation that forced expression of, for instance, the GM-CSF receptor not usually found on erythroid-committed progenitors leads to the expansion of erythroid progenitors and cells following stimulation with GM-CSF supports this model.[198] Overexpression of bcl-2 in hematopoietic cells prevents apoptosis of cells upon withdrawl of cytokines. The finding that differentiation of immature progenitor cells was seen in the absence of cytokines supports the contention that external factors may only serve to prevent cell death but that commitment and differentiation are governed by cell intrinsic factors.[200] More recent studies have shown that overexpression of the homeobox gene Hox-B4,[201] already highly expressed in immature hematopoietic progenitors[202] results in the expansion of murine long-term repopulating cells whereas overexpression of Hox-A5,[203] Hox-A9,[204] Hox-A10[205] and Hox-B3,[206] present in more differentiated progenitors, leads to the expansion of myeloid lineage-committed progenitors. Although this too can be seen as cell intrinsic control of decision making, the factors that regulate expression of Hox transcription factors are unknown and may well be extrinsic to the hematopoietic cell.

A second model of hematopoiesis is the 'deterministic' or the 'instructive' model, in which all decisions made by stem and progenitor cells are influenced by external conditions.[195,207] Support for this model comes from studies demonstrating that the nature of colonies generated *in vitro* can be influenced by the cytokine mixture added to the culture system. The same arguments used in the studies described above favoring a 'stochastic' model of hematopoiesis have been used to support the notion of a 'deterministic' model. For instance, mice transgenic for the human GM-CSF receptor, treated with GM-CSF demonstrate expanded myelopoiesis, but normal numbers of erythroid and megakaryocytic elements. These results, though different than seen in the study quoted above, favor a deterministic hematopoietic model.[208] Further, it was previously thought that thymic selection is stochastic.[199] However, our understanding of the notch signaling system has now provided evidence to suggest that the thymic selection process may be determined by extrinsic rather than thymocyte-intrinsic factors. Thus, there is now mounting evidence that non-cytokine interactions between hematopoietic cells and stromal cells, stromal matrix molecules and other hematopoietic cells influence the effect of cytokines on progenitors.[209] The combined effect of these non-cytokine interactions and cytokine-mediated signals is ultimately responsible for dictating the fate of hematopoietic stem and progenitor cells, essentially independent of factors intrinsic to stem cells.

As follows from studies described in the previous sections, it is believed that the marrow microenvironment is subdivided in specialized areas, also termed 'niches'[56,57,75] that will support for instance proliferation of stem cells, yet others will support terminal differentiation of committed progenitors (see Fig. 4.1). Although presence of such 'niches' has not been proven, this model helps us to conceptualize regulation of the normal hematopoietic process.

The putative stem cell niche would for instance be generated around myo-fibroblast cells or endosteal cells.[62,63,65,82] These cells can produce the vast majority of cytokines active in hematopoiesis. However, only few cytokines are needed to maintain the population of stem cells and to allow these cells to undergo self-renewing cell divisions. Cytokine access to the stem cells may be restricted by stem cell-specific glycosaminoglycans[75,116,117] also secreted by the myo-fibroblasts or endosteal cells in the stem cell niche. The task of such glycosaminoglycans would be to present and protect only those cytokines that are suitable for the stem cell population. Myo-fibroblasts or endosteal cells also produce fibronectin and express VCAM-1 to which the stem cell binds through β1-integrins.[131,132] Engagement of β1-integrins on the stem cells helps protect them from apoptotic cell death[121,122] and from excessive proliferation.[124,125] Finally, molecules that can affect cell fate decisions, such as the Notch ligands Jagged 1,[188,189,210] delta,[190] and dlk,[71] or members from the Wnt-family,[180,181] are being produced by stem cell supportive stromal cells. These then help the stem cell interpret cytokines as signals to induce a self-renewing rather than differentiating cell division.

In contrast, an erythroid differentiation niche would consist of erythroid-committed progenitors that grow and differentiate surrounding a 'nurse' macrophage.[51] To allow terminal differentiation, such a niche would contain fibronectin to which erythroid progenitors adhere[151,211] and cadherins would transfer the necessary signals from the macrophage to adjacent erythroid progenitors.[212,213]

To complicate matters further, there is also new evidence to suggest that stromal cells are influenced by the presence of mature or immature progenitors.[115,214,215] For instance, coculture of CD34+ cells with either mixed stromal feeders or osteoblast feeders causes increases in production of IL6 and G-CSF by the feeder layers. This happens through a soluble factor secreted by the hematopoietic cells. Of interest, when more mature myeloid precursors are added to stromal feeders no such effect is seen.

Further, addition of an excess number of CD15+ cells to CD34+/stromal cell cocultures prevents increased secretion of cytokines. The mechanisms underlying this cross-talk are not known. Also not known is whether the cross-talk seen for these two cytokines also exists for the production/expression of ECM components, Notch-ligands, Wnt molecules or other yet to identify factors.

Conclusions

The marrow microenvironment is a complex organ in which mesenchymal and hematopoietic 'stromal' cells express adhesive ligands, transmembrane cytokines and other intercellular ligands, and produce soluble cytokines and extracellular matrix components. Interaction of stem cells, committed progenitors and more mature precursors with the 'correct' combination of these signals results in the well-orchestrated generation of mature blood elements for the life time of an individual. A large number of signals that are necessary and sufficient for the expansion and terminal differentiation of more mature lineage-committed progenitors and precursors have been identified. However, our knowledge of signals required for the regulated production of stem cells vs committed progenitors vs differentiated progeny remains limited. It is likely that in the next few years the number of components present in the putative niches depicted above will become much more numerous. Increased understanding of factors in the microenvironment that regulate growth and differentiation of hematopoietic progenitors will decrease the apparent stochastic behavior of stem cells. Further studies will unravel the signals provided by stromal cells for the hematopoietic process and will examine the potential therapeutic use of these cells.

REFERENCES

1. Tavian M, Coulombel L, Luton D et al 1996 Aorta-associated CD34$^+$ hematopoietic cells in the early human embryo. Blood 87: 67–76
2. Medvinsky A, Dzierzak E 1996 Definitive hematopoiesis is autonomously initiated by the AGM region. Cell 86: 897–903
3. Sanchez M, Holmes A, Miles C, Dzierzak E 1996 Characterization of the first definitive hematopoietic stem cells in the AGM and liver of the mouse embryo. Immunity 5: 513–520
4. Yoder M, Hiatt K, Mukherjee P 1997 *In vivo* repopulating hematopoietic stem cells are present in the murine yolk sac at day 9.0 postcoitus. Proceedings of the National Academy of Science USA 94: 6776–6781
5. Yoder M, Papaioannou V, Breitfeld P, Williams D 1994 Murine yolk sac endoderm- and mesoderm-derived cell lines support *in vitro* growth and differentiation of hematopoietic cells. Blood 83: 2436–2447
6. Rebel VI, Miller CL, Eaves CJ, Lansdorp PM 1996 The repopulation potential of fetal liver hematopoietic stem cells in mice exceeds that of their liver adult bone marrow counterparts. Blood 87: 3500–3507
7. Zanjani ED, Flake AW, Rice H et al 1994 Long-term repopulating ability of xenogeneic transplanted human fetal liver hematopoietic stem cells in sheep. Journal of Clinical Investigation 93: 1051–1055
8. Clark BR, Keating A 1995 Biology of bone marrow stroma. Annals of the New York Academy of Science 770: 70–78
9. Lemischka IR 1997 Microenvironmental regulation of hematopoietic stem cells. Stem Cells 15 (suppl 1): 63–68
10. Verfaillie C, Hurley R, Bhatia R, McCarthy J 1994 Role of bone marrow matrix in normal and abnormal hematopoiesis. Critical Reviews in Oncology and Hematology 16: 201–223
11. Yoder M, Williams D 1995 Matrix molecule interactions with hematopoietic stem cells. Experimental Hematology 23: 961–967
12. Huang S, Terstappen L 1994 Lymphoid and myeloid differentiation of single human CD34+/HLA-DR+/CD38- hematopoietic stem cells. Blood 83: 1515–1524
13. Baum C, Weissman I, Tsukamoto A et al 1992 Isolation of a candidate human hematopoietic stem cell population. Proceedings of the National Academy of Sciences USA 89: 2804–2809
14. Larochelle A, Vormoor J, Hanenberg H et al 1996 Identification of primitive human hematopoietic cells capable of repopulating NOD/SCID mouse bone marrow: implications for gene therapy. Nature Medicine 2: 1329–1337
15. Sutherland H, Eaves C, Eaves A et al 1989 Characterization and partial purification of human marrow cells capable of initiating long-term hematopoiesis *in vitro*. Blood 74: 1563–1570
16. Terstappen L, Huang S, Safford M et al 1991 Sequential generations of hematopoietic colonies derived from single nonlineage-committed CD34+CD38– progenitor cells. Blood 77: 1218–1227
17. Galy A, Travis M, Cen D, Chen B 1995 Human TB natural killer and dendritic cells arise from a common bone marrow progenitor cell subset. Immunity 3: 459–473
18. Robin C, Pflumio F, Tourino C, Coloumbel L 1998 Single cells with multiple lymphoid (T B NK) and myeloid potentials are identified in fresh cord blood and in NOD-SCID mice transplanted with cord blood CD34+ cells. Experimental Hematology 26: 40a
19. Miller J, Alley K, McGlave P 1994 Differentiation of human natural killer (NK) cells from human primitive marrow progenitors in a stroma-based long-term culture system: identification of a CD34+ 7+ NK progenitor. Blood 83: 2594–2603
20. LeBien T 1998 B-cell lymphopoiesis in mouse and man. Current Opinion in Immunology 10: 188–193
21. Hodgson G, Bradley T 1979 Properties of hematopoietic stem cells surviving 5-fluorouracil treatment. Nature 281: 381–384
22. Randall TD, Weissman IL 1997 Phenotypic and functional changes induced at the clonal level in hematopoietic stem cells after 5-fluorouracil treatment. Blood 89: 3596–3606
23. Chaudhary PM, Roninson IB 1991 Expression and activity of P-glycoprotein a multidrug efflux pump in human hematopoietic stem cells. Cell 66: 85–94
24. Gothot A, Pyatt R, McMahel J et al 1997 Functional heterogeneity of human CD34(+) cells isolated in subcompartments of the G0/G1 phase of the cell cycle. Blood 90: 4384–4393
25. Zijlmans JM, Visser JW, Kleiverda K et al 1995 Modification of rhodamine staining allows identification of hematopoietic stem cells with preferential short-term or long-term bone marrow-repopulating ability. Proceedings of the National Academy of Sciences USA 92: 8901–8905
26. Bhatia M, Bonnet D, Dick JE 1997 Identification of a novel CD34 negative population of primitive human hematopoietic cells capable of repopulating NOD/SCID mice. Blood 90: 1134a
27. Zanjani ED, Almeida-Porada G, Livingston AG et al 1998 Human bone marrow CD34– cells engraft *in vivo* and undergo multilineage expression that includes giving rise to CD34+ cells. Experimental Hematology 26: 353–360
28. Sato T, Laver J, Ogawa M 1999 Reversible expression of CD34 by murine hematopoietic stem cells. Blood 94: 2548–2554
29. Goodell M, Brose K, Paradis G et al 1996 Isolation and functional properties of murine hematopoietic stem cells that are replicating *in vivo*. Journal of Experimental Medicine 183: 1797–1806
30. Goodell M, Rosenzweig M, Kim H et al 1997 Dye efflux studies suggest that hematopoietic stem cells expressing low or undetectable levels of 34 antigen exist in multiple species. Nature Medicine 3: 1337–1345
31. McNiece K, Robinson BE, Quesenberry PJ 1988 Stimulation of murine colony-forming cells with high proliferative potential by the combination of GM-CSF and CSF-1. Blood 72: 191–195
32. Dexter TM 1979 Haemopoiesis in long-term bone marrow cultures. A review. Acta Haematologica 62: 299–305
33. Fraser C, Szilvassy S, Eaves C, Humphries R 1992 Proliferation of totipotent hematopoietic stem cells culture at limiting dilution on supportive marrow stroma. Proceedings of the National Academy of Sciences USA 89: 1968–1972
34. Hao QL, Thiemann FT, Petersen D et al 1996 Extended long-term culture reveals a highly quiescent and primitive human hematopoietic progenitor population. Blood 88: 3306–3313
35. Berardi A, Meffre E, Pflumio F et al 1997 Individual CD34+CD38lowCD19-CD10– progenitor cells from human cord blood generate B lymphocytes and granulocytes. Blood 89: 3554–3563
36. Robin C, Pflumio F, Vainchenker W, Coulombel L 1999 Identification of lymphomyeloid primitive progenitor cells in fresh human cord blood and in the marrow of nonobese diabetic-severe combined immunodeficient (NOD-SCID) mice transplanted with human CD34(+) cord blood cells. Journal of Experimental Medicine 189: 1601–1610
37. Robin C, Bennaceur-Griscelli A, Louache F et al 1999 Identification of human T-lymphoid progenitor cells in CD34+ CD38low and CD34+ CD38+ subsets of human cord blood and bone marrow cells using

NOD-SCID fetal thymus organ cultures. British Journal of Haematology 104: 809–819

38. Whitlock C, Witte O 1982 Long-term culture of B-lymphocytes and their precursors from murine bone marrow. Proceedings of the National Academy of Sciences USA 79: 3608–3613

39. Hao Q, Smogorzewska E, Barsky L, Crooks G 1998 *In vitro* identification of single CD34+/CD38– cells with both lymphoid and myeloid potential. Blood 91: 4145–4152

40. Punzel M, Wissink S, Aselson K et al 1999 Development of an *in vitro* assay that can enumerate Myeloid-Lymphoid Initiating Cells (ML-IC) in adult human bone marrow. Blood 93: 3750–3756

41. Spangrude G, Heimfeld S, Weissman I 1988 Purification and characterization of mouse hematopoietic stem cells. Science 241: 58–63

42. Lemischka IR, Raulet DH, Mulligan RC 1986 Developmental potential and dynamic behavior of hematopoietic stem cells. Cell 45: 917–927

43. Jordan C, McKearn J, Lemischka I 1990 Cellular and developmental properties of fetal hematopoietic stem cells. Cell 61: 953–963

44. Szilvassy SJ, Fraser CC, Eaves CJ et al 1989 Retrovirus-mediated gene transfer to purified hemopoietic stem cells with long-term lympho-myelopoietic repopulating ability. Proceedings of the National Academy of Sciences USA 86: 8798–8802

45. McCune JM, Namikawa R, Kaneshima H et al 1988 The SCID-hu mouse: murine model for the analysis of human hematolymphoid differentiation and function. Science 24: 1632–1639

46. Nolta JA, Hanley MB, Kohn DB 1994 Sustained human hematopoiesis in immunodeficient mice by cotransplantation of marrow stroma expressing human interleukin-3: analysis of gene transduction of long-lived progenitors. Blood 83: 3041–3051

47. Srour EF, Zanjani ED, Cornetta K et al 1993 Persistence of human multilineage self-renewing lymphohematopoietic stem cells in chimeric sheep. Blood 82: 3333–3342

48. Andrews RG, Bryant EM, Bartelmez SH et al 1992 CD34+ marrow cells devoid of T and B lymphocytes reconstitute stable lymphopoiesis and myelopoiesis in lethally irradiated allogeneic baboons. Blood 80: 1693–1701

49. Tisdale JF, Hanazono Y, Sellers SE et al 1998 *Ex vivo* expansion of genetically marked rhesus peripheral blood progenitor cells results in diminished long-term repopulating ability. Blood 92: 1131–1141

50. Charbord P, Tavian M, Humeau L, Peault B 1996 Early ontogeny of the human marrow from long bones: an immunohistochemical study of hematopoiesis and its microenvironment. Blood 87: 4109–4118

51. Barbe E, Huitinga I, Dopp E et al 1993 A novel bone marrow frozen section assay for studying hematopoietic interactions *in situ*: the role of stroma bone marrow macrophages in erythroblast binding. Journal of Cell Sciencec 109: 2937

52. Thiele J, Galle R, Sander C, Fischer R 1991 Interactions between megakaryocytes and sinus wall. An ultrastructural study on bone marrow tissue in primary (essential) thrombocythemia. Journal of Submicroscopic Cytology and Pathology 23: 595–603

53. Rafii S, Shapiro F, Pettengell R et al 1995 Human bone marrow microvascular endothelial cells support long-term proliferation and differentiation of myeloid and megakaryocytic progenitors. Blood 86: 3353

54. Coloumbel L, Eaves A, Eaves C 1983 Enzymatic treatment of long-term marrow cultures reveals the preferential location of primitive hematopoietic progenitors in the adherent layer. Blood 62: 291–299

55. Moore KA, Hideo E, Lemischka IR 1997 *In vitro* maintenance of highly purified transplantable hematopoietic stem cells. Blood 89: 4337–4437

56. Shofield R 1978 The relationship between the spleen colony-forming cell and the hematopoietic stem cell: a hypothesis. Blood Cells 4: 7–14

57. Quesenberry PJ, Crittenden RB, Lowry P et al 1994 *In vitro* and *in vivo* studies of stromal niches. Blood Cells 2: 97–106

58. Xu M, Tsuji K, Ueda T et al 1998 Stimulation of mouse and human primitive hematopoiesis by murine embryonic aorta-gonad-mesonephros-derived stromal cell lines. Blood 92: 2032

59. Ohneda O, Fennie C, Zheng Z et al 1998 Hematopoietic stem cell maintenance and differentiation are supported by embryonic aorta-gonad-mesonephros region-derived endothelium. Blood 92: 908–916

60. Auerbach R, Wang S, Yu D et al 1998 Role of endothelium in the control of mouse yolk sac stem cell differentiation. Developmental and Comparative Immunology 22: 333–341

61. Lu L, Wang S, Auerbach R 1998 *In vitro* and *in vivo* differentiation into B cells T cells and myeloid cells of primitive yolk sac hematopoietic precursor cells expanded > 100-fold by coculture with a clonal yolk

sac endothelial cell line. Proceedings of the National Academy of Sciences USA 93: 14782–14787

62. Wineman J, Moore K, Lemischka I, Muller-Sieburg C 1996 Functional heterogeneity of the hematopoietic microenvironment: rare stromal elements maintain long-term repopulating stem cells. Blood 87: 4082–4090

63. Aiuti A, Friedrich C, Sieff CA, Gutierrez-Ramos C 1998 Identification of distinct elements of the stromal microenvironment that control human hematopoietic stem/progenitor cell growth and differentiation. Experimental Hematology 26: 143–151

64. Burroughs J, Gupta P, Blazar B, Verfaillie C 1994 Diffusible factors from the murine cell line M2-10B4 support human *in vitro* hematopoiesis. Experimental Hematology 22: 1095–1104

65. Moreau I, Duvert V, Caux C et al 1993 Myofibroblastic stromal cells isolated from human bone marrow induce the proliferation of both early myeloid and B-lymphoid cells. Blood 82: 2396

66. Li J, Sensebe L, Herve P, Charbord P 1995 Nontransformed colony-derived stromal cell lines from normal human marrows. II. Phenotypic characterization and differentiation pathway. Experimental Hematology 23: 133

67. Li J, Sensebe L, Herve P, Charbord P 1997 Nontransformed colony-derived stromal cell lines from normal human marrows. III. The maintenance of hematopoiesis from CD34+ cell populations. Experimental Hematology 25: 582

68. Sensebe L, Li J, Lilly M et al 1995 Nontransformed colony-derived stromal cell lines from normal human marrows. I. Growth requirement and myelopoiesis supportive ability. Experimental Hematology 23: 507

69. Roecklein B, Torok-Storb B 1995 Functionally distinct human marrow stromal cell lines immortalized by transduction with the human papilloma virus E6/E7 genes. Blood 85: 997

70. Henderson A, Johnson A, Dorshkind K 1990 Functional characterization of two stromal cell lines that support B lymphopoiesis. Immunology 145: 423–429

71. Moore K, Pytowski B, Witte L et al 1997 Hematopoietic activity of a stromal cell transmembrane protein containing epidermal growth factor-like repeat motifs. Proceedings of the National Academy of Sciences USA 94: 4011–4016

72. Li L, Milner LA, Deng Y et al 1998 The human homologue of rat Jagged 1 expressed by marrow stroma inhibits differentiation of 32D cells through interaction with Notch 1. Immunity 8: 43–55

73. Bigas A, Martin D, Milner L 1998 Notch 1 and Notch2 inhibit myeloid differentiation in response to different cytokines. Molecular and Cell Biology 18: 2324–2331

74. Gupta P, McCarthy J, Verfaillie C 1996 Marrow stroma derived proteoglycans combined with physiological concentrations of cytokines are required for LTC-IC maintenance. Blood 87: 3229–3237

75. Gupta P, Oegema TJ, Brazil J et al 1998 Structurally specific heparan sulfates support primitive human hematopoiesis by formation of a multimolecular stem cell niche. Journal of Experimental Medicine 92: 4641–4651

76. Rafii S, Shapiro F, Rimarachin J et al 1994 Isolation and characterization of human bone marrow microvascular endothelial cells: hematopoietic progenitor cell adhesion. Blood 84: 10–17

77. Schweitzer K, Vicart P, Delouis C et al 1997 Characterization of a newly established human bone marrow endothelial cell line: distinct adhesive properties for hematopoietic progenitors compared with human umbilical vein endothelial cells. Laboratory Investigations 76: 25–32

78. Jo DY, Rafii S, Hamada T, Moore MA 2000 Chemotaxis of primitive hematopoietic cells in response to stromal cell-derived factor-1. Journal of Clinical Investigation 105: 101–111

79. Peled A, Petit I, Kollet O et al 1999 Dependence of human stem cell engraftment and repopulation of NOD/SCID mice on CXCR4. Science 283: 845–848

80. Mohle R, Bautz F, Rafii S et al 1998 The chemokine receptor CXCR-4 is expressed on CD34+ hematopoietic progenitors and leukemic cells and mediates transendothelial migration induced by stromal cell-derived factor-1. Blood 91: 4523–4530

81. Mazo I, Gutierrez-Ramos J, Frenette P et al 1998 Hematopoietic progenitor cell rolling in bone marrow microvessels: parallel contributions by endothelial selectins and vascular cell adhesion molecule 1. Journal of Experimental Medicine 188: 465–472

82. Taichman R, Emerson S 1994 Human osteoblasts support hematopoiesis through the production of granulocyte colony-stimulating factor. Journal of Experimental Medicine 179: 1677.

83. Fridenshtein A 1982 Stromal bone marrow cells and the hematopoietic microenvironment. Arkhiv Patologii 44: 3–11

84. Gronthos S, Graves S, Ohta S, Simmons P 1994 The STRO-1+ fraction of adult human bone marrow contains the osteogenic precursors. Blood 84: 4164–4173

85. Wakitani S, Saito T, Caplan A 1995 Myogenic cells derived from rat bone marrow mesenchymal stem cells exposed to 5-azacytidine. Muscle Nerve 18: 1417–1426

86. Pittenger MF, Mackay AM, Beck SC et al 1999 Multilineage potential of adult human mesenchymal stem cells. Science 284: 143–147

87. Koc ON, Gerson SL, Cooper BW et al 2000 Rapid hematopoietic recovery after coinfusion of autologous-blood stem cells and culture-expanded marrow mesenchymal stem cells in advanced breast cancer patients receiving high-dose chemotherapy. Journal of Clinical Oncology 18: 307–316

88. Liechty KW, MacKenzie TC, Shaaban AF et al 2000 Human mesenchymal stem cells engraft and demonstrate site-specific differentiation after *in utero* transplantation in sheep. Nature Medicine 6: 1282–1286

89. Reyes M, Lund T, Lenvik T et al 2001 Purification and *ex vivo* expansion of post-natal human marrow mesodermal progenitor cells. Blood: in press 98: 2615–2625

90. Bagley C, Woodcock J, Stomski F 1997 The structural and functional basis of cytokine receptor activation: lessons from the common beta subunit of the granulocyte-macrophage colony-stimulating factor interleukin-3 (IL-3) and IL-5 receptors. Blood 89: 1471–1482

91. Liu KD, Gaffen SL, Goldsmith MA 1998 JAK/STAT signaling by cytokine receptors. Current Opinion in Immunology 10: 271–278

92. Hamel W, Westphal M 1997 The road less travelled: c-kit and stem cell factor. Journal of Neurooncology 35: 327–333

93. Lyman SD, Williams DE 1995 Biology and potential clinical applications of flt3 ligand. Current Opinion in Hematology 2: 177–181

94. Wendlin F, Cohen-Solal K, Villeval JL et al 1998 Mpl ligand or thrombopoietin: biological activities. Biotherapy 10: 269–276

95. Petzer A, Zandstra P, Piret J, Eaves C 1996 Differential cytokine effects on primitive (CD34+/CD38–) human hematopoietic cells: novel responses to Flt3-ligand and thrombopoietin. Journal of Experimental Medicine 183: 2551

96. Petzer A, Hogge D, Lansdrop P et al 1996 Self-renewal of primitive hematopoietic cells (long-term-culture-initiating-cells) *in vitro* and their expansion in defined medium. Proceedings of the National Academy of Sciences USA 93: 1470–1475

97. Peters M, Muller AM, Rose-John S 1998 Interleukin-6 and soluble interleukin-6 receptor: direct stimulation of gp130 and hematopoiesis. Blood 92: 3495–3504

98. Nandurkar HH, Robb L, Begley CG 1998 The role of IL-II in hematopoiesis as revealed by a targeted mutation of its receptor. Stem Cells 16 (suppl 2): 53–65

99. Miyajima A, Kinoshita T, Tanaka M et al 2000 Role of Oncostatin M in hematopoiesis and liver development. Cytokine and Growth Factor Reviews 11: 177–183

100. Taupin JL, Pitard V, Dechanet J et al 1998 Leukemia inhibitory factor: part of a large ingathering family. International Review in Immunology 16: 397–426

101. Taga T, Kishimoto T 1997 Gp 130 and the interleukin-6 family of cytokines. Annual Review in Immunology 15: 797–819

102. Peters M, Muller AM, Rose-John S 1998 Interleukin-6 and soluble interleukin-6 receptor: direct stimulation of gp 130 and hematopoiesis. Blood 92: 3495–3504

103. Eaves C, Cashman J, Kay R et al 1991 Mechanisms that regulate the cell cycle status of very primitive hematopoietic cells in long-term human marrow cultures. II. Analysis of positive and negative regulators produced by stromal cells within the adherent layer. Blood 78: 110–117

104. Fortunel N, Hatzfeld A, Hatzfeld JA 2000 Transforming growth factor-beta: pleiotropic role in the regulation of hematopoiesis. Blood 96: 2022–2036

105. Jacobsen SE, Jacobsen FW, Fahlman C 1998 TNF-alpha, the great imitator: role of p55 and p75 TNF receptors in hematopoiesis. Stem Cells 12 (suppl1): 126–128

106. Selleri C, Maciejewski JP, Sato T, Young NS 1996 Interferon-gamma constitutively expressed in the stromal microenvironment of human marrow cultures mediates potent hematopoietic inhibition. Blood 89: 4149–4157

107. Ahuja SK, Gao JL, Murphy PM 1994 Chemokine receptors and molecular mimicry. Immunology Today 15: 281–287

108. Campbell JJ, Butcher EC 2000 Chemokines in tissue-specific and microenvironment-specific lymphocyte homing. Current Opinion Immunology 12: 336–341

109. Ganju RK, Brubaker SA, Meyer J et al 1998 The α-chemokine, stromal cell-derived factor-1α, binds to the transmembrane G-protein-coupled CXCR-4 receptor and activates multiple signal transduction pathways. Journal of Biological Chemistry 273: 23169–23175

110. Nagasawa T, Hirota S, Tachibana K et al 1996 Defects of B-cell lymphopoiesis and bone marrow myelopoiesis in mice lacking the CXC chemokine PBSF/SDF-1. Nature 382: 635–638

111. Ma Q, Jones D, Borghesani P et al 1998 Impaired B-lymphopoiesis myelopoiesis and derailed cerebellar neuron migration in CXCR4-and SDF-1-deficient mice. Proceedings of the National Academy of Sciences USA 95: 9448–9453

112. Naiyer AJ, Jo DY, Ahn J et al 1999 Stromal derived factor-1-induced chemokinesis of cord blood CD34(+) cells (long-term culture-initiating cells) through endothelial cells is mediated by E-selectin. Blood 94: 4011–4019

113. Weber C, Alon R, Moser B, Springer TA 1996 Sequential regulation of alpha 4 beta 1 and alpha 5 beta 1 integrin avidity by CC chemokines in monocytes: implications for transendothelial chemotaxis. Journal of Cell Biology 134: 1063–1073

114. Kittler E, McGrath H, Temeles D et al 1992 Biologic significance of constitutive and subliminal growth factor production by bone marrow stroma. Blood 79: 3168–3175

115. Punzel M, Gupta P, Roodell A et al 1999 Factor(s) secreted by AFT024 fetal liver cells following stimulation with human cytokines are important for human LTC-IC growth. Leukemia 13: 1079–1084

116. Gordon M, Riley G, Watt S, Greaves M 1987 Compartmentalization of a haematopoietic growth factor (GM-CSF) by glycosaminoglycans in the bone marrow microenvironment. Nature 326: 403–407

117. Roberts R, Gallagher J, Spooncer E et al 1988 Heparan sulphate bound growth factors: a mechanism for stromal cell mediated haemopoiesis. Nature 332: 376–379

118. Spooncer E, Gallagher JT, Krizsa F, Dexter TM 1983 Regulation of haemopoiesis in long-term bone marrow cultures. IV. Glycosaminoglycan synthesis and the stimulation of haemopoiesis by beta-D-xylosides. Journal of Cell Biology 96: 510–514

119. Rapraeger AC, Guimond S, Krufka A, Olwin BB 1994 Regulation by heparan sulfate in fibroblast growth factor signaling. Methods in Enzymology 245: 219–227

120. Friel J, Heberlein C, Itoh K, Ostertag W 1997 Role of the stem cell factor (SCF) receptor and the alternative forms of its ligand (SCF) in the induction of long-term growth by stroma cells. Leukemia 11 (1): 493–495

121. Dao MA, Hashino K, Kato I, Nolta JA 1998 Adhesion to fibronectin maintains regenerative capacity during *ex vivo* culture and transduction of human hematopoietic stem and progenitor cells. Blood 92: 4612–4621

122. Moritz T, Dutt P, Xiao X et al 1996 Fibronectin improves transduction of reconstituting hematopoietic stem cells by retroviral vectors: evidence of direct viral binding to chymotryptic carboxy-terminal fragments. Blood 88: 855–862

123. Levesque J, Haylock D, Simmons P 1996 Cytokine regulation of proliferation and cell adhesion are correlated events in human CD34+ hemopoietic progenitors. Blood 88: 1168–1175

124. Hurley RW, McCarthy JB, Verfaillie CM 1995 Direct adhesion to bone marrow stroma via fibronectin receptors inhibits hematopoietic progenitor proliferation. Journal of Clinical Investigation 96: 511–521

125. Jiang Y, Zhao RCH, Verfaillie CM 2000 Inactivation of the cyclin-dependent kinase inhibitor, p27, is responsible for overriding the integrin-mediated inhibition of CML CD34+ cells. Proceedings of the National Academy of Sciences USA 97: 10538–10543

126. Prosper F, Verfaillie CM 2001 Regulation of hematopoiesis through adhesion receptors. Journal of Leukocyte Biology 69: 307–316

127. Whetton AD, Spooncer E 1998 Role of cytokines and extracellular matrix in the regulation of haemopoietic stem cells. Current Opinion in Cell Biology 10: 721–726

128. Coulombel L, Auffray I, Gaugler M, Rosemblatt M 1997 Expression and function of integrins on hematopoietic progenitor cells. Acta Haematologica 97: 13–21

129. Papayannopoulou T, Craddock C 1997 Homing and trafficking of hemopoietic progenitor cells. Acta Haematologica 97: 97–104

130. Simmons P, Levesque J, Zannettino A 1997 Adhesion molecules in haemopoiesis. Baillière's Clinical Haematology 10: 485–499
131. Verfaillie C, McCarthy J, McGlave P 1991 Differentiation of primitive human multipotent hematopoietic progenitors into single lineage clonogenic progenitors is accompanied by alterations in their interaction with FN. Journal of Experimental Medicine 174: 693–703
132. Williams D, Rios M, Stephens C, Patel V 1991 Fibronectin and VLA-4 in haematopoietic stem cell–microenvironment interactions. Nature 352: 438
133. Simmons P, Masinovsky B, Longenecker B et al 1992 Vascular cell adhesion molecule-1 expressed by bone marrow stromal cells mediates the binding of hematopoietic progenitor cells. Blood 80: 388–396
134. Hurley R, McCarthy J, Verfaillie C 1997 Monoclonal antibody crosslinking of the alpha 4 or beta 1 integrin inhibits committed clonogenic hematopoietic progenitor proliferation. Experimental Hematology 25: 321–328
135. Jiang Y, Prosper F, Verfaillie CM 2000 Opposing effects of engagement of integrins and stimulation of cytokine receptors on cell cycle progression of normal human hematopoietic progenitors. Blood 95: 846–854
136. Levesque JP, Leavesley DI, Niutta S et al 1995 Cytokines increase human hemopoietic cell adhesiveness by activation of very late antigen (VLA)-4 and VLA-5 integrins. Journal of Experimental Medicine 181: 1805–1812
137. Schofield K, Rushton G, Humphries M et al 1997 Influence of interleukin-3 and other growth factors on alpha4beta1 integrin-mediated adhesion and migration of human hematopoietic progenitor cells. Blood 90: 1858–1866
138. Schofield K, Humphries M, de Wynter E et al 1998 The effect of alpha4 beta1-integrin binding sequences of FN on growth of cells from human hematopoietic progenitors. Blood 91: 3230–3238
139. Bazzoni G, Carlesso N, Griffin J, Hemler ME 1996 Bcr/Abl expression stimulates integrin function in hematopoietic cell lines. Journal of Clinical Investigation 98: 52–61
140. Hannigan G, Dedhar S 1997 Protein kinase mediators of integrin signal transduction. Journal of Molecular Medicine 75: 35–44
141. Guan J 1997 Focal adhesion kinase in integrin signaling. Matrix Biology 16: 195–200
142. LaFlamme S, Homan S, Bodeau A, Mastrangelo A 1997 Integrin cytoplasmic domains as connectors to the cell's signal transduction apparatus. Matrix Biology 16: 153–161
143. Zeng C, Xing Z, Bian ZC et al 1998 Differential regulation of Pyk2 and focal adhesion kinase (FAK). Journal of Biological Chemistry 273: 2384–2389
144. Sieg DJ, Llic D, Jones KC et al 1998 Pyk2 and Src-family protein-tyrosine kinases compensate for the loss of FAK in fibronectin-stimulated signaling events but Pyk2 does not fully function to enhance FAK-cell migration. EMBO 17: 5933–5947
145. Vuori K, Hirai H, Aizawa S, Ruoslahti E 1996 Induction of p130cas signaling complex formation upon integrin-mediated cell adhesion: a role for Src family kinases. Molecular and Cellular Biology 16: 2606–2613
146. Hildebrand J, Schaller M, Parsons J 1995 Paxillin a tyrosine phosphorylated focal adhesion-associated protein binds to the carboxyl terminal domain of focal adhesion kinase. Molecular Biology of the Cell 6: 637–645
147. Chen H, Appeddu P, Parsons J et al 1995 Interaction of focal adhesion kinase with cytoskeletal protein talin. Journal of Biological Chemistry 270: 16995–17003
148. Sattler M, Salgia R, Shrikhande G et al 1997 Differential signaling after β1 integrin ligation is mediated through binding of CRKL to p120CBL and p110HEF1. Journal of Biological Chemistry 272: 14320–14326
149. Morino N, Mimura T, Hamasaki K et al 1995 Matrix/integrin interaction activates the mitogen-activated protein kinase p44erk-1 and p42erk-2. Journal of Biological Chemistry 270: 269–276
150. Shimizu Y, Hunt SI 1996 Regulating integrin-mediated adhesion: one more function for PI3-kinase? Immunology Today 17–20
151. Papayannopoulou T, Brice M 1992 Integrin expression profiles during erythroid differentiation. Blood 79: 1686–1694
152. Patel V, Lodish H 1986 The fibronectin receptor on mammalian erythroid precursor cells: characterization and developmental regulation. Journal of Cell Biology 102: 449–460
153. Patel V, Lodish H 1987 A fibronectin matrix is required for differentiation of murine erythroleukemia cells into reticulocytes. Journal of Cell Biology 105: 3105
154. Michigami T, Shimizu N, Williams PJ 2000 Cell–cell contact between marrow stromal cells and myeloma cells via VCAM-1 and alpha(4)beta(1)-integrin enhances production of osteoclast-stimulating activity. Blood 96: 1953–1960
155. Vincent AM, Cawley JC, Burthem J 1996 Integrin function in chronic lymphocytic leukemia. Blood 87: 4780–4788
156. de Ia Fuente M T, Casanova M, Garcia-Gila M et al 1999 Fibronectin interaction with alpha4beta1 integrin prevents apoptosis in B cell chronic lymphocytic leukemia: correlation with Bcl-2 and Bax. Leukemia 13: 266–274
157. Young P, Baumhueter S, Lasky L 1995 The sialomucin CD34 is expressed on hematopoietic cells and blood vessels during murine development. Blood 85: 96–104
158. Healy L, May G, Gale K et al 1995 The stem cell antigen CD34 functions as a regulator of hemopoietic cell adhesion. Proceeding of the National Academy of Sciences USA 92: 12240–12245
159. Bhatia M, Bonnet D, Murdoch B et al 1998 A newly discovered class of human hematopoietic cells with SCID-repopulating activity. Nature Medicine 4: 1038–1045
160. Verfaillie CM, Almeida-Porada G, Wissink S, Zanjani ED 2000 Kinetics of engraftment of CD34(−) and CD34(+) cells from mobilized blood differs from that of CD34(−) and CD34(+) cells from bone marrow. Experimental Hematology 28: 1071–1079
161. Fackler MJ, Krause DM, Smith OM et al 1995 Full-length but not truncated CD34 inhibits hematopoietic cell differentiation of M1 cells. Blood 85: 3040–3047
162. Cheng J, Baumhueter S, Cacalano G 1996 Hematopoietic defects in mice lacking the sialomucin CD34. Blood 87: 479–486
163. Bazil V, Brandt J, Chen S et al 1996 A monoclonal antibody recognizing CD34 (leukosialin) initiates apoptosis of human hematopoietic progenitor cells but not stem cells. Blood 87: 1272–1279
164. Serrador J, Nieto M, Alonso-Lebrero J et al 1998 CD43 interacts with moesin and ezrin and regulates its redistribution to the uropods of T lymphocytes at the cell–cell contacts. Blood 91: 4632–4641
165. Bazil V, Brandt J, Tsukamoto A, Hoffman R 1995 Apoptosis of human hematopoietic progenitor cells induced by crosslinking of surface CD43 the major sialoglycoprotein of leukocytes. Blood 86: 502–510
166. Zannettino A, Buhring H, Niutta S et al 1998 The sialomucin CD164 (MGC-24v) is an adhesive glycoprotein expressed by human hematopoietic progenitors and bone marrow stromal cells that serves as a potent negative regulator of hematopoiesis. Blood 92: 2613–2621
167. Watt S, Buhring H, Rappold I et al 1998 CD164 a novel sialomucin on CD34(+) and erythroid subsets is located on human chromosome 6q21. Blood 92: 849–866
168. Doyonnas R, Yi-Hsin Chan J, Butler LH et al 2000 CD164 monoclonal antibodies that block hemopoietic progenitor cell adhesion and proliferation interact with the first mucin domain of the CD164 receptor. Journal of Immunology 165: 840–851
169. Watt SM, Butler LH, Tavian M et al 2000 Functionally defined CD164 epitopes are expressed on CD34(+) cells throughout ontogeny but display distinct distribution patterns in adult hematopoietic and nonhematopoietic tissues. Blood 95: 3113–3124
170. Levesque JP, Zannettino AC, Pudney M 1999 PSGL-1-mediated adhesion of human hematopoietic progenitors to P-selectin results in suppression of hematopoiesis. I. Immunity 11: 369–378
171. Devine P, McKenzie I 1992 Mucins: structure function and associations with malignancy. Bioessays 14: 619–627
172. Simmons P, Zannettino A, Levesque J et al 1998 Mucin-like molecules as regulators of hematopoiesis. Experimental Hematology 26: 69a
173. Wright T, Kinsella M, Keating A, Singer J 1986 Proteoglycans in human long-term bone marrow cultures: biochemical and ultrastructural analyses. Blood 67: 1333–1341
174. Fedarko N 1994 Isolation and purification of proteoglycans. EXS 70: 9–14
175. Gupta P, Oegema T, Verfaillie C 1998 Differences in the LTC-IC maintaining capacity of stromal cells correlates with patterns of sulfation of their heparan sulfate glycosaminoglycans. Blood 92: 4641–4651
176. Clarke D, Katoh O, Gibbs R et al 1995 Interaction of interleukin 7 (IL-7) with glycosaminoglycans and its biological relevance. Cytokine 7: 325–334
177. Tanaka Y, Adams DH, Hubscher S et al 1993 T-cell adhesion induced by proteoglycan-immobilized cytokine MIP-1 beta. Nature 361: 79–82
178. Han ZC, Lu M, Li J et al 1997 Platelet factor 4 and other CXC chemokines support the survival of normal hematopoietic cells and

reduce the chemosensitivity of cells to cytotoxic agents. Blood 89: 2328–2335

179. Milner LA, Kopan R, Martin DI, Bernstein ID 1994 A human homologue of the *Drosophila* developmental gene Notch is expressed in CD34+ hematopoietic precursors. Blood 83: 2057–2062

180. Austin T, Solar G, Ziegler F et al 1997 A role for the Wnt gene family in hematopoiesis: expansion of multilineage progenitor cells. Blood 89: 3624–3631

181. Van Den Berg D, Sharma A, Bruno E, Hoffman 1998 Role of members of the Wnt gene family in human hematopoiesis. Blood 92: 3189–3197

182. Weinmaster G 1997 The ins and outs of notch signaling. Molecular and Cellular Neuroscience 9: 91–102

183. Simpson P 1997 Notch signaling in development: on equivalence groups and asymmetric developmental potential. Current Opinion in Genetics and Development 7: 537–548

184. Muskavitch M 1994 Delta-notch signaling and drosophila cell fate choice. Developmental Biology 166: 415

185. Dale T 1998 Signal transduction by the Wnt family of ligands. Biochemical Journal 329: 209–215

186. Wodarz A, Nusse R 1998 Mechanisms of Wnt signaling in development. Annual Review of Cellular and Developmental Biology 14: 59–88

187. Pear W, Aster J, Scott M et al 1996 Exclusive development of T cell neoplasms in mice transplanted with bone marrow expressing activated Notch alleles. Journal of Experimental Medicine 183: 2283–2293

188. Varnum-Finney B, Purton L, Yu M et al 1998 The Notch ligand Jagged-1 influences the development of primitive hematopoietic precursor cells. Blood 91: 4084–4093

189. Karanu FN, Murdoch B, Gallacher L et al 2000 The notch ligand jagged-1 represents a novel growth factor of human hematopoietic stem cells. Journal of Experimental Medicine 192: 1365–1372

190. Karanu FN, Murdoch B, Miyabayashi T et al 2001 Human homologues of Delta-1 and Delta-4 function as mitogenic regulators of primitive human hematopoietic cells. Blood 97: 1960–1967

191. Barnes M, Duckworth D, Beeley L 1998 Frizzled proteins constitute a novel family of G protein-coupled receptors most closely related to the secretin family. Trends in Pharmacological Sciences 19: 399–406

192. Willert K, Nusse R 1998 Beta-catenin: a key mediator of Wnt signaling. Current Opinion in Genetics and Development 8: 95–104

193. Hsu S, Galceran J, Grosschedl R 1998 Modulation of transcriptional regulation by LEF-1 in response to Wnt-1 signaling and association with beta-catenin. Molecular and Cellular Biology 18: 4807–4815

194. Brandon C, Eisenberg LM, Eisenberg CA 2000 WNT signaling modulates the diversification of hematopoietic cells. Blood 96: 4132–4141

195. Busslinger M, Nutt SL, Rolink AG 2000 Lineage commitment in lymphopoiesis. Current Opinion in Immunology 12: 151–258

196. Ogawa M 1999 Stochastic model revisited. International Journal of Hematology 69: 2–5

197. Mayani H, Dragowska W, Lansdorp P 1993 Lineage commitment in human hemopoiesis involves asymmetric cell division of multipotent progenitors and does not appear to be influenced by cytokines. Journal of Cellular Physiology 157: 579–586

198. Kinashi T, Lee KH, Ogawa M et al 1991 Premature expression of the macrophage colony-stimulating factor receptor on a multipotential stem cell line does not alter differentiation lineages controlled by

stromal cells used for coculture. Journal of Experimental Medicine 173: 1267–1278

199. Crump A, Grusby M, Glimcher L, Cantor H 1993 Thymocyte development in major histocompatibility complex-deficient mice: evidence for stochastic commitment to the CD4 and CD8 lineages. Proceedings of the National Academy of Sciences USA 90: 10739–10744

200. Cowling G, Dexter T 1993 Apoptosis in the haemopoietic system. Philosophical Transactions of the Royal Society of London Series B-Biological Sciences 345: 257–264

201. Sauvageau G, Thorsteinsdottir U, Hough M et al 1997 Overexpression of HOXB3 in hematopoietic cells causes defective lymphoid development and progressive myeloproliferation. Immunity 6: 13–19

202. Thorsteinsdottir U, Sauvageau G, Humphries R 1997 Hox homeobox genes as regulators of normal and leukemic hematopoiesis. Hematology-Oncology Clinics of North America 11: 1221–1234

203. Crooks GM, Fuller J, Petersen D et al 1999 Constitutive HOXA5 expression inhibits erythropoiesis and increases myelopoiesis from human hematopoietic progenitors. Blood 94: 519–528

204. Lawrence H, Helgason C, Sauvageau G et al 1997 Mice bearing a targeted interruption of the homeobox gene HOXA9 have defects in myeloid erythroid and lymphoid hematopoiesis. Blood 89: 1922–1930

205. Thorsteinsdottir U, Sauvageau G, Hough M et al 1997 Overexpression of HOXA10 in murine hematopoietic cells perturbs both myeloid and lymphoid differentiation and leads to acute myeloid leukemia. Molecular and Cellular Biology 17: 495–508

206. Sauvageau G, Thorsteinsdottir U, Hough MR et al 1997 Overexpression of HOXB3 in hematopoietic cells causes defective lymphoid development and progressive myeloproliferation. Immunity 6: 13–21

207. Metcalf D 1998 Lineage commitment and maturation in hematopoietic cells: the case for extrinsic regulation. Blood 92: 345–352

208. Nishijima I, Watanabe S, Nakahata T, Arai K 1997 Human granulocyte-macrophage colony-stimulating factor (hGM-CSF)-dependent *in vitro* and *in vivo* proliferation and differentiation of all hematopoietic progenitor cells in hGM-CSF receptor transgenic mice. Journal of Allergy and Clinical Immunology 100: S79

209. Robey E, Fowlkes B, Gordon J et al 1991 Thymic selection in CD8 transgenic mice supports an instructive model for commitment to a CD4 or CD8 lineage. Cell 64: 99–112

210. Jones P, May G, Healy L et al 1998 Stromal expression of Jagged 1 promotes colony formation by fetal hematopoietic progenitor cells. Blood 92: 1505–1514

211. Weinstein R, Riordan M, Wemc K et al 1989 Dual role of fibronectin in hematopoietic differentiation. Blood 73: 111–120

212. Armeanu S, Buhring H, Reuss-Borst M et al 1995 E-cadherin is functionally involved in the maturation of the erythroid lineage. Journal of Cell Biology 131–138

213. Hanspal M 1997 Importance of cell–cell interactions in regulation of erythropoiesis. Current Opinion in Hematology 4: 142–149

214. Taichman R, Reilly M, Verma R et al Emerson S 1997 Augmented production of interleukin-6 by normal human osteoblasts in response to CD34+ hematopoietic bone marrow cells *in vitro*. Blood 89: 1165–1172

215. Gupta P, Blazar B, Gupta K et al Verfaillie C 1998 Human CD34(+) bone marrow cells regulate stromal production of interleukin-6 and granulocyte colony-stimulating factor and increase the colony-stimulating activity of stroma. Blood 92: 3724–3733

Pathology of the marrow

General considerations   128

Pathology of the marrow: general considerations

5

SN Wickramasinghe   BJ Bain

Examination of the marrow

Examination post mortem

Alterations of the marrow in disease

Alterations in cellularity

Alterations in the frequency and morphology of various types of marrow cells
Erythroblasts and neutrophil precursors
Eosinophil series
Basophils
Mast cells
Megakaryocytes
Lymphocytes
Plasma cells
Macrophages (histiocytes)
Osteoblasts and osteoclasts

Changes in iron stores and intraerythroblastic iron
Iron stores
Alterations in stainable non-hemoglobin iron within erythroblasts

Infections and the bone marrow
HIV infection

Bone marrow granulomas
Lipid granulomas
Granuloma-like lesions

Metastatic tumors in bone marrow
Value of histologic sections

Bone marrow fibrosis including idiopathic myelofibrosis
Idiopathic myelofibrosis (myelosclerosis, agnogenic myeloid metaplasia)

Storage cells in lysosomal storage diseases
Sphingolipidoses
Mucopolysaccharidoses
Other storage diseases and hyperlipidemias

Bone marrow necrosis

Gelatinous transformation

Amyloidosis

Vascular and embolic lesions

Aluminum deposition

Bone marrow function is altered in a large number of pathologic states. However, there is a relatively limited range of cytologic and histologic changes that can be detected in the marrow in disease. This chapter provides a summary of the various types of physiologic or pathologic alterations that may be seen. Details of abnormalities encountered in particular diseases are given in subsequent chapters.

Examination of the marrow

The bone marrow may be examined after aspiration through a special wide-bore needle. The usual sites of aspiration are the posterior or anterior iliac crest or manubrium sterni in adults, the posterior superior iliac spine in infants and children and the medial aspect of the upper end of the tibia in neonates. The aspirate, which consists of fragments of marrow tissue, individual nucleated marrow cells and a variable quantity of blood, is spread on glass slides and examined after fixation and staining. Marrow smears are regularly stained by a Romanowsky method and by Perls' acid ferrocyanide method for hemosiderin. In appropriate cases smears can also be stained for specific cellular constituents such as lipids (using Sudan black B or Oil red O), glycogen (periodic acid-Schiff [PAS] reaction), DNA (Feulgen reaction), RNA and various enzymes; the diagnostic value of hematologic cytochemistry has been reviewed.[1] Examination of marrow smears allows a detailed analysis of the morphology and cytochemistry of cells and the percentages of various cell types. However, differential counts performed on marrow smears do not give accurate data on the prevalence of some cell types, such as megakaryocytes and macrophages, which are relatively resistant to aspiration or have a tendency to remain attached to the aspirated marrow fragments during the preparation of the smears. This drawback may be overcome, to a large extent, by examining preparations obtained by crushing marrow fragments between two glass slides and pulling the slides apart.

Apart from its use for cytologic studies with the light microscope, aspirated marrow can be used for immunophenotypic, cytogenetic, molecular genetic, biochemical and electron microscope studies.

The histology of the marrow is investigated by examining sections of aspirated marrow particles (either in clotted aspirates or after concentration of the particles in various ways) or by examining sections of a cylinder of bone obtained using a specially-constructed trephine needle. The usual site of trephine biopsy is the posterior superior iliac spine. Unlike marrow smears, histologic sections of trephine biopsies permit an appreciation of intercellular relationships and particularly of the relationship between hemopoietic cells, non-hemopoietic cells, the blood vessels and bone. Such sections are therefore useful for the detection of granulomas and focal accumulations of malignant cells. They also allow a study of the quantity and distribution of reticulin and collagen in marrow and make possible the diagnosis of myelofibrosis. Histologic sections are usefully stained with hematoxylin and eosin (H&E), Giemsa stain and stains for hemosiderin and reticulin. The PAS stain is applied selectively. The Leder stain for α-naphthyl AS-D chloroacetate esterase in the granules of cells of the neutrophil series and mast cells can be applied to sections of marrow particles and to sections of plastic-embedded trephine biopsy specimens. However, some methods of decalcification impair the reaction when the Leder stain is applied to sections of paraffin-embedded trephine biopsy specimens.[2] The various types of hemopoietic cells can be distinguished in histologic sections of paraffin-embedded decalcified trephine biopsies but not as easily as in marrow smears. However, cytologic detail is considerably improved if semi-thin (3 μm) sections of plastic-embedded undecalcified trephine biopsies are studied.[3] It is useful to pick up the freshly obtained biopsy specimen gently with forceps and lightly touch a slide with the specimen before placing it in fixative. Such 'touch preparations' may be useful in the identification of abnormal cells seen in histologic preparations. They may also reveal abnormal cells that were not detected in an aspirate because they remained trapped within particles.

Examination post mortem

A variety of morphologic changes occur fairly rapidly in marrow cells post mortem[4,5] (Fig. 5.1). This applies particularly to the neutrophil metamyelocytes and granulocytes which are rich in hydrolytic enzymes. Postmortem marrow aspirations and tissue sampling with a trephine needle should therefore be performed as soon after death as possible and preferably not more than 3 h after death. Vacuolation of the cytoplasm of granulocytes may be first seen in smears of marrow aspirated 1.5–7 h after death and the vacuolation increases progressively thereafter. Swelling of the nuclei of neutrophil metamyelocytes and granulocytes may be detected as early as 2 h after death; the swelling causes the affected metamyelocytes to look like myelocytes. By 8–12 h post mortem, most of the nuclei of the neutrophil metamyelocytes and granulocytes appear rounded, with a

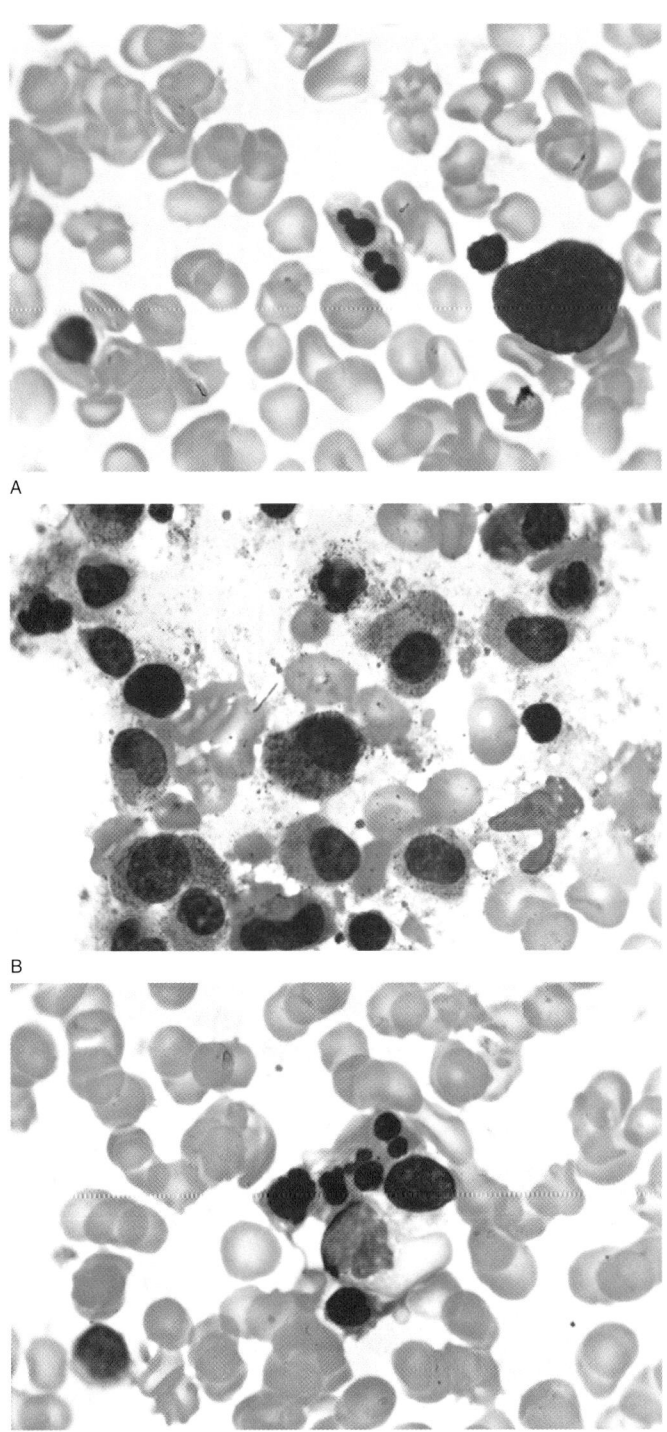

A

B

C

Fig. 5.1 (A–C) Marrow smear prepared from aspirates taken 30 and 82 h post mortem. (A) Two erythroblasts showing dumb-bell-shaped nuclei. (B) Normal-looking and degenerating cells of the neutrophil series. The latter have many coarse cytoplasmic granules and round nuclei. (C) Five erythroblasts. Two of these show nuclear budding, one has a dumb-bell-shaped nucleus and another shows lobulation of the nucleus. May–Grünwald–Giemsa stain. Courtesy of Dr N Francis.

loosening of the nuclear chromatin and the appearance of structures resembling small nucleoli. The nuclear membrane is ruptured and many of the cells have indistinct

cell membranes. The neutrophil myelocytes begin to lyse after 7–12 h. Karyorrhexis and budding, lobulation or segmentation of erythroblast nuclei may begin as an agonal event or during the first 2 h after death; in occasional cases, over 20% of erythroblasts show nuclear abnormalities 25 min post mortem, but in others marked changes do not develop in less than 3 h. Macrophages are greatly increased in number in aspirates taken within hours of death, probably mainly because they are released into the aspirate more readily than from living marrow. The post-mortem appearances of marrow aspirated 10–20 h after death differ markedly from those obtained during life and are sufficiently confusing to have led to the incorrect diagnosis of leukemia or malignant infiltration.

Alterations of the marrow in disease

The alterations that may be seen in the marrow include changes in cellularity, alterations in the proportions or morphology of various types of marrow cells, hemophagocytosis, changes in iron stores and intraerythroblastic iron, the presence of specific microorganisms and the formation of granulomas, infiltration by malignant cells, fibrosis, presence of storage cells, necrosis, gelatinous transformation, deposition of amyloid, and vascular and embolic lesions. Marrow cells may also show various cytogenetic abnormalities in some diseases and these are discussed in sections dealing with specific disorders.

Alterations in cellularity

The method of assessing the proportion of the marrow tissue that is composed of hemopoietic cells as opposed to fat cells (percentage cellularity) and the normal values for this parameter are discussed in Chapters 2 and 3. Hypocellularity (i.e. cellularity <25%) is seen in the acquired aplastic or hypoplastic anemias, Fanconi's syndrome, paroxysmal nocturnal hemoglobinuria, rare cases of acute leukemia, and in normal adults over the age of 70 years. Hypercellularity (cellularity >75%) may be seen in a variety of conditions, including hemolytic anemia, hemorrhage, megaloblastic and sideroblastic anemias, the congenital dyserythropoietic anemias, polycythemia rubra vera and other chronic myeloproliferative disorders, infections, malignant disease, myelodysplastic syndromes, the leukemias and in normal infants and young children.

Alterations in the frequency and morphology of various types of marrow cells

Erythroblasts and neutrophil precursors

Myeloid/erythroid ratio

The myeloid/erythroid ratio (M/E ratio) is often defined as the ratio between the number of cells of the neutrophil granulocyte series (including mature granulocytes) and the number of erythroblasts. The normal range for this ratio in adults has been reported as 2.0–8.3[6] and 1.1–5.2[7] in marrow smears and 1.5–3.0 in histologic sections. Some hematologists include eosinophils, basophils and monocytes, and their precursors in the 'myeloid' figure but this has only a slight effect on the values for the M/E ratio in normal subjects. The M/E ratio can be used as an index of total erythropoietic activity in patients in whom there is reason to assume that the total number of marrow granulocytes and their precursors is normal (e.g. in patients with normal counts of circulating granulocytes). Conversely, the M/E ratio may be used as an index of total granulocytopoietic activity, provided that the total number of erythroblasts in the body may be assumed to be normal. Some causes of a reduced or increased M/E ratio are listed in Table 5.1.

Morphologic changes in erythroblasts

Most of the erythroblasts in normal bone marrow are uninucleate, show synchrony between nuclear and cytoplasmic maturity and do not display any peculiar cytologic features. In one study of normal marrow, only 0.136 ± 0.04 ($\pm$ s.d.)% erythroblasts were binucleate[8] and in a more recent study this figure was 0.31% (range 0–0.57%).[9] In the latter study, 0.24% (range 0–0.91%) of normal erythroblasts showed basophilic stippling of the cytoplasm, up to 0.7% had vacuolated cytoplasm, 2.38% (range 0.72–4.77%) had intererythroblastic cytoplasmic bridges and 0.22% (range 0–0.55%) possessed markedly irregular or karyorrhectic nuclei (see Fig. 2.5C). Howell–Jolly bodies were found in 0.18% (range 0–0.39%) and asynchrony between nuclear and cytoplasmic maturation was found very infrequently. In various diseases accompanied by a disturbance of erythropoiesis, the frequency with which such cytologic features ('dysplastic' changes) are found is increased (Table 5.2); hence these cytologic 'aberrations' are described as dyserythropoietic changes. Morphologic abnormalities which are not encountered in normal marrow such as internuclear chromatin bridges and giant erythroblasts may also be found in a few diseases

(Table 5.2). Dyserythropoiesis occurs in a number of congenital and acquired disorders. The congenital disorders include some thalassemia syndromes, homozygosity for hemoglobin C or E, some unstable hemoglobins, hereditary sideroblastic anemias, thiamine-responsive anemia, homozygosity for pyruvate kinase deficiency, congenital myelodysplasia and the congenital dyserythropoietic anemias. The acquired disorders include vitamin B_{12} and folate deficiency, iron-deficiency anemia, alcohol abuse, acquired myelodysplastic syndromes, acute myeloid leukemia, aplastic anemia, paroxysmal nocturnal

Table 5.1 Causes of alterations in myeloid/erythroid (M/E) ratio

Reduced M/E ratio due to erythroid hyperplasia:
Hemorrhagic and hemolytic states
Megaloblastic anemias
Sideroblastic anemias
Congenital dyserythropoietic anemias
Polycythemia rubra vera
Secondary polycythemia
Myelodysplastic syndromes
Erythroleukemia

Reduced M/E ratio due to decreased total granulocytopoiesis:
Certain drugs
Radiotherapy
Some cases of aplastic anemia

Increased M/E ratio due to erythroid hypoplasia:
Pure red cell aplasia
Some cases of anemia of chronic disorders

Increased M/E ratio due to increased total granulocytopoiesis:
Infections
Malignant disease
Tissue necrosis
Non-infective inflammatory disease
Hypersplenism
Severe congenital neutropenia
During recovery from marrow suppression

Table 5.2 Morphologic abnormalities in erythroblasts that may be detected in pathologic states using the light microscope

Increased proportion of cells with:
Irregularly shaped nuclei
Karyorrhexis
Howell–Jolly bodies
Binuclearity or multinuclearity
Intercellular cytoplasmic bridges
Basophilic stippling of cytoplasm
Orthochromatic cytoplasm
Vacuolation of cytoplasm

Internuclear chromatin bridges

Megaloblasts

Excess of coarse acid-ferrocyanide-positive siderotic granules (abnormal sideroblasts)

Ringed sideroblasts

Gigantoblasts (mononucleate or multinucleate)

hemoglobinuria, acquired immunodeficiency syndrome (AIDS), *Plasmodium falciparum* and *P. vivax* malaria, kala azar and liver disease. Dyserythropietic changes have also been reported after excess ingestion of kelp and after bone marrow transplantation.

Increased vacuolation of the cytoplasm of erythropoietic cells has been observed during treatment with chloramphenicol and as an effect of taking excess ethanol. It has also been reported in aplastic anemia associated with glue sniffing, in protein-energy malnutrition, riboflavin and phenylalanine deficiency, acute myeloid leukemia and hyperosmolar diabetic coma.[10] Increased vacuolation of both erythroid cells and granulocyte precursors is observed in Pearson's syndrome (a mitochondrial cytopathy).

When there is asynchrony between nuclear and cytoplasmic maturation in a substantial proportion of erythroblasts, erythropoiesis is described as being megaloblastic. A detailed description and the causes of megaloblastic erythropoiesis are given in Chapter 12.

Minor ultrastructural peculiarities are seen in some of the erythroblasts of normal individuals (Fig. 5.2). Thus, small autophagic vacuoles are found in 22% of erythroblast profiles, slight to substantial degrees of myelinization of the nuclear membrane in 12%, short (250–910 nm) stretches of 'duplication' of the nuclear membrane in 2%, short (260–520 nm) intranuclear clefts in 1.7% and iron-laden mitochondria in less than 0.2%.[11] Although all of the above-mentioned ultrastructural features are sometimes described as dyserythropoietic, it is likely that at least the autophagic vacuoles and the myelinization of membranes are the morphologic manifestations of degradative processes which play an important physiologic role during normal erythropoiesis.

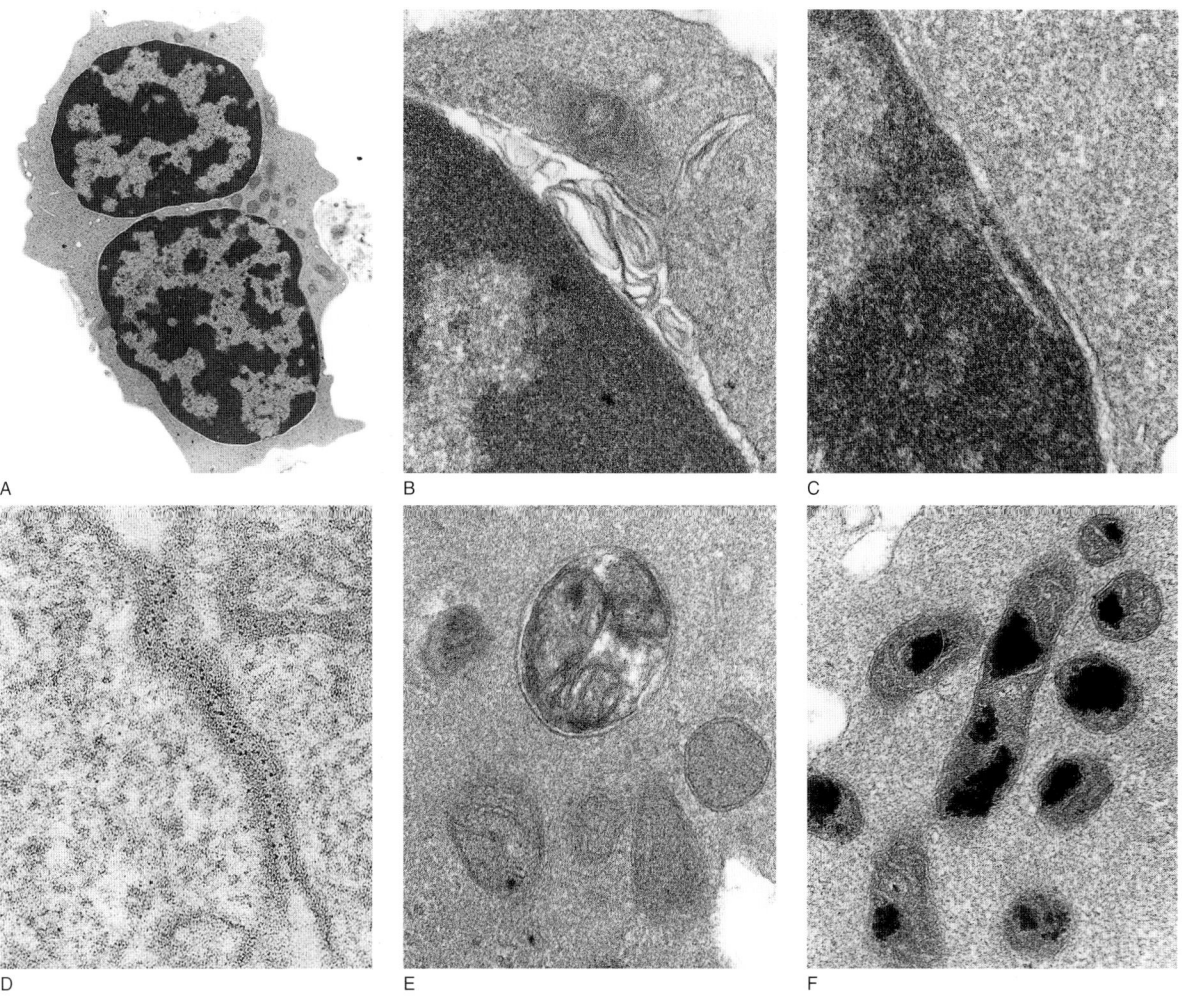

Fig. 5.2 (A–F) Ultrastructural peculiarities affecting some normal erythropoietic cells. (A) Binucleate polychromatic erythroblast. (B) Myelination of a short stretch of the nuclear membrane. (C) Short intranuclear cleft. (D) Area of intercellular interaction with ferritin molecules between the opposing cell membranes. (E) Autophagic vacuole containing three mitochondria. (F) Iron-laden mitochondria (rare). Uranyl acetate and lead citrate. (A) × 7050; (B) × 55 850; (C) × 54 450; (D) × 82 300; (E) × 45 375; (F) × 39 725.

Various ultrastructural abnormalities are seen in the erythropoietic cells of patients with disturbed erythropoiesis;[12] these are listed in Table 5.3 and illustrated in Figs 5.3 and 5.4. Although most of these are not specific for any particular disease, certain patterns of abnormality are characteristic of specific diseases or groups of diseases. For example, although a short stretch of double membrane may be found parallel to the cell membrane in an occasional erythroblast in other diseases, the presence of long stretches of double membrane 40–60 nm away from and parallel to one quarter or more of the cell membrane in a substantial proportion of the erythroblasts is a characteristic feature of congenital dyserythropoietic anemia type II.

Morphologic changes in the neutrophil series

These include the absence of specific granules in the myelocytes and metamyelocytes in acute leukemia and myelodysplastic syndromes, the reduction of nuclear segmentation in the marrow granulocytes in cases of the inherited and acquired Pelger–Huët anomaly and the formation of giant metamyelocytes and macropolycytes in vitamin B_{12} or folate deficiency. Giant metamyelocytes may also be found, usually in small numbers, in the absence of evidence of vitamin B_{12} or folate deficiency, in iron deficiency, infections, malignant disease, falciparum malaria (especially chronic falciparum malaria) and

protein-energy malnutrition. They are seen quite often in the bone marrow of patients with AIDS.[13] Macropolycytes are also not specific for vitamin B_{12} or folate deficiency, being found in infections, chronic myeloproliferative disorders, drug-induced marrow damage and protein-energy malnutrition. Increased numbers of binucleate cells of the neutrophil series occur in protein-energy malnutrition and to a lesser extent in vitamin B_{12} or folate deficiency. Macropolycytes and binucleate cells are sometimes seen in myelodysplastic syndromes. An increased proportion of neutrophils with ring- or doughnut-shaped nuclei may be seen in chronic granulocytic leukemia, acute myeloid leukemia, chronic neutrophilic leukemia, the myelodysplastic syndromes, AIDS and falciparum malaria.

Vacuolation of the neutrophil precursors, usually from the promyelocyte/myelocyte stage onwards, may be seen in patients with acute alcoholic intoxication, severe infections, drug-induced marrow damage (e.g. chloramphenicol toxicity), protein-energy malnutrition and certain rare conditions such as the Chédiak–Higashi syndrome, severe congenital neutropenia, hereditary transcobalamin II deficiency[14] and Jordans' anomaly (familial vacuolation of leukocytes).[15] Giant metamyelocytes, whatever the condition with which they are associated, may also be vacuolated.

Detached nuclear fragments in neutrophils, resembling Howell–Jolly bodies in erythrocytes, are occasionally

Table 5.3 Ultrastructural abnormalities that may be detected in erythroblasts in pathologic states

Non-specific abnormalities; of little diagnostic value
Long membrane-bound intranuclear clefts (> 600 nm)
Absence, extensive myelinization or reduplication of large parts of the nuclear membrane
Separation of the nuclear membrane from the heterochromatin
Widening of the space between the two layers of the nuclear membrane
Intranuclear inclusions (mitochondria, myelin figures)
Different ultrastructural appearance of different nuclei within the same multinucleate cell
Fusion of two or more nuclei in a multinucleate cell
Deposition of ribosomes on the cytoplasmic surface of the nuclear membrane
Mitochondrial degeneration (swelling, loss of cristae, iron loading in a small proportion of cells)
Abnormally large siderosomes (diameter > 300 nm)
Large intracytoplasmic autophagic vacuoles (diameter ≥ 290 nm), sometimes containing degenerating mitochondria or myelin figures
Large myelin figures lying free within the cytoplasm
Intracytoplasmic lipid droplets
Annulate lamellae
Clustering of degenerating cytoplasmic organelles near the nucleus
Scarcity of ribosomes
Reduction in electron-density of cytoplasmic matrix
Specialized regions of contact between erythroblasts

Abnormalities of diagnostic value
Iron-laden mitochondria in many erythroblasts (sideroblastic anemias)
Intracytoplasmic inclusions consisting of precipitated α- or β-globin chains (thalassemia syndromes)
Large rhomboidal crystals of deoxygenated HbC within red cells (HbC disease)
'Swiss-cheese' appearance of the heterochromatin in many erythroblasts (CDA type I)
Presence of a double membrane 40–60 nm away from and parallel to the cell membrane in several cells (CDA type II)

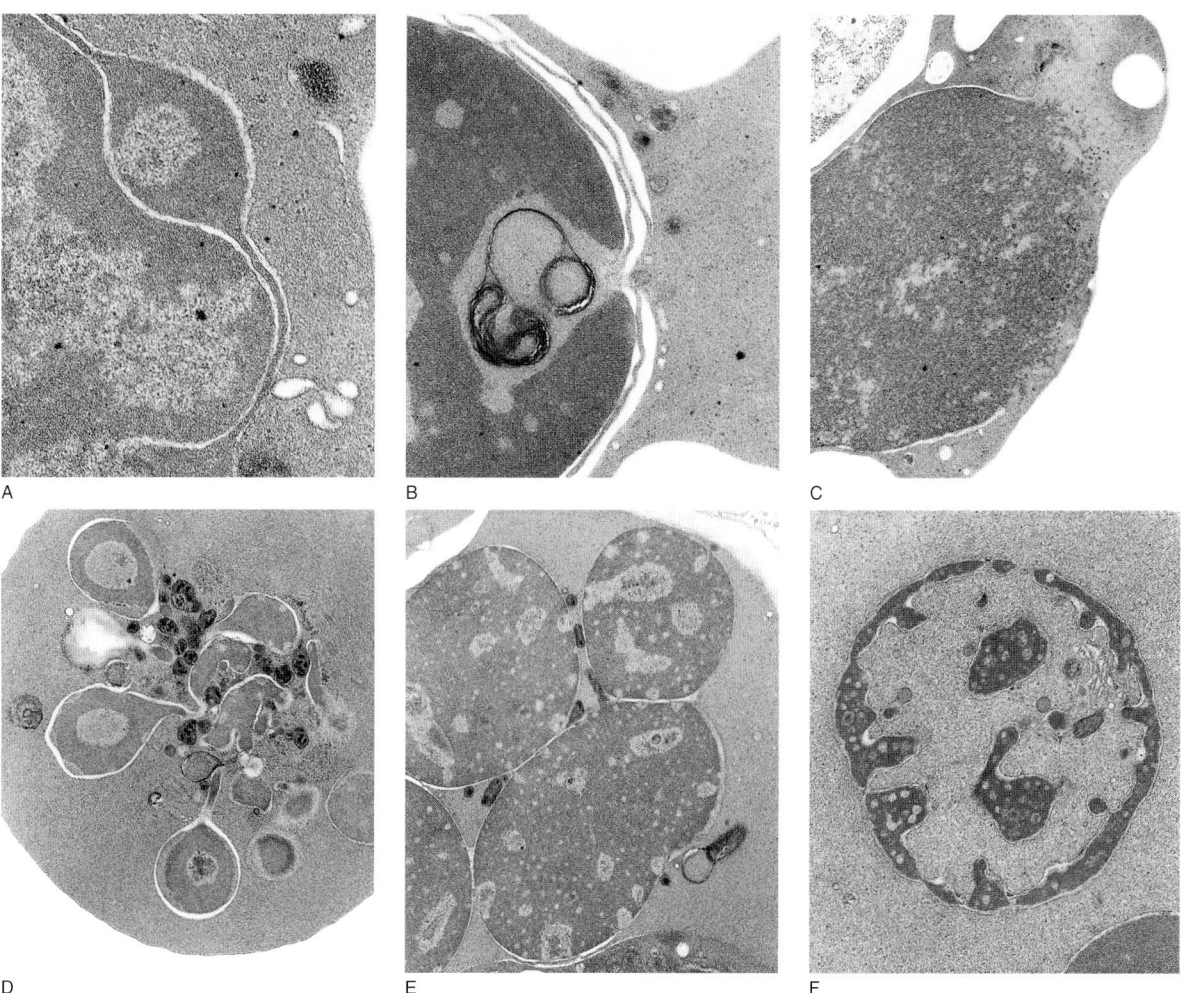

Fig. 5.3 (A–F) Examples of ultrastructural abnormalities affecting the nuclei of erythroblasts in disorders of erythropoiesis. (A) Large intranuclear cleft (megaloblastic anemia due to vitamin B_{12} deficiency). (B) Duplication of the nuclear membrane and an intranuclear myelin figure (HbS/β-thalassemia). (C) Loss of part of the nuclear membrane and oozing of nuclear material into the cytoplasm (HbC disease). (D) Karyorrhexis and clumping of iron-laden mitochondria at the center of the cell (congenital dyserythropoietic anemia, type III). (E) Fusion of nuclei within a multinucleate erythroblast (congenital dyserythropoietic anemia, type III). (F) 'Swiss-cheese' nucleus (congenital dyserythropoietic anemia, type III). This type of nuclear abnormality is diagnostic of congenital dyserythropoietic anemia (CDA), type I, when found in about half the erythroblasts, but may also be found in occasional erythroblasts in other forms of CDA and in other diseases associated with dyserythropoiesis such as hemoglobin Q-H disease, megaloblastic anemias, *Plasmodium vivax* malaria and AIDS. Uranyl acetate and lead citrate. (A) × 36 500; (B) × 23 100; (C) × 13 300; (D) × 8300; (E) × 8700; (F) × 10 000.

seen as a reversible drug-induced anomaly but more often they are indicative of HIV infection. Other morphologic abnormalities that may be seen in the neutrophil series in HIV infection are listed in Table 5.9.

Eosinophil series

An increase of eosinophils and their precursors, sometimes without an associated eosinophilia in the peripheral blood, may be seen in parasitic infections, allergic disorders, certain skin diseases, Hodgkin's disease, carcinoma and collagen vascular diseases. A marrow and

peripheral blood eosinophilia is also seen in the idiopathic hypereosinophilic syndrome, chronic granulocytic leukemia, other chronic myeloproliferative disorders and eosinophilic leukemia.

Basophils

An increase of basophils in the marrow may be seen in chronic granulocytic leukemia and myelofibrosis. Basophils are generally not detected in formalin-fixed tissues, since basophil granules are water-soluble.

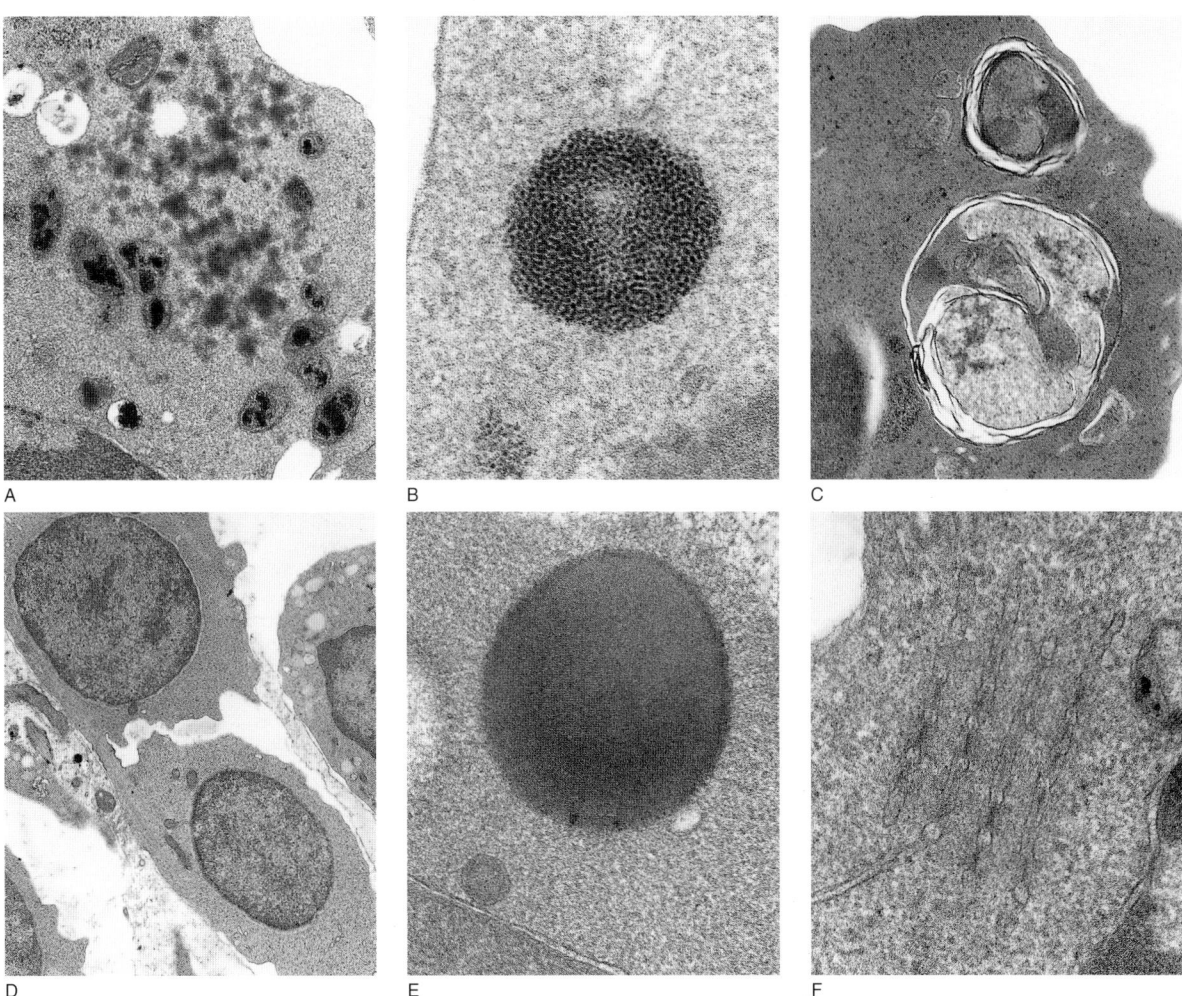

Fig. 5.4 (A–F) Examples of ultrastructural abnormalities affecting the cytoplasm of erythroblasts in disorders of erythropoiesis. (A) Multiple small electron-dense inclusions of precipitated α-globin chains associated with iron-laden mitochondria (HbE/β-thalassemia). (B) Large siderosome that is not enclosed within a membrane; note that the individual ferritin molecules within the siderosome can be readily identified (HbS/β-thalassemia). (C) Two large autophagic vacuoles containing myelin figures (HbC disease). (D) Intercellular cytoplasmic bridge containing microtubules of the mitotic spindle (homozygosity for HbE). (E) Intracytoplasmic lipid droplet (congenital dyserythropoietic anemia, type III). (F) Annulate lamellae (thiamine-responsive anemia). Uranyl acetate and lead citrate. (A) × 22 750; (B) × 99 000; (C) × 24 400; (D) × 7200; (E) × 47 500; (F) × 51 000.

Mast cells

Mast cells may be increased in the marrow in infection and inflammation, renal failure, aplastic anemia, paroxysmal nocturnal hemoglobinuria, Waldenström's macroglobulinemia, chronic lymphocytic leukemia, non-Hodgkin's lymphoma, myelodysplastic states, scleroderma, systemic mastocytosis (in which the mast cells are neoplastic) and less often in a variety of other conditions.[16–18] Mast cells are difficult to recognize in sections stained with H&E but are detectable when stained with a Giemsa stain, which stains the granules purple. The granules also stain by the PAS reaction, are α-naphthyl AS-D chloroacetate esterase-positive[19] (positive Leder stain) and stain metachromatically with toluidine blue.

Megakaryocytes

Conditions associated with an increased number of megakaryocytes include chronic granulocytic leukemia, polycythemia rubra vera, essential thrombocythemia, myelofibrosis, infections, chronic alcoholism, malignant disease, Hodgkin's disease, other lymphomas and hemorrhage. They also include diseases such as 'idiopathic' (autoimmune) thrombocytopenic purpura and thrombotic thrombocytopenic purpura in which thrombocytopenia is primarily caused by a reduced platelet life span (Chapter 26). In sections of normal marrow there are clusters of megakaryocytes with up to three cells per cluster. Larger clusters are seen in essential thrombocythemia but not reactive thrombocytosis as well as during regeneration of the marrow after chemotherapy and bone marrow transplantation.

A decreased number of megakaryocytes is seen in acute leukemia, Fanconi's anemia and other constitutional aplastic anemias, the syndrome of thrombocytopenia with absent radii, and acquired aplastic anemia. The morphological abnormalities which may affect megakaryocytes in HIV infection are described later in this Chapter and those found in inherited disorders are reviewed in Chapter 25.

Lymphocytes

Lymphocytes are more numerous in the bone marrow in children than in adults (Chapter 2). An artifactual increase in the percentage of lymphocytes occurs if a bone marrow aspirate is much diluted with peripheral blood. Bone marrow lymphocytes are increased in many reactive and malignant conditions in which there is a peripheral blood lymphocytosis (e.g. infectious mononucleosis, chronic lymphocytic leukemia). In addition, bone marrow lymphocytes may be increased in the absence of a peripheral blood lymphocytosis in Waldenström's macroglobulinemia and non-Hodgkin's lymphoma. The majority of lymphocytes in normal bone marrow are T-cells (usually CD8[+]), and bone marrow infiltration is more likely to be seen in B-lymphoproliferative disorders.

A trephine biopsy will show whether a lymphocytic infiltrate is diffuse or focal and whether there is any follicle formation (see Chapter 3). In normal marrow, lymphocytes are spread diffusely through the marrow but small aggregates or nodules also develop, and rarely they may have germinal centers.[20–22] The incidence of such lymphoid aggregates rises with age,[19] and an increased incidence is seen in pernicious anemia,[21] chronic myeloproliferative disorders, hemolytic states, inflammatory reactions[18] and autoimmune conditions such as rheumatoid arthritis. Bone marrow biopsies showing lymphoid aggregates are more likely than other bone marrow biopsies to show lipid granulomas and plasmacytosis.[21] A malignant lymphocytic infiltrate may be diffuse or focal and occasionally a follicular pattern is seen (detailed in Chapters 21 and 22). A paratrabecular pattern of infiltration is characteristic of certain non-Hodgkin's lymphomas. It may be difficult to distinguish focal lymphomatous infiltrates from benign hyperplasia of lymphoid follicles. The latter tend to be more circumscribed and smaller with some admixture of histiocytes, eosinophils and plasma cells [21,23] and, unless a germinal center is present, consist of well-differentiated cells (also see Chapter 22).[21]

Plasma cells

There are less than 1–2% of plasma cells in normal bone marrow. An increased percentage of plasma cells may be found in the marrow in a wide range of pathologic conditions (Table 5.4). In various non-neoplastic conditions, up to 50% of nucleated marrow cells may be plasma cells (reactive plasmacytosis).[24–26] It is sometimes difficult to distinguish between reactive plasmacytosis and multiple myeloma on the basis of the morphologic characteristics of the plasma cells. Some differences are shown in Table 5.5. Russell bodies, Mott cells (see Chapter 2) and intranuclear inclusions resembling Russell bodies (Dutcher–Fahey bodies) may be seen in both reactive conditions and multiple myeloma but intranuclear inclusions are more often seen in myeloma. Cells with flaming cytoplasm may be found in both reactive plasmacytosis and myeloma but a substantial proportion of such cells is more likely in myeloma. Examination of the distribution of plasma cells in histologic sections of bone marrow is of considerable value in elucidating the cause of plasmacytosis since homogeneous nodules of these cells, with little supporting stroma, are found in myeloma but not in reactive plasmacytosis (Table 5.5). Myeloma cells may show hemophagocytosis.[29] Hemosiderin-containing granules are sometimes found in the cytoplasm of plasma cells in alcoholics and in porphyria cutanea tarda, megaloblastic anemia, refractory normoblastic anemia and iron overload.[30,31]

Macrophages (histiocytes)

An increase of macrophages in the bone marrow is common in a wide variety of hematologic and non-

Table 5.4 Causes of plasmacytosis in the bone marrow

Reactive polyclonal plasmacytosis[24,25]	
Infection and inflammation	*Immunologic disorders*
Viral infection including AIDS	Hypersensitivity states
Bacterial infection	Autoimmune disorders
Pyrexia of unknown origin	including AITP
Chronic inflammatory disorders	
	Miscellaneous
Malignant disease	Iron-deficiency anemia
Carcinoma	Megaloblastic anemia
Hodgkin's disease	Marrow hypoplasia
Non-Hodgkin's lymphoma	Cirrhosis
Chronic granulocytic leukemia	

Monoclonal plasmacytosis
Monoclonal gammopathy of uncertain significance
Light-chain-derived amyloidosis
Systemic light chain disease
Multiple myeloma

AITP, autoimmune thrombocytopenic purpura.

Table 5.5 Characteristics of bone marrow plasma cells in reactive plasmacytosis and multiple myeloma[25–27]

	Reactive plasmacytosis	Multiple myeloma
Number	Up to 10–20%, rarely 50%	Usually 30–90%
Cytology	Most cells are mature and look like normal plasma cells	More cells show features of immaturity; cells are either pleomorphic or monomorphic; occasionally lymphoid
	Majority of cells are mononucleate; 4 nuclei per cell rare	Multinuclearity common
	Nucleoli only in occasional cells	Nucleoli common
	Nucleocytoplasmic asynchrony usually not a prominent feature	Nucleocytoplasmic asynchrony common
Distribution	Interstitial infiltrate, especially perivascular; some cells may be aggregated around macrophages	Commonly near endosteal surface as well as perivascular
	Small clusters of plasma cells may be present but large homogeneous nodules are absent	Large homogeneous nodules of plasma cells with little intervening hemopoietic tissue common
	Broad band-like infiltrates very rare	Broad band-like infiltrates common
Immunocytochemistry	κ:λ ratio about 2:1[28]	Monotypic κ- or λ-chains

hematologic conditions. These include various infective and inflammatory disorders, conditions associated with increased blood cell destruction or increased ineffective hemopoiesis and post-granulocyte–macrophage colony-stimulating factor (GM-CSF) therapy. The macrophages range from immature cells showing little phagocytic activity to mature cells containing phagocytosed material or foamy cytoplasm. In most instances the increase in macrophages is reactive. However, in malignant histiocytosis the increase results from the proliferation of a malignant clone. The two features that distinguish malignant histiocytosis from reactive macrophage hyperplasia are: (1) pleomorphism of macrophages, with immature and atypical features such as a prominent nucleolus, distinct and thick nuclear membrane, irregular nuclear chromatin and multinuclearity;[32,33] and (2) the presence amongst the macrophages and large multinucleate cells of many monoblasts and promonocytes[34] (Fig. 5.5). Cytochemical reactions of the malignant cells are similar to those of monocytes and macrophages; they are positive for non-specific esterase, acid phosphatase and lysozyme. The number of malignant cells in the bone marrow varies from 5 to 90%[34] and the infiltration of the marrow may be focal or diffuse (Fig. 5.6). The blood count may show anemia, leukopenia, thrombocytopenia and eosinophilia and the peripheral blood film may contain macrophages and small numbers of monoblasts. A minor degree of hemophagocytosis is common (Fig. 5.7); when malignant histiocytosis is associated with marked erythrophagocytosis, the designation 'histiocytic medullary reticulosis' is sometimes used. However, it is now apparent that the majority of patients initially

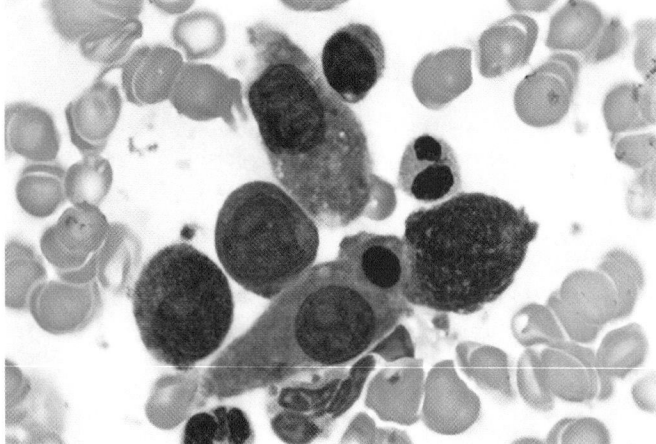

Fig. 5.5 Marrow smear from a patient with malignant histiocytosis showing a monoblast, a promonocyte and two macrophages. May–Grünwald–Giemsa stain.

described as having 'histiocytic medullary reticulosis' actually had a reactive hemophagocytic syndrome and the observation of striking erythrophagocytosis should raise the suspicion of a reactive rather than malignant condition.

Hemophagocytic syndromes[35]

In the hemophagocytic syndrome, there is a deregulation of T-lymphocytes and excessive production of cytokines leading to macrophage hyperplasia, enhanced macrophage activity and increased phagocytosis by macrophages of red cells, granulocytes, platelets and hemopoietic cells. The clinico-pathologic features of the syndrome include fever,

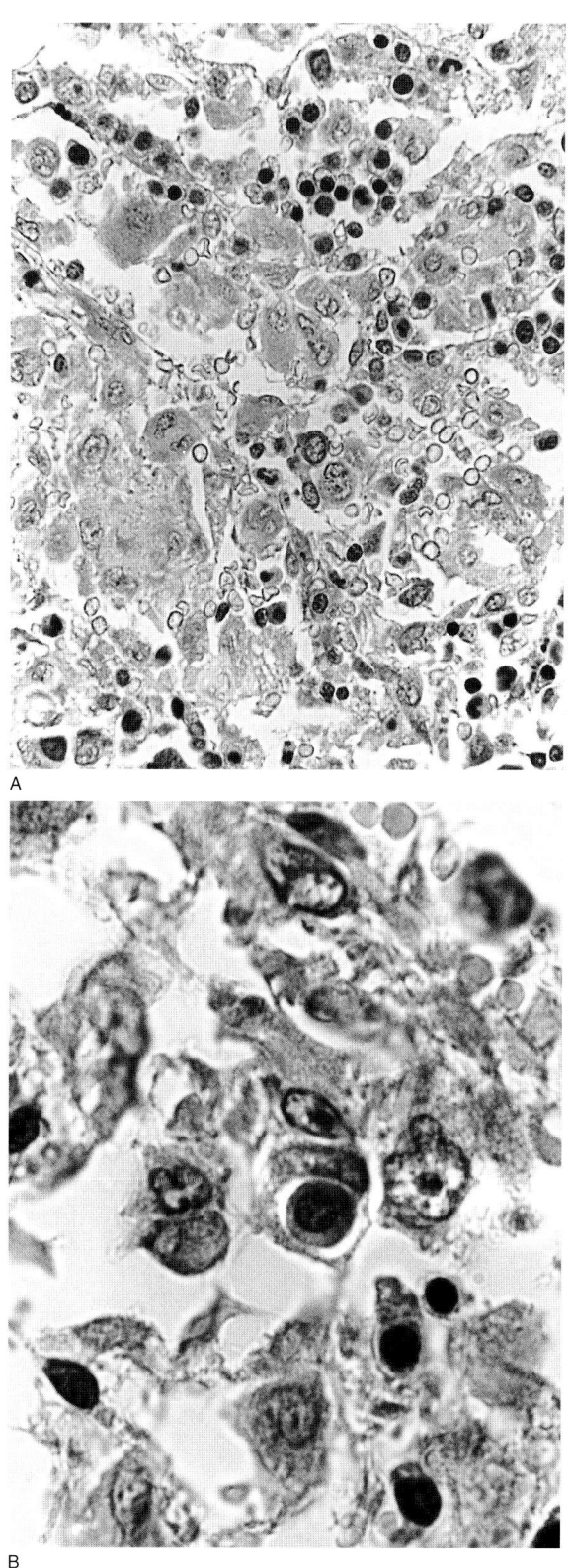

A

B

Fig. 5.6 (A,B) Trephine biopsy of the bone marrow of a patient with malignant histiocytosis. (A) The marrow is diffusely infiltrated with large malignant histiocytes. (B) Higher-power view of the section shown in (A). The malignant histiocyte in the centre contains a phagocytosed hemopoietic cell. H&E. (A) × 94; (B) × 940.

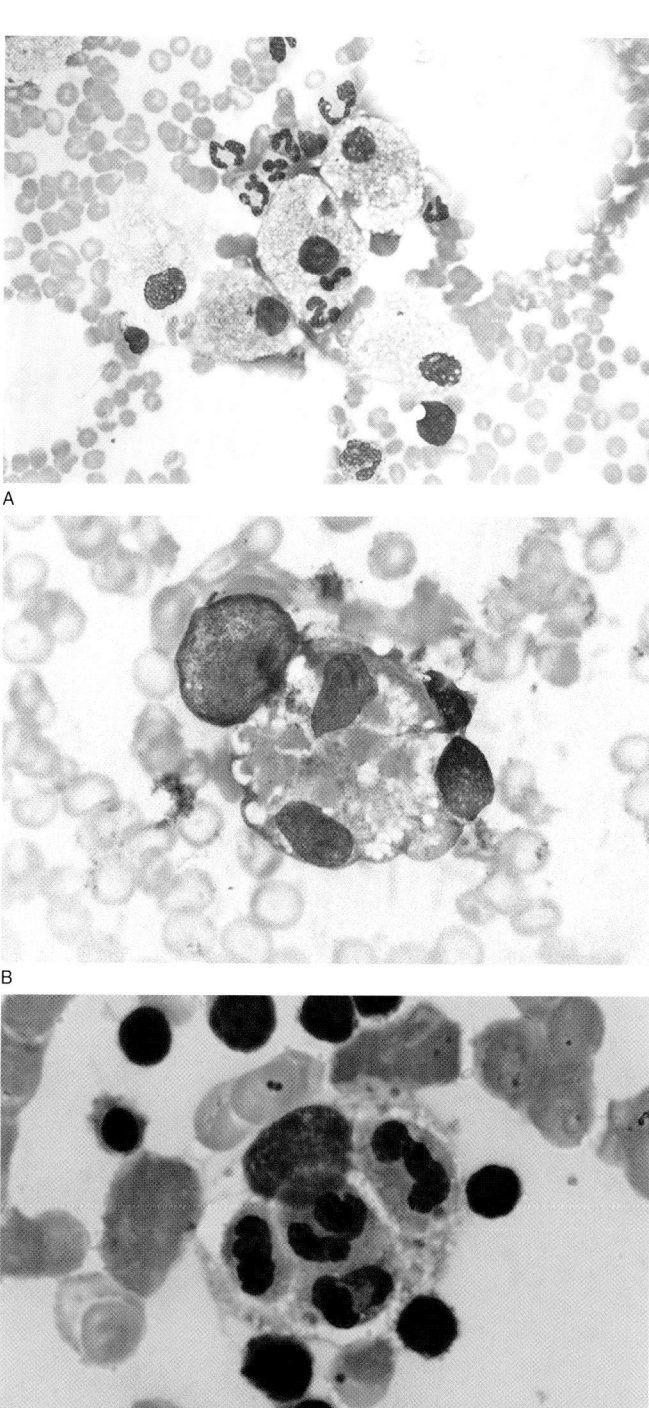

A

B

C

Fig. 5.7 Marrow smears from patients with infection-associated hemophagocytic syndromes. (A) Gram-negative septicemia. (B) Tuberculosis. (C) Acute *P. falciparum* malaria. The central foamy macrophage in (A) contains two ingested neutrophils and an ingested red cell. The macrophage in (B) contains several red cells and that in (C) contains four granulocytes. May–Grünwald–Giemsa stain.

hepatosplenomegaly, lymphadenopathy, skin rash, neurologic abnormalities, cytopenias, hypertriglyceridemia, high serum ferritin level and coagulopathy. Conditions associated with the hemophagocytic syndrome are listed in Table 5.6. In the 'primary' hemophagocytic syndrome, there is an inherited immune defect. Many cases of acquired hemophagocytic syndrome have an underlying predisposing condition leading to immunosuppression such as HIV infection, renal transplantation, malignant disease and autoimmune disease.[38] The most frequent cause of a virus-associated hemophagocytic syndrome is the Epstein–Barr (EB) virus. The many other causes of infection-associated hemophagocytic syndrome include tuberculosis and falciparum malaria (Fig. 5.7). Reactive macrophages containing phagocytosed blood or marrow cells can be distinguished on the basis of cytologic and cytochemical characteristics, from other malignant cells showing hemophagocytic activity such as cells of carcinomas of lung or breast,[67] medulloblastoma,[68] prolymphocytic leukemia,[69] acute lymphoblastic leukemia,[70] T-cell lymphoma[71] and multiple myeloma.[29]

Increased phagocytosis only of granulocyte lineage cells may be seen in drug-induced agranulocytosis[72] and increased erythrophagocytosis may be observed in hemolytic states such as autoimmune hemolytic anemia, malaria and sickle cell anemia.

An increase of bone marrow macrophages that do not show excessive hemophagocytic activity is commonly seen in reactive conditions such as viral infections, bacterial endocarditis, mycobacterial infections[73] and histoplasmosis.[74]

In lysosomal storage diseases, bone marrow macrophages are laden with lipid or mucopolysaccharide.

Osteoblasts and osteoclasts

Marrow smears contain increased numbers of osteoblasts and osteoclasts when there is enhanced bone remodeling. An increase is often seen in bone marrow aspirates containing metastatic malignant cells. Strongly PAS-positive, vacuolated osteoblasts have been reported in Pompe's disease (type II glycogen storage disease).[75]

Table 5.6 Conditions associated with the hemophagocytic syndrome

1. Familial hemophagocytic lymphohistiocytosis[36,37]	
2. Other reactive hemophagocytic syndromes	**3. Malignant histiocytosis**
Infection-associated[35]	Rickettsial infection
Viral infection[38,39]	Rocky Mountain spotted fever[53]
EB virus[40]	Q fever[54]
Other herpes viruses e.g. herpes simplex,[41]	*Rickettsia tsutsugamushi* infection[55]
varicella zoster	Fungal infection
Cytomegalovirus (CMV)	Histoplasmosis[39]
Human herpesvirus-6 (HHV-6)	Candidiasis[56]
Human herpesvirus-7 (HHV-7)	*Cryptococcus*
Human herpesvirus-8 (HHV-8)	Trichosporonosis[57]
Parvovirus B19[42]	Parasitic infection
Hepatitis viruses B,C or A	*Leishmania donovani*
Hantavirus	*Babesia microti*[58]
Adenovirus[38]	*Toxoplasma gondii*[59]
Parainfluenza type III[43,44]	*Pneumocystis carinii*
Rubella[45]	Malaria
Measles	*Disease-associated*[a]
Dengue[46]	Malignant disease
Coxsackie	Lymphomas, particularly T- and NK-cell
Influenza A	lymphomas[60–65]
Bacterial infection	Acute leukemia
Pyogenic bacteria	Breast cancer, gastric cancer[66]
Mycobacterium tuberculosis[47]	Non-malignant disease
Atypical mycobacterial infection	AIDS
Brucellosis[48]	Autoimmune disease (SLE)
Salmonella typhi[49]	Chediak–Higashi syndrome
Mycoplasma pneumoniae[50]	Weber–Christian disease
Legionella pneumophila[51]	*Drug-associated*
Ehrlichia[52]	Phenytoin
Chlamydiae	

[a] The association with these diseases is likely to be the result of disease- or treatment-related immune deficiency.

Changes in iron stores and intraerythroblastic iron

Iron stores

In the bone marrow, storage iron is normally present in the form of ferritin and hemosiderin and is mainly within the macrophages but also in endothelial cells. The stores of hemosiderin can be assessed by examining marrow smears or histologic sections of either trephine biopsies or aspirated marrow fragments. In unstained smears and sections and in H&E-stained sections, hemosiderin granules appear as golden-yellow or brown refractile particles. In preparations stained by Perls' acid ferrocyanide method (Prussian blue method), the hemosiderin appears as blue or bluish-black granules that may vary considerably in size. Various methods of grading hemosiderin stores semiquantitatively have been employed by different authors and one such method used in the study of both marrow smears and histologic sections is given in Table 5.7. In practice, it is adequate to grade hemosiderin iron as absent (or greatly reduced), present or increased. The average size of individual hemosiderin granules increases with increasing iron stores from small (diameter 0.5–2 μm) to large (diameter >4 μm); in subjects with normal erythropoiesis most marrow hemosiderin granules are medium-sized (2–4 μm) or small. There have been conflicting reports regarding the relative merits of the use of smears and histologic sections of bone marrow for the assessment of iron stores.[76–78] The discrepancies in the published data may have resulted at least partly from technical differences in the processing of the material for histology in the different studies because prolonged treatment of trephine biopsies in decalcifying solutions may cause leaching of hemosiderin. In view of this possibility, the best methods for the assessment of iron stores in the marrow would appear to be the study (after staining for iron) of: (1) a large number of aspirated marrow fragments in smears;

(2) semi-thin sections of plastic-embedded (and un-decalcified) trephine biopsy specimens; or (3) histologic sections of adequate numbers of aspirated marrow fragments. Marrow hemosiderin stores are either absent or virtually absent in iron-deficiency anemia from any cause. Rarely, patients recently treated with large doses of iron dextran may develop iron-deficiency anemia in the presence of stainable iron in the marrow; in this situation the stainable iron is in a form that is unavailable for rapid mobilization.

Increased marrow hemosiderin may be found in hereditary hemochromatosis, transfusion-induced hemosiderosis, anemia of chronic disorders, hemolytic anemias with predominantly extravascular hemolysis (e.g. sickle cell anemia, pyruvate kinase deficiency, glucose-6-phosphate dehydrogenase [G6PD] deficiency), aplastic anemia and anemias associated with increased ineffective erythropoiesis. The latter include megaloblastic and sideroblastic anemias, certain thalassemia syndromes even in the absence of repeated transfusions, congenital dyserythropoietic anemia and erythremic myelosis. A number of mechanisms operate to increase marrow hemosiderin stores in various types of anemia. As two-thirds of the total body iron is normally present as hemoglobin within circulating erythrocytes, an anemia that is not primarily due to iron deficiency and is unassociated with hemorrhage will result in a redistribution of body iron with some increase of storage iron. In addition, because iron absorption via the gut is proportional to total erythropoiesis, patients with anemia associated with increased effective or ineffective erythropoiesis have an absolute increase in their total body iron due to increased iron absorption. The increase in iron absorption may, even in untransfused patients, eventually lead to hemosiderosis. Repeated transfusion for chronic anemia also causes a progressive increase of iron stores as the body has no effective mechanism for getting rid of excess iron. Signs and symptoms of hepatic, cardiac and endocrine dysfunction due to hemosiderosis are usually

Table 5.7 Criteria for grading iron stores in squashed marrow fragments or histological sections of marrow. The grading is based on examining the preparations at high magnification (× 1200). After Lundin *et al*[76]

Grade	Quantity of hemosiderin	Predominant hemosiderin particle size
0	None in whole preparation	–
Trace	One or few granules in whole preparation	–
1+	Few granules in every third or fourth field	Small (0.5–2 μm)
2+	Several granules in every second or third field	Small (0.5–2 μm) and medium (2–4 μm)
3+	Granules in every field, in one or more cells	Medium (2–4 μm)
4+	Massive hemosiderin deposits	Large (> 4 μm); granules often clumped

only seen after the transfusion of about 50 l of blood (equivalent to a total of about 25 g of iron).

There is a reasonable correlation between the cytochemical assessment of iron stores in stained preparations of marrow and biochemical determinations such as the iron content of the marrow or liver[79] or, with certain exceptions, the serum ferritin level. The causes of alterations in the serum ferritin level are given elsewhere (Chapter 11).

Alterations in stainable non-hemoglobin iron within erythroblasts

When normal marrow smears are stained by Perls' acid ferrocyanide method and examined at high magnification (e.g. × 950) using an oil immersion lens, 20–90% of the polychromatic erythroblasts are found to contain a few (one to five) very small (usually, barely visible) blue-staining granules randomly distributed in the cytoplasm.[80–82] Such granules are termed siderotic granules and the cells containing them sideroblasts. Ultrastructural studies indicate that the siderotic granules present in normal erythroblasts correspond to intracytoplasmic aggregates of altered ferritin molecules

(siderosomes or ferritin bodies) that may be membrane-bound (Fig. 5.8). In iron-deficiency anemia and the anemia of chronic disorders, the percentage of sideroblasts is decreased. By contrast, in a wide variety of diseases associated with an increase in the percentage saturation of transferrin (e.g hemolytic anemia, megaloblastic anemia, thalassemia, hereditary and secondary hemochromatosis), the number (per erythroblast) and size of siderotic granules are increased, but the granules remain randomly distributed. Erythroblasts showing this phenomenon are described as abnormal sideroblasts. Most of the siderotic granules of such erythroblasts also consist of siderosomes (albeit abnormally large ones) but a few consist of iron-laden mitochondria. In the sideroblastic anemias, there is an increase in both the coarseness and number (per erythroblast) of siderotic granules but additionally the majority of the granules tend to be distributed in either a partial or complete perinuclear ring; cells showing such perinuclear rings are termed ringed or ring sideroblasts; some authors require a ringed sideroblast to contain at least six perinuclear or paranuclear granules. Ultrastructural studies indicate that most of the siderotic granules within a ringed sideroblast consist of iron-laden mitochondria. The sideroblastic anemias are discussed in Chapter 14.

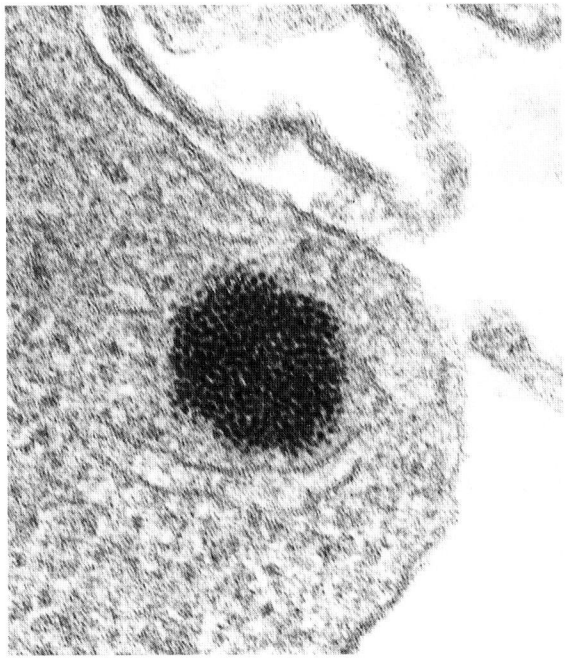
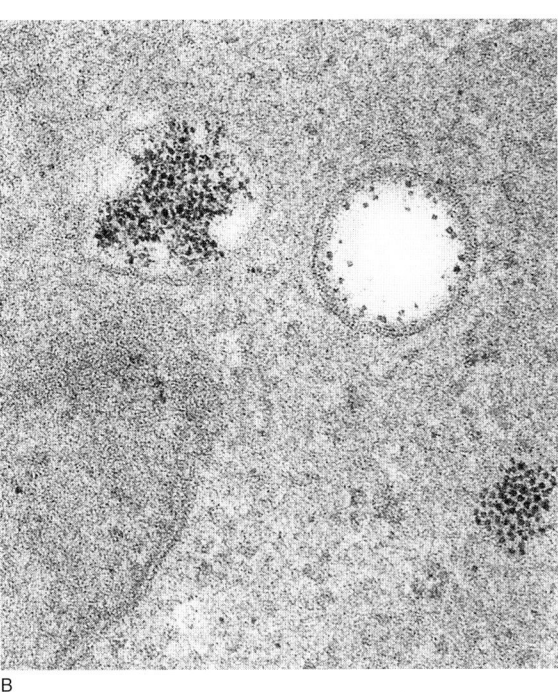

A   B

Fig. 5.8 (A, B) Different ultrastructural appearances of siderosomes in two erythroblasts from normal bone marrow. (A) Siderosome consisting of a densely packed aggregate of hemosiderin molecules. The aggregate does not appear to be enclosed within a membrane. (B) Siderosome consisting of a membrane-bound collection of hemosiderin granules (top left). The electron micrograph also shows a smaller aggregate of ferritin molecules (bottom right) and a rhopheocytotic vesicle lined by ferritin molecules. Uranyl acetate and lead citrate. (A) × 113 300; (B) × 120 400.

Infections and the bone marrow

In acute bacterial infections the bone marrow shows increased cellularity and an increased M/E ratio due to increased neutrophil granulocytopoiesis. Even when the cellularity of the marrow is greatly increased, some fat cells persist. The neutrophil series may show toxic granulation and the formation of Döhle bodies. The marrow may also contain occasional giant metamyelocytes. In severe infections there may be a marked reduction of the proportion of neutrophil granulocytes. In histologic sections of marrow, the spatial distribution of the granulocyte precursors is normal, with myeloblasts and promyelocytes located near the bone trabeculae. Some degree of erythroid hypoplasia is frequent in many infections and there are reduced numbers of siderotic granules within erythroblasts.

In microbial infections associated with monocytosis, the marrow may show an increased proportion of cells of the mononuclear phagocyte system. In occasional patients with some types of infection the macrophages show prominent hemophagocytosis (see Table 5.6 and Fig. 5.7). Certain infections are characterized by granulomatous lesions in the bone marrow (see below).

Microscopic examination of marrow smears and sections after staining with specific stains may be useful in diagnosing certain mycobacterial and fungal infections, especially but not exclusively in patients with granulomas. Fungi are usually seen in the marrow in immunocompromised patients and may be found extracellularly and within macrophages. In Whipple's disease, *Tropheryma whippelii*, which stain violet with Romanowsky stains and black with methenamine-silver, may be seen within bone marrow macrophages.[83]

In certain bacterial and fungal infections, the organisms can be cultured from marrow. In histoplasmosis, cryptococcosis, candidosis, blastomycosis and coccidioidomycosis, organisms may be demonstrated both by microscopy of smears or histologic sections and by culture.[74,84–86]

Chronic *Plasmodium falciparum* malaria in young children is associated with a marked increase of dyserythropoiesis and ineffective erythropoiesis.[87] Dyserythropoiesis is also seen in severe acute falciparum malaria, especially cerebral malaria. Bone marrow aspiration is not usually performed for the diagnosis of malaria and there is limited information on its value.[88] A bone marrow aspirate is helpful in making a retrospective diagnosis of *Plasmodium falciparum* malaria in an undiagnosed but treated patient; in this situation, malarial pigment will be present in marrow macrophages (Fig. 5.9). In post-mortem examinations of patients who have had recurrent attacks of falciparum malaria, malarial pigment is found in the marrow, spleen and liver.

Leishmaniasis may be diagnosed by studies of bone marrow smears or sections although culture of the bone marrow aspirate is more sensitive (Figs 5.10 and 5.11); occasionally, the organisms may also be seen in peripheral blood monocytes. As in the case of chronic falciparum malaria, the erythroblasts of patients with leishmaniasis show non-specific morphologic abnormalities indicative of dyserythropoiesis (Fig. 5.12).[89]

In viral infections, the bone marrow contains an increased number of normal or atypical lymphocytes. Especially in herpes virus infections, macrophages may show hemophagocytosis. In cytomegalovirus (CMV) infection the marrow may contain the typical giant cells with eosinophilic intranuclear inclusions.[90] Infection by

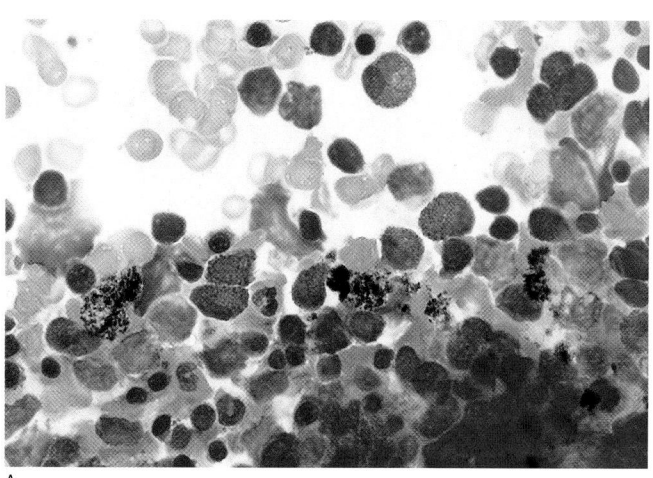
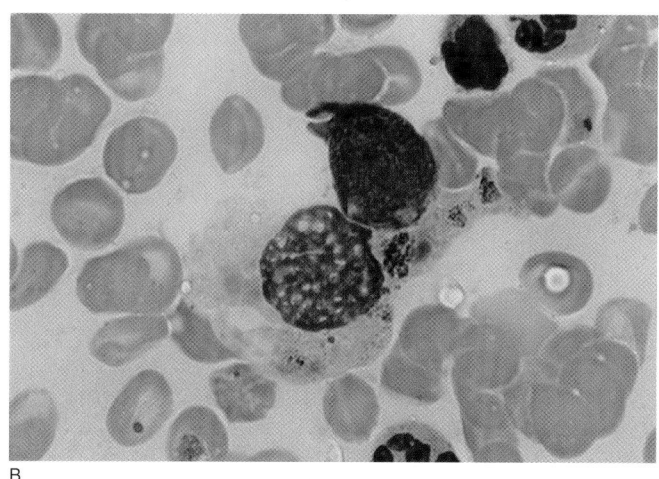

A B

Fig. 5.9 Bone marrow smear from a patient with acute *P. falciparum* malaria. (A) Edge of a marrow fragment showing three macrophages laden with malarial pigment. (B) Higher power view of a macrophage with pigment. May–Grünwald–Giemsa stain.

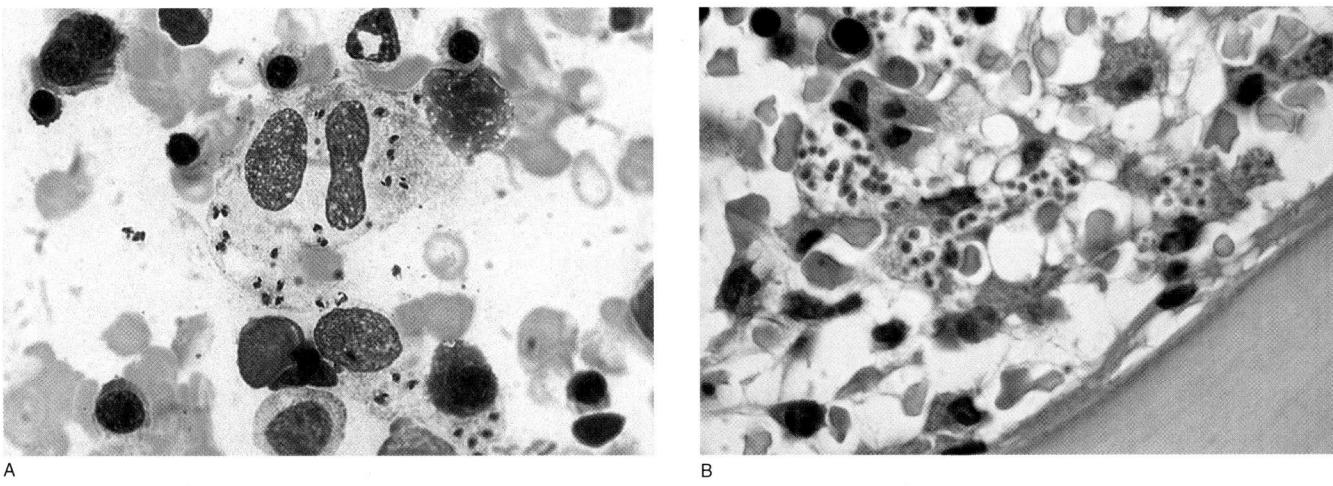

A

B

Fig. 5.10 (A) Macrophages containing several Leishman–Donovan bodies, from a marrow smear of a patient with kala-azar. Each parasite contains a large ovoid or rounded nucleus and a rod-like kinetoplast situated more or less at right-angles to the nucleus. Both the nucleus and the kinetoplast stain reddish-violet. May–Grünwald–Giemsa stain. (B) Trephine biopsy of the bone marrow of a case of AIDS, showing Leishman–Donovan bodies within macrophage cytoplasm. H&E.

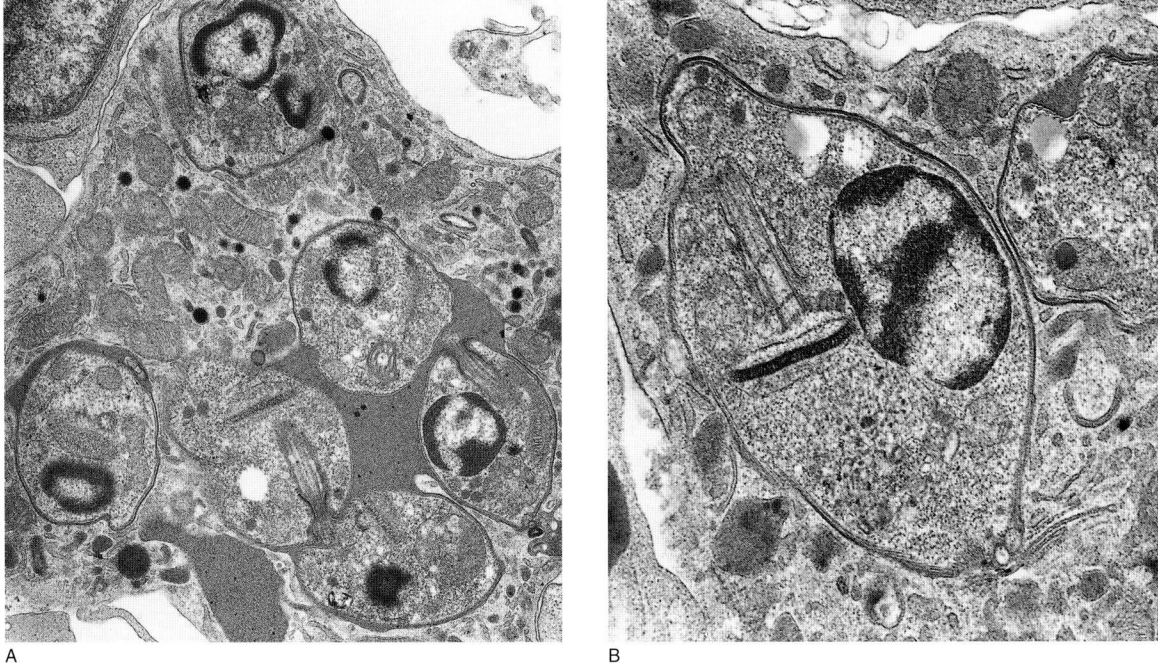

A

B

Fig. 5.11 (A, B) Electron micrograph showing *Leishmania donovani* within the bone marrow macrophages of a patient with kala-azar. (A) Part of the cytoplasm of a macrophage containing six intracellular parasites. (B) Higher-power view of a single parasite. The periplast covering the organism, the large ovoid nucleus and the sausage-shaped kinetoplast (arranged at right angles to the nucleus) can be recognized. The kinetoplast contains an electron-dense band which runs parallel to its long axis and which contains nucleic acid. Uranyl acetate and lead citrate. (A) × 13 200; (B) × 25 800.

parvovirus B19 causes transient red cell aplasia and, consequently, severe anemia occurs in patients with an underlying hemolytic state (e.g. sickle cell anemia, thalassemia intermedia, hereditary spherocytosis and pyruvate kinase deficiency) (see Chapter 14).[91, 92] In some cases of the congenital rubella syndrome thrombocytopenia is at least partly due to reduced numbers of megakaryocytes in the marrow. In other cases the thrombocytopenia is mainly caused by a decreased platelet life span and is associated with normal or increased numbers of megakaryocytes in the marrow.

HIV infection[93]

A variety of hematologic abnormalities may be found in HIV infection, especially at the later stages of infection.

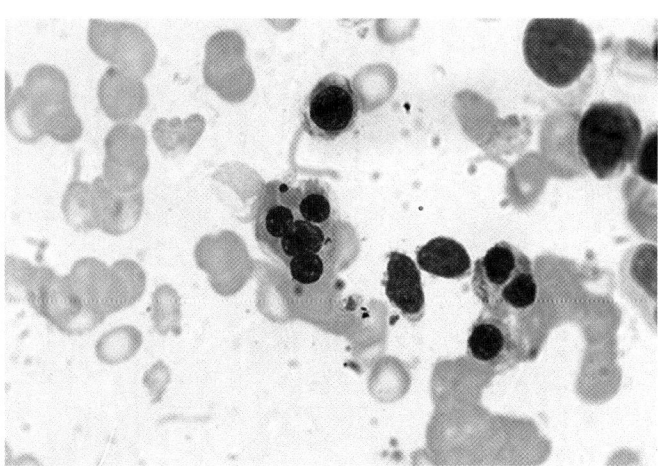

Fig. 5.12 Erythroblast with four nuclei and a micronucleus in a marrow smear from a case of kala-azar. May–Grünwald–Giemsa stain.

These include cytopenias, dysplastic changes affecting all hemopoietic cell lineages and changes in the bone marrow resulting from opportunistic infections.

Changes in the peripheral blood

During the primary infection with HIV, which is associated with fever, sore throat and cervical lymphadenopathy, there is an initial lymphopenia followed by lymphocytosis.[94,95] Atypical lymphocytes are present in the blood film and false-positive results may be obtained in tests for glandular fever.[95] Other changes may include a mild normocytic normochromic anemia, with or without neutropenia or thrombocytopenia, and pancytopenia. The blood picture returns to normal after seroconversion.

During the phase of clinically latent infection that follows the primary infection there is a slowly progressive CD4+ lymphopenia. The total lymphocyte count may be initially normal because of a CD8+ lymphocytosis. The prevalence of various cytopenias increases with progression of infection (i.e. increasing viral load). In CDC category II, lymphopenia, anemia, neutropenia and thrombocytopenia have been reported in 0–15%, 17%, 0–30% and 5–20% of cases, respectively.[96] The corre-

sponding figures in patients with AIDS (CDC category IV B–E) are 70–83%, 71–83%, 20–65% and 25–50%. In a recent study of over 32 000 HIV-infected patients in the USA, an Hb < 10 g/dl was found in 37% of patients with AIDS and 12% of patients without AIDS but with a CD4+ lymphocyte count < 0.2×10^9/l.[97] When isolated thrombocytopenia occurs during the clinically latent phase, platelet-associated immune-complexes are frequently present and the antibody in some such complexes may have specificity against HIV antigens.

The blood film in AIDS may show various changes. The red cells are normocytic and normochromic or macrocytic; macrocytosis may occur even in the absence of zidovudine therapy. There may be reticulocytopenia, monocytopenia and atypical lymphocytes with lobulated nuclei. Some neutrophils may show various dysplastic changes including Howell–Jolly-body-like nuclear fragments,[98] hypogranularity, the acquired Pelger–Huët anomaly, a high nucleocytoplasmic ratio, bizarre nuclear shapes and binuclearity.[99] There may also occasionally be circulating giant metamyelocytes and giant neutrophils. Neutrophils may also show changes related to infection, such as toxic granulation, vacuolation, Döhle bodies and a 'left-shift'.

Changes in the bone marrow

The various abnormalities found in trephine biopsies from patients with AIDS and their prevalence are shown in Table 5.8. The bone marrow is hypercellular at the early stages and hypocellular in advanced AIDS. Polymorphous lymphoid aggregates are seen in the absence of lymphoma or opportunistic infections and appear to be at least partly a manifestation of the HIV infection itself; they are aggravated by opportunistic infections. The reticulin fibrosis is usually mild or moderate and leads to the marrow sinusoids being held open in paraffin-embedded trephine biopsy sections.

Gelatinous transformation occurs late in the disease and affects patients with considerable weight loss. The gelatinous material, which is composed of hyaluronic

Table 5.8 Various abnormalities[a] found in trephine biopsies from patients with AIDS. From Wickramasinghe[96]

Abnormality	% Cases affected	Abnormality	% Cases affected
Hypercellular	35–55	Gelatinous transformation	9–20
Hypocellular	13–33	Granulomas	11–16
Plasmacytosis	25–98	Burkitt's lymphoma	1–5
Lymphoid aggregates	16–32	Hodgkin's disease	< 1–3
Reticulin fibrosis	20–55	Acid-fast bacilli	1–7

[a] Other malignant diseases encountered include other non-Hodgkin's lymphomas and Kaposi's sarcoma.

acid and sulfated glycosaminoglycan, first appears around the fat cells as these decrease in size but eventually appears in between hemopoietic cells, presumably because of the replacement of the fat cells by this extracellular material.

Trilineage myelodysplasia. This is seen more frequently in AIDS (38–86% of cases) than in AIDS-related complex (18%). The many dysplastic changes that may be observed are summarized in Table 5.9. These changes may be seen in patients without current opportunistic infections. Some of the ultrastructural abnormalities encountered in hemopoietic cells are illustrated in Figs 5.13 and 5.14.

Opportunistic infections in AIDS. The important organisms responsible for opportunistic infections in AIDS are as follows:

Table 5.9 Dysplastic changes affecting hemopoietic cells in AIDS

Erythroid series
Light microscopy: megaloblastic change, abnormal nuclear shape, Howell–Jolly bodies, karyorrhexis, multinuclearity, cytoplasmic stippling and vacuolation, internuclear chromatin bridges, ring sideroblasts (uncommon)
Electron microscopy: intranuclear clefts, loss or duplication or myelinisation of parts of the nuclear membrane, multinuclearity, autophagic vacuoles, iron-laden mitochondria

Neutrophil series
Light microscopy: isolated nuclear fragments, hypogranularity, aquired Pelger–Huët anomaly, bizarre nuclear shapes, ring-shaped nuclei, high nucleo-cytoplasmic ratio, giant metamyelocytes, giant granulocytes, binuclearity, excessive chromatin clumping in 'immature' cells, open chromatin pattern in 'mature' cells
Electron microscopy: myelination of the nuclear membrane, hypogranularity, autophagic vacuoles, multivesicular bodies

Megakaryocyte series
Light microscopy: bizarre nuclear shapes, hypolobulated nuclei, many 'bare' megakaryocyte nuclei, clustering of megakaryocytes (trephine biopsy), abnormal location adjacent to bone trabeculae
Electron microscopy: 'bare' megakaryocyte nuclei, ballooning or blebbing of the peripheral zone of the cytoplasm, marked cytoplasmic vacuolation

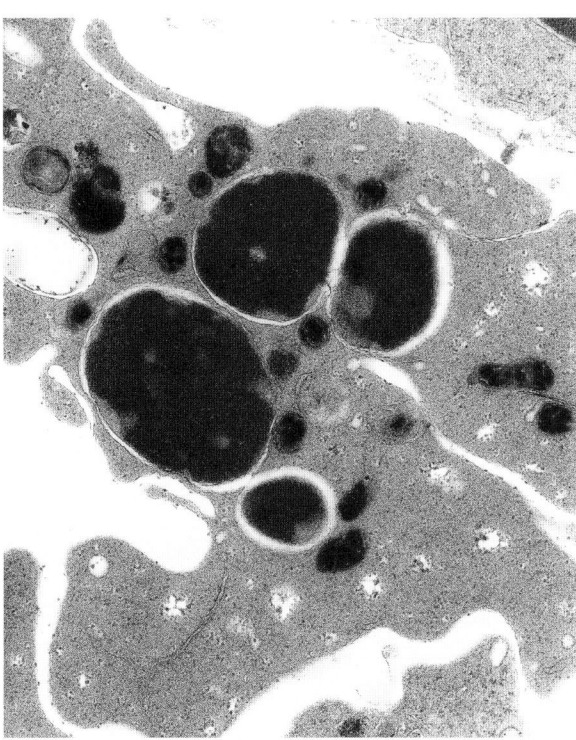
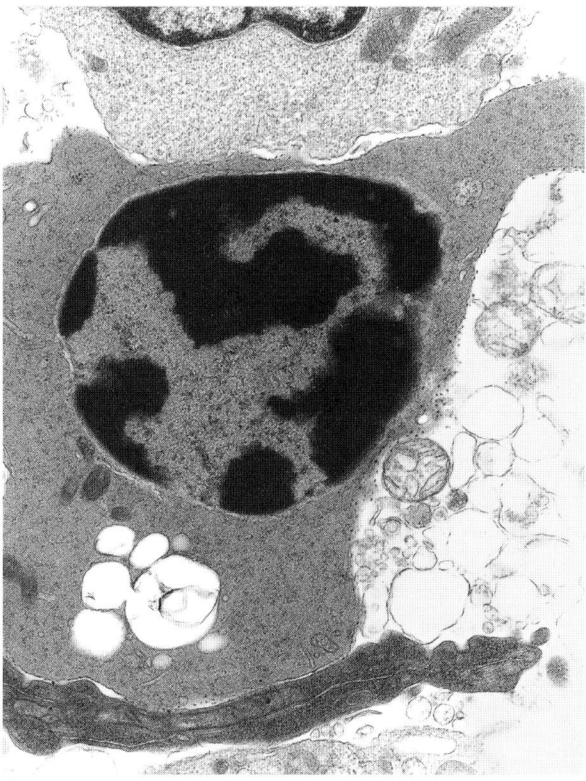

A   B

Fig. 5.13 (A, B) Electron micrographs of erythroblasts from the bone marrow of a case of AIDS. (A) Bizarre multinucleate erythroblast. (B) Erythroblast showing large intracytoplasmic vacuoles. Uranyl acetate and lead citrate.

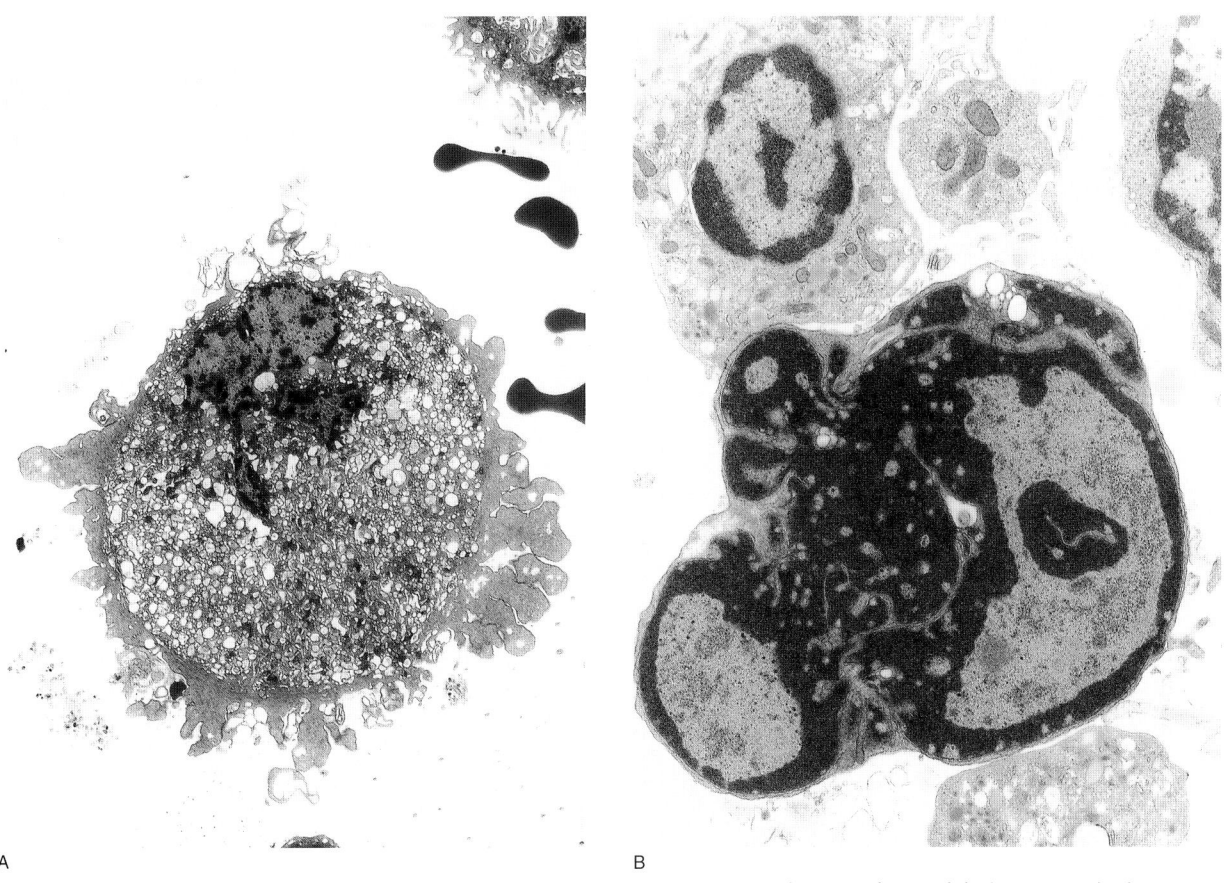

A   B

Fig. 5.14 (A, B) Electron micrographs of megakaryocytes from the bone marrow of a case of AIDS. (A) There is marked blebbing of the peripheral zone of the cytoplasm and extensive vacuolation of the intermediate zone. (B) A 'bare' megakaryocyte nucleus with a narrow rim of cytoplasm around it. Uranyl acetate and lead citrate.

1. Bacteria: *Mycobacterium tuberculosis* (common in Africa), *Mycobacterium avium intracellulare* and other atypical mycobacterial infections (common in UK), rarely *Bartonella* species (causing focal epithelioid angiomatosis).[100]
2. Viruses: CMV, Epstein–Barr virus (EBV), parvovirus B19.
3. Fungi: *Cryptococcus neoformans*, *Histoplasma capsulatum* (reported especially from USA, Central and South America), *Candida* species, *Penicillium marneffei* (reported from the Far East).[101]
4. Parasites: leishmaniasis, toxoplasmosis, histoplasmosis, American trypanosomiasis.

In keeping with the virulence of *Mycobacterium tuberculosis*, this organism becomes disseminated in patients whose CD4⁺ lymphocyte count is not severely reduced and, consequently, well-formed granulomas may be found in the marrow. However, less-virulent opportunistic organisms (e.g. atypical mycobacteria and fungi) generally provoke poorly formed granulomas (Fig. 5.15). Trephine biopsies of marrow are more useful than marrow smears in detecting such infections.[102] Sections should be stained

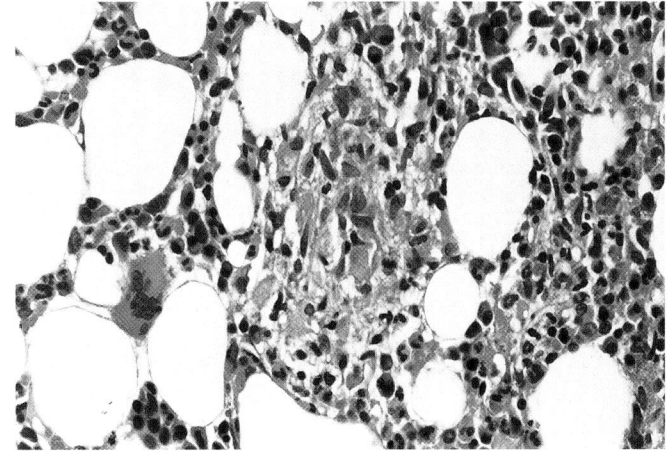

Fig. 5.15 Granuloma in a trephine biopsy of bone marrow from a patient with AIDS and disseminated atypical mycobacterial infection. H&E.

by the Ziehl–Neelsen stain to look for mycobacteria (Fig. 5.16), by the PAS stain or Grocott's methenamine silver stain to look for fungi such as *Cryptococcus neoformans* (Fig. 5.17), *Histoplasma capsulatum* and *Candida albicans* and the Giemsa stain, to look for protozoa such as

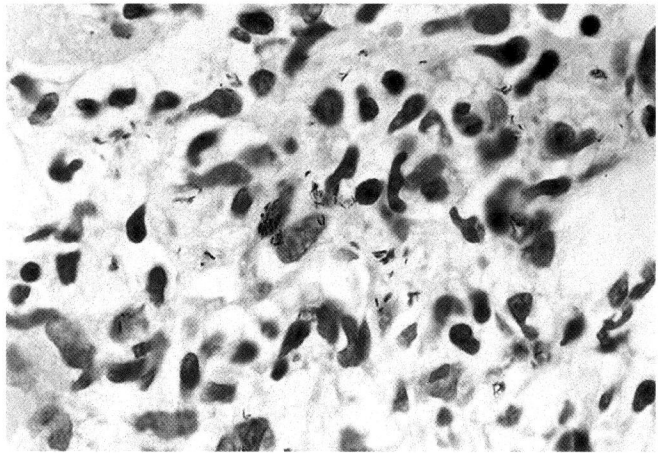

Fig. 5.16 Bone marrow granuloma from a patient with AIDS and disseminated *Mycobacterium avium intracellulare* infection. The macrophages contain many acid-fast bacillli. Ziehl–Neelsen stain.

Toxoplasma gondii and *Leishmania donovani*. These organisms may be found within poorly formed granulomas or diffusely in the marrow, within macrophages.

Mechanisms underlying the hematologic abnormalities in HIV infection

A number of different mechanisms operate together to cause the hematologic abnormalities in HIV infection[93,96,103] and the relative importance of the different mechanisms may vary from patient to patient. The possible mechanisms are outlined below.

Infection by HIV of hemopoietic stem cells or progenitor cells and hemopoietic cells. Many studies have been performed to investigate the possibility that the dysplastic changes in the hemopoietic and blood cells are a consequence of *in vivo* infection of the stem cells, progenitor cells or hemopoietic cells by HIV. Such studies have produced conflicting data and the discrepancies have not yet been fully resolved. However, hemopoietic progenitor cells, mononuclear phagocytes and megakaryocyte precursors have been shown to express CD4, the major HIV receptor, on their cell surface, and to be susceptible to infection *in vitro* by T-cell tropic HIV-1 strains. The CXCR4 and CCR5 co-receptors are also expressed in quiescent progenitor cells and progenitor-cell-derived mononuclear phagocytes and CXCR4 is expressed on megakaryocyte precursors.[104] The CXCR4 coreceptor is required for infection by T-cell-tropic HIV strains and the CCR5 coreceptor for infection by the macrophage-tropic HIV strain.

Disordered regulation of hemopoiesis due to stromal cell damage. The data supporting this possibility are:

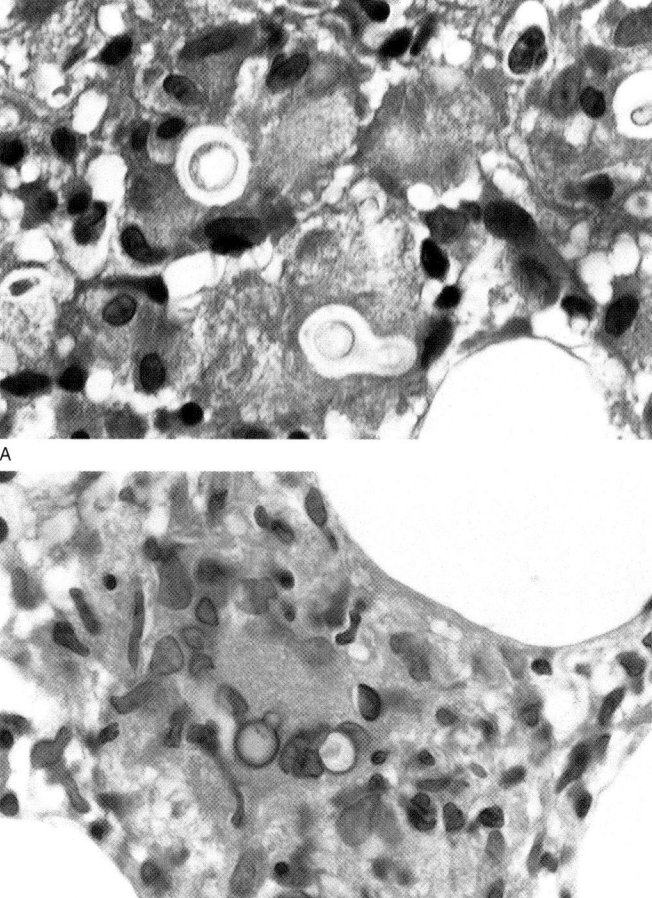

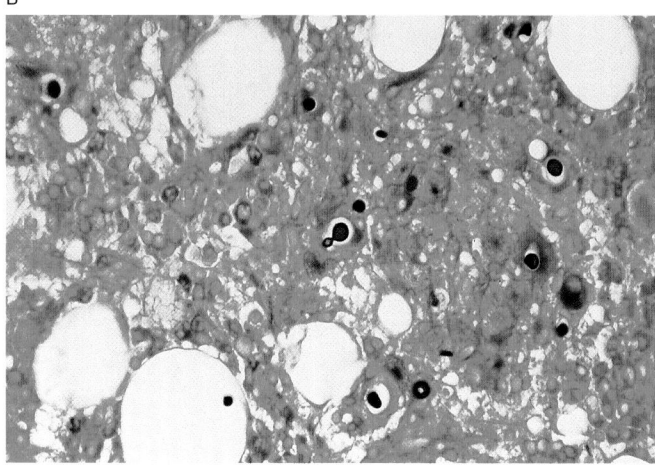

Fig. 5.17 (A–C) Poorly formed granuloma in trephine biopsies of bone marrow from patients with AIDS, showing budding yeast forms of *Cryptococcus neoformans*. (A) H&E; (B) PAS stain; (C) Grocott's methenamine silver stain.

(1) the technique of *in-situ* hybridization has shown HIV nucleic acid in endothelial cells and reticular cells; (2) immunohistochemical studies have shown *gag*-coded HIV proteins in CD68⁺ phagocytic and non-phagocytic reticular cells; (3) human marrow fibroblasts may be

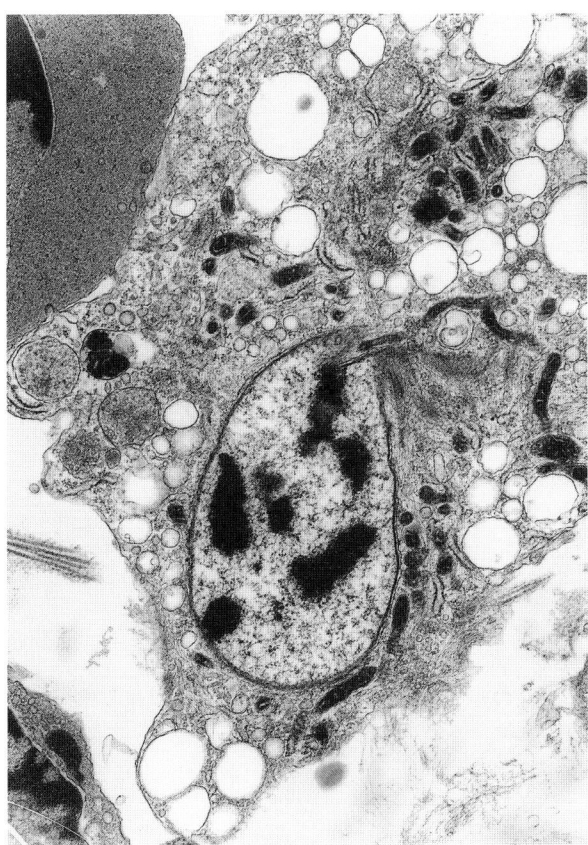

Fig. 5.18 Bone marrow stromal cell from a patient with AIDS. The cytoplasm is extensively vacuolated. Much of the condensed chromatin has detached from the membrane, leaving only a thin adherent layer at the areas of detachment. Uranyl acetate and lead citrate.

infected with HIV *in vitro;* and (4) bone marrow stromal cells show ultrastructural abnormalities indicative of cellular damage. Furthermore, the bone marrow shows gelatinous transformation (in advanced infection) and reticulin fibrosis.

The ultrastructural abnormalities affecting stromal cells are the detachment of much of the heterochromatin from the nuclear membrane and extensive cytoplasmic vacuolation[105,106] (Fig. 5.18).

Opportunistic-infection-related disturbances. The most important of these is the anemia of chronic disorder, characterized by a low serum iron and transferrin concentration, a high serum ferritin level, a suboptimal erythropoietin response and elevated levels of tumor necrosis factor. Other abnormalities associated with opportunistic infections include chronic pure red cell aplasia due to parvovirus B19 infection, and the hemophagocytic syndrome that may complicate infection with mycobacteria or herpes viruses. In this syndrome, the bone marrow macrophages contain increased numbers of phagocytosed red cells, platelets and granulocytes and,

sometimes, may even contain phagocytosed hemopoietic cells.

Drug-related hematological disturbances. Bone marrow suppression may result from antiretroviral drugs (e.g zidovudine), drugs against opportunistic viral infections (e.g. ganciclovir for CMV infection) and drugs against HIV-associated neoplasms. Oxidant-drug-induced hemolysis may occur in patients with or without G6PD deficiency and may be caused by dapsone given for the prevention of pneumocystis infection. Oxidant drugs may also cause methemoglobinemia. More rarely, some drugs cause immune hemolysis.[107,108]

Bone marrow infiltration by neoplastic cells. Marrow dysfunction may result from infiltration of this tissue by various neoplasms that develop with an unusually high prevalence in AIDS.[109] These are Hodgkin's disease, B-lineage non-Hodgkin's lymphomas such as Burkitt's lymphoma, Burkitt's-like lymphoma and diffuse large B-cell lymphoma, and Kaposi's sarcoma. Rarely, myeloma may develop.

Other mechanisms. Reduced serum levels of vitamin B_{12} and other hematinics and abnormal Schilling test results may be found in AIDS secondary to an HIV-induced gastropathy and enteropathy; however, treatment with vitamin B_{12} does not usually result in substantial clinical improvement. Rarely, an immune thrombocytopenia and autoimmune hemolysis may develop as may a microangiopathic hemolytic anemia and thrombocytopenia resembling that seen in the hemolytic uremic syndrome or thrombotic thrombocytopenic purpura.[110]

Bone marrow granulomas

A granuloma is a compact collection of mature cells of the mononuclear phagocyte system.[111] The types of monocyte-derived cells that may be found in granulomas include epithelioid cells, macrophages, Langhans'-type giant cells (containing numerous small nuclei situated around the periphery of the cell) and foreign-body type giant cells (containing a smaller number of nuclei scattered throughout the cell). Granulomas may also contain lymphocytes, plasma cells, neutrophils, eosinophils, fibroblasts and necrotic or caseating areas. Bone marrow granulomas are seen in many conditions characterized by the formation of granulomas in other tissues (Table 5.10).[112] Immunodeficient patients may fail to generate granulomas in response to organisms that evoke granuloma formation in immunocompetent subjects.[122] This is

Table 5.10 Causes of bone marrow granulomas

Bacterial infections
  Tuberculosis,[86] atypical mycobacterial infection[113]
  Brucellosis[114,115]
  Leprosy[116]
  Syphilis
  Typhoid fever[49]
  Legionnaires' disease[51]
  Ehrlichiosis[117]
  Tularemia
  Cat-scratch disease
Rickettsial infections
  Q fever[118,119]
  Rocky Mountain spotted fever
Fungal infections
  Histoplasmosis[74,120–122]
  Cryptococcosis[123,124]
  Blastomycosis
  Saccharomyces cerevisiae
  Coccidioidomycosis[125]
  Paracoccidioidomycosis
Viral infections
  Infectious mononucleosis[126,127]
  Varicella-zoster infection[120]
  Cytomegalovirus infection[128]
  Hantaan virus infection
Protozoal infections
  Leishmaniasis
  Toxoplasmosis
Sarcoidosis[129]
Malignant disease
  Hodgkin's disease[120,130]
  Non-Hodgkin's lymphoma[131]
  Multiple myeloma[132]
  Mycosis fungoides[133]
  Acute lymphoblastic leukemia[133–135]
  Acute myeloid leukemia and hairy cell leukemia on
    therapy[136,137]
  Metastatic carcinoma
Myelodysplastic syndrome[134]
Drug hypersensitivity[138–142]
Reaction to particulate material
  Anthracosis, silicosis, berylliosis, talc[134,135,143–145]
Eosinophilic interstitial nephritis[146]

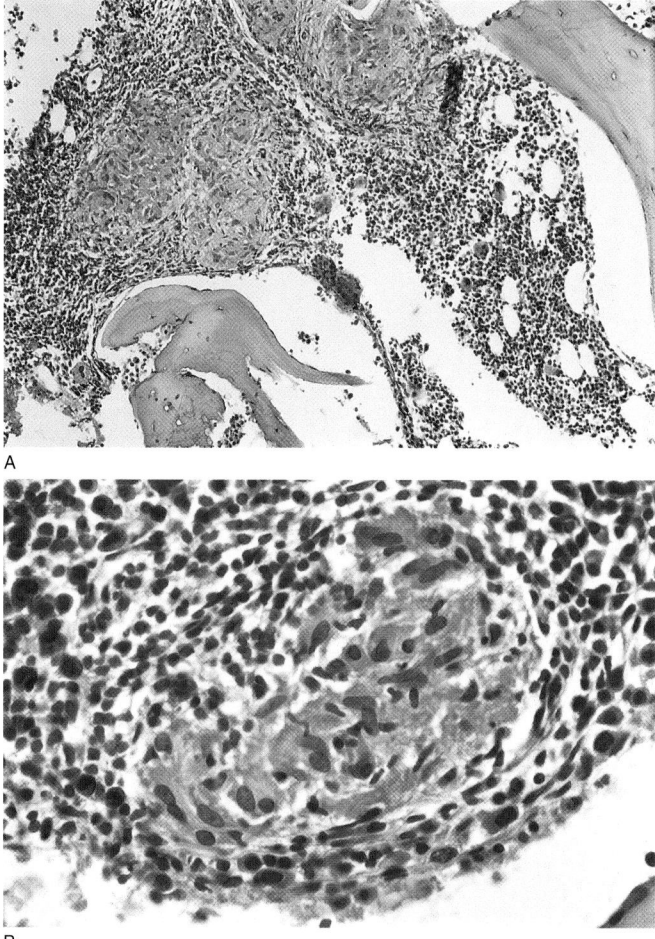

Fig. 5.19 (A, B) Trephine biopsies of bone marrow showing sarcoid granulomas. H&E. (A) × 94; (B) × 375.

because the development of granulomas requires normal lymphocyte functions; in experimental animals granuloma formation is suppressed by neonatal thymectomy and antilymphocyte serum.

Epithelioid cells may rarely be seen in Romanowsky-stained marrow smears suggesting the possibility of granuloma formation. In marrow smears, epithelioid cells tend to occur in groups and have abundant blue-gray to dark blue cytoplasm and round, oval or reniform nuclei. However, bone marrow granulomas are best detected in histologic sections of trephine biopsies or clot sections of aspirated marrow (Fig. 5.19).

Patients being investigated for infections that generate granulomas, for example those with pyrexia of unknown origin, should not only have a trephine biopsy for histo-

logic studies but also a marrow aspiration for culture of mycobacteria and fungi and, if they have visited or lived in an endemic area, leishmaniasis. If granulomas are found, sections should be stained by the Ziehl–Neelsen stain for mycobacteria and the PAS and silver stains for fungi.

Bone marrow granulomas are found in 15–40% of patients with miliary tuberculosis, including some patients with normal chest radiology.[86] In tuberculous granulomas, Langhans'-type giant cells are usually found, caseation is present in about 50% of patients and acid-fast bacilli are usually absent or, when present, found in small numbers. In disseminated *Mycobacterium avium intracellulare* infection, granulomas of variable size and appearance are seen in about half the cases.[113] Giant cells and necrosis are uncommon and macrophages are packed with organisms and may appear foamy. The organisms are best demonstrated using the Ziehl–Neelsen stain; they are acid-fast but longer, more curved and more coarsely beaded than *Mycobacterium tuberculosis* and unlike the latter are PAS-positive. *Mycobacterium tuberculosis* and atypical mycobacteria may be cultured from the bone marrow sometimes even in patients in whom the Ziehl–Neelsen stain has not revealed organisms. Patients with hairy cell leukemia and those with AIDS may have absent or impaired granuloma formation with mycobacterial infection of the bone marrow.[147,148]

Granulomas with large foamy macrophages may be found in typhoid fever and the bacilli may be seen within macrophages;[19] the organisms can usually be cultured from the bone marrow. In leprosy, the *Mycobacterium leprae* may appear as bacilliform 'ghosts' within macrophages in Romanowsky-stained marrow smears, and the acid-fast organisms can be demonstrated by the Fite stain.[116] Bone marrow granulomas are frequently found in brucellosis. In one study, 15 of 22 patients with brucellosis had granulomas in sections of sternal marrow aspirates[115] and in another study, 17 of 18 patients had granulomas in sections of iliac crest aspirates.[114] In brucellosis, the granulomas tend to be smaller and less distinct than those in tuberculosis or sarcoidosis.[115] *Brucella* may be cultured from the marrow and bone marrow cultures may sometimes be positive when simultaneous blood cultures are negative.[114]

Large granulomas, often with Langhans' giant cells and scanty organisms and sometimes with caseation, may occur in patients with histoplasmosis and reasonably normal immunity.[86] By contrast, patients with immune suppression usually have a marked and diffuse increase in macrophages and bone marrow necrosis.[74,122] In both types of patient, the yeast form of the organism is found within macrophages. The yeast forms appear blue in Romanowsky-stained films and are 2–5 μm in diameter. In histologic sections, they may be seen after staining with H&E but are best demonstrated when stained by the PAS reaction and by Gomori's methenamine-silver stain. The fungi can be cultured from marrow aspirates in 60–75% of patients with disseminated infection.[86] Granulomas may also be seen in the marrow in disseminated *Cryptococcus neoformans* infection.[123,124] The organisms (yeasts) are 5–10 μm in diameter, have a thick capsule that appears as a clear halo in sections stained with H&E and show unequal budding (see Fig. 5.17). The capsule is PAS-positive and also stains with mucicarmine (red) and Alcian blue.

Small bone marrow granulomas are fairly frequently seen in infectious mononucleosis, being found, for example, in 8 of 18 cases in which particles of sternal marrow were examined by sectioning.[126] Giant cells are uncommon and caseation does not occur but there may be focal necrosis.[127] Similar granulomas are less commonly found in varicella-zoster infection, CMV infection[128] and some other viral infections.

Granulomas may also be seen in the marrow in infections with the protozoa, *Leishmania donovani* and *Toxoplasma gondii*.

Bone marrow granulomas are found in some cases of sarcoidosis (Fig. 5.19) and in one-third of cases the granulomas contain Langhans' giant cells.[129] Granulomas are found more frequently at autopsy than by biopsy. It is not always possible to distinguish between granulomas in sarcoidosis and tuberculosis or other microbial infections on histologic features alone. Caseation is characteristic of tuberculosis but is neither invariably present nor restricted to it. Furthermore, non-caseating granulomas with no detectable acid-fast bacilli may sometimes be due to tuberculosis rather than sarcoidosis. Both tuberculous and sarcoid granulomas may have associated eosinophils and lymphocytes and these features are not helpful in making a distinction between them. Although sarcoid granulomas do not caseate they may show eosinophilic coagulative necrosis and, in the healing stage, hyaline fibrosis.[130]

In Hodgkin's disease and non-Hodgkin's lymphoma, malignant infiltration of the marrow may be accompanied by granuloma formation.[131] In these conditions, bone marrow granulomas (or liver or spleen granulomas) may also be found in the absence of malignant infiltration of the tissue either as a reaction to an infection or as a non-infiltrative manifestation of the disease.[130]

Poorly circumscribed bone marrow granulomas may occur as part of a hypersensitivity reaction to drugs such as phenytoin, procainamide, oxyphenbutazone, chlorpropamide, sulphasalazine, ibuprofen, indomethacin, allopurinol and amiodarone.[120,133,138–142] The granulomas may coexist with other adverse reactions such as neutropenia, eosinophilia, rash and fever.

Lipid granulomas

Lipid granulomas in which fat globules are present both within macrophages and extracellularly do not have any diagnostic significance.[149] They may contain plasma cells, lymphocytes and eosinophils and frequently occur near sinusoids or lymphoid nodules.

Granuloma-like lesions

Lesions seen in the bone marrow in systemic mastocytosis and in angioimmunoblastic lymphadenopathy need to be distinguished from granulomas. In systemic mastocytosis the lesions are composed of mast cells, eosinophils, lymphocytes and collagen fibers[150] and in angioimmunoblastic lymphadenopathy of immunoblasts, plasma cells, lymphocytes, histiocytes, eosinophils, arborizing capillaries[3] and reticulin fibers.

Metastatic tumors in bone marrow

Patients with metastatic tumor cells in the bone marrow usually have a normochromic normocytic anemia and, less commonly, thrombocytopenia or neutropenia. In less than half the patients with bone marrow metastases, the blood film contains some erythroblasts and neutrophil precursors (leukoerythroblastic anemia)[151–153] and the presence of such cells reflects the extent of myelofibrosis. Circulating malignant cells may occasionally be seen, especially in children with small cell tumors and, more rarely, in adults with carcinoma. The peripheral blood may also show abnormalities not directly related to the marrow infiltration such as the anemia of chronic disease, iron deficiency anemia, red cell fragmentation, neutrophilia, thrombocytosis and eosinophilia.

In adults, the tumors that most commonly metastasize to the marrow are carcinomas of the prostate, breast, lung, thyroid and kidney[153,154] and in children they are neuroblastoma, rhabdomyosarcoma, Ewing's tumor and retinoblastoma.[155,156]

Metastatic carcinoma cells can usually be readily recognized in bone marrow smears because they are larger than all hemopoietic cells other than megakaryocytes and tend to occur in clumps (Fig. 5.20A). Generally, carcinoma cells are markedly pleomorphic and have a moderate quantity of slightly or moderately basophilic cytoplasm, sometimes with vacuoles. Some cells are multinucleate and there may be a high mitotic index. Usually, it is not possible to identify the primary tumor on the basis of the morphologic features of the metastatic cells in marrow smears. However, some melanomas can be identified by the presence of intracytoplasmic melanin pigment (which stains positively with the Masson–Fontana or Schmorl stains for melanin) and renal carcinoma may be suspected if the cells have abundant foamy cytoplasm and small nuclei. Mucin-secreting adenocarcinoma cells possess foamy or vacuolated cytoplasm. The mucin may push the nucleus to the periphery, thus giving the cell a 'signet-ring' appearance. Stains for mucin (combined diastase-treated PAS/Alcian blue stain) can be used to identify mucin-secreting carcinoma cells. Patients with metastatic carcinoma frequently have increased numbers of macrophages and plasma cells in their marrow. When there is associated osteosclerosis, the marrow smears may also contain increased numbers of osteoblasts and osteoclasts. Sometimes, there may be necrosis of the infiltrated bone

marrow and necrotic material may be seen in both smears and histologic sections.

Information on the nature of malignant cells may be obtained by immunocytochemistry and immunohistochemistry. Monoclonal antibodies against antigens such as human milk fat globulin, epithelial membrane antigen (an antigen found in carcinoma of the breast but also in other adenocarcinomas) or cytokeratin[157,158] have proved most useful in detecting carcinoma cells either in histologic sections of biopsies or bone marrow smears.[159–162] Antibody against S100 protein reacts with most malignant melanomas, including amelanotic melanomas.[163] The detection of metastatic prostate carcinoma cells requires the use of antibodies against both prostate-specific antigen and prostatic acid phosphatase.[164,165]

Metastatic tumor cells of neuroblastoma (Fig. 5.20B), medulloblastoma, retinoblastoma, rhabdomyosarcoma and Ewing's sarcoma are small and round with relatively little cytoplasm and may be difficult to distinguish from the blast cells of acute lymphoblastic leukemia (ALL)

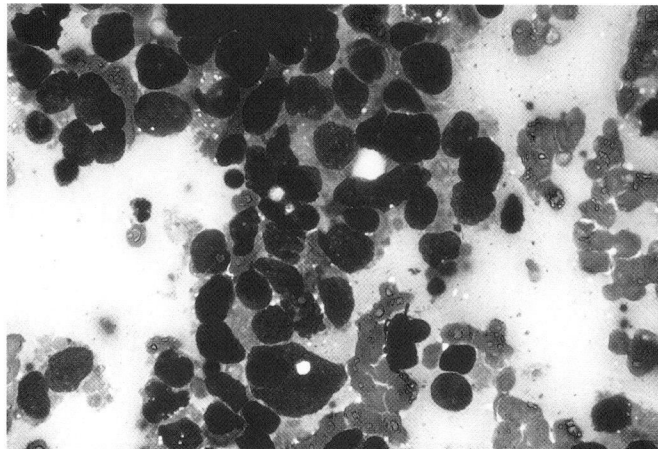

A

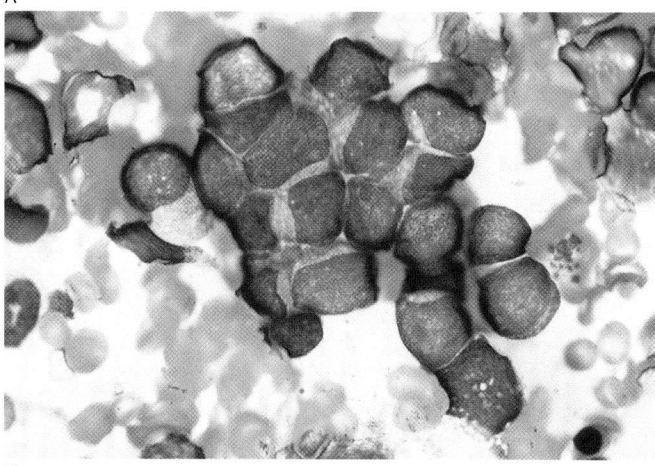

B

Fig. 5.20 (A, B) Clumps of metastatic tumor cells in bone marrow smears. (A) Carcinoma of the bronchus. (B) Neuroblastoma. May–Grünwald–Giemsa stain.

and lymphoblastic lymphoma. In some cases of neuro-blastoma, medulloblastoma and rhabdomyosarcoma, the small tumor cells may circulate.[166] Metastatic small round cell tumors can sometimes be distinguished from acute leukemia on morphologic criteria alone. However, in other cases this distinction requires cytochemical, ultra-structural and immunochemical studies. In neuro-blastoma, both bone marrow smears and sections may show characteristic rosettes of tumor cells near fibrillar extracellular material that stains blue gray by Romanowsky methods and eosinophilic by H&E.[167,168] However, these features are often absent[169] and the diagnosis may then be made by demonstrating the outgrowth of neurites on tissue culture,[170] and by the detection of neurone-specific enolase, protein gene product 9.5, chromogranin and other neuroectodermal antigens by immunohisto-chemistry.[171–174] Rhabdomyosarcoma cells are usually heavily vacuolated, reflecting glycogen in the cytoplasm, and can be identified by electron microscopy on the basis of the presence of cross-striated myofibrils and by the immunohistochemical demonstration of myosin, desmin or myoglobin.[175,176] In Ewing's sarcoma histologic sections may show small numbers of 'pseudorosettes' around blood vessels.[168] In medulloblastoma, tumor cells may display hemophagocytosis and autophagocytosis. The malignant cells of acute lymphoblastic leukemia give positive reactions with monoclonal antibodies against the common leukocyte antigen (CD45) and HLA-DR antigen whereas the malignant cells from neuroblastoma, rhabdomyosarcoma and Ewing's sarcoma give negative reactions.[177,178] The blasts of acute leukemia also have terminal deoxynucleotidyl transferase (TdT) activity while neuroblastoma and retinoblastoma cells do not.[179]

Value of histologic sections

A bone marrow trephine biopsy is generally more useful in detecting metastatic tumor cells in the marrow than a section of aspirated bone marrow and the latter is more useful than a marrow smear.[153,180] However, the three procedures should be regarded as complementary.[154,181,182] Another advantage of histologic sections (either particle sections or trephine biopsies) over smears is that they can better reveal intercellular organization such as the formation of rosettes in neuroblastoma or acini in adeno-carcinoma (Fig. 5.21) and can demonstrate fibrosis and osteoblastic reactions that may be associated with tumor metastases (Fig. 5.22). Bone marrow fibrosis in response to tumor metastases is particularly marked in carcinomas of the breast, stomach and prostate and correlates with the occurrence of a leukoerythroblastic anemia.[152]

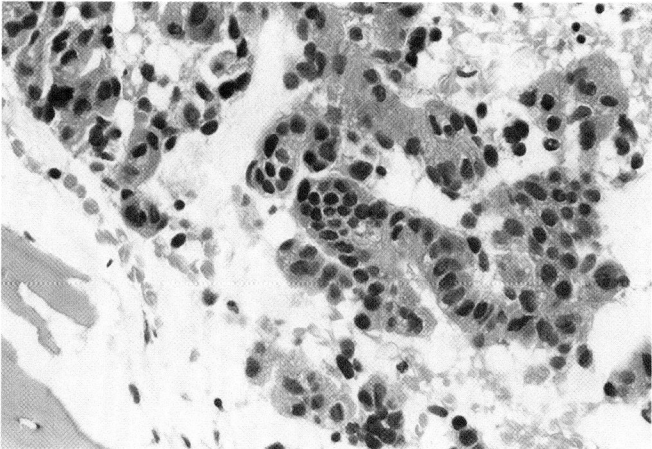

Fig. 5.21 Trephine biopsy of bone marrow showing metastases from an adenocarcinoma. The carcinoma cells are arranged in a well-defined tubular pattern. H&E. × 94.

Bone marrow fibrosis including idiopathic myelofibrosis[183]

An increase in the reticulin or reticulin and collagen in bone marrow is referred to as bone marrow fibrosis. Reticulin fibers are collagen precursors and are produced by fibroblasts. A scheme for grading bone marrow reticulin and collagen is shown in Table 5.11. Grades 0–1 and possibly 2 are considered normal. The term myelo-fibrosis is best restricted to an increase in mature collagen in bone marrow tissue (i.e. to grade 4 fibrosis). Some patients with myelofibrosis also have osteosclerosis.

Increased reticulin deposition (reticulin fibrosis) (detected by silver stains) is a common abnormality which does not help to make a specific diagnosis. It is seen in a variety of conditions, including chronic granulocytic leukemia, acute myeloid leukemia, multiple myeloma, chronic lymphocytic leukemia, acute lym-phoblastic leukemia, malignant mastocytosis, hairy cell leukemia, Waldenström's macroglobulinemia[184] and kala-azar.[185] Although reticulin fibrosis does not help to make a specific diagnosis it may serve to attract attention to an area of abnormal bone marrow, for example the site of a granuloma or a malignant infiltrate, so the corresponding area in an H&E-stained section should be re-examined.

Myelofibrosis may be generalized or focal. Generalized myelofibrosis occurs as an apparently idiopathic con-dition and also in association with a number of diseases with widely differing etiology (Table 5.12 and Fig. 5.22). 'Idiopathic' myelofibrosis is now known to represent a myeloproliferative disorder with reactive fibrosis and there is no essential difference between the fibrosis seen in 'idiopathic' myelofibrosis and that associated with

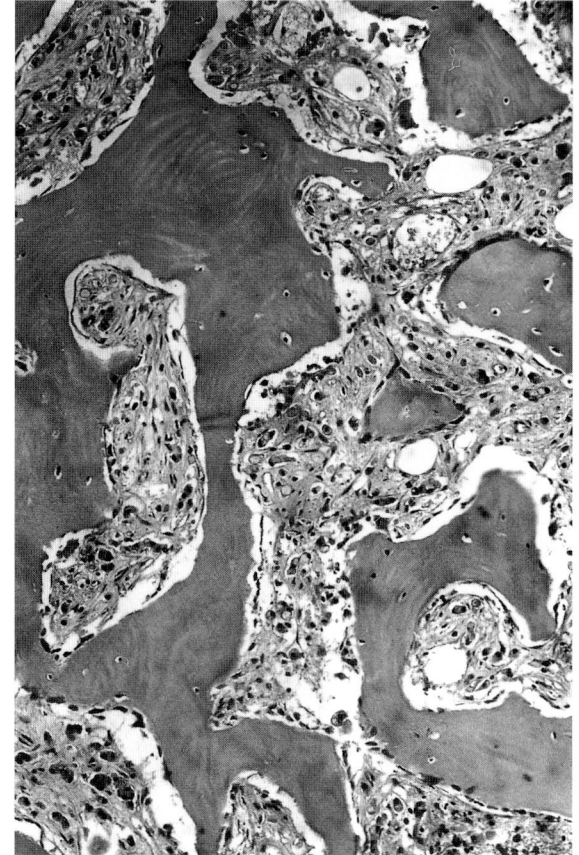

A

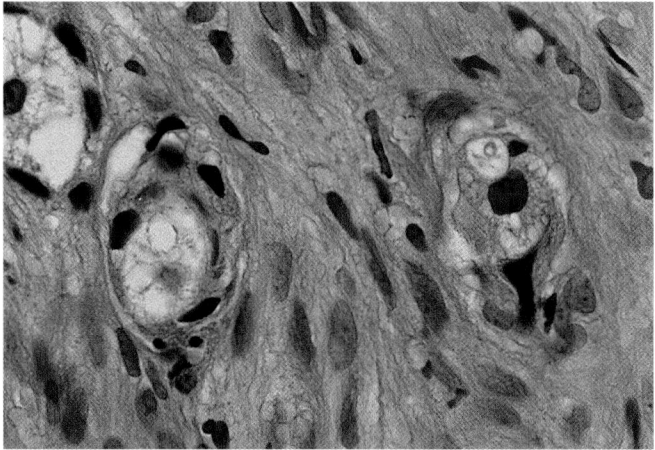

B

Fig. 5.22 (A, B) Trephine biopsy of bone marrow showing myelofibrosis and osteosclerosis secondary to the presence in the marrow of scattered metastatic tumor cells from an unidentified primary tumor. Tumor cells with secretory products and surrounding fibroblasts are shown at higher power in (B). H&E. (A) × 94; (B) × 940.

Table 5.11 Grading of bone marrow reticulin and collagen

Grade	Features
0	No reticulin fibers seen
1	Few scattered fine reticulin fibers
2	Network of fine reticulin fibers in most of the section; coarse reticulin fibers absent
3	As in (2), with coarse reticulin fibers; collagen fibers absent
4	Diffuse network of mainly coarse reticulin fibers; collagen fibers present in some areas

Table 5.12 Causes of myelofibrosis

Generalized:
Chronic myeloproliferative disorders
  'Idiopathic' myelofibrosis
  (agnogenic myeloid metaplasia)[a]
  Polycythemia rubra vera
  Essential thrombocythemia
  Chronic granulocytic leukemia
Acute leukemias
  Acute myeloid leukemia
   (particularly acute
   megakaryoblastic leukemia[186]
   and acute panmyelosis)
  Acute lymphoblastic leukemia[187]
Other malignant diseases
  Secondary carcinoma[a188,189]
  Hodgkin's disease[152]
  Non-Hodgkin's lymphoma[152]
  Multiple myeloma[190]
  Systemic mastocytosis[a150]
  Waldenström's macroglobulinemia
Bone diseases
  Nutritional and renal rickets[191–193]
  Primary hyperparathyroidism[194]
  Marble bone disease – osteopetrosis
  Osteomalacia
  Primary hypertrophic osteoarthropathy[195]
Miscellaneous
  Tuberculosis
  Other granulomatous disorders
  Myelodysplastic syndrome (especially secondary)[196,197]
  Paroxysmal nocturnal hemoglobinuria[198]
  Gaucher's disease
  Gray platelet syndrome[199]
  Systemic lupus erythematosus[200,201]
  Systemic sclerosis

Focal or localized:
Osteomyelitis
Paget's disease
Following bone
  marrow necrosis[202]
Following irradiation
  of bone marrow
Adult T-cell leukemia/
  lymphoma[203]
Healing fracture site
Old trephine biopsy
  site

[a] There may also be osteosclerosis.

other chronic myeloproliferative disorders. Thus studies of cytogenetic and G6PD isoenzyme markers and *N-RAS* mutations have shown that in idiopathic myelofibrosis, as in chronic granulocytic leukemia and polycythemia rubra vera,[204,205] the hemopoietic cells belong to a single abnormal clone whereas the fibroblasts are polyclonal.

The underlying hemopoietic stem cell defect in 'idiopathic' myelofibrosis is also reflected in the high incidence of a 'paroxysmal-nocturnal hemoglobinuria like' defect in the red cells[206] which is not seen when myelofibrosis is secondary to non-hemopoietic malignancy. However, it is still convenient to distinguish a disorder termed 'idiopathic' myelofibrosis from the other well-defined chronic myeloproliferatve disorders.

The development of myelofibrosis in patients with myeloproliferative disorders may be related to secretion of platelet-derived growth factor, transforming growth factor β and platelet factor 4 (which inhibits collagenase) by megakaryocytes. Myelofibrosis is commonly found in acute megakaryoblastic leukemia and acute panmyelosis, which often present with the clinical picture of 'acute myelofibrosis'.[186] In idiopathic myelofibrosis, necrotic megakaryocytes have been noted in fibrotic areas.[207] In chronic granulocytic leukemia and polycythemia rubra vera the degree of fibrosis has been related to the total number of megakaryocytes and the number of atypical megakaryocytes respectively.[207] In the congenital defect, the gray platelet syndrome, it has been hypothesized that associated myelofibrosis may be consequent on the release of granule contents (which could include platelet-derived growth factor) from abnormal megakaryocytes. When myelofibrosis is secondary to non-hemopoietic malignancy it is likely that the tumor cells themselves promote fibrosis, since they may do so in sites other than the bone marrow. When myelofibrosis is secondary to a non-hemopoietic disorder, reversal of the fibrosis may occur when the primary condition is effectively treated. This is also true if effective treatment can be given for a hematological malignancy with associated fibrosis.

Whenever extensive dense fibrosis occurs, for example in patients with metastatic carcinoma, the hematological findings may mimic those of idiopathic myelofibrosis. Extramedullary hemopoiesis may occur in secondary as well as in 'idiopathic' myelofibrosis.[188,189]

Idiopathic myelofibrosis (myelosclerosis, agnogenic myeloid metaplasia)[208–210]

This disorder usually affects the middle-aged and elderly. It is characterized by leukoerythroblastic anemia, progressive fibrosis of the bone marrow, moderate to gross splenomegaly and extramedullary hemopoiesis. The liver may be enlarged. There is radiologic evidence of osteosclerosis, particularly in the axial skeleton and the upper ends of the humeri and femora in about 50% of cases. A similar clinico-pathologic syndrome can occur following polycythemia rubra vera, essential thrombocythemia and Ph-positive chronic granulocytic leukemia and the diagnosis of idiopathic myelofibrosis is only made in the absence of these disorders.

Patients diagnosed early may have a normal hemoglobin (Hb). At diagnosis, most patients are anemic and the severity of the anemia increases with disease progression. Occasional patients have a high Hb and hematocrit, without a preceding history of polycythemia

rubra vera. The anemia is caused by a combination of a reduced rate of effective erythropoiesis, an expanded plasma volume due to splenomegaly, increased pooling of red cells within the large spleen and some reduction in red cell life span. The circulating red cells show marked anisocytosis and poikilocytosis, often with frequent tear-drop-shaped poikilocytes (Fig. 5.23). The number of poikilocytes decreases after splenectomy, suggesting that the spleen plays a role in the production of such cells. The blood film contains at least a few erythroblasts. The total white cell and platelet counts vary; they may be raised (in about 50% of cases) or normal but with disease progression they fall. There may be abnormally large platelets and increased numbers of circulating megakaryocytes. Several patients have been reported to become folate deficient due to an increased requirement for folate: such patients may show macrocytosis and megaloblastic erythropoiesis. Serum uric acid and serum vitamin B_{12} levels may be raised, as in polycythemia rubra vera; serum lactate dehydrogenase and bilirubin levels may be increased, reflecting ineffective erythropoiesis, and serum lysozyme may be elevated, indicating increased (often ineffective) granulocytopoiesis. About half the patients show a polyclonal increase of serum immunoglobulins. Other abnormalities found in some patients include positive tests for rheumatoid factor, antinuclear or anti-smooth-muscle antibodies, a positive direct antiglobulin test, anti-I autoantibody, decreased levels of immunoglobulins or a monoclonal immunoglobin.

Some patients present with hypercellularity of all hemopoietic cell lines and minimal fibrosis of the marrow (hypercellular panmyelosis phase)[184] and show progressively increasing fibrosis thereafter. Others present with established fibrosis. In the hypercellular phase, large

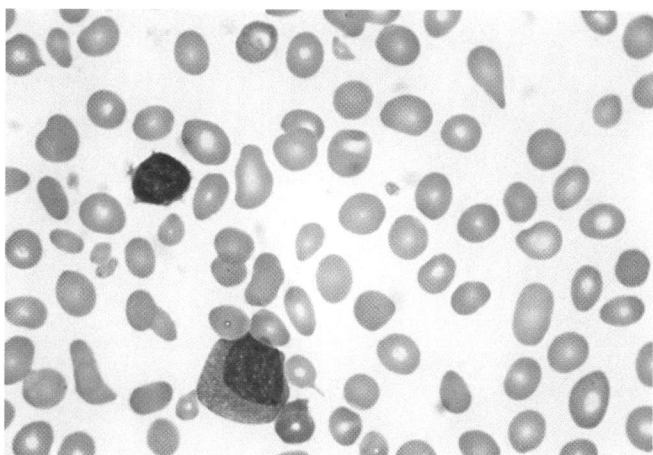

Fig. 5.23 Photomicrograph of a blood film from a patient with idiopathic myelofibrosis, showing two tear-drop-shaped poikilocytes and several other poikilocytes. May–Grünwald–Giemsa stain.

clusters of erythroblasts and many large megakaryocytes are present, reticulin fibers are slightly increased and bone marrow aspiration may be possible. With established fibrosis, bone marrow aspiration is difficult and frequently yields only a little blood ('blood tap') or no aspirate ('dry tap'). Trephine biopsy shows a reduction of hemopoietic tissue and the presence of many fibroblasts and greatly increased quantities of reticulin and collagen (Figs 5.24 and 5.25). The reticulin fibers are abnormally coarse and tend to run in parallel bundles. All types of hemopoietic cells may be present in the fibrotic marrow but megakaryocytes are particularly prominent. There may also be patches of hyperplastic hemopoietic marrow between the fibrosed areas. In some patients there is a considerable increase in the amount of bone (osteosclerosis); this results from appositional bone formation leading to trabecular thickening and formation of woven bone in intertrabecular spaces. Osteolytic lesions and pathologic fractures occur uncommonly. The proliferating fibroblasts are not part of the neoplastic clone. It is now thought that the fibroblastic reaction is induced by mitogenic factors secreted by the increased number of (possibly functionally-abnormal) megakaryocytes and that a similar explanation might underly the lesser degrees of myelofibrosis which may occur in polycythemia rubra vera, essential thrombocythemia and chronic granulocytic leukemia.

Patients show a slow clinical and hematologic deterioration with increasing splenomegaly. Complications during the course of the disease include splenic infarction, splenic rupture (rare), portal hypertension with esophageal varices (sometimes secondary to the Budd–Chiari syndrome), infection, hemorrhage (due to thrombocytopenia and impaired platelet function) and pressure on the spinal cord and other organs by tumors composed of extramedullary hemopoietic tissue (rare). Average survival from the time of diagnosis is about 5–7 years but some patients survive much longer. From 10 to 20% of patients eventually develop acute myeloblastic or acute megakaryoblastic leukemia. Other causes of death include infection, congestive cardiac failure, bleeding and thrombosis.

Treatment is largely directed at alleviating symptoms and includes blood transfusion and folate supplementation when necessary, low-dose busulfan or hydroxyurea to decrease the size of a large spleen causing discomfort and splenectomy to reduce transfusion requirements or improve troublesome thrombocytopenia. Allogeneic stem cell transplantation prolongs survival in some patients under 55 years.[210]

At post mortem, the spleen is very large and may show recent or old infarcts. Extramedullary hemopoiesis is seen in the spleen and liver and may also be seen in many other sites including lymph nodes, kidneys, adrenals, peritoneum, gut, pleura, lungs, fatty tissue, skin, breasts, ovaries and thymus; proliferating myeloid cells may form tumor masses. Extramedullary hemopoiesis in the liver may result in cramming of sinusoids with hemopoietic cells;[211] it may be accompanied by periportal fibrosis. Portal hypertension and ascites are not uncommon.[211] Osteosclerosis may be evident.

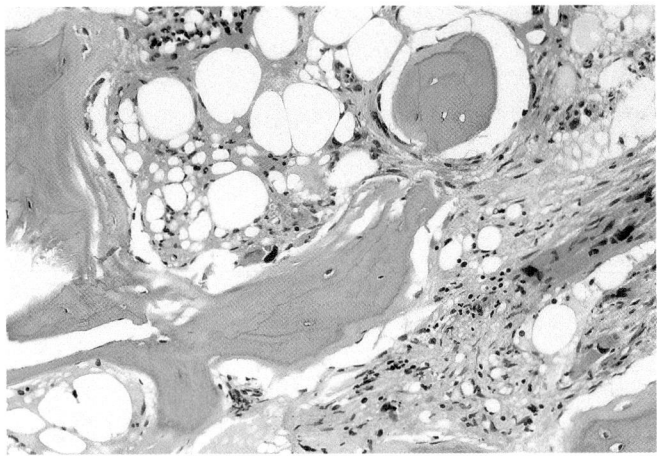

Fig. 5.24 Trephine biopsy of bone marrow from a patient with idiopathic myelofibrosis at the end-stage of the disease. The marrow cells are markedly reduced in number and replaced by fibroblasts and collagen. The bony trabeculae are sclerotic. H&E. × 350.

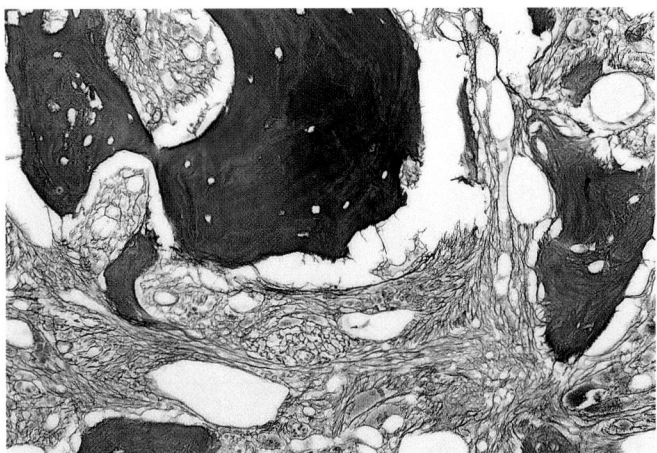

Fig. 5.25 Trephine biopsy of bone marrow from a patient with idiopathic myelofibrosis. There is a marked increase in the quantity of reticulin fibers. Silver impregnation of reticulin. × 375.

Storage cells in lysosomal storage diseases[212,213]

Lysosomes catabolize lipids, carbohydrates, proteins and nucleotides. In a group of inherited diseases, mutations in one of the genes encoding a lysosomal hydrolytic enzyme lead to the intracellular accumulation of abnormal amounts of various substances and consequent clinical manifestations.

Sphingolipidoses

Gaucher's disease[214]

In Gaucher's disease, which is usually inherited as an autosomal recessive character, there is defective production of the lysosomal enzyme glucocerebroside β-glucosidase leading to the intracellular accumulation of abnormal quantities of glucocerebrosides.[215] Typical storage cells are seen in the bone marrow (Fig. 5.26) as well as in other tissues; these cells are macrophages distended by glucocerebrosides. Gaucher's cells are large, round or oval, and have pale blue cytoplasm with a wrinkled appearance due to the presence of many fibrillar structures (Romanowsky stain). The cytoplasm is Sudan black B- and PAS-positive. Gaucher cells also stain positively for non-specific esterase and tartrate-resistant acid phosphatase. Stains for iron give weak positive reactions. In histologic sections, Gaucher cells are often found in clumps or sheets and their abundant cytoplasm has a crumpled appearance (Fig. 5.27). The affected marrow may show an increase in reticulin and collagen. Electron microscopy reveals that the cytoplasm is packed with large elongated sacs containing characteristic tubes, 30–40 nm wide, each of which is made up of spirally arranged fibrils. Occasionally, particularly after splenectomy, Gaucher cells may be seen in the peripheral blood. Cells resembling Gaucher cells under the light microscope are seen in the marrow in a variety of

hematologic disorders including chronic granulocytic leukemia,[216] acute leukemia,[217] thalassemia major,[218] the congenital dyserythropoietic anemias (Fig. 5.28),[219] Hodgkin's disease,[220] non-Hodgkin's lymphoma,[221] multiple myeloma[222] and *Mycobacterium avium intracellulare* infection[223] and after many platelet transfusions.[224] However, such cells (pseudo-Gaucher cells) are ultrastructurally different from Gaucher cells.[216,225] Pseudo-Gaucher cells, with the exception of those in mycobacterial infection, are caused by an increased phagocytic load (e.g. of abnormal red cells or erythroblasts or leukemic cells) on the macrophages resulting in the production of lipid in excess of that which can be metabolized, with consequent intracellular accumulation. In mycobacterial infection the abnormal staining characteristics of the macrophages ('pseudo-pseudo-Gaucher's cells') result from the presence of very large numbers of mycobacteria within the macrophages.

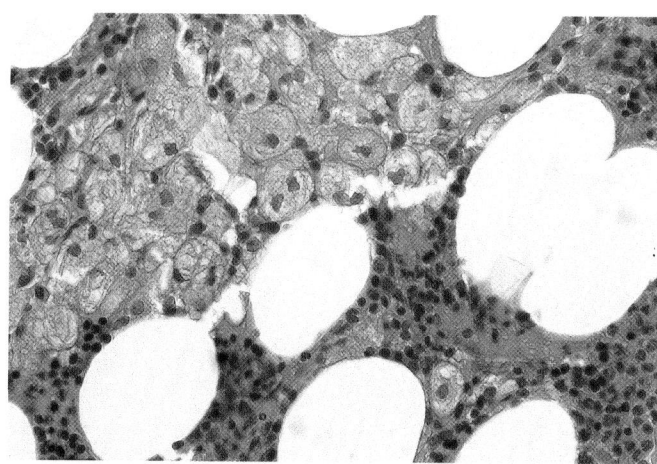

Fig. 5.27 Trephine biopsy from a case of Gaucher's disease. H&E.

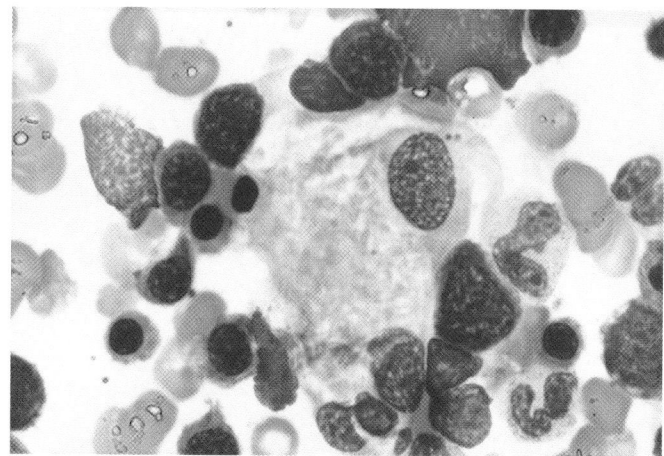

Fig. 5.26 Gaucher cell from the marrow smear of a patient with Gaucher's disease. May–Grünwald–Giemsa stain. × 940.

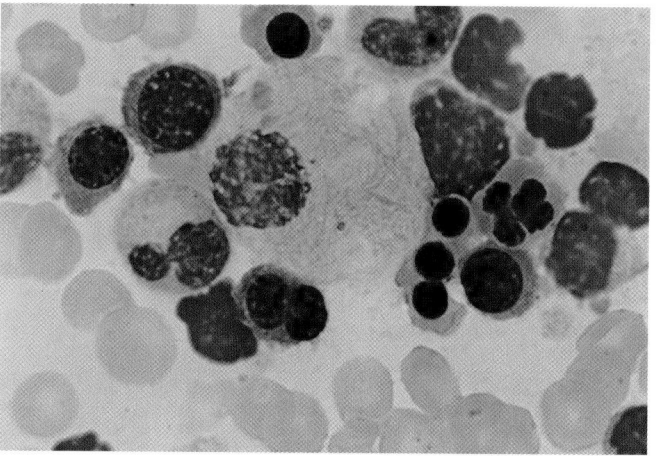

Fig. 5.28 Pseudo-Gaucher cell from the marrow smear of a patient with congenital dyserythropoietic anemia, type II. May–Grünwald–Giemsa stain. × 940.

Sea-blue histiocyte syndrome[226]

Sea-blue histiocytosis is an inherited group of disorders in which large macrophages containing coarse granules that stain sea-blue or blue-green (Romanowsky stain) are seen in the spleen, liver, bone marrow and other organs. The characteristic color of these granules after Romanowsky staining is attributed to the presence of ceroid; when unstained the granules are yellow or brown. The granules stain with oil red O and Sudan black B; as the pigment ages it develops autofluorescence and, subsequently, PAS-positivity followed by acid-fast positivity.[227] Ceroid is histochemically similar to lipofuscin. Ultrastructural studies have revealed that the granules are pleomorphic and that some of them contain concentric arrangements of membrane (myelin figures).[226] Sea-blue histiocytes have also been observed in the bone marrow in conditions other than the inherited sea-blue histiocyte syndrome (Fig. 5.29). These include acquired disorders such as chronic granulocytic leukemia, polycythemia rubra vera, multiple myeloma, lymphoproliferative disorders (including Hodgkin's disease), idiopathic thrombocytopenic purpura and rheumatoid arthritis as well as various inherited disorders such as sickle cell anemia, thalassemia, chronic granulomatous disease, Niemann–Pick disease, Tay–Sachs disease, Fabry's disease, Hurler's disease, Wolman's disease, lecithin-cholesterol acyltransferase deficiency, type V hyperlipidemia, and Hermansky–Pudlak syndrome.[226,228,229]

Niemann–Pick disease[212]

Niemann–Pick disease is usually inherited as an autosomal recessive condition and is often due to a deficiency of sphingomyelinase. This leads to the accumulation of excess sphingomyelin within the macrophages of the bone marrow and other organs. The cytoplasm of affected macrophages appears foamy, being filled with rounded lipid-containing inclusions (Fig. 5.30). The inclusions stain faint blue with Romanowsky stains and variably with the PAS reaction and lipid stains. Some sea-blue histiocytes are present. The cytoplasm of the foamy cells appears pale-yellow to yellow-brown in sections stained with H&E. The inclusions within these cells vary in their ultrastructure but often show myelin figures towards their periphery. Blood monocytes and lymphocytes in cases of Niemann–Pick disease have lipid-containing inclusions similar to those in macrophages.

Foamy macrophages are not specific for Niemann–Pick disease. They are also seen in some other storage diseases and in hyperlipidemias. They may also be found in certain infections, fat necrosis,[230,231] bone marrow infarction and in the Langerhans cell histiocytoses (eosinophilic granuloma, Letterer–Siwe disease and Hand–Schüller–Christian disease).

Fabry's disease

Fabry's disease is an X-linked recessive disorder due to deficiency of α-galactosidase. This leads to the accumulation of globotriaosylceramide and other neutral glycolipids in bone marrow macrophages. The cytoplasm of the abnormal macrophages appears foamy, being crowded with small globular structures staining pale blue with Romanowsky stains and strongly with PAS, Sudan black B, Luxol fast blue, oil red O, and stains for acid phosphatase.[75,232] In sections stained with H&E, the cytoplasmic globules appear pink.

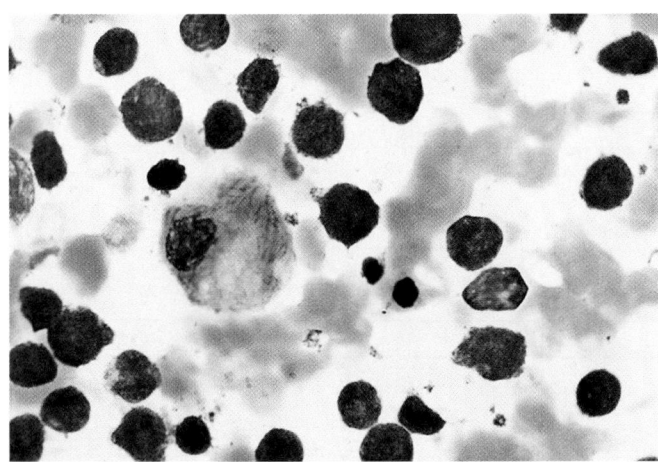

Fig. 5.29 Sea-blue histiocyte from a patient with chronic lymphocytic leukemia. May–Grünwald–Giemsa stain.

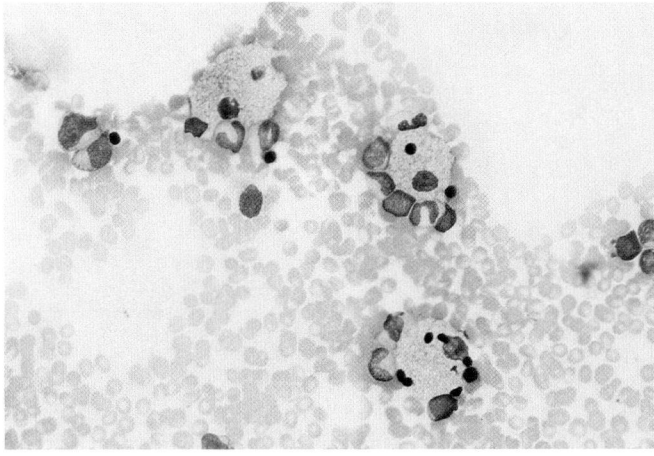

Fig. 5.30 Three foamy macrophages from the marrow smear of a patient with Niemann–Pick disease. May–Grünwald–Giemsa stain.

Mucopolysaccharidoses[75]

In Hurler's syndrome and other mucopolysaccharidoses, there is a deficiency of enzymes involved in the metabolism of the carbohydrate component of glycoproteins leading to an accumulation within lysosomes of mucopolysaccharides and glycolipids. The abnormal lysosomes inside bone marrow macrophages, plasma cells and lymphocytes may appear as metachromatic granules; the granules stain lilac or purple with Romanowsky stains (Alder–Reilly bodies). The cytoplasm of macrophages may be packed with basophilic inclusions of varying size which are surrounded by a clear halo. In histologic sections, the macrophage cytoplasm appears foamy due to extraction of the mucopolysaccharides.

Other storage diseases and hyperlipidemias[75]

Foamy histiocytes resembling those seen in Niemann–Pick disease and Fabry's disease may also be seen in the bone marrow in Wolman's disease, neuronal ceroid lipofuscinosis, hypercholesterolemia, hyperchylomicronemia, late-onset cholesterol ester storage disease and in Tangier disease (familial high-density lipoprotein deficiency).

Bone marrow necrosis[233–235]

In some pathologic conditions, there is necrosis of both the hemopoietic and the non-hemopoietic cells of the red marrow and there may also be necrosis of adjacent bone. Bone marrow necrosis is a common finding at autopsy[236] but is less often diagnosed during life. It may be widespread and can recur. The necrosis may be caused by interference with the blood supply or a failure to meet increased metabolic demands from a hypercellular marrow, or both, and may sometimes be related to high concentrations of tumor necrosis factor in the blood.[237]

The conditions associated with bone marrow necrosis are given in Table 5.13. In sickle cell anemia, Hb SC disease (heterozygous state for both hemoglobin S and hemoglobin C), hemoglobin S/β+-thalassemia and, rarely, heterozygosity for both hemoglobins S and E (plus parvovirus infection), necrosis may occur due to occlusion of the microvasculature of the bone marrow by sickled cells. In sickle cell disease pregnancy increases the degree of bone marrow hyperplasia and, thereby, further increases the likelihood of bone marrow infarction and also of death from the embolism of necrotic marrow to the lungs. In mucormycosis, the mucorales invade vessel

Table 5.13 Conditions associated with bone marrow necrosis

Relatively common:
Sickle cell anemia[a,233,238]
Hemoglobin SC disease,[a,239] hemoglobin S/β+-thalassemia[b,240,241]
Acute myeloid leukemia[234,242–245]
Acute lymphoblastic leukemia[202,233,246–248]
Metastatic carcinoma[233,234]
Caisson disease

Uncommon:
Essential thrombocythemia[249]
Chronic granulocytic leukemia[233,250]
Idiopathic myelofibrosis[234,235]
Lymphoma, both non-Hodgkin's lymphoma and Hodgkin's disease[234,251–253]
Chronic lymphocytic leukemia[254]
Multiple myeloma[236,255]
Malignant histiocytosis
Other hemoglobinopathies (Hb SD, hemoglobin SE,[b,256] sickle cell trait)[234]
Disseminated intravascular coagulation[257,258]
Antiphospholipid syndrome[259,260]
Tumor embolism of the marrow
Embolism from vegetations on cardiac valves[233,261]
Systemic lupus erythematosus[262]
Hyperparathyroidism[263]
Megaloblastic anemia[233]
Infections:
    Cytomegalovirus[264]
    Parvovirus[265]
    HIV infection (AIDS)
    Miliary tuberculosis[266]
    Gram-positive infections (e.g. streptococcus, staphylococcus)
    Gram-negative infections (e.g. *Escherichia coli*)[267]
    Typhoid fever[233]
    Fusobacterium necrophorum[268]
    Diphtheria[233]
    Q fever[269]
    Histoplasmosis[74]
    Mucormycosis[270]

[a] Particularly during pregnancy.
[b] With parvovirus infection.

walls and cause thrombosis and infarction.[270] In caisson disease (acute decompression illness) and disseminated intravascular coagulation (DIC) the microvasculature is occluded by bubbles of nitrogen and thrombi, respectively. In acute leukemia, carcinomatous infiltration of the marrow and megaloblastic anemia plus infection, the increased metabolic needs of a hyperplastic marrow may play a role in the pathogenesis of the bone marrow necrosis. In addition, in leukemia and carcinomatosis, the malignant cells may compress vessels, invade vessel walls and occlude their lumina or cause thrombosis.[202,242]

Bone marrow necrosis is accompanied by bone pain and fever. Extensive necrosis causes a leukoerythroblastic blood picture and pancytopenia. The macroscopic appearance of the aspirated bone marrow fragments may be abnormal with the fragments appearing opaque and white/pale yellow, or plum-colored. In a Romanowsky-stained smear of necrotic marrow, little cellular detail is discernible (Fig. 5.31); the blurred outlines of cells are seen in a background of amorphous pink material. In some patients with bone marrow necrosis secondary to metastatic carcinoma, an aspirate may show a mixture of intact tumor cells and necrotic tumor and hemopoietic cells. If bone marrow aspirated from one site shows only bone marrow necrosis and leukemia or metastatic carcinoma is suspected, a second aspiration from another site may be useful in demonstrating infiltration by malignant cells. The appearance of the trephine biopsy depends on the time after infarction as well as the underlying disorder. Initially, the cells have indistinct margins, granular cytoplasm and pyknotic nuclei. Later, cell outlines are unrecognizable and there is karyorrhexis. Necrosis of the adjacent bone is common, with loss of

osteoclasts, osteoblasts and osteocytes (Fig. 5.32). Recovery is accompanied by repopulation with hemopoietic tissue but small fibrotic scars[271] or, rarely, large areas of fibrous tissue may develop (Fig. 5.33); new bone is laid down on the spicules of dead bone. Radiologic examination shows no abnormality initially and may show sclerotic changes after some time. However, in the acute phase, bone scanning with ^{99m}Tc-sulfur-colloid shows lack of reticuloendothelial function in the infarcted area. The scan gradually returns to normal. Extramedullary hemopoiesis may develop in patients with extensive bone marrow necrosis.[251]

Gelatinous transformation[272–284]

The bone marrow of most patients with severe anorexia nervosa, some patients with cachexia secondary to AIDS and chronic disorders (e.g. tuberculosis, carcinoma) and occasional cases of leukemia post-chemotherapy and of systemic lupus erythematosus (SLE) contains a gelatinous material which appears to consist of acid mucopolysaccharide. Gelatinous transformation has also been reported in other conditions including severe hypothyroidism, intestinal lymphangiectasia (Waldman's disease) and leishmaniasis. The gelatinous material is amorphous, granular or fibrillar, stains pink-purple with Romanowsky stains or H&E (Figs 5.34 and 5.35) and stains positively with Alcian blue (particularly at a high pH) and the PAS stain. The hemopoietic cells are reduced in number and embedded within the gelatinous material and there is an absence or marked reduction of fat cells. Marrow fragments showing gelatinous transformation do not smear properly. A deficiency of carbohydrates and calories may underlie the gelatinous transformation and

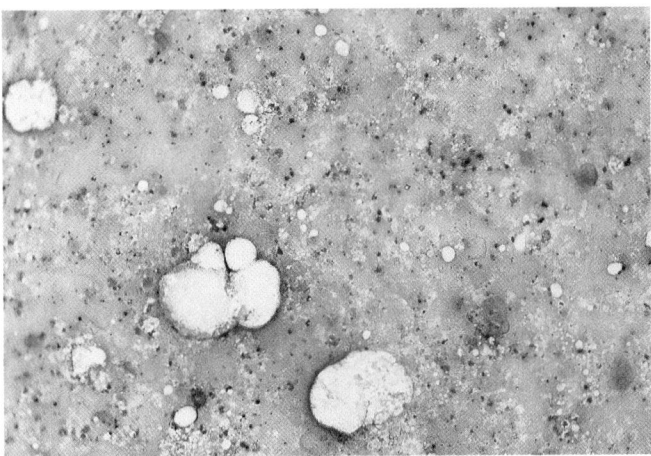

Fig. 5.31 Bone marrow smear showing necrosis of the marrow cells. May–Grünwald–Giemsa stain. × 940.

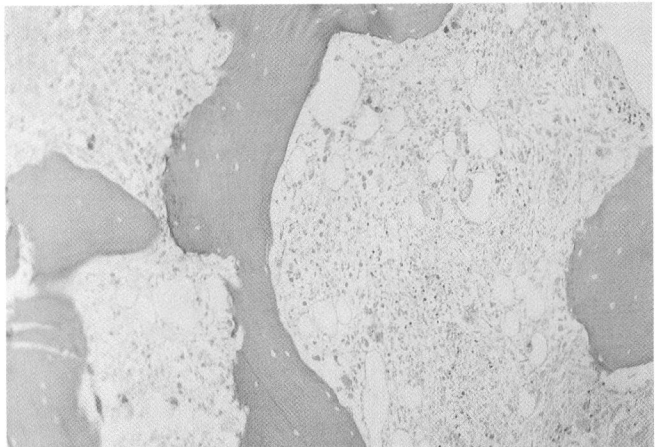

Fig. 5.32 Trephine biopsy of bone marrow showing necrosis of both the bone and the marrow. The lacunae within the bone do not contain osteocytes and appear empty. H&E. × 375.

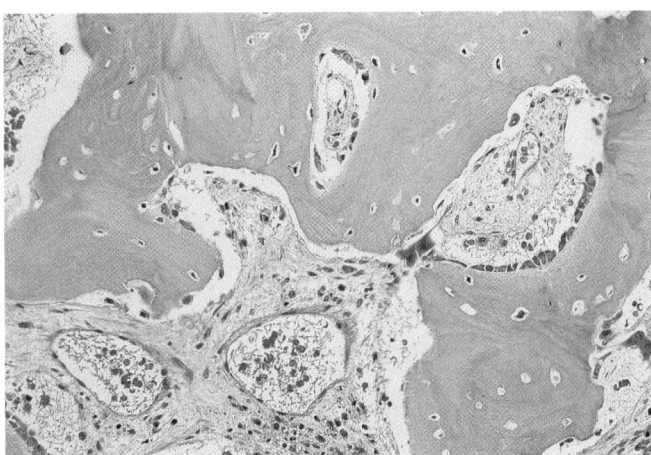

Fig. 5.33 Bone marrow fibrosis and osteosclerosis following bone marrow necrosis in a case of Ph[+] chronic granulocytic leukemia. H&E.

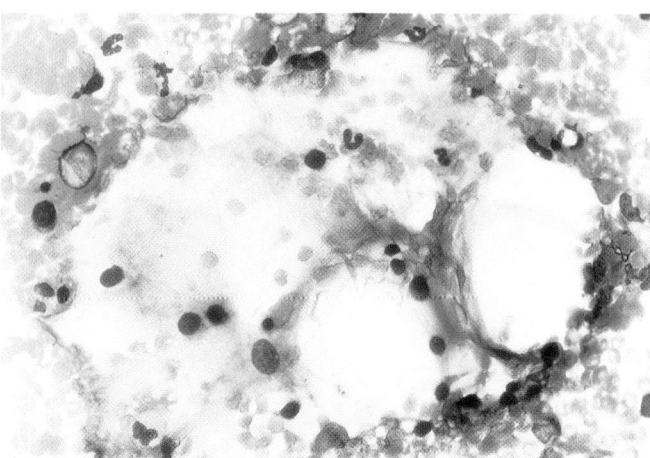

Fig. 5.34 Very small marrow fragment from a bone marrow smear of a patient with AIDS showing gelatinous transformation. In this photomicrograph, the pink-purple gelatinous material is mainly found in between the fat cells. May–Grünwald–Giemsa stain. × 94.

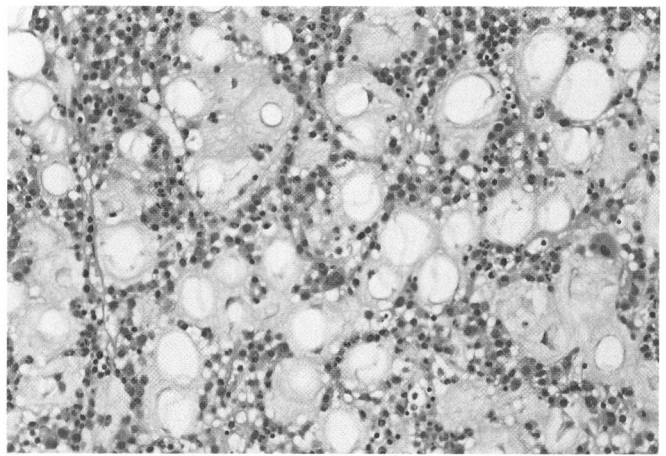

Fig. 5.35 Trephine biopsy of bone marrow from a patient with AIDS showing gelatinous transformation. H&E. × 375.

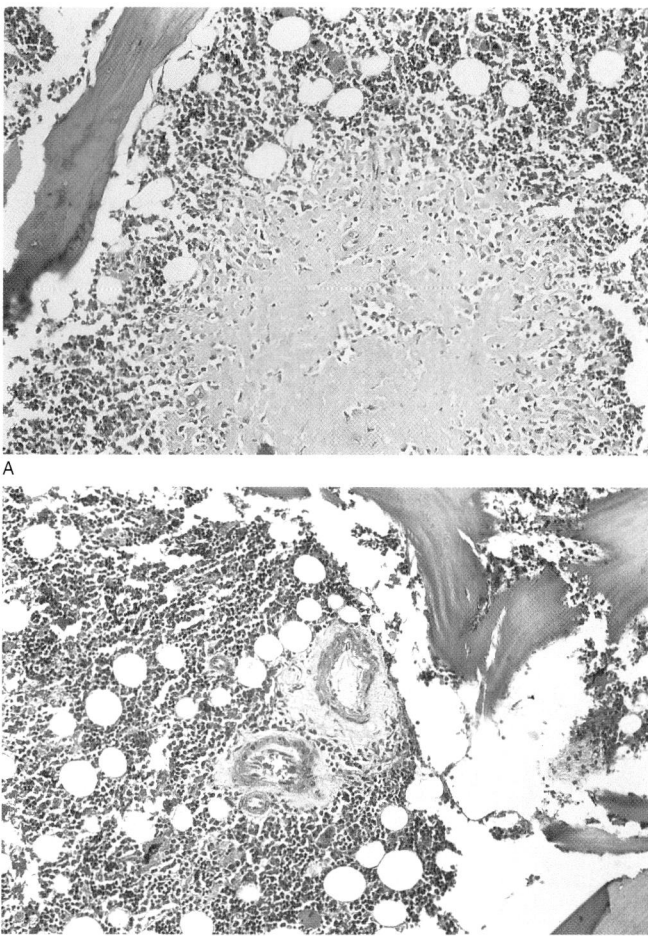

A

B

Fig. 5.36 (A–B) Amyloid deposition in the bone marrow. (A) Much of the normal hemopoietic tissue is replaced by a nodule of amyloid that appears faintly eosinophilic and homogeneous. (B) Two arterioles showing advanced amyloid deposition in their walls and occlusion of their lumina with amyloid. In arterioles and small arteries, amyloid deposition commences in the subendothelial tissues and gradually spreads outwards. H&E. (A) × 90; (B) × 90.

the excessive accumulation of acid mucopolysaccharide may serve to fill the marrow space normally occupied by fat cells. Interestingly, young children with protein-energy malnutrition do not show gelatinous transformation.

Amyloidosis

Amyloid deposits may be seen in the bone marrow both in smears of aspirated material, infrequently, and in histologic sections. In Romanowsky-stained smears amyloid appears pink to purple, waxy to transparent, and has been described as resembling a cumulus cloud.[285] In histologic sections of marrow, amyloid has the same appearance and staining characteristics as in other tissues (Fig. 5.36). It is seen most often in vessel walls but sometimes in the interstitium. Bone marrow amyloid is observed most frequently in light-chain-associated amyloidosis[286] (sometimes referred to as primary amyloidosis) but is also observed in secondary amyloidosis, for example in familial Mediterranean fever and secondary to chronic inflammatory conditions such as rheumatoid arthritis. In light-chain-associated amyloidosis the marrow may show, in additon, a slight to moderate increase in monotypic plasma cells or overt multiple myeloma.

Vascular and embolic lesions

The marrow may show arteritis and arteriolitis in any form of generalized arteritis, including giant cell arteritis.[287] Hypersensitivity reactions to drugs may cause granulomatous vasculitis[288] and in polyarteritis nodosa there may be vasculitic lesions with fibrinoid necrosis.

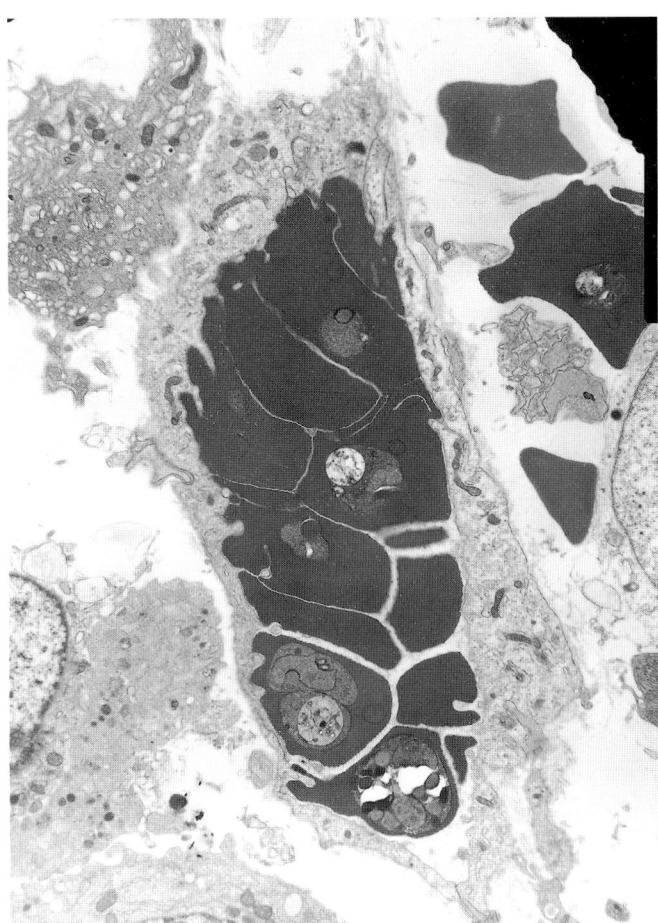

Fig. 5.37 Bone marrow sinusoid from a patient with cerebral malaria. The lumen is occluded by parasitized red cells. Uranyl acetate and lead citrate. × 4900.

Trephine biopsies may reveal arteriosclerotic and thromboembolic lesions. Emboli that are acellular or composed of hyaline material or cholesterol crystals may be derived from atheromatous plaques and cause a multisystem disease characterized by anemia, leukocytosis, eosinophilia and elevated erythrocyte sedimentation rate.[289–291] Bone marrow emboli are found in 20% of these cases at autopsy and may also be seen in biopsy material.[290] Vessels are partly or completely occluded by acellular material with cholesterol clefts and there may be intimal hyperplasia and infiltration of vessel walls initially with granulocytes and subsequently with mononuclear cells and giant cells.

Tumor emboli may be seen in patients with carcinoma and may be accompanied by microangiopathic hemolytic anemia. In thrombotic thrombocytopenic purpura, intravascular and subendothelial hyaline deposits and platelet thrombi may be seen in bone marrow vessels.[292]

In cerebral malaria, some bone marrow sinusoids are packed with parasitized red cells (Fig. 5.37). These red cells attach to the endothelial cells and to each other via surface knobs.[293]

Aluminum deposition[294,295]

In patients on hemodialysis and other patients with chronic renal failure aluminum may be deposited both in bone (at the osteoid/mineralized tissue junction) and in marrow cells as coarse granules. The aluminum is derived from oral intake and dialysis fluids and may cause dementia. Aluminum may be demonstrated by a specific stain (Irwin stain on an undecalcified trephine biopsy). The marrow cell that contains the aluminum may be the macrophage.

REFERENCES

1. Hayhoe FGJ, Quaglino D 1980 Haematological cytochemistry. Churchill Livingstone, Edinburgh
2. Rywlin AM 1976 Histopathology of the bone marrow. Little, Brown, Boston, 10
3. Burkhardt R, Frisch B, Bartl R 1982 Bone biopsy in haematological disorders. Journal of Clinical Pathology 35: 257–284
4. Rohr K, Hafter E 1937 Untersuchungen über postmortale Veränderungen des menschlichen Knochenmarks. Folia Haematologica 58: 38–50
5. Findlay AB 1977 Bone marrow changes in the post mortem interval. Journal of Forensic Science Society 16: 213–218
6. Young RH, Osgood EE 1935 Sternal marrow aspirated during life. Cytology in health and in disease. Archives of Internal Medicine 55: 186–203
7. Bain BJ 1996 The bone marrow aspirate of healthy subjects. British Journal of Haematology 94: 206–209
8. Nemec J, Polak H 1964 Erythropoietic polyploidy. I. The morphology of polyploid erythroid elements and their incidence in healthy subjects. Folia Haematologica (Leipzig) 84: 24–40
9. Wickramasinghe SN, Lee MJ, Furukawa T et al 1996 Composition of intra-erythroblastic precipitates in thalassaemia and congenital dyserythropoietic anaemia (CDA): identification of a new type of CDA with intra-erythroblastic precipitates not reacting with monoclonal antibodies to α– and β-globin chains. British Journal of Haematology 93: 576–585
10. Lehane DE 1974 Vacuolated erythroblasts in hyperosmolar coma. Archives of Internal Medicine 134: 763–765
11. Wickramasinghe SN, Hughes M 1984 Globin chain precipitation, deranged iron metabolism and dyserythropoiesis in some thalassaemia syndromes. Haematologia (Budapest) 17: 35–55
12. Lewis SM, Verwilghen RL (eds) 1977 Dyserythropoiesis. Academic Press, New York
13. Bain BJ 1997 The haematological features of HIV infection. British Journal of Haematology 99: 1–8
14. Niebrugge DJ, Benjamin DR, Christie D, Scott CR 1982 Hereditary transcobalamin II deficiency presenting as red cell hypoplasia. Journal of Pediatrics 101: 732–735
15. Rozensajn L, Klajman A, Yaffe D, Efrati P 1966 Jordan's anomaly in white blood cells. Report of case. Blood 28: 258–265
16. Rywlin AM 1976 Histopathology of the bone marrow. Little, Brown, Boston, 13
17. Yoo D, Lessin LS, Jensen WN 1978 Bone marrow mast cells in lymphoproliferative disorders. Annals of Internal Medicine 88: 753–757
18. Burkhardt R, Zettl K, Bartl R 1978 Significance of non-specific changes of the bone marrow tissues from the bioptic viewpoint. Bibl Haematologica 45: 38–49
19. Prokocimer M, Polliack A 1980 Increased bone marrow mast cells in preleukemic syndromes, acute leukemia, and lymphoproliferative syndromes. American Journal of Clinical Pathology 75: 34–38
20. Rywlin AM, Ortega RS, Dominguez CJ 1974 Lymphoid nodules of bone marrow: normal and abnormal. Blood 43: 389–400
21. Maeda K, Hyun BH, Rebuck JW 1977 Lymphoid follicles in bone marrow aspirates. American Journal of Clinical Pathology 67: 41–48
22. Faulkner-Jones BE, Howie AJ, Boughton BJ, Franklin IM 1988

Lymphoid aggregates in bone marrow: study of eventual outcome. Journal of Clinical Pathology 41: 768–775

23. Dick F, Bloomfield CD, Brunning RD 1974 Incidence, cytology, and histopathology of non-Hodgkin's lymphomas in the bone marrow. Cancer 33: 1382–1398

24. Klein H, Block M 1953 Bone marrow plasmacytosis. Blood 8: 1034–1041

25. Hyun BH, Kwa D, Gabaldon H, Ashton JK 1976 Reactive plasmacytic lesions in the bone marrow. American Journal of Clinical Pathology 65: 921–928

26. Canale DD Jr, Collins RD 1974 Use of bone marrow particle sections in the diagnosis of multiple myeloma. American Journal of Clinical Pathology 61: 382–392

27. Kyle RA, Bayrd ED 1976 The monoclonal gammopathies: multiple myeloma and related plasma cell disorders. Thomas, Springfield

28. Crocker J, Curran RC 1981 Quantitative study of the immunoglobulin-containing cells in trephine samples of bone marrow. Journal of Clinical Pathology 34: 1080–1082

29. Fitchen JH, Lee S 1979 Phagocytic myeloma cells. American Journal of Clinical Pathology 71: 722–723

30. Cook MK, Madden M 1982 Iron granules in plasma cells. Journal of Clinical Pathology 35: 172–181

31. Karcioglu GL, Hardison JE 1978 Iron-containing plasma cells. Archives of Internal Medicine 138: 97–100

32. Lombardi L, Carbone A, Pilotti S, Rilke F 1978 Malignant histiocytosis: a histological and ultrastructural study of lymph nodes in six cases. Histopathology 2: 315–328

33. Carbone A, Micheau C, Caillaud JM, Carlu C 1981 A cytochemical and immunochemical approach to malignant histiocytosis. Cancer 47: 2862–2871

34. Lampert IA, Catovsky D, Bergier N 1978 Malignant histiocytosis: a clinicopathological study of 12 cases. British Journal of Haematology 40: 65–77

35. Tiab M, Mechinaud F, Harousseau J-L 2000 Haemophagocytic syndromes associated with infections. Baillière's Clinical Haematology 13(2): 163–178

36. Perry MC, Harrison EG Jr, Burgert EO Jr, Gilchrist GS 1976 Familial erythrophagocytic lymphohistiocytosis. Report of two cases and clinicopathological review. Cancer 38: 209–218

37. Arico M, Caselli D, Burgio GR 1989 Familial hemophagocytic lymphohistiocytosis: clinical features. Pediatric Hematology and Oncology 6: 247–251

38. Risdall RJ, McKenna RW, Nesbit ME et al 1979 Virus-associated hemophagocytic syndrome: a benign histiocytic proliferation distinct from malignant histiocytosis. Cancer 44: 993–1002

39. Daneshbod K, Kissane JM 1978 Idiopathic differentiated histiocytosis. American Journal of Clinical Pathology 70: 381–389

40. Mills MJ 1982 Post-viral haemophagocytic syndrome. Journal of the Royal Society of Medicine 75: 555–557

41. Wilson ER, Malluh A, Stagno S, Crist WM 1981 Fatal Epstein–Barr virus associated hemophagocytic syndrome. Journal of Pediatrics 98: 260–262

42. Muir K, Todd WTA, Watson WH, Fitzsimons E 1992 Viral associated haemophagocytosis with parvovirus-B19-related pancytopenia. Lancet 339: 1139–1140

43. Yin JA, Kumaran TO, Marsh GW et al 1983 Complete recovery of histiocytic medullary reticulosis-like syndrome in a child with acute lymphoblastic leukemia. Cancer 51: 200–202

44. Imashuku S 1997 Differential diagnosis of hemophagocytic syndrome: underlying disorders and selection of most effective treatment. International Journal of Hematology 66: 135–151

45. Zinkham WH, Medearis DN Jr, Osborn JE 1967 Blood and bone marrow findings in congenital rubella. Journal of Pediatrics 71: 512–524

46. Wong KF, Chan JK, Chan JC et al 1991 Dengue virus infection-associated hemophagocytic syndrome. American Journal of Hematology 38: 339–340

47. Chandra P, Chaudhery SA, Rosner F, Kagen M 1975 Transient histiocytosis with striking phagocytosis of platelets, leukocytes, and erythrocytes. Archives of Internal Medicine 135: 989–991

48. Zuazu JP, Duran JW, Julia AF 1979 Hemophagocytosis in acute brucellosis. New England Journal of Medicine 301: 1185–1186

49. Macias EG 1975 Typhoidal cells. Lancet ii: 927–928

50. Gill K, Marrie TJ 1987 Hemophagocytosis secondary to *Mycoplasma pneumoniae* infection. American Journal of Medicine 82: 668–670

51. Weisenburger DD, Rappaport H, Ahluwalia MS et al 1980 Legionnaires' disease. American Journal of Medicine 69: 476–482

52. Abbott KC, Vakelja ST, Smith CE et al 1991 Hemophagocytic syndrome: a cause of pancytopenia in human Ehrlichiosis. American Journal of Hematology 38: 230–234

53. Woodard BH, Farnham R, Bradford WD 1981 Fatal Rocky Mountain spotted fever. Hematologic and lymphoreticular observations. Archives of Pathology and Laboratory Medicine 105: 452–453

54. Estrov Z, Bruck R, Shtalrid M et al (1983) Histiocytic hemophagocytosis in Q-fever. Archives of Pathology and Laboratory Medicine 108: 7

55. Wong K-F, Chan JKC 1992 Reactive haemophagocytic syndrome – a clinico-pathologic study of 40 patients in an Oriental population. American Journal of Medicine 93, 177–180

56. Reiner AP, Spivak JL 1988 Hematophagic histiocytosis: a report of 23 new patients and a review of the literature. Medicine 67: 369–388

57. Higgins EM, Layton DM, Arya R et al 1994 Disseminated *Trichosporon beigelii* infection in an immunosuppressed child. Journal of the Royal Society of Medicine 87: 292–293

58. Auerbach M. Haubenstock A, Soloman G 1980 Systemic babesiosis. Another cause of the hemophagocytic syndrome. American Journal of Medicine 80: 301–303

59. Krause JR, Kaplan SS 1982 Bone marrow findings in infectious mononucleosis and mononucleosis-like diseases in the older adult. Scandinavian Journal of Haematology 28: 15–22

60. Korman LY, Smith JR, Landaw SA, Davey FR 1979 Hodgkin's disease: intramedullary phagocytosis with pancytopenia. Annals of Internal Medicine 91: 60–61

61. Jaffe ES, Costa J, Fauci AS 1981 Erythrophagocytic Tγ lymphoma. New England Journal of Medicine 305: 103–104

62. Chan EY, Pi D, Chan GT et al 1989 Peripheral T-cell lymphoma presenting as hemophagocytic syndrome. Hematological Oncology 7: 275–285

63. Sonneveld P, van Lom K, Kappers-Klunne M et al 1990 Clinico-pathological diagnosis and treatment of malignant histiocytosis. British Journal of Haematology 75: 511–516

64. Takeshita M, Kikuchi M, Ohshima K et al 1993 Bone marrow findings in malignant histiocytosis, and/or malignant lymphoma with concurrent hemophagocytic syndrome. Leukemia and Lymphoma 12: 79–89

65. Okuda T, Sakamoto S, Deguchi T et al 1991 Hemophagocytic syndrome associated with natural killer cell leukemia. American Journal of Hematology 38, 321–323

66. James LP, Stass SA, Peterson V, Schumacher HR 1979 Abnormalities of bone marrow simulating histiocytic medullary reticulosis in a patient with gastric carcinoma. American Journal of Clinical Pathology 71: 600–602

67. Falini B, Bucciarelli E, Grignani F, Martelli MF 1980 Erythrophagocytosis by undifferentiated lung carcinoma cells. Cancer 46: 1140–1145

68. Youness E, Barlogie B, Ahearn M, Trujillo JM 1980 Tumor cell phagocytosis. Its occurrence in a patient with medulloblastoma. Archives of Pathology and Laboratory Medicine 104: 651–653

69. Martelli MF, Falini B, Tabilio A et al 1980 Prolymphocytic leukaemia with erythrophagocytic activity. British Journal of Haematology 46: 141–142

70. Foadi MD, Slater AM, Pegrum GD 1978 Erythrophagocytosis by acute lymphoblastic leukaemia cells. Scandinavian Journal of Haematology 20: 85–88

71. Kadin ME, Kamoun M, Lamberg J 1981 Erythrophagocytic Tγ lymphoma: a clinicopathologic entity resembling malignant histiocytosis. New England Journal of Medicine 304: 648–653

72. Tsan MF, Mehlman DJ, Green RS, Bell WR 1976 Dilantin, agranulocytosis, and phagocytic marrow histiocytes. Annals of Internal Medicine 84: 710–711

73. Miranda D, Vuletin JC, Kauffman SL 1979 Disseminated histiocytosis and intestinal melakoplakia. Occurrence due to *Mycobacterium intracellulare* infection. Archives of Pathology and Laboratory Medicine 103: 302–305

74. Davies SF, McKenna RW, Sarosi GA 1979 Trephine biopsy of the bone marrow in disseminated histoplasmosis. American Journal of Medicine 67: 617–622

75. Brunning RD 1970 Morphological alterations in nucleated blood and marrow cells in genetic disorders. Human Pathology 1: 99–124

76. Lundin P, Persson B, Weinfeld A 1964 Comparison of hemosiderin estimation in bone marrow sections and bone marrow smears. Acta Medica Scandinavica 175: 383–390

77. Fong TP, Okafor LA, Thomas W Jr, Westerman MP 1977 Stainable iron in aspirated and needle-biopsy specimens of bone marrow. American Journal of Hematology 2: 47–51

78. Krause JR, Brubaker D, Kaplan S 1979 Comparison of stainable iron in aspirated and needle-biopsy specimens of bone marrow. American Journal of Clinical Pathology 72: 68–70

79. Gale E, Torrance J, Bothwell T 1963 The quantitative estimation of total iron stores in human bone marrow. Journal of Clinical Investigation 42: 1076–1082

80. Dacie JV, Mollin DL 1966 Siderocytes, sideroblasts and sideroblastic anaemia. Acta Medica Scandinavica 445 (suppl): 237–248

81. Douglas AS, Dacie JV 1953 The incidence and significance of iron-containing granules in human erythrocytes and their precursors. Journal of Clinical Pathology 6: 307–313

82. Kaplan E, Zuelzer WW, Mouriquand C 1954 Sideroblasts. A study of stainable nonhemoglobin iron in marrow normoblasts. Blood 9: 203

83. Rausing A 1973 Bone marrow biopsy in diagnosis of Whipple's disease. Acta Medica Scandinavica 193: 5–8

84. Robert F, Durant JR, Gams RA 1977 Demonstration of *Cryptococcus neoformans* in a stained bone marrow specimen. Archives of Internal Medicine 137: 688–690

85. Pasternak J, Bolivar R 1983 Histoplasmosis in acquired immunodeficiency syndrome (AIDS): diagnosis by bone marrow examination. Archives of Internal Medicine 143: 2024

86. Elman L 1976 Bone marrow biopsy in the evaluation of lymphoma, carcinoma and granulomatous disorders. American Journal of Medicine 60: 1–7

87. Wickramasinghe SN, Abdalla SH 2000 Blood and bone marrow changes in malaria. Baillière's Clinical Haematology 13(2): 277–299

88. Cuartas F, Rothenberg J, Fecci C, Gutterman J 1972 Diagnosis of malaria by bone marrow aspiration. Southern Medical Journal 65: 523

89. Wickramasinghe SN, Abdalla SH, Kasili EG 1987 Ultrastructure of bone marrow in patients with visceral leishmaniasis. Journal of Clinical Pathology 40: 267–275

90. Penchansky L, Krause JR 1979 Identification of cytomegalovirus in bone marrow biopsy. Southern Medical Journal 72: 500–501

91. Rao KR, Patel AR, Anderson MJ et al 1983 Infection with parvovirus-like virus and aplastic crisis in chronic hemolytic anemia. Annals of Internal Medicine 98: 930–932

92. Brown KE 2000 Haematological consequences of parvovirus B19 infection. Baillière's Clinical Haematology 13(2): 245–259

93. Evans RH, Scadden DT 2000 Haematological aspects of HIV infection. Baillière's Clinical Haematology 13(2): 215–230

94. Cooper DA, Gold J, Maclean P et al 1985 Acute AIDS retrovirus infection: definition of a clinical syndrome associated with seroconversion. Lancet i: 537–545

95. Van Essen GG, Lieverse AG, Sprenger HG et al 1988 False positive Paul-Bunnel test in HIV seroconversion. Lancet ii: 747–748

96. Wickramasinghe SN 1994 Bone marrow damage in AIDS. In: Bhatt HR, James VHT, Besser GM et al (eds) Advances in Thomas Addison's diseases, vol 1. Journal of Endocrinology, Bristol, 339–355

97. Sullivan PS, Hanson DL, Chu SY et al and the Adult/Adolescent Spectrum of Disease Group 1998 Epidemiology of anemia in human immunodeficiency virus (HIV)-infected persons; results from the multistate adult and adolescent spectrum of HIV disease surveillance project. Blood 91: 301–308

98. Slagel DD, Lager DJ, Dick FR 1994 Howell–Jolly body-like inclusions in the neutrophils of patients with acquired immunodeficiency syndrome. American Journal of Clinical Pathology 101: 429–431

99. Candido A, Rossi P, Menichella G et al 1990 Indicative morphological myelodysplastic alterations of bone marrow in overt AIDS. Haematologica 75: 327–333

100. Milam MW, Balerdi MJ, Toney JF et al 1990 Epithelioid angiomatosis secondary to disseminated cat scratch disease involving the bone marrow and skin in a patient with acquired immune deficiency syndrome: a case report. American Journal of Medicine 88: 180–183

101. Wong KF, Tsang DN, Chan JK 1994 Bone marrow diagnosis of penicilliosis. New England Journal of Medicine 330: 717–718

102. Nichols L, Florentine B, Lewis W et al 1991 Bone marrow examination for the diagnosis of mycobacterial and fungal infections in the acquired immunodeficiency syndrome. Archives of Pathology and Laboratory Medicine 115: 1125–1132

103. Moses A, Nelson J, Bagby GC Jr 1998 The influence of human immunodeficiency virus-1 on hematopoiesis. Blood 91: 1479–1495

104. Chelucci C, Casella M, Federico M et al 1999 Lineage-specific expression of human immunodeficiency virus (HIV) receptor/coreceptors in differentiating hematopoietic precursors: correlation with susceptibility to T- and M-tropic HIV and chemokine-mediated HIV resistance. Blood 94: 1590–1600

105. Wickramasinghe SN, Beatty C, Shiels S et al 1992 Ultrastructure of the bone marrow in HIV infection: evidence of dyshaemopoiesis and stromal cell damage. Clinical and Laboratory Haematology 14: 213–229

106. Wickramasinghe SN, Shiels S 1993 Bone marrow stromal cell damage in HIV infection. Clinical and Laboratory Haematology 15: 236–237

107. Prazuck T, Semaille C, Roques S 1998 Fatal acute haemolysis in AIDS patients treated with indinavir. AIDS 12: 531–533

108. Moallem HJ, Garraty G, Wakeham M et al 1998 Ceftriaxone-related fatal hemolysis in an adolescent with perinatally acquired human immunodeficiency virus infection. Journal of Pediatrics 133: 279–281

109. Bain BJ 1998 Lymphomas and reactive lymphoid lesions in HIV infection. Blood Reviews 12: 154–162

110. Nair JMG, Bellevue R, Bertoni M, Dosik H 1988 Thrombotic thrombocytopenia in patients with acquired immunodeficiency syndrome (AIDS)-related complex: a report of two cases. Annals of Internal Medicine 109: 242–243

111. Adams DO 1976 The granulomatous inflammatory response. A review. American Journal of Pathology 84: 164–191

112. Eid A, Carion W, Nystrom JS 1996 Differential diagnoses of bone marrow granuloma. Western Journal of Medicine 164: 510–515

113. Farhi DC, Mason UG, Horsburgh CR 1984 The bone marrow in disseminated *Mycobacterium avium intracellulare* infection. American Journal of Clinical Pathology 83: 463–468

114. Hamilton PK 1954 The bone marrow in brucellosis. American Journal of Clinical Pathology 34: 580–587

115. Gormsen H 1948 The occurrence of epithelioid cell granulomas in human bone marrow with special reference to the diagnostic value of sternal puncture in Boeck's sarcoid and the differential diagnosis of sarcoidosis, miliary tuberculosis and brucellosis. Acta Medica Scandinavica 213 (suppl): 154–164

116. Lawrence C, Schreiber AJ 1979 Leprosy's footprints in bone marrow histiocytes. New England Journal of Medicine 300: 834–835

117. Dumler JS, Dawson JE, Walker DH 1993 Human ehrlichiosis: hematopathology and immunohistologic detection of *Ehrlichia chaffeensis*. Human Pathology 24: 391–396

118. Delsol G, Pellegrin M, Familiades J, Auvergnat JC 1978 Bone marrow lesions in Q fever. Blood 52: 637–638

119. Okun DB, Sun NCJ, Tanaka KR 1979 Bone marrow granulomas in Q-fever. American Journal of Clinical Pathology 71: 117–121

120. Pease GL 1956 Granulomatous lesions in bone marrow. Blood 11: 720–734

121. Walsh TJ, Catchatourian R, Cohen H 1983 Disseminated histoplasmosis complicating bone marrow transplantation. American Journal of Clinical Pathology 79: 509–511

122. Kurtin PJ, McKinsey DS, Gupta MR, Driks M 1989 Histoplasmosis in patients with acquired immunodeficiency syndrome. Hematologic and bone marrow manifestation. American Journal of Clinical Pathology 93: 367–372

123. Rywlin AM 1976 Histopathology of the bone marrow. Little, Brown, Boston, 170

124. Pantanowitz L, Omar T, Sonnendecker H, Karstaedt AS 2000 Bone marrow cryptococcal infection in the acquired immunodeficiency syndrome. Journal of Infection 41: 92–94

125. Ampel NM, Ryan KJ, Carry PJ et al 1986 Fungemia due to *Coccidioides immitis*. An analysis of 16 episodes in 15 patients and a review of the literature. Medicine (Baltimore) 65: 312–321

126. Hovde RF, Sundberg RD 1950 Granulomatous lesions in the bone marrow in infectious mononucleosis. Blood 5: 209–232

127. Martin MF 1977 Atypical infectious mononucleosis with bone marrow granulomas and pancytopenia. British Medical Journal ii: 300–301

128. Young JF, Goulian M 1993 Bone marrow fibrin ring granulomas and cytomegalovirus infection. American Journal of Clinical Pathology 99: 65–68

129. Browne PM, Shanna OP, Salkin D (1978) Bone marrow sarcoidosis. Journal of the American Medical Association 240: 2654–2655

130. Kadin ME, Donaldson SS, Dorfman RF 1970 Isolated granulomas in Hodgkin's Disease. New England Journal of Medicine 283: 859–861

131. Yu NC, Rywlin AM 1982 Granulomatous lesions of the bone marrow in non-Hodgkin's lymphoma. Human Pathology 13: 905–910

132. Falini B, Tabilio A, Velardi A et al 1982 Multiple myeloma with a sarcoidosis-like reaction. Scandinavian Journal of Haematology 29: 211–216

133. Bodem CR, Hamory BH, Taylor HM, Kleopfer L 1983 Granulomatous bone marrow disease. A review of the literature and clinicopathological analysis of 58 cases. Medicine (Baltimore) 62: 372–383

134. Vilalta-Castel E, Valdes-Sanchez MD, Guerra-Vales JM et al 1988 Significance of granulomas in bone marrow: a study of 40 cases. European Journal of Haematology 41: 12–14

135. Hyun BH 1986 Colour atlas of clinical hematology. Igaku-Shoin Med US, New York

136. Franco V, Florena AM, Quintini G, Musso M 1994 Bone marrow granulomas in hairy cell leukaemia following 2-chloro-deoxyadenosine therapy. Histopathology 24: 271–273

137. O'Brien DV, Boon AP, Boughton BJ 1992 Bone marrow granulomas in acute myeloid leukaemia following interleukin 2 and lymphokine-activated killer cells. Histopathology 20: 271–272

138. Wu HV, Kosmin M 1977 Bone marrow granulomata and phenytoin. Annals of Internal Medicine 86: 663

139. Riker J, Baker J, Swanson M 1978 Bone marrow granulomas and neutropenia associated with procainamide. Report of a case. Archives of Internal Medicine 138: 1731–1732

140. Andersson DE, Langworth S, Newman HC, Ost A 1980 Reversible bone marrow granulomas – adverse effect of oxyphenbutazone therapy. Acta Medica Scandinavica 207: 131–133

141. Poland GA, Love KR 1986 Marked atypical lymphocytosis, hepatitis, and skin rash in sulfasalazine drug allergy. American Journal of Medicine 81: 707–708

142. Rosenbaum H, Ben-Arie Y, Azzam ZS, Krivoy N 1998 Amiodarone-associated granuloma in bone marrow. Annals of Pharmacotherapy 32: 60–62

143. Pelstring RJ, Kim K, Lower EE, Swerdlow SH 1988 Marrow granulomas in coal workers' pneumoconiosis. American Journal of Clinical Pathology 89: 553–556

144. Lewis JH, Sundeen JT, Simon GL et al 1985 Disseminated talc granulomatosis: acquired immunodeficiency syndrome and fatal cytomegalovirus infection. Archives of Pathology and Laboratory Medicine 109: 147–150

145. Davis S, Trubowitz S 1982 Pathologic reactions involving the bone marrow. In: Trubowitz S, Davis S (eds), The human bone marrow: anatomy, physiology, and pathophysiology, vol II. CRC Press, Boca Raton, FL, 255

146. Dobrin RS, Vernier RL, Fish AL 1975 Acute eosinophilic interstitial nephritis and renal failure with bone marrow-lymph node granulomas and anterior uveitis. A new syndrome. American Journal of Medicine 59: 325–333

147. Rice L, Shenkenberg T, Lynch EC, Wheeler TM 1982 Granulomatous infections complicating hairy cell leukemia. Cancer 49: 1924–1928

148. Cohen RJ, Samoszuk MK, Busch D, Lagios M 1983 Occult infections with *M. intracellulare* in bone marrow biopsy specimens from patients with AIDS. New England Journal of Medicine 308: 1475–1476

149. Rywlin AM, Ortega R 1972 Lipid granulomas of the bone marrow. American Journal of Clinical Pathology 57: 457–462

150. Sawers AH, Davson J, Braganza J, Geary CG 1982 Systemic mastocytosis, myelofibrosis and portal hypertension. Journal of Clinical Pathology 35: 617–619

151. Ingle JN, Tormey DC, Tan HK 1978 The bone marrow examination in breast cancer. Cancer 41: 670–674

152. Rubins JM 1983 The role of myelofibrosis in malignant leukoerythroblastosis. Cancer 51: 308–311

153. Singh G, Krause JR, Breitfeld V 1977 Bone marrow examination for metastatic tumor: aspirate and biopsy. Cancer 40: 2317–2321

154. Anner RM, Drewinko B 1977 Frequency and significance of bone marrow involvement by metastatic solid tumors. Cancer 39: 1337–1344

155. Finkelstein JZ, Ekert H, Isaacs H, Higgins G 1970 Bone marrow metastases in children with solid tumours. American Journal of Diseases of Children 119: 49–52

156. Delta BG, Pinkel D 1964 Bone marrow aspiration in children with malignant tumours. Journal of Paediatrics 64: 542–546

157. Gatter KC, Abdulaziz Z, Beverley P et al 1982 Use of monoclonal antibodies for the histopathological diagnosis of human malignancy. Journal of Clinical Pathology 35: 1253–1267

158. Athanasou NA, Quinn J, Heryet A et al 1987 The effect of decalcification on cellular antigens. Journal of Clinical Pathology 40: 874–878

159. Mansi JL, Berger U, Easton D et al 1987 Micrometastases in bone marrow in patients with breast cancer: evaluation as an early predictor of bone metastases. British Medical Journal 295: 1093–1096

160. Berger U, Bettelheim R, Mansi JL et al 1988 The relationship between micrometastases in the bone marrow, histopathologic features of the primary tumor in breast cancer and prognosis. American Journal of Clinical Pathology 90: 1–6

161. Ellis G, Ferguson M, Yamanaka E et al 1989 Monoclonal antibodies for detection of occult carcinoma cells in bone marrow of breast cancer patients. Cancer 63: 2509–2514

162. Untch M, Harbeck N, Eiermann W 1988 Micrometastases in bone marrow in patients with breast cancer. British Medical Journal 296: 290

163. Gatter KC, Ralfkiaer E, Skinner J et al 1985 An immunohistochemical study of malignant melanoma and its differential diagnosis from other malignant tumours. Journal of Clinical Pathology 38: 1353–1357

164. Nadji M, Tabel SZ, Castro A et al 1984 Prostate specific antigen. An immunohistologic marker for prostatic neoplasms. Cancer 48: 1229–1239

165. Wilbur DC, Krenzer K, Bonfiglio TA 1987 Prostate specific antigen (PSA) staining in carcinomas of non-prostatic origin. American Journal of Clinical Pathology 88: 530

166. Nunez C, Abboud SL, Lemon NC, Kemp JA 1983 Ovarian rhabdomyosarcoma presenting as leukemia. Case report. Cancer 52: 297–300

167. Head DR, Kennedy PS, Goyette RE 1979 Metastatic neuroblastoma in bone marrow aspirate smears. American Journal of Clinical Pathology 72: 1008–1011

168. Smith SR, Reid MM 1994 Neuroblastoma rosettes in aspirated bone marrow. British Journal of Haematology 88: 445–447

169. Franklin IM, Pritchard J 1983 Detection of bone marrow invasion by neuroblastoma is improved by sampling at two sites with both aspirates and trephine biopsies. Journal of Clinical Pathology 36: 1215–1218

170. Reynolds CP, Smith RG, Frenkel EP 1981 The diagnostic dilemma of the 'small round cell neoplasm': catecholamine fluorescence and tissue culture morphology as markers for neuroblastoma. Cancer 48: 2088–2094

171. Rogers DW, Treleavan JG, Kemshead JT, Pritchard J 1989 Monoclonal antibodies for detecting bone marrow invasion by neuroblastoma. Journal of Clinical Pathology 42: 422–426

172. Carey PJ, Thomas L, Buckle G, Reid MM 1990 Immunocytochemical examination of bone marrow in disseminated neuroblastoma. Journal of Clinical Pathology 43: 9–12

173. Reid MM, Wallis JP, McGuckin AG et al 1991 Routine histological compared with immunohistological examination of bone marrow trephine biopsy specimens in disseminated neuroblastoma. Journal of Clinical Pathology 44: 485–486

174. Lloyd RV, Cano M, Rosa P et al 1988 Distribution of chromogranin A and secretogranin I (chromogranin B) in neuroendocrine cells and tumour. American Journal of Pathology 130: 296–304

175. Brooks JJ 1982 Immunohistochemistry of soft tissue tumors: progress and prospects. Human Pathology 13: 969–974

176. Variend S 1985 Small cell tumours in childhood: a review. Journal of Pathology 145: 1–27

177. Andres TL, Kadin ME 1983 Immunologic markers in the differential diagnosis of small round cell tumors from lymphocytic lymphoma and leukemia. American Journal of Clinical Pathology 79: 546–552

178. Kemshead JT, Goldman A, Fritschy J et al 1983 Use of panels of monoclonal antibodies in the differential diagnosis of neuroblastoma and lymphoblastic disorders. Lancet i: 12–15

179. Muehleck SD, McKenna RW, Gale PF, Brunning RD 1983 Terminal deoxynucleotidyl transferase (TdT)-positive cells in bone marrow in the absence of hematologic malignancy. American Journal of Clinical Pathology 79: 277–284

180. Savage RA, Hoffman GC, Shaker K 1978 Diagnostic problems involved in detection of metastatic neoplasms by bone marrow aspirate compared with needle biopsy. American Journal of Clinical Pathology 70: 623–627

181. Frey U, Senn HJ 1978 Demonstration of osseous tumor micrometastasis: comparison of the value of bone marrow cytology and histology. Schweiz Med Wochenschr 108: 82–91

182. Ihde DC, Simms EB, Matthews MJ et al 1979 Bone marrow metastases in small cell carcinomas of the lung: frequency, description, and influence on chemotherapeutic toxicity and prognosis. Blood 53: 677–686

183. McCarthy DM 1985 Fibrosis of the bone marrow: content and causes. British Journal of Haematology 59: 1–7

184. Lennert K, Nagai K, Schwarze EW 1975 Patho-anatomical features of the bone marrow. Clinics in Haematology 4: 331–351

185. Rocha-Filho FD, Ferreira FV, Mendes F-de-O et al 2000 Bone marrow fibrosis (pseudo-myelofibrosis) in human kala-azar. Revista da Sociedade Brasileira de Medicina Tropical 33: 363–366

186. Bain BJ, Catovsky D, O'Brien M et al 1981 Megakaryoblastic leukemia presenting as acute myelofibrosis – a study of four cases with the platelet-peroxidase reaction. Blood 58: 206–213

187. Hann IM, Evans DIK, Marsden HB et al 1978 Bone marrow fibrosis in acute lymphoblastic leukaemia of childhood. Journal of Clinical Pathology 31: 313–315

188. Kiely JM, Silverstein MN 1969 Metastatic carcinoma simulating agnogenic myeloid metaplasia. Cancer 24: 1041–1044

189. Spector JI, Levine PH 1973 Carcinomatous bone marrow invasion simulating acute myelofibrosis. American Journal of Medical Science 266: 145–148

190. Abildgaard N, Bendix-Hansen K, Kristensen JE et al 1997 Bone marrow fibrosis and disease activity in multiple myeloma monitored by the aminoterminal propeptide of procollagen III in serum. British Journal of Haematology 99: 641–648

191. Weinberg SG, Lubin A, Wiener SN et al 1977 Myelofibrosis and renal osteodystrophy. American Journal of Medicine 63: 755–764

192. Yetgin S, Ozsoylu S 1982 Myeloid metaplasia in vitamin D deficiency rickets. Scandinavian Journal of Haematology 28: 180–185

193. Kim CD, Kim SH, Kim YL et al 1998 Bone marrow immunoscintigraphy (BMIS): a new and important tool for the assessment of marrow fibrosis in renal osteodystrophy? Advances in Peritoneal Dialysis 14: 183–187

194. Boxer M, Ellman L, Geller R, Wang CA 1977 Anemia in primary hyperparathyroidism. Archives of Internal Medicine 137: 588–593

195. Fontenay-Roupie M, Dupuy E, Berrou E et al 1995 Increased proliferation of bone marrow derived fibroblasts in primary hypertrophic osteoarthropathy with severe myelofibrosis. Blood 85: 3229–3238

196. Fukuda S, Nagai H, Kotani S et al 1998 Myelodysplastic syndrome resembling chronic myeloproliferative disorders in clinicopathological aspects. International Journal of Hematology 68: 79–85

197. Antillon F, Raimondi SC, Fairman J et al 1998 5q- in a child with refractory anemia with excess blasts: similarities to 5q- syndrome in adults. Cancer Genetics and Cytogenetics 105: 119–122

198. Hansen NE, Kilmnann SA 1970 Paroxysmal nocturnal hemoglobinuria in myelofibrosis. Blood 36: 428–431

199. Breton-Gorius J, Vainchenker W, Nurden A et al 1981 Defective α granule production in megakaryocytes in gray platelet syndrome: ultrastructural studies of bone marrow cells and megakaryocytes growing in culture from blood precursors. American Journal of Pathology 102: 10–19

200. Konstantopoulos K, Terpos E, Prinolakis H et al 1998 Systemic lupus erythematosus presenting as myelofibrosis. Haematologia (Budapest) 29: 153–156

201. Aharon A, Levy Y, Bar-Dayan Y et al 1997 Successful treatment of early secondary myelofibrosis in SLE with IVIG. Lupus 6: 408–411

202. Kundel DW, Brecher G, Bodey GP, Brittin GM 1964 Reticulin fibrosis and bone infarction in acute leukemia. Implications for prognosis. Blood 23: 526–544

203. Blayney DW, Jaffe ES, Blattner WA et al 1983 The human T-cell leukemia/lymphoma virus associated with American adult T-cell leukemia/lymphoma. Blood 62: 401–405

204. Fialkow PJ, Jacobson RJ, Papayannopoulou T 1977 Chronic myelocytic leukemia: clonal origin in a stem cell common to the granulocyte, erythrocyte, platelet and monocyte/macrophage. American Journal of Medicine 63: 125–130

205. Jacobson RJ, Salo A, Fialkow PJ 1978 Agnogenic myeloid metaplasia: a clonal proliferation of hematopoietic stem cells with secondary myelofibrosis. Blood 51: 189–194

206. Kuo C, Van Voolen GA, Morrison AN 1972 Primary and secondary myelofibrosis: its relationship to 'PNH-like defect'. Blood 40: 875–880

207. Burkhardt R 1981 Bone marrow histology. In: Catovsky D (ed), Methods in haematology. The leukaemic cell. Churchill Livingstone, Edinburgh, 49–86

208. Bouroncle BA, Doan CA 1962 Myelofibrosis: clinical, hematologic and pathologic study of 110 patients. American Journal of Medical Science 243: 697

209. Ward HP, Block MH 1971 The natural history of agnogenic myeloid metaplasia (AMM) and a critical evaluation of its relationship with the myeloproliferative syndrome. Medicine 50: 357

210. Barosi G 1999 Myelofibrosis with myeloid metaplasia: diagnostic definition and prognostic classification. Journal of Clinical Oncology 17: 2954–2970

211. Ligumski M, Polliack A, Benbassat J 1978 Nature and incidence of liver involvement in agnogenic myeloid metaplasia. Scandinavian Journal of Haematology 21: 81–93

212. Savage RA 1984 Specific and not-so-specific histiocytes in bone marrow. Laboratory Medicine 13: 467–471

213. Lee RE 1988 Histiocytic diseases of the bone marrow. Hematology and Oncology Clinics of North America 2: 657–667

214. Beutler E 1988 Gaucher disease. Blood Reviews 2: 59–70

215. Beutler E, Saven A 1990 Misuse of marrow examination in the diagnosis of Gaucher's disease. Blood 76: 646–648

216. Lee RE, Ellis LD 1971 The storage cells of chronic myelogenous leukemia. Laboratory Investigation 24: 261–264

217. Rosner F, Dosik H, Kaiser SS et al 1969 Gaucher cells in leukemia. Journal of the American Medical Association 209: 935–937

218. Zaino EC, Rossi MB, Pham TD, Azar HA 1971 Gaucher's cells in thalassemia. Blood 38: 457–462

219. Van Dorpe A, Broeckaert-van-Orshoven A, Desmet V, Verwilghen RL 1973 Gaucher-like cells and congenital dyserythropoietic anaemia, type II (HEMPAS). British Journal of Haematology 25: 165–170

220. Lee KS, Tobin MS, Chen KT et al 1982 Acquired Gaucher's cells in Hodgkin's disease. American Journal of Medicine 73: 290–294

221. Papadimitriou JC, Chakravarthy A, Heyman MR 1988 Pseudo-Gaucher cells preceding the appearance of immunoblastic lymphoma. American Journal of Clinical Pathology 90: 454–458

222. Scullin DC, Shelburne JD, Cohen HJ 1979 Pseudo-Gaucher cells in multiple myeloma. American Journal of Medicine 67: 347–352

223. Solis OG, Belmonte AH, Ramaswamy G, Tchertkoff V 1986 Pseudogaucher cells in *Mycobacterium avium intracellulare* infections in acquired immune deficiency syndrome (AIDS). American Journal of Clinical Pathology 85: 233–235

224. Yamauchi K, Shimamura K 1995 Mild thrombocytopenia induced by phagocytosis of marrow pseudo-Gaucher cells in a patient with chronic myelogenous leukaemia. European Journal of Haematology 54: 55–56

225. Wickramasinghe SN, Hughes M 1978 Some features of bone marrow macrophages in patients with homozygous β-thalassaemia. British Journal of Haematology 38: 23–28

226. Varela-Duran J, Roholt PC, Ratliff NB Jr 1980 Sea-blue histiocyte syndrome. A secondary degenerative process of macrophages? Archives of Pathology and Laboratory Medicine 104: 30–34

227. Rywlin AM 1976 Histopathology of the bone marrow. Little, Brown, Boston 976: 145

228. Burns DA, Sarkany I 1979 Chronic granulomatous disease in an adult. Journal of the Royal Society of Medicine 72: 139–142

229. Tadmor R, Aghai E, Sarova-Pinhas I, Braham J 1976 Sea-blue histiocytes in a case of Takayasu arteritis. Journal of the American Medical Association 235: 2852–2853

230. Rywlin AM 1976 Histopathology of the bone marrow. Little, Brown, Boston, 142.

231. Wong KF, Chan JKC 1989 Foamy histiocytes in repeat marrow aspirates. Pathology 21: 153–154

232. Brunning RD 1996 Bone marrow. In: Rosai J (ed), Ackerman's surgical pathology, 8th edn, vol 2. CV Mosby, St Louis, 1895

233. Brown CH 1972 Bone marrow necrosis. A study of seventy cases. Bulletin of the Johns Hopkins Medical School 131: 189–203

234. Kiraly JF, Wheby MS 1976 Bone marrow necrosis. American Journal of Medicine 60: 361–368

235. Janssens AM, Offner FC, Van-Hove WZ 2000 Bone marrow necrosis. Cancer 88: 1769–1780

236. Norgard MJ, Carpenter JT Jr, Conrad ME 1979 Bone marrow necrosis and degeneration. Archives of Internal Medicine 139: 905–911

237. Knupp C, Pekela PH, Cornelius P 1988 Extensive bone marrow necrosis in patients with cancer and tumor necrosis factor activity in plasma. American Journal of Hematology 29: 215–221

238. Eckardt P, Raez LE, Restrepo A, Temple JD 1999 Pulmonary bone marrow embolism in sickle cell disease. Southern Medical Journal 92: 245–247

239. Ballas SK, Pindzola A, Chang CD et al 1998 Postmortem diagnosis of hemoglobin SC disease complicated by fat embolism. Annals of Clinical and Laboratory Science 28: 144–149

240. Kolquist KA, Vnencak-Jones CL, Swift L et al 1996 Fatal fat embolism syndrome in a child with undiagnosed hemoglobin S/β⁺ thalassemia: a complication of acute parvovirus B19 infection. Pediatric Pathology and Laboratory Medicine 16: 71–82
241. Zaidi Y, Sivakumaran M, Graham C, Hutchinson RM 1996 Fatal bone marrow embolism in a patient with sickle cell β⁺ thalassaemia. Journal of Clinical Pathology 49: 774–775
242. Bernard C, Sick H, Boilletot A, Oberling F 1978 Bone marrow necrosis. Acute microcirculation failure in myelomonocytic leukemia. Archives of Internal Medicine 138: 1567–1569
243. Markovic SN, Phyliky RL, Li CY 1998 Pancytopenia due to bone marrow necrosis in acute myelogenous leukemia: role of reactive CD8 cells. American Journal of Hematology 59: 74–78
244. Katayama Y, Deguchi S, Shinagawa K et al 1998 Bone marrow necrosis in a patient with acute myeloblastic leukemia during administration of G-CSF and rapid hematologic recovery after allotransplantation of peripheral blood stem cells. American Journal of Hematology 57: 238–240
245. Limentani SA, Pretell JO, Potter D et al 1994 Bone marrow necrosis in two patients with acute promyelocytic leukemia during treatment with all-trans retinoic acid. American Journal of Hematology 47: 50–55
246. Shibata K, Shimamoto Y, Watanabe M et al 1994 Two cases of acute lymphocytic leukaemia associated with bone marrow necrosis – a brief review of recent literature. European Journal of Haematology 52: 115–116
247. Chim CS, Ooi C, Ma SK, Lam C 1998 Bone marrow necrosis in bone marrow transplantation: the role of MR imaging. Bone Marrow Transplantation 22: 1125–1128
248. Eguiguren JM, Pui CH 1992 Bone marrow necrosis and thrombotic complications in childhood acute lymphoblastic leukemia. Medical and Pediatric Oncology 20: 58–60
249. Majumdar G, Phillips JK, Pearson TC 1994 Massive bone marrow necrosis and post-necrotic myelofibrosis in a patient with primary thrombocythaemia. Journal of Clinical Pathology 47: 674–676
250. Macheta AT, Cinkotai KI, Love EM et al 1991 Bone marrow necrosis complicating chronic myeloid leukaemia. Clinical and Laboratory Haematology 13: 163–167
251. Carloss H, Winslow D, Kastan L, Yam LT 1977 Bone marrow necrosis. Diagnosis and assessment of extent of involvement by radioisotope studies. Archives of Internal Medicine 137: 863–866
252. Majumdar G 1997 Massive bone marrow necrosis as the presenting feature in a case of primary bone marrow high grade non-Hodgkin's lymphoma. Leukemia and Lymphoma 26: 409–412
253. Weirich G, Sandherr M, Fellbaum C et al 1998 Molecular evidence of bone marrow involvement in advanced case of Tγδ lymphoma with secondary myelofibrosis. Human Pathology 29: 761–765
254. Hughes RG, Islam A, Lewis SM, Catovsky D 1981 Spontaneous remission following bone marrow necrosis in chronic lymphocytic leukaemia. Clinical and Laboratory Haematology 3: 173–183
255. Zhu AX, Niesvizky R, Hedrick E et al 1999 Extensive bone marrow necrosis associated with multiple myeloma. Leukemia 13: 2118–2120
256. Eichhorn RF, Buurke EJ, Blok P et al 1999 Sickle cell-like crisis and bone marrow necrosis associated with parvovirus B19 infection and heterozygosity for haemoglobins S and E. Journal of Internal Medicine 245: 103–106
257. Rose MS 1973 Apparent necrosis of bone marrow in a patient with disseminated intravascular coagulation, post-partum. Lancet ii: 730–731
258. Harigaya K, Watanabe S, Watanabe Y et al 1977 Multiple bone marrow necrosis and disseminated intravascular coagulation. Archives of Pathology and Laboratory Medicine 101: 652–654
259. Schaar CG, Ronday KH, Boets EP et al 1999 Catastrophic manifestation of the antiphospholipid syndrome. Journal of Rheumatology 26: 2261–2264
260. Paydas S, Kocak R, Zorludemir S, Baslamisli F 1997 Bone marrow necrosis in antiphospholipid syndrome. Journal of Clinical Pathology 50: 261–262
261. Laso F-J, Gonzalez-Diaz M, Paz J-I, De Castro S 1983 Bone marrow necrosis associated with tumor emboli and disseminated intravascular coagulation. Archives of Internal Medicine 143, 2220
262. Upchurch KS 1988 Case records of the Massachusetts General Hospital. Case 38–1988. New England Journal of Medicine 319: 768–781

263. Tavassoli M 1983 Bone marrow necrosis secondary to hyperparathyroidism. Journal of the Mississippi State Medical Association 24: 39–41
264. Rustgi VK, Sacher RA, O'Brien P, Garagusi VF 1983 Fatal disseminated cytomegalovirus infection in an apparently normal adult. Archives of Internal Medicine 143: 372–373
265. Petrella T, Bailly F, Mugneret F et al 1992 Bone marrow necrosis and human parvovirus associated infection preceding a Ph1+ acute lymphoblastic leukemia. Leukemia and Lymphoma 8: 415–419
266. Katzen H, Spagnolo SV 1980 Bone marrow necrosis from miliary tuberculosis. Journal of the American Medical Association 244: 2438–2439
267. Garewal G, Marwaha N, Marwaha RK, Das KC 1991 Bone marrow necrosis and pancytopenia associated with gram negative septicemia. Indian Journal of Pediatrics 28: 79–81
268. Epstein M, Pearson ADJ, Hudson SJ et al 1992 Necrobacillosis with pancytopenia. Archives of Diseases of Childhood 67: 958–959
269. Brada M, Bellingham AJ 1980 Bone marrow necrosis and Q fever. British Medical Journal 281: 1108–1109
270. Caraveo J, Trowbridge AA, Amaral BW et al 1977 Bone marrow necrosis associated with a *Mucor* infection. American Journal of Medicine 62: 404–408
271. Kiraly JF, Wheby MS 1976 Bone marrow necrosis. American Journal of Medicine 60: 361–368
272. Mant MJ, Faragher BS 1972 The haematology of anorexia nervosa. British Journal of Haematology 23: 737–749
273. Tavassoli M, Eastlund DT, Yam LT et al 1976 Gelatinous transformation of bone marrow in prolonged self-induced starvation. Scandinavian Journal of Haematology 16: 311–319
274. Amos RJ, Deane M, Ferguson C et al 1990 Observations on the haemopoietic response to critical illness. Journal of Clinical Pathology 43: 850–856
275. Clarke BE, Brown DJ, Xipell JM 1983 Gelatinous transformation of the bone marrow. Pathology 15: 85–88
276. Bohm J 2000 Gelatinous transformation of the bone marrow: the spectrum of underlying diseases. American Journal of Surgical Pathology 24: 56–65
277. Savage RA, Sipple C 1987 Marrow myxedema: gelatinous transformation of marrow ground substance in patient with severe hypothyroidism. Archives of Pathology and Laboratory Medicine 111: 375–377
278. Nonaka D, Tanaka M, Takaki K et al 1998 Gelatinous bone marrow transformation complicated by self-induced malnutrition. Acta Haematologica 100: 88–90
279. Sicard D, Casadevall N, Wyplosz B et al 1994 Anorexia nervosa and gelatinous transformation of bone marrow. Nouvelle Revue Francaise d'Hematologie 36 suppl 1: S85–86
280. Feng CS 1993 A variant of gelatinous transformation of marrow in leukemic patients post-chemotherapy. Pathology 25: 294–296
281. Feng CS 1991 Gelatinous transformation of marrow in a case of acute myelogenous leukemia post-chemotherapy. American Journal of Hematology 38: 220–222
282. Feng CS, Ng MH, Szeto RS, Li EK 1991 Bone marrow findings in lupus patients with pancytopenia. Pathology 23: 5–7
283. Marie I, Levesque H, Heron F et al 1999 Gelatinous transformation of the bone marrow: an uncommon manifestation of intestinal lymphangiectasia (Waldmann's disease). American Journal of Medicine 107: 99–100
284. Varma N, Bhoria U, Bambery P, Dash S 1991 Gelatinous transformation of the bone marrow and Leishmania donovani infection. Journal of Tropical Medicine and Hygiene 94: 310–312
285. Stavem P, Larsen IF, Ly B, Rorvik TO 1980 Amyloid deposits in bone marrow aspirates in primary amyloidosis. Acta Medica Scandinavica 208: 111–113
286. Feiner HD 1988 Pathology of dysproteinemia: light chain amyloidosis, non-amyloid immunoglobulin deposition disease, cryoglobulinemia syndromes and macroglobulinemia of Waldenstrom. Human Pathology 11: 1255–1272
287. Enos WF, Pierre RV, Rosenblatt JE 1981 Giant cell arteritis detected by bone marrow biopsy. Mayo Clinic Proceedings 56: 381–383
288. Rywlin AM 1976 Histopathology of the bone marrow. Little, Brown, Boston, 180
289. Retan JW, Miller RE 1966 Microembolic complications of atherosclerosis. Archives of Internal Medicine 118: 534–543
290. Pierce JR, Wren MV, Cousar JB 1978 Cholesterol embolism: diagnosis

antemortem by bone marrow biopsy. Annals of Internal Medicine 89: 937–938

291. Muretto P, Carnevali A, Ansini AL (1991) Cholesterol embolism of bone marrow clinically masquerading as systemic or metastatic tumor. Haematologica 76: 248–250

292. Myers TJ 1981 Treatment of thrombotic thrombocytopenic purpura with combined exchange plasmapheresis and anti-platelet agents. Seminars in Thrombosis and Hemostasis 7: 37–42

293. Wickramasinghe SN, Phillips RE, Looareesuwan S et al 1987 The bone marrow in cerebral malaria: parasite sequestration within sinusoids. British Journal of Haematology 66: 295–306

294. Kaye M 1983 Bone marrow aluminium storage in renal failure. Journal of Clinical Pathology 36: 1288–1291

295. Mc Clure J, Fazzalari NL, Fassett RG, Pugsley DG 1983 Bone histoquantitative findings and histochemical staining reactions for aluminium in chronic renal failure patients treated with haemodialysis fluids containing high and low concentrations of aluminium. Journal of Clinical Pathology 36: 1281–1287

Recommended reading

Bain BJ, Clark DM, Lampert IA, Wilkins BS 2001 Bone Marrow pathology, 3rd edn. Blackwell Science, Oxford

Rywlin AM 1976 Histopathology of the bone marrow. Little, Brown, Boston

Disorders affecting erythroid cells

Investigation and classification of anemia	131
Abnormalities of the red cell membrane	141
Inherited abnormalities of red cell enzymes	149
Abnormalities of the structure and synthesis of hemoglobin	159
Acquired hemolytic anemias	185
Iron deficiency anemia, anemia of chronic disorder and iron overload	203
Macrocytic anemia	229
Aplastic anemia	249
Pure red cell aplasia and sideroblastic anemia	265
Congenital dyserythropoietic anemias	273
Polycythemia (the erythrocytoses)	283

Investigation and classification of anemia

6

SN Wickramasinghe

Abnormalities of red cell morphology

Assessment of erythropoiesis

Anemia

Blood loss

Hemolytic anemia: general considerations
Extravascular and intravascular hemolysis
Hematologic changes
Changes in other tissues
Causes of hemolytic anemia

Abnormalities of red cell morphology

Red cell morphology should be examined in an area of the blood film in which only occasional red cells overlap. In such an area normal red cells show a central area of pallor which occupies less than a third of the diameter of the cell. They also show some variation in diameter (Fig. 6.1a). Most normal red cells have a circular outline but occasional cells may be oval or have other shapes. Abnormalities of red cell morphology may be seen in disease.

The terms *anisocytosis* and *poikilocytosis* describe an increased degree of variation in cell diameter (size) and cell shape respectively. Poikilocytes may be oval, pear- or tear-drop-shaped, sickle-shaped or irregularly contracted.

The terms *normochromic* and *hypochromic* are applied to red cells in which the central area of pallor is, respectively, normal in size and larger than normal. Severely hypochromic red cells have a very large central area of pallor surrounded by a narrow rim of eosinophilic cytoplasm. An erythrocyte is described as a *normocyte, microcyte* or *macrocyte* (Fig. 6.1b,c) when its diameter (size) appears to be normal, smaller than normal or larger than normal, respectively. *Target cells* are abnormally thin red cells with a well-stained zone in the middle of the usual central area of pallor (Fig. 6.2e,f,i). *Microspherocytes* are small, rounded, deeply-staining cells without a central area of pallor (Fig. 6.2g). These cells show a varying degree of loss of their central concavities and are sometimes completely spherical.[1] *Schistocytes* (helmet cells, triangular cells and small cells with other peculiar shapes) seem to arise from

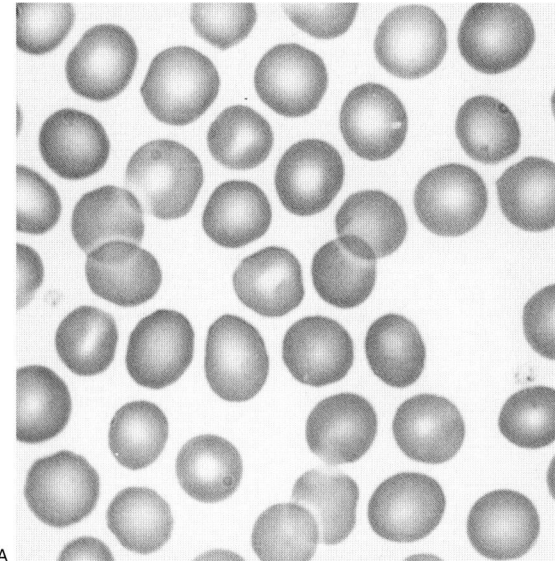

A

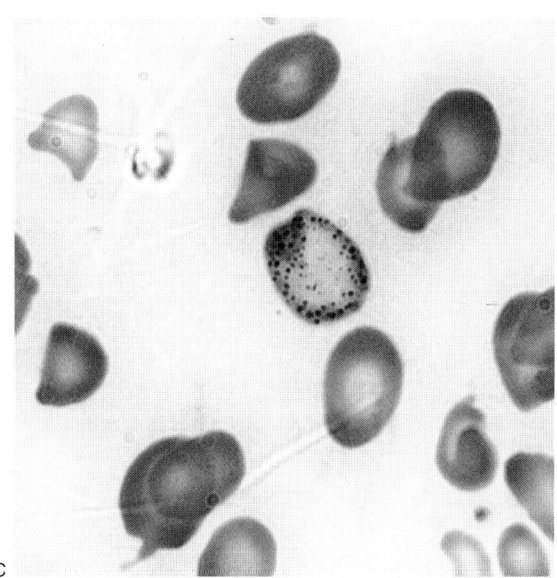

C

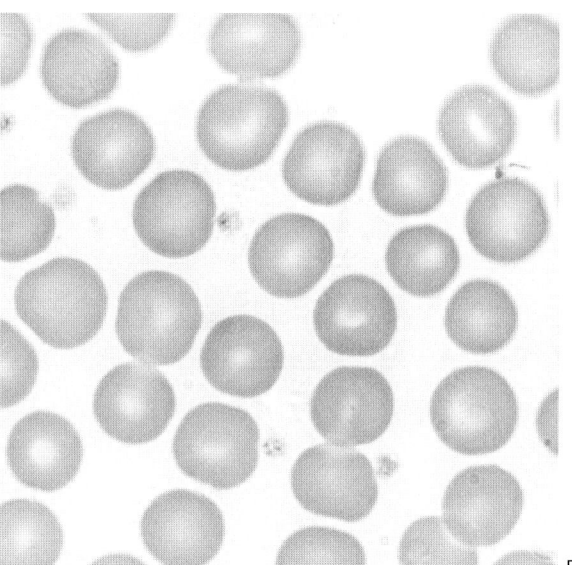

B

Fig. 6.1 (A–C) Some abnormalities of red cell morphology that may be seen on examination of peripheral blood smears. (A) Normal blood film (for comparison). (B) Macrocytosis induced by chronic alcoholism. The majority of the red cells have a rounded outline, as is typical of alcohol-induced macrocytosis. (C) Oval macrocytes, marked anisocytosis and poikilocytes in severe anemia due to vitamin B_{12} deficiency. One of the macrocytes displays coarse basophilic stippling. May–Grünwald–Giemsa stain.

the fragmentation of erythrocytes as a result of their interaction with fibrin strands, diseased vessel walls or foreign surfaces (e.g. cardiac valve prostheses).

Red cells may sometimes have projections (spicules) on their surface.[1,2] Such cells are grouped into two main categories: *echinocytes* (crenated red cells) and *acanthocytes* (spur cells) (Fig. 6.2a,b). When examined in the scanning electron microscope (SEM), echinocytes are flat or spherical with 10–30 spicules of similar length distributed evenly over the surface. By contrast, acanthocytes have

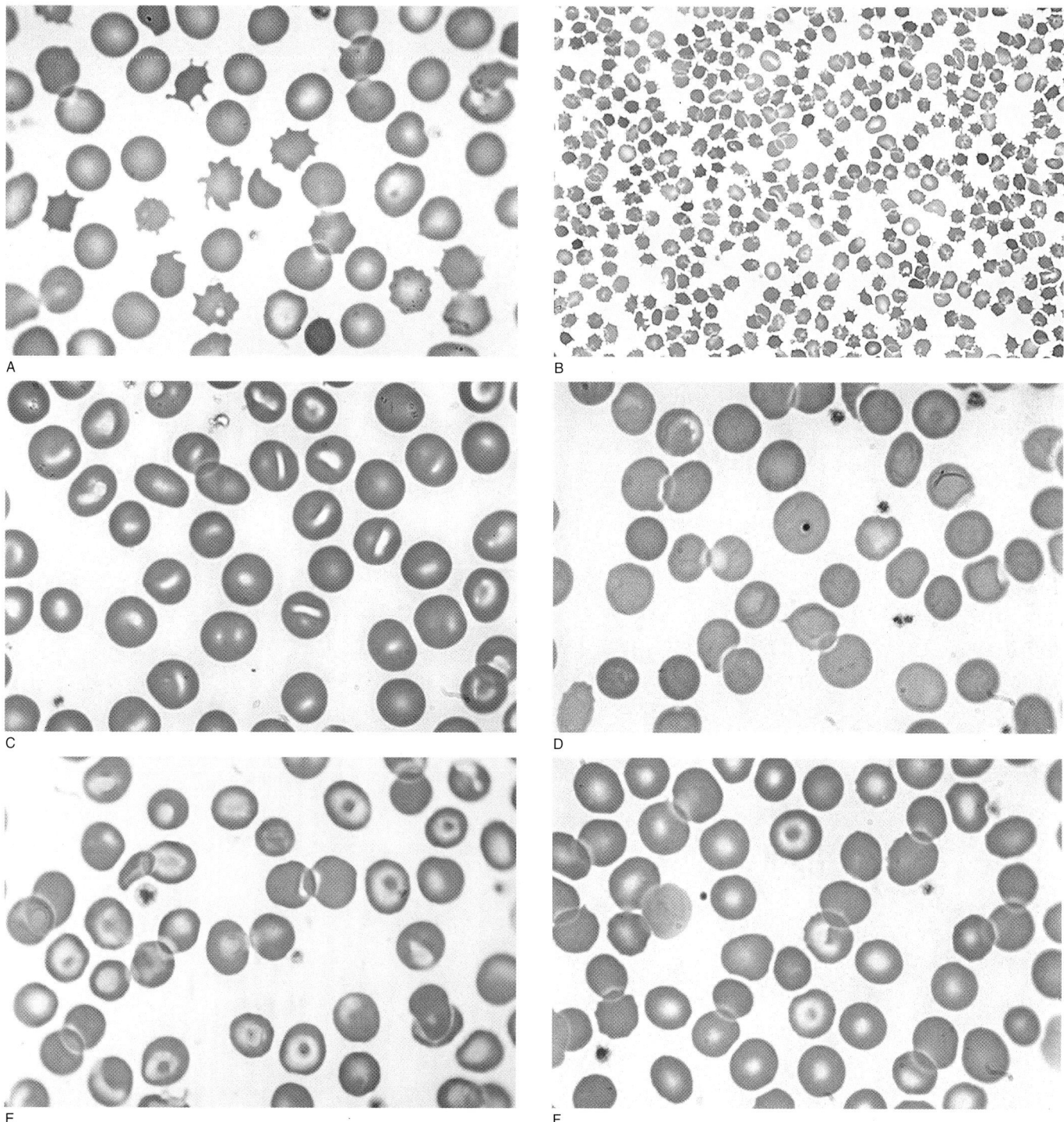

Fig. 6.2 (A–J) Some abnormalities of red cell morphology that may be seen on examination of peripheral blood smears. (A) Acanthocytes in a hematologically normal patient subjected to splenectomy. (B) Echinocytes and acanthocytes in blood mixed with citrate-phosphate-dextrose solution (CPD) containing adenine and stored at 4°C for 4 weeks. (C) Stomatocytes induced by acute alcoholism. (D) Howell–Jolly body within an erythrocyte of a splenectomized patient. (E) High proportion of target cells in a patient with obstructive jaundice. (F) Target cells post-splenectomy.

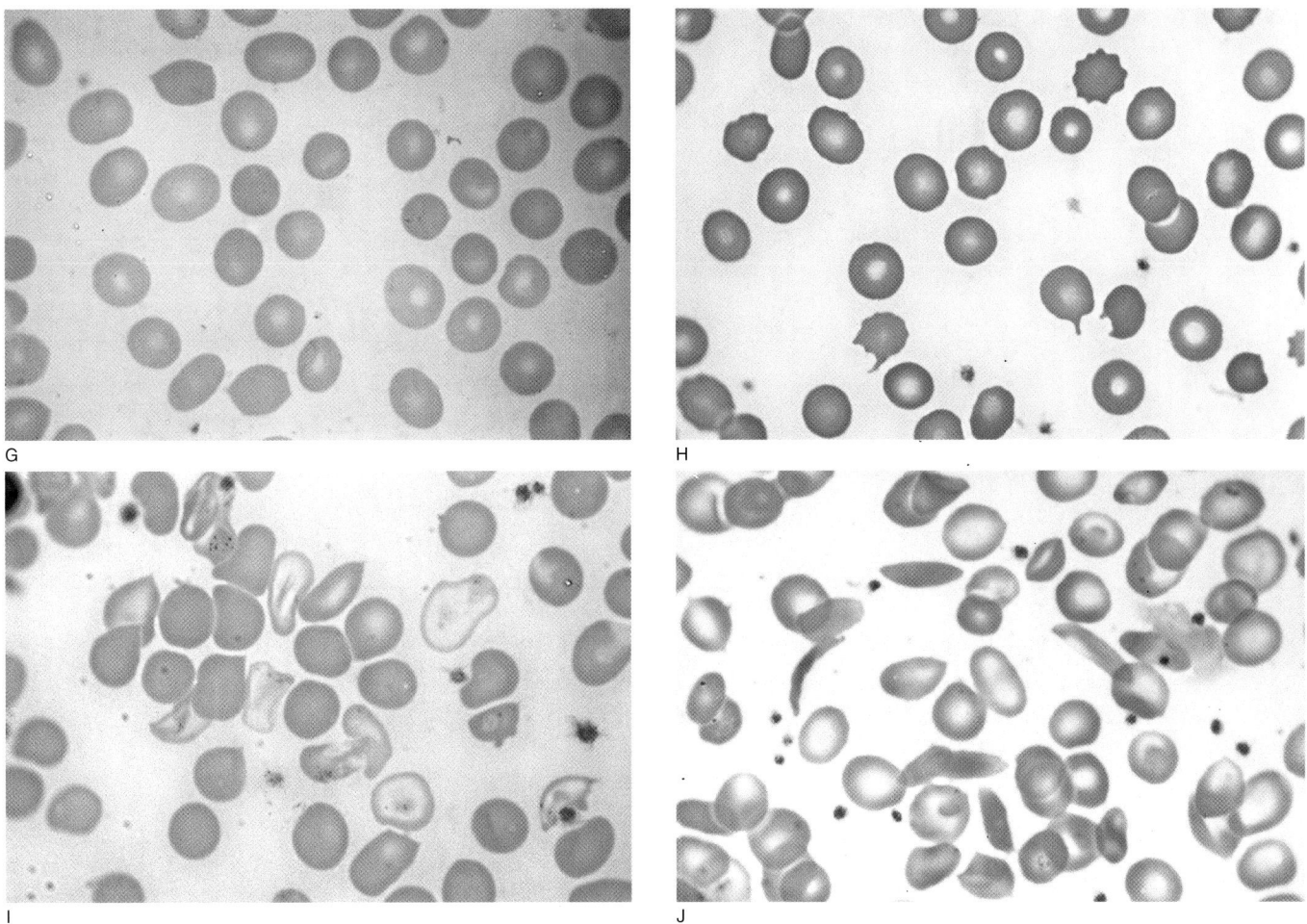

Fig. 6.2 *(Cont'd)* (G) Spherocytes in hereditary spherocytosis. (H) Keratocytes in renal failure. (I) Hypochromic red cells, including hypochromic target cells, alongside many transfused normochromic normocytic red cells in homozygous β-thalassemia. (J) Sickle cells and target cells in sickle cell anemia. May–Grünwald–Giemsa stain.

5–10 spicules of varying length irregularly distributed over the surface. In addition, the spicules of acanthocytes have knobby ends. In Romanowsky-stained smears, echinocytes have a serrated outline with small projections more or less evenly distributed over their circumference and acanthocytes have a few spicules of varying length and thickness projecting irregularly from the circumference.

When red cells have a slit-like appearance across the middle instead of the circular area of pallor, they are called *stomatocytes* (Fig. 6.2c). The term *keratocyte* is used to describe a cell with two pointed projections ('horns') that are thought to result from the rupture of a vacuole at the cell's periphery (Fig. 6.2h).

Sickle-shaped red cells are found in homozygotes for hemoglobin S (Fig. 6.2j) and in patients who are double heterozygotes for hemoglobin S and either β-thalassemia or certain abnormal hemoglobins such as hemoglobin C, E, O-Arab, D-Punjab or Lepore. In sickle cell anemia, the characteristic sickle shape results from the fact that de-

oxygenated hemoglobin S is about 50 times less soluble than deoxygenated hemoglobin A and, under appropriate conditions, form long fibers (tactoids) which deform the red cell (Fig. 6.3) In several disorders, the ribosomes within reticulocytes form clumps of various sizes during the preparation of a Romanowsky-stained smear. Such cells show many fine or coarse basophilic dots distributed uniformly throughout the cell and are described as displaying *basophilic stippling* (Fig. 6.1c). Another type of basophilic inclusion that may be seen within erythrocytes is a *Pappenheimer body*. These vary markedly in size from 1 μm downwards, may be single or multiple, are unevenly distributed and stain positively with the Prussian blue reaction for iron. Red cells containing iron-positive granules are called *siderocytes*. In some circumstances, one or more rounded, dark purple inclusions known as *Howell–Jolly bodies* are found within red cells (Fig. 6.2d). These consist of nuclear material and are formed within erythroblasts either by karyorrhexis or from chromosome

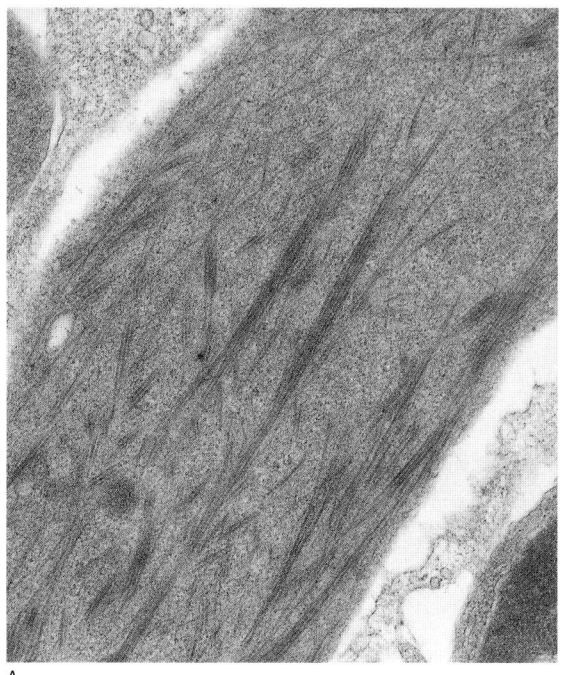
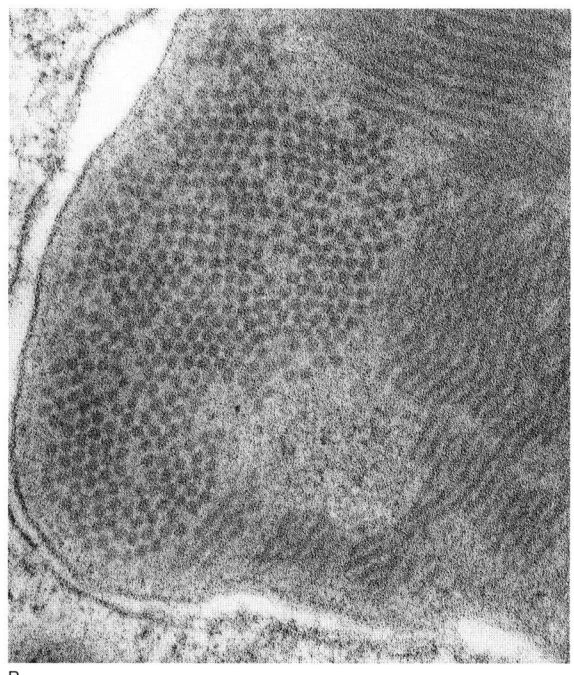

A   B

Fig. 6.3 (A,B) Electron micrographs of two red cells from the bone marrow of a patient homozygous for hemoglobin S. The cell profiles contain fibers of polymerized deoxyhemoglobin S, many of which have been sectioned longitudinally in (A) and transversely in (B). Uranyl acetate and lead citrate. (A) x 29 100; (B) x 97 200.

fragments which become isolated outside the nucleus when the nuclear membrane is reformed during telophase.

The conditions in which the above-mentioned abnormalities of red cell morphology may be found as a prominent feature of the blood film are summarized in Table 6.1. In malaria, babesiosis and bartonellosis (Oroya fever) the causative organism may be found inside red cells.

Assessment of erythropoiesis

A proper understanding of red cell production in a patient requires information on effective erythropoiesis, ineffective erythropoiesis and total erythropoiesis. Effective erythropoiesis is the rate of release of newly-formed red cells from the marrow and ineffective erythropoiesis is the rate of loss of potential erythrocytes as a result of the phagocytosis of defective erythropoietic cells by bone marrow macrophages. Total erythropoiesis is the overall erythropoietic activity, effective and ineffective. Various indices of these three aspects of erythropoietic activity are summarized in Table 6.2. The absolute reticulocyte count, myeloid/erythroid (M/E) ratio and morphologic evidence of dyserythropoiesis or of erythroblast phagocytosis are more easily and, therefore, more frequently determined than the other indices listed in the table. The scientific

basis and the limitations of various indices of erythropoiesis have been reviewed previously.[11,12]

Anemia[13]

The term anemia is used when there is a reduction in the hemoglobin concentration in the peripheral blood below the reference range for the age and sex of an individual. The reference ranges at different ages are given in Chapter 1.

Anemia may cause numerous symptoms and signs. These result both from decreased tissue oxygenation leading to widespread organ dysfunction as well as from adaptive changes, particularly in the cardiovascular system. The nature and severity of symptoms is influenced by the rapidity of development of anemia and the health of the cardiovascular and respiratory systems. For example, patients with significant coronary artery or chronic obstructive airways disease may develop symptoms with only a mild degree of anemia. Symptoms of anemia include lassitude, easy fatiguability, dyspnea on exertion, palpitation, angina or intermittent claudication (in older patients with degenerative arterial disease), headache, vertigo, light-headedness, visual disturbances, drowsiness, anorexia, nausea, bowel disturbances, menstrual disturbances and loss of libido. Physical signs include pallor, signs of a hyperkinetic circulation (tachy-

Table 6.1 Some causes of various abnormalities of red cell morphology

Abnormality	Significance
Hypochromia and microcytosis (Fig. 6.2i)	Impaired synthesis of heme or globin: iron deficiency anemia, thalassemia syndromes, sideroblastic anemia, congenital atransferrinemia,[3] aluminum-induced anemia (dialysis patients)[4]
Macrocytosis (Figs 6.1b,c)	Dyserythropoiesis or accelerated release of reticulocytes: megaloblastic erythropoiesis (e.g. vitamin B_{12} or folate deficiency, congenital dyserythropoietic anemia types I and III) or macronormoblastic erythropoiesis (e.g. chronic alcoholism, chronic hemolysis)
Anisocytosis	Non-specific evidence of a perturbation of erythropoiesis
Target cells (Figs 6.2e,f,i)	Increased surface area relative to volume: thalassemia syndromes, iron deficiency anemia, some hemoglobinopathies (HbAC, HbCC, HbEE), liver disease, obstructive jaundice, hyposplenism, post-splenectomy, familial lecithin-cholesterol-acyltransferase deficiency[5]
Stomatocytes (Fig. 6.2c)	Hereditary stomatocytosis, the Rh null phenotype,[6] acute alcoholism,[7] phenothiazines and other drugs
Spherocytosis (Fig. 6.2g)	Abnormality of cell membrane: hereditary spherocytosis, membrane damage mediated by antibodies, heat, certain chemicals, hypophosphatemia
Elliptocytosis (Fig. 6.1c)	Abnormality of cell membrane: usually hereditary; also acquired defect in various anemias (megaloblastic anemia, iron deficiency)
Acanthocytes (Fig. 6.2a)	Hemolytic anemia in liver disease,[8] hypothyroidism, anorexia nervosa, post-splenectomy, abetalipoproteinemia,[9] hemolysis with McLeod blood type[10]
Echinocytes (Fig. 6.2b)	Neonates, recently transfused red cells, *in vitro* storage changes
Keratocytes (Fig. 6.2h)	Uremia
Sickle cells (Fig. 6.2j)	Sickle cell anemia, HbS/β-thalassemia, HbSC disease, HbS/O-Arab, HbS/D-Punjab, HbS/Lepore
Schistocytes	Red cell fragmentation: cardiac valve prostheses, micro-angiopathic hemolytic anemias including that due to malignant hypertension
Tear-drop cell	Prominent in myelofibrosis, also present in various anemias (e.g. thalassemia)
Basophilic stippling (Fig. 6.1c)	Lead poisoning, thalassemia syndromes, pyrimidine 5′-nucleotidase deficiency, homozygosity for Hb Constant Spring, accelerated erythropoiesis, dyserythropoiesis
Pappenheimer bodies	Lead poisoning, sideroblastic anemias, hemolytic anemias, post-splenectomy
Howell–Jolly bodies (Fig. 6.2d)	Post-splenectomy, hyposplenism, megaloblastic hemopoiesis

Table 6.2 Indices of erythropoietic activity

Effective erythropoiesis
Absolute reticulocyte count
Red cell turnover calculated from the mean cell life span, red cell count and total blood volume
Red cell ^{59}Fe utilization
Red cell iron turnover

Total erythropoiesis
M/E ratio (see Chapter 5)
Plasma iron turnover
Total marrow iron turnover
Fecal urobilinogen excretion
Carbon monoxide production

Ineffective erythropoiesis
Discrepancy between indices of total and effective erythropoiesis
Morphologic evidence of increased dyserythropoiesis (see Chapter 5) and erythroblast phagocytosis
Early-labeled bilirubin production after administration of labeled glycine

cardia, wide pulse pressure with capillary pulsation, hemic murmurs), signs of congestive cardiac failure, and hemorrhages and occasional exudates in the retina. Severe anemia may also cause slight proteinuria, mild impairment of renal function and low-grade fever.

A moderate degree of chronic anemia is usually associated with only mild symptoms and only slight increases in cardiac output at rest and slight decreases in mixed venous Po_2. This is because there is a substantial shift of the oxygen dissociation curve to the right (see Chapter 1), mainly due to an adaptive increase in the levels of 2,3-diphosphoglycerate within red cells. When the hemoglobin falls below 7–8 g/dl symptoms usually become more marked. The intraerythrocytic adaptation cannot by itself maintain an adequate oxygen delivery to the tissues and other compensatory mechanisms come into operation. These include: (1) an increase of stroke volume, heart rate and cardiac output at rest; (2) redistribution of blood flow

Table 6.3 Morphologic classification of anemia

Type	Mean cell volume (MCV)
Normochromic, normocytic anemia	Within reference range
Hypochromic, microcytic anemia	Low
Macrocytic anemia	High

Table 6.4 Mechanisms of anemia

Blood loss

Increased red cell destruction (hemolytic anemia)

Impaired red cell formation
   Decreased or inadequately increased total erythropoiesis
   Greatly increased ineffective erythropoiesis

Splenic pooling and sequestration

Increased plasma volume

with vasoconstriction in the skin and kidneys and increased perfusion of the heart, brain and muscle; and (3) reduction of the mixed venous P_{O_2} (which increases the arterial–venous oxygen difference).

Two useful classifications of anemia are based on: (1) the mean cell volume (MCV) and an assessment of the size and hemoglobin content (intensity of staining) of the red cells in a Romanowsky-stained blood smear (Table 6.3); and (2) the main pathogenetic mechanisms underlying the anemia (Table 6.4). In most cases of anemia more than one of the mechanisms listed in Table 6.4 are involved. Useful clues regarding the etiology of an anemia may be provided by various abnormalities of red cell morphology other than abnormalities of size.

Blood loss[14]

Acute hemorrhage results in an acute reduction of blood volume. Restoration of the blood volume occurs slowly over the next 36–72 h by an expansion of the plasma volume: the rate of recovery of the blood volume appears to be determined by the rate of addition of protein to the plasma. A gradual fall in hemoglobin level accompanies the expansion in plasma volume. Thus, the hemoglobin level is normal soon after the hemorrhage, is slightly decreased about 3 h later and gradually falls to reach its lowest value between 36 and 72 h after the bleed. The anemia is normochromic and normocytic in type. The reticulocyte count is slightly increased 1–2 days after the hemorrhage, reaches a peak at about 7–10 days and returns to normal by about 2 weeks. The extent of the reticulocytosis is proportional to the amount of blood lost

but seldom exceeds 10–15%. A few normoblasts appear in the blood after a severe hemorrhage. The leukocyte count increases within 1–2 h of acute hemorrhage, usually to the range $12–20 \times 10^9/l$ and remains elevated for several days. This leukocytosis is caused by a raised neutrophil count associated with a few neutrophil metamyelocytes and an occasional myelocyte. There is also a temporary increase in the platelet count.

The rapid loss of 500 ml of blood within a few minutes usually causes a slight fall in central venous pressure but no significant changes in the blood pressure or pulse rate. When 750 ml or more are lost rapidly, there is a substantial fall in central venous pressure, a fall in cardiac output, a fall in blood pressure and peripheral vasoconstriction. The rapid loss of 1.5–2 l may cause unconsciousness.[15]

Chronic blood loss, such as results from chronic peptic ulcers or neoplasms of the large bowel, eventually causes the development of a hypochromic microcytic anemia due to iron deficiency (see Chapter 11).

Hemolytic anemia: general considerations[16–18]

A hemolytic state is said to exist when the survival of a patient's red cells in the circulation is reduced below the normal value of 110–120 days due to lysis within the vascular tree (intravascular hemolysis), premature phagocytosis and destruction by cells of the mononuclear phagocyte system (extravascular hemolysis), or both. As normal individuals can increase the rate of red cell production to six to eight times the basal rate in response to anemia, patients whose mean red cell life span is reduced to one-sixth of normal (i.e. to about 20 days) do not suffer from anemia provided there is no impairment of bone marrow function. Such patients are said to suffer from a compensated hemolytic state. Anemia develops when the bone marrow cannot adequately compensate for the degree of reduction of red cell life span.

Extravascular and intravascular hemolysis[13,19]

In the majority of hemolytic anemias, hemolysis occurs extravascularly in the spleen, liver and bone marrow. The cells of the mononuclear phagocyte system present in these organs remove abnormal erythrocytes and red cell fragments from the circulation. The fate of these prematurely removed red cells is similar to that of normal red cells that are removed at the end of their life span.

The degradation of 1 mol of heme within these phago-cytes leads to the production of 1 mol of bilirubin and 1 mol of carbon monoxide. The bilirubin enters the plasma and is transported to the liver bound to albumin. In the liver the water-insoluble bilirubin is converted to soluble glucuronides and excreted in the bile. The bilirubin is then converted by the bacterial flora of the bowel to unrobilingen and eliminated in the feces. Some of the urobilinogen is reabsorbed from the gut and excreted in the urine. In normal adults about 1% of the circulating red cells (i.e. about 20 ml of red cells) are destroyed extravascularly per day and, provided liver function is unimpaired, this results in a serum bilirubin level of 5–17 μmol/l (0.3–1.0 mg/dl) and a daily fecal urobilinogen excretion of 50–265 mg. Patients with hemolytic anemia usually show mild to moderate jaundice, slight hyper-bilirubinemia and an increased excretion of fecal and urinary urobilinogen. The serum bilirubin level is usually in the range 20–50 μmol/l (1–3 mg/dl). The exact level depends not only on the rate of hemolysis but also on the capacity of the liver to cope with an increased bilirubin load. In hemolytic states the body attempts to cope with the increased rate of red cell destruction both by an increase in the number of macrophages involved in erythrophagocytosis and by increasing the capacity of the liver to conjugate and excrete bilirubin. For this reason, an occasional patient with hemolytic anemia may have a normal serum bilirubin level and may not be jaundiced.

The hemoglobin released from intravascular lysis of red cells is bound to haptoglobins, a family of hemoglobin-binding α globulins present in the plasma. The resulting hemoglobin–haptoglobin complex is rapidly cleared from the circulation by hepatocytes. The concentration of haptoglobin is usually expressed in terms of its hemoglobin-binding capacity and in normal individuals there is sufficient to bind 0.4–2.1 g of hemoglobin per liter of plasma. A reduction in the plasma haptoglobin level is a feature of intravascular hemolysis but is also seen in extravascular hemolysis, possibly because of a leak of some free hemoglobin into the circulation. When the amount of hemoglobin released during intravascular hemolysis exceeds the hemoglobin-binding capacity of the haptoglobins, free hemoglobin appears in the plasma. Heme is released from the free hemoglobin and binds to a specific heme-binding plasma β glycoprotein called hemopexin; the heme–hemopexin complex is removed by the liver. When the heme-binding capacity of the hemopexin is exceeded, hematin is formed and binds to albumin to produce methemalbumin which gives the plasma a dirty brown color. In severe intravascular hemolysis, tetrameric hemoglobin ($\alpha_2\beta_2$) and αβ dimers are present in the plasma (hemoglobinemia). The dimers

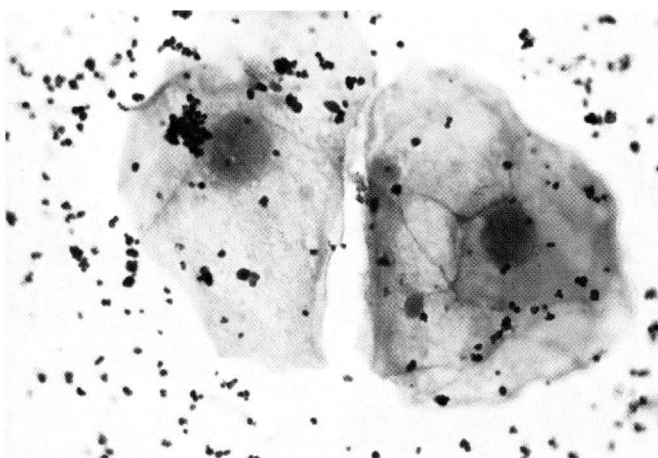

Fig. 6.4 Urinary deposit stained by Perls' acid ferrocyanide method for hemosiderin. The deposit was obtained by centrifugation of the urine of a patient with chronic intravascular hemolysis due to a malfunctioning aortic valve prosthesis and shows the presence of hemosiderin granules.

pass through the glomerular filter and when the hemo-globin level exceeds about 0.3 g/l, appear in the urine (hemoglobinuria). Some of the αβ dimers are metabolized in the renal tubular cells with the formation of hemosiderin granules. These granules may be seen both within shed tubular cells and extracellularly when the urine is spun and the deposit examined after staining by Perls' acid ferrocyanide method (Fig. 6.4). Thus, apart from the reduction of haptoglobin levels, the other biochemical changes of intravascular hemolysis include reduced hemopexin levels, methemalbuminemia (detected by Schumm's test), hemoglobinemia (serum level > 4 mg/dl), hemoglobinuria (Fig. 6.5) and hemosiderinuria.

Hematologic changes

These consist of morphologic abnormalities in the red cells (e.g. spherocytosis, fragmentation of red cells) resulting from the disorder underlying the hemolysis and changes caused by a compensatory increase of erythro-poietic activity. The latter include reticulocytosis, erythro-blastemia, macrocytosis, and erythroid hyperplasia. Most patients have a clearly increased reticulocyte percentage and absolute reticulocyte count. Reticulocyte percentages of 5–20% are usual but values as high as 50–70% may occasionally be seen. In general, the extent of the increase in the reticulocyte count is proportional to the severity of the anemia. Small numbers of erythroblasts may be present in the circulation (less than 1 per 100 leukocytes). The degree of erythroblastemia is higher in patients with higher reticulocyte counts and may increase considerably if the hemolysis continues following splenectomy. The anemia is generally normochromic and normocytic in type but may be macrocytic. The macrocytosis is usually associated with macronormoblastic erythropoiesis and in such cases is the result of alterations in the kinetics of erythropoiesis; the reticulocytes formed during accelerated erythropoiesis are considerably larger than normal and mature into macrocytes. Occasionally, the macrocytosis may be partly or wholly due to a secondary folate deficiency and in these cases erythropoiesis is megaloblastic. The bone marrow of subjects with hemolysis shows increased cellularity due to erythroid hyperplasia, and a corresponding decrease in fat cells. The myeloid–erythroid ratio is reduced and may be as low as 0.5 (normal range, 2.0–8.3). There may be an extension of hemopoietic marrow down the long bones.

Patients with chronic hemolytic anemias suffer from temporary aplastic crises in which morphologically recognizable erythropoietic cells virtually disappear from

the marrow, the reticulocyte count falls, sometimes to zero, and the hemoglobin level falls very rapidly. Neutropenia and thrombocytopenia may also be occasionally present. Reticulocytes reappear after about 7–10 days. The aplastic crises are often associated with 'trivial' infections and may affect more than one member of a family at about the same time. Recent studies indicate that such infections are frequently caused by a parvovirus (see Chapter 14).[20–22]

There may be a substantial loss of iron in the urine of patients with chronic hemoglobinuria and hemosiderinuria and this may lead to iron deficiency.

Changes in other tissues

The increased hemolysis leads to an increased rate of production and excretion of bilirubin and, consequently, to an increased frequency of pigment gall stones. Cholecystitis or deep jaundice due to obstruction of the common bile duct may follow. The persistence of stones in the gall bladder for long periods may be associated with the subsequent development of carcinoma.

Particularly in severe congenital hemolytic anemia, the erythroid hyperplasia may be so marked that it causes an increase in the volume of the marrow cavity, thinning of cortical bone and deformities of the bones (Fig. 6.6). Furthermore, extramedullary hemopoiesis may occur in the liver, spleen and lymph nodes.

Splenomegaly is common and is associated with an increase in phagocytic cells to cope with the high rate of

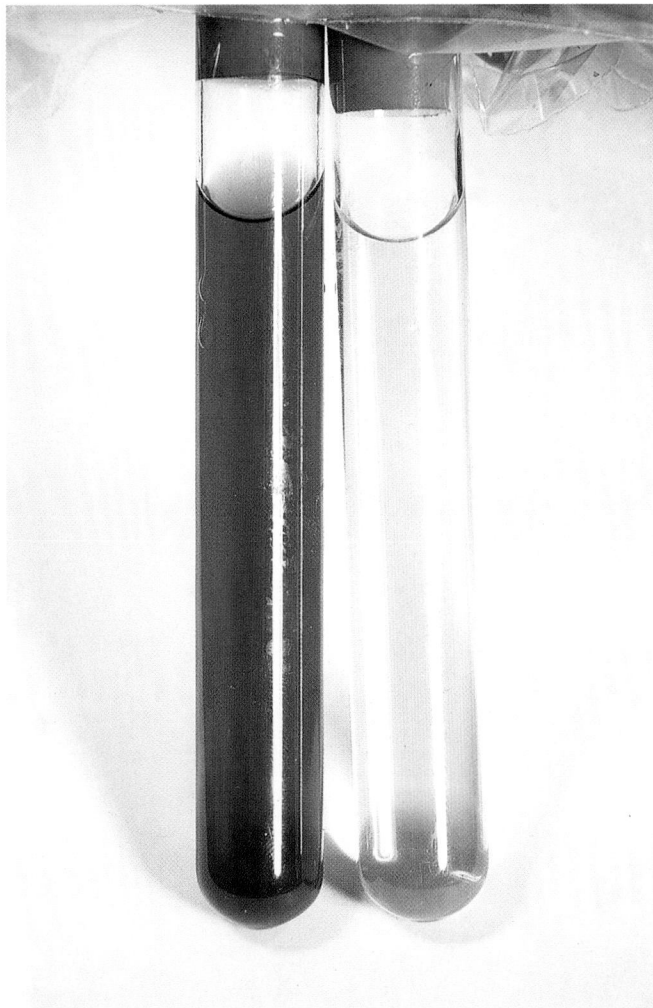

Fig. 6.5 Sample of urine showing hemoglobinuria from a patient with acute intravascular hemolysis caused by an overdose of phenacetin, photographed alongside a normal urine sample for comparison.

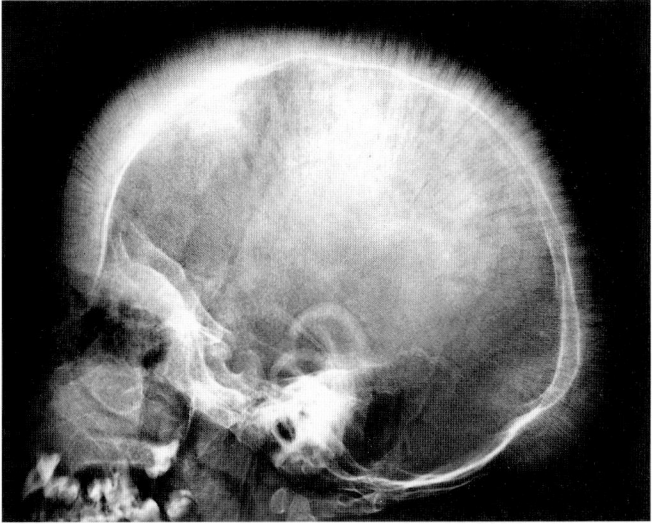

Fig. 6.6 X-ray of the skull of a patient with sickle cell anemia. There is a thickening of the parietal and frontal bones due to widening of the marrow-containing diploic space. Both tables of these bones, particularly the outer table, are abnormally thin and bony trabeculae have developed at right angles to the tables, giving a 'hair-on-end' appearance.

Table 6.5 Classification of the hemolytic anemias

Hereditary hemolytic anemia
  Abnormalities of the red cell membrane
  Abnormalities of the red cell enzymes
  Abnormalities of the structure or synthesis of hemoglobin

Acquired hemolytic anemia
  Immune
  Non-immune

destruction of abnormal red cells in this organ. In some conditions, the spleen also shows foci of extramedullary hemopoiesis. Retardation of growth may occur in children with gross splenomegaly.

Hemosiderosis may develop as a consequence of recurrent blood transfusions, an increased absorption of iron (secondary to the erythroid hyperplasia) or both.

Chronic leg ulcers over the malleoli have been occasionally observed in various types of hemolytic anemia.

Causes of hemolytic anemia

Hemolytic anemia may be due to: (1) inherited abnormalities of the cell membrane, energy-generating and other metabolic pathways, or hemoglobin constitution of the red cell; or (2) various acquired abnormalities. A classification of the causes of hemolytic anemia is given in Table 6.5.

REFERENCES

1. Bessis M 1973 Living blood cells and their ultrastructure. Springer, Berlin, 197
2. Brecher G, Bessis M 1972 Present status of spiculed red cells and their relationship to the discocyte–echinocyte transformation: a critical review. Blood 40: 333–344
3. Hamill RL, Woods JC, Cook BA 1991 Congenital atransferrinemia. A case report and review of the literature. American Journal of Clinical Pathology 96: 215–218
4. O'Hare JA, Murnaghan DJ 1982 Reversal of aluminum-induced hemodialysis anemia by a low-aluminum dialysate. New England Journal of Medicine 306: 654–656
5. Gjone E, Torsvik H, Norum KR 1968 Familial plasma cholesterol ester deficiency. A study of the erythrocytes. Scandinavian Journal of Clinical and Laboratory Investigation 21: 327–332
6. Sturgeon P 1970 Hematological observations on the anemia associated with blood type Rhnull. Blood 36: 310–320
7. Davidson RJ, How J, Lessels S 1977 Acquired stomatocytosis: its prevalence and significance in routine haematology. Scandinavian Journal of Haematology 19: 47–53
8. Morse EE 1990 Mechanisms of hemolysis in liver disease. Annals of Clinical and Laboratory Science 20: 169–174
9. Cooper RA, Gulbrandsen CL 1971 The relationship between serum lipoproteins and red cell membranes in abetalipoproteinemia: deficiency of lecithin: cholesterol acyltransferase. Journal of Laboratory and Clinical Medicine 78: 323–335
10. Symmans WA, Shepherd CS, March WL et al 1979 Hereditary acanthocytosis associated with the McLeod phenotype of the Kell blood group system. British Journal of Haematology 42: 575–583
11. Finch CA, Deubelbeiss K, Cook JD et al 1970 Ferrokinetics in man. Medicine (Baltimore) 49: 17–53
12. Wickramasinghe SN 1975 Human bone marrow. Blackwell Scientific Publications, Oxford
13. Wickramasinghe SN, Weatherall DJ 1982 The pathophysiology of erythropoiesis. In: Hardisty RM, Weatherall DJ (eds), Blood and its disorders, 2nd edn. Blackwell Scientific Publications, Oxford, 101
14. Adamson J, Hillman RS 1968 Blood volume and plasma protein replacement following acute blood loss in normal man. Journal of the American Medical Association 205: 609–612
15. Wallace J, Sharpey-Shafer EP 1941 Blood changes following controlled haemorrhage in man. Lancet ii: 393
16. Dacie JV 1985 The haemolytic anaemias, vol 1: The hereditary haemolytic anaemias, part 1, 3rd edn. Churchill Livingstone, Edinburgh
17. Dacie JV 1988 The haemolytic anaemias, vol 2: The hereditary haemolytic anaemias, part 2, 3rd edn. Churchill Livingstone, Edinburgh
18. Dacie JV 1992 The haemolytic anaemias, vol 3: The auto-immune haemolytic anaemias, 3rd edn. Churchill Livingstone, Edinburgh
19. Bunn HF 1972 Erythrocyte destruction and hemoglobin catabolism. Seminars in Hematology 9: 3–17
20. Mortimer PP 1983 Hypothesis: the aplastic crisis of hereditary spherocytosis is due to a single transmissible agent. Journal of Clinical Pathology 36: 445–448
21. Duncan JR, Potter CB, Cappellini MD et al 1983 Aplastic crisis due to parvovirus infection in pyruvate kinase deficiency. Lancet ii: 14–16
22. Kelleher JF Jr, Luban NL, Cohen BJ, Mortimer PP 1984 Human serum parvovirus as the cause of aplastic crisis in sickle cell disease. American Journal of Diseases of Children 138: 401–403

Abnormalities of the red cell membrane

7

J Delaunay

Hereditary spherocytosis
ANKI gene mutations
SLC4A1 gene mutations
EPB42 gene mutations
SPTB gene mutations
SPTA1 gene mutations

Hereditary elliptocytosis and poikilocytosis
SPTA1 gene mutations
SPTB gene mutations
EBP41 gene mutations

Southeast Asian ovalocytosis

Genetically leaky red cells
Overhydrated hereditary stomatocytosis
Dehydrated hereditary stomatocytosis

Others

Conclusions

A number of hereditary hemolytic anemias have been related to genes encoding proteins that belong to the red cell membrane. The membrane is comprised of the lipid bilayer and the skeleton that laminates the inner surface of the bilayer (Table 7.1 and Fig. 7.1). Many proteins of interest are also expressed in nonerythroid cell types through a variety of isoforms.

Hereditary spherocytosis

Hereditary spherocytosis (HS) is the most frequent congenital hemolytic anemia. At a rough estimate, it affects one family in about 2000. Although described in all ethnic groups, HS seems to be less common among Black people. The clinical presentation of HS varies from a nearly symptomless picture to death *in utero*. The usual manifestations are anemia, jaundice and splenomegaly. Common complications include biliary obstruction and parvovirus B19 infections. Blood smears display spherocytes (Fig. 7.2) which can be scarce, however. The decreased osmotic resistance of red cells is sometimes difficult to assess based on usual techniques. When available, osmotic gradient ektacytometry provides a straightforward and highly reliable test. The treatment includes blood transfusions. In infancy, transfusions can be replaced by the administration of human recombinant erythropoietin. Splenectomy corrects the anemia of HS and increases red cell life span. Early in life, partial splenectomy is useful, to be completed later on. HS will be considered according to the five genes likely to be involved. Whatever the genetic origin, the stability of the membrane skeleton is

Table 7.1 Characteristics of the main membrane proteins, and their genes, involved in hereditary disorders of the red cell membrane

Proteins	Number of amino acids; molecular weights (kDa)	Number of monomers per red cell	Genes and their chromosomal locations	Gene sizes (kb) and number of their exons	Sizes of the messenger RNAs (kb)
Spectrin α-chain	2429; 281	242 000	*SPTA1;* 1q22-q23	80; 52	8.0
Spectrin β-chain	2137; 246	242 000	*SPTB;* 14q23–q24.1	>100; 36	7.0
Ankyrin	1880; 206	124 000	*ANK1;* 8p11.2	>120; 42	6.8; 7.2
AE1[a]	911; 102	1 200 000	*SLC4A1;* 17q12–q21	17; 20	4.7
Protein 4.1	588; 66	200 000	*EPB41;* 1p33–p34.2	>250; >23	5.6
Protein 4.2	691; 77	200 000	*EPB42;* 15q15–q21	20; 13	2.4

AE1[a]: anion exchanger 1, or band 3 (in the red cell).

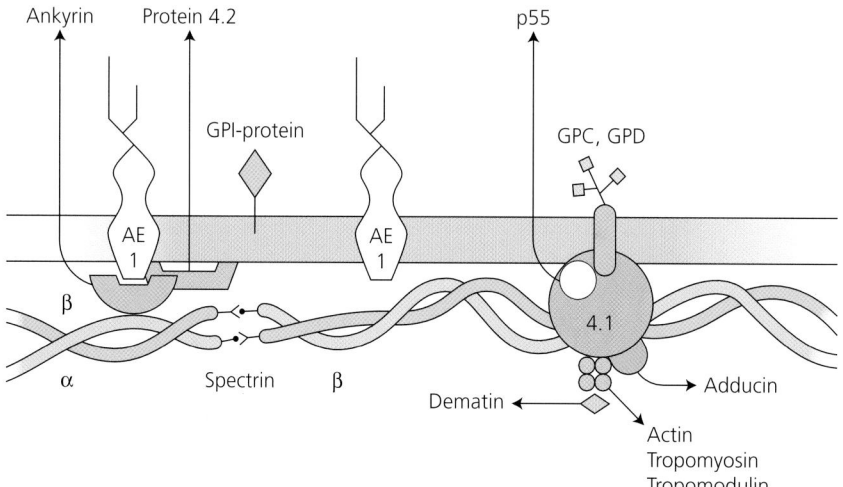

Fig. 7.1 *Cross-section of the red cell membrane.* Only the main proteins are represented. Spectrin, actin and protein 4.1 are skeleton proteins. They combine into a two-dimensional network, the membrane skeleton. Spectrin is an $\alpha_2\beta_2$ tetramer. To form a dimer, an α-chain and a β-chain combine side-by-side through complementary nucleation sites, one on the α-chain (*C*-terminus region), one on the β-chain (*N*-terminus region). To form a tetramer, two dimers then interact head-to-head through complementary sites, one on each α-chain (*N*-terminus) and one on each β-chain (*C*-terminus). Skeletal proteins are connected to transmembrane proteins. Spectrin next to its self-association site binds to band 3 (that is, the anion exchanger 1, or AE1) through ankyrin, with the participation of protein 4.2 ; protein 4.1 (at the ends of spectrin tetramers) binds to glycophorin C/D and protein p55.

decreased (Fig. 7.1) and causes microvesicles to swarm out and reduce the surface area of the erythrocyte.

ANKI gene mutations (OMIM 182900)

ANK1 gene mutations (for recent listing, see Ref.1) account for about 60% of HS, but this percentage may be lower in some populations. The inheritance pattern is dominant. There is a primary decrease in ankyrin and a secondary reduction in spectrin and protein 4.2. On average, the clinical presentation is relatively severe.

In 20% of *ANKI*-related HS, the mutation arises *de novo*.[2] The inheritance of HS has long been viewed mistakenly as recessive when the proband 'inaugurating' the mutation in a family is first examined. Genuine recessive HS and homozygous cases of HS have not been unequivocally described in humans with *ANKI* gene mutations.

SLC4A1 gene mutations (OMIM 109270)

SLC4A1 (or *EPB3*) gene mutations (for recent listing, see Ref. 3) account for about 20% of HS. The inheritance pattern is dominant. In the heterozygous state, the encoded protein, band 3 (or the anion exchanger 1, AE1), part of which spans the lipid bilayer, and secondarily band 4.2 are reduced by about 20%. *SLC4A1* gene mutations are essentially sporadic, except for some that change arginine into other amino acids. This applies to arginine at position 760 (hot spot: CGG). In the heterozygous state, the clinical manifestations are mild to moderate. The occurrence, *in trans* to common *SLC4A1* HS alleles, of low expression alleles that are symptomless by themselves in the heterozygous state, may result in a substantial aggravation of HS.[4] Two known homozygous cases have been documented in detail. In one Portuguese patient, the AE1 was completely missing, yielding a dramatic, transfusion-dependent anemia which was lethal if not attended to. The electrophoretic pattern was markedly altered: absence of band 3 and protein 4.2, reduction to various extents of band 6, spectrin, ankyrin and glycophorin A. This case was associated with distal renal tubular acidosis, for the mutation also affected (and, presumably, abolished) the band 3 isoform found in tubular α-intercalated cells. One patient who survived (now three and a half years of age) was heavily transfused and has recently been splenectomized.[5] In an Italian patient, a comparable yet not quite as dramatic picture was seen. The absence of the AE1 was not complete (Perrotta *et al*, personal communication). Distal renal

tubular acidosis was absent because the mutation stood upstream of the renal promoter within the *SLC4A1* gene and therefore spared the expression of the AE1 renal isoform.[6]

EPB42 gene mutations (OMIM 177070)

EPB42 gene mutations are uncommon (for recent listing, see Ref. 3). Eight different mutations have been described. One is protein 4.2 Nippon which has been found in several cases in Japan, but may be encountered elsewhere sporadically[7] due, presumably, to independent mutational events. The inheritance pattern is strictly recessive. In the homozygous state, protein 4.2 is absent (or present in vanishingly low amounts). The quantity of band 3 is unchanged. The corresponding type of HS is atypical, and splenectomy has only a partial efficacy.

SPTB gene mutations (OMIM 182870)

SPTB gene mutations (for recent listing, see Ref. 1) are responsible for about 20% of HS in Europe. Their inheritance pattern is dominant, in keeping with the limiting synthesis of spectrin β-chains with respect to its partner α-chains. *De novo* mutations are common. Many mutations are null and abolish the output of the β-chain (splicing, frameshift or nonsense mutations).

SPTA1 gene mutations (OMIM 182860)

SPTA1 gene mutations are rare, since clinical expression requires homozygosity or compound heterozygosity (for recent listing, see Ref. 1). Their inheritance pattern is recessive. Among the low-expression *SPTA1* alleles, allele α^{LEPRA} (-99 c→t in intron 30, yielding a disturbed splicing) is encountered in a recurrent manner.

Hereditary elliptocytosis and poikilocytosis

Hereditary elliptocytosis (HE) and poikilocytosis (HP) are two aspects of the same entity. Whereas HE is often mild and may go undetected, HP is highly symptomatic. There is a continuum between both of them. They affect one family in 5000, approximately. HE and HP are found in all populations; however, spectrin α-chain related forms have a higher incidence among Black Africans conferring, presumably, some resistance against malaria in the latter. The usual manifestations are anemia, jaundice and splenomegaly. Biliary obstruction is a common complication. Blood smears display elliptocytes which vary in percentage and degree of elongation (Fig. 7.2). As the presentation becomes more severe, elliptocytes are associated with an increasing proportion of poikilocytes, and the pattern eventually shifts towards complete poikilocytosis. Again, osmotic gradient ektacytometry provides a straightforward and highly reliable diagnostic test. The treatment includes blood transfusions. Splenectomy has a beneficial effect, though not as marked as in HS. Mutations in three genes may cause HE or HP. These mutations alter the elastic deformability of the red cells. The abnormal red cells are adversely affected by collision against the walls of the main arteries, and have difficulty in negotiating passage through narrow capillaries, especially in the spleen.

SPTA1 gene mutations (OMIM 182860)

SPTA1 gene mutations account for at least 60% of HE or HP cases (for recent listing, see Refs. 8 and 9). Mutations lie in or near the binding site of spectrin α-chain (*N*-terminus) for spectrin β-chain (*C*-terminus), as part of the spectrin tetramerization site.

In virtually all kindreds with any particular *SPTA1* gene mutation, some members are mildly affected, if at all (depending on the *SPTA1* mutation intrinsic severity), and others are more or less severely affected. This dual presentation suggests the frequent involvement of some aggravating factor likely to occur *in trans*. The latter remains silent in both the heterozygous and the homozygous states (because of the large excess of α-chains normally synthesized over the β-chains). This aggravating factor has been termed allele α^{LELY}. Half of the α^{LELY} transcripts lose exon 46 due to a mutation in intron 45 (−12c→t). It is noteworthy that this mutation is in linkage disequilibrium with the 1857 Leu→Val amino acid change (CTA→GTA, in exon 40), which is functionally neutral.[10] The absence of exon 46 hampers the initiation of the dimerization process, favoring the incorporation

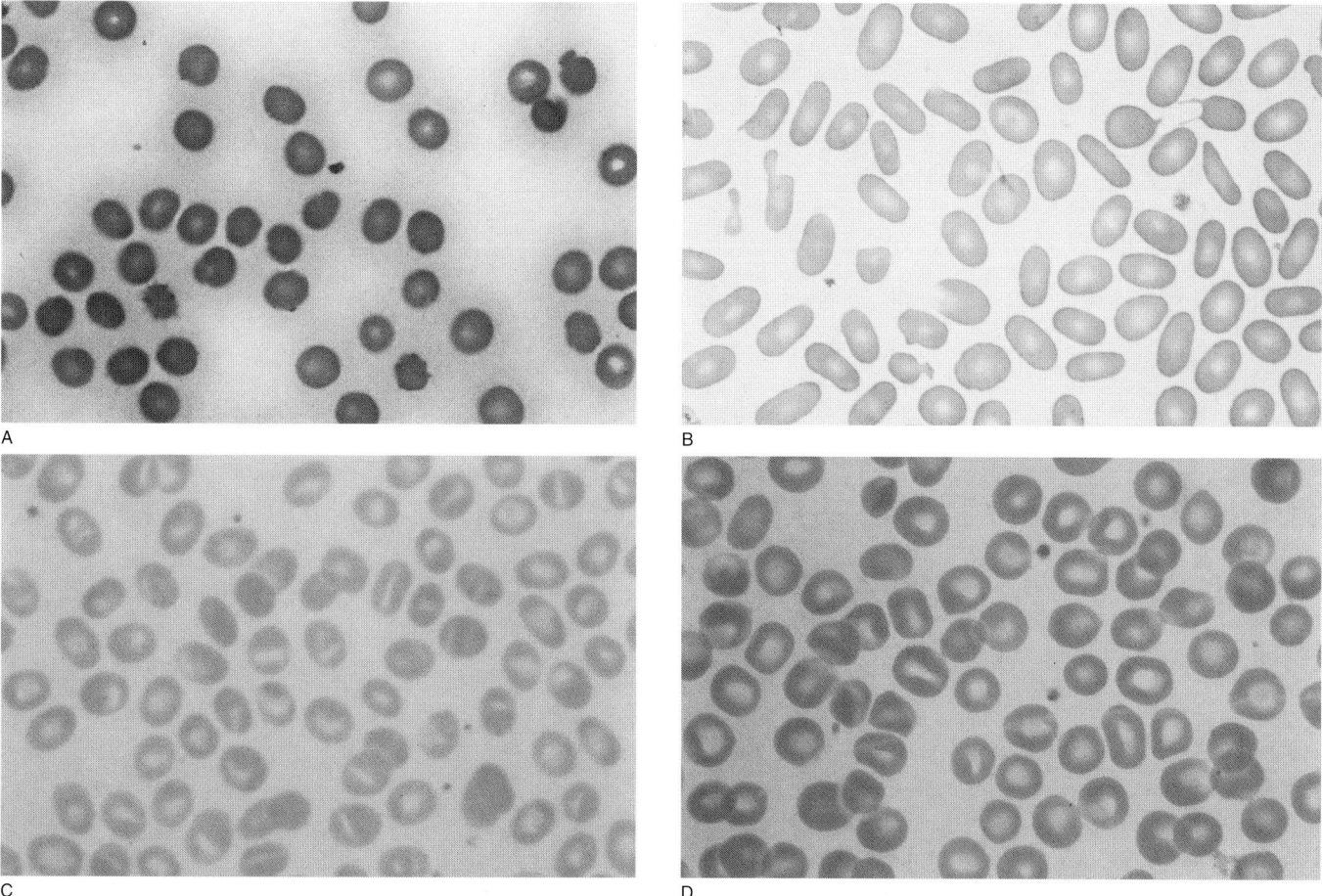

Fig. 7.2 *A gallery of abnormally shaped red cells.* (A) Spherocytes. In this particular example, the presence of some mushroom-red cells indicates a mutation in the AE1 in the heterozygous state. (B) Elliptocytes and a few poikilocytes in a patient with a mutation in the α-chain of spectrin. Some elliptocytes start fragmenting, because of the instability of the red cell skeleton. (C) Ovalo-stomatocytes that constitute the signature of Southeast Asian ovalocytosis. (D) Stomatocytes, seen in a patient presenting with dehydrated hereditary stomatocytosis, pseudohyperkalemia and, at birth fetal edema.

of more α^{HE} chains (*in trans*) into dimers. Such $\alpha^{HE}\beta$ dimers, however, will prove unable to self-associate into tetramers. $\alpha^{LELY}/\alpha^{HE}$ compound heterozygosity is as severe as α^{HE}/α^{HE} homozygosity or $\alpha^{HE}/\alpha^{HE'}$ compound heterozygosity.

Allele α^{LELY} occurs with about the same frequency in all the ethnic groups that have been investigated.[11–13] The leucine→valine change at position 1857 is constantly present and no recombination event has been found that would dissociate this mutation from the intron 45 mutation.

Mutations at position 28 appear in a recurrent manner (hot spot: CGT). One HE *SPTA1* allele (encoding an additional leucine at position 153) has some incidence in people who originate from Central West Africa, in fact from the same area as hemoglobin S ('Benin haplotype'). It is a mild mutation, and even homozygosity, or compound heterozygosity with allele α^{LELY}, results in moderate clinical effects. This allele provides some protection against malaria and followed trans-Saharan migrations towards North Africa. The migration trail went on through the Straits of Sicily toward Italy,[14] but apparently not through the Gibraltar Sound towards Spain. One may speculate that the mutation was brought to North Africa after the Moors had invaded Spain (8th century AD).

SPTB gene mutations (OMIM 182870)

SPTB gene mutations are less common (for recent listing, see Refs. 8 and 9). They stand in or near the binding site of spectrin β-chain (*C*-terminus) for spectrin-α chain (*N*-terminus), as part of the spectrin tetramerization site. Like their α-counterpart, they impede the self-association process.

EBP41 gene mutations (OMIM 130500)

The mutations in the *EBP41* gene, encoding protein 4.1R, account for 20–30% of HE in Caucasians. They cause an asymptomatic trait, which none the less produces the most numerous, the smoothest and the most elongated of all elliptocytes ever observed. The inheritance pattern is dominant. Owing to the very large size of the *EBP41* gene and the complex splicing pattern of its transcript, less than 10 mutations have been elucidated to date. For example, 4.1R Aravis bears a deletion of lysine 447, which abolishes its ability to bind the β-spectrin-actin complex.[15]

Incidentally, 4.1R Aravis exemplifies a genetic isolate. Endogamy, imposed upon some populations by geographical constraints, made the frequency of 4.1 (–) HE at least a 100-fold higher than normal in a neatly demar-cated area of French Northern Alps. The frequency of 4.1R mutations in the heterozygous state leads one to expect a relatively high frequency of homozygous cases. Actually, only three of them are known. The reason for this may be that homozygous mutations in 4.1R are viable as long as the damage is confined to the red cell membrane, the effects of the mutations being more harmful in nonerythroid cell types than in red cells. Protein 4.1 Madrid in the homozygous state[16] brings support to this view. A mutation cancels the 'downstream' initiation codon (AUG→AGG), which is the only initiation codon to remain in the erythroid precursors by the time 4.1R is synthesized. The red cells are devoid of any 4.1R. On the other hand, nonerythroid cell types can synthesize a longer isoform of 4.1R using the 'upstream' initiation codon.

Southeast Asian ovalocytosis

Southeast Asian ovalocytosis (SAO) is a dominantly inherited, asymptomatic trait which alters the morphology and mechanical properties of red cells in the heterozygous state. Homozygosity for the SAO allele has never been encountered and is thought to be lethal; however, the reason for this is not understood. SAO is widespread among various ethnic groups in Papua New Guinea, the Philippines and Indonesia, due to its protective effects against malaria, and has diffused round the Indian Ocean shore in the wake of migration trails. From there, a few carriers reached Europe. Smears display unmistakable ovalo-stomatocytes (Fig. 7.2). The genetic alteration is a 27 nucleotide deletion in the *SLC4A1* gene. As a consequence, amino acids 400 to 408 which stand at the junction of the cytoplasmic and membrane domains of the AE1 are missing.[17,18] Such a molecular defect is likely to account for the cellular rigidity associated with ovalocytosis. The deletion is in linkage disequilibrium with the so-called Memphis I polymorphisms (AAG→GAG; K56E).

Genetically leaky red cells

A rare category of genetic conditions of the red cell is associated with an abnormal shape, that is stomatocytosis[19] (Fig. 7.2). However, this conspicuous morphologic abnormality is not the most significant feature. The important defect is an increase of the passive leak of monovalent cations. The conditions are dominantly transmitted. The presentation includes anemia, jaundice and splenomegaly. Additional symptoms, which have been overlooked until recently, are also encountered in dehydrated hereditary stomatocytosis (see below). Osmotic gradient ektacytometry is a powerful tool to establish the diagnosis of each of the conditions considered. Generally speaking, conditions with leaky red cells frequently cause biliary complications. An important recent discovery is that splenectomy, which is moderately effective in increasing the hemoglobin, is indeed strongly contra-indicated because it dramatically increases the risk of thromboembolic accidents.[20]

Overhydrated hereditary stomatocytosis (OMIM 185000)

Overhydrated hereditary stomatocytosis (OHS) is rare. Less than 20 cases have been reported. Kindreds have a small size because the mutations are often de novo and the patients fail to have many children. As a result, genetic studies have been hindered. The main features of the phenotype are a macrocytosis, a reduced mean cell hemoglobin concentration (MCHC) and a rightward shift of the osmotic gradient ektacytometric curve. Stomatin is lacking, completely or nearly so, but this is a secondary event. The primary missing protein is unknown. The monovalent cation leak (i.e. the K^+ efflux in the presence of ouabain + bumetanide) is increased, sometimes 'torrentially'. The curve: *log* (leak) vs temperature, dis-plays a steep downward slope. In some kindreds, the curve reascends as temperature draws near 0°C (cryo-OHS). The otherwise total resemblance between OHS and cryo-OHS suggests that both stem from mutations within the same locus.

Dehydrated hereditary stomatocytosis (OMIM 194380)

Dehydrated hereditary stomatocytosis (DHS) is much less infrequent than OHS, but remains 10–100 times rarer than hereditary spherocytosis. There is a tendency toward macrocytosis, an increased MCHC, and a leftward shift of the osmotic gradient ektacytometric curve. DHS, which appears as a well-compensated hemolytic anemia, causes marked iron loading. The monovalent cation leak is increased, though much less than in OHS. The curve: *log* (leak) vs temperature, is simply shifted up the y-axis compared to normal.

Quite unexpectedly, DHS must now be viewed as part of a broader, pleiotropic syndrome.[21,22] This new syn-drome (OMIM 603528) includes fetal edema and pseudo-hyperkalemia. Fetal edema is a transient manifestation which disappears before or soon after birth. It may be lethal, though, if not attended to. Pseudohyperkalemia

may exist on its own: this trait was indeed discovered as such and called familial pseudohyperkalemia by Stewart *et al* in 1979[23] (OMIM 177720). The different mani-festations of the pleiotropic syndrome can combine in any fashion. Even within a given kindred (i.e. for a given mutation) different affected members can have distinct combinations.

The gene responsible for DHS, reported in a large Irish family, was mapped to 16q23-q24.[24] The gene responsible for familial pseudohyperkalemia, recorded in a large Scottish family, was mapped to 16q23-q24 also.[25] In 10 different smaller families (8 French and 2 American) with various presentations of the pleiotropic syndrome, mapping led again to 16q23-q24.[26]

Others

The list of the genetic syndromes with leaky red cells is likely to lengthen:

1. A unique case of DHS noticeably departing from the common DHS has been described. In particular, the curve: *log* (leak) vs temperature had a shallow downhill slope.[27] It did not map to chromosome 16.[28]
2. We recently found a large Flemish family with familial pseudohyperkalemia which, likewise, failed to map to chromosome 16. In those two instances, genome-wide searches are underway.

Conclusions

Over the past 15 years, the genetic disorders of the red cell skeleton have yielded a wealth of molecular infor-mation, putting these disorders on a par with hemo-globinopathies and red cell enzyme defects. The mutations discovered have not only provided diagnostic help, but also have illuminated in many instances the genotype–phenotype or the structure–function relationships. More recently, interest has shifted towards conditions that render the red cell membrane leaky to monovalent cations. The corresponding proteins are unknown. Positional cloning has proved a fruitful approach. Eventually, a number of new proteins involved in this abnormality will come into sight.

REFERENCES

1. Gallagher PG, Forget BG 1998 Hematologically important mutations: spectrin and ankyrin variants in hereditary spherocytosis. Blood Cells, Molecules and Diseases 24: 539–543 (review article)
2. Miraglia del Giudice E, Francese M, Nobili B et al 1998 High frequency of the *de novo* mutations in ankyrin gene (ANK1) in children with hereditary spherocytosis. Journal of Pediatrics 132: 117–120

3. Gallagher PG, Forget B 1997 Hematologically important mutations: band 3 and protein 4.2 in hereditary spherocytosis. Blood Cells, Molecules and Diseases 23: 417–421 (review article)
4. Alloisio N, Texier P, Vallier A et al 1997 Modulation of clinical expression and band 3 deficiency in hereditary spherocytosis. Blood 90: 414–420
5. Ribeiro L, Alloisio N, Almeida H et al 2000 Near lethal hereditary spherocytosis and distal tubular acidosis associated with the total absence of band 3. Blood 96: 1602–1604
6. Perrotta S. Nigro V, Iolascon et al 1998 Dominant hereditary spherocytosis due to band 3 Neapolis produces a life-threatrning anemia at the homozygous state. Blood 92: 9a, (abstr, suppl)
7. Perrotta S, Iolascon A, Polito R et al 1999 4.2 Nippon mutation in a non-Japanese patient with hereditary spherocytosis. Haematologica 84: 660–662 (correspondence)
8. Maillet P, Alloisio N, Morlé L et al 1996 Spectrin mutations in hereditary elliptocytosis and hereditary spherocytosis. Human Mutation 8: 97–107 (review article)
9. Delaunay J 1998 Genetic disorders of the red cell membrane. In: Jameson JL (ed), Principles of molecular medicine. Humana Press, Totawa, NJ, 191–195 (review article)
10. Wilmotte R, Maréchal J, Morlé L et al 1993 Low expression allele α^{LELY} of red cell spectrin is associated with mutations in exon 40 ($\alpha^{V/41}$ polymorphism) and intron 45 and with partial skipping of exon 46. Journal of Clinical Investigation 91: 2091–2096
11. Maréchal J, Wilmotte R, Kanzaki A et al 1995 Ethnic distribution of allele α^{LELY}, a low expression allele of red cell spectrin α-gene. British Journal of Haematology: 90, 553–556
12. Basseres DS, Salles TSI, Costa FF, Saad STO 1998 Presence of allele α^{LELY} in an Amazonian population. American Journal of Hematology 57: 212–214
13. Papassideri I, Antonelou M, Karababa F et al 1999 The frequency of allele α^{LELY}, a low expression allele of the gene encoding erythroid spectrin α-chain, in the Greek population. Haematologica 84: 754–755 (correspondence)
14. Miraglia del Giudice E, Ducluzeau MT, Alloisio N et al 1992 $\alpha^{I/65}$ Hereditary elliptocytosis in Southern Italy: Evidence for an African origin. Human Genetics 89: 553–556
15. Lorenzo F, Dalla Venezia N, Morlé L et al 1994 Protein 4.1 deficiency associated with an altered binding to the spectrin–actin complex of the red cell membrane skeleton. Journal of Clinical Investigation 94: 1651–1656
16. Dalla Venezia N, Gilsanz F, Alloisio N et al Homozygous 4.1(–)
17. Jarolim P, Palek J, Amato D et al 1991 Deletion of erythrocyte band 3 gene in malaria-resistant Southeast Asian ovalocytosis. Proceedings of the National Academy of Sciences of the United States of America 88: 11022–11026
18. Schofield AE, Tanner MJA, Pinder JC et al 1992 Basis of unique red cell membrane properties in hereditary ovalocytosis. Journal of Molecular Biology 223: 949–958
19. Delaunay J, Stewart G, Iolascon A 1999 Hereditary dehydrated and overhydrated stomatocytosis: recent advances. In: Narla M (ed) Current Opinion in Hematology. William & Wilkins, Lippincott, PA, 6: 110–114
20. Stewart GW, Amess JAL, Eber SW et al Thrombo-embolic disease after splenectomy for hereditary stomatocytosis. British Journal of Haematology 93: 303–310
21. Entezami M, Becker R, Menssen H et al 1996 Xerocytosis with concomitant intrauterine ascites: first description and therapeutic approach. Blood 87: 5392–5393 (correspondence)
22. Grootenboer S, Schischmanoff PO, Cynober T et al 1998 A genetic syndrome associating dehydrated hereditary stomatocytosis, pseudohyperkalaemia and perinatal oedema. British Journal of Haematology 103: 383–386
23. Stewart GW, Corral RJM, Fyffe JA et al 1979 Familial pseudohyperkalaemia. The Lancet ii: 175–177
24. Carella M, Stewart G, Ajetunmobi JF et al 1998 Genomewide search for dehydrated hereditary stomatocytosis (hereditary xerocytosis): mapping of locus to chromosome 16 (16q23-qter). American Journal of Human Genetics 63: 810–816
25. Iolascon A, Stewart G, Ajetunmobi JF et al 1999 Familial pseudohyperkalemia maps to the same locus as dehydrated hereditary stomatocytosis (hereditary xerocytosis). Blood 93: 3120–3123
26. Grootenboer S, Schischmanoff PO, Laurendeau I et al 2000 Pleiotropic syndrome of dehydrated hereditary stomatocytosis, pseudohyperkalemia and perinatal edema maps to 16q23-q24. Blood 96: 2599–2605
27. Coles SE, Ho MH, Chetty MC et al 1999 A variant of hereditary stomatocytosis with marked pseudohyperkalaemia. British Journal of Haematology 104: 275–283
28. Carella M, Stewart G, Ajetunmobi JF et al 1999 Genetic heterogeneity of hereditary stomatocytosis syndrome showing pseudohyperkalaemia. Haematologica 84: 862–863

Erythroenzyme disorders

8

DM Layton   DR Roper

Introduction

Clinical features

Blood cell morphology

Biochemical investigation of erythroenzyme disorders

Molecular basis of erythroenzyme disorders

Introduction

To achieve optimal performance as an oxygen transporter during its life span in circulation the mature red cell has sacrificed metabolic versatility.[1] Its structural and functional integrity depend on catabolism of glucose via the anerobic Embden–Meyerhof pathway to replenish adenosine triphosphate (ATP) required for cation homeostasis and other energy-dependent processes in conjunction with the oxidative pentose phosphate pathway (hexose monophosphate shunt) to maintain redox capacity. In the resting state 90% of glucose is catabolized anerobically through the Embden–Meyerhof pathway,

which also serves to generate nicotinamide adenine dinucleotide in its reduced form (NADH) required as a cofactor for cytochrome b5 reductase for the conversion of methemoglobin to hemoglobin (Fig. 8.1). The pentose phosphate pathway serves mainly to supply the reduced form of nicotinamide adenine dinucleotide phosphate (NADPH) necessary to regenerate reduced glutathione (GSH), which acts as a sacrificial reductant to protect the membrane and contents of the red cell against oxidative damage (Fig. 8.2). Glucose-6-phosphate dehydrogenase (G6PD) catalyses the first and rate limiting step, the conversion of glucose-6-phosphate (G6P) to 6-phosphogluconate (6PG) in this pathway. Synthesis of the tripeptide glutathione from its constituent amino acids and nucleotide salvage complete the essential metabolic repertoire of the red cell cytosol. Conservation of adenine nucleotides to maintain intracellular ATP and elimination of pyrimidine nucleotides is facilitated through the action of pyrimidine 5'-nucleotidase (P5N) which specifically dephosphorylates pyrimidine nucleoside-5'-monophosphates formed by RNA breakdown. This permits removal of toxic pyrimidines by passive diffusion and prevents their accumulation within the red cell. Defects in each of these key pathways may produce hemolytic anemia.

With the exception of polymorphic G6PD variants (Fig. 8.3) estimated to affect up to 400 million people worldwide, most inherited disorders of red cell metabolism are uncommon. Pyruvate kinase (PK) deficiency is the most commonly encountered defect of the Embden–Meyerhof pathway with heterozygote frequencies based on biochemical population studies that vary from 0.14% in the United States[2] to 6% in Saudi Arabia.[3] After PK the most common enzyme deficiencies implicated in hemolytic anemia are in approximate order of frequency: glucosephosphate isomerase (GPI); class I G6PD variants (associated with chronic hemolytic anemia); phosphofructokinase (PFK), triosephosphate isomerase (TPI), phosphoglycerate kinase (PGK) and hexokinase (HK). Deficiencies of P5N,[4] which has been described in

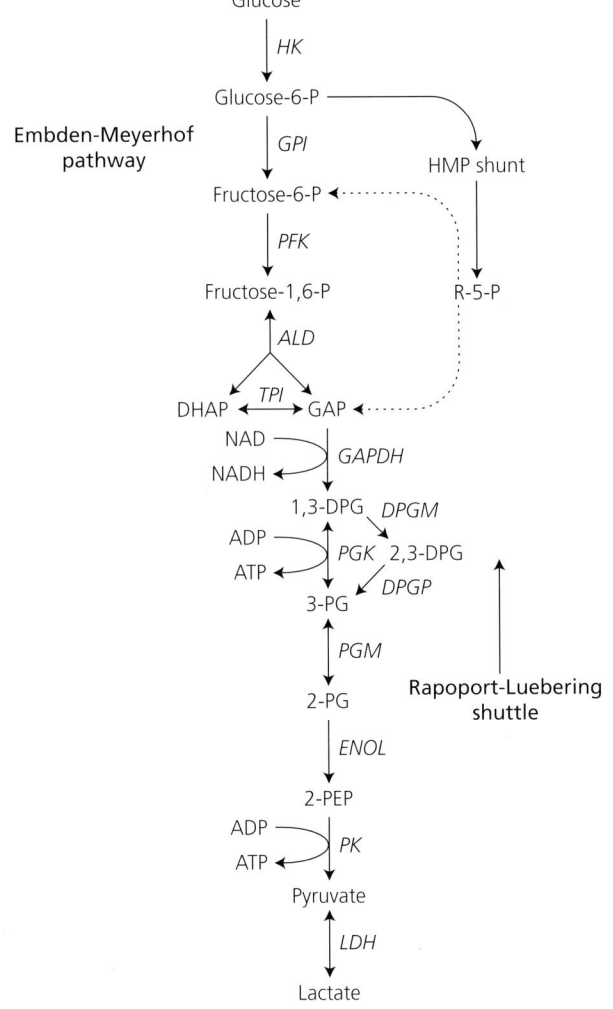

Fig. 8.1 Glycolytic pathways in the human red cell. HK, hexokinase; GPI, glucosephosphate kinase; PFK, phosphofructokinase; ALD, aldolase; TPI, triosephosphate isomerase; DPGM, diphosphoglycerate mutase; PGM, phosphoglycerate mutase; GAPDH, glyceraldehyde-3-phosphate dehydrogenase; PGK, phosphoglycerate kinase; 2,3-DPG, 2,3-diphosphoglycerate; DPGP, diphosphoglycerate phosphatase; ENOL, enolase; PK, pyruvate kinase; LDH, lactate dehydrogenase; HMP, hexose monophosphate pathway.

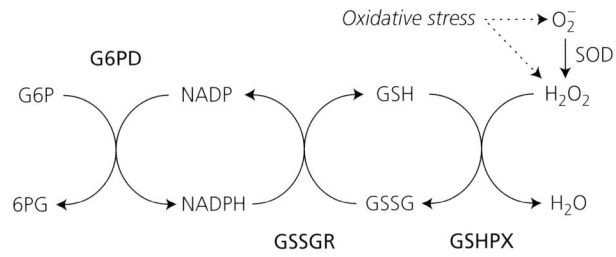

Fig. 8.2 Role of glucose-6-phosphate dehydrogenase (G6PD) in defense against oxidative damage. GSSGR, glutathione reductase; GSHPX, glutathione peroxidase; SOD, superoxide desmutase, H_2O_2, hydrogen peroxide; GSH, glutathione; GSSG, oxidized glutathione.

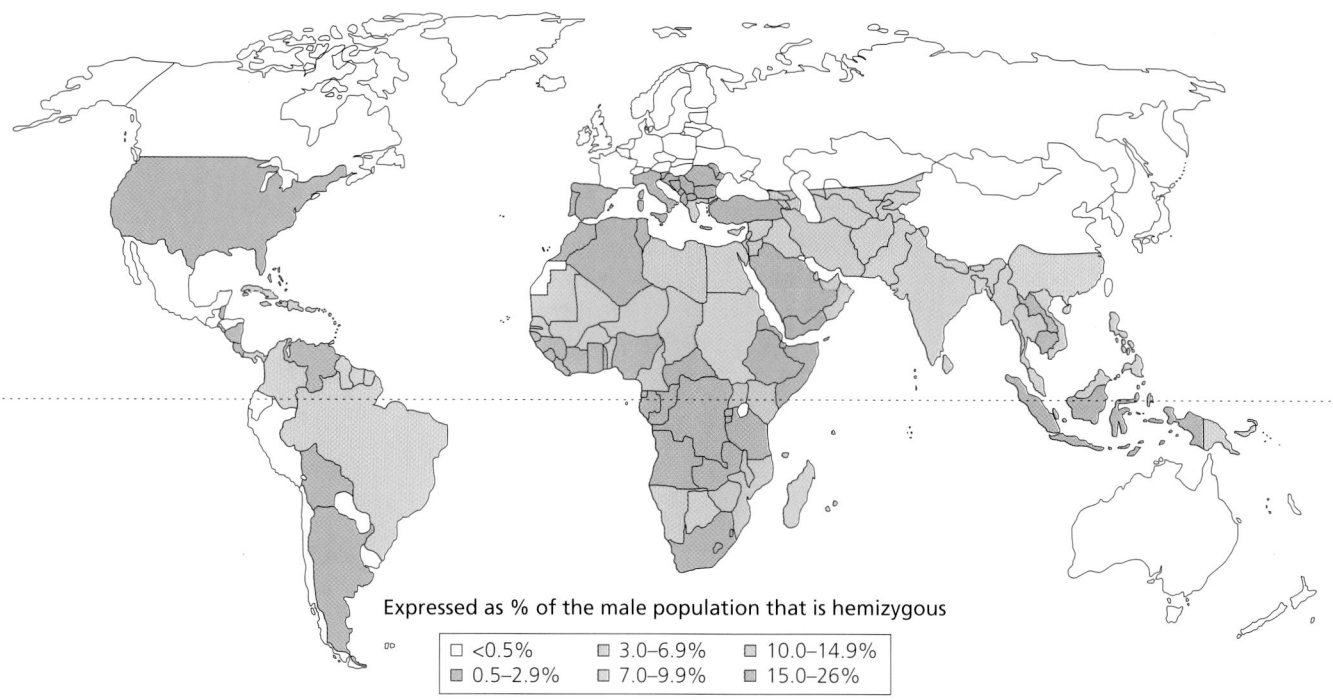

Fig. 8.3 World distribution of glucose-6-phosphate dehydrogenase (G6PD) deficiency.

Expressed as % of the male population that is hemizygous

□ <0.5%	▨ 3.0–6.9%	▨ 10.0–14.9%
▨ 0.5–2.9%	▨ 7.0–9.9%	▨ 15.0–26%

populations of diverse geographic origin, and glutathione synthetase[5] also occur at appreciable frequency. Other erythroenzyme disorders are rare.

Clinical features

Several features may aid the clinical diagnosis of an underlying enzyme disorder in a patient with hemolytic anemia. The pattern of hemolysis, whether episodic or chronic, and likely mode of inheritance discerned from a family history is often informative. In general, defects of the Embden–Meyerhof glycolytic pathway, essential for energy (ATP) generation in the steady state, result in chronic hemolytic anemia, whereas those of the pentose phosphate and glutathione pathways typically are associated with acute hemolysis after oxidative challenge. Overlap in the pattern of hemolysis renders this a useful though fallible distinction. The presence of neurological, myopathic or other non-hematologic manifestations is of considerable diagnostic value. Neurodevelopmental abnormalities should be interpreted with caution as severe neonatal hyperbilirubinemia sufficient to cause kernicterus has been described in deficiency of several red cell enzymes including G6PD and PK. Distinctive features of erythroenzymopathies are summarized in Table 8.1.

The somatic manifestations of individual enzyme disorders are determined by several factors. Deficiency of a red cell isoenzyme, expression of which is restricted (e.g. pyruvate kinase-L/R) generally causes isolated hemolysis. Conversely, defects of ubiquitously expressed enzymes (e.g. triosephosphate isomerase) result in a more generalized phenotype. The physiochemical properties of a mutant enzyme also influence clinical expression. Enzyme variants associated with impaired catalytic efficiency produce greater metabolic perturbance than those resulting in structural instability, the consequences of which are offset in tissues which possess the capacity for protein synthesis. This is reflected in a correspondingly more severe clinical phenotype. Examples include stable GPI mutants associated with multisystem[6] disease and high Km class I G6PD variants which in addition to hemolysis manifest impaired leukocyte function or cataract due to reduction of enzyme activity in non-erythroid tissues.[7]

Blood cell morphology

Red cell enzyme defects have traditionally been grouped under the heading congenital non-spherocytic hemolytic anemia. While red cell atypia are usually apparent these overlap with other causes of hemolysis and are seldom exclusive to a specific enzyme defect. A notable exception is the striking basophilic stippling associated with P5N deficiency which may be seen in up to 5% of red cells on a freshly stained blood film prepared from an ethylenediamine tetra-acetic acid (EDTA) sample (Fig.

151

Table 8.1 Distinctive clinical features associated with erythroenzymopathies

Enzyme	Inheritance	Neurological	Myopathy	Other
Glycolytic pathway				
Hexokinase	AR			Poor effort tolerance, erythrocytosis
Glucosephosphate isomerase	AR	+ rare	+ rare	Fetal hydrops, recurrent infection, priapism
Phosphofructokinase	AR		+/−	Myoglobinuria, hyperuricemia, erythrocytosis
Aldolase	AR	(+)	+/−	
Triosephosphate isomerase	AR	+	+	Recurrent infection, sudden cardiac death
Phosphoglycerate kinase	XL	+/−	+/−	Myoglobinuria
Diphosphoglycerate mutase	AR			Erythrocytosis
Enolase	AD?			Spherocytosis
Pyruvate kinase L/R	AR, rarely AD			Fetal hydrops, iron overload
Lactate dehydrogenase M (B)	AR		+	
Glutathione biosynthesis or regeneration				
γ-glutamylcysteine synthetase	AR	+/−		
Glutathione synthetase	AR	+/−		Acidosis, 5-oxoprolinuria, recurrent infection
Glutathione reductase	AR			Favism, cataract
Nucleotide metabolism				
Pyrimidine 5′ – nucleotidase	AR	(+)		Basophilic stippling. Acquired deficiency in plumbism, transient erythroblastopenia of childhood and thalassemia
CDP–choline phosphotransferase	AR			Basophilic stippling
Adenosine deaminase	AD			
Adenylate kinase	AR	+/−		

AR, autosomal recessive; XL, X-linked; AD, autosomal dominant.
Parenthesis denote link unproven.

8.4). Stippling may disappear if the stain is delayed by more than a few hours, presumably because EDTA chelates metal ions required for ribonucleoprotein aggregation. This problem may be circumvented by examination of blood taken into lithium heparin. Conspicuous punctate basophilia such as occurs in P5N deficiency accompanies unstable hemoglobins and CDP-choline phosphotransferase deficiency,[8] a putative defect of nucleotide metabolism described in only a few families. Inhibition of P5N by lead in plumbism produces a similar morphological picture though the presence of other clinical and morphologic stigmata, the latter including red cell hypochromia and microcytosis, reticulocytosis or sideroblastic erythropoiesis, usually render distinction from primary P5N deficiency straightforward. Basophilic stippling may also be found in a wide range of congenital and acquired dyserythropoietic states including thalassemia and occasionally in some glycolytic defects (e.g. pyruvate kinase or phosphofructokinase deficiency).

Features of oxidative damage to red cells are most commonly associated with, though not confined to, G6PD deficiency. These are most remarkable during hemolytic crises following exposure to oxidant drugs (Table 8.2) or fava bean (broad bean) consumption and include

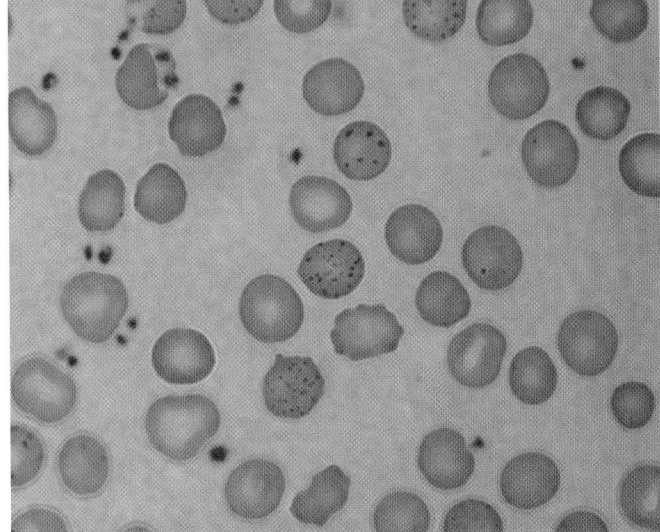

Fig. 8.4 Coarse basophilic stippling in pyrimidine 5′-nucleotidase deficiency.

irregularly contracted hyperchromic erythrocytes, some of which display a characteristic 'bite' or 'hemighost' appearance (Fig. 8.5). 'Bite' cells in which the surface of the erythrocyte is breached producing an irregular gap are thought to be generated by removal of Heinz bodies during transit through the spleen. Erythrocyte 'hemighosts' are forms in which the hemoglobin appears condensed and is retracted to one side leaving an empty space in the cell. In common G6PD variants (e.g. G6PD A⁻ or Med) these morphologic abnormalities are declared only during hemolytic episodes. Following acute hemolysis in G6PD deficiency rapid clearance of damaged cells by the spleen ensues and during the recovery phase polychromasia and macrocytosis predominate. Similar though

usually less marked features of oxidative damage may be seen in defects which impair glutathione biosynthesis (Fig. 8.6) or regeneration due to deficiency of γ-glutamylcysteine synthetase,[9] glutathione synthetase[5,10] or glutathione reductase[11] as well as neonatal hemolysis due to deficiency of glutathione peroxidase (Fig. 8.7).[12] The latter phenomenon appears to reflect transient deficiency of selenium required as a cofactor for glutathione peroxidase which serves to detoxify harmful peroxides in the red cell. This produces an acute and usually self-limiting hemolytic anemia in the newborn period. The diagnosis may be confirmed by assay of neonatal and maternal selenium levels and red cell

Table 8.2 Drugs and chemicals associated with hemolysis in glucose-6-phosphate dehydrogenase (G6PD) deficiency

Class of drug	Examples
Antimalarials	Primaquine, pentaquine, pamaquine, chloroquine*
Sulfonamides and sulfones	Sulfanilamide, sulfacetamide, sulfapyridine, sulfamethoxazole (including co-trimoxazole), dapsone
Other antibacterial agents	Nitrofurantoin, nalidixic acid, chloramphenicol, ciprofloxacin*
Analgesic/antipyretic	Acetanilid, acetylsalicylic acid (Aspirin)†, paracetamol (Acetominophen)†
Miscellaneous	Probenecid Dimercaprol Vitamin K analogs Naphthalene (moth balls) Methylene blue Ascorbic acid Trinitrotoluene

* Possible association.
† Only after high doses or overdose.

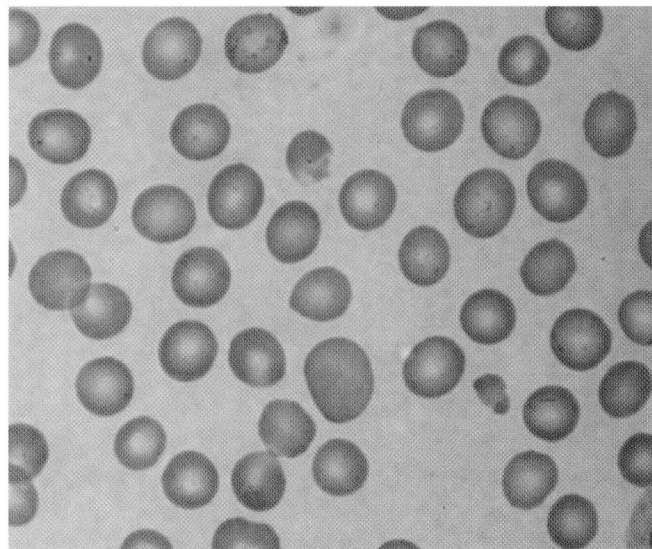

Fig. 8.6 Glutathione synthetase deficiency.

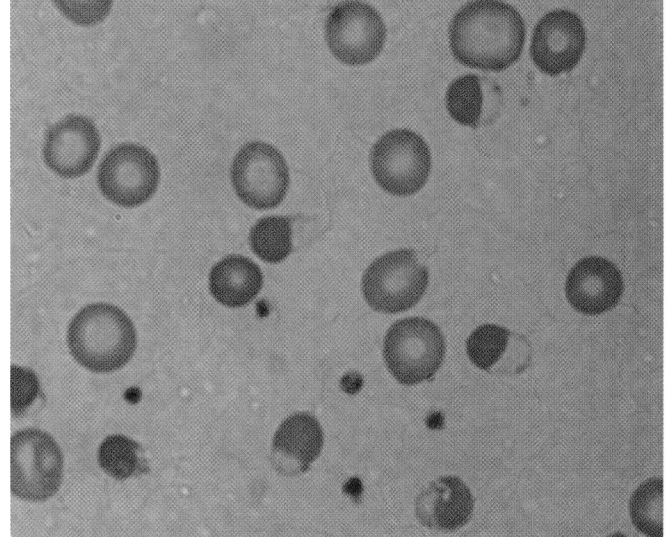

Fig. 8.5 Blood film during acute hemolytic episode in G6PD deficiency.

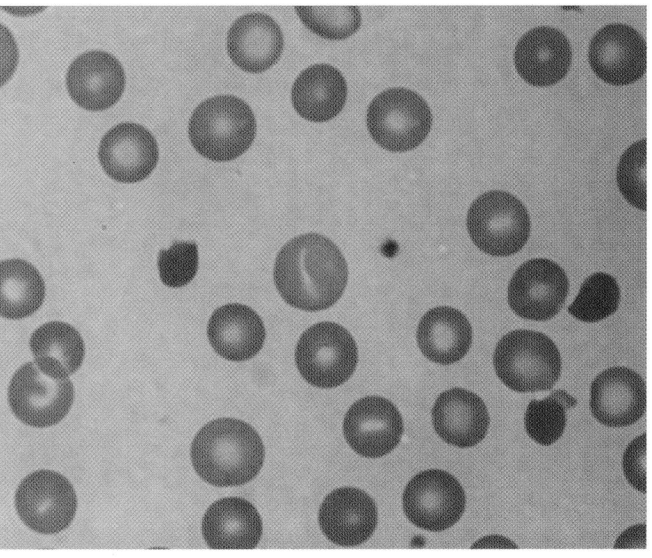

Fig. 8.7 Glutathione peroxidase deficiency.

glutathione peroxidase. Defects of other enzymes in the pentose phosphate pathway, 6-phosphogluconolactonase[13] and phosphogluconate dehydrogenase[14] have been described and should be considered if changes suggestive of oxidative damage are evident and other causes excluded. Examination of a blood film for Heinz bodies should be performed in cases of suspected oxidative hemolysis. These intraerythrocytic inclusions first characterized in experimental studies of acetylphenylhydrazine toxicity are visualized after staining supravitally with the basic dyes methyl violet or brilliant cresyl blue (Fig. 8.8). Heinz bodies are formed from denatured globin which attaches to the inner surface of the erythrocyte membrane and develop either spontaneously in the case of unstable hemoglobin variants or after oxidative challenge in susceptible (e.g. G6PD-deficient) red cells. The numbers increase dramatically after splenectomy. Similar inclusions due to precipitation of surplus α-globin chains may be visible in some thalassemia syndromes. It should be emphasized that unstable hemoglobin variants which produce a Heinz-body hemolytic anemia often escape detection by conventional separation techniques either because they result from structural alteration within the interior of the hemoglobin molecule and therefore do not alter surface charge or are so unstable as to undergo rapid degradation *ex vivo*. Stability tests in combination with mass spectrometry[15] provide a reliable approach to the detection of unstable hemoglobins which should be undertaken in cases where oxidative changes or Heinz bodies are present before detailed studies of red cell metabolism are embarked upon. Similarly, if there is a history of drug or toxin ingestion, screening for sulphemoglobin and methemoglobin by absorbance at 620 and 630 nm respectively is indicated to exclude drug- or chemical-induced hemolysis which may follow severe oxidant stress in the absence of any intrinsic red cell defect.

True spherocytes such as seen in hereditary spherocytosis in which both the normal discoid shape of the erythrocyte is lost and cell volume reduced are generally not seen in erythroenzymopathies with the possible exception of enolase 1 deficiency, a disorder hitherto described in only a single kindred in which a dominant mode of inheritance and spherocytosis but normal acidified glycerol lysis test were evident. Morphologic vatiants, particularly spheroechinocytes, derived from the Greek for sea urchin (*Echinus*), are frequently present in variable numbers in glycolytic disorders (Fig. 8.9). These crenated cells have multiple short spicules of uniform appearance and represent effete red cells in which ATP depletion has led to failure of cation homeostasis and cellular dehydration. They are most striking in, though not specific to, PK deficiency where the number of such

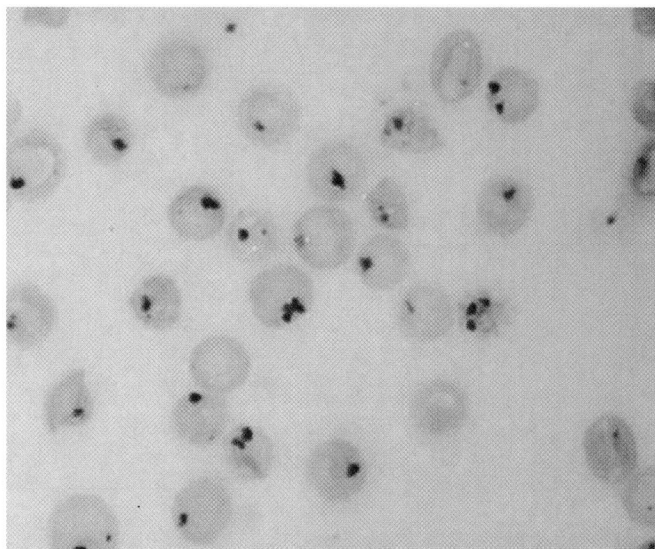
Fig. 8.8 Methyl violet stain showing numerous Heinz bodies.

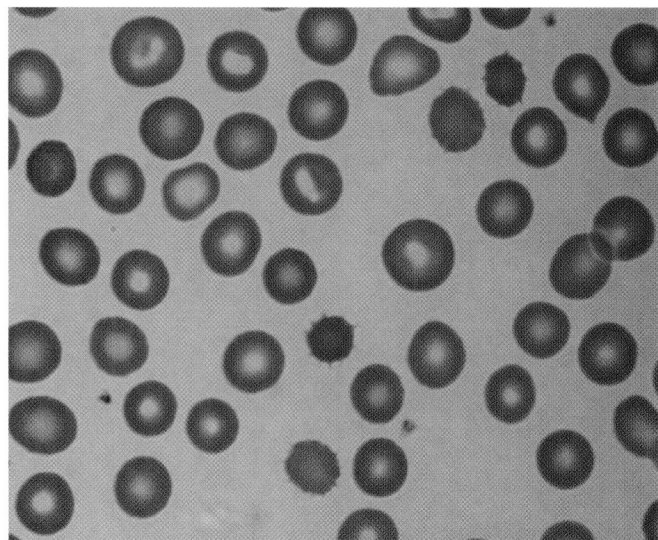
Fig. 8.9 Triosephosphate isomerase deficiency.

cells often increases dramatically (up to 30% of red cells) after splenectomy (Fig. 8.10). Poikilocytosis with elliptocytic, ovalocytic and dacrocytic (tear-drop) forms may also be seen in PK deficiency (Fig. 8.11). These findings are non-specific and probably attributable to dyserythropoiesis, a conclusion supported by evidence of ineffective erythropoiesis with defective utilization of ^{59}Fe in some cases.

Biochemical investigation of erythroenzyme disorders

Initial investigation of a patient in whom enzymopathy is suspected usually necessitates the exclusion of other

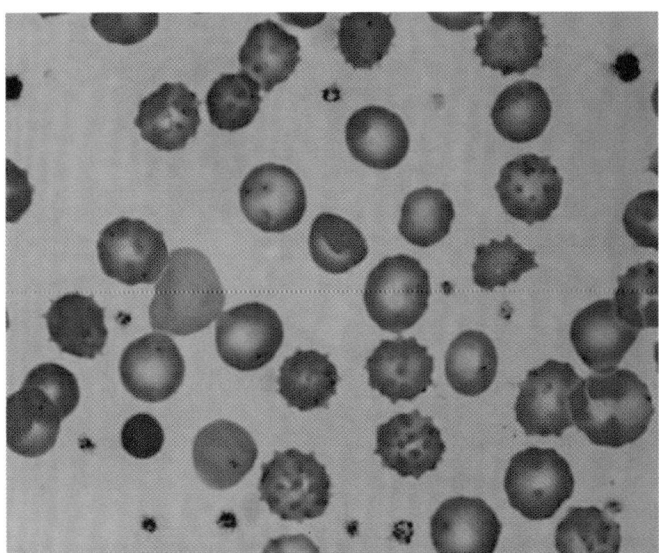

Fig. 8.10 Pyruvate kinase deficiency post-splenectomy.

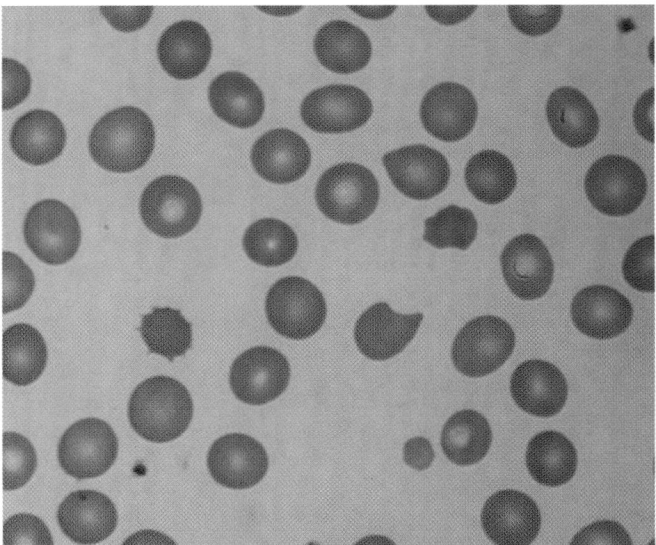

Fig. 8.11 Dyerythropoietic features in pyruvate kinase deficiency.

mechanisms of shortened red cell survival specifically immune hemolysis, a membrane cytoskeleton defect, unstable or thalassemic hemoglobinopathies and paroxysmal nocturnal hemoglobinuria. An increased rate of autohemolysis not corrected by exogenous glucose (type 2) first recognized by Dacie is a characteristic though not consistent feature of glycolytic disorders. Autohemolysis pattern and osmotic fragility, though both abnormal in some enzyme disorders, have been largely superseded by direct estimation of enzyme activity or intermediate metabolites and their utility lies mainly in the exclusion of membrane defects as a cause of unexplained hemolytic anemia.

While useful screening methods[16] exist for detection of some more common enzyme defects (e.g. G6PD and PK

deficiency) definitive diagnosis relies on quantitation of enzyme activity in red cells in conjunction with physiochemical properties of the mutant enzyme.[17] Rigorous removal of leukocytes in which residual enzyme activity is substantially higher or reflects expression of a different isoenzyme to that in red cells potentially masking deficiency and correction for the higher activity of some enzymes (HK, PK, aldolase, G6PD and P5N) by comparison with a control matched for a reticulocyte count or another age-dependent enzyme is essential. In most clinical erythroenzymopathies residual enzyme activity in red cells is 5–40% of normal. Higher levels do not exclude an erythroenzyme disorder and particular care must be taken in interpretation of studies performed in patients who have received transfusion due to interference from donor red cells and neonates. Significant differences in erythrocyte metabolism have been observed between neonatal and adult red cells. These include a higher activity for some enzymes (PK, GPI, G6PD) and lower activity for others (PFK, glutathione peroxidase, adenylate kinase) in erythrocytes from cord blood. Under the saturating substrate conditions employed for quantitation of enzyme activity *in vitro* catalytic mutants may elude detection. If a strong suspicion of enzymopathy remains, measurement of enzyme activity at low substrate concentration or studies of enzyme kinetics and response to physiologic modulators may be necessary (Fig. 8.12A, B).

Quantitation of the major red cell metabolites 2,3-diphosphoglycerate (2,3-DPG) and GSH by spectrophotometry is of value in the diagnosis of glycolytic disorders and hemolytic anemias due to impaired defence against oxidative damage to the red cell. The ratio of 2,3-DPG to ATP specifically may localize a defect in glycolysis to the proximal or distal part of the Embden–Meyerhof pathway (Table 8.3). A reduced GSH concentration is found in G6PD deficiency, other pentose phosphate pathway defects and enzyme disorders directly affecting glutathione biosynthesis or regeneration. A low red cell GSH level is, however, a relatively non-specific finding which may be seen in other causes of hemolytic anemia particularly unstable hemoglobins as well as some glycolytic (e.g. GPI deficiency) and membrane defects. Marked reduction in GSH implies a defect in glutathione biosynthesis due to γ-glutamylcysteine synthetase or glutathione synthetase deficiency.

To overcome the limitation of *in vitro* measurement of enzyme activity under conditions which may not accurately reflect enzyme function *in vivo*, defects in the Embden–Meyerhof pathway may be identified by measurement of the concentration of intermediate metabolites in a deproteinized red cell extract. Typically, metabolic block is indicated by accumulation of intermediates

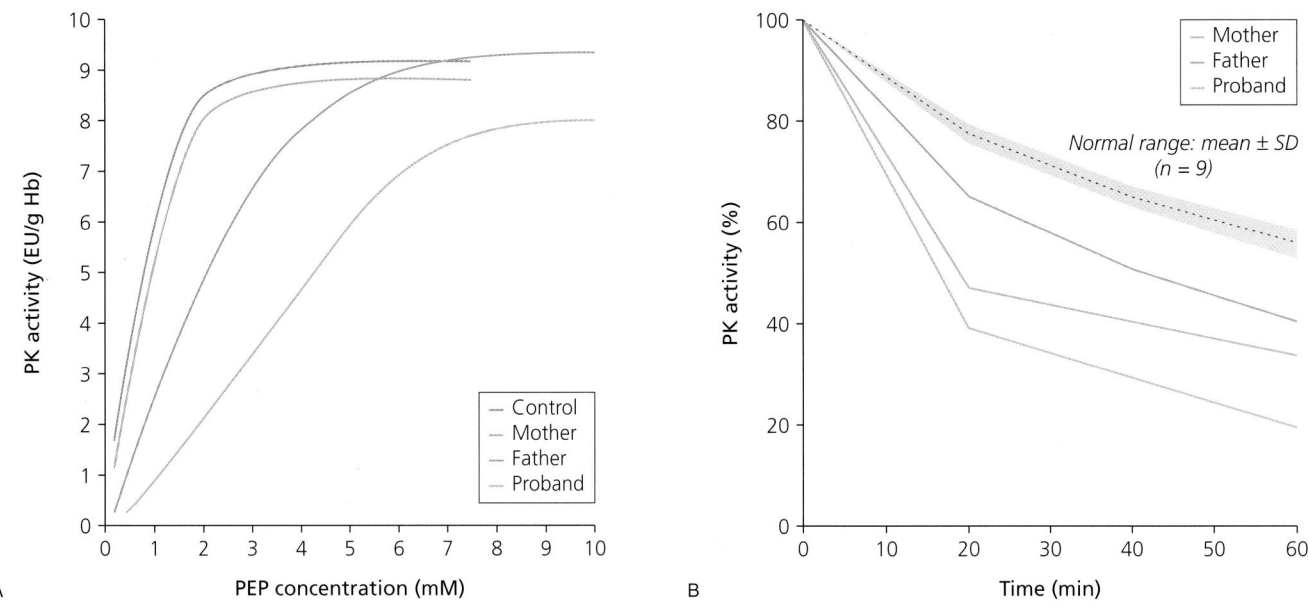

A   PEP concentration (mM)   B   Time (min)

Fig. 8.12 Pyruvate kinase (PK) kinetics. (A) Although the maximum PK activity is normal enzyme activity at 50% phosphoenolpyruvate (PEP) saturation is reduced in the proband and father. Residual PK activity after incubation at 55°C. The results indicate both the parents and proband have an unstable enzyme variant.

Table 8.3 2,3-diphosphoglycerate (2,-DPG) and ATP patterns in some hereditary hemolytic anemias

Defect	2,3-DPG	ATP	Comments
Proximal glycolytic HK GPI PFK	N or ↓	N or ↓	Variable ↓2,3-DPG also seen in DPGM deficiency Stomatocytosis ADA overexpression and some cases of HS before splenectomy
Distal glycolytic PGK PK	↑↑	N or ↓	↑2,3-DPG:ATP useful in PK deficiency. Also seen in Zieve's syndrome

DPGM, diphosphoglycerate mutase; GPI, glucosephosphate isomerase; HK, hexokinase; HS, hereditary spherocytosis; N, normal; PFK, phosphofructokinase; PGK, phosphoglycerate kinase; PK, pyruvate kinase

proximal and depletion distal to the step catalyzed by the deficient enzyme. In some instances substrate accumulation may be dramatic and the resulting intermediate profile pathognomonic of a specific disorder (Fig. 8.13). Prenatal diagnosis by biochemical or molecular analysis has been undertaken for several severe erythroenzymopathies including deficiencies of TPI, GPI, PK and G6PD.[18–21]

Molecular basis of erythroenzyme disorders

Over the past decade the molecular defects that underlie hematologically important erythroenzyme disorders have been elucidated. This has revealed a striking bias towards missense mutation mainly affecting conserved residues in the encoded protein (Fig. 8.14).[22–24] The paucity of null mutations found among patients with

clinical enzyme deficiencies is consistent with evidence from murine models that complete disruption of the Embden–Meyerhof, pentose phosphate or glutathione biosynthetic pathways is lethal during embryogenesis. Exceptions to this are severe forms of PK deficiency due to mutations that abolish PK-L/R expression, for example the PK Gypsy deletion. In these cases homozygotes are rescued from what would otherwise be a lethal phenotype by persistence of the muscle isoenzyme PK-M2, normally expressed during early erythroid differentiation, which is encoded by a separate genetic locus.[25] Although few examples of regulatory mutations have been described in erythroenzyme disorders, sequence variation within the TATA box and other essential promoter elements of the TPI gene is widely distributed in human populations and has been linked to a reduction of enzyme activity *in vivo*.[26] In certain populations individual mutations account for a high proportion of deficient alleles. This applies not only to

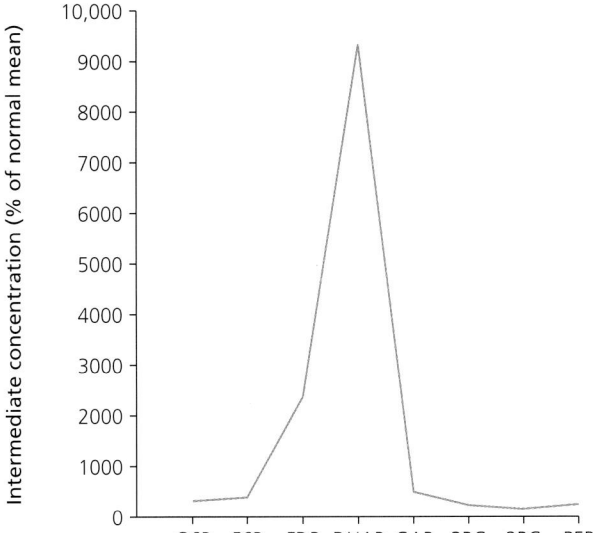

Fig. 8.13 Pattern of glycolytic intermediates in a patient with triosephosphate isomerase (TPI) deficiency demonstrating markedly elevated dihydroxyacetone phosphate (DHAP) concentration. Values are expressed as a percentage of the normal mean. G6P, glucose-6-phosphate; F6P, fructose-6-phosphate; FDP, fructose-1,6-diphosphate; GAP, glyceraldehyde-3-phosphate; 3PG, 3-phosphoglycerate; 2PG, 2-phosphoglycerate; PEP, phosphoenolpyruvate.

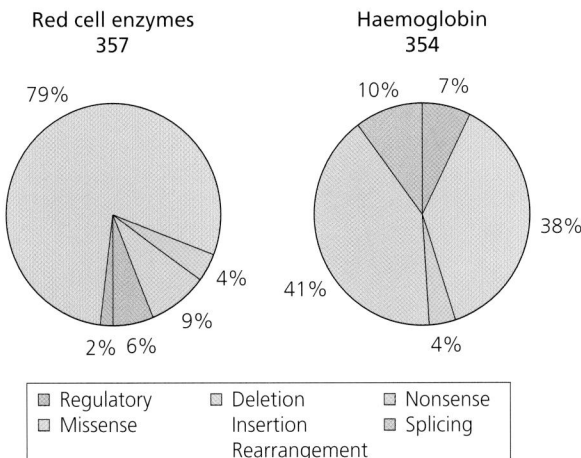

Fig. 8.14 Distribution of gene mutations in human erythroenzyme (n = 357) and hemoglobin (n = 354) disorders.

G6PD deficiency where the prevalence of variants reflects selective advantage in the form of resistance to malaria but is also evident among patients of European descent with PK deficiency in whom 1529A and 1456T substitutions together account for over 40% of mutations. Even greater homogeneity is evident in TPI deficiency where a single missense mutation Glu 105 Asp accounts for the majority of reported cases. Haplotype studies support a single origin for these mutations. Distant genetic factors may also exert an influence on the clinical course

of erythroenzyme disorders. The level of unconjugated bilirubin in G6PD[26] and PK[25] deficiency correlates with inheritance of the (TA)$_7$ allele of the uridinine diphosphate glucuronosyltransferase gene (UGT1A1) promoter associated with Gilbert syndrome which has been shown to potentiate gall-stone formation in other hemolytic states. Coinheritance of hereditary hemochromatosis may accelerate iron loading though the high prevalence of this complication in pyruvate kinase deficiency suggests the contribution of other mechanisms, for example ineffective erythropoiesis may be more important.

REFERENCES

1. Beutler E 1978 The red cell. In: (eds), Haemolytic anemia in disorders of red cell metabolism. Plenum, New York, 1–21
2. Mohrenweiser HW 1981 Frequency of enzyme deficiency variants in erythrocytes of newborn infants. Proceedings of the National Academy of Sciences USA 78: 5046–5050
3. El-Hazmi MAF, Al-Swailem AR, Al-Faleh FZ, Warsy AS 1986 Frequency of glucose-6-phosphate dehydrogenase, pyruvate kinase and hexokinase deficiency in the Saudi population. Human Hereditory 36: 45–49
4. Vives Corrons JL 2000 Chronic non-spherocytic haemolytic anaemia due to congenital pyrimidine 5' nucleotidase deficiency: 25 years later. Baillière's Best Practice and Research in Clinical Haematology 13: 103–118
5. Ristoff E, Mayatepek E, Larsson A 2001 Long-term clinical outcome in patients with glutathione synthetase deficiency. Journal of Pediatrics 139: 79–84
6. Schroter W, Eber SW, Bardosi A et al 1985 Generalized glucosephosphate isomerase (GPI) deficiency causing hemolytic anemia, neuromuscular symptoms and impairment of granulocytic function: a new syndrome due to a new stable GPI variant and diminished specific activity (GPI Homburg). European Journal of Pediatrics 144: 301–305
7. Luzzatto L, Mehta A, Vulliamy T 2001 Glucose-6-phosphate dehydrogenase deficiency. In: Scriver CR, Beaudet AL, Sly WS, Valle D (eds), The metabolic and molecular basis of inherited disease. McGraw-Hill, 4517–4553
8. Paglia DE, Valentine WN, Nakatani M et al 1983 Selective accumulation of cytosol CDP-choline as an isolated erythrocyte defect in chronic haemolysis. Proceedings of the National Academy of Sciences USA 80: 3081–3085
9. Konrad PN, Richards F II, Valentine WN, Paglia DE 1972 Gammaglutamyl-cysteine synthetase deficiency. New England Journal of Medicine 1972; 286: 557–561
10. Hirono A, Iyori H, Skine I et al 1996 Three cases of hereditary non-spherocytic haemolytic anemia associated with red blood cell glutathione deficiency. Blood 1996; 87: 2071–2074
11. Loos H, Roos D, Weening R, Houwerzijl J 1976 Familial deficiency of glutathione reductase in human blood cells. Blood 48: 53–62
12. Necheles TF, Steinberg MH, Cameron D 1970 Erythrocyte glutathione-peroxidase deficiency. British Journal of Haematology 19: 605–612
13. Beutler E, Kuhl W, Gelbert T 1985 6-Phosphogluconolactonase deficiency, a hereditary erythrocyte enzyme deficiency: possible interaction with glucose-6-phosphate dehydrogenase deficiency. Proceedings of the National Academy of Sciences USA 82: 3876–3878
14. Vives Corrons JL, Colomer D, Pujades A et al 1996 Congenital 6-phosphogluconate dehydrogenase (6PGD) deficiency associated with chronic hemolytic anemia in a Spanish family. American Journal of Hematology 53: 221–227
15. Wild BJ, Green BN, Cooper EK et al 2001 Rapid identification of hemoglobin variants by electrospray ionization mass spectrometry. Blood Cells, Molecules and Diseases 27: 691–704
16. Beutler E, Blume KG, Kaplan JC et al 1979 International committee for standardization in haematology: Recommended screening test for glucose-6-phosphate dehydrogenase (G-6-PD) deficiency. British Journal of Haematology 43: 469–477

17. Beutler E 1984 Red cell metabolism. A manual of biochemical methods, 2nd edn. Grune & Stratton, Orlando, FL

18. Ayra R, Lalloz MRA, Nicolaides KH et al 1996 Prenatal diagnosis of triosephosphate isomerase deficiency. Blood 87: 4507–4509

19. Whitelaw AGL, Rogers PA, Hopkinson DA et al 1979 Congenital haemolytic anaemia resulting from glucose phosphate isomerase deficiency: genetics, clinical picture and prenatal diagnosis. Journal of Medical Genetics 16: 189–196

20. Baronciani L, Beutler E 1994 Prenatal diagnosis of pyruvate kinase deficiency. Blood 84: 2354–2356

21. Beutler E, Kuhl W, Fox M et al 1992 Prenatal diagnosis of glucose-6-phosphate dehydrogenase deficiency. Acta Haematologica 87: 103–104

22. Krawczak M, Ball EV, Fenton I et al 2000 Human gene mutation database-a biomedical information and research resource. Human Mutation 15: 45–51

23. Mehta A, Mason PJ, Vulliamy TJ Glucose-6-phosphate dehydrogenase deficiency 2000 Baillières Best Practice and Research in Clinical Haematology 13: 21–38

24. Marinaki AM, Escuredo E, Duley JA et al 2001 Genetic basis of hemolytic anemia caused by pyrimidine 5′ nucleotidase deficiency. Blood 97: 3327–3332

25. Zanella A, Bianchi P 2000 Red cell pyruvate kinase deficiency: from genetics to clinical manifestations. Baillières Best Practice and Research in Clinical Haematology 13: 57–81

26. Samipietro M, Lupica L, Perrero L, Comino A et al 1997 The expression of uridine diphosphate glucuronsyltransferase gene is a major determinant of bilirubin level in heterozygous thalassaemia and in glucose-6-phosphate dehydrogenase deficiency. British Journal of Haematology 99: 437–439

Abnormalities of the structure and synthesis of hemoglobin

SL Thein

9

Introduction

Normal human hemoglobin

The inherited disorders of hemoglobin

The thalassemias
The β thalassemias
Hb E/β thalassemia
The δβ, γδβ thalassemias and HPFH syndromes
Intermediate forms of β thalassemia
The α thalassemias
α thalassemia with mental retardation (ATR) syndromes
Acquired α thalassemia
Management

Structural hemoglobin variants
Sickle cell disease
Other sickling disorders
Other hemoglobin variants
The unstable hemoglobin disorders
Hemoglobin variants with abnormal oxygen binding
Hemoglobins M

The thalassaemic hemoglobinopathies

Introduction

Hemoglobin is the protein in red blood cells that is responsible for the delivery of oxygen from the lungs to the tissues and the transport of carbon dioxide from the tissues back to the lungs. All human hemoglobins have a tetrameric structure consisting of two identical α-like (α and ζ) and two β-like (ε, γ, δ or β) globin chains, each linked to a heme group, the moiety that is responsible for the reversible binding and transfer of oxygen.[1] At different stages of development, different types of hemoglobin are expressed. In the human embryo, the main hemoglobins include Hb Portland (ζ$_2$ γ^2), Hb Gower I (ζ$_2$ε$_2$) and Hb Gower II (α$_2$ε$_2$); in the fetus, Hb F (α$_2$γ$_2$) predominates and in adults, Hb A (α$_2$β$_2$) comprises over 95% of the total hemoglobin in the red cells. These different types of hemoglobin have been adapted to the changes in physiologic requirements that occur during development. Fetal hemoglobin (Hb F) exhibits a higher oxygen affinity than adult hemoglobins *in vivo;* the higher oxygen affinity of Hb F relative to adult hemoglobin facilitates the transfer of oxygen across the placenta from the maternal to the fetal circulation.

Normal human hemoglobin

Human hemoglobin production is characterized by two 'switches'; the switch from embryonic to fetal hemoglobin production begins as early as week 5 of gestation and is completed by week 10 (Fig. 9.1). β-globin expression starts as early as week 8 but the synthesis remains low, increases to approximately 10% at weeks 30–35 of gestation with a dramatic upregulation of β-globin synthesis just before birth, coinciding with a decrease in γ-globin expression. At birth, Hb F (α$_2$γ$_2$) comprises 60–80% of the total hemoglobin, falling to ~5% at 6 months of age and eventually reaching the adult level of 0.5–1.0% at 2 years. The switch from fetal to adult hemoglobin production is not complete in that variable levels of Hb F continue to be produced throughout adult life, and is restricted to a subset of erythrocytes termed F cells.[2]

Much interest has focused on the mechanisms underlying hemoglobin switching by which the different globins are produced in a tissue- and development-stage-specific manner. Each of the α-like and β-like globin chains are encoded by genetically distinct loci, the α-like cluster on the tip of chromosome 16p, and the β-like

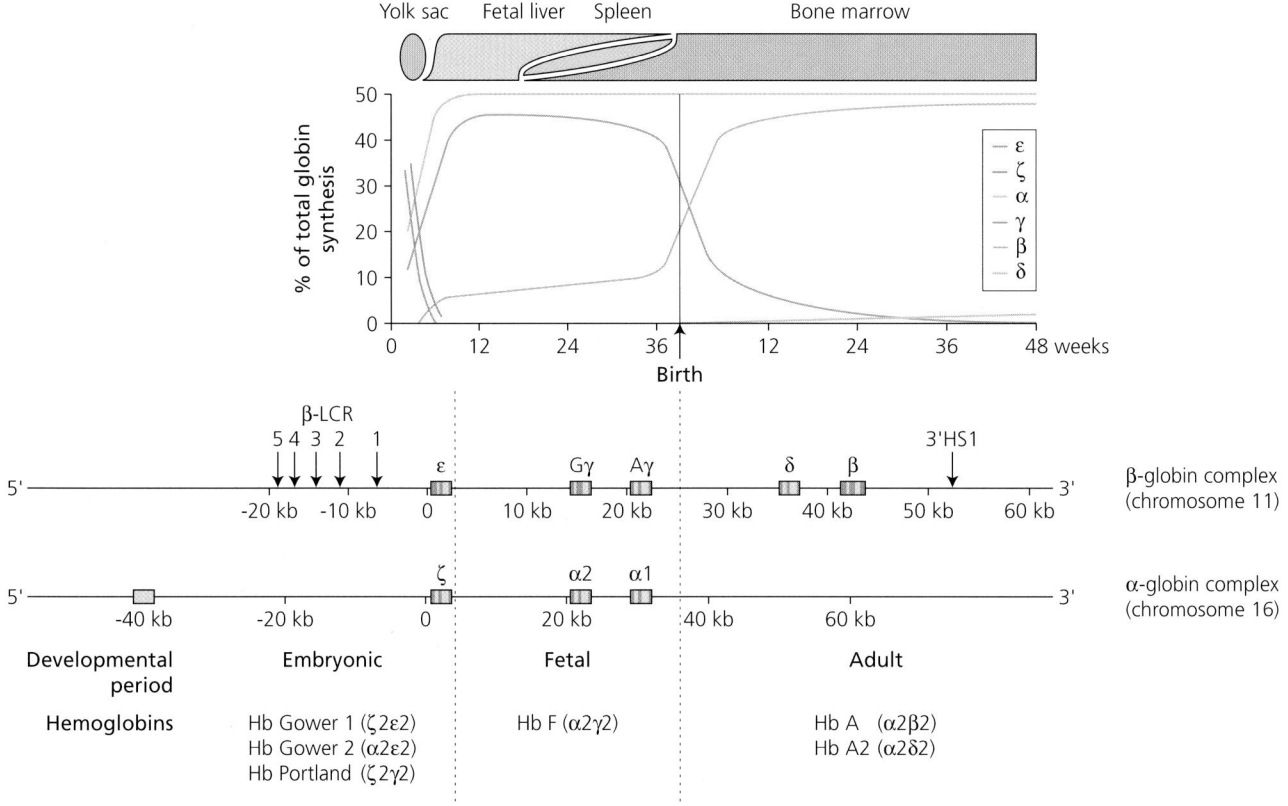

Fig. 9.1 Sequence of human hemoglobin synthesis (above) and the organization of the globin gene clusters on chromosome 11p and 16p (below) with the types of hemoglobin synthesized during the different developmental periods. Solid arrows represent the deoxyribonuclease I hypersensitive sites (HSs) in the β cluster. HSs 1 to 5 upstream of the β cluster form the β-LCR; the 3'HS1 site is a downstream enhancer. HS -40 form the equivalent of the β-LCR in the α-globin complex.

cluster on chromosome 11p15.5 (Fig.9.1). In both clusters, the genes are arranged along the chromosome in the order in which they are expressed during development, 5′-ε-^{G}γ-^{A}γ-δ-β-3′; and 5′-ζ-α$_2$-α$_1$-3′; suggesting that gene order may be important in the program of their expression. The β-like globin genes contain three exons (coding regions) interrupted by two intervening sequences (IVSs) or introns of 122–130 and 850–900 bp, respectively; IVS1 interrupts the sequence between codons 30 and 31, and IVS2, between codons 104 and 105. The α-like globin genes contain similar but smaller introns between codons 30 and 31, and between codons 99 and 100. In addition to the primary *cis*-determinants of individual globin gene expression, which are found in the promoter region immediately upstream of each gene, there are other local regulatory elements known as enhancers, which are located at variable distances from the individual genes.[3]

Throughout development, the appropriate genes of the α- and β-globin gene clusters are co-ordinately expressed, maintaining a balance in the production of α- and β-like globins needed for the synthesis of normal hemoglobin. Expression of the individual genes within each cluster is controlled by complex interactions between the local regulatory sequences within each gene and regulatory elements upstream of the cluster, mediated by a series of transcription factors. In the β cluster, the upstream element is referred to as the β locus control region (β-LCR), which consists of five DNase I hypersensitive sites (designated HSs1–5) distributed between 5 and 25 kb 5′ of the ε globin gene (Fig. 9.1). The corresponding element in the α globin cluster is the HS-40 which encompasses 0.4 kb and consists of a single DNase hypersensitive site, 40 kb upstream of the cluster. The β-LCR establishes a transcriptionally active chromatin domain that encompasses the whole β globin cluster and acts as a unique enhancer while the α globin HS-40 is most similar to HS2 of the β-LCR and acts as an enhancer. In both clusters, however, full expression of the respective genes is critically dependent on the presence of the upstream regulatory elements.

The precise molecular mechanisms by which the globin genes are expressed in a tissue- and developmental-stage-specific manner are still poorly understood. Each cluster contains various binding sites for both erythroid-specific and more ubiquitous DNA-binding proteins in the upstream regulatory elements as well as in the local promoters of the genes. Tissue-specific expression may be explained by the presence of the binding sites for the erythroid-specific transcription factors. These motifs include 'GATA', 'CACCC' and 'TGA(C/G)TCA' (NF-E2/AP-1 like) elements binding the tissue-restricted zinc finger proteins (GATA-1 and GATA-2), their cofactors (FOG1 and FOG2), the erythroid Krüppel-like factors (EKLF and FLKL), and the b-Zip family of proteins (NF-E2, Nrf1, Nrf2, Nrf3, Bach 1 and Bach2).[4,5] It seems likely that these erythroid-specific transcription factors form part of a network of factors that commit hemopoietic cells to erythroid differentiation. The mechanisms by which developmental regulation is controlled are less clear and rely on two mechanisms: autonomous gene silencing and gene competition. It appears that the ε and ζ genes are switched on in embryonic cells and autonomously switched off in definitive cells (liver and bone marrow) in which they cannot be substantially reactivated. The second switch from γ- to β-gene expression is more complex and involves both autonomous silencing of the γ genes and competition between the γ and β genes for the β-LCR. The balance between the γ- and β-gene expression is thought to be mediated by changes in the repertoire and/or abundance of various nuclear factors (with or without post-translational modifications) favoring particular promoter – LCR interactions. So far, the best defined example of a developmental-stage-specific regulatory factor is the erythroid Krüppel-like factor (EKLF) without which the β genes cannot be fully activated in the definitive cells.[6,7] Not only is EKLF restricted mainly to erythroid cells but it is also a highly promoter-specific activator, binding with high affinity to the β-globin CACCC box.[8] Its greater affinity for the β- than the γ-globin promoter accelerates the shutoff of γ in transgenic mice overexpressing EKLF, which suggests a role for EKLF in the γ- to β-globin switching process.[9] However, EKLF is unlikely to be the only factor because: (1) γ-globin silencing can also occur in the absence of a competing β-globin promoter; and (2) EKLF expression is equivalent at all developmental stages.[10]

The inherited disorders of hemoglobin

The vast majority of disorders affecting hemoglobin are inherited; it is estimated that ~7% of the world's population are carriers for different inherited disorders of hemoglobin making them the commonest monogenic diseases.[11] They can be divided into two main groups, those in which there is a structural change in a globin chain (hemoglobin variants) and the thalassemias, which result from a quantitative deficiency in one or more of the globin chains of hemoglobin (for review see (Ref. 1)). There is also a third group which is characterized by a persistent increase of fetal hemoglobin of various levels into adult life, referred to as hereditary persistence of fetal hemoglobin (HPFH). This classification of the inherited hemoglobin disorders is complicated by the existence of some structural hemoglobin variants that are synthesized at a reduced rate, or are highly unstable so that they result in a deficiency of the globin chain and a phenotype of thalassemia. The former subgroup is also referred to as thalassemic hemoglobinopathies and includes the δβ fusion variants (Hb Lepore) and Hb E, β26 (Glu→Lys), in which the substitution at β-codon 26 (GAG→AAG) also causes alternative splicing of the β-globin mRNA, leading to a reduction of the normally spliced β message encoding the variant. The hyper-unstable globin-chain variants act in a dominant negative fashion causing a disease phenotype even when present in a single copy; for example, Hb Geneva, a dominantly inherited β thalassemia.[12] Some hemoglobin disorders are acquired, these can also be classified into those characterized by a reduced synthesis of the globin chain (e.g. acquired Hb H disease) and those that alter the structure and function of hemoglobin so that oxygen transport is affected (e.g. carboxyhemoglobinemia, methemoglobinemia).

The thalassemias

Background

Thalassemia was first recognized by Cooley and Lee in 1925[13] as a form of severe anemia associated with splenomegaly and bone changes in children. The term thalassemia is derived from the Greek θαλασσα (the sea) since many of the early cases came from the Mediterranean region. However, it is now clear that the disorder is not just limited to the Mediterranean region but occurs throughout the world, prevalent in the tropical and subtropical regions including the Middle East, parts of Africa, Indian subcontinent and Southeast Asia. It appears that heterozygotes for thalassemia are protected from the severe effects of falciparum malaria and natural selection has increased and maintained their gene frequencies in these malarious regions.

The thalassemias are classified into α, β, δβ, γδβ, δ, γ and εγδβ thalassemias according to the type of globin chain(s) that is produced in reduced amounts. The two major categories are the α and β thalassemias while the rare forms include the γ, δ and εγδβ thalassemias. HPFH syndromes refer to the group of disorders in which the switch from fetal to adult hemoglobin production is incomplete and the fetal hemoglobin levels are variably increased in otherwise normal individuals. Because of their concomitant increased Hb F levels, the δβ and γδβ

thalassemias are often considered with the HPFH syndromes. In many populations the α and β thalassemias coexist with a variety of different structural hemoglobin variants. In these populations it is quite common to inherit a combination of genes; these complex interactions give rise to an extremely wide spectrum of clinical phenotypes which together constitute the thalassemia syndromes.[14] It has been estimated that about 300 000 individuals severely affected with thalassemia are born each year, posing a heavy burden on the health services.[15] Owing to population movements in the past 200 years, these hemoglobin disorders have become an important part of clinical practice in all countries, including the UK.[16]

The β thalassemias

The β thalassemias pose by far the most important public health problem.

Clinical features

The clinical phenotypes of β thalassemia range from very severe (major) to mild (minor) or a completely silent carrier state, with a huge range of intermediate phenotypes between the two ends of the spectrum.[17]

Infants affected with β thalassemia major are well at birth.[18] Anemia usually develops during the first few months of life when the switch from fetal to adult hemoglobin synthesis becomes established. There are no specific clinical signs and further clinical manifestations of the disease depend on whether the child is maintained on an adequate transfusion regime.

The inadequately transfused child develops the typical features of Cooley's anemia. They show marked retardation of growth and development with progressive hepatosplenomegaly. A typical 'thalassemic' facies develops with frontal bossing, prominent cheek bones and protruding upper jaw due to extension of the marrow in the skull and facial bones. Radiography of the skull shows the typical 'hair-on-end' appearance. The long bones and phalanges become rarefied from marrow expansion and show a lacy, trabecular pattern on radiography. These changes may be associated with repeated pathologic fractures. Occasionally, the expanding marrow extends from the rib or vertebrae and forms large paraspinal extramedullary masses. The massive marrow expansion causes a hypermetabolic state accompanied by intermittent fevers and weight loss. Gall stones and leg ulcers are common complications. Without any transfusion, death occurs within the first 2 years. 'Palliative' transfusion allows the child to live somewhat longer but the bony deformities remain unchanged and the child normally succumbs to an overwhelming infection. If these children survive to puberty, they develop complications of iron overload. Iron accumulation results from an increased rate of gastrointestinal absorption as well as that derived from the blood transfusions.

When transfused adequately to maintain a hemoglobin level of > 11 g/dl, these children grow and develop normally until early puberty. Progress of their disease then depends on whether they have received regular iron chelation. If not, they begin to show signs of progressive hepatic, cardiac and endocrine disturbances including liver failure, diabetes, hypoparathyroidism, and delayed or absent secondary sexual development. These changes are due largely to tissue siderosis from the progressive accumulation of iron derived from transfusions. Throughout their teenage life these children suffer from a variety of complications due to different endocrine deficiencies. Unless iron overload is controlled by regular chelation therapy, death results in the second or third decade, from acute or intractable congestive cardiac failure. Children who are adequately transfused and fully compliant with iron chelation therapy may grow and develop normally, and achieve sexual maturity. Even within this group there is a high frequency of growth retardation and retarded sexual maturity, with variable complications relating to iron metabolism, bone disease, endocrine abnormalities and liver disease. Recent studies have suggested that such complications may be related to variability at loci involved in iron metabolism (such as *HFE* gene, and genes involved in iron hemostasis),[19–21] bilirubin metabolism (UDP-glucuronosyltransferase or UGT1 gene),[22–24] and bone disease (genes for vitamin D receptor, collagen and estrogen receptor).[25,26]

Individuals with β thalassemia minor are typically asymptomatic. Splenomegaly is rare.

Diagnosis

Untransfused hemoglobin levels in β thalassemia major can be as low as 2–3 g/dl. The red cells show severe hypochromia, marked anisopoikilocytosis, target-cell formation, and basophilic stippling (see Fig. 6.2I). Poorly hemoglobinized nucleated red cells are frequently found in the peripheral blood, and may reach very high levels after splenectomy. Despite the severe anemia, the reticulocyte count is usually not very high because of the massive destruction of erythroid precursor cells in the bone marrow (i.e. ineffective erythropoiesis). The bone marrow shows marked erythroid hyperplasia characterized by poorly hemoglobinized normoblasts. Ragged inclusions (α-chain aggregates) in the normoblasts are revealed under phase microscopy or after supravital staining (e.g. methyl violet). Increased iron deposition is also seen in the bone marrow, the majority of the iron granules are randomly distributed. Biochemical evidence of hemolysis and progressive iron loading is observed. Other biochemical changes may include evidence of diabetes, and endocrine dysfunction such as parathyroid insufficiency.

The findings on Hb electrophoresis vary with the β-thalassemia genotype and is informative only in the previously untransfused patient. In homozygous β° thalassemia, Hb A is completely absent, and the hemoglobin consists of F and A_2 only. In β⁺ thalassemia (homozygous or compound heterozygotes), a variable amount of Hb A is present. The Hb F is usually elevated and varies from 10 to 90% of the total hemoglobin. The Hb A_2 level is of no diagnostic value. *In vitro* globin-chain biosynthesis of peripheral blood reticulocytes or bone marrow shows globin-chain imbalance with a marked excess of α- over β- and γ-chain production. In β° thalassemia there is a complete absence of β-chain synthesis.

The heterozygous state for β thalassemia (β° or β⁺) is remarkably uniform hematologically. Anemia, if present, is mild and the diagnosis is based on a low mean cell volume (MCV) and mean cell hemoglobin (MCH) accompanied by an increased proportion of Hb A_2 from 3.5 to 5.5%, with the exception of a subgroup that has a normal level of Hb A_2.

Globin-chain biosynthesis shows α chains in excess of about two-fold.

Normal A_2 heterozygous β thalassemia may be difficult to distinguish hematologically from heterozygous α thalassemia since both cases are characterized by hypochromic microcytic red cells and a normal Hb A_2 level. The distinction is made by globin-chain biosynthesis and DNA analysis. Type I normal A_2 β thalassemia is 'silent' in that the red cell indices are almost normal and the phenotype is due to very mild mutations which cause only a minimal deficit in β-chain production (e.g. C-T mutation in position-101 of the β gene).[17] Other cases (type 2 normal Hb A_2 β thalassemia) are due to the coinheritance of δ thalassemia in *cis* or in *trans* to the β-thalassemia gene.

Genetic basis of disease

The β thalassemias are considered to be autosomal recessive disorders since individuals who have inherited one abnormal β gene (carrier) are asymptomatic and the inheritance of two abnormal β-globin genes is required to produce a clinically detectable phenotype. Molecular analysis of the β-thalassemia genes has demonstrated a striking heterogeneity. Although almost 200 β-thalassemia alleles have been characterized, population studies indicate that probably only 20 β-thalassemia alleles account for > 80% of the β-thalassemia mutations in the whole world.[27] This is because in each of the high-frequency areas, only a few (4–6) mutations are common with a varying number of rare ones and each of these populations has its own unique group of mutations. This is particularly relevant to prenatal diagnosis because direct detection of these mutations by DNA analysis becomes feasible.

DNA analysis frequently shows the β-globin cluster to be intact with point mutations within the β gene or its immediate flanking regions.[17,28]

The vast majority of β-thalassemia mutations are single base substitutions, small insertions or deletions of 1–2 bases involving the critical sequences that interfere with gene function either at the transcriptional, translational or posttranslational stages (Fig. 9.2). Approximately half of these mutations completely inactivate the β gene with no β-globin production and cause a phenotype of β° thalassemia. Mutations that allow the production of some β globin lead to the phenotype of β+ or β++ thalassemia depending on whether there is a marked or mild reduction in the output of the β chains, respectively. Mutations affecting the conserved sequences in the 5′ promoter (i.e. TATA box, proximal CACCC and distal CACCC box) typically cause a 70–80% reduction in promoter activity and are often very mild. Mutations affecting the polyadenylation signal (AATAAA) at the 3′ end, also generally result in a mild β+ thalassemia phenotype.

A few β thalassemia mutations are 'silent'; carriers do not have any evident hematologic phenotypes with red cell indices and Hb A$_2$ levels within the normal range, the only abnormality being an imbalanced globin chain synthesis. These β thalassemia mutations have usually been ascertained by finding individuals with intermediate forms of β thalassemia resulting from compound heterozygosity for one typical β thalassemia mutation in combination with mild β++-thalassemia allele. In this case, one parent has typical β-thalassemia trait and the other, apparently normal. Overall, the 'silent' β-thalassaemia alleles are uncommon except for the −101 C→T mutation which has been observed fairly frequently in the Mediterranean region where it interacts with a variety of more severe β-thalassemia mutations to produce milder forms of β thalassemia.[29]

About half of the β-thalassemia alleles completely inactivate the gene mostly by premature termination of translation, either by single base substitution to a non-

sense codon, or through a frameshift mutation. Studies show that the different in-phase termination mutants exhibit a 'positional' effect and are subjected to a surveillance mechanism (nonsense mediated RNA decay or NMD) to prevent the accumulation of mutant mRNAs coding for truncated peptides.[30,31] Frameshifts and nonsense mutations that result in premature termination early in the sequence (in exon 1 and 2) are associated with minimal amounts of mutant β mRNA. In such cases, no β chain is produced from the mutant allele and only half the normal β globin is present, resulting in a phenotype of typical heterozygous β thalassemia. In contrast, mutations that produce in-phase terminations later in the β sequence, in exon 3,[32] are associated with substantial amounts of mutant β-mRNA leading to a synthesis of β-chain variants that are highly unstable and damage the red cell precursors.[33] Such mutations, even when present in a single copy, result in a moderately severe anemia and are said to be 'dominantly inherited'.[34] Small amounts of truncated β-variant chains have been isolated in one case (heterozygous β codon 121).[35] These truncated β chains, however, are non-functional and not able to form viable tetramers. They precipitate in the erythroid precursors causing premature death of these cells, accentuating the ineffective erythropoiesis and resulting in clinical disease even in the heterozygous state. For a detailed review of the dominantly inherited β thalassemias, see Thein.[36]

β thalassemia is rarely caused by deletions. Of these, only the 619 bp deletion at the 3′ end of the β gene is common, but even that is restricted to the Sind populations of India and Pakistan where it constitutes ~ 30% of the β-thalassemia alleles.[37,38] The other deletions, although extremely rare, are of particular phenotypic interest because they are associated with an unusually high level of Hb A$_2$ in heterozygotes.[17] The mechanism underlying the markedly elevated levels of Hb A$_2$ and the variable increases in Hb F in heterozygotes for these deletions is related to the removal of the 5′-promoter region of the β-globin gene which removes competition for the upstream β-LCR leading to an increased interaction of the LCR with the γ and δ genes in *cis*, thus enhancing their expression (Fig. 9.2b). In this regard the promoter mutations at positions −88 and −29, are also associated with unusually high Hb A$_2$ levels. Even more rare are three upstream deletions which remove all or part of the β-LCR but leave the β gene itself intact, and yet downregulate the β-globin gene as part of εγδβ thalassemia. Other extensive deletions which cause εγδβ thalassemia remove all, or substantial regions of, the cluster including the β gene. Clinically, the εγδβ thalassemias are characterized in newborns by anemia and hemolysis which is self-limiting, often necessitating

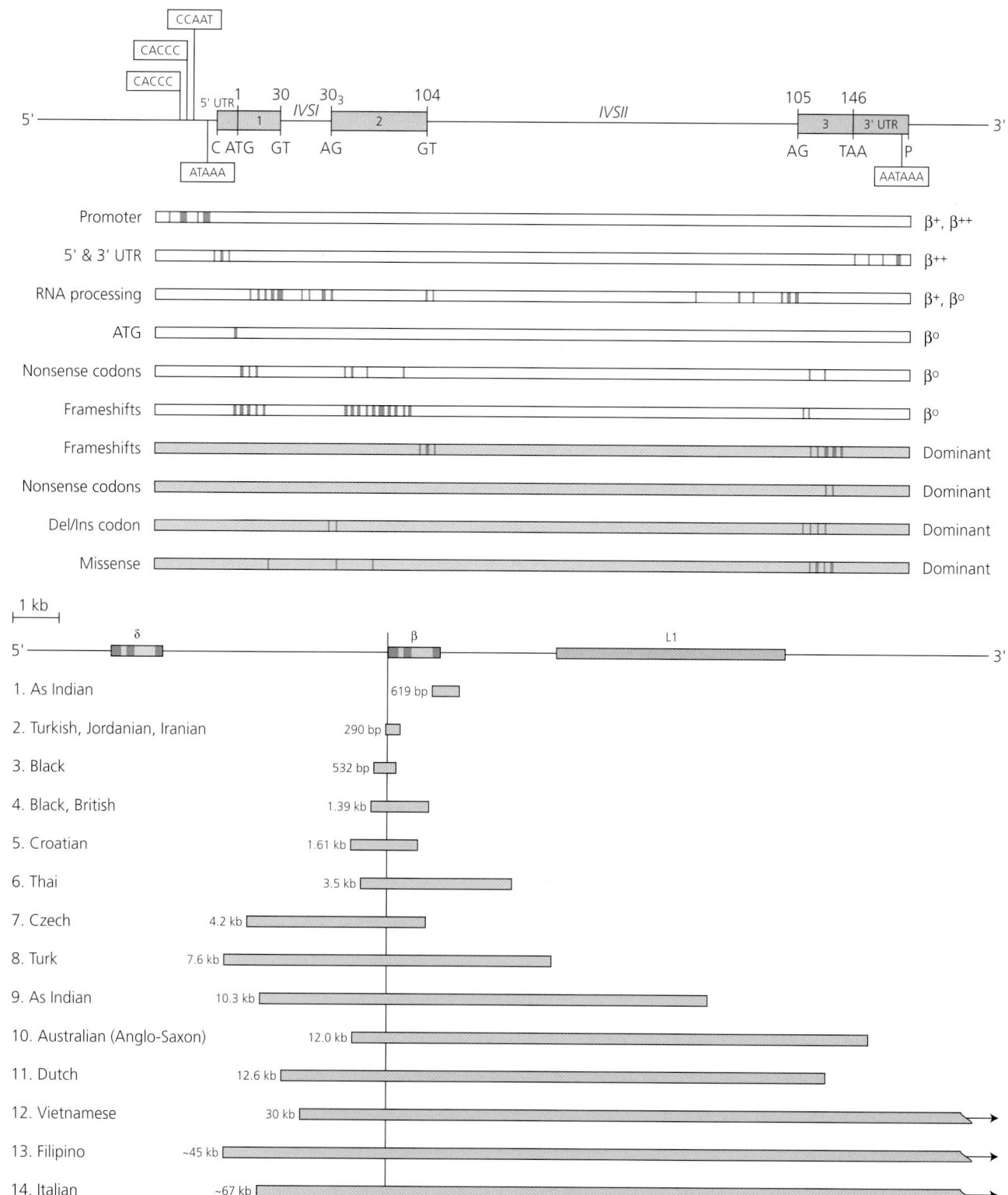

Fig. 9.2 (A) Point mutations causing β thalassemia. The β-globin gene is represented by 3 exons (gray) interrupted by 2 introns with the 5′ and 3′ untranslated regions (UTRs, striped boxes). The vertical lines within the open rectangular boxes represent the sites of the different mutations which can be found in the UTRs, exons and introns, and causing typical recessively inherited β thalassemia. Mutations in the hatched rectangular boxes are dominantly inherited. They include mutations that lead to premature termination due to frameshifts or nonsense codons, insertions or deletions of intact codons and amino acid substitutions. (B) Deletions causing β thalassemia. These deletions remove part or all of the β gene, and range from 290 bp to > 45 kb in size. The 619 bp deletion remove the 3′ end of the β gene but leave the 5′ end intact while the other deletions remove, in common, the 5′ promoter region of the β gene including sequences from positions −125 to +78 (relative to the β mRNA cap site). The latter mutations which remove the promoter region are associated with unusually high Hb A_2 levels and variably increased Hb F levels in the heterozygous state.

blood transfusions.[39] After this initial period, they have a hematologic phenotype of heterozygous thalassemia with normal levels of Hb A_2 and Hb F (as the δ and γ genes are also removed on one chromosome).

Owing to the vast number of different β-thalassemia mutations, many patients with thalassemia major are compound heterozygotes for two different molecular lesions.

Pathophysiology

The molecular defects in β thalassemias result in absent or reduced β-chain production while α-chain synthesis proceeds at a normal rate. This imbalance in globin synthesis in β thalassemia gives rise to excess α chains which are extremely unstable and precipitate in the red cell precursors forming inclusion bodies (Figs 9.3 and 9.4). These inclusions interfere with the red cell maturation and are responsible for the intramedullary destruction of the erythroid precursors and hence the ineffective erythropoiesis that characterizes all β thalassemias (Fig. 9.5). The anemia of β thalassemia results from a combination of underproduction of hemoglobin and ineffective erythropoiesis and, ultimately, is related to the degree of imbalance between the α- and non α-globin chains. The complications of splenomegaly, bone disease, endocrine and cardiac damage are related to the severity of anemia and the subsequent degree of iron loading resulting from the increased iron absorption and from recurrent blood transfusion.

Hb E/β thalassemia

Hb E is probably the commonest structural hemoglobin variant, occurring at a very high frequency in parts of the Indian subcontinent and throughout Southeast Asia. Since β thalassemia is also prevalent in these regions, it is

not uncommon to encounter individuals who are compound heterozygotes for Hb E and β thalassemia.[40]

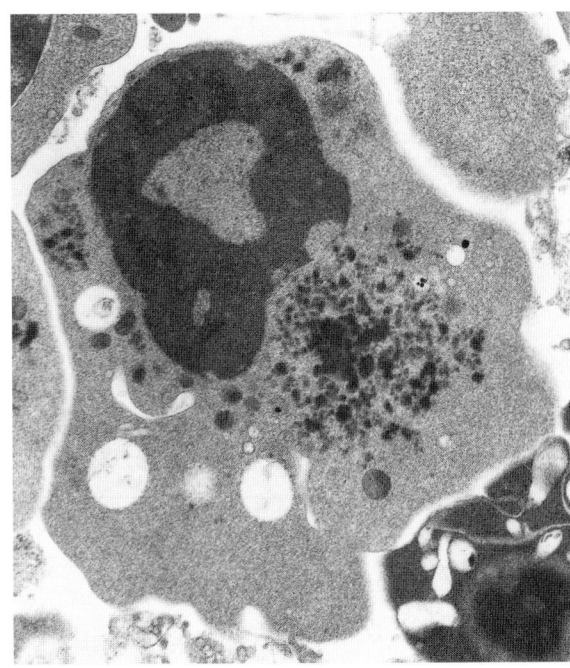

Fig. 9.4 Electron micrograph of a late erythroblast from a homozygote for β thalassemia. The cytoplasm contains multiple small rounded masses of electron-dense material, some of which have fused together to form larger masses. The masses probably consist of precipitated α chains. Uranyl acetate and lead citrate. × 11 625. Courtesy of Professor S N Wickramasinghe.

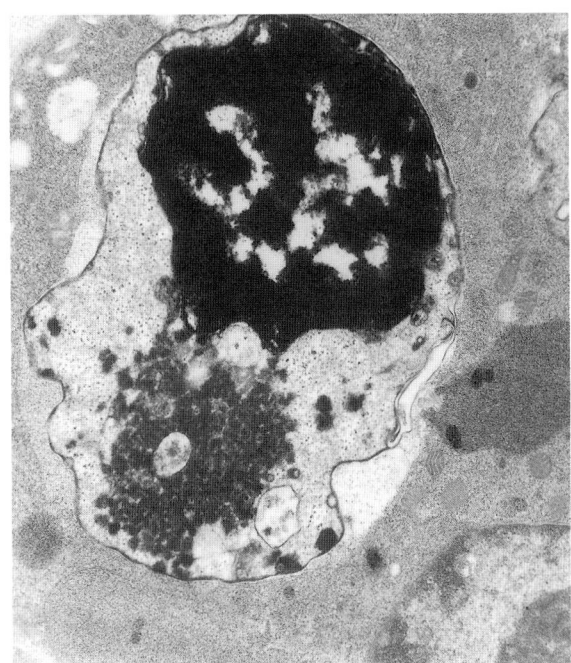

Fig. 9.5 Bone marrow macrophage from a case of homozygous β thalassemia. The macrophage contains a phagocytosed late erythroblast within which intracytoplasmic α-chain precipitates can be recognized. Uranyl acetate and lead citrate. × 11 150. Courtesy of Professor S N Wickramasinghe.

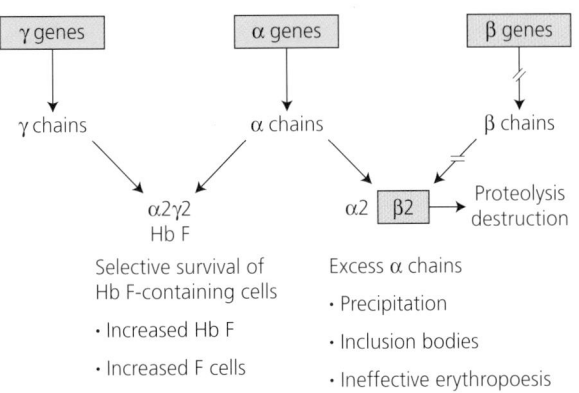

Fig. 9.3 Diagrammatic representation of the pathophysiology of: (A) β thalassemia; (B) α thalassemia.

The mutation at β-codon 26 (GAC→AAG) that gives rise to Hb E, β26 (Glu→Lys), also activates a cryptic splice site causing abnormal mRNA processing such that normal splicing that produces the Hb E variant is reduced. Since Hb E production is also quantitatively reduced, the compound heterozygous state, Hb E/β thalassemia, results in a clinical picture closely resembling homozygous β thalassemia ranging from severe anemia and transfusion dependency to thalassemia intermedia.

While a large part of this phenotypic variability can be explained by the severity of the β-thalassemia alleles, this cannot be the only answer since an equally broad range of clinical phenotypes has been encountered in Hb E/β-thalassemic individuals who carry identical β-thalassemia mutations.[41] The diagnosis of Hb E/β thalassemia is confirmed by finding Hb E and F (with or without Hb A, depending on whether it is β+ or β° thalassemia) on hemoglobin electrophoresis and by demonstrating Hb E trait in one parent and β-thalassemia trait in the other.

It can be difficult to differentiate homozygous Hb E (Hb E/Hb E) from Hb E/β° thalassemia on Hb electrophoresis alone since only Hb E and F are observed in both cases. Genetic studies would be definitive since both parents would be Hb E carriers in Hb E/E, but Hb E trait in one and β-thalassemia trait in Hb E/β thalassemia. Clinically, homozygotes for Hb E are very mild while Hb E/β°-thalassemic individuals have a more severe disease ranging from thalassemia intermedia to total transfusion dependence.

The δβ, γδβ thalassemias and HPFH syndromes

This group of disorders is characterized by a reduced or absent synthesis of β- and δ-globin chains and a variable compensatory increase in γ-chain production.[42] The distinction between δβ thalassemias and the HPFH syndromes is subtle and originally made on what appeared to be clear-cut clinical and hematological phenotypes. However, with the elucidation of the molecular basis of these conditions, it became increasingly clear that this broad classification is rather arbitrary, and that there is considerable overlap in many of the parameters that were initially used to differentiate them. Heterozygotes for δβ thalassemia have a red cell picture similar to β thalassemia, with hypochromic microcytic red cells, but a normal level of Hb A$_2$ (< 3.0%). In addition, however, there is an increased level of Hb F (5–15%) that was unevenly distributed (heterocellular) among the erythrocytes. Homozygotes for δβ thalassemia or compound

heterozygotes with β thalassemias are not common but have been reported to have clinical phenotypes ranging from mild anemia to thalassemia major, the α/γ-globin chain synthesis ratios ranging from 2.5 to 5.1.[43] In contrast, HPFH heterozygotes have essentially normal red cell indices, a normal level of Hb A$_2$, and even higher levels of Hb F (15–30%) with a homogeneous pancellular distribution of the Hb F. HPFH homozygotes are clinically normal, their hemoglobin levels may be increased with mildly hyochromic microcytic red cells. Compound heterozygotes with β thalassemia may have a mild anemia but are clinically asymptomatic.

These conditions are remarkably heterogeneous genotypically; at the molecular level they can be classified into two groups:

1. Those due to varying deletions of the β-globin cluster removing the β and δ, or the β, δ and Aγ genes producing an increase of both ${}^{G}\gamma$ and ${}^{A}\gamma$ chains [${}^{G}_{\gamma}{}^{A}_{\gamma}$ (δβ)° thalassemia or HPFH] or only ${}^{G}_{\gamma}$ chain [${}^{G}_{\gamma}$(${}^{A}_{\gamma}$δβ)° thalassemia], respectively.
2. Non-deletional type in which there is an increase of only the ${}^{G}_{\gamma}$- or ${}^{A}_{\gamma}$- globin chains and usually due to mutation in the respective promoters.

The increases in Hb F levels in such non-deletion HPFHs are variable and the Hb F distribution among the red cells is pancellular. A non-deletion form of δβ thalassemia due to a point mutation inactivating the β gene, in *cis* with a point mutation in the γ-gene promoter upregulating Hb F production has also been described.[44] These forms of δβ thalassemia and HPFH are clearly defined on a molecular basis and are inherited in a Mendelian fashion as alleles of the β-globin complex.

There is another form of non-deletion HPFH conditions characterized by modest increases of Hb F (1–5%) in which the inheritance patterns are less clear cut. Because the Hb F is unevenly distributed among the erythrocytes, this form is referred to as heterocellular HPFH, previously known as Swiss-type HPFH, after the original report in which some members of a group of Swiss soldiers were found to have slight increases in Hb F levels.[45] The β-globin cluster is intact in heterocellular HPFH and no mutations can be found in the γ promoters. Heterocellular HPFH is probably present in 10–15% of the normal population, representing the high values of Hb F and F cells at the upper tail of the continuous skewed trait distribution. It should be considered as a multifactorial discrete trait, but the number of loci or genes contributing to this trait is not known, although quantitative trait loci (QTLs) controlling Hb F and F cells have been mapped to chromosomes 6q23 and Xp22.[46,47] The clinical significance of heterocellular HPFH lies in its interaction with sickle cell disease and β thalassemia in which coinheritance of a determinant for heterocellular HPFH can increase Hb F production to clinically beneficial levels.

Intermediate forms of β thalassemia

Thalassemia intermedia is a descriptive clinical term used to describe patients with a diverse collection of phenotypes that range from only being less severe than the transfusion-dependent major through a spectrum of decreasing severity of anemia to one that is just mildly anemic and detected through routine blood examination.[18] The criteria on which the diagnosis is based is that patients present later in life relative to thalassemia major and that they are capable of maintaining a reasonable level of hemoglobin (6 g/dl or more) without regular transfusion. At the severe end of the spectrum, patients present between the ages of 2 and 6 years, and although they are just capable of surviving without blood transfusion, it is clear that growth and development are retarded. Many will show the skeletal and facial changes and progressive splenomegaly as seen in untreated thalassemia major. As they become older they develop iron-overload because of increased gastrointestinal absorption of iron, a modifying factor here is the presence of genetic variants involved in iron homeostasis, for example *HFE* gene.[19,21] At the other end of the spectrum, patients are completely asymptomatic until adult life and are transfusion independent with hemoglobin levels of 10–12 g/dl. Such patients are diagnosed either during episodes of infection when they become anemic or by a chance hematological examination. There is usually some degree of splenomegaly.

Because of the extreme variability of these disorders, these patients should be regularly followed from early childhood and the disease carefully monitored in terms of the growth charts and iron accumulation.

The underlying genotypes are equally heterogeneous, resulting from the interactions of other genetic variables with the inheritance of a single, or two β-thalassemia alleles (Table 9.1). At the primary level, the severity of the deficit of β globin is a critical determinant but this is complicated by the 'dominantly-inherited' β-thalassemia alleles which leads to the production of β-chain variants that are highly unstable and non-functional for one reason or another (see Thein).[36] The secondary level relates to the variants involving the α- and γ-globin genes that can redress the globin-chain imbalance. The tertiary level involves loci that are not directly involved in globin-chain balance but might modify the complications of the

Table 9.1 Molecular basis of β thalassemia intermedia

I   Homozygous or compound heterozygous state for β thalassemia
  1. inheritance of mild β⁺ thalassemia alleles e.g. β-promoter mutations and 'silent' β-thalassemia alleles
  2. coinheritance of α thalassemia
     • effect more evident in β⁺ thalassemia
  3. β thalassemia with elevated γ-chain production
     • polymorphism at position -158^{G_γ} gene (Xmn I-$^{G_\gamma}$ site)
     • β-promoter mutations
     • coinheritance of heterocellular HPFH e.g. 6q-linked, Xp-linked

II Compound heterozygotes for β thalassemia and deletion forms of HPFH or δβ thalassemia

III Compound heterozygotes for β thalassemia and β-chain variants e.g. Hb E/β thalassemia

IV Heterozygotes for β thalassemia
  1. coinheritance of extra α-globin genes e.g. ααα/αα, ααα/ααα, αα/αααα
     • effect more evident with more severe β thalassemia
  2. dominantly inherited forms of β thalassemia (including some thalassemic hemoglobinopathies)

HPFH, hereditary persistence of fetal hemaglobin.

disease in many ways. The latter group is likely to include a whole host of genetic variants, some of which have been recently elucidated, for example genes involved in iron metabolism (see Clinical features of β thalassemia).

Given the differences in the spectrum of β-thalassemia mutations and differences in the frequency of the different α-thalassemia variants and other genetic modifiers, the relative importance of these genetic factors would vary accordingly in different population groups. It is also important to note that the genotypic factors are not mutually exclusive. Analysis of the thalassemia intermedia patients has revealed that ~ 75% of these patients have inherited two β-thalassemia alleles (homozygous or compound heterozygous) and that in two-thirds of the patients (i.e. 50% of all thalassemia intermedia patients), one or two of these alleles are mild β⁺-thalassemia mutations.[48-50] Coinheritance of α thalassemia can ameliorate the severity of β thalassemia; the effect is not so evident in the homozygous or compound heterozygous states for β° thalassemia but it can convert the severe forms of β⁺ thalassemia into milder, non-transfusion-dependent conditions. The role of increased Hb F response as an ameliorating factor becomes evident in the group of β° thalassemia intermedia patients who have a very mild disorder and are able to maintain hemoglobin levels of 11–12 g/dl, all of which is Hb F, without α thalassemia and independent of blood transfusion.[48] In some cases the individuals are compound heterozygotes for δβ thalassemia or one of the HPFH determinants but these genetic interactions are not common. Much more common is the C→T polymorphism at position -158 in the $^G_\gamma$-globin gene, referred to as the *Xmn*1-$^G/_\gamma$ site (the substitution creates a cutting site for the restriction enzyme *Xmn*1). This polymorphism seems to have little effect in normal people but clinical studies have shown that under erythropoietic stress (such as in homozygous β thalassemia and sickle cell disease), presence of the *Xmn*1-$^G_\gamma$ site is associated with higher levels of Hb F and a milder disease.[51,52] As this sequence variant is widely distributed and occurs in *cis* to many β°-thalassemia alleles, it is an important modifying factor in the disease severity of the disorder. Other genetic determinants responsible for increased levels of Hb F are not encoded in the β-globin gene cluster and are transmitted in the group of heterocellular HPFH conditions.[53,54]

Thalassemia intermedia can also result from an increase in the severity of the heterozygous state for β thalassemia. In the majority of cases this is related to increase α-globin production from the coinheritance of triplicated or quadruplicated α-globin genes (i.e. ααα/ or αααα/).[55-57] The additional α-globin genes have no phenotype in normal people but the small excess of α chains in heterozygous β thalassemia appears to tip the balance, crossing the critical threshold of α globin excess with phenotypic consequences. In other heterozygotes with β thalassemia intermedia, the β thalassemia mutation itself leads to the synthesis of highly unstable β variants which are non-functional and deleterious posing a dominant negative effect.[33,36] Such β-thalassemia alleles are dominantly inherited since presence of a single copy causes a clinical phenotype of moderately severe dyserythropoietic anemia. Coinheritance of extra α-globin genes accentuates the disease severity.

The α thalassemias

α thalassemia can be regarded as α^+- or α°-, reflecting either a reduction or complete absence of α-globin synthesis from the affected chromosome.[58] The geographical distribution of α thalassemia is very similar to that of β thalassemia; in some parts of the tropical and subtropical regions where it is prevalent, carrier frequency for the mild form (α^+) reaches 90%. The more severe defect, α° thalassemia, is prevalent in the Mediterranean region and Southeast Asia where carrier frequency can reach 10%. Although the α thalassemias are more common than β thalassemias, they pose less of a public-health problem since the severe homozygous states cause death *in utero* and the milder forms that survive into adulthood do not cause a major disability.

Clinical features

The clinical disorders resulting from α thalassemia range from death *in utero* (Hb Bart's hydrops syndrome) to a completely silent carrier state.[59] Hemoglobin Bart's hydrops is a frequent cause of stillbirths in Southeast Asia. Affected infants are usually stillborn with gross pallor, generalized edema and massive hepatosplenomegaly. The placenta is enlarged and friable and frequently causes obstetric difficulties. The intermediate form of α thalassemia is Hb H disease, commonly seen in the Mediterranean, Middle East and Southeast Asia. A broad spectrum of disease severity is also encountered in Hb H disease. Generally, these individuals have a moderately severe anemia and splenomegaly but are usually transfusion independent except during episodes of hemolysis associated with infection. The skeletal deformities and growth retardation characterstic of β thalassemia are not unusually seen. Rarely, the very severe forms of Hb H disease can present with hydrops fetalis.[59]

Diagnosis

Diagnosis is based on the hemoglobin level, red cell indices, examination of the peripheral blood smear and hemoglobin analysis. Infants with Hb Bart's hydrops are severely anemic with hemoglobin levels of 6–8 g/dl. The blood film shows severe thalassemic changes with numerous hypochromic nucleated red cells. There is no Hb A or F, the hemoglobin consists mainly of Hb Bart's (γ_4 tetramers) with small amounts of embryonic hemoglobin and Hb H (β_4 tetramers). Biosynthetic studies confirm the complete absence of α chains. Patients with Hb H disease run an hemoglobin level of 7–10 g/dl with moderate reticulocytosis. Again, typical thalassemic changes are seen in the blood film. On incubation of the red cells with brilliant cresyl blue, numerous inclusion bodies are generated by precipitation of the Hb H which are tetramers of β chain (β^4), forming typical 'golf balls' (Figs 9.6 and 9.7). Hemoglobin analysis shows 5–40% Hb H, with the major component being Hb A and a normal or reduced level of Hb A$_2$. Sometimes, there is also a small amount of Hb Bart's. Carriers for α thalassemia may be slightly anemic with hypochromic microcytic red cells or 'silent' with minimal hematologic changes. The Hb electrophoretic pattern is normal and globin biosynthetic studies show a deficit of α-chain production.

Diagnosis of α thalassemia is confirmed by DNA analysis which commonly reveals deletions of the α-gene cluster, removing one or both α genes. Less commonly, the genes are present and DNA sequence analysis reveals point changes within the α$_2$ gene or its immediate flanking regions.

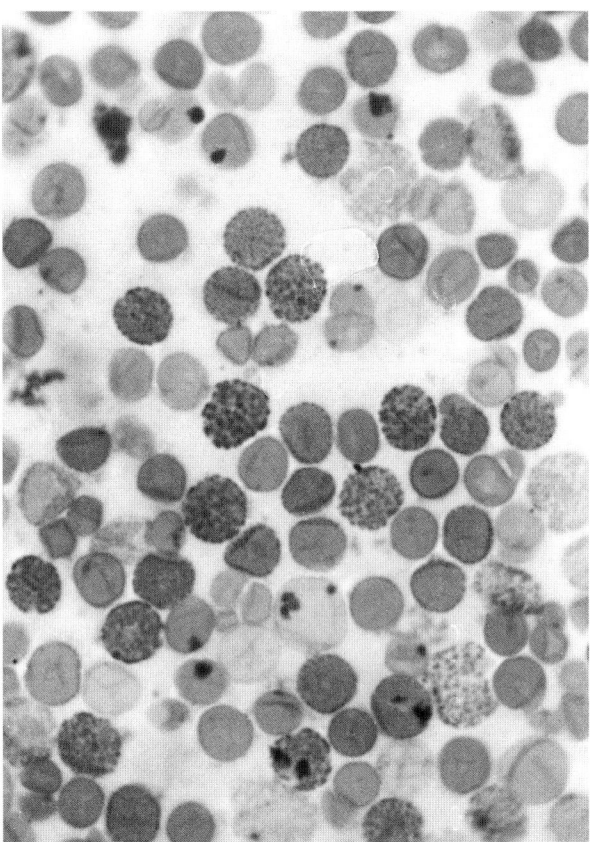

Fig. 9.6 Golf-ball-like appearance of many of the red cells of a case of HbH disease after supravital staining with brilliant cresyl blue. Courtesy of Professor S N Wickramasinghe.

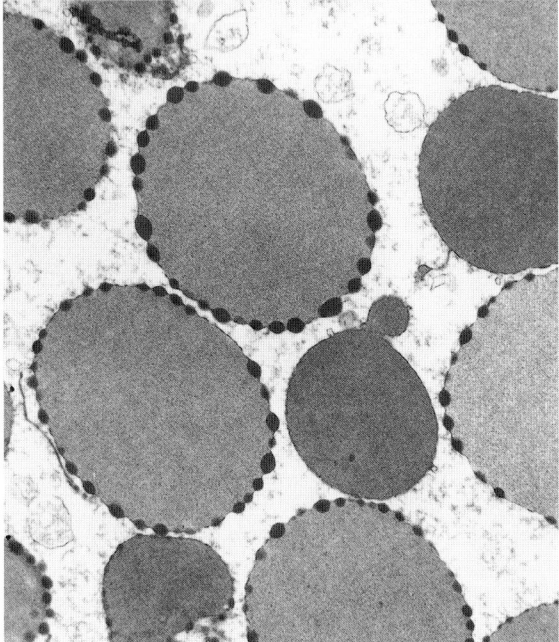

Fig. 9.7 Ultrastructure of red cells from a case of HbH disease after incubation with brilliant cresyl blue for 1 h. The HbH-containing cells show membrane-bound, redox-dye-induced masses of denatured HbH. Uranyl acetate and lead citrate. × 6650. Courtesy of Professor S N Wickramasinghe.

Genetic basis of disease

Normal individuals have four α-globin genes arranged as linked pairs, α_2 and α_1, at the tip of each chromosome 16, the normal α genotype being written as αα/αα.[60] The α thalassemias usually result from deletion of one (/-α) or both (/—) α genes of the linked pair from chromosome 16, causing a reduction (α^+) or absence (α°) of α globin from the affected chromosome, respectively. The extensive deletions which remove both the linked α_1 and α_2 genes tend to be geographically isolated and are often referred to by their geographical origin, for example /—SEA and /—MED. Although more than 30 such deletions have been characterized, the majority of α thalassemia is caused by six deletions (/-α$^{3.7}$, /-α$^{4.2}$, /—SEA, /—MED, /-(α)$^{20.5}$, and /—FIL). Less commonly, α thalassemia results from point mutations involving the critical sequences that control the various stages of gene expression as encountered in the β thalassemias. With the exception of one phenotypically mild α-thalassemia mutant, all of these non-deletional mutations affect the dominant α_2-globin gene. In general, the non-deletion α^+-thalassemia variants (/$\alpha^T\alpha$) gives rise to a more severe reduction in α-chain synthesis than the single α-gene deletion (/-α). A common non-deletion α-thalassemia variant in Southeast Asia is Hb Constant Spring (Hb CS, /$\alpha^{CS}\alpha$), which is due to a single base substitution (TAA→CAA) in the α_2-globin termination codon. This results in readthrough of the 3'-untranslated sequence until another in-phase termination codon is encountered 31 codons later. Three other variants (Hb Icaria, Hb Seal Rock and Hb Koya Dora) involving different base substitutions in the α2-termination codon have been identified. Non-deletional α thalassemia can also arise from single base substitutions causing structural α-globin variants that are highly unstable, for example Hb Quong Sze α125 Leu→Pro (/$\alpha^{QS}\alpha$). More rarely, α thalassemia is caused by upstream deletions which remove the α-globin regulatory element (HS -40) but leave the α genes themselves intact. It is the characterization of these natural deletions that led to the identification of the α-globin HS-40 element.[61]

Loss of one functioning α gene (αα/-α) is almost completely silent with normal or only slightly hypochromic red cells. Loss of two α genes (—/αα or-α/-α) produces a mild hypochromic microcytic anemia, the α-thalassemia trait. Homozygotes for α° thalassemia (—/—) have a lethal condition with intrauterine hemolytic anemia called the Hb Bart's hydrops fetalis syndrome. Deficiency of α chains gives rise to an excess of γ chains (in fetal life) or β chains (in adult life) which form γ_4-tetramers (Hb Bart's) and β_4-tetramers (Hb H), respectively. The presence of Hb Bart's or Hb H is thus diagnostic of α thalassemia.

Hb H disease lies between the two ends of the clinical spectrum, the asymptomatic α thalassemia trait and Hb Bart's hydrops fetalis. As in β-thalassemia intermedia, Hb H disease spans a wide range of clinical and hematological phenotypes, the diagnostic feature being the presence of Hb H inclusions in the peripheral red-blood cells. The most severe forms can be lethal late in gestation or in the perinatal period (Hb H hydrops fetalis). The molecular basis of this order is equally heterogeneous, varying with the geographic distribution of the different α thalassemia variants.[62] Hb H disease most commonly results from the interaction of α° and α^+ thalassemia (—/-α). Less often it can result from the interaction of α° thalassemia with non-deletional forms of α thalassemia (—/$\alpha^T\alpha$) or from homozygous non-deletional α thalassemia ($\alpha^T\alpha/\alpha^T\alpha$). A less severe form of Hb H disease in Southeast Asia commonly arises from homozygosity or compound heterozygosity for Hb Constant Spring ($\alpha^{CS}\alpha/\alpha^{CS}\alpha$) or ($\alpha^{CS}\alpha/$—). Very low levels of this elongated α-globin chain (5–8% of the total hemoglobin in homozygotes) are found; the defective α^{CS}-chain production is a consequence of the instability of the α^{CS}-mRNA.[63]

Pathophysiology

There is a fundamental difference in the pathophysiology of the α and β thalassemias (Fig. 9.8). Because γ^4 and β^4 tetramers are soluble, they do not precipitate to a significant degree in the bone marrow and those erythroblasts containing precipitated β-globin chains (Fig. 9.9) appear to be functionally less disturbed than the precipitate-containing cells in β thalassemia (i.e. erythropoiesis is more effective than in β thalassemia). However, these β^4 tetramers do precipitate as the red cells age, forming inclusion bodies in the mature erythrocytes (Fig. 9.10). Peripheral hemolysis occurs due to the red cell membrane damage and obstruction in the spleen. The degree of anemia and the amount of the tetramers (Hb H and Bart's) produced reflects the severity of the reduction in the output of the α-globin chain.

α thalassemia with mental retardation (ATR) syndromes

These are rare forms of the α thalassemias found in association with a variety of developmental abnormalities, in particular with mental retardation and hence they are often referred to as α thalassemia with mental retardation (ATR) syndromes.[64] One group, ATR-16 results from extensive deletions and rearrangements of 1–2 Mb from the tip of chromosome 16 including the α-globin genes.[65]

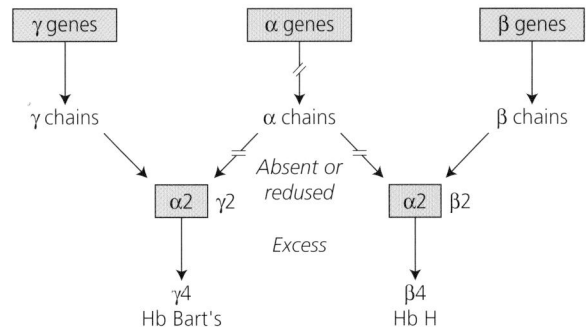

Fig. 9.8 Diagrammatic representation of the pathophysiology of α thalassemia.

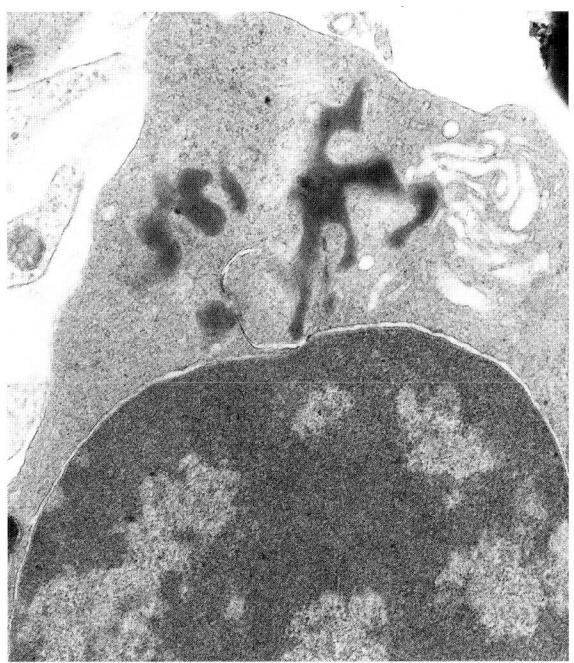

Fig. 9.9 Electron micrograph of a late erythroblast from a patient with HbH disease. The cell contains an electron-dense stellate intracytoplasmic inclusion, probably consisting of precipitated β chains. Uranyl acetate and lead citrate. × 21 875. Courtesy of Professor S N Wickramasinghe.

Although in some cases, one of the parents may have α thalassemia, the rearrangement in all cases is *de novo*. Several of the patients have similar degrees of mild, mental retardation and share common developmental and dysmorphic features. The mechanisms by which these deletions cause the developmental abnormalities is still not clear; there is no clear association between the extent of deletion and the degree of phenotypic severity, the critical genes involved have yet to be identified. ATR-X is also characterized by α thalassemia, but the mental retardation is much more severe, accompanied by remarkably characteristic dysmorphic facies and urogenital anomalies.[66] More than 100 cases of the ATR-X syndrome

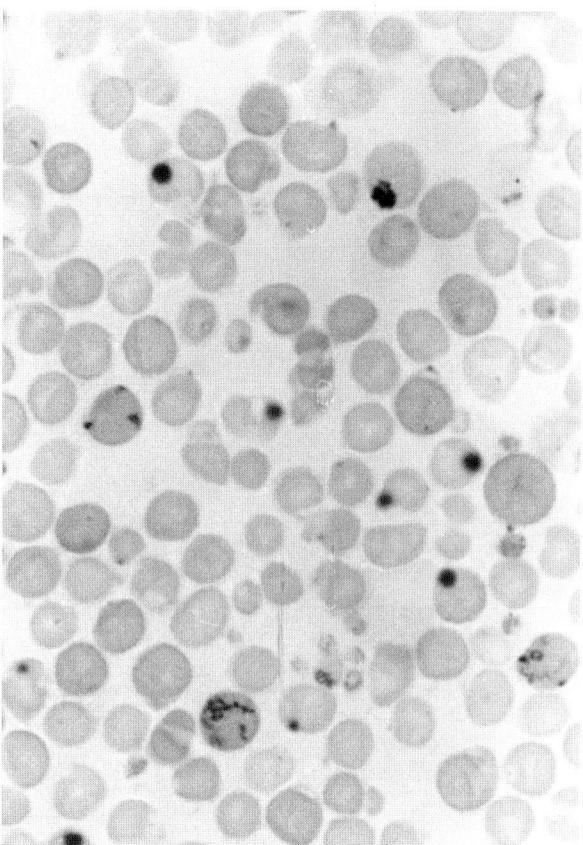

Fig. 9.10 Blood film of a splenectomized patient with HbH disease. The smears were made after supravital staining of venous blood with an equal volume of 0.5% methyl violet in normal saline for 10 min. Several of the red cells in the photomicrograph contain a membrane-bound Heinz body which had formed *in vivo*. × 1500. Courtesy of Professor S N Wickramasinghe.

from more than 70 families have been characterized and in all cases the affected individuals are males.[64] In these cases, the α-globin cluster is intact and the underlying mutations reside in a *trans*-acting gene encoded on the X-chromosome (Xq131-q21.1). The ATR-X gene contains 36 exons spanning 300 kb. It is a member of the SNF2 subgroup of a superfamily of proteins involved in a variety of cellular functions including transcription, cell cycle control and DNA repair. ATR-X is likely to perturb the expression of multiple 'target' genes including the α-globin genes. Although detailed genotype/phenotype correlations have elucidated the critical functional domains of the protein, the relationship with α thalassemia is less clear. There is no consistent relationship between the severity of α thalassemia and the predicted severity of the ATR-X mutations.

Acquired α thalassemia

Very rarely, α thalassemia can be encountered as an acquired mutation in patients with a variety of hemato-logic disorders within the myelodysplastic syndromes (MDS).[59] These individuals are predominantly males of North European origin with a mean age of 66 years at presentation. They have a normal complement of α-globin genes (αα/αα) and in all cases where data are available, there is no evidence of pre-existing α thalassemia and thus the α thalassemia and abnormal erythropoeisis is presumably acquired as a clonal genetic abnormality of the MDS. The marked hypochromic microcytic anemia associated with an almost absent α-globin chain synthesis and classical Hb H inclusions is likely to be due to a *trans*-acting mutation downregulating the α genes but the nature and location of the specific defect remains unknown.

Management

The thalassemias are a major health problem in many populations and because there is no definitive treatment, major efforts are concentrated on prevention.

Preventive programs in the past were based on education, population screening, heterozygote detection and genetic counseling but were not entirely effective. Most countries now combine this approach with screening programs at antenatal clinics.[67] When heterozygous mothers are detected, their partners are tested and if they are also carriers, the couples are offered prenatal diagnosis and selective termination of pregnancy.

Regular transfusion and iron chelation remain the cornerstones of treatment for severe β thalassemia and are primarily palliative.[18] Currently, the most useful chelating agent is desferrioxamine (Desferal). Unfortunately, Desferal is not only expensive but has to be administered parenterally via an infusion pump. It is not surprising that non-compliance becomes a problem, particularly during adolescence. Considerable effort is directed towards the development of a safe and effective oral iron chelator. The most promising of these is deferipone (L1) but its long-term effectiveness and toxicity still need to be evaluated.[68]

Before embarking on a transfusion regime, it is essential to assess the patient carefully over a period of a few months. Many patients with thalassemia intermedia may not need regular transfusion and have been locked into a transfusion program simply because they happen to present with an unusually low hemoglobin during an infection. On the other hand, blood transfusions have been known to be withheld simply on the basis of a steady-state hemoglobin even though the child's growth is retarded, in an attempt to reduce iron loading. However, it is worth remembering that an increase in body iron can still occur via increased gastrointestinal absorption due to the increased erythropoeitic activity. In this regard, blood transfusion not only corrects the anemia but also dampens erythropoeisis and the increased iron absorption. The main indications for transfusion, therefore, are based on growth and development of the child, and preventing the irreversible facial and skeletal changes and not the hemoglobin level.

The development of hypersplenism as shown by the falling platelet and white-cell counts, increasing spleen size and increasing blood transfusion requirements is an indication for splenectomy. Prior to splenectomy, patients should be vaccinated with pneumonococcal and *Haemophilus influenzae* type B vaccine, followed, post-splenectomy by daily prophylactic penicillin during childhood and probably indefinitely.[18]

Bone marrow transplantation is the only form of treatment that can cure the severe forms of β thalassemia but is dependent on the availability of an HLA-compatible related donor.[69] Young, well-chelated patients without evidence of liver disease are the best candidates with a 90% chance of cure. Following transplantation, there is a small but significant probability of graft-versus-host disease (GVHD). Mixed chimerism which is present in ~ 25% of patients increases graft failure. Post-transplant, iron chelation by desferrioxamine or phlebotomy have been shown to be quite effective in reducing hepatic iron loading and arresting or reversing the hepatic and cardiac complications related to iron overload.[70]

With increasing knowledge of cell and molecular biology a long-term aim would be the replacement of the defective β gene with its normal counterpart. While significant progress has been made in addressing the problems of gene transfer and expression, major biological problems remain.[71] It has long been known that the severity of disease in β thalassemia can be ameliorated by coinheritance of genetic factors that increase Hb F production. Thus, activation of the normal γ genes in patients with β thalassemia represents a potentially important approach of therapy for this disorder.[72] Several compounds, including 5-azacytidine, hydroxyurea, butyrate and butyrate analogs, have been tried. To date, the compounds that show most promise are hydroxyurea and butyric acid analogs but to achieve the therapeutic levels of Hb F needed, significant toxic side-effects are still encountered. Combination therapies such as hydroxyurea with erythropoeitin and butyrate with hydroxyurea have resulted in substantial increases in fetal hemoglobin but there is a marked variability of response among the different individuals which could relate to an underlying genetic variability.

The group of patients who fall into the thalassemia intermedia category is probably the most difficult to manage due to the diversity in their clinical severity.

Although the underlying thalassemic genotypes could predict the phenotypic severity to some extent, management should always be dictated by the well-being of the child and not by the type of β-thalassemia mutations. This group of patients should be maintained on folate supplements. Although these patients are not on a regular transfusion regimen, iron overload can still occur due to the increased gastrointestinal absorption and hence their iron status should be regularly assessed and iron chelation started if necessary. Splenectomy may be indicated when the hemoglobin levels start to fall and the spleen enlarges. Extramedullary hemopoeisis may be a problem; treatments include hypertransfusion, X-ray therapy and hydroxyurea.

For most patients with β thalassemia in the emerging countries, however, blood transfusion, iron chelation, bone marrow transplantation and treatment with expensive drugs for therapeutic augmentation of Hb F are only remotely possible, and prevention remains the main management of the disease.

Structural hemoglobin variants

More than 700 structurally different hemoglobin variants have been described,[73] but only three, sickle hemoglobin (Hb S), Hb C and Hb E, occur at a high frequency in different populations.[27] Many of them are harmless and have been discovered in population surveys using electrophoretic analyses of human hemoglobin. Since only variants that alter the charge of the hemoglobin molecule are detectable in routine electrophoresis, this number is probably an underestimate. Diseases resulting from structural abnormalities of hemoglobin are shown in Table 9.2. In this section only those abnormal hemoglobins of clinical importance are described.

Table 9.2 Clinical disorders due to structural hemoglobin variants

1. Sickle syndromes causing hemolysis and tissue damage HbS and interaction of HbS with other Hb variants (Hbs S/C, S/O-Arab and S/D-Punjab) and β thalassemia (S/β thal)

2. Chronic hemolysis – unstable hemoglobin variants (congenital Heinz body anemia, CHBA) e.g. Hb Köln, Hb Bristol

3. Congenital polycythemia – high-oxygen-affinity Hb variants

4. Congenital cyanosis – low-oxygen-affinity Hb variants M hemoglobins

5. Hypochromic microcytic anemia (thalassemic hemoglobinopathy)
   e.g. HbE – β structural variant
   Hb Constant Spring – α structural variant
   δβ fusion variants – e.g. Hb Lepore

6. Drug-induced hemolysis e.g. Hb Zurich

Sickle cell disease

Background

Sickle cell disease (SCD) was first described by James Herrick from Chicago in 1910 in a West Indian student.[74] Peculiar elongated and sickle-shaped red blood cells were observed in the peripheral blood films (see Fig. 6.2J) and suggested the term sickle cell anemia. In 1949 Pauling *et al* demonstrated that this sickling phenomenon was related to an abnormal hemoglobin present in all patients with sickle cell anemia;[75] this hemoglobin had an abnormally slow electrophoretic migration. Subsequently, in 1956 the sickle hemoglobin was chemically characterized by Ingram and was shown to differ from normal adult hemoglobin (Hb A, $\alpha_2\beta_2$) by the single substitution of glutamic acid to valine at position 6 in the β subunit.[76] Since then, molecular characterization has shown that, apart from the homozygous state for the β^S gene, the syndrome of sickle cell disease can also arise from the compound heterozygous state for Hb S and β thalassemias (Hb S/β thalassemia) and other structural variants such as Hbs C (Hb SC disease) and D (Hb SD) (Table 9.3).[77,78]

The sickling disorders occur predominantly in Black African populations but are also prevalent throughout the Mediterranean, Middle East and parts of India. It appears that heterozygotes for the β^S gene are protected from the severe effects of *Plasmodium falciparum* thus explaining the high gene frequencies in those malarious regions. The β^S gene in these diverse population groups is caused by the same molecular defect (β codon 6 G<u>A</u>G to G<u>T</u>G).

Investigations using β haplotypes constructed from the linked-groupings of DNA sequence polymorphisms in the β-globin cluster have provided some insights into the origins and migration of the β^S gene.[79] The β^S gene occurs on four different β haplotypes in Africa, known as the Senegal, Benin, Central African Republic (or Bantu) and the Cameroon types. In addition, it is associated with a different β haplotype in Saudi Arabian and Asian Indian sickle patients. The evidence suggests multiple independent origins of the β^S mutation although gene conversion on regionally specific β haplotypes cannot be excluded.

Clinical features

Sickle cell trait (carrier status) is a benign condition and generally does not cause any clinical disability. However, under certain extreme conditions, such as severe pneumonia, flying in unpressurized aircraft, and exercise at high altitude, vasoocclusive episodes can occur.[78]

Homozygous state for the β^S gene causes SCD with clinical manifestations that range from a chronic hemolytic anemia interrupted by acute and recurrent painful crises to a completely asymptomatic state, detected only by chance on routine hematological examination. Most patients fall between these two extremes and are relatively asymptomatic except for the occasional clinical crisis.

Sickle cell anemia normally presents in infancy after 6 months of life when adult-type hemoglobin becomes the predominant hemoglobin, with attacks of dactylitis, manifested as painful swelling of the fingers and feet, the

Table 9.3 The major sickling disorders

	β Genotype	α Genotype	Hb electrophoresis
Sickle cell trait	β^A/β^S	$\alpha\alpha/\alpha\alpha$	HbS ~ 45%; HbA$_2$ normal; rest HbA
Sickle cell trait[a]	β^A/β^S	$-\alpha/\alpha\alpha$ $-\alpha/-\alpha$	HbS ~ 25–30%; HbA$_2$ increased (3.2–3.7%)
Sickle cell anemia	β^S/β^S	$\alpha\alpha/\alpha\alpha$	HbS 80–100%; HbF 0–20%, No Hb A
Sickle cell disease	β^S/β^C	$\alpha\alpha/\alpha\alpha$	HbS 50%; HbC 50%
SO-Arab disease[b]	$\beta^S/\beta^{D\text{-}Punjab}$	$\alpha\alpha/\alpha\alpha$	HbS, HbO Arab
SD-Punjab disease[c]	β^S/β^C		HbS 50%; HbD Punjab 50%
Sβ^+ thal	β^S/β^{Th}	$\alpha\alpha/\alpha\alpha$	HbS 50–80%; HbF 0–20%; HbA 1–30%; HbA$_2$ 3–6%
Sβ° thal	β^S/β^{Th}		HbS 75–100%; HbF 0–20%; HbA$_2$ 3–6%; no HbA
S HPFH	$\beta^S/\beta*$	$\alpha\alpha/\alpha\alpha$	HbS 70–80%; HbF 20–30%; HbA$_2$ decreased; no HbA

[a] Coinheritance of α thalassemia ($-\alpha/-\alpha$ or $\alpha\alpha/-\alpha$) with sickle cell trait can be difficult to differentiate from HbS/mild β^+ thal; both demonstrate hypochromic microcytic red cells and raised A$_2$ levels.
[b] HbC, HbO-Arab and HbE are not separated on routine alkaline electrophoresis.
[c] Quantitation based on agar gel electrophoresis.
$\beta*$Deletion of β-globin cluster.
HPFH, hereditary persistence of fetal hemoglobin.

so-called 'hand–foot syndrome'. At this stage, the infant is usually anemic with mild jaundice and the spleen palpable. Splenomegaly usually resolves due to repeated infarctions of the spleen, the 'autosplenectomy' manifested by typical post-splenectomy changes in the peripheral blood film. It is unusual to feel the spleen after the first decade of life. Typically, these children have a chronic hemolytic anemia with a hemoglobin level that varies between 6 and 8 g/dl and a reticulocyte count of 10–20%. There is a slight elevation of the serum bilirubin level and increased urinary urobilinogen and examination of the peripheral blood smear shows polychromasia and poikilocytosis with a variable number of sickled erythrocytes.

The chronic hemolysis of sickle cell anemia is punctuated by acute exacerbations of the illness termed sickling crises traditionally classified as vaso-occlusive, sequestration, aplastic or hemolytic. The most common are the vaso-occlusive crises characterized by acute painful episodes due to blockage of small vessels with sickled erythrocytes and tissue infarction. Commonly, the patient experiences a rapid onset of deep, throbbing bone pain in the lumbosacral spine and limb bones, usually without physical findings but sometimes accompanied by local tenderness, warmth and swelling. Marrow aspirated from areas of bone tenderness has revealed infarction of the marrow tissue. Occasionally, abdominal pain is the major symptom and can pose a difficult problem in differential diagnosis. The abdominal crisis is accompanied by distension and rigidity with loss of bowel sounds, findings typical of an acute surgical abdomen.

Vaso-occlusion in the lung, acute chest syndrome, is characterized by acute dyspnea and pleuritic pain and often accompanied by a significant fall in the hemocrit which may reflect sequestration of the sickled cells in the pulmonary vessels. The distinction from pulmonary infection is often very difficult, particularly as infection and infarction usually coexist. Acute chest syndrome is the commonest cause of death after 2 years of age; the patient with acute chest syndrome is extremely vulnerable because hypoxia has a profound effect on sickling. Acute vaso-occlusion in the CNS usually presents in childhood, either as fits, transient neurologic symptoms resembling ischemia attacks, or with a fully developed stroke.[80] Recurrent attacks are common, 70% of patients experience a recurrence within 3 years and many are left with permanent motor and intellectual disabilities. Cerebrovascular injury probably occurs in 6–12% of patients with SCD with a peak between the ages of 2 and 5 years, being rare in infants less than 1 year of age. Children with Hb SS are at highest risk followed by Hb S/β° thalassemia and Hb SC disease. Priapism is a distressing problem resulting from vaso-occlusion of the outflow vessels from the corpora cavernosa by sickled erythrocytes. This complication may present as multiple short-lived episodes ('stuttering' priapism) which may progress to 'severe prolonged' priapism lasting several days and leading to permanent sexual dysfunction.

Temporary marrow aplasia can have a profound effect with reticulocytopenia and a very sudden drop in hematocrit. These aplastic crises appear to result from intercurrent infections, particularly due to parvovirus B19 and often occur in epidemics, frequently involving more than one sibling in the same family (see Chapter 14).

Sequestration crises are the most serious of the acute crises, and commonly involve the spleen in the first 2 years of life. Acute splenic sequestration is characterized by sudden, rapid, massive enlargement of the spleen that becomes engorged with sickled erythrocytes. As the crisis progresses, a large proportion of the circulating red cell mass may be trapped in the spleen leading to profound anemia and death. Splenic sequestration shows a tendency to recur in the same individual. A similar type of sequestration may occur in the liver in adult life, causing a dramatic fall in the hematocrit.

Patients with SCD are particularly susceptible to infection, due to *Streptococcus pneumoniae*, salmonella, *Escherichia coli* and *Hemophilus influenza*. Osteomyelitis is common and results from infection of bone infarcts. Pneumococcal pneumonia and overwhelming septicemia are particularly important causes of death in infancy and childhood because of hyposplenism.

Repeated vaso-occlusive events ultimately result in end-organ damage and almost any organ can be affected. The vertebral bodies and femoral heads are particularly prone to infarction. Avascular necrosis of the femoral head may lead to total disability, frequently requiring a total hip prosthesis. Virtually every patient with sickle cell anemia has some form of renal impairment. Sickling of the erythrocytes is enhanced in the hypertonic, hypoxic and acidotic environment of the renal medulla leading to progressive infarction of the medullary papillae. There is progressive inability to concentrate urine, polyuria, nocturia and enuresis, which is common in children. Eventually the glomerular damage causes chronic renal failure, particularly in patients over 40 years of age. Owing to the chronic hemolysis, gallstones are very common and are seen in one-third of SS patients by the age of 10 years. However, it is difficult to assess its clinical significance since only a minority develops clear-cut cholecystitis. Recurrent chronic leg ulceration is common and can be a major handicap (Fig. 9.11). The lesions normally occur just above the medial malleoli and seem to be more common in those patients with severe

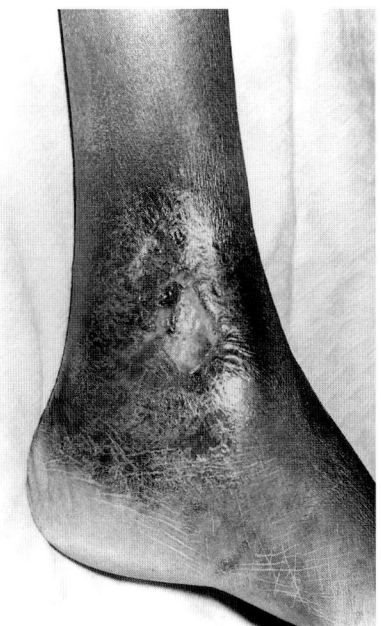

Fig. 9.11 Chronic leg ulcer in an adult with sickle cell anemia. Note the increased pigmentation of the skin around the ulcer. Courtesy of Professor S N Wickramasinghe.

anemia. Proliferative retinopathy leading to progressive visual loss is an important ocular complication, although this is more common in Hb SC disease.

Infection is the major cause of death in children. During the course of the disease, repeated infections lead to hyposplenism increasing the susceptibility to encapsulated bacteria, in particular *Steptococcus pneumonia*. Causes of death in adults are more variable and include infection, acute chest syndrome, liver failure, and stroke and heart failure. In Jamaica, a life expectancy of 58 years for men and 66 years for women has been estimated, while in the USA a median age of death of 42 years for men and 48 years for women was reported in 1994.

Diagnosis

Diagnosis is established by a combination of several tests for the detection and quantification of Hb S plus the other Hbs for the elucidation of the different genetic interactions: hemoglobin electrophoresis on cellulose acetate (pH 8.6) and agar (pH 6.2) and positive sickling or solubility tests.[1] In sickle cell anemia (Hb SS), it is usual to see sickled cells, Howell–Jolly bodies and changes typical of hyposplenism. In Hb SC disease target cells are prominent and Hb C crystals may be present and in Hb S/β thalassemia (or Hb S with α thalassemia) hypochromic microcytic target cells are present.

Because the gene for Hb S (and the structural hemoglobin variants, Hb C and Hb E) and the thalassemias (both α and β) occur together at high frequency in many populations, it is not uncommon for an individual to inherit genes for both types of condition posing difficulties in diagnosis. Although these diagnostic difficulties can normally be resolved by family studies, often family members may not be accessible and one has to rely on a careful assessment of the hemoglobin electrophoresis and the red cell indices. In sickle cell trait (Table 9.3), uncomplicated by α or β thalassemia, the level of Hb S varies between 40 and 45% and is always less than 50%. This is because the β^S chain is positively charged and is less able to compete with the negatively charged β^A chains for the positively charged α-globin subunits.[81,82] In the presence of α thalassemia, in which limiting amounts of α chains are synthesized in the red cells, the effects are exaggerated and the Hb S varies from ~ 25% (in –α/–α) to ~ 35% (in αα/–α). Electrophoretically there may be little difference between Hb SS with high levels of Hb F and Hb S/β^O thalassemia but the latter is accompanied by hypochromic microcytic red cells and an elevated Hb A_2 level. These features are also present in Hb S/β^+ thalassemia, but in this case, there is some Hb A and the Hb S is, of course, more than 50%. However, the increased levels of Hb A_2 does not always reflect the coexistence of β thalassemia. In terms of electrostatic attraction for the α-globin subunit, the δ-globin subunit lies between that of the β^A and β^S. Since the δ-globin chain has a greater affinity for the α subunit compared to β^S, coinheritance of α thalassemia with Hb S can mimic Hb S/β thalassemia. In both scenarios, the Hb S level is lower than expected, the red cells hypochromic microcytic and the level of Hb A_2 increased.

Genetic basis and molecular pathophysiology of disease

Fundamental to the pathophysiology of SCD is the polymerization of the sickle hemoglobin (Hb S) under conditions of deoxygenation.[83] The sickled red cells become less pliable and this leads to vaso-occlusion and all its complications. Polymerization of the Hb S is dependent on several factors – concentration of the Hb S itself, oxygen saturation, pH, temperature and other factors such as the 2, 3-diphosphoglycerate concentration (2,3-DPG). Fully oxygenated Hb S cannot enter the polymer phase whereas partially oxygenated or deoxygenated Hb S can.[84] Mixed hybrids of Hb S with non-S hemoglobins, for example Hb A ($\alpha_2\beta\beta^S$) and Hb C ($\alpha_2\beta^C\beta^S$), have a 0.5 probability of entering the polymer phase while those from Hb F, that is ($\alpha_2\gamma\beta^S$), and Hb A_2 ($\alpha_2\delta\beta^S$) cannot enter the polymer phase.

To understand the pathophysiology of the disease, one should consider the process of polymer formation. When a polymer-free solution is deoxygenated, there is a delay time before any polymer is detected. The delay time is exquisitely dependent on the concentration of the deoxy Hb S, and also pH and temperature. Delay time shortens as deoxy Hb S increases, pH falls and temperature rises. This explains the harmful effects of over-exercise, fever and dehydration. Although polymerization of Hb S is critical, the irreversibly sickled red cells alone are not sufficient for initiating or maintaining the vaso-occlusion that underlies all the complications of SCD. Vaso-occlusion is also dependent on factors extrinsic to the cell, such as the state of the vascular endothelium, vascular tone (balance of vasoconstrictors and vasodilators) and activation of platelets and white cells involving cytokines and adhesion molecules.

The anemia in SCD is primarily hemolytic, a consequence of the shortened survival of the damaged sickled red cells. Survival of the red cells is indirectly related to the level of Hb F since red cells containing Hb F are less likely to sickle. At the molecular level, the sickle mutation is identical in all patients, yet SCD has long been appreciated to exhibit extraordinary phenotypic variability, ranging from mild to very severe. This is, perhaps, not too surprising given that the disease has multiple pleiotropic effects and now occurs against a variety of genetic and environmental backgrounds.[85] Investigations on the genetic modulators concentrated on Hb F levels and its genetic determinants, β-globin gene cluster polymorphisms (β haplotypes) and coinheritance of α thalassemia, which are factors involved at the primary level of the Hb S polymer formation.

These investigations should be interpreted in the context of the different geographical and environmental backgrounds but in general, coinheritance of α thalassemia and high Hb F levels are associated with higher hemoglobin levels, and its complications such as painful bone crises, a lower incidence of leg ulceration, acute chest syndrome and priapism, and persistence of splenomegaly. At the secondary level, it is likely that genetic variants controlling differences in vascular hemodynamics, endothelial adhesion, red cell membrane proteins and cytokine response account for much of the individual variability in vaso-occlusive complications. Environmental factors are less documented but include infection, climate, nutrition, socioeconomic status and medical care.

Management

Currently, there is no specific treatment that is useful in SCD. Management consists of continuous general medical care, attention to good nutrition, immunization, avoidance of extremes of temperature and dehydration, and treatment of complications as they arise.[86] In high-risk populations, neonatal screening programs should be established to identify babies with sickle cell anemia as soon as possible. These babies should be started on prophylactic penicillin at 3–4 months of age followed by polyvalent pneumococcal vaccine at the age of 6–12 months. Once the patient is enrolled in a comprehensive program of care, and if pneumococcal disease has not occurred, prophylactic penicillin can be discontinued at 5 years of age.

Folate supplements should be given during pregnancy and in patients with severe anemia. Transfusions are not usually required except in special circumstances. Episodes of infection should be treated early and sudden exposure to cold and high altitudes avoided. All but the mildest crises should be managed in hospital. The patient should be examined for any underlying infection, kept warm and adequately hydrated, orally or intravenously, and given appropriate antibiotics. Prompt and adequate relief of pain is of prime importance. In selected patients, exchange transfusion may be effective in preventing recurrent painful crises.

Most patients with sickle cell anemia tolerate the relatively low levels of hemoglobin quite well and blood transfusion is usually not required. However, a blood transfusion is indicated when there is a sharp fall in the hemoglobin level due to bone marrow failure (aplastic crisis) or increased hemolysis. A sequestration crisis requires very close surveillance and urgent transfusion is usually indicated due to the prompt development of profound anemia. 'Acute chest syndrome' and cerebrovascular accidents should be treated by partial exchange transfusion, to maintain a level of sickle hemoglobin of < 30% of the total hemoglobin.

Proliferative retinopathy may require photocoagulation or diathermy to reduce the risk of vitreous hemorrhage. Chronic leg ulcers may respond to conservative treatment such as rest and elevation of the affected limb and zinc sulphate dressings. Occasionally, a regime of regular blood transfusion is helpful. Priapism occurs in ~40% of SS male patients. Preliminary data suggest that stilboesterol (5 mg daily) may be effective in preventing a major episode in patients with 'stuttering' priapism. Initial management should be conservative and include sedation, adequate hydration and analgesia and partial exchange transfusion to maintain the level of Hb S at < 30%. Failure to respond after 24 h requires immediate surgical intervention rather than waiting in hope of resolution. Patients who develop a long-standing impotence may benefit from a penile prosthesis.

There is no special treatment during pregnancy except for close supervision and folate supplementation. Blood transfusions are not normally indicated except when there is a significant drop in hemoglobin level or recurrent crises. In such cases a regular transfusion regime should be started to maintain the Hb S level below 30% throughout pregnancy and delivery. Although there is no evidence that oral contraceptives increase the risk of veno-occlusive episodes, it may be prudent to use a low estrogen preparation. Any surgical procedure should be undertaken with caution and scrupulous care taken to avoid factors known to precipitate crisis, including hypoxia, dehydration, cold, acidosis and circulatory stasis. Major surgical procedures may be best carried out after exchange transfusions.

Prenatal diagnosis. Despite the advances in prenatal diagnosis, there has been little uptake of these services with little impact on the prevention of SS disease.[16] The situation may be a reflection of the extreme clinical variability of disease and the ineffective genetic counseling.

Anti-sickling therapy. Treatment for SCD is constantly evolving.[87] Currently, treatment to prevent sickling follow three approaches: chemical inhibition of Hb S polymerization itself, reduction of mean cell hemoglobin concentration (MCHC) and pharmacologic induction of fetal hemoglobin.

Numerous chemical anti-sickling agents have been promoted but none can be regarded as safe and effective. The rationale of reducing MCHC by inducing hyponatremia thereby causing an osmotic swelling of red cells is sound but too cumbersome and risky. Agents that inhibit potassium and water loss from sickle cell erythrocytes by inhibiting the Gardos channel include clotrimazole. Although clotrimazole shows promise in sickle mouse models, further studies to address its therapeutic effects in SCD patients are clearly needed.

Induction of Hb F as a form of therapy was initially based on clinical and epidemiologic observations which showed that even slight elevations of fetal Hb have an ameliorating effect on the clinical severity.[88,89] These observations were subsequently supported by biophysical studies. An increase in intracellular Hb F effectively reduces the concentration of Hb S and mixed hybrids of Hb S and Hb F ($\alpha_2\gamma\beta^S$) do not form polymers. Pharmacologic agents used include 5-azacytidine, a potent inhibitor of DNA methylation, arabinosylcytosine (Ara-C), hydroxyurea, erythropoietin and the butyrate analogs.[90] Hydroxyurea is currently the agent of choice. It is relatively non-toxic, its myelosuppressive effects are reversible and it is not known to induce secondary

malignancies. A recent trial in the USA suggests that hydroxyurea reduced the frequency of hospitalization and the incidence of painful crises, acute chest syndromes and blood transfusion by almost 50% in SS patients given daily hydroxyurea.[91] Hydroxyurea has also been shown to be highly effective in a group of Greek sickle/β thalassemia patients[92] with promising results in children with Hb SS.[93]

Not all patients, however, respond to hydroxyurea. In the multicenter USA trial, the best Hb F responders have the highest baseline neutrophil and reticulocyte counts, which prompted the suggestion that the ability to respond to hydroxyurea is dependent on the capacity of the bone marrow to withstand moderate doses of the agent.[94] Indeed, the clinical benefits of hydroxyurea is not solely dependent on Hb F increases but likely to be associated with the accompanying reduction in the levels of neutrophils, monocytes and reticulocytes, and improved red-cellular hydration, all of which are mitigating factors of vaso-occlusion. Recent trials of pulse intravenous treatment (once or twice monthly) with arginine butyrate have been encouraging. Increases of 7–21% were observed in 11/15 of Hb SS patients and in some individuals, the level was maintained for 1–2 years.[95] A baseline level of 2% Hb F appeared to be critical, only patients who had baseline levels of Hb F above 2% responded.

Bone marrow transplant. Bone marrow transplant (BMT) is currently the only cure for SCD. Because it carries its own mortality, the risk of BMT should always be weighed against the risks of having SCD. The primary barrier to BMT in SCD is the lack of an HLA-identical donor.[96] Until more is known about the natural history of the disease and the ability to predict the disease severity, BMT as a form of curative treatment for all cases is not recommended.

Other sickling disorders

These include mainly the compound heterozygous states for Hb S together with Hbs C, O-Arab, and D-Punjab as well as the inheritance of the β^S gene with the different forms of thalassemia (see Table 9.3).[1]

Sickle/β thalassemia is the most common sickling disorder in individuals of Mediterranean origin. The severity of disease ranges from a completely asymptomatic state to one similar to that seen in sickle cell anemia. Much of this heterogeneity depends on the type of β-thalassemia mutation and the amount of Hb A produced. Because the majority of the β-thalassemia alleles in Africans cause a minimal deficit in β-chain production, sickle/β thalassemia in Africans is generally milder than in the Mediterranean populations. The presence of β thalassemia is indicated by the presence of hypochromic microcytic red cells, a Hb S level of more than 50% on electrophoresis and an elevated level of Hb A_2. Family studies are often crucial in distinguishing between the two disorders. Globin-chain biosynthetic studies are also useful, in S/β thalassemia the $β^S/α$ ratio is 0.5 while in SS disease, it is close to 1.

Other hemoglobin variants

The other hemoglobin variants that are encountered commonly are Hbs C and E (Table 9.4). Hb C is the second most common variant among individuals of African ancestry. Hb C is less soluble than Hb A and tends to crystallize within the red cells leading to their reduced deformability. The important interactions of Hb C are with Hb S (to produce Hb SC disease)[97] and β thalassemia. Individuals with Hb C/$β^O$ thalassemia have a mild to moderate hemolytic anemia.

Hb E (β26 Glu→Lys) is probably the most common hemoglobin variant in the world, occurring in a region extending from Bangladesh through to China, including Southeast Asia. Like SCD and the thalassemias, Hb E carriers have been selected by endemic malaria. Gene frequencies of 50–70% have been recorded in parts of Thailand, Laos and Kampuchea. The pathophysiology of Hb E is thought to result from a combination of inefficient synthesis of Hb E due to activation of a cryptic site in exon 1 of the β-globin gene and reduced stability of Hb E itself. The overall reduction in splicing is the molecular basis for the mild $β^+$-thalassemia phenotype of Hb E.

Hence, when Hb E is coinherited with β thalassemia, Hb E/β thalassemia, a syndrome with the phenotype of β thalassemia intermedia or β thalassemia major results (see section on Hb E/β thalassemia). Other symptomatic forms of Hb E-associated conditions encountered in Southeast Asia include its interaction with the different genotypic forms of Hb H disease.[41] However, inclusions and Hb H ($β^4$) are present only in Hb AE but not Hb E/E or Hb E/$β^0$ thalassemia, presumably the abnormal $β^E$ subunits do not form tetramers.

The diagnosis of Hb E is based on detection or quantitation of the variant by electrophoretic or chromatographic separation of the hemoglobin in peripheral blood. Blood smear shows hypochromic microcytic erythrocytes and target cells. Separation of hemoglobins using routine techniques, including HPLC columns, cannot differentiate Hb E from Hb A_2. In uncomplicated heterozygous Hb E, the variant forms ~ 35% of the total hemoglobin. As with $β^S$, the $β^E$ globin variant is positively charged and is less able to compete with the negatively-charged β globin for the positively-charged α subunits.[82] Hence, when α thalassemia is coinherited with heterozygous Hb E, the proportion of Hb E varies from ~ 10% (in —/-α), 20–22% (in —/-αα or -α/-α) to 27–30% (in αα/-α).

The unstable hemoglobin disorders

Structural changes in the globin subunits can lead to instability of the hemoglobin molecule causing it to precipitate intracellularly, detectable by supravital staining as globular aggregates known as Heinz bodies. These inclusions reduce the life span of the erythrocytes and cause variable hemolysis, an integral part of the syndrome of congenital Heinz body hemolytic anemia (CHBA).[1] The true incidence of CHBA is not known; according to the Globin Gene Server (http://globin.cse.psu.edu), more than 25% of the 800 hemoglobin variants were designated 'unstable' and associated with varying degrees of reticulocytosis and hemolytic anemia. Many of the unstable variants are also associated with a thalassemic phenotype.[33,36] A basis for the phenotypic variation of these disorders lies in the variable instability of the abnormal globin subunits. Those at the severe end

Table 9.4 Molecular abnormalities observed in thalassemic hemoglobinopathies

Unstable variants	e.g. Hb Suan Dok ($α2^{109\ Leu→Arg}$)
Hyperunstable variants	Hb Quong Sze ($α2^{125\ Leu→Pro}$) Hb Showa Yakushiji ($β^{110\ Leu→Pro}$)
Variants that cause abnormal splicing	HbE ($β^{26\ Leu→Lys}$) Hb Knossos ($β^{27\ Ala→Ser}$)
Variants with mutations in the termination codon	Hb Constant Spring ($α2^{142\ Term→Gln}$)a
Variants linked to thalassemic mutation	Hb G-Philadelphia (/-$α^{G-Phil}$)
δ/β fusion globin subunits	Hb Lepore

a Hb Constant Spring is a particularly common form of non-deletion α thalassemia in Thailand.

of the spectrum are not able to form functional tetramers and precipitate in the red cell precursors causing a functional deficiency and a thalassemic phenotype, while the less-unstable globin variants are able to form a hemoglobin tetramer that survives the different stages of red cell maturation only to precipitate in the mature red cell causing hemolysis in the peripheral circulation.

The majority of CHBA follows an autosomal dominant pattern of inheritance; affected individuals are almost exclusively heterozygotes.[1] Unstable hemoglobins are not common, generally limited to single families, and only the proband is affected suggesting that the mutation has arisen by a *de novo* mutation. There are two exceptions: Hb Koln (β98 Val→Met) has been reported in various ethnic groups and often observed as a *de novo* mutation;[73] and Hb Hasharon (α47 Asp→His) is found in Italian families and Ashkenazi Jews, and causes hemolytic anemia in newborns.[73]

Hemolytic anemia, the main feature of the unstable hemoglobins, is highly variable in intensity and often precipitated by infections and exposure to chemical oxidants. Instability of the hemoglobin can be demonstrated by the presence of flocculent precipitates on heating a dilute hemoglobin solution at 50°C for 15 min or by the addition of isopropanol. However, a single test may be negative and multiple tests are often needed.

Blood films are not specific; features include prominent reticulocytosis and basophilic stippling, Howell–Jolly bodies, presence of nucleated red cells, anisocytosis and hypochromia. Heinz bodies can be detected by incubating the erythrocytes with a supravital stain such as new methyline blue or crystal violet. Hb electrophoresis can detect ~ 70% of the unstable hemoglobin, which often appears as a diffuse band.

Most patients with CHBA do not require treatment. General supportive measures include folic-acid supplements, prompt treatment of infection and reduction of fever. Oxidant drugs should be avoided. Transfusions are indicated only rarely, such as during an aplastic crisis. In cases with very severe hemolysis, splenectomy can reduce hemolysis and anemia.

Hemoglobin variants with abnormal oxygen binding

The 1998 Syllabus of Human Hemoglobin Variants (Huismann 1998 #1882) lists 750 human hemoglobin variants, of which 73 have a high oxygen affinity and 26 have a decreased oxygen affinity. The molecular basis underlying the abnormal oxygen binding of these structural hemoglobin variants lies in the perturbation of the transitional state between hemoglobin conformations – R or 'relaxed' in which it has a high affinity for oxygen, and low affinity for effectors such as 2,3-DPG, and T or 'tense' when it has a relatively low affinity for oxygen and high affinity for the allosteric affectors.[98]

The transition between these two conformations requires 'heme–heme interaction', which involves a series of structural changes. Thus, mutations that result in a structural alteration which affects the equilibrium between the R and T states would have a marked effect on hemoglobin binding of oxygen. Both high- and low-oxygen affinity variants have been described.

Mutations for high-oxygen affinity variants have been described only in the heterozygous form with the exception of one α-chain variant, Hb Tarrent (α126 Asp→Asn) in which, on the basis of the Hb electrophoresis quantitation, two of the four α-globin genes were affected.[99] Since most of the affected individuals are likely to have four α-globin genes (αα/αα), α-globin variants cause a less clinically significant condition compared to those of the β subunit.

The first high-affinity mutant to be described was Hb Chesapeake (α92 Arg→Leu) in an 81-year-old man who presented with erythrocytosis and mild angina.[100] The fast-moving electrophoretic variant comprises ~ 20% of the total hemoglobin and was associated with a whole blood P50 of 19 mmHg (normal, 26 mmHg). Molecular basis of the high affinity for oxygen lies in the stabilization of the R state at the α1β2 as a result of the α92 Leu mutation.

High-affinity hemoglobin variants follow an autosomal dominant inheritance pattern; all affected individuals are heterozygotes.[1] A positive family history is useful but occasionally the variants arise from *de novo* mutations. The majority of patients with high-affinity hemoglobins have a benign clinical course and no apparent complications apart from a ruddy complexion. The red cell mass is increased as shown by the increased hemoglobin concentration and hematocrit but the white cell and platelet counts are within normal limits, and splenomegaly is absent. Diagnosis is made by excluding other causes for erythrocytosis (such as primary, inappropriate, increase of erythropoeitin; cardiopulmonary shunt, carbon monoxide poisoning, mutations of the erythropoeitin receptor, etc.), by demonstrating a left-shifted oxygen dissociation curve with a reduced P50 value, a normal 2,3-DPG value and by DNA sequence analysis. A normal hemoglobin electrophoresis or HPLC does not exclude a diagnosis of high-affinity hemoglobin. Mass spectrometry, if available, is an extremely valuable tool for the identification of these variants. The mutation is then confirmed by DNA sequence analysis of the appropriate globin gene.

Most patients with high-affinity hemoglobins require no medical intervention, although rare individuals appear to have benefitted from phlebotomy.

Far fewer hemoglobin variants with low oxygen affinity have been described but should always be considered in any patient with unexplained congenital cyanosis, the differential diagnosis being methemoglobinemia. Cyanosis is present from birth in some carriers of α-globin variants, while cyanosis associated with the β-globin variants presents in the second half of the first year of life when β-globin gene expression predominates.

Diagnosis of a low-oxygen-affinity hemoglobin is made by excluding other causes of cyanosis, especially cardiopulmonary, and differentiation of the cyanosis from that of methemoglobinemia.[101] A simple test is to expose the individual's blood to pure oxygen when it will turn bright red in cases of low-oxygen-affinity hemoglobin and cardiopulmonary disease. In contrast, blood of patients with methemoglobinemia, M hemoglobins and sulfhemoglobinemia retain their abnormal color despite exposure to pure oxygen. Most of the low-oxygen-affinity hemoglobin variants are unstable, and determination of the whole blood P50 is not always reliable. Hemoglobin electrophoresis, mass spectrometry of hemoglobin and DNA sequence analysis are useful tools for diagnosis.

Hemoglobins M

A striking clinical feature of the M hemoglobins is the dusky blue appearance of the skin and mucous membranes.[1] In the vast majority of cases, the cyanosis is due to an excess of deoxyhemoglobin in the blood from a congenital cardiopulmonary defect. Rarely, it can be caused by a low-oxygen-affinity hemoglobin variant. Next in the differential diagnosis are the methemoglobinemias or sulfhemoglobinemias usually caused by a deficiency of the enzyme cytochrome b5 reductase. The enzyme enables red cell hemoglobin to be maintained in a reduced form and deficiency of the enzyme results in oxidized hemoglobin and a cyanotic appearance. A much rarer cause of methemoglobinemia is the presence of one of the M hemoglobins. The M hemoglobins are inherited in an autosomal dominant pattern. Affected individuals present with cyanosis that varies from brownish to slate gray but are otherwise asymptomatic. If cyanosis is present from birth, it is normally due to an α-chain variant, whereas β-chain Hb M produces cyanosis after the first few months of life when adult hemoglobin ($\alpha_2\beta_2$) synthesis becomes established.

Seven M hemoglobins have been described, of which two affect the α-, three the β-, and two, the γ-globin subunit. Six of the seven subunits have substitutions of tyrosine for the proximal (F8) or distal (E7) histidine, creating an abnormal microenvironment for stabilization of the heme iron in the ferric form. As a result of these substitutions, these Hbs M are resistant to reduction by methemoglobin reductase. The M hemoglobins are also functionally abnormal with a decreased oxygen affinity and they are mildly unstable.

The most reliable diagnostic test is based on examination of the hemolysate by recording spectrophotometry which shows an abnormal pattern that is similar to, but not identical with, that of methemoglobin.

Hb electrophoresis is of limited value unless the entire hemolysate is converted to methemoglobin prior to electrophoresis. Diagnosis is confirmed by mass spectrometry and DNA sequence analysis of the globin genes.

The thalassemic hemoglobinopathies

This group of hemoglobin disorders includes structural hemoglobin mutants associated with a thalassemia phenotype (i.e. hypochromia, microcytosis and basophilic stippling).[102] The phenotype ranges from the mild forms of heterozygous thalassemia to that resembling thalassemia intermedia. In some cases, chronic severe hemolytic anemia with splenomegaly is a feature. The molecular abnormalities are remarkably heterogeneous and includes single amino-acid mutations causing hemoglobin variants such as Hbs E and Knossos with abnormal splicing, amino-acid deletions, elongated or truncated globin chains and fusion globins such as Hb Lepore (Table 9.5).

Some of the α-globin mutants are invariably linked to a tandem α-globin gene deletion and hence the concomitant deficiency, for example Hb G-Philadelphia (/-$\alpha^{G\text{-Phil}}$). Thalassemic hemoglobinopathies also include an increasing number of α- and β- structural variants in which the amino-acid substitutions confer such instability that they are readily degraded in the bone marrow erythroid precursors resulting in an ineffective erythropoiesis and a thalassemic phenotype.[33] The hyperunstable β-globin-chain variants cause a disease phenotype even in heterozygotes who produce normal chains as well – hence, the alternative term 'dominantly inherited β thalassemia'.[36] As information accumulates on the hemoglobin variants, it is becoming clear that there is a continuum that blurs the distinction between those producing a thalassemia phenotype and those that give rise to CHBA. The critical determinant appears to be the degree of instability of the globin subunit (see section on CHBA).

Acknowledgment

I thank Claire Steward for preparation of the manuscript.

REFERENCES

1. Bunn HF, Forget BG 1986 Hemoglobin: Molecular, genetic and clinical aspects. WB Saunders Philadelphia
2. Stamatoyannopoulos G, Nienhuis AW 1994 Hemoglobin switching. In: Stamatoyannopoulos G, Nienhuis AW, Majerus PW, Varmus H (eds), The molecular basis of blood diseases 2nd edn. WB Saunders Philadelphia, 107–155
3. Forget BG, Molecular genetics of the human globin genes. In: Steinberg MH, Forget BG, Higgs DR, Nagel RL (eds), Disorders of hemoglobin: genetics, pathophysiology, and clinical management. Cambridge University Press, Cambridge, 117–130
4. Blobel GA, Weiss MJ 2001 Nuclear factors that regulate erythropoeisis. In: Steinberg MH, Forget BG, Higgs DR, Nagel RL (eds), Disorders of hemoglobin: genetics, pathophysiology, and clinical management. Cambridge University Press, Cambridge, 72–94
5. Orkin SH 1995 Regulation of globin gene expression in erythroid cells. European Journal of Biochemistry 231: 271–281
6. Perkins AC, Sharpe AH, Orkin SH 1995 Lethal β-thalassaemia in mice lacking the erythroid CACCC-transcription factor EKLF. Nature 375: 318–322
7. Nuez B, Michalovich D, Bygrave A et al 1995 Defective haematopoiesis in fetal liver resulting from inactivation of the EKLF gene. Nature 375: 316–318
8. Feng WC, Southwood CM, Bieker JJ 1994 Analyses of β-thalassemia mutant DNA interactions with erythroid Krüppel-like factor (EKLF), an erythroid cell-specific transcription factor. Journal of Biological Chemistry 269: 1493–1500
9. Tewari R, Gillemans N, Wijgerde M et al 1998 Erythroid krüppel-like factor (EKLF) is active in primitive and definitive erythroid cells and is required for the function of 5'HS3 of the β-globin locus control region. EMBO Journal 17: 2334–2341
10. Guy L-G, Mei Q, Perkins AC et al 1998 Erythroid Krüppel-like factor is essential for β-globin gene expression even in absence of gene competition, but is not sufficient to induce the switch from γ-globin to β-globin gene expression. Blood 91: 2259–2263
11. Weatherall DJ, Clegg JB 1996 Thalassemia – a global public health problem. Nature Medicine 2(8): 847–849
12. Beris P, Miescher PA, Diaz-Chico JC et al 1988 Inclusion-body β-thalassemia trait in a Swiss family is caused by an abnormal hemoglobin (Geneva) with an altered and extended β chain carboxy-terminus due to a modification in codon β114. Blood 72: 801–805
13. Cooley TB, Lee P. 1925 A series of cases of splenomegaly in children with anemia and peculiar bone changes. Trans Am Pediatr Soc 37: 29
14. Weatherall DJ, Clegg JB 1981 The thalassaemia syndromes. Oxford: Blackwell Scientific
15. Angastiniotis M, Modell B, Englezos P, Boulyjenkov V 1995 Prevention and control of haemoglobinopathies. Bulletin of the World Health Organization 73: 375–386
16. Modell B, Petrou M, Layton M et al 1997 Audit of prenatal diagnosis for haemoglobin disorders in the United Kingdom: the first 20 years. British Medical Journal 315: 779–784
17. Thein SL 1998 Baillières clinical haematology: beta thalassaemia in sickle cell disease and thalassaemia. In: Rodgers GP (ed), Sickle cell disease and thalassaemia. London: Baillière Tindall; p. 91–126
18. Olivieri N, Weatherall DJ 2001 Clinical aspects of β thalassemia. In: Steinberg MH, Forget BG, Higgs DR, Nagel RL, editors. Disorders of Hemoglobin: Genetics, Pathophysiology, and Clinical Management. Cambridge University Press, Cambridge 277–341
19. Rees DC, Luo LY, Thein SL et al 1997 Nontransfusional iron overload in thalassemia: association with hereditary hemochromatosis. Blood 90: 3234–3236
20. Piperno A, Mariani R, Arosio C et al 2000 Haemochromatosis in patients with beta-thalassaemia trait. British Journal of Haematology 111(3): 908–14
21. Andrews N 2000 Iron homeostasis: insights from genetics and animal models. Nature Reviews Genetics 1: 208–216
22. Galanello R, Perseu L, Melis MA et al 1997 Hyperbilirubinaemia in heterozygous β-thalassaemia is related to co-inherited Gilbert's syndrome. British Journal of Haematology 99: 433–436
23. Galanello R, Cipollina MD, Dessì C et al 1999 Co-inherited Gilbert's syndrome: a factor determining hyperbilirubinemia in homozygous β-thalassemia. Haematologica 84: 103–105
24. Sampietro M, Lupica L, Perrero L, Comino A, Martinez di Montemuros F 1997 The expression of uridine diphosphate glucuronosyltransferase gene is a major determinant of bilirubin level in heterozygous β-thalassaemia and in glucose-6-phosphate. British Journal of Haematology 99: 437–439
25. Wonke B 1998 Bone disease in β-thalassaemia major. British Journal of Haematology 103: 897–901
26. Dresner Pollack R, Rachmilewitz E, Blumenfeld A, Idelson M, Goldfarb AW 2000 Bone mineral metabolism in adults with beta-thalassaemia major and intermedia. British Journal of Haematology 111(3): 902–907
27. Flint J, Harding RM, Boyce AJ, Clegg JB 1998 The population genetics of the haemoglobinopathies. In: Rodgers GP (ed), Baillière's clinical haematology. London: Baillière Tindall; p. 1–52
28. Huisman THJ, Carver MFH, Baysal E 1997 A syllabus of thalassemia mutations The Sickle Cell Anemia Foundation, Augusta, GA
29. Maragoudaki E, Kanavakis E, Trager-Synodinos J et al 1999 Molecular, haematological and clinical studies of the -101 C→T substitution in the β-globin gene promoter in 25 β-thalassaemia intermedia patients and 45 heterozygotes. British Journal of Haematology 107: 699–706
30. Frischmeyer PA, Dietz HC. 1999 Nonsense-mediated mRNA decay in health and disease. Human Molecular Genetics 8: 1893–1900
31. Hentze MW, Kulozik AE 1999 A perfect message: RNA surveillance and nonsense-mediated decay. Cell 96: 307–310
32. Nagy E, Maquat LE 1998 A rule for termination-codon position within intron-containing genes: when nonsense affects RNA abundance. Trends in Biological Sciences 23: 198–199
33. Thein SL 2001 Structural variants with a β-thalassemia phenotype. In: Steinberg MH, Forget BG, Higgs DR, Nagel RL, (eds), Disorders of hemoglobin: genetics, pathophysiology, and clinical management. Cambridge University Press, Cambridge, 342–355
34. Thein SL, Hesketh C, Taylor P et al 1990 Molecular basis for dominantly inherited inclusion body β-thalassaemia. Proceedings of the National Academy of Sciences, USA 87: 3924–3928
35. Adams JG, III, Morrison WT, Steinberg MH et al 1986 Isolation of the protein product of β°-thalassaemia gene containing a nonsense mutation. Blood 64: 69a
36. Thein SL 1999 Is it dominantly inherited β thalassaemia or just a β-chain variant that is highly unstable? British Journal of Haematology 107: 12–21
37. Thein SL, Old JM, Wainscost JS et al 1984 Population and genetic studies suggest a single origin for the Indian deletion β° thalassaemia. British Journal of Haematology 57: 271–278
38. Varawalla NY, Old JM, Sarkar R et al 1991 The spectrum of β-thalassaemia mutations on the Indian subcontinent: the basis for prenatal diagnosis. British Journal of Haematology 78: 242–247
39. Trent RJ, Williams BG, Kearney A et al 1990 Molecular and hematologic characterization of Scottish–Irish type (εγδβ)° thalassaemia. Blood 76: 2132–2138
40. Weatherall DJ, Clegg JB, (eds) 2001 The thalassaemia syndromes, 4th edn. Oxford: Blackwell Science
41. Fucharoen S 2001 Hemoglobin E disorders. In: Steinberg MH, Forget BG, Higgs DR, Nagel RL (eds). Disorders of hemoglobin: genetics, pathophysiology, and clinical management. Cambridge University Press, Cambridge, 1139–1154
42. Wood WG 2001 Hereditary persistence of fetal hemoglobin and δβ thalassemia. In: Steinberg MH, Forget BG, Higgs DR, Nagel RL, (eds). Disorders of Hemoglobin: Genetics, Pathophysiology, and Clinical Management. Cambridge University Press, Cambridge, p. 356–388
43. Rochette J, Craig JE, Thein SL 1994 Fetal hemoglobin levels in adults. Blood Reviews 8: 213–224
44. Ottolenghi S, Giglioni B, Pulazzini A et al 1987 Sardinian δβ°-thalassemia: a further example of a C to T substitution at position -196 of the $^{A}\gamma$ globin gene promoter. Blood 69: 1058–1061
45. Thein SL, Craig JE 1998 Genetics of Hb F/F cell variance in adults and heterocellular hereditary persistence of fetal hemoglobin. Hemoglobin 22: 401–414
46. Craig JE, Rochette J, Fisher CA et al 1996 Dissecting the loci controlling fetal haemoglobin production on chromosomes 11p and 6q by the regressive approach. Nature Genetics 12: 58–64

47. Dover GJ, Smith KD, Chang YC et al 1992 Fetal hemoglobin levels in sickle cell disease and normal individuals are partially controlled by an X-linked gene located at Xp22.2. Blood 80: 816–824
48. Ho PJ, Hall GW, Luo LY et al 1998 Beta thalassemia intermedia: is it possible to consistently predict phenotype from genotype? British Journal of Haematology 100: 70–78
49. Camaschella C, Maza U, Roetto A et al 1995 Genetic interactions in thalassemia intermedia: analysis of β-mutations, α-genotype, γ-promoters, and β-LCR hypersensitive sites 2 and 4 in Italian patients. American Journal of Hematology 48: 82–87
50. Rund D, Oron-Karni V, Filon D et al 1997 Genetic analysis of β-thalassaemia intermedia in Israel: diversity of mechanisms and unpredictability of phenotype. American Journal of Hematology 54: 16–22
51. Labie D, Pagnier J, Lapoumeroulie C et al 1985 Common haplotype dependency of high $^G\gamma$-globin gene expression and high Hb F levels in β-thalassemia and sickle cell anemia patients. Proceedings of the National Academy of Sciences, USA 82: 2111–2114
52. Thein SL, Wainscoat JS, Sampietro M et al 1987 Association of thalassaemia intermedia with a beta-globin gene haplotype. British Journal of Haematology 65: 367–373
53. Gianni AM, Bregni M, Cappellini MD et al 1983 A gene controlling fetal hemoglobin expression in adults is not linked to the non-α globin cluster. EMBO Journal 2: 921–925
54. Thein SL, Weatherall DJ 1989 A non-deletion hereditary persistence of fetal hemoglobin (HPFH) determinant not linked to the β-globin gene complex. In: Stamatoyannopoulos G, Nienhuis AW, (eds). Hemoglobin Switching, Part B: Cellular and Molecular Mechanisms. New York: Alan R Liss, p. 97–111
55. Thein SL, Al-Hakim I, Hoffbrand AV 1984 Thalassaemia intermedia: a new molecular basis. British Journal of Haematology 56: 333–337
56. Camaschella C, Kattamis AC, Petroni D et al 1997 Different hematological phenotypes caused by the interaction of triplicated α-globin genes and heterozygous β-thalassemia. American Journal of Hematology 55: 83–88
57. Traeger-Synodinos J, Kanavakis E, Vrettou C et al 1996 The triplicated α-globin gene locus in β-thalassaemia heterozygotes: clinical, haematological, biosynthetic and molecular studies. British Journal of Haematology 95: 467–471
58. Higgs DR, 1993 α-thalassaemia. In: Higgs DR, Weatherall DJ, (eds). Baillière's clinical haematology. International practice and research: the haemoglobinopathies. London: Baillière Tindall; p. 117–150
59. Higgs DR, DK B 2001 Clinical and laboratory features of the α-thalassaemia syndromes. In: Steinberg MH, Forget BG, Higgs DR, Nagel RL, (eds). Disorders of hemoglobin: genetics, pathophysiology, and clinical management. Cambridge University Press, Cambridge, p. 431–469
60. Higgs DR 2001 Molecular Mechanisms of α Thalassaemia. In: Steinberg MH, Forget BG, Higgs DR, Nagel RL, (eds). Disorders of Hemoglobin: Genetics, Pathophysiology, and Clinical Management. Cambridge University Press, Cambridge, p. 405–430
61. Higgs DR, Wood WG, Jarman AP et al 1990 A major positive regulatory region located far upstream of the human α-globin gene locus. Genes and Development 4: 1588–1601
62. Kanavakis E, Papassotiriou I, Karagiorga M et al 2000 Phenotypic and molecular diversity of haemoglobin H disease: a Greek experience. British Journal of Haematology 111(3): 915–923
63. Liebhaber SA, Schrier SL 2001 Pathophysiology of α Thalassaemia. In: Steinberg MH, Forget BG, Higgs DR, Nagel RL, (eds). Disorders of Hemoglobin: Genetics, Pathophysiology, and Clinical Management. Cambridge University Press, Cambridge, p. 391–404
64. Gibbons RJ, Higgs DR 2001 The Alpha Thalassaemia/Mental Retardation Syndromes. In: Steinberg MH, Forget BG, Higgs DR, Nagel RL, (eds). Disorders of Hemoglobin: Genetics, Pathophysiology, and Clinical Management. Cambridge University Press, Cambridge, p. 470–488
65. Wilkie AOM, Buckle VJ, Harris PC et al 1990 Clinical features and molecular analysis of the α thalassaemia/mental retardation syndromes. I. Cases due to deletions involving chromosome band 16p 13.3. American Journal of Human Genetics 46: 1112–1126
66. Wilkie AOM, Zeitlin HC, Lindenbaum RH et al 1990 Clinical features and molecular analysis of the α thalassaemia/mental retardation syndromes. II. Cases without detectable abnormality of the α globin complex. American Journal of Human Genetics 46: 1127–1140
67. Cao A, Galanello R, Rosatelli MC 1998 Prenatal diagnosis and screening of the haemoglobinopathies. In: Rodgers GP, (ed). Baillière's Clinical Haematology. London: Baillière Tindall; p. 215–238
68. Oliveri NF, Brittenham GM, McLaren CE et al 1998 Long-term safety and effectiveness of iron-chelation therapy with deferiprone for thalassemia major. New England Journal of Medicine 339: 417–423
69. Angelucci E, Lucarelli G 2001 Bone Marrow Transplantation in β Thalassaemia. In: Steinberg MH, Forget BG, Higgs DR, Nagel RL, (eds). Disorders of Hemoglobin: Genetics, Pathophysiology, and Clinical Management. Cambridge University Press, Cambridge, p. 1052–1072.
70. Mariotti E, Angelucci E, Agostini A et al 1998 Evaluation of cardiac status in iron-loaded thalassaemia patients following bone marrow transplantation: improvement in cardiac function during reduction in body iron burden. British Journal of Haematology 103: 916–921
71. Sorrentino BP, Nienhuis AW 2001 Prospects for Gene Therapy of Sickle Cell Disease and β Thalassemia. In: Steinberg MH, Forget BG, Higgs DR, Nagel RL, (eds). Disorders of Hemoglobin: Genetics, Pathophysiology, and Clinical Management. Cambridge University Press; Cambridge p. 1084–1118
72. Rodgers GP, Steinberg MH 2001 Pharmacologic Treatment of Sickle Cell Disease and Thalassemia: The Augmentation of Fetal Hemoglobin. In: Steinberg MH, Forget BG, Higgs DR, Nagel RL, (eds). Disorders of Hemoglobin: Genetics, Pathophysiology, and Clinical Management. Cambridge University Press; Cambridge p. 1028–1051
73. Huisman THJ, Carver MFH, Efremov GD 1998 A Syllabus of Human Hemoglobin Variants. 2nd ed. Augusta, GA, The Sickle Cell Anemia Foundation.
74. Herrick JB 1910 Peculiar elongated and sickle-shaped red blood corpuscles in a case of severe anemia. Archives of Internal Medicine 6: 517–521
75. Pauling L, Itano HA, Singer SJ, Wells IC 1949 Sickle cell anemia: a Molecular Disease. Science 110: 543–548
76. Ingram VM 1956 A specific chemical difference between the globins of normal human and sickle cell anaemia haemoglobin. Nature 178: 792–794
77. Serjeant GR 1997 Sickle cell disease. Lancet 350: 725–730
78. Embury SH, Hebbel RP, Mohandas N, Steinberg MH 1994 Sickle Cell Disease: Basic Principles and Clinical Practice. New York: Raven Press.
79. Nagel RL, Steinberg MH 2001 Genetics of the β^S Gene: Origins, Genetic Epidemiology, and Epistasis in sickle cell Anemia. In: Steinberg MH, Forget BG, Higgs DR, Nagel RL, (eds). Disorders of Hemoglobin: Genetics, Pathophysiology, and Clinical Management. Cambridge University Press, Cambridge, p. 711–755
80. Ohene-Frempong K 1991 Stroke in sickle cell disease: demographic, clinical, and therapeutic considerations. Seminars in Hematology 28(3): 213–219
81. Bunn HF, McDonald MJ 1983 Electrostatic interactions in the assembly of human hemoglobin. Nature 306: 498–500
82. Bunn HF 1987 Subunit assembly of hemoglobin: an important determinant of hematologic phenotype. Blood 69: 1–6
83. Nagel RL, Platt OS 2001 General Pathophysiology of Sickle Cell Anemia. In: Steinberg MH, Forget BG, Higgs DR, Nagel RL, (eds). Disorders of Hemoglobin: Genetics, Pathophysiology, and Clinical Management. Cambridge University Press, Cambridge, p. 494–526
84. Noguchi C, Schechter AN, Rodgers GP 1993 Sickle cell disease pathophysiology. In: Higgs DR, Weatherall DJ, (eds). Baillière's Clinical Haematology: The Haemoglobinopathies. London: Baillière Tindall p. 57–91
85. Serjeant G 2001 Geographic Heterogeneity of Sickle Cell Disease. In: Steinberg MH, Forget BG, Higgs DR, Nagel RL, (eds). Disorders of Hemoglobin: Genetics, Pathophysiology, and Clinical Management. Cambridge University Press; Cambridge p. 895–905
86. Steinberg MH 1999 Management of sickle cell disease. New England Journal of Medicine 340(13): 1021–1030
87. Beuzard Y, De Franceschi L 2001 Experimental Therapies for Sickle Cell Anemia and β Thalassaemia. In: Steinberg MH, Forget BG, Higgs DR, Nagel RL, (eds). Disorders of Hemoglobin: Genetics, Pathophysiology, and Clinical Management. Cambridge University Press, Cambridge, p. 1119–1135
88. Platt OS, Thorington BD, Brambilla DJ et al 1991 Pain in sickle cell disease: Rates and risk factor. New England Journal of Medicine 325: 11–16

89. Platt OS, Brambilla DJ, Rosse WF et al 1994 Mortality in sickle cell disease: Life expectancy and risk factors for early death. New England Journal of Medicine 330: 1639–1644

90. Bunn HF 1999 Induction of fetal hemoglobin in sickle cell disease. Blood 93: 1787–1789

91. Charache S, Terrin ML, Moore RD, et al 1995 Effect of hydroxyurea on the frequency of painful crises in sickle cell anemia. New England Journal of Medicine 332: 1317–1322

92. Voskaridou E, Kalotychou V, Loukopoulos D 1995 Clinical and laboratory effects of long-term administration of hydroxyurea to patients with sickle cell/β-thalassaemia. British Journal of Haematology 89(3): 479–484

93. Kinney TR, Helms RW, O'Branski EE et al 1999 Safety of hydroxyurea in children with sickle cell anemia: results of the HUG-KIDS study, a phase I/II trial. Blood 94: 1550–1554

94. Steinberg MH, Lu Z-H, Barton FB et al 1997 Fetal hemoglobin in sickle cell anemia: Determinants of response to hydroxyurea. Blood 89(3): 1078–1088

95. Atweh GF, Sutton M, Nassif I et al 1999 Sustained induction of fetal hemoglobin by pulse butyrate therapy in sickle cell disease. Blood 93(6): 1790–1797

96. Vermylen C 2001 Bone Marrow Transplantation in Sickle Cell Anemia. In: Steinberg MH, Forget BG, Higgs DR, Nagel RL, (eds). Disorders of Hemoglobin: Genetics, Pathophysiology, and Clinical Management. Cambridge University Press, Cambridge, p. 1073–1083

97. Nagel RL, Steinberg MH 2001 Hemoglobin SC Disease and HbC Disorders. In: Steinberg MH, Forget BG, Higgs DR, Nagel RL, (eds). Disorders of Hemoglobin: Genetics, Pathophysiology, and Clinical Management. Cambridge University Press, Cambridge, p. 756–785

98. Perutz MF 2001 Molecular anatomy and physiology of hemoglobin. In: Steinberg MH, Forget BG, Higgs DR, Nagel RL (eds), Disorders of hemoglobin: genetics, pathophysiology, and clinical management. Cambridge University Press, Cambridge, 174–196

99. Ibarra B, Vaca G, Cantu JM et al 1981 Heterozygosity and homozygosity for the high oxygen affinity hemoglobin Tarrant or alpha 126 (H9) Asp replaced by Asn in two Mexican families. Hemoglobin 5(4): 337–48

100. Charache S, Weatherall DJ, Clegg JB 1966 Polycythemia associated with a hemoglobinopathy. Journal of Clinical Investigation 45: 813–822

101. Nagel RL 2001 Disorders of Hemoglobin Function and Stability. In: Steinberg MH, Forget BG, Higgs DR, Nagel RL, (eds). Disorders of Hemoglobin. Genetics, Pathophysiology, and Clinical Management. Cambridge University Press, Cambridge, p. 1155–1194

102. Steinberg MH, Adams JG 1983 Thalassemic hemoglobinopathies. American Journal of Pathology 113: 396–409

Acquired hemolytic anemia

10

JG Kelton   H Chan   N Heddle   S Whittaker

Introduction

Clinical presentation and laboratory features

Pathogenesis of immune and non-immune hemolytic anemias

Immune hemolytic anemia

Autoimmune hemolytic anemia
Warm autoimmune hemolytic anemia (WAHA)
Immune specificity of WAHA
The diagnostic evaluation of a patient with suspected WAHA
Management of patients with WAHA
Cold autoimmune hemolytic anemia
Paroxysmal cold hemoglobinuria

Alloimmune hemolytic anemia
Transfusion reactions due to immune-mediated hemolysis
Hemolytic disease of the newborn

Drug-induced hemolytic anemia
Drug-induced autoantibody
Drug (hapten) dependent antibody
Innocent bystander
Oxidative injury to red cells

Non-immune hemolytic anemia

Infection-induced hemolytic anemia

Mechanical trauma to red cells
Thrombotic thrombocytopenic purpura – hemolytic uremic syndrome
Cardiac hemolysis
External impact on the red cells
Thermal damage of red cells
Osmotic damage of red cells

Miscellaneous causes of hemolytic anemia
Paroxysmal nocturnal hemoglobinuria
Venom-induced hemolytic anemia
Toxin-induced hemolytic anemia
Hemolytic anemia in organ dysfunction

Introduction

As described earlier, hemolysis is a process characterized by accelerated red cell destruction, which can be compensated for if the body steps up production of new red blood cells. However, if red cell destruction surpasses production, hemolytic anemia could result. Hemolytic anemia is traditionally categorized by cause as either congenital or acquired. Congenital hemolytic anemia has previously been presented in detail; therefore, this chapter is restricted to a discussion of acquired hemolytic anemia.

The term 'acquired hemolytic anemia' was first coined in the early 1900s[1] and it is now commonly used to describe hemolytic anemia triggered by extrinsic factors such as immune disorders, drugs, infections, mechanical trauma to red cells, exposure to toxins, and other miscellaneous causes. Generally, acquired hemolytic anemia can be classified as immune hemolytic anemia (auto-immune, alloimmune or drug-induced) and non-immune hemolytic anemia (infection-induced, mechanical trauma, and other miscellaneous causes, including paroxysmal nocturnal hemoglobinuria). In this chapter, the various categories of acquired hemolytic anemia are reviewed including pathogenesis, clinical presentation, treatment and management.

Clinical presentation and laboratory features

Similar to other anemia, the symptoms of acquired hemolytic anemia generally include: fever, abdominal pain, back pain or pain in the limbs (which may mimic acute abdominal conditions or musculoskeletal diseases); cardiovascular symptoms such as dyspnea, angina and tachycardia; or non-specific complaints of generalized malaise or dizziness. In some cases, patients can be asymptomatic and their pallor is detected by family members or other individuals. Jaundice and brownish discolored urine are also typical of acute hemolysis. Sometimes, in massive acute hemolysis, shock and renal failure can occur.

Determining whether the hemolytic anemia has an intravascular or extravascular origin can be helpful when establishing the diagnosis. The differential diagnosis of extravascular hemolysis is more extensive than that of intravascular hemolysis with the five most common intravascular hemolytic disorders being: cold autoimmune hemolysis; malaria; drug-induced hemolysis; major ABO blood group incompatibility; and paroxysmal nocturnal hemoglobinuria. Table 10.1 provides a summary of the laboratory results typically seen in intravascular and extravascular hemolysis.

The diagnostic pathway and related laboratory tests used to determine whether a patient has a hemolytic anemia are presented in Chapter 6 of this book. Laboratory test information is discussed in this section as they pertain to specific acquired hemolytic anemia. The laboratory tests that are typically reviewed when diagnosing acquired hemolytic anemia are: peripheral blood film examination, reticulocyte count, bilirubin, haptoglobin, hemoglobinemia, methemalbumin and hemopexin, hemoglobinuria and hemosiderinuria, lactate dehydrogenase (LDH) and aspartate aminotransferase (AST), bone marrow examination, direct antiglobulin test (Coombs' test), and determination of red cell lifespan using radioactive isotope-labeled red cells.

Table 10.1 Typical features that distinguish between intravascular and extravascular hemolysis

		Intravascular hemolysis	Extravascular hemolysis
Mechanism		Red cell destruction in the intravascular compartment resulting in hemoglobin being released into the plasma	Red cells are recognized as foreign or become more rigid and are sequestered in the spleen with subsequent phagocytosis
Possible causes		Complement, toxins, membrane defects, enzyme deficiencies, drugs	Immunoglobulin, complement, membrane defects
Laboratory feature			
Hemoglobinemia		Present	Absent/present in severe cases
Hemoglobinuria		Present	Absent/present in severe cases
Haptoglobin		Reduced or absent	Normal or reduced
Methemalbumin		Present	Absent
Hemosidinuria		Present	Absent
LDH		Grossly elevated	Elevated
Jaundice		Present	Present
Splenomegaly		Absent	Present
Blood film		Schistocytes, helmet cells, fragmented red cells	Spherocytes, erythrophagocytosis

LDH, lactate dehydrogenase.

Pathogenesis of immune and non-immune hemolytic anemias

In this chapter, immune hemolytic anemia is classified as autoimmune, alloimmune and drug-induced; whereas, non-immune hemolytic anemia is presented under the headings of infection-induced, mechanical trauma and other miscellaneous causes. Note that different causes of hemolytic anemia can overlap. For example, drug-induced hemolysis often overlaps with immune hemolysis because drugs can cause hemolysis either by immune mechanism or by direct damage to the red cells.

Immune hemolytic anemia

Immune hemolytic anemia is the most common form of acquired hemolytic anemia and it can be classified as autoimmune, alloimmune or drug-induced. Irrespective of the etiology, the typical feature in the peripheral blood smear is microspherocytosis (Fig. 10.1).

Autoimmune hemolytic anemia

Autoimmune hemolytic anemia (AIHA) involves the premature destruction of red blood cells by autoantibodies. AIHA may be idiopathic (no underlying cause identified) or secondary to underlying malignancy or disorder such as lymphoid malignancy, connective tissue disorders, infection, medication, vaccinations, HIV-induced, myelodys-

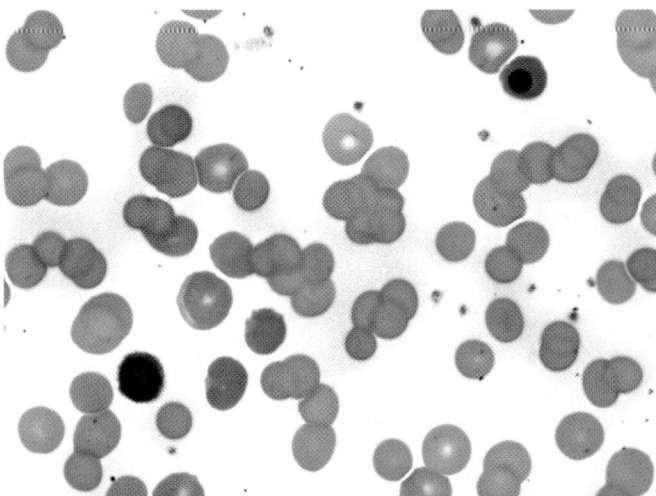

Fig. 10.1 Peripheral blood smear showing microspherocytosis, nucleated red cell, and red cell clumps in a patient with immune mediated hemolysis. The spherocytes lack central halo of normal red cells and they are smaller than the nucleus of a normal lymphocyte. Wright stain, × 1000, oil field.

plastic syndrome,[2] or graft-versus-host disease. In one study, neoplasia-related AIHA was the most common secondary cause (233/1834 patients; 2.7%) followed by drug-induced hemolysis (140/1834 patients; 7.6%).[2] For diagnostic evaluations, it is important to determine the autoantibody idiotype. Autoantibodies may readily be separated into warm antibody or cold antibody based on the thermal range of the antibody and this classification serves as the framework of the following discussion.

Warm autoimmune hemolytic anemia (WAHA)

Warm autoimmune hemolytic anemia (WAHA) accounts for more than 70% of AIHAs[3] and it is caused by production of an autoantibody directed against the patient's red cells. Most frequently, the autoantibody is IgG (particularly IgG1 and IgG3 subclass),[4] although IgM and IgA can be detected in addition to IgG.[5] IgA warm autoantibody is rare, and most antiglobulin reagents are unable to detect this immunoglobulin. Warm autoantibody (IgG) may cause extravascular hemolysis through one of two mechanisms: (1) Fc receptor-mediated immune adherence; and (2) complement mediated hemolysis. Most warm autoantibodies do not cause autoagglutination or intravascular hemolysis.

Fc receptor (FcR)-mediated immune adherence

Antibody-coated red cells can be removed from the circulation by two different mechanisms: phagocytosis and cell lysis. During the phagocytic process, macrophages engulf and lyse red cells by formation of oxygen radicals in the cytoplasm; whereas, for cytotoxic cell lysis, the target cell is destroyed by the lysosomal enzyme released by the phagocytic cells.[6]

The phagocytic process is facilitated by the deposition of opsonins, including antibody or C3b, on the antigen. The immune effector cells have receptors (FcR) on the cell surface for the Fc portion of antibodies. There are at least three different classes of IgG FcR on the macrophages (FcγRI, FcγRII and FcγRIII). FcγRII and FcγRIII bind to IgG oligomer[7,8] but FcγRI binds only to monomeric IgG.[9,10] FcγRII and FcγRIII binds IgG3 oligomer and IgG1 oligomer with the highest affinity.[9] The high affinity of IgG3 to FcRs might explain why IgG3 is the most efficient warm antibody in extravascular hemolysis *in vivo*.[3,11] The *in vivo* functions of FcγRIII include phagocytosis, endocytosis and antibody-dependent cell-mediated cytotoxicity.[12,13] FcγRII is an inhibitory receptor and acts as a negative regulator of B-cell and mast cell activation.[14,15] On the other hand, FcγRI exclusively mediates *in vitro* cytotoxic activity.[16]

Apart from IgG, the presence of other classes of anti-red cell antibodies (IgM and IgA) is a major determining factor of hemolysis.[4] IgM, apart from complement activation, may synergistically enhance IgG-mediated hemolysis. It has been demonstrated that patients with red cells coated with IgG and IgM have more severe hemolysis than those with IgG alone as these patients have lower level of haptoglobin.[5] IgA autoantibodies, although rare, probably induce hemolysis via FcR in the same way as IgG.[2] However, the exact relationship between FcR and the different combinations of immunoglobulin classes remains unclear. Circulating monocytes, K-cells and granulocytes also have FcR; however, the role of these cells in the pathogenesis of hemolysis is uncertain, although it has been postulated that they may play a role in patients with immune hemolytic anemia refractory to splenectomy.[17]

The amount of antibody bounded on the red cell surface also determines the mechanism of FcR-mediated hemolysis. When the amount of antibody on the red cell membrane is low, the phagocytic process is predominant.[2] However, because IgG1 is a less efficient mediator of phagocytosis than IgG3, IgG1 coated red cells are not always rapidly destroyed.

Under normal conditions, a typical splenic macrophage has 30 000–40 000 FcR per cell.[18] Concomitant infection or immunization worsens the hemolysis by increasing the number and affinity of FcR, possibly through cytokines such as gamma interferon.[19] Circulating neutrophils probably have only a marginal role in autoimmune phagocytosis, however, they may become important during infection.[20]

In summary, the FcR-mediated cell destruction processes depend on a number of factors: the specific immune characteristics of the immunoglobulins; the amount of antibody bound to the red cells; and the overall activity of the macrophages in the reticuloendothelial system.

Complement-mediated hemolysis

The activation of the complement cascade, up to and including the terminal pathway, brings about the formation of a membrane attack complex and intravascular hemolysis. To activate the complement pathways, two FcRs must be spatially close together. IgM is the most efficient antibody class in the activation of complement; however, in warm autoimmune hemolysis, IgG on the red cell membrane occasionally may be of sufficient density to activate complement. Of the IgG subclass, IgG3 and IgG1 bind readily to C1q, but not IgG4.

Complement activation is controlled by a number of regulatory mechanisms. Some complement fragments can become enzymatically cleaved and the cleavage products, such as C3d or C4d, are incapable of further activation. The complement inhibitors on cell membrane include decay accelerating factor (DAF),[21] C8-binding protein,[22,23] membrane cofactor protein, CR1/CD35 protein and P18/CD59 protein.[24] Other proteins such as C1 inhibitors, C4 binding protein, factor H and factor I are circulating in the plasma. The complement cascade is arrested and early complement protein fragments are bound to the red cell membrane. The complement-coated red cells are then recognized by complement receptors on hepatic Kupffer's cells. It has been demonstrated that about 550–800 bound C3b molecules are required to trigger hepatic clearance of red cells. As these receptors are less efficient than the splenic macrophage FcRs, complement-sensitized red cells often escape the phagocytic or cytotoxic process and circulate in the peripheral blood with normal or slight reduction in red cell survival. Because C3d or C4d coated red cells have less binding sites for other complement proteins, these cells are in fact protected from further hemolysis. However, C3d and C4d coated cells are less deformable than normal erythrocytes; hence, the complement proteins may augment IgG-mediated phagocytosis.[25–27] Consequently, the extravascular hemolytic process may be enhanced by the presence of complement on the cell, whereby complement acts as an opsonin to facilitate the phagocytic process.

Immune specificity of WAHA

In initial serologic testing, most warm autoantibodies are panagglutinins reacting with all red cells. These panagglutinins can be classified into different categories based on the agglutinating pattern with certain Rh phenotypes: (1) the antibodies react with all red cells with a normal Rh phenotype but not with those having Rh_{null} phenotype, or with those having partially deleted Rh antigens; (2) the antibodies are specific to part of the Rh antigen system (i.e. react with normal Rh phenotype and cells with partially deleted antigens); and (3) the antibodies react to all cells including Rh_{null} cells.[28] The first two categories, which are specific to the Rh antigen system, account for 50–70% of warm autoantibodies[29] as most warm autoantibodies react with all red cells except those of the Rh_{null} phenotype. In one series of 150 persons with warm autoantibodies, only four were specific to only a single Rh antigen (i.e. anti-e or anti-c specificity).[30] Because Rh antigens have a relatively low density on the red cell membrane, autoantibodies against Rh antigens do not activate complement.

Autoantibodies not showing Rh specificity can sometimes show specificity for other red cell antigens. Using immunoprecipitation methods, up to 50% of warm autoantibodies precipitate band 3 and glycophorin A.[31,32] Band 3, an anion transport protein, requires a portion of glycophorin A to form Wr^b antigen. Interestingly, Di^b, an alloimmune antigen of Diego system, is also carried on protein band 3. Compared with antigen Wr^b, Di^b is a rare target for autoantibodies.[30] The glycosylation and the complexity of the Wr^b and Rh antigen system may implicate their immunogenicity.[30]

Autoantibody formation can also impact red cell antigenic expression.[33] Decreased expression of blood group antigens in the following systems have been described: Kell, Rh, MNS, Duffy, and the Kidd system.[33,34] The mechanism of this phenomenon is unknown, but it may be an effect to protect against hemolysis.

Some warm autoantibodies appear to have specificity against certain red cell antigens on initial testing, but the antibodies can still be absorbed by red cells lacking the corresponding antigen. In addition, elutes made from the red cells used for this absorption procedure again demonstrate immune specificity against that particular antigen. The cause of pseudo-specificity of warm autoantibodies is unclear. Clinically, the pseudo-specificity of the autoantibodies is not directly associated with the severity of hemolysis, although the serologic results may lead to diagnostic confusion. Sometimes, autoantibodies of real specificity and of pseudo-specificity may coexist in the same patient.[33,35] This is of practical importance in selecting compatible blood for transfusing patients with warm autoimmune hemolytic anemia. Autoantibodies of pseudo-specificity have been described in blood group systems such as Kell, Duffy, Kidd and MNS systems.[33]

The diagnostic evaluation of a patient with suspected WAHA

With suspected WAHA, the most useful test to detect warm antibodies is the direct antiglobulin test (DAT) with polyclonal or monoclonal antibodies specific for IgG or C3d (also called the Coombs' test). However, the presence of antibodies and/or complement on the red cell membrane does not necessarily result in hemolysis and the strength of reactivity of the DAT is not directly related to the clinical severity of hemolysis. A positive DAT without evidence of hemolysis occurs in about one per 10 000 healthy blood donors.

IgG and C3 are detected on the red cells in 50% of the cases; IgG alone in 23% of cases and C3 in 27% of the cases. When IgG is detected on red cells of normal individuals,

IgG1 appears to be the predominant IgG subclass detected. IgG1 has been shown to be less efficient than IgG3 for activating complement,[36] which may explain the lack of hemolysis. In about 2% of patients with WAHA, the DAT is negative (i.e. Coomb's negative autoimmune hemolytic anemia). There are at least two possible explanations: (1) the level of red cell antibody sensitization is below the sensitivity of the DAT; or (2) hemolytic anemia caused by IgA or other immunoglobulins[37–39] that would not be detected by conventional antiglobulin reagents. Variable expression of red cell antigen during the course of disease[40] may also play a role in Coomb's negative autoimmune hemolytic anemia.

The lower limit of immunoglobulin detection using the DAT is estimated to be about 100–300 antibody molecules per red cell.[41] Tests such as ^{125}I-radioimmune direct antiglobulin test,[42] enzyme-linked direct antiglobulin test,[43,44] and two-stage immunoradiometric assay with ^{125}I-staphylococcal protein A[45] may increase the sensitivity of detecting antibodies on the red cells of patients with DAT-negative autoimmune hemolytic anemia.[3] However, the significance of these findings is uncertain as it has been shown that clinical hemolysis is unlikely to occur if the number of IgG1 molecules is less than 1000 per cell.[46] Special techniques for detecting IgG, such as assays using staphylococcal protein A or functional assays (e.g. the monocyte-phagocytic test), are sometimes useful in these cases; however, these assays are difficult to perform and they are not routinely available. In some cases, concentrated elutes may demonstrate the presence of antibody even though the DAT is negative. Before the diagnosis of Coombs' negative autoimmune hemolytic anemia is made, other non-immune causes of hemolysis must be excluded.

The indirect antiglobulin test (IDAT) will detect autoantibody in the patient's serum in 57.4% of patients with a routine antibody screen, and up to 88.9% of cases when enzyme-treated red cells are used.[47] If the patient requires transfusion, the challenge for the laboratory is the detection of alloantibodies when warm autoantibodies are present. A warm autoabsorption technique will remove autoantibody and leave alloantibody to be detected. Alternatively, a titration technique can be useful if the alloantibody has a higher titer than the autoantibody.

Management of patients with WAHA

The fundamental therapy for WAHA is to suppress autoantibody production. However, it usually takes time for immunosuppressive therapy to exert its full therapeutic effect. Hence, acute supportive measures may be required in patients with acute hemolytic events. Treatment of

WAHA can be broadly divided into supportive and more definite treatments.

There should be no difficulty in finding compatible blood for transfusion if patients have a negative DAT. However, many patients with severe hemolysis have detectable plasma antibody (panagglutinins); hence, it may be impossible to find compatible blood for these patients. In this case, if clinically indicated, incompatible blood can be transfused if the laboratory takes special care to ensure it is ABO and Rh compatible. It has been reported that blood transfusion may adversely affect the patient by introducing more alloimmune antigens that further activate the immune system.[33] None the less, transfusion therapy is still an important supportive measure in patients whose anemia has put them at risk of serious complications or death.

Corticosteroid therapy, initiated with the blood transfusion, may suppress the immune destruction of the transfused red cells.[3] Rarely, other adjunct supportive measures such as oxygen, sedation, ventilator support, and hypothermia therapy may be needed.

High-dose intravenous gamma-globulin (IVIgG) has been investigated as an acute treatment of WAHA.[48–59] This therapy causes blockage of the reticuloendothelial system and reduces the clearance of the IgG-sensitized red blood cells. The use of IVIgG is well described in the treatment of hemolysis associated with Evan's syndrome and lymphoproliferative diseases, and during an acute phase of hemolytic crisis.[60] However, the use of IVIgG is consistently less effective for AIHA compared to immune thrombocytopenia. Consequently, a higher dose of gamma globulin may be needed because patients with autoimmune hemolytic anemia may have an expanded reticuloendothelial system.[60] The mechanism of action of IVIgG therapy is likely due to FcR blockade,[61–67] although other mechanisms such as the presence of anti-idiotype in the IVIgG,[61,68–72] interference with T-cell signals to B-cells,[73–76] activation of T-suppressor cells, and inhibition of B-cell maturation[77–82] have been described.[33] Because the therapeutic effect of IVIgG is usually short-lived, further immunosuppressive therapy is required to maintain clinical remission.

Treatment with high-dose steroids, usually in the form of prednisone at 1–1.5 mg/kg/day, is initiated once the diagnosis of WAHA has been confirmed. The median time of response is 7–10 days. The mechanism of action of steroid therapy include: suppression of red cell clearance by the reticuloendothelial system;[83] downregulation of the number of FcR;[84] inhibition of the release of lysosomal enzymes by macrophages; and suppression of autoantibody production.[85] Steroid therapy can reduce the concentration of autoantibody, but has no effect on alloantibody production.[33] When hematologic improvement is seen, the dose of steroid should be gradually tapered over the next several months to minimize the side-effects of long-term steroid therapy. In 60–70% of patients, complete remission can be achieved, but for some patients, maintenance therapy is required. Among these patients, 50% may relapse and further treatment with higher doses of steroid therapy may be beneficial. If there is a nonresponse to steroid by the end of the first 3 weeks, continued therapy with steroid alone is usually ineffective. Up to 40% of patients with WAHA become either steroid-dependent or steroid-resistant.[86,87]

Splenectomy is effective in about half of patients with WAHA.[88] Splenectomy removes the major site of antigen presentation and, in turn, reduces antibody production.[33,89,90] With the advance of laparoscopic splenectomy, the incidence of severe surgical complications has been reduced.[91,92] The major long-term complication of splenectomy is infection, particularly of encapsulated organisms. Therefore, all patients undergoing splenectomy should receive vaccine immunization against *Streptococcus pneumoniae*, *Meningococcus* and possibly *Hemophilus influenzae*.

Immunosuppressive therapies, including vinca alkaloids,[93] azathioprine and cyclophosphamide, have been reported to be beneficial in the treatment of WAHA, although the therapeutic effect may be delayed for 3–6 months after the initiation of treatments. In a small case series, the response rate was reported to be about 50%.[86] Patients who do experience a clinical response to this therapy may require maintenance therapy for up to 12 months to induce remission.

A recent study has suggested that Danazol may induce long-lasting remission in patients with refractory WAHA.[94–97] The possible mechanisms include: reduction in red cell bound C3d;[98] immunomodulation by alteration of T-cell subsets;[99] and reduction of FcR in the reticuloendothelial (RE) system.[100] Side-effects from Danazol include virilization effects and dose-dependant hepatic toxicity.

Cold autoimmune hemolytic anemia

Cold autoimmune hemolytic anemia (CAHA), also known as cold hemagglutinin disease, is much less common than WAHA. In a large prospective series,[3] 391/2390 patients (16.4%) undergoing investigations for red cell autoantibodies presented with cold autoantibodies while another 10 patients (0.4%) had both warm and cold autoantibodies. In another series AIHA,[101] a combination of warm and cold autoantibodies was reported in 8% of patients with AIHA. These antibodies react best at cold

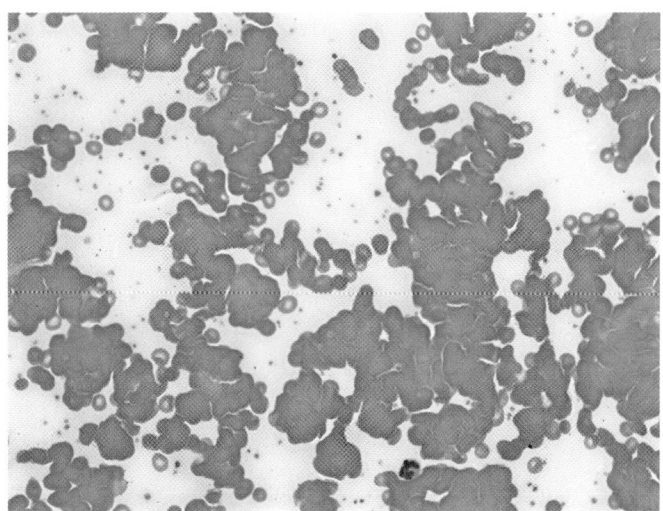

Fig. 10.2 Peripheral blood smear showing agglutination of red cells in a patient with Waldenström's macroglobulinemia. The background of the smear is bluish because of high protein content, which contains IgM hemagglutinin. Wright stain, × 400.

temperatures (below 30°C). When the peripheral blood of patients with cold hemagglutinin examined at room temperature, it typically shows agglutination of red cells (Fig. 10.2). This temperature-dependent reactivity of the cold autoantibodies is of clinical significance because hemolysis is unlikely to occur if the thermal reactivity is below 30°C. Cold autoantibodies are mainly IgM (85%);[3] however, the IgG biphasic Donath–Landsteiner antibody accounts for approximately 15% of the cases, especially in the pediatric age group.[3,102]

Red cell sensitization by cold IgM usually occurs in the body extremities (e.g. fingers, ears, nose) where temperatures may fall below 30°C allowing antibody binding to the red cells. The complement cascade is activated, and if the cascade proceeds to activation of the membrane attack complex, hemolysis will occur. This gives rise to the characteristic clinical features of Raynaud's phenomenon, acrocyanosis or gangrene. If the inhibitors of complement stop the cascade, the red cells (now coated with C3b) can be removed through extravascular phagocytosis. Eventually C3b is degraded to C3d on the cell surface. As macrophages do not have receptors for C3d, these red cells will not be cleared from the circulation. It is this component of complement that is detected by the DAT. The most common autoantibody specificity in CAHA is to the 'I' blood group antigen. Auto-anti-I typically occurs during or after *Mycoplasma pneumoniae* infection. In contrast, anti-I may be formed during or following infectious mononucleosis. Other less frequent autoantibody specificities include: P, Pr, A1, D, Vo, Gd (glycolipid dependent gangliosides),[103,104] -Lud,[105] F1,[106] Ju and IA[3,107] antigens. Specificity will be apparent at

temperatures between 15 and 20°C. Clinically, the specificity of cold antibody is less important than the thermal amplitude.

The presence of a cold hemagglutinin is readily demonstrated using the cold agglutinin test. When determining the thermal range of the antibody using this procedure, albumin should be added as this improves the clinical correlation. The cold agglutinin often causes problems with ABO and Rh phenotype cross-match. To overcome this dilemma, the red cells should be washed with warm saline to remove the cold agglutinin. The cross-match and antibody screen should be done using a prewarmed sample and using monospecific anti-IgG to avoid false-positive reactions. The DAT, using monoclonal reagents, is usually negative for IgG, but positive for C3d when using an ethylene diamine tetra-acetic acid (EDTA) sample.

Most patients with CAHA have mild symptoms or none at all. Patients are warned to avoid exposure to cold. During a severe acute hemolytic episode, plasmapheresis can be used to reduce the level of IgM cold autoantibody. Plasmapheresis is especially effective in CAHA because IgM is confined to the intravascular space. This procedure is best performed in a warm environment and the tubing of the plasmapheresis machine may have to be prewarmed. Blood transfusion, when needed, is infused at room temperature with a controlled rate. It is still controversial whether the use of a blood warmer offers additional benefits. If CAHA is secondary to an underlying neoplastic disease, chemotherapy including alkylating agents may reduce the production of cold autoantibody.

Paroxysmal cold hemoglobinuria

Paroxysmal cold hemoglobinuria (PCH) was one of the first recognized anemias when described in the mid-1800s[107] and, for years, it was commonly believed to be a rare acquired AIHA associated with congenital syphilis. However, it is now recognized that PCH causes up to 40% of acute transient hemolytic anemia in young children[108] during viral infections such as measles, mumps, chickenpox and influenza; however, due to the transient nature of the disease, the diagnosis of PCH may be difficult after acute episodes. The cold biphasic IgG antibody (Donath–Landsteiner antibody) directs against globoside glycosphingolipid (P antigen) and causes hemolysis by a unique mechanism. The antibody binds to red cells at cooler temperatures in the peripheral circulation. The complement pathway is activated and intravascular hemolysis occurs when red cells return to the warmer core body temperature. The Donath–Landsteiner antibody is more potent than IgM cold agglutinin in its ability to initiate intravascular hemolysis, mainly because antigen/antibody affinity of the cold IgM antibody decreases when red cells return to core temperatures.[2,109] It has been demonstrated that IgG3 is the major immunoglobulin subclass for Donath–Landsteiner antibody.[110]

The definitive test for PCH is the Donath–Landsteiner test, which can be performed as a direct or indirect procedure.[111] The direct test is conducted by incubating a test sample at 0°C for 1 h, and then at 37°C for an additional 30 min. If the Donath–Landsteiner antibody is present, it will bind to the red cells during the cold incubation phase and hemolyse the cells during the warm phase. A positive test result is not considered validated unless a control tube, maintained at 37°C throughout the test, shows no hemolysis. The indirect test is done by mixing the patient's serum with ABO compatible P-positive red cells of a normal person in the presence of fresh serum as a source of complements. The indirect test has a much higher sensitivity than the direct test for several reasons: (1) complement proteins are present in fresh normal serum; (2) the serum-to-cell ratio can be adjusted to increase sensitivity; and (3) the indicator cells from an allogenic donor are more susceptible to lysis than the patient's own red cells as the indicator cells are not coated with C3d. The sensitivity of the test can be increased further by using enzyme-treated red cells. False-positive results can occur due to IgM hemolytic antibody with a high thermal range. False negatives occur less frequently in the indirect Donath–Landsteiner test, although they can occur when the antibody titer is low or if soluble globoside (P antigen) present in the fresh normal serum causes inhibition of the antibody.[102]

The management of PCH may require urgent blood transfusions depending on the level of anemia and whether the patient is symptomatic. Theoretically, donor cells from P-negative patients may minimize *in vivo* hemolysis; however, P-negative blood is usually not available and in most cases, transfusion with P-positive blood can be beneficial. Patients with PCH can be successfully transfused if the transfusion rate is slow and the patient is kept warm and closely monitored.[112] The use of a blood warmer may be beneficial for some patients. It has been shown that the removal of complement proteins from donor plasma by washing red cells[113] and by using steroid therapy have not been beneficial.[102,108,112]

Alloimmune hemolytic anemia

Alloimmune hemolytic anemia occurs when the immune system is sensitized and antibodies form in response to red cell alloantigens. Typically, this occurs following a blood transfusion, during or after pregnancy, or following bone marrow or stem cell transplantation. Apart from another individual's red cells, the sources of alloantigen also can be from environmental antigens unrelated to erythrocytes.

Transfusion reactions due to immune-mediated hemolysis

The first transfusion reaction was recorded in 1667 by Denis.[114] Today, the incidence of clinically relevant immune-mediated hemolytic reactions is estimated to be around one reaction per 20 000 units of blood transfused.[115–119] The spectrum of clinical presentations can range from life-threatening ABO incompatibility to subclinical hemolysis depending on the magnitude of antigen–antibody interactions, the degree of complement activation, and the activity of the reticuloendothelial system.

There are two major types of immune-mediated hemolysis following blood transfusion: acute and delayed. More than 80% of acute hemolytic transfusion reactions are due to ABO incompatibility.[116] The mortality rates of up to 40% seen in the past[115] have declined to 10%, probably reflecting improved management and support. Transfusion reactions due to intravascular hemolysis are generally more severe than with extravascular hemolysis because of the side-effects associated with complement activation which may be triggered by alloantibodies to Kell, Kidd and Duffy antigen systems.[114–116] Patients may experience fever, chills, joint pain, shock, renal failure and/or disseminated intravascular coagulation.

Delayed hemolytic transfusion reactions may be caused by primary alloimmunization but, more frequently, the transfused red cells trigger a delayed (anamnestic) IgG-mediated transfusion reaction 7–14 days after the blood transfusion. Although most patients have been previously alloimmunized, over time, their antibody level falls below detectability and it can be difficult to prevent this form of transfusion reaction.[33] Sometimes, the only clinical evidence of this reaction is a positive DAT.

One of the major dilemmas for clinicians in the management of post-transfusion reactions is how to differentiate immune-mediated transfusion reactions from pseudo-hemolytic transfusion reactions. Non-immune hemolytic anemia can occur if transfused red cells are subject to excessive thermal, osmotic, mechanical or chemical insults. Clinically, febrile symptoms secondary to hemolysis may have other causes including: (1) febrile reactions due to non-hemolytic transfusion reactions; (2) bacterially contaminated blood products; (3) transfusion-related acute lung injury; or (4) severe allergic symptoms (hypotension and shock) that mimic acute hemolytic transfusion reactions. However, the presence of cutaneous manifestations suggest an allergic pathophysiology.

Hemolytic disease of the newborn

Hemolytic disease of the newborn (HDN), also called erythroblastosis fetalis, is hemolysis in the fetus caused by transplacental transfer of maternal IgG. During pregnancy, maternal IgG is transferred via specific FcRs on the placental cells.[120–123] Alloimmune hemolytic anemia may occur in the fetus if there is a blood group incompatibility between the mother and the fetus. Generally, by 12 weeks, maternal IgG is detectable in the fetal circulation[33] and the rate of IgG transfer progressively increases across the pregnancy so that, at term, the fetal IgG level may be equal to[124] or higher[33,120] than that of the mother's. The antibodies against the Rh and the ABO antigen systems are the two major causes of hemolytic disease of the newborn, with anti-D causing the most severe cases.[33] With the routine use of Rh immune globulin, HDN is now seen more often with antibodies of other blood group antigens.

During pregnancy, most women are exposed to less than 0.1 ml of fetal blood, and this small volume does not cause alloimmunization. However, in a subsequent pregnancy, the secondary immune response may trigger the production of large amounts of IgG antibody and this could cause severe hemolysis of the fetal red cells. Hence, Rh HDN seldom affects the first pregnancy. With Rh antibodies, the severity of the disease is progressive in each subsequent pregnancy. The risk of stillbirth in a woman with a previous history of mild Rh HDN is about 2% compared to a 70% risk in a woman with a previous history of Rh alloimmunization.[125] Conversely, ABO HDN may affect a firstborn infant as the antibodies are already preformed due to environmental stimulation. The severity of ABO HDN in a previously born fetus does not predict the severity in the next infant.[33]

Stillbirth and hydrops occur in the severest cases of HDN. Severe fetal anemia can result in extramedullary erythropoiesis, gross hepatosplenomegaly, portal hypertension and hepatic failure. More commonly, the affected fetus may present with anemia and hyperbilirubinemia within the first 24 h of life. Without proper treatment, kernicterus may develop. On the other end of the spectrum, positive serologic tests with no clinical findings may be the only indication of antibody transfer to the fetus. Since HDN cannot be diagnosed solely by serologic tests, it has been suggested that laboratory evidence of disease without clinical findings should be described simply as maternal–fetal blood group incompatibility.[33]

With the advance of modern medicine, hydrops fetalis due to Rh HDN is rarely seen. Primary prevention is the cornerstone of the management of Rh HDN. First, Rh-negative women who can bear children should receive Rh-negative blood. Second, Rh-negative pregnant woman should receive passive immunization with Rh immune globulin at 28-weeks' gestation and within 72 h of exposure to fetal D-positive red cells due to either delivery or an invasive procedure such as an abortion. Although the dose regimens are slightly different between North America and Europe, the rule of thumb is that 10 μg of anti-D should be given for each ml of Rh D positive whole blood. This dose can be decreased if intravenous anti-D is used. Kleihauer–Betke tests or flow cytometry can be useful in determining the amount of fetal cells in the maternal circulation so that the dose of Rh immune globulin can be adjusted. The successful rate associated with Rh immune globulin prophylaxis is estimated to be 98–99%.

The prenatal management of women at risk of HDN varies. All pregnant women should be typed for ABO and Rh D and have an antibody screen performed during the first trimester, usually at the first visit to the obstetrician. For D-negative women without detectable antibody, an antibody screening should be repeated at the 28th–30th week at the time that Rh immune globulin is given. If alloantibody is detected, titration studies should be performed at regular intervals. The antibodies titer may be used to guide the timing of fetal monitoring and further interventions;[126] however, it must be emphasized that the titer is only a semi-quantitative indicator. Once the titer reaches a certain level (1:16–1:32), other measurements should be considered to estimate the risk of severe HDN. The severity of HDN may be predicted by various methods including: (1) amniocentesis with measurement of total bile pigment in the amniotic fluid;[127] (2) ultrasonography to detect the evidence of extramedullary hematopoiesis;[128,129] and (3) percutaneous umbilical blood sampling.[130] However, there is no available test to identify women whose infants are at risk of ABO HDN. ABO alloimmunization does not affect the fetus *in utero*; however, symptoms of hemolysis occur 12–24 hours after birth.

There are several therapeutic interventions to reduce fetal death due to severe HDN. IVIG, started at the 10th–12th gestational week at 1 g/kg every 1–3 weeks until delivery, is moderately effective with multifactorial effects including blockage of FcRs on the placenta and fetal RE system. Anecdotal reports describe that intense maternal plasmapheresis with IVIG replacement and/or plasma replacement from a D-negative donor may be a useful treatment between the 10th and 24th weeks, after which intrauterine transfusion can be performed. As intrauterine transfusion requires specialized trained personnel and some risk of maternal/fetal hemorrhage, it should only be used in the case where fetal survival is at risk. Donor blood should be fresh, irradiated, cytomegalovirus (CMV)-negative, and lacking the antigen specific for the mother's antibody.[33] Some blood centers use group O blood whereas others use ABO-specific blood. Preterm delivery usually occurs around the 35th week gestation given the risk associated with HDN. After delivery, phototherapy and/or exchange transfusion may be used to reduce hyperbilirubinemia and the risk of kernicterus. Intravenous immunoglobulin (IVIg), directly infused to the newborn, has been shown to be beneficial in reducing the need of exchange transfusion.[131] If the infant is severely anemic, small volume transfusion may be required during the first few months of life.

Drug-induced hemolytic anemia

Drug-induced hemolysis can be immune mediated or non-immune mediated. The former is categorized into three major groups based on different mechanisms of action. Drugs, such as α-methyldopa, may induce true autoantibody production similar to warm autoimmune hemolytic anemia. Penicillin (hapten) binds to the red cell membrane and stimulates antibodies that are directed at the drug bound to the red cell. Drugs, such as quinine and quinidine, bind to plasma proteins, antibody, and then to the red cell. The last two categories illustrate the immunologic principle that a small chemical with a molecular weight under 500–1000 is unable to induce an immunologic response unless it is tightly bound to a macromolecule such as a protein. As the antibodies cannot bind to red cells in the absence of a drug, they are also called drug-dependent antibodies. On the other hand, some drugs may directly damage the red cells or induce oxidative changes in the cells. The former mainly occurs with industrial toxins such as copper and arsine, and do not involve antibodies (non-immune).

Drug-induced autoantibody

True autoantibody induction by α-methyldopa provides a human model for studying the mechanism underlying autoimmune disorders. It is one of the most extensively studied drug-induced autoimmune hemolytic anemia. None the less, the exact mechanism of autoantibody formation is still unclear. Up to 20% of patients on methyldopa therapy develop a positive direct antiglobulin

test;[132] however, only 0.3–0.8% of patients develop hemolytic anemia.[133,134] Kelton[135] showed that patients with a positive DAT, but without hemolysis, have significant impaired RE function. The development of a positive DAT in patients on α-methyldopa depends on the dose[132] and the duration of the therapy. It typically occurs in patients after 3 or more years of continuous treatment.[136] Hemolysis resolves after discontinuation of the drug although serologic abnormalities usually resolve more gradually and this can last for up to 24 months.[137] The autoantibody induced by α-methyldopa is IgG,[138] and is directed against Rh antigens in many patients.[139,140] The antibody does not activate complement; hence, the DAT is positive only with IgG detected on the cells. The pattern of antibody specificities is similar to that in idiopathic autoimmune hemolytic anemia. Besides a positive direct antiglobulin test, patients may have positive antinuclear factor,[136,141,142] lupus erythematosis (LE) cells,[136,142–145] rheumatoid factor[142,145] and factor III inhibitor.[146] The underlying pathogenesis is still unknown but α-methyldopa is demonstrated to produce an aberration in lymphocyte proliferation by increasing lymphocyte c-AMP that inhibits suppressor T-cell function.[147] Other drugs including levodopa, procainamide and NSAIDs (e.g. mefenamic acid and diclofenac) may also induce autoantibody similar to α-methyldopa.[148]

Drug (hapten) dependent antibody

A number of drugs bind firmly to red cell membranes, possibly via covalent bonds[149] and they elicit the production of IgG specific for that drug. As a rule, the antibody binds to red cells in the presence of the drug and this causes a positive DAT result. Usually the positive DAT is a coincidental finding and only rarely will these antibodies cause overt hemolysis, which is usually extravascular and, very infrequently, intravascular.[150] Penicillin and cephalosporin are the most common drugs that stimulate antibody production by this mechanism. They share a common benzyl-penicillol group that acts as a hapten.[151] It should be noted that up to 97% of normal healthy adults have antipenicillin antibody; however, this is an IgM antibody that can be present even without prior treatment with penicillin or cephalosporin.[152] The occurrence of hemolytic anemia depends on the appropriate ratio of antigen and antibody. Therefore, penicillin-induced hemolytic anemia typically occurs in patients treated with high-dose penicillin for 7–14 days via intravenous route, or in patients with renal failure resulting in reduced drug clearance.[33,152] Hemolysis stops promptly when the drug is stopped.

Innocent bystander

Instead of binding to red cell membranes, this group of drugs (haptens) binds to plasma proteins, and the drug–protein complex becomes sufficiently large to trigger an immune response.[153] The drug–protein complex binds to the surface of red cells and is further stabilized by the drug-dependent antibodies that also have immune specificities against alloantigens on the red cell membrane. The antibody can be IgM, IgG or both. The antibody–drug–protein complex activates the complement pathway and triggers red cell clearance. Sometimes, other cell lines in the blood are also involved producing neutropenia or thrombocytopenia.[33,152] Examples of drugs in this category include quinine, quinidine, sulfonamides, sulphonylurea and thiazide.

It is likely that the pathophysiology of drug-induced hemolysis is more complex than noted previously. For example, Phenacetin, Streptomycin, and non-steroidal anti-inflammatory drugs can cause hemolysis by both autoantibodies (drug-independent antibodies) and drug-dependent antibodies.[138,154–156]

Oxidative injury to red cells

Hemoglobin binds oxygen and, consequently, it is prone to oxidation and denaturation by oxidative agents, particularly if the anti-oxidative protective mechanisms in the red cell are overwhelmed. The amount of oxidative hemolysis is determined by the strength and the blood level of the oxidant, and congenital deficiency of the G6PD or glutathione-dependant pathways. Older red cells are more prone to oxidative injury by oxidants than are young red cells. The characteristic features of oxidative hemolysis include the formation of methemoglobin, sulfhemoglobin and Heinz bodies. Clinically, methemoglobin and sulfhemoglobin may present as bluish discoloration indistinguishable from cyanosis. Heinz bodies are the microscopic appearance of denatured hemoglobin. Moreover, examination of a peripheral blood smear may also reveal 'bite cells',[118,119] blister cells,[114] and eccentrocytes[119] (Fig. 10.3). 'Bite cells' are semicircular remnants of red cells after being partially phagocytosed or after extrusion of the Heinz body from the red cells.[117] If the denatured hemoglobin shifts to one side of the red cell, the red cell may appear as a blister cell and this is usually an indicator of brisk hemolysis.

Drugs that can cause oxidative hemolysis include nitrofurantoin, amniosalicylic acid, dapsone and pyridium (phenazopyridine). Very rarely, high-dose oxygen therapy can result in oxidative injury to the red cells, particularly in patients with vitamin E deficiency.[115,116,149,157]

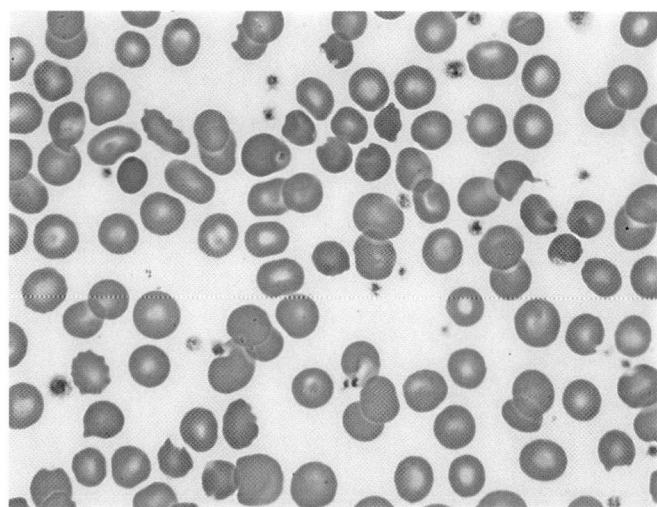

Fig. 10.3 Peripheral blood smear showing spherocytosis, bite cells and blister cells (ghost cells) in a patient with drug-induced oxidative hemolysis. Wright stain, × 1000, oil field.

Diagnosis of drug-induced hemolytic anemia depends on a detailed drug history. Demonstration of drug-dependent hemagglutination in the indirect antiglobulin test is confirmatory. However, sometimes, the diagnosis may only be established by resolution of the hemolysis on removal of the offending drug.

Non-immune hemolytic anemia

Infection-induced hemolytic anemia

Microorganisms may cause injury to red cells through different mechanisms such as: (1) physical invasion of red cells (e.g. malaria); (2) hemolysin secretions to damage the red cells directly (e.g. *Clostridium perfringen*) (Fig. 10.4); (3) infection that triggers formation of antibody (anti-I) against red cells (e.g. mycoplasma); (4) microangiopathic hemolysis caused by disseminated intravascular coagulation associated with infection; or (5) antibiotic therapy may cause hemolysis. In some cases, multiple mechanisms of hemolysis coexist, which often poses a diagnostic challenge to the clinician.

Mechanical trauma to red cells

Mechanical trauma to red cells can occur in three conditions: excessive shearing forces due to high-pressure gradient in the circulation; direct external impact; and microangiopathic thrombotic hemolysis.[158] On examination of a peripheral blood smear, burr cells

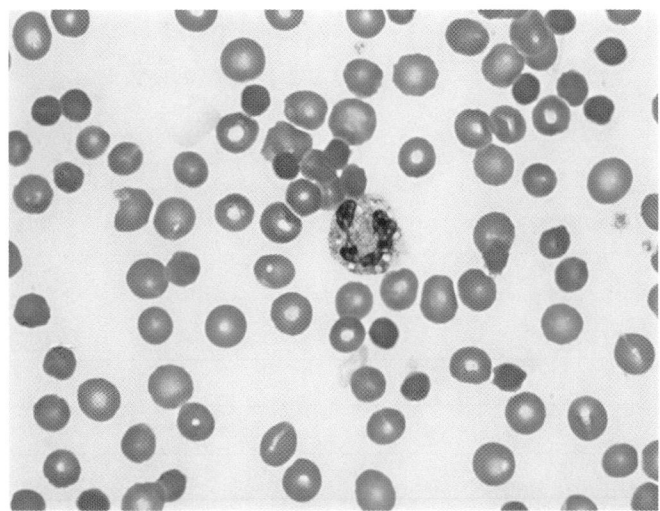

Fig. 10.4 Peripheral blood smear showing micro-spherocytosis and cytoplasmic vacuolation in neutrophils in a patient with clostridia infection. Wright stain, × 1000, oil field.

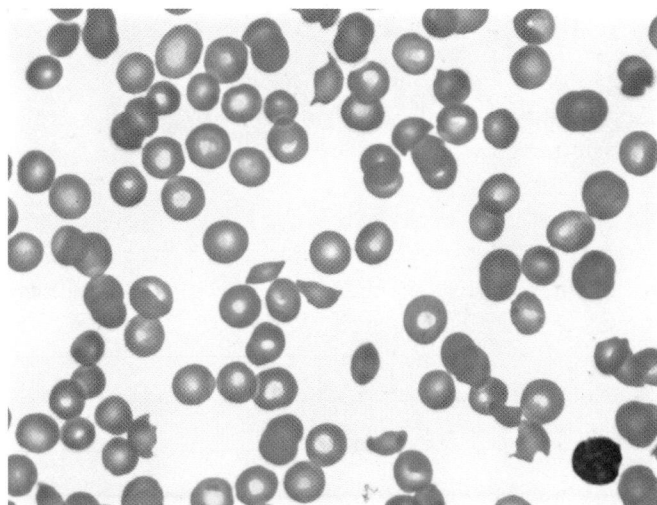

Fig. 10.5 Peripheral blood smear showing fragments of red cells and thrombocytopenia in a patient with thrombotic thrombocytopenic purpura. The size of red cells is approximately equal to the size of the nucleus in a non-reactive lymphocyte. Similar features may be present in patients with hemolytic uremic syndrome or microangiopathic hemolysis. Wright stain, × 1000, oil field.

and schistocytes of variable shapes such as crescents, helmets, micro-spherocytes and fragments are apparent. Therefore, this is commonly called schistocytic hemolytic anemia. Other non-specific features include aniso-poikilocytosis, polychromatic macrocytosis, thrombocytopenia and/or procoagulants activation. Extravascular hemolysis is the predominant feature, although intra-vascular hemolysis occurs in severe cases.

Schistocytic hemolytic anemia (SHA) is classified according to the size of the blood vessels where hemolysis occurs. Large-vessel SHA includes hemolysis in malignant hypertension and in patients with prosthetic heart valves. Small-vessel SHA occurs in march hemoglobinuria, autoimmune vasculitis, disseminated intravascular hemolysis, and thrombotic thrombocytopenic purpura – hemolytic uremic syndrome (TTP/HUS).

Thrombotic thrombocytopenic purpura – hemolytic uremic syndrome

In 1924, Moschowitz identified thrombotic thrombocytopenic purpura (TTP) as observed in a 16-year-old girl, while hemolytic uremic syndrome (HUS) was first described by Gasser in 1955. They are characterized by the triad of thrombocytopenia, anemia and renal dysfunction. Fever and neurological symptoms such as hemiparesis, aphasia, seizure, fluctuating mental function and coma are less common manifestations. Only about half of the patients present with full pentad symptoms (anemia, thrombocytopenia, renal dysfunction, fever and neurological dysfunction).[159] Because of the overlap in the clinical and pathologic features, TTP and HUS may

actually be a different spectrum of the same disorder. Most adult cases of TTP/HUS syndrome are idiopathic. However, TTP/HUS syndrome may be triggered or associated with other disorders or conditions such as: (1) vaccination; (2) infection such as enterotoxin-producing *Escherichia coli* and *Shigella dysenteriae*; (3) human immunodeficiency virus (HIV); (4) drugs (e.g. quinine, quinidine, ticlopidine and mithramycin); (5) malignancy such as adenocarcinoma; (6) bone marrow transplantation; (7) pregnancy; and (8) collagen vascular disease.

The pathogenesis of TTP/HUS syndrome is unknown. Disseminated platelet-rich thrombi are the key pathology and endothelial cell apoptosis induced by plasma from TTP patients,[160] disseminated platelet activation triggered by protein p37[161] or calpain,[162] and abnormally large multimers of von Willebrand factor (vWF)[163] have been shown. Recently, mutations in zinc metalloproteinase genes (ADAMTS13) have been found in familial TTP patients.[164]

Laboratory abnormalities of a TTP patient may include thrombocytopenia, fragmented red cells (Fig. 10.5), elevated LDH and renal impairment. Serial measurements of platelet counts using a phase contrast microscope are important because platelet count and LDH are the markers of TTP activity. In contrast, hemolysis indicates neither the severity nor the activity of TTP.

The primary treatment of TTP or HUS is plasma exchange with vWF-poor plasma, and 1–1.5 times the plasma volume should be exchanged with fresh-frozen plasma (FFP).[165] On-going trials comparing cryosupernatant or detergent-treated FFP may provide evidence on the choice of replacement fluids. Plasma infusion is less effective than plasma exchange[166] because less plasma volume is being replaced.[167] However, plasma infusion has been used in familial TTP patients. Neurological symptoms may recover within hours after plasmapheresis. LDH and thrombocytopenia usually normalize within days. If possible, platelet transfusions should be avoided in patients with TTP or HUS. Antiplatelet therapy such as aspirin, ticlopidine or dipyridamole may be considered when the platelet count is above $50 \times 10^9/l$. Evidence of the value of corticosteroid therapy exists only from anecdotal studies and one retrospective study.[168] Intravenous IgG, splenectomy and vincristine should be reserved for refractory or resistant TTP patients. Without definitive treatment, the mortality of TTP exceeds 90%. However, if treated promptly, TTP has a relatively low mortality.

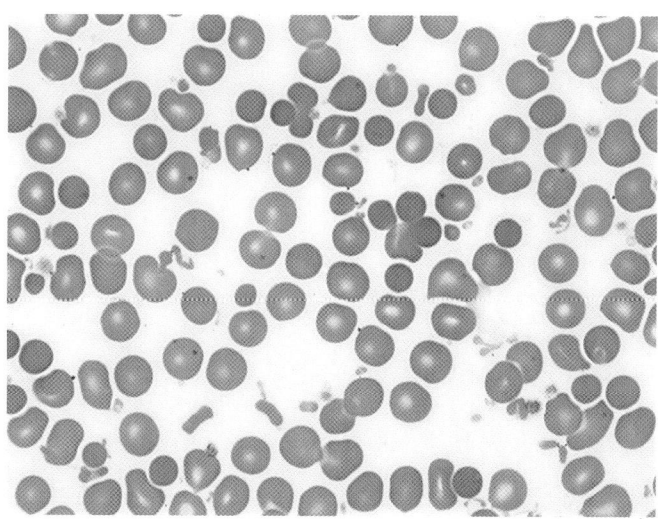

Fig. 10.6 Peripheral blood smear showing spherocytes of variable sizes in a patient with burn injury. The red cells have also formed micro-vesicles and fine filamentous structures. Wright stain, × 1000, oil field.

Cardiac hemolysis

Almost any intracardiac lesion that alters the hemo-dynamics and generates excessive shear force to the red cells can cause intravascular hemolysis. Traumatic hemolysis may occur after cardiac surgeries such as heart valve replacement or heart valve repair. Synthetic material, small valvular area, and complications such as thrombotic valve and perivalvular leaks are particularly at the risk of significant hemolysis. Hemolysis also occurs in patients with native valvular lesion including severe aortic stenosis, coarctation of aorta and ruptured aneurysm of the sinus of Valsalva. In addition, aortofemoral bypass has been described as being associated with traumatic hemolysis because of the same pathophysiology.[158]

External impact on the red cells

When red cells flow through small vessels over the surface of bony prominences, they are prone to external impact. March hemoglobinuria, a well-described but uncommon condition of intravascular hemolysis, typically occurs after strenuous marching or running on a hard surface in susceptible individuals who wear thin-soled shoes. There is usually no underlying intrinsic erythrocyte abnormality. This condition can be prevented by insertion of a soft inner sole.

Thermal damage of red cells

In patients with extensive burn injury, red cell denatu-ration and fragmentation occur (Fig. 10.6). Less commonly,

a similar mechanism of hemolysis occurs in patients with heat stroke.

Osmotic damage of red cells

Fresh water or salt water drowning can cause hemolysis because of abrupt osmotic changes in the pulmonary circulation.

Miscellaneous causes of hemolytic anemia

Paroxysmal nocturnal hemoglobinuria

Paroxysmal nocturnal hemoglobinuria (PNH) is a rare type of intravascular hemolysis, caused by an abnormal membrane protein. The disease arises from abnormal clones of red cells with increased sensitivity to com-plements, particularly in an acidic environment. It is a disease of pluripotent stem cells and, therefore, other hematopoietic cells are affected. Patients with PNH can progress to aplastic anemia and acute myeloid leukemia. For uncertain reasons, it is sometimes complicated by thrombotic episodes at unusual sites.

More than 20 different proteins, including complement proteins, enzymes and various other receptors, are missing from the surface of PNH red cells.[169] Ferguson *et al*[170] identified glycosyl-phosphatidyl-inositol (GPI anchor) as the key glycolipid structure to hold the proteins on to the red cell membrane. The defect of GPI synthesis has been mapped to the mutation of *pig-a* gene on the X chromosome (Xp22.1). However, it is still unclear why the abnormal PNH clone proliferates preferentially as compared with other normal hematopoietic stem cells.

The screening test of PNH is the Ham's test. This test demonstrates that the abnormal red cells are abnormally sensitive to be hemolysed by the complements in acidified serum. Although the Ham's test was the gold standard for PNH, it is semi-quantitative and not sensitive enough to detect small numbers of PNH clones. In addition, the sensitivity of the test is affected by recent hemolysis or blood transfusion. Flow cytometry with a combination of monoclonal antibodies has contributed significantly to the diagnosis of PNH. CD55 and CD59 are the best-studied monoclonal antibodies to detect GPI-linked proteins on the red cells from peripheral blood sample. Based on the extent of GPI deficiency, it is possible to classify the abnormal clones into partially deficient cells and completely deficient cells.[169] Characteristically, patients with PNH have a hypoplastic bone marrow in spite of significant hemolysis.

Immunosuppressive therapy using corticosteroids, antilymphocyte globulin or cyclosporin A has been used to treat patients with progressive pancytopenia.[171] Supportive treatment, such as blood transfusion with washed red cells, not only relieves the symptoms of anemia, but also suppresses the production of abnormal clones. Anticoagulation with Warfarin is required to prevent thrombosis. Bone marrow transplantation is considered in young patients and in patients with bone marrow failure. Up to 15% of the patients with PNH may have a spontaneous recovery.[172]

Venom-induced hemolytic anemia

Cobras, pit vipers, spiders such as *Loxosceles* (also known as violin spider), and black widow spiders (belonging to *Latrodectus* genus), produce a hemolytic venom that activates coagulation and causes disseminated intravascular hemolysis, although the cases are rarely fatal.[173]

Toxin-induced hemolytic anemia

A condition such as Wilson's disease causes an accumulation of copper in body organs and this can damage red cells by interference with glucose metabolism. The diagnosis of Wilson's disease should be considered when a patient presents with neurological symptoms and severe acute hemolysis. A pathognomonic physical sign is a Kayser–Fleischer ring in the eye. Treatment with Penicillamine can halt the hemolysis

Hemolytic anemia in organ dysfunction

Hemolysis may occur in patients with renal failure or hepatic failure. Hemolytic anemia in these conditions is of less importance than other causes of anemia.

Acknowledgments

We thank Neame P. for help with figures and Horsewood P. for critical comments of the manuscript on the section of Fc receptors.

REFERENCES

1. Mack P, Freedman J 2000 Autoimmune hemolytic anemia: a history. Transfusion Medicine Review 14(3): 223–233
2. Sokol RJ, Booker DJ, Stamps R et al 1992 The pathology of autoimmune haemolytic anaemia. Journal of Clinical Pathology 45(12): 1047–1052
3. Engelfriet CP, Overbeeke MA, dem Borne AE et al 1992 Autoimmune hemolytic anemia. Seminars in Hematology 29(1): 3–12
4. Sokol RJ, Hewitt S, Booker DJ et al 1990 Erythrocyte autoantibodies, subclasses of IgG and autoimmune haemolysis. Autoimmunity 6(1–2): 99–104
5. Sokol RJ, Hewitt S, Booker DJ *et al* 1990 Red cell autoantibodies, multiple immunoglobulin classes, and autoimmune hemolysis. Transfusion 30(8): 714–717
6. Fleer A, van Schaik ML, dem Borne AE et al 1978 Destruction of sensitized erythrocytes by human monocytes *in vitro*: effects of cytochalasin B, hydrocortisone and colchicine. Scandinavian Journal of Immunology 8(6): 515–524
7. Hulett MD, Witort E, Brinkworth RI et al 1994 Identification of the IgG binding site of the human low affinity receptor for IgG Fc gamma RII. Enhancement and ablation of binding by site-directed mutagenesis. Journal of Biological Chemistry 269(21): 15287–15293
8. Ghirlando R, Keown MB, Mackay GA et al 1995 Stoichiometry and thermodynamics of the interaction between the Fc fragment of human IgG1 and its low-affinity receptor Fc gamma RIII. Biochemistry 34(41): 13320–13327
9. Huizinga TW, Kerst M, Nuyens JH et al 1989 Binding characteristics of dimeric IgG subclass complexes to human neutrophils. Journal of Immunology 142(7): 2359–2364
10. Allen JM, Seed B 1989 Isolation and expression of functional high-affinity Fc receptor complementary DNAs. Science 243(4889): 378–381
11. dem Borne AE, Beckers D, van der Meulen FW et al 1977 IgG4 autoantibodies against erythrocytes, without increased haemolysis: a case report. British Journal of Haematology 37(1): 137–144
12. Takai T, Li M, Sylvestre D et al 1994 FcR gamma chain deletion results in pleiotrophic effector cell defects. Cell 76(3): 519–529
13. Van de Winkel JG, Anderson CL. 1991 Biology of human immunoglobulin G Fc receptors. Journal of Leukocyte Biology 49(5): 511–524.
14. Muta T, Kurosaki T, Misulovin Z et al. 1994 A 13-amino-acid motif in the cytoplasmic domain of Fc gamma RIIB modulates B-cell receptor signalling. Nature 369(6478): 340
15. Daeron M, Latour S, Malbec O et al 1995 The same tyrosine-based inhibition motif, in the intracytoplasmic domain of Fc gamma RIIB, regulates negatively BCR-, TCR-, and FcR-dependent cell activation. Immunity 3(5): 635–646
16. Davis W, Harrison PT, Hutchinson MJ et al 1995 Two distinct regions of FC gamma RI initiate separate signalling pathways involved in endocytosis and phagocytosis. EMBO Journal 14(3): 432–441
17. Urbaniak SJ 1976 Lymphoid cell dependent (K-cell) lysis of human erythrocytes sensitized with Rhesus alloantibodies. British Journal of Haematology 33(3): 409–413
18. Hunt JS, Beck ML, Tegtmeier GE et al 1982 Factors influencing monocyte recognition of human erythrocyte autoantibodies *in vitro*. Transfusion 22(5): 355–358

19. Unanue ER 1984 Antigen-presenting function of the macrophage. Annual Review of Immunology 2: 395–428
20. Sokol RJ, Hewitt S 1985 Autoimmune hemolysis: a critical review. Critical Reviews in Oncology and Hematology 4(2): 125–154
21. Nicholson-Weller A, Burge J, Fearon DT et al 1982 Isolation of a human erythrocyte membrane glycoprotein with decay-accelerating activity for C3 convertases of the complement system. Journal of Immunology 129(1): 184–189
22. Schonermark S, Rauterberg EW, Shin ML et al 1986 Homologous species restriction in lysis of human erythrocytes: a membrane-derived protein with C8-binding capacity functions as an inhibitor. Journal of Immunology 136(5): 1772–1776
23. Zalman LS, Wood LM, Frank MM et al 1987 Deficiency of the homologous restriction factor in paroxysmal nocturnal hemoglobinuria. Journal of Experimental Medicine 165(2): 572–577
24. Sugita Y, Nakano Y, Tomita M et al 1988 Isolation from human erythrocytes of a new membrane protein which inhibits the formation of complement transmembrane channels. Journal of Biochemistry (Tokyo) 104(4): 633–637
25. Ehlenberger AG, Nussenzweig V 1977 The role of membrane receptors for C3b and C3d in phagocytosis. Journal of Experimental Medicine 145(2): 357–371
26. Gaither TA, Vargas I, Inada S et al 1987 The complement fragment C3d facilitates phagocytosis by monocytes [published erratum appears in Immunology 1988 Mar; 63(3): 559]. Immunology 62(3): 405–411
27. Wellek B, Hahn HH, Opferkuch W et al 1975 Evidence for macrophage C3d-receptor active in phagocytosis. Journal of Immunology 114(5): 1643–1645
28. Vos GH, Weiner W 1963 Serology of acquired hemolytic anemia. Blood 22, 606–613
29. Vos GH, Petz LD, Fudenberg HH et al 1971 Specificity and immunoglobulin characteristics of autoantibodies in acquired hemolytic anemia. Journal of Immunology 106(5): 1172–1176
30. Issitt PD, Pavone BG, Goldfinger D et al 1976 Anti-Wrb, and other autoantibodies responsible for positive direct antiglobulin tests in 150 individuals. British Journal of Haematology 34(1): 5–18
31. Leddy JP, Falany JL, Kissel GE et al 1993 Erythrocyte membrane proteins reactive with human (warm-reacting) anti-red cell autoantibodies Journal of Clinical Investigation 91(4): 1672–1680
32. Leddy JP, Wilkinson SL, Kissel GE et al 1994 Erythrocyte membrane proteins reactive with IgG (warm-reacting) anti-red blood cell autoantibodies: II. Antibodies coprecipitating band 3 and glycophorin A. Blood 84(2): 650–656
33. Issitt PD, Anstee DJ 1998 Applied blood group serology, 4th edn. Montgomery Scientific Publications, Durham, North Carolina
34. Seyfried H, Gorska B, Maj S et al 1972 Apparent depression of antigens of the Kell blood group system associated with autoimmune acquired haemolytic anaemia. Vox Sanguinis 23(6): 528–536
35. Issitt PD, Pavone BG 1978 Critical re-examination of the specificity of auto-anti-Rh antibodies in patients with a positive direct antiglobulin test. British Journal of Haematology 38(1): 63–74
36. Gorst DW, Rawlinson VI, Merry AH et al 1980 Positive direct antiglobulin test in normal individuals. Vox Sanguinis 38(2): 99–105
37. Clark DA, Dessypris EN, Jenkins DE, Jr et al 1984 Acquired immune hemolytic anemia associated with IgA erythrocyte coating: investigation of hemolytic mechanisms. Blood 64(5): 1000–1005
38. Suzuki S, Amano T, Mitsunaga M et al 1981 autoimmune hemolytic anemia associated with IgA autoantibody. Clinical Immunology and Immunopathology 21(2): 247–256
39. Wolf CF, Wolf DJ, Peterson P et al 1982 Autoimmune hemolytic anemia with predominance of IgA autoantibody. Transfusion 22(3): 238–240
40. Issitt PD, Wilkinson SL, Gruppo RA et al 1983 Depression of Rh antigen expression in antibody-induced haemolytic anaemia [letter]. British Journal of Haematology 53(4): 688
41. Merry AH, Thomson EE, Rawlinson VI et al 1984 Quantitation of IgG on erythrocytes: correlation of number of IgG molecules per cell with the strength of the direct and indirect antiglobulin tests. Vox Sanguinis 47(1): 73–81
42. Schmitz N, Djibey I, Kretschmer V et al 1981 Assessment of red cell autoantibodies in autoimmune hemolytic anemia of warm type by a radioactive anti-IgG test. Vox Sanguinis 41(4): 224–230
43. Sokol RJ, Hewitt S, Booker DJ et al 1985 Enzyme linked direct antiglobulin tests in patients with autoimmune haemolysis. Journal of Clinical Pathology 38(8): 912–914
44. Sokol RJ, Hewitt S, Booker DJ et al 1987 Small quantities of erythrocyte bound immunoglobulins and autoimmune haemolysis. Journal of Clinical Pathology 40(3): 254–257
45. Salama A, Mueller-Eckhardt C, Bhakdi S et al 1985 A two-stage immunoradiometric assay with 125I-staphylococcal protein A for the detection of antibodies and complement on human blood cells. Vox Sanguinis 48(4): 239–245
46. Stratton F, Rawlinson VI, Merry AH et al 1983 Positive direct antiglobulin test in normal individuals. II. Clinical and Laboratory Haematology 5(1): 17–21
47. Petz LD, Garratty G 1980 Acquired immune hemolytic anemias. Churchill Livingstone, New York
48. Argiolu F, Diana G, Arnone M et al 1990 High-dose intravenous immunoglobulin in the management of autoimmune hemolytic anemia complicating thalassemia major. Acta Haematologica 83(2): 65–68.
49. Besa EC 1988 Rapid transient reversal of anemia and long-term effects of maintenance intravenous immunoglobulin for autoimmune hemolytic anemia in patients with lymphoproliferative disorders. American Journal of Medicine 84(4): 691–698
50. Bolis S, Marozzi A, Rossini F et al 1991 High dose intravenous immunoglobulin (IVIgG) in Evans' syndrome. Allergology and Immunopathology 19(5): 186
51. Hilgartner MW, Bussel J 1987 Use of intravenous gamma globulin for the treatment of autoimmune neutropenia of childhood and autoimmune hemolytic anemia. American Journal of Medicine 83(4A): 25–29
52. Macintyre EA, Linch DC, Macey MG et al 1985 Successful response to intravenous immunoglobulin in autoimmune haemolytic anaemia. British Journal of Haematology 60(2): 387–388
53. Mitchell CA, Van der Weyden MB, Firkin BG et al 1987 High dose intravenous gammaglobulin in Coombs positive hemolytic anemia. Australian and New Zealand Journal of Medicine 17(3): 290–294
54. Oda H, Honda A, Sugita K et al 1985 High-dose intravenous intact IgG infusion in refractory autoimmune hemolytic anemia (Evans syndrome). Journal of Pediatrics 107(5): 744–746
55. Petrides PE, Hiller E 1992 Autoimmune hemolytic anemia combined with idiopathic thrombocytopenia (Evans syndrome). Sustained remission in a patient following high-dose intravenous gamma-globulin therapy. Clinical Investigation 70(1): 38–39
56. Pocecco M, Ventura A, Tamaro P et al 1986 High-dose IVIgG in autoimmune hemolytic anemia [letter]. Journal of Pediatrics 109(4): 726
57. Pui CH, Wilimas J, Wang W et al 1980 Evans syndrome in childhood. Journal of Pediatrics 97(5): 754–758
58. Ritch PS, Anderson T 1987 Reversal of autoimmune hemolytic anemia associated with chronic lymphocytic leukemia following high-dose immunoglobulin. Cancer 60(11): 2637–2640
59. Roldan R, Roman J, Lopez D et al 1994 Treatment of hemolytic anemia and severe thrombocytopenia with high-dose methylprednisolone and intravenous immunoglobulins in SLE [letter]. Scandinavian Journal of Rheumatology 23(4): 218–219
60. Telen MJ, Rao N 1994 Recent advances in immunohematology. Current Opinion in Hematology 1(2): 143–150
61. Blanchette VS, Kirby MA, Turner C et al 1992 Role of intravenous immunoglobulin G in autoimmune hematologic disorders. Seminars in Hematology 29(3 Suppl 2): 72–82.
62. Kimberly RP, Salmon JE, Bussel JB et al 1984 Modulation of mononuclear phagocyte function by intravenous gamma-globulin. Journal of Immunology 132(2): 745–750
63. Morfini M, Vannucchi AM, Grossi A et al 1985 Direct evidence that high dose intravenous gammaglobulin blocks splenic and hepatic sequestration of 51Cr-labeled platelets in ITP [letter]. Thrombosis and Haemostasis 54(2): 554
64. Nugent DJ 1992 IVIG in the treatment of children with acute and chronic idiopathic thrombocytopenic purpura and the autoimmune cytopenias. Clinical Reviews in Allergy 10(1–2): 59–71
65. Smiley JD, Talbert MG 1995 Southwestern Internal Medicine Conference: high-dose intravenous gamma globulin therapy: how does it work? American Journal of Medical Science 309(5): 295–303
66. Templeton JG, Cocker JE, Crawford RJ et al 1985 Fc gamma-receptor blocking antibodies in hyperimmune and normal pooled gammaglobulin [letter]. Lancet 1(8441): 1337
67. Wordell CJ 1991 Use of intravenous immune globulin therapy: an overview. DICP 25(7–8): 805–817

68. Dietrich G, Pereira P, Algiman M et al 1990 A monoclonal anti-idiotypic antibody against the antigen-combining site of anti-factor VIII autoantibodies defines and idiotope that is recognized by normal human polyspecific immunoglobulins for therapeutic use (IVIg). Journal of Autoimmunity 3(5): 547–557

69. Dietrich G, Kaveri SV, Kazatchkine MD et al 1992 Modulation of autoimmunity by intravenous immune globulin through interaction with the function of the immune/idiotypic network. Clinical Immunology and Immunopathology 62(1 Pt 2): S73–S81

70. Rossi F, Dietrich G, Kazatchkine MD et al 1989 Antiidiotypic suppression of autoantibodies with normal polyspecific immunoglobulins. Research in Immunology 140(1): 19–31

71. Roux KH, Tankersley DL 1990 A view of the human idiotypic repertoire. Electron microscopic and immunologic analyses of spontaneous idiotype-anti-idiotype dimers in pooled human IgG. Journal of Immunology 144(4): 1387–1395

72. Sultan Y, Kazatchkine MD, Maisonneuve P et al 1984 Anti-idiotypic suppression of autoantibodies to factor VIII (antihaemophilic factor) by high-dose intravenous gammaglobulin. Lancet 2(8406): 765–768

73. Andersson JP, Andersson UG 1990 Human intravenous immunoglobulin modulates monokine production *in vitro*. Immunology 71(3): 372–376

74. Andersson UG, Bjork L, Skansen-Saphir U et al 1993 Down-regulation of cytokine production and interleukin-2 receptor expression by pooled human IgG. Immunology 79(2): 211–216

75. Aukrust P, Froland SS, Liabakk NB et al 1994 Release of cytokines, soluble cytokine receptors, and interleukin-1 receptor antagonist fter intravenous immunoglobulin administration *in vivo*. Blood 84(7): 2136–2143

76. Shimozato T, Iwata M, Kawada H et al 1991 Human immunoglobulin preparation for intravenous use induces elevation of cellular cyclic adenosine 3′:5′-monophosphate levels, resulting in suppression of tumour necrosis factor alpha and interleukin-1 production. Immunology 72(4): 497–501

77. Dammacco F, Iodice G, Campobasso N et al 1986 Treatment of adult patients with idiopathic thrombocytopenic purpura with intravenous immunoglobulin: effects on circulating T cell subsets and PWM-induced antibody synthesis *in vitro*. British Journal of Haematology 62(1): 125–135

78. Delfraissy JF, Tchernia G, Laurian Y et al 1985 Suppressor cell function after intravenous gammaglobulin treatment in adult chronic idiopathic thrombocytopenic purpura. British Journal of Haematology 60(2): 315–322

79. Dwyer JM 1992 Manipulating the immune system with immune globulin. New England Journal of Medicine 326(2): 107–116

80. Macey MG, Newland AC 1990 CD4 and CD8 subpopulation changes during high dose intravenous immunoglobulin treatment. British Journal of Haematology 76(4): 513–520

81. Pogliani EM, Della VA, Casaroli I et al 1991 Lymphocyte subsets in patients with idiopathic thrombocytopenic purpura during high-dose gamma globulin therapy. Allergology and Immunopathology 19(3): 113–116

82. Tsubakio T, Kurata Y, Katagiri S et al 1983 Alteration of T cell subsets and immunoglobulin synthesis *in vitro* during high dose gamma-globulin therapy in patients with idiopathic thrombocytopenic purpura. Clinical and Experimental Immunology 53(3): 697–702

83. Atkinson JP, Schreiber AD, Frank MM 1973 Effects of corticosteroids and splenectomy on the immune clearance and destruction of erythrocytes. Journal of Clinical Investigation 52(6): 1509–1517

84. Fries LF, Brickman CM, Frank et al MM 1983 Monocyte receptors for the Fc portion of IgG increase in number in autoimmune hemolytic anemia and other hemolytic states and are decreased by glucocorticoid therapy. Journal of Immunology 131(3): 1240–1245

85. Gibson J 1988 Autoimmune hemolytic anemia: current concepts. Australian and New Zealand Journal of Medicine 18(4): 625–637

86. Murphy S, LoBuglio AF 1976 Drug therapy of autoimmune hemolytic anemia. Seminars in Hematology 13(4): 323–334

87. Rosse WF 1985 Autoimmune hemolytic anemia. Hospital Practice (Off Ed) 20(8): 105–109

88. Bowdler AJ 1976 The role of the spleen and splenectomy in autoimmune hemolytic disease. Seminars in Hematology 13(4): 335–348

89. Hosea SW, Burch CG, Brown EJ et al 1981 Impaired immune response of splenectomised patients to polyvalent pneumococcal vaccine. Lancet 1(8224): 804–807

90. Ruben FL, Hankins WA, Zeigler Z et al 1984 Antibody responses to meningococcal polysaccharide vaccine in adults without a spleen. American Journal of Medicine 76(1): 115–121

91. Targarona EM, Espert JJ, Bombuy E et al 2000 Complications of laparoscopic splenectomy [In Process Citation]. Archives of Surgery 135(10): 1137–1140

92. Katkhouda N, Mavor E 2000 Laparoscopic splenectomy. Surgical Clinics of North America 80(4): 1285–1297

93. Ahn YS, Harrington WJ 1980 Clinical uses of macrophage inhibitors. Advances in Internal Medicine 25: 453–473

94. Pignon JM, Poirson E, Rochant H 1993 Danazol in autoimmune haemolytic anaemia. British Journal of Haematology 83(2): 343–345

95. Cervera H, Jara LJ, Pizarro S et al 1995 Danazol for systemic lupus erythematosus with refractory autoimmune thrombocytopenia or Evans' syndrome. Journal of Rheumatology 22(10): 1867–1871

96. Tan AM, Lou J, Cheng HK 1989 Danazol for treatment of refractory autoimmune hemolytic anaemia. Annals/Academy of Medicine Singapore 18(6): 707–709

97. Ahn YS, Harrington WJ, Mylvaganam R et al 1985 Danazol therapy for autoimmune hemolytic anemia. Annals of Internal Medicine 102(3): 298–301

98. Ahn YS, Harrington WJ, Mylvaganam R et al 1985 Danazol therapy for autoimmune hemolytic anemia. Annals of Internal Medicine 102(3): 298–301

99. Mylvaganam R, Ahn YS, Harrington WJ et al 1987 Immune modulation by danazol in autoimmune thrombocytopenia. Clinical Immunology and Immunopathology 42(3): 281–287

100. Schreiber AD, Chien P, Tomaski A et al 1987 Effect of danazol in immune thrombocytopenic purpura. New England Journal of Medicine 316(9): 503–508

101. Sokol RJ, Hewitt S, Stamps BK et al 1983 Autoimmune hemolysis: mixed warm and cold antibody type. Acta Haematologica 69(4): 266–274

102. Heddle NM 1989 Acute paroxysmal cold hemoglobinuria. Transfusion Medicine Reviews 3(3): 219–229

103. Roelcke D, Riesen W, Geisen HP et al 1977 Serological identification of the new cold agglutinin specificity anti- Gd. Vox Sanguinis 33(5): 304–306

104. Roelcke D, Pruzanski W, Ebert W et al 1980 A new human monoclonal cold agglutinin Sa recognizing terminal N-acetylneuraminyl groups on the cell surface. Blood 55(4): 677–681

105. Roelcke D 1981 The Lud cold agglutinin: a further antibody recognizing N- acetylneuraminic acid-determined antigens not fully expressed at birth. Vox Sanguinis 41(5–6): 316–318

106. Roelcke D 1981 A further cold agglutinin, F1, recognizing a N-acetylneuraminic acid- determined antigen. Vox Sanguinis 41(2): 98–101

107. Silberstein LE 1993 Natural and pathologic human autoimmune responses to carbohydrate antigens on red blood cells. Springer Seminars in Immunopathology 15(2–3): 139–153

108. Sokol RJ, Hewitt S, Stamps BK et al 1984 Autoimmune haemolysis in childhood and adolescence. Acta haematologica 72(4): 245–257

109. Kurlander RJ, Rosse WF, Logue GL 1978 Quantitative influence of antibody and complement coating of red cells on monocyte-mediated cell lysis. Journal of Clinical Investigation 61(5): 1309–1319

110. Gelfand EW, Abramson N, Segel GB et al 1971 Buffy-coat observations and red cell antibodies in acquired hemolytic anemia. New England Journal of Medicine 284(22): 1250–1252

111. Dacie JV, Lewis SM 1975 Practical haematology, 5th edn Churchill Livingstone, Edinburgh

112. Wolach B, Heddle N, Barr RD et al 1981 Transient Donath–Landsteiner haemolytic anaemia. British Journal of Haematology 48(3): 425–434

113. Nordhagen R, Stensvold K, Winsnes A et al 1984 Paroxysmal cold haemoglobinuria. The most frequent acute autoimmune haemolytic anaemia in children? Acta Paediatrica Scandinavica 73(2): 258–262

114. Beauregard P, Blajchman MA 1994 Hemolytic and pseudo-hemolytic transfusion reactions: an overview of the hemolytic transfusion reactions and the clinical conditions that mimic them. Transfusion Medicine Reviews 8(3): 184–199

115. Pineda AA, Brzica SM, Jr, Taswell HF et al 1978 Hemolytic transfusion reaction. Recent experience in a large blood bank. Mayo Clinic Proceedings 53(6): 378–390

116. Sazama K 1990 Reports of 355 transfusion-associated deaths: 1976 through 1985. Transfusion 30(7): 583–590

117. Pineda AA, Taswell HF, Brzica SM, Jr. 1978 Transfusion reaction. An immunologic hazard of blood transfusion. Transfusion 18(1): 1–7

118. Baker RJ, Moinichen SL, Nyhus LM et al 1969 Transfusion reaction: a reappraisal of surgical incidence and significance. Annals of Surgery 169(5): 684–693

119. Moore SB, Taswell HF, Pineda AA et al 1980 Delayed hemolytic transfusion reactions. Evidence of the need for an improved pretransfusion compatibility test. American Journal of Clinical Pathology 74(1): 94–97

120. Kohler PF, Farr RS 1966 Elevation of cord over maternal IgG immunoglobulin: evidence for an active placental IgG transport. Nature 210(40): 1070–1071

121. Matre R, Tonder O, Endresen C et al 1975 Fc receptors in human placenta. Scandinavian Journal of Immunology 4(7): 741–745

122. McNabb T, Koh TY, Dorrington KJ et al 1976 Structure and function of immunoglobulin domains. V. Binding, University of immunoglobulin G and fragments to placental membrane preparations. Journal of Immunology 117(3): 882–888

123. van der Meulen JA, McNabb TC, Haeffner-Cavaillon N et al 1980 The Fc gamma receptor on human placental plasma membrane. I. Studies on the binding of homologous and heterologous immunoglobulin G1. Journal of Immunology 124(2): 500–507

124. Lee SI, Heiner DC, Wara D 1986 Development of serum IgG subclass levels in children. Monographs of Allergy 19: 108–121

125. Walker W, Murray S, Russel JK 1957 Stillbirth due to haemolytic disease of the newborn. British Journal of Obstetrics and Gynaecology, Symposium, 573–581

126. Judd WJ, Luban NL, Ness PM et al 1990 Prenatal and perinatal immunohematology: recommendations for serologic management of the fetus, newborn infant, and obstetric patient. Transfusion 30(2): 175–183

127. Morris ED, Murray J, Ruthven CR 1967 Liquor bilirubin levels in normal pregnancy: a basis for accurate prediction of haemolytic disease. British Medical Journal 2(548): 352–354

128. Nicolaides KH, Rodeck CH. 1985 Rhesus disease: the model for fetal therapy. British Journal of Hospital Medicine 34(3): 141–148.

129. Frigoletto FD, Greene MF, Benacerraf BR et al 1986 Ultrasonographic fetal surveillance in the management of the isoimmunized pregnancy. New England Journal of Medicine 315(7): 430–432.

130. Weiner CP. 1992 Human fetal bilirubin levels and fetal hemolytic disease. American Journal of Obstetrics and Gynecology 166(5): 1449–1454.

131. Rubo J, Wahn V. 1991 High-dose intravenous gammaglobulin in rhesus-haemolytic disease. Lancet 337(8746): 914.

132. Carstairs KC, Breckenridge A, Dollery CT et al 1966 Incidence of a positive direct coombs test in patients on alpha-methyldopa. Lancet 2(7455): 133–135.

133. Worlledge SM 1969 Autoantibody formation associated with methyldopa (aldomet) therapy. British Journal of Haematology 16(1): 5–8.

134. Worlledge SM 1978 The interpretation of a positive direct antiglobulin test. British Journal of Haematology 39(2): 157–162.

135. Kelton JG 1985 Impaired reticuloendothelial function in patients treated with methyldopa. New England Journal of Medicine 313(10): 596–600.

136. Hunter E, Raik E, Gordon S et al 1971 Incidence of positive Coombs' test, LE cells and antinuclear factor in patients on alpha-methyldopa ('Aldomet') therapy. Medical Journal of Australia 2(16): 810–812.

137. Worlledge SM, Carstairs KC, Dacie JV 1966 Autoimmune haemolytic anaemia associated with alpha-methyldopa therapy. Lancet 2(7455): 135–139.

138. Petz LD 1993 Drug-induced autoimmune hemolytic anemia. Transfusion Medicine Reviews 7(4): 242–254.

139. LoBuglio AF, Jandl JH 1967 The nature of the alpha-methyldopa red cell antibody. New England Journal of Medicine 276(12): 658–665.

140. Bakemeier RF, Leddy JP 1968 Erythrocyte autoantibody associated with alpha-methyldopa: heterogeneity of structure and specificity. Blood 32(1): 1–14.

141. Breckenridge A, Dollery CT, Worlledge SM et al 1967 Positive direct Coombs tests and antinuclear factor in patients treated with methyldopa. Lancet 2(7529): 1265–1267.

142. Perry HM, Jr, Chaplin H, Jr, Carmody S et al 1971 Immunologic findings in patients receiving methyldopa: a prospective study. Journal of Laboratory and Clinical Medicine 78(6): 905–917.

143. Harth M L.E, 1968 cells and positive direct Coombs' test induced by methyldopa. Canadian Medical Association Journal 99(6): 277–280.

144. Mackay IR, Cowling DC, Hurley TH et al 1968 Drug-induced autoimmune disease: haemolytic anaemia and lupus cells after treatment with methyldopa. Medical Journal of Australia 2(23): 1047–1050.

145. Sherman JD, Love DE, Harrington JF et al 1967 Anemia, positive lupus and rheumatoid factors with methyldopa. A report of three cases. Archives of Internal Medicine 120(3): 321–326.

146. Devereux S, Fisher DM, Roter BL et al 1983 Factor VIII inhibitor and raised platelet IgG levels associated with methyldopa therapy. British Journal of Haematology 54(3): 485–488.

147. Kirtland HH, III, Mohler DN, Horwitz DA et al 1980 Methyldopa inhibition of suppressor-lymphocyte function: a proposed cause of autoimmune hemolytic anemia. New England Journal of Medicine 302(15): 825–832.

148. Petz LD 1980 Drug-induced immune haemolytic anaemia. Clinical Haematology 9(3): 455–482.

149. Levine B, Redmond A 1967 Immunochemical mechanisms of penicillin induced Coombs positivity and hemolytic anemia in man. Internal Archives of Allergy and Applied Immunology 31(6): 594–606.

150. Kerr RO, Cardamone J, Dalmasso AP et al 1972 Two mechanisms of erythrocyte destruction in penicillin-induced hemolytic anemia. New England Journal of Medicine 287(26): 1322–1325.

151. Garratty G, Petz LD 1975 Drug-induced immune hemolytic anemia. American Journal of Medicine 58(3): 398–407.

152. Levine BB, Fellner MJ, Levytska V et al 1966 Benzylpenicilloyl-specific serum antibodies to penicillin in man. II. Sensitivity of the hemagglutination assay method, molecular classes of the antibodies detected, and antibody titers of randomly selected patients. Journal of Immunology 96(4): 719–726.

153. Lee GR, Bithell TC, Foerster J et al 1993 Wintrobe's clinical hematology, 9th edn. Lea & Febiger, Philadelphia.

154. Florendo NT, MacFarland D, Painter M et al 1980 Streptomycin-specific antibody coincident with a developing warm autoantibody. Transfusion 20(6): 662–668.

155. Hart MN, Mesara BW 1969 Phenacetin antibody cross-reactive with autoimmune erythrocyte antibody. American Journal of Clinical Pathology 52(6): 695–701.

156. Wright MS 1999 Drug-induced hemolytic anemias: increasing complications to therapeutic interventions. Clinical Laboratory Sciences 12(2): 115–118.

157. Mollison PL 1993 Blood transfusion in clinical medicine. Blackwell, Oxford.

158. Cooper RA, Bunn HF 1991 Hemolytic anemia. In: Braunwald E, Fauci AS, Isselbacher KJ et al (eds), Harrison's online, McGraw-Hill, New York, 1531–1537.

159. McCrae KR, Cines D 2000 Thrombotic thrombocytopenic purpura and hemolytic uremic syndrome. In: Hoffman R, Benz EJ, Jr, Shattil SJ et al eds, Hematology, basic principles and practice. Churchill Livingstone, Philadelphia, 2126–2154.

160. Laurence J, Mitra D 1997 Apoptosis of microvascular endothelial cells in the pathophysiology of thrombotic thrombocytopenic purpura/sporadic hemolytic uremic syndrome. Seminars in Hematology 34(2): 98–105.

161. Siddiqui FA, Lian EC 1993 Characterization of platelet agglutinating protein p37 purified from the plasma of a patient with thrombotic thrombocytopenic purpura. Biochemistry and Molecular Biology International 30(2): 385–395.

162. Kelton JG, Moore JC, Warkentin TE et al 1996 Isolation and characterization of cysteine proteinase in thrombotic thrombocytopenic purpura. British Journal of Haematology 93(2): 421–426.

163. Moake JL, Rudy CK, Troll JH et al 1982 Unusually large plasma factor VIII:von Willebrand factor multimers in chronic relapsing thrombotic thrombocytopenic purpura. New England Journal of Medicine 307(23): 1432–1435.

164. Levy GG, Nichols WC, Lian EC et al 2001 Mutations in a member of the ADAMTS gene family cause thrombotic thrombocytopenic purpura. Nature 413(6855): 488–494.

165. Rock G, Shumak KH, Sutton DM et al 1996 Cryosupernatant as replacement fluid for plasma exchange in thrombotic thrombocytopenic purpura. Members of the Canadian Apheresis Group. British Journal of Haematology 94(2): 383–386.

166. Rock GA, Shumak KH, Buskard NA et al 1991 Comparison of plasma exchange with plasma infusion in the treatment of thrombotic thrombocytopenic purpura. Canadian Apheresis Study Group. New England Journal of Medicine 325(6): 393–397.

167. Novitzky N, Jacobs P, Rosenstrauch W 1994 The treatment of thrombotic thrombocytopenic purpura: plasma infusion or exchange? British Journal of Haematology 87(2): 317–320.

168. Bell WR, Braine HG, Ness PM et al 1991 Improved survival in thrombotic thrombocytopenic purpura-hemolytic uremic syndrome. Clinical experience in 108 patients. New England Journal of Medicine 325(6): 398–403.

169. Hillmen P, Richards SJ 2000 Implications of recent insights into the pathophysiology of paroxysmal nocturnal haemoglobinuria. British Journal of Haematology 108(3): 470–479.

170. Ferguson MA 1992 Colworth Medal Lecture. Glycosyl-phosphatidylinositol membrane anchors: the tale of a tail. Biochemical Society Transactions 20(2): 243–256.

171. Schubert J, Scholz C, Geissler RG et al 1997 G-CSF and cyclosporin induce an increase of normal cells in hypoplastic paroxysmal nocturnal hemoglobinuria. Annals of Hematology 74(5): 225–230.

172. Hillmen P, Lewis SM, Bessler M et al 1995 Natural history of paroxysmal nocturnal hemoglobinuria. New England Journal of Medicine 333(19): 1253–1258.

173. Schrier SL 2000 Extrinsic Nonimmune hemolytic anemias. In: Hoffman R, Benz EJ, Jr, Shattil SJ et al (eds), Hematology: basic principles and practice. Churchill Livingstone New York, 630–638.

Iron-deficiency anemia, anemia of chronic disorders, and iron overload

MJ Pippard

Introduction

Spectrum of pathology related to disorders of iron metabolism
Iron deficiency
Iron mal-distribution
Iron overload

Major pathways of iron exchange

Molecular mechanisms in iron metabolism

Cellular uptake of iron from transferrin

Regulation of cellular iron homeostasis

Regulation of iron uptake in specific tissues
Role of HFE protein
Development (transcriptional) regulation of iron uptake in the erythron
Hepatocyte iron uptake
Macrophage iron uptake
Uptake of iron by duodenal mucosal cells

Iron release from 'donor' cells

Regulation of iron absorption and internal iron exchange

Pathophysiology

Molecular mechanisms

Assessment of iron status

Serum transferrin receptors

Serum ferritin

Tissue biopsy

Iron deficiency

Causes of iron deficiency

Clinical features of iron-deficiency anemia

Development and pathologic effects of iron deficiency
Exhaustion of iron stores
Iron-deficient erythropoiesis
Iron-deficiency anemia

Mechanism of iron-deficiency anemia

Non-hematologic effects of iron deficiency

Diagnosis of iron deficiency

Treatment of iron deficiency

Functional iron deficiency
Pathophysiology
Treatment

Anemia of chronic disorders

Pathogenesis
Impaired production of erythropoietin
Inhibition of erythropoiesis
Decreased red cell survival
Reduction in iron supply to the erythroid marrow

Diagnosis

Treatment

Iron overload

Iron-overload disorders
Primary iron overload

HFE-related hereditary hemochromatosis
Non-HFE-related hereditary hemochromatosis
Ferroportin mutations
Neonatal hemochromatosis
Congenital atransferrinemia
Aceruloplasminemia

Secondary iron overload
Parenteral iron loading
Increased iron absorption
Pathogenesis of iron-induced damage
Treatment

Introduction

Disturbances of iron metabolism are among the commonest disorders affecting human populations. This high frequency reflects the combination of an essential requirement for iron by all living organisms, with a relatively precarious human iron balance. Iron is required for oxygen carriage, the cellular heme and iron–sulfur enzymes that are responsible for electron transport and energy generation in mitochondrial respiration and the citric acid cycle, and for ribonucleotide reductase, responsible for DNA synthesis.[1] To be available for absorption, dietary iron needs to be in a soluble form, but in an oxygen-rich environment it is readily converted to insoluble ferric hydroxide ('rust'),[2] or bound as insoluble ferric iron complexes, particularly where the diet is predominantly vegetarian. This places an upper limit on the capacity of dietary iron to meet increased iron needs, whether physiologic or due to blood loss. As a result, iron-deficiency anemia affects, at a conservative estimate, at least 500 million of the world's population,[3] and this takes no account of the additional, greater numbers of people who will have borderline iron status with depleted iron stores.[4,5] This is despite the abundance of iron in the earth's crust (which contains approximately 4% of iron). In this context it is perhaps not surprising that humans conserve iron rigorously, with no mechanisms for active iron excretion.[6] However, it does mean that if the normal regulation of iron status through control of iron absorption breaks down, or there is a non-physiologic parenteral source of iron, such as red cell transfusion in chronic anemias, iron overload results. Such iron-loading disorders are less common than iron deficiency, affecting perhaps 5 million of the world's population. However, they are potentially fatal: the very feature that makes iron essential to living organisms – its ability to undergo reversible oxidation–reduction between ferrous and ferric states – is responsible for generating toxic oxygen free radicals, and eventually results in the tissue damage associated with iron overload that characterizes hemochromatosis.

Spectrum of pathology related to disorders of iron metabolism

Iron deficiency

A persistent negative iron balance leads eventually to exhaustion of iron stores, the development of iron-deficient erythropoiesis and eventually anemia. Lack of iron thus has major direct effects on the bone marrow and blood, though other tissues are also affected by the impaired iron supply. This chapter reviews these changes and their accompanying diagnostic features.

Iron mal-distribution

Anemia secondary to a variety of inflammatory illnesses is the commonest form of anemia encountered in hospital practice. Here, disturbances of iron metabolism, leading to retention of iron within the macrophages of the reticuloendothelial system, play a variable part in the pathophysiology of the anemia, other factors usually being of either equal or greater importance. Nevertheless, the diagnosis may depend upon assessment of the changes in iron metabolism, and the hematologist may be involved in excluding more specific causes for anemia, including iron deficiency.

Much less commonly, impaired iron supply to the erythron may occur in association with other causes of localized tissue iron overload, for example in pulmonary hemosiderosis, and the renal tubular iron loading that is associated with paroxysmal nocturnal hemoglobinuria.

Iron overload

Iron overload has no clear direct effects on bone marrow function, but through iron-induced damage to other organs, including liver damage and cirrhosis, it may have indirect effects on blood cells (e.g. red cell macrocytosis, or cytopenias related to hypersplenism). Furthermore, disturbed bone marrow function, particularly with massive ineffective erythropoiesis (e.g. in the β-thalassemia intermedia syndromes, and some patients with congenital dyserythropoietic or sideroblastic anemias – see Chapters 9, 14 and 15), may be associated with inappropriately increased iron absorption and eventual iron overload. The hematologist is likely to be involved in the diagnosis of iron overload, and in its treatment, including phlebotomy in hereditary hemochromatosis and iron chelation therapy in iron-loading anemias.

Major pathways of iron exchange

These were delineated many years ago by use of ferrokinetic studies, following the tissue uptake of ^{59}Fe after its intravenous injection bound to plasma transferrin.[7] The pathways (Fig. 11.1) are dominated (80–90% of plasma iron turnover) by the supply of plasma iron, bound to the circulating transport protein, transferrin, to bone marrow erythroid precursors. There, within mito-chondria, the iron is incorporated into a protoporphyrin ring by the enzyme ferrochelatase in the final step of

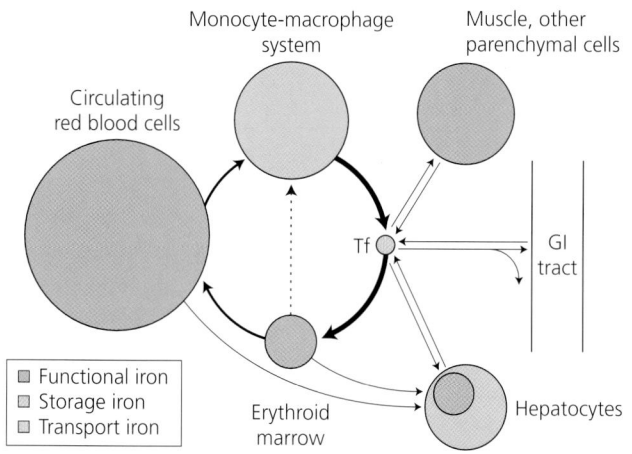

Fig. 11.1 Pathways of iron exchange in an adult. The area of each circle is proportional to the amount of iron within the compartment, and the width of the arrows represents the relative size of the iron fluxes between compartments. Iron supply for erythropoiesis, and the recycling of iron from senescent red cells by macrophages, dominate internal iron exchange. The dotted line represents iron released from the normal 'wastage' of erythroblasts which die before reaching maturation. Tf, transferrin. After Brittenham, 1994,[33] with permission.

heme synthesis.[8] At the end of their life span, the senescent red cells are phagocytosed by tissue macrophages. Heme oxygenase releases the iron from heme for recycling back to plasma transferrin or, alternatively, diversion to stores in the intracellular iron-storage protein, ferritin. A smaller uptake by the liver hepatocytes is the main alternative site of transferrin iron uptake (approximately 10%), and reflects the expression of transferrin receptors on hepatocytes as well as erythroblasts. Whereas macrophages gain nearly all their iron in the unidirectional flow from senescent red cells, hepatocytes are able both to take up iron in a variety of forms (including the non-transferrin-bound iron which is found in many iron-loaded patients with increased saturation of the plasma transferrin) and to release the iron in times of increased need. This makes the liver the major 'buffer' within the system, and a prime target for iron loading and damage in iron-overload conditions. There is very limited exchange of iron with the exterior. Obligatory losses (skin and gastrointestinal mucosal cell loss) of approximately 1 mg/day in males (rather more in women of child-bearing age with the additional losses of menstruation, pregnancy and lactation) are normally balanced by absorption of a similar amount from the diet. The regulation of iron absorption is considered in a later section.

Over recent years, understanding of the processes of cellular iron uptake through transferrin receptors, and regulation of intracellular iron homeostasis, has greatly increased. Identification of a range of additional proteins involved in regulating iron fluxes has been driven by molecular genetic studies of animal models with altered iron metabolism or erythropoiesis.[9,10] The current understanding of the molecular processes involved in iron metabolism is now outlined, since these underpin any discussion of the pathophysiology of the iron disorders and their diagnosis.

Molecular mechanisms in iron metabolism

Cellular uptake of iron from transferrin

Cell-surface transferrin receptors (coded for by a gene at 3q21) have a greater affinity for fully saturated, diferic, transferrin than for monoferric transferrin,[11,12] and do not bind apotransferrin at the neutral pH of plasma. These affinities in part account for the importance of measuring the transferrin saturation as a vital part of a screen for the risk of an iron-loading condition,[13] and the fact that transferrin saturation is a better guide to iron supply to the tissues in iron deficiency than the serum iron value.[14] At a high-transferrin saturation most of the iron is present as diferric transferrin, and iron uptake via transferrin receptors is enhanced. By contrast, the increased concentrations of serum transferrin which are found in iron deficiency mean that the small amount of iron present is in the form of monoferric transferrin, with its reduced rate of uptake by transferrin receptors. After receptor-mediated endocytosis of the transferrin/receptor complex (Fig. 11.2), acidification of the endosome releases the iron from the transferrin, which at low pH even after releasing its iron still has a high affinity for the receptor.[15] The apotransferrin thus recycles with the receptor back to the cell membrane, where it dissociates and is released into the plasma to continue its role in iron delivery to the tissues. The iron is transported into the cell from the endosome by divalent metal transporter, DMT1 (also known as NRAMP2, or DCT1).[16,17] Within the cell it is used in a variety of functional iron compounds, including heme proteins, or is taken up by the iron-storage protein, ferritin.

Regulation of cellular iron homeostasis

The intracellular iron content is finely regulated at the level of translation of the mRNA of several key iron-

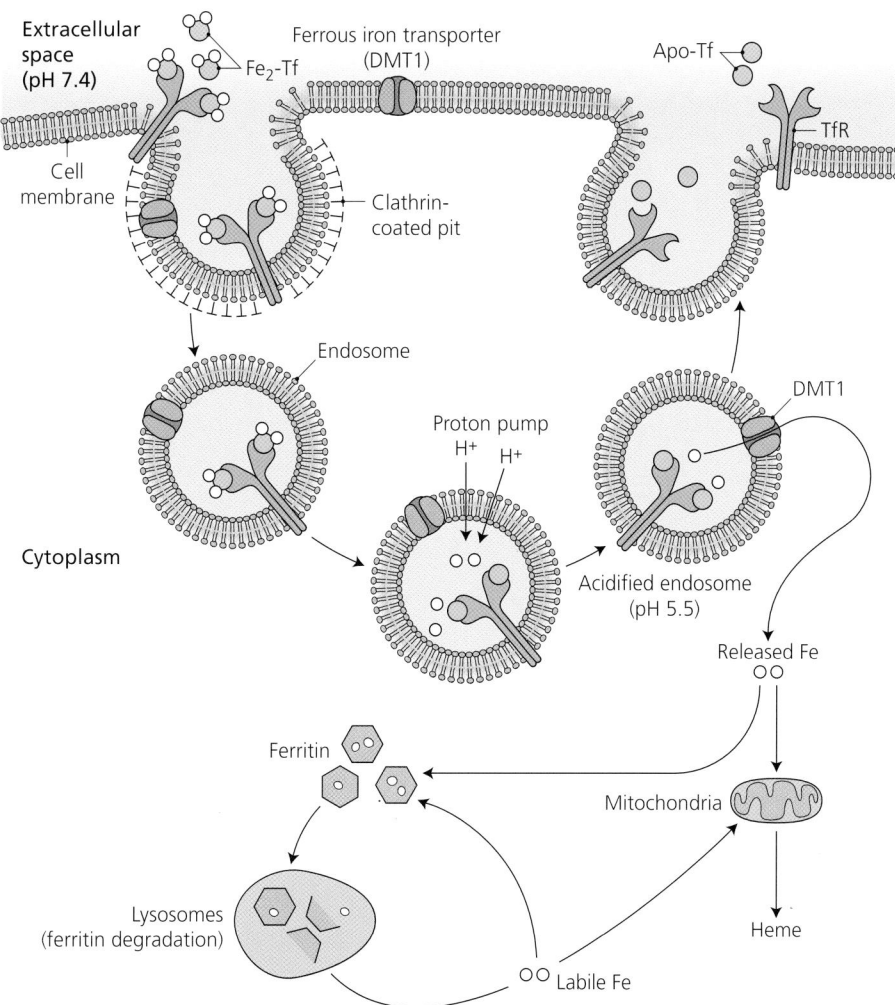

Fig. 11.2 Cellular uptake of transferrin iron and its intracellular utilization. The iron released into the cytoplasm plays a role in the translational regulation of transferrin receptor, ferritin and erythroid ALAS (see text and Fig. 11.3). Ferritin is constantly being catabolized within lysosomes, and the iron is either released back to the cytosolic pool, or remains as hemosiderin (insoluble, partially degraded, ferritin). DMT, divalent metal transporter; Tf, transferrin; TfR, transferrin receptor. Adapted with permission from Andrews, 1999. Copyright © 1999 Massachusetts Medical Society. All rights reserved.[65]

related proteins.[18] Two iron-regulatory proteins (IRP-1, coded on chromosome 9, and IRP-2, coded on chromosome 15), are able to bind to sequences which form stem loop structures called iron-responsive elements (IREs) in the untranslated regions of mRNAs for transferrin receptor and ferritin (Fig. 11.3). When IRP-1 contains an iron–sulfur (4Fe-4S) cluster it has a low affinity for the IRE (and functions as cytoplasmic aconitase), while IRP-2 is unstable in the presence of iron. However, when intracellular 'labile' iron is at a low level, the absence of the iron–sulfur cluster leads to binding of IRP to IREs. IRP binding to IREs that are present in the 3′ untranslated region of the mRNA for transferrin receptor protects the message from cytoplasmic degradation and allows its translation: at the same time, binding of IRP to the single

stem loop in the 5′ untranslated region of the ferritin mRNA inhibits ferritin protein synthesis. The relative rates of synthesis of the two proteins are reversed in conditions of iron excess, and this reciprocal relationship serves to stabilize the intracellular iron content. Other iron-related proteins also have IRE structures in their mRNA.[19] These include erythroid delta-aminolevulinic acid synthase (ALAS), where IRP binding to an IRE in the 5′ untranslated region helps to match iron supply to heme synthesis, and DMT1, where IRP binding to an IRE in the 3′ untranslated region may lead to stabilization of the mRNA in an iron-depleted cell and thus enhanced iron uptake.

Disturbances of intracellular iron distribution result-ing from abnormal mitochondrial iron homeostasis are associated with a number of diseases. Mutations in

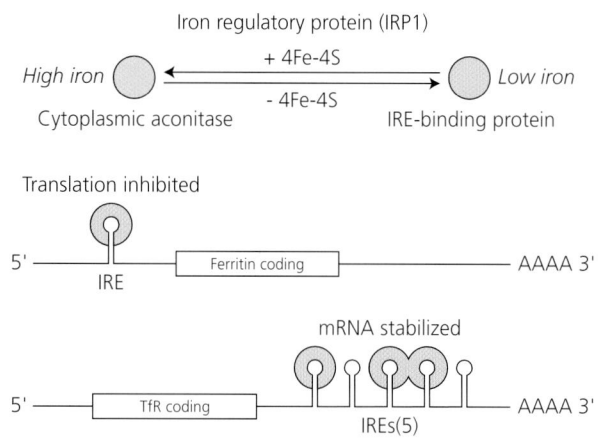

Fig. 11.3 Coordinate regulation of the synthesis of ferritin and transferrin receptor-1 (TfR) by the interaction of iron-binding protein (IRP) with the mRNA iron-responsive element (IRE). When cytoplasmic 'labile' iron (see Fig. 11.2) is low, IRP binds to the IRE stem-loop structures to inhibit ferritin translation, but increases translation of transferrin receptor (TfR) by preventing degradation of the mRNA. When iron levels are high, the IRP functions as a cytoplasmic aconitase and no longer binds to the IREs. This allows increased ferritin synthesis but reduced TfR synthesis. From Postgraduate Haematology 4/e by Hoffbrand, Lewis & Tuddenham.[171] Reprinted by permission of Elsevier Science Ltd.

erythroid ALAS are responsible for X-linked sideroblastic anemia, with iron accumulation within mitochondria related to impaired protoporphyrin synthesis (see Chapter 14).[20] Mutations in two other mitochondrial proteins give rise to mitochondrial iron accumulation and decreased cytosolic iron with defects in iron–sulfur protein maturation. Mutations in the gene for ATP-binding cassette 7 (ABC7) underlie the sideroblastic anemia with spinocerebellar ataxia that is linked to Xq13.[21,22] Autosomal recessive inheritance of mutations in the frataxin gene are responsible for defective mitochondrial export of iron, and the neurological and cardiac problems of Friederich's ataxia.[23,24]

Regulation of iron uptake in specific tissues

Superimposed upon the general mechanisms of the regulation of cellular iron uptake described above are more specific mechanisms related to the different functions of the main 'iron user' cells (in the erythron, and to a lesser extent all other tissues, to support their need for 'functional' iron compounds), and the 'iron donor' cells that are involved in recycling iron to plasma transferrin and iron storage in intracellular ferritin (the macrophages and hepatocytes) or in iron absorption (duodenal mucosal cells).

Role of HFE protein

Of particular interest is the role of the normal HFE protein, produced from the *HFE* gene that is mutated in the common north-European form of hereditary hemochromatosis.[25] This is a membrane protein that is structurally similar to major histocompatibility complex (MHC) class 1 proteins, and which is complexed to β_2-microglobulin to allow its transport to the cell surface. There it binds with the transferrin receptor (TfR1) in competition with diferric transferrin,[26] reducing the affinity of the latter for its receptor. In cultured cell lines transfected with the wild-type *HFE* gene, iron uptake and cellular ferritin content is reduced.[27] Loss of HFE function, as in HFE-related hereditary hemochromatosis (where the C282Y mutation impairs the association of the mutant HFE with β_2-microglobulin and reduces its cell-surface expression,[28] might therefore be expected to *increase* cellular uptake of iron. However, the cells that normally express HFE (macrophages and crypt duodenal mucosal cells,[29,30] but not erythroid cells or hepatocytes) contain *reduced* amounts of iron in hereditary hemo-chromatosis. The precise role(s) of HFE in regulating iron metabolism in the different cell types are thus still unclear.[31] Its putative role in regulating iron absorption by duodenal mucosal cells is discussed elsewhere.

Developmental (transcriptional) regulation of iron uptake in the erythron

Committed erythroid progenitors express erythropoietin receptors maximally at the late erythroid burst-forming unit (BFU-E) and erythroid colony-forming unit (CFU-E) stages, declining from the proerythroblast stage. Erythropoietin prevents apoptosis of these progenitors and allows their proliferation. It also activates IRP and thus upregulates synthesis of transferrin receptor[32]: maximum expression of transferrin receptors reaches a peak in the basophilic erythroblasts. Uptake of iron thus precedes the onset of maximum heme synthesis in the later poly-chromatic erythroblasts.[33] Any iron not subsequently used appears in cytoplasmic ferritin and siderotic granules (giving rise to normal sideroblasts on Perls' staining of marrow smears, or to Pappenheimer bodies in mature red cells on Romanowsky staining of peripheral blood films). These are more prominent where transferrin saturation, and thus the proportion of diferric transferrin, which has a high affinity for the receptor (see above), is increased, and are absent when a low saturation gives rise to iron-deficient erythropoiesis.

Hepatocyte iron uptake

As previously discussed, the hepatocyte is able to take up iron in many forms, including transferrin- and non-transferrin-bound iron, hemoglobin–haptoglobin and heme–hemopexin complexes (which provide a potential direct shunt from the erythron to the hepatocyte in conditions associated with hemolysis or ineffective erythropoiesis), and any tissue ferritin which has been released into the circulation. The hepatocyte has a low level of expression of classical transferrin receptors (TfR1), but these are replaced by a homolog, transferrin receptor 2 (TfR2), coded on chromosome 7.[34,35] This differs from TfR1 in having no IRE in its mRNA, and it is thus not downregulated in the presence of iron overload.[36] Homozygous inheritance of a mutation in the TfR2 gene underlies some cases of non-HFE hemochromatosis, implicating this receptor in the pathway that regulates iron absorption in relation to iron stores (see section below).[37] Iron uptake by hepatocytes from transferrin may occur by the receptor-mediated endocytosis described above or, following release of the iron at the hepatocyte surface, by the route taken by non-transferrin-bound iron. A stimulator of iron transport (STR) coded on chromosome 10q1 may have some role in uptake of both transferrin-bound-, and non-transferrin-bound iron. It is reciprocally regulated in response to cellular iron levels but may be aberrantly upregulated in hereditary hemochromatosis.[38] Clearly, the liver may continue to take in iron from various sources, even when there are high iron stores, and it is thus highly vulnerable to damage in iron-loading disorders.

Macrophage iron uptake

The phagocytic cells of the reticuloendothelial system normally recycle approximately 20 mg iron a day from senescent red cells and the normal small proportion of ineffective erythropoiesis,[7,33] hemoglobin iron thus being their main source of iron. Although they express transferrin receptors, these are at a low level, and do not account for a significant proportion of the plasma iron turnover derived from transferrin. Increased uptake of iron from lactoferrin produced by neutrophils is no longer thought to be a significant source of the increased macrophage storage iron that is seen in inflammatory conditions.[39]

Uptake of iron by duodenal mucosal cells

Duodenal mucosal cells are specialized in relation to iron metabolism to take up iron that has been solubilized in the gut lumen, and to transfer this across their basolateral membrane to circulating plasma transferrin (Fig. 11.4). However, they also express TfRs (both TfR1 and TfR2) at their basolateral membrane, and iron uptake by this route during their cellular maturation from duodenal cells into absorptive enterocytes is believed to set the program for the subsequent level of iron absorption (see below).

Essential initial steps in the uptake of dietary non-heme iron are solubilization (in which stomach acid has an important role) and reduction from ferric (Fe^{3+}) to ferrous (Fe^{2+}) iron.[40] The latter is mediated by a heme-containing enzyme, duodenal cytochrome b (Dcytb), which is expressed in the apical brush-border membrane of duodenal enterocytes.[41] Ascorbate could have a role as an electron donor in this process, accounting, at least in part, for its ability to promote the availability of iron for absorption. An apical transporter, DMT1, then transfers the ferrous iron into the enterocyte.[42,43] Dietary heme iron

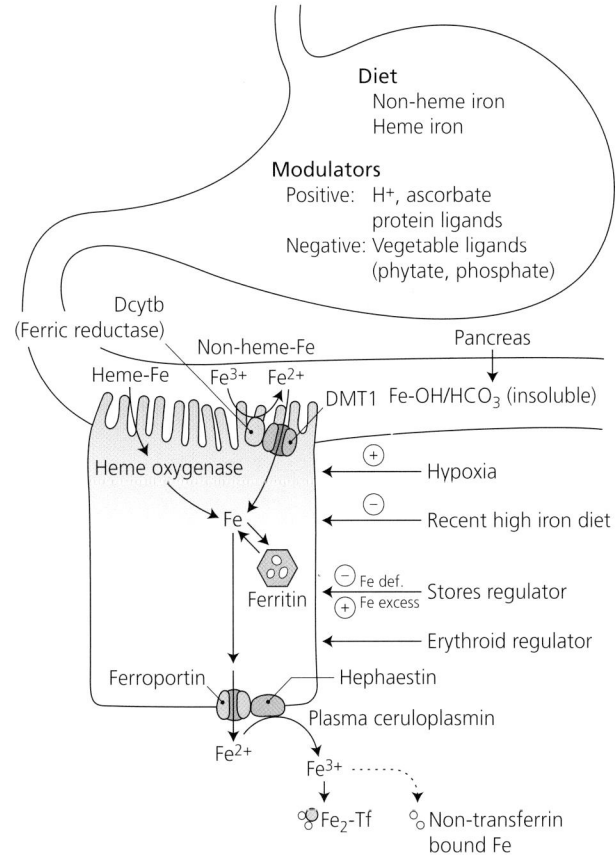

Fig. 11.4 Gastrointestinal and duodenal enterocyte pathways for iron absorption. Iron status is thought to program the subsequent absorptive capacity of the mature enterocyte by altering iron uptake by the early crypt cells. Hepcidin produced by the liver in response to iron may play an important signaling role in this 'stores' regulator. The stimulatory effects of hypoxia and increased erythropoiesis link iron absorption to the main iron-user tissue, the erythron, but the mechanism remains unknown. DMT, divalent metal transporter; Tf, transferrin

is taken up at the apical surface by an independent mechanism and, after release by intracellular heme oxygenase, it joins the same metabolic pool as that derived from inorganic iron.[44] The iron may either be incorporated into ferritin iron stores (to be shed with the enterocyte into the gut lumen at the end of the cell's life span) or transferred across the basolateral membrane by another transport protein, ferroportin (also known as Ireg1).[45]

Iron release from 'donor' cells

Until recently there were few data on the mechanism(s) by which iron is released from cells. This has changed with the identification of the transmembrane transporter, ferroportin,[45] found in the basolateral membrane of the duodenal enterocyte (as discussed above), in the macrophage cytoplasm, and in the hepatocyte sinusoidal membrane.[46] Ferroportin requires oxidation of the iron from Fe^{2+} to Fe^{3+}, and is coupled to the copper oxidases, hephaestin,[47] found within the membrane, and plasma ceruloplasmin,:[48] the released ferric iron is taken up by plasma transferrin. A ceruloplasmin defect may impair hepatocyte iron release, giving rise to liver iron overload that is resistant to phlebotomy,[49] but direct evidence that ferroportin is essential for liver iron release is not yet available. However, transferrin does not appear to be essential for release of iron at the plasma membrane, since in rare cases of congenital atransferrinemia, absence of plasma transferrin does not prevent increased iron uptake from the duodenal enterocyte, and subsequent development of liver parenchymal iron overload.[50]

Regulation of iron absorption and internal iron exchange

Pathophysiology

Iron absorption is normally extremely sensitive to changes in body iron status, and both heme and non-heme iron absorption show an inverse relationship to iron stores.[51] However, it has long been recognized that greatly expanded erythropoiesis, particularly when the latter is ineffective as, for example, in the thalassemia disorders, is associated with increased iron absorption, even in the face of pre-existing iron overload.[52,53] Some have sought to explain these relationships by considering how the overall requirement for iron by the erythron (reflected in the plasma iron turnover) is met in proportion to the iron that is available at the different sites (hepatocytes, macrophages and duodenal enterocytes).[54]

Any increased demand for iron by an expanded erythron that could not be met from recycled hemoglobin iron (from macrophages), or mobilization of iron stores (from macrophages and hepatocytes) would then be met by increased iron absorption from the gut. However, it has remained unclear how such an essentially passive process could account for upregulation of iron uptake and transfer from the duodenal enterocyte, particularly when transferrin saturation was commonly increased in iron-loading anemias such as the thalassemia disorders. The concept of 'store' and 'erythroid' regulators of iron absorption therefore gained currency.[55] To these factors the effect of hypoxia, including that related to anemia, should be added, since this is known to potentiate mucosal uptake[56] (see Fig. 11.4).

An opportunity to examine the relative effects of these three factors was provided by the introduction of recombinant erythropoietin. In normal subjects, stimulation of erythropoiesis by injection of erythropoietin markedly enhanced non heme iron absorption.[57] By contrast, in iron-loaded patients with chronic renal failure who had received multiple red cell transfusions in the past, initial stimulation of erythropoiesis had no effect on mucosal iron uptake or transfer to the plasma at the basolateral membrane. However, after erythropoietin therapy had corrected the anemia, there was a marked decrease in overall iron absorption, due mainly to a reduction in mucosal iron uptake. Repeated phlebotomy to reduce iron stores during continued erythropoietin therapy was accompanied by a tendency for the mucosal transfer of iron to increase, while cessation of erythropoietin treatment after removal of the excess iron was accompanied by a marked drop in overall iron retention due to a reduction in mucosal transfer.[58] These results suggest that anemic hypoxia may play a role in enhancing mucosal iron uptake, while changes in iron stores and erythropoiesis have their main effect on transfer of iron from the enterocyte to the plasma. Furthermore, at the modest levels of increased erythropoiesis achieved in these studies, the upregulation by the 'erythroid regulator' appeared subordinate to downregulation by the 'stores regulator', at least until iron stores had been reduced to a low level. This contrasts with the apparently limited capacity of the stores regulator to upregulate iron absorption when iron stores are low,[59] and the capacity for much greater increases in iron absorption, in the face of increased iron stores, when there is massive ineffective erythropoiesis.

Molecular mechanisms

The complex molecular basis for the physiologic regulation and pathophysiologic changes in iron absorption is slowly emerging. In iron deficiency and hypoxia, expression of essential components of mucosal iron uptake (Dcytb and DMT1) and transfer (ferroportin) is increased at both mRNA and protein level.[41,45,60,61] Expression of DMT1 and ferroportin was inversely related to measures of iron stores, except in hereditary hemochromatosis, where paradoxical increases in DMT1 and ferroportin were observed.[61] The latter are likely to be accompanied by a functional increase in iron uptake, as was seen in HFE-knockout mice.[62] It is thought that the β_2-microglobulin/HFE/TfR1 complex may modulate the uptake of iron from transferrin at the basolateral surface of duodenal mucosal cells, and that loss of this function with mutated HFE in hereditary hemochromatosis could then result in reduced uptake or retention of iron in the developing crypt cells. Maturation within a low-iron environment may program the enterocytes for increased expression of the membrane iron-transporter proteins[63,64] and thus a higher set point for the 'stores' regulator of iron absorption.[65]

Macrophages are the main iron donor cells for internal iron exchange (see Fig. 11.1) and in hereditary hemochromatosis, like the duodenal enterocyte, they appear more ready to release their iron, with subsequent hepatic iron uptake and loading.[66] By contrast, as discussed in relation to the pathophysiology of the anemia of chronic diseases, macrophage iron retention and reduced iron absorption are characteristic of inflammatory or infective diseases. Recent studies suggest that an antimicrobial peptide, hepcidin, produced in the liver in response both to inflammation and to increased storage iron levels,[67] may be an integral part of a stores regulatory mechanism. Knock-out mice that fail to express hepcidin develop hepatic iron overload associated with increased iron absorption and macrophage iron depletion.[68] These authors speculate that iron in hepatocytes stimulates production of a hepcidin signal, which interacts with a sensor, the HFE/β_2-microglobulin/TfR1 complex in the duodenal crypt cells and macrophages, to downregulate iron absorption or increase iron retention respectively.

Assessment of iron status

There is no single measure of iron status that is applicable in every situation. Combinations of measures of iron stores (macrophage and hepatocyte), iron supply to the tissues, and functional iron are often needed to arrive at a clear assessment of iron status.[69] The measures used are summarized in Table 11.1. All are subject to potential confounding factors.

Serum transferrin receptors

Serum transferrin receptors are truncated soluble receptors that are shed into the circulation mainly from the erythroblasts in the marrow.[70] The measurement reflects both the iron status of individual erythroblasts and the total mass of the erythron.[71] It is likely to be of most value in distinguishing iron deficiency from the anemia of chronic disorders,[72] but may also have a role in predicting the risk of iron loading from excessive gastrointestinal iron absorption in the iron-loading anemias.[73]

Serum ferritin

Serum ferritin is apoferritin made up from glycosylated ferritin light chains, the release of which from cells reflects their current rate of ferritin protein synthesis.[74] It is thus related to the metabolically active iron within the cells that determines the activity of IRP-1 and IRP-2, and only indirectly to the ferritin iron stores – the latter are continually being catabolized through lysosomal degradation to release metabolically active iron transiently before it is reincorporated within newly synthesized ferritin or other iron-dependent proteins (see Fig. 11.2). Ferritin protein synthesis also increases in response to inflammatory cytokines, and thus behaves as an acute phase protein independently of iron stores. Damage to ferritin-rich tissues may also release iron-containing ferritin into the circulation and produce high ferritin values, for example in hepatitis, splenic infarction, or bone marrow infarction in sickle cell disease. It is therefore of only limited use as a guide to the presence of increased iron stores,[75,76] though a low serum ferritin is a clear indication that iron stores are absent. Finally, the dependence of ferritin protein synthesis on translational regulation by the IRP/IRE mechanism is illustrated by the hereditary hyperferritinemia/cataract syndrome, where mutations in critical parts of the IRE stem loop are accompanied by uncontrolled synthesis of ferritin light chain. High serum ferritin values are seen with the development of cataracts being directly related to the degree of hyperferritinemia, but there is no iron overload and transferrin saturations are not increased.[77,78]

The reciprocal relationship between the synthesis of transferrin receptors and ferritin within cells (see above) has its counterpart in measurements of serum transferrin receptors and serum ferritin at different stages in the development of phlebotomy-induced iron deficiency (Fig. 11.5). The sensitivity of these measures for assessing iron status is increased by expressing them as a receptor/ferritin ratio[79] or receptor/log ferritin index.[80]

Table 11.1 Assessment of body iron status and confounding factors

Measurement	Representative reference range (adults)	Confounding factors	Diagnostic use
Functional iron			
Hemoglobin concentration		Other causes for anemia besides iron deficiency; a reciprocal relationship with iron stores should be expected in all anemias except in iron-deficiency anemia	Assess severity of IDA (iron deficiency anemia); response to a therapeutic trial of iron confirms IDA. Not aplicable to assessment of iron overload
Males	13–18 g/dl		
Females	12–16 g/dl		
Red cell indices		May be reduced in other disorders of hemoglobin synthesis (e.g. thalassemia, sideroblastic anemias) in addition to iron deficiency	
MCV	80–94 fl		
MCH	27–32 pg		
Tissue iron supply			
Serum iron	10–30 µmol/l	Labile measures: normal short-term fluctuations mean that a single value may not reflect iron supply over a longer period	Raised saturation of TIBC used to assess risk of tissue iron loading (e.g. in hemochromatosis or iron-loading anemias)
Saturation of TIBC	16–50%		
Serum transferrin receptor	2.8–8.5 mg/l	Directly related to extent of erythroid activity as well as being inversely related to iron supply to cells	Decreased saturation of TIBC, reduced red cell ferritin, increased zinc protoporphyrin, and increased serum transferrin receptors indicate impaired iron supply to the erythroid marrow. Particular value in identifying early iron deficiency and, in conjunction with a measure or iron stores, distinguishing this from anemia of chronic disorders
Red cell zinc protoporphyrin	< 80 µmol/mol Hb (< 70 µg/dl red cells)	Stable measures: reduced iron supply at time of red cell formation leads to increases in free protoporphyrin and hypochromic red cells, and reduced red cell ferritin. However, values may not reflect current iron supply. May be increased by other causes of impaired iron incorporation into heme (e.g. lead poisoning, aluminum toxicity in chronic renal failure, sideroblastic anemias)	
Red cell ferritin (basic)	3–40 ag/cell		
% hypochromic red cells	< 10%		
Iron stores			
Serum ferritin	15–300 µg/l	Increased: as an acute phase protein and by release of tissue ferritins after organ damage Decreased: by ascorbate deficiency	All measures are positively correlated with iron stores except TIBC which is negatively correlated. Serum ferritin is of value throughout the range of iron stores. Quantitative phlebotomy, liver iron concentration, chelatable iron and MRI are of value only in iron overload
Tissue biopsy iron			
Liver (chemical assay)	3–33 µmol/g dry wt	Potential for sampling error on needle biopsy, especially when this is < 0.5 mg, or liver is nodular, but remains the 'gold standard' in iron overload	
Bone marrow (Perls' stain)			Bone marrow iron may be graded as absent, normal or increased and is most commonly used to differentiate ACD from IDA
Quantitative phlebotomy	< 2 g iron		In IDA, a raised TIBC is characteristic
Serum TIBC/Transferrin	47–70 µmol/l		
Urine chelatable iron (after 0.5 g im desferrioxamine)	< 2 mg/24 h		
Non-invasive imaging e.g. MRI	–		

IDA, iron deficiency anemia; MCH, mean corpuscular hemoglobin; MCV, mean corpuscular volume; MRI, magnetic resonance imaging; TIBC, total iron-binding capacity.

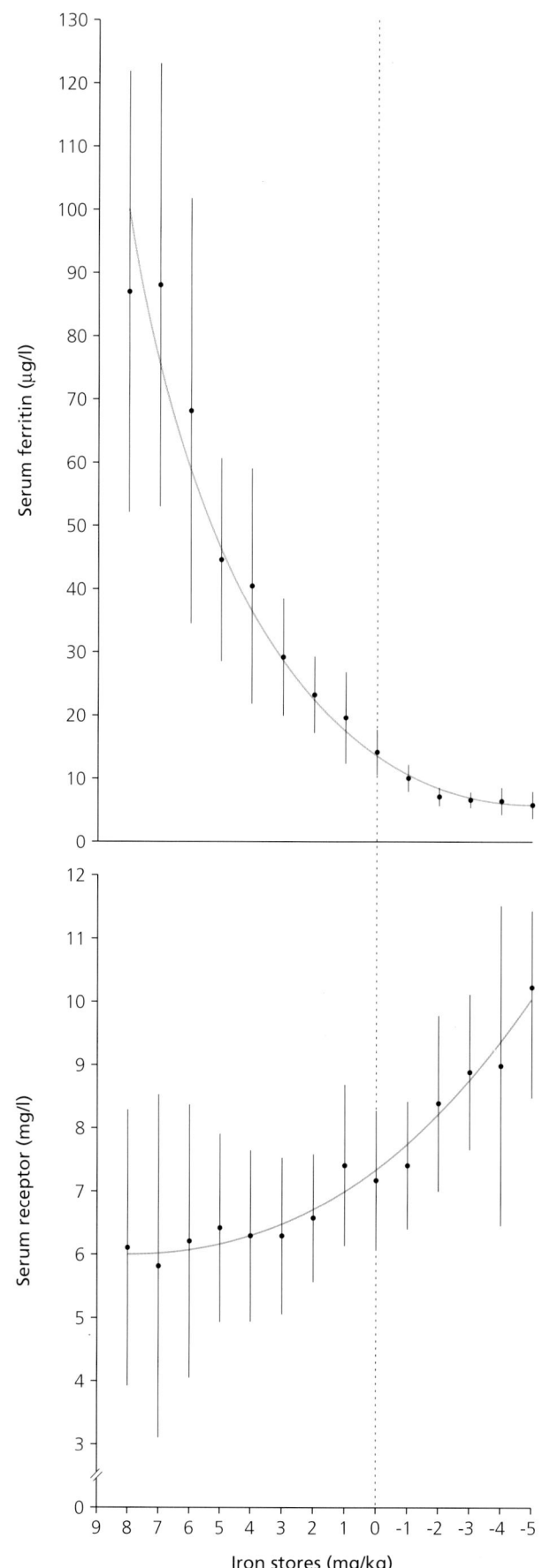

Tissue biopsy

Bone marrow biopsy is used in the assessment of iron status for examining macrophage iron stores. It is thus primarily used in the identification of iron deficiency or for supporting a diagnosis of the anemia of chronic disorders. Bone marrow biopsy touch preparations may give results comparable to aspirates,[81] and positive identification of the absence of iron stores may be inaccurate[82] unless careful examination of macrophages is made.

Liver biopsy provides the opportunity for histologic examination of parenchymal liver iron stores and any fibrotic or cirrhotic changes. In addition, chemical iron determination allows the calculation of a hepatic iron index (μmol iron/g dry liver weight ÷ patient's age in years[83]) values in excess of 1.9 are characteristic of hereditary hemochromatosis, and the measure may help in separating the modest iron overload that sometimes accompanies alcoholic liver disease from the iron-induced liver disease of hemochromatosis. Recent studies using quantitative phlebotomy in patients with thalassemia major who had undergone curative allogeneic bone marrow transplantation, have confirmed that the liver iron concentration is a reliable indicator of total body iron stores in secondary iron overload resulting from red cell transfusions.[84]

Iron deficiency

Iron supply to the erythron may be impaired as a result of an overall deficiency of body iron (absolute iron deficiency), or as a result of a functional defect associated with malutilization of iron. The latter is characteristic of the anemia of chronic disorders (see below), and of patients with chronic renal failure receiving erythropoietin therapy, where the demands of new erythropoiesis can outstrip the rate at which otherwise adequate iron stores can be mobilized.[85] Absolute iron deficiency eventually develops when the ability of the diet and iron absorption to keep pace with requirements or losses is exceeded. The identification of iron-deficiency anemia is not usually difficult (see below), and the main clinical diagnostic task is to determine the cause of the negative iron balance.

Fig. 11.5 Relationship between serum ferritin and soluble transferrin receptor concentrations in volunteers undergoing quantitative phlebotomy. The dotted line shows the point at which iron stores are exhausted, and further phlebotomy produces a loss of functional hemoglobin iron. From: Skikne BS, Flowers CH, Cook JD. Serum transferrin receptor: a quantitative measure of tissue iron deficiency. *Blood* 1990; 75:1870–1876. Copyright American Society of Hematology, used by permission.

Causes of iron deficiency (Table 11.2)

Iron-deficiency anemia is extremely common[3] particularly among women of child-bearing age, and preschool children (who have increased physiologic requirements for iron) and in populations dependent upon largely vegetarian diets. The latter lack more readily absorbable heme iron and the peptide ligands derived from animal foods that help to keep non-heme iron in a soluble form, and contain phytates and phosphates that tend to produce insoluble iron complexes (see Fig. 11.4). In the UK, the diet contains between 5 and 6 mg iron/1000 kcal and the average daily intake of iron has fallen from around 12 mg to 10 mg/day over the last 25 years, as energy intake has fallen.[86] For adult men the mean daily intake was 14.1 mg, and for women 12.3 mg, in 1986–87,[87] and can be compared with the estimated average requirements of 6.7 mg for men and 11.4 mg for the majority of premenopausal women.[88]

The combination of a diet with poorly available iron and physiologic increased iron requirements is probably the commonest cause of iron deficiency on a world scale. However, diet alone is very seldom the cause of iron deficiency in men or postmenopausal women in whom pathologic blood loss should be suspected. Blood loss of more than about 6 ml (3 mg iron)/day, added to obligatory losses of about 1 mg/day through shedding of skin and intestinal cells, is likely to exceed the maximum absorptive capacity from the gastrointestinal tract, hookworm infestation being a major cause in many parts of the world. In women of reproductive age, menstruation adds an average of 20 mg/month, and menorrhagia is very likely where anemia develops. In men or postmenopausal women, occult gastrointestinal blood loss must be considered, and in these patients, as well as younger women who have symptoms suggestive of gastrointestinal disease, endoscopic and/or radiologic investigation of the gut is likely to be required.[89] This should be considered whether or not fecal occult blood tests are positive, since otherwise unexplained iron deficiency is itself a sufficient pointer to occult bleeding, which may be intermittent and undetected by fecal testing. Less commonly, malabsorption of iron may be responsible for negative iron balance. Iron deficiency is a predictable complication after gastrectomy, where loss of the stomach acid and more rapid transit past the duodenal absorptive area of the gut, combine to reduce dietary iron availability. Gastric atrophy and achlorhydria in pernicious anemia also lead to an increased risk of iron deficiency.[90] Coeliac disease may present with isolated iron deficiency, and features of hyposplenism on the blood film.

Though a cause for iron deficiency can usually be identified there remain a few patients in whom the cause remains uncertain. In older patients, bleeding from angiodysplastic lesions in the gut may be suspected, but careful follow-up is required since reinvestigation may be needed if there are new symptoms or worsening of the negative iron balance. In occasional younger patients in whom other causes of hypochromic anemia have been excluded, a failure to respond to iron therapy may lead to a suspicion of malabsorption of iron.[91] A possible defect in one of the proteins involved in iron metabolism may be suspected, though failure to take the iron therapy, or continued occult blood loss are far more likely explanations. Many polymorphisms of the transferrin gene have been described, and at least one may be associated with an increased risk of iron deficiency.[92] Autoimmune

Table 11.2 Causes of iron deficiency

Increased physiologic requirements	
Growth	Preterm and low birthweight
	Preschool children
	Adolescents
Reproduction	Menstruation
	Pregnancy
	Lactation
Dietary insufficiency or poor bioavailability	
	Early introduction of cow milk (low iron content) in infancy
	Vegetarian diet (insoluble phytate iron complexes)
	Antacids/protein pump inhibitors
	Clay eating (pica)
Blood loss	
Gastrointestinal	Epistaxes
	Varices
	Erosive gastritis
	Peptic ulcer
	Aspirin or other NSAIDs
	Carcinoma of stomach, colon
	Mekel's diverticulum
	Angiodysplasia
	Inflammatory bowel disease
	Diverticulosis
	Hemorrhoids
Pulmonary	Hemoptysis
	Pulmonary hemosiderosis
Genitourinary	Menorrhagia
	Postmenopausal bleeding
	Parturition
	Hematuria (e.g. renal or bladder origin)
	Hemoglobinuria (e.g. paroxysmal nocturnal hemoglobinuria)
Other blood loss	Trauma
	Widespread bleeding disorder
	Self-inflicted
Malabsorption	
	Post-gastrectomy
	Atrophic gastritis
	Chronic systemic inflammatory disease
	Gluten-induced enteropathy

antibodies directed against the transferrin receptor were thought to account for iron deficiency in one report.[93] The possibility that mutations/polymorphisms in one or other of the recently identified proteins involved in transmembrane iron transport may underlie some cases of unexplained iron deficiency that are refractory to iron therapy[94,95] has yet to be explored systematically.

Clinical features of iron-deficiency anemia

The symptoms of iron-deficiency anemia are non-specific, and where the anemia has developed over a prolonged period of negative iron balance the patient may be well adapted even at low concentrations of hemoglobin. Tiredness and shortness of breath are common complaints, while in the elderly with pre-existing cardiovascular pathology, angina or heart failure may develop. Other symptoms may be related to effects of iron deficiency on epithelial tissues or the gastrointestinal tract. For example, a sore mouth may be due to glossitis and/or angular cheilosis, and brittle nails may reflect the atrophic skin and nail changes, though frank koilonychia is uncommon now that severe iron deficiency is much less likely to go untreated for prolonged periods. Difficulty in swallowing may be related to an esophageal or pharyngeal web: this is still seen occasionally, particularly in middle-aged women with a history of chronic iron deficiency, and is a premalignant condition. Pica is sometimes a feature, and where this involves ingestion of clay or chalk this may be the cause rather than the result of iron deficiency, through the formation of insoluble iron complexes in the gut lumen.

Development and pathologic effects of iron deficiency

The development of iron deficiency can be considered in three stages,[96] corresponding to the sequential involvement of storage iron, iron supply to the tissues, and the functional compartment of hemoglobin iron.

Exhaustion of iron stores

The first response to a negative iron balance is the mobilization of any iron stores from macrophages or hepatocytes, and an upregulation of iron absorption (see earlier discussion). Assessment of iron stores will show declining values (see Table 11.1 and Fig. 11.5), but there is no evidence that depletion of iron stores has any harmful effects apart from reducing the ability to respond to

increased demands for iron whether these are physiologic (e.g. pregnancy) or pathologic (e.g. hemorrhage). Erythropoiesis remains unaffected at this stage.

Iron-deficient erythropoiesis

A continued negative iron balance after iron stores are exhausted leads to a decline in serum iron concentration and transferrin saturation to below the value of 16% found necessary to support normal erythropoiesis.[14] The reduced iron supply to the erythron leads to upregulation of the expression of transferrin receptors on the erythroblasts, with a rise in serum transferrin receptor concentration (see Table 11.1 and Fig. 11.5). Other measures also begin to reflect the impaired iron supply, with increase in red cell protoporphyrin,[97] and detection of poorly hemoglobinized reticulocytes[98] and hypochromic red cells.[99] At this stage the hemoglobin concentration, mean red cell volume (MCV) and mean corpuscular hemoglobin (MCH) may still be in the reference range, though the blood film may show occasional hypochromic red cells.

Iron-deficiency anemia

Further depletion of body iron leads to the development of iron-deficiency anemia. The hemoglobin concentration drops below the threshold for definition of anemia (13.0 g/dl in men and 12.0 g/dl in women), and the red cell MCV and MCH are reduced. On the blood film, the red cells become more obviously hypochromic and variable in size, and poikilocytosis may be marked (Fig. 11.6) often with elongated 'pencil' forms. Target cells may be visible. Reticulocytes are not increased appropriately

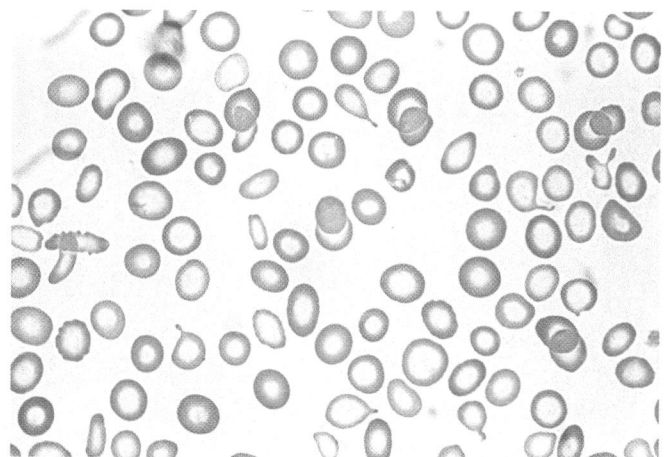

Fig. 11.6 Peripheral blood film from an iron-deficient preschool child (Hb of 5.5 g/dl and MCV of 50 fl). Microcytes and poikilocytes are prominent, as well as poor hemoglobinization of the red cells.

for the degree of anemia, though serum erythropoietin concentrations are markedly raised. Platelet counts are usually increased, but there are case reports of associated thrombocytopenia,[100] and even the development of transient thrombocytopenia a few days after starting oral replacement iron therapy.[101] The serum transferrin saturation is likely to be very low: this effect is exacerbated by a rising serum transferrin concentration – transcriptional regulation of transferrin synthesis by the liver is inhibited by iron excess and stimulated by its absence.[102]

A bone marrow examination is rarely needed to confirm the diagnosis. Marrow sideroblasts disappear early in the development of iron-deficient erythropoiesis.[14] Erythroblasts show delayed hemoglobinization with a ragged, vacuolated cytoplasm, and relatively pyknotic nucleus for the stage of hemoglobinization. The white cell series is usually normal. Absence of stainable marrow iron stores in a randomly selected population of 38-year-old women could be predicted by a serum ferritin concentration of $< 16\,\mu g/l$ (specificity 98%; sensitivity 75%).[103] However, iron-deficient erythropoiesis may have already begun at values above this, consistent with the pattern of increasing serum transferrin receptor before iron stores are completely exhausted[79] (see Fig. 11.5).

Mechanism of iron-deficiency anemia

Impaired heme synthesis within individual erythroid precursors clearly accounts for many of the marrow and peripheral blood findings. However, this does not account for why the anemia is hypoproliferative, with an inappropriately low reticulocyte count despite raised erythropoietin concentrations. Studies in iron-deficient rats[104] show normal numbers of BFU-E, a markedly increased number of CFU-E, and only mildly increased numbers of erythroblasts, suggesting that the iron deficiency is responsible for a maturation defect between the CFU-E and early normoblasts.

Non-hematologic effects of iron deficiency

These are less well defined than the effects on the erythron, and it has been difficult to disentangle the effects of anemia from those of tissue iron deficiency: anemia and depletion of tissue iron-containing enzymes usually develop in parallel.

The epithelial abnormalities described above are poorly correlated with tissue enzyme levels[105] and may respond slowly or not at all to iron-replacement therapy.

Gastric atrophy and esophageal webs are also associated with circulating parietal cell antibodies, achlorhydria and an increased risk of pernicious anemia,[106] suggesting that additional environmental or genetic factors may predispose to these effects.

Iron deficiency may impair immune function, with reduced T-cell and neutrophil function,[107] but the data are conflicting about the role for iron in protecting against or potentiating the risk of infection.[39]

Work performance is impaired in the presence of iron-deficiency anemia.[108,109] The major effect can be attributed to the anemia, with additional effects of tissue iron depletion on muscle oxidative metabolism and function (e.g. increased lactate production[110]) being likely.

Iron-deficiency anemia in young children is associated with impaired performance in a number of developmental and psychological tests. However, iron deficiency without anemia does not seem to affect psychomotor functions.[111] There is some suggestion that the deficit may not be restored by iron treatment. Since iron deficiency is common in preschool children even in developed nations, there is a need to determine whether the impairment is long-lasting.

Diagnosis of iron deficiency

The identification of a microcytic hypochromic anemia in a patient with a good reason for iron deficiency (e.g. menorrhagia) may require no further immediate investigation, diagnosis being confirmed by the correction of the hematologic abnormalities with iron therapy. Where there are other potential reasons for red cell microcytosis (e.g. defects of globin chain synthesis, severe and chronic underlying inflammatory disease, or sideroblastic anemia) a low serum ferritin combined with anemia will confirm the presence of depleted total body iron. However, because the serum ferritin is an acute-phase protein, it may be within the reference range in the presence of an inflammatory disorder, even when there is coexistent depletion of iron stores (see discussion of the diagnosis of anemia of chronic disorders on page 219). Mild iron-deficiency anemia may still have a red cell MCV within the reference range, and here the main differential diagnosis is with the anemia of chronic disease.

Treatment of iron deficiency

Treatment is usually readily achieved with an oral preparation of a simple iron salt, preferably ferrous sulfate (200 mg three times daily provides 180 mg elemental iron per day). Adverse effects such as nausea, epigastric pain, diarrhea and constipation are related to the amount of available iron, and can usually be ameliorated by reducing the dose of ferrous sulfate, switching to ferrous gluconate (which contains only 35 mg iron in each 300 mg tablet), and/or taking the iron with food. Although these measures reduce the amount of iron available to be absorbed, the speed of regeneration of the hemoglobin concentration is not usually critical. Slow-release preparations should be avoided – they are an expensive way of avoiding adverse gastrointestinal effects by giving iron which is less available (it tends to be carried past the main absorption site in the duodenum).

Failure to respond to oral iron therapy is usually due to poor compliance, but may be due to continuing blood loss. It should lead to a reassessment of the diagnosis before considering alternative forms of iron therapy.

Parenteral iron is rarely needed, and should be restricted to patients with proven iron deficiency who cannot tolerate even small doses of oral iron, or in whom continuing blood loss is so great that the oral therapy cannot keep pace. Iron sucrose (Venofer®) and iron dextran (Cosmofer®) preparations are available for iv use, while iron sorbitol (Jectofer) has to be given as a course of deep intramuscular injections. Adverse effects include anaphylaxis, and fever and arthropathy may occur particularly when large doses are given intravenously: this underscores the preference for oral iron therapy whenever possible.

Functional iron deficiency

Pathophysiology

A functional iron deficiency develops when the demands of the erythron for iron outstrip the ability to deliver iron to the marrow. This balance is disturbed in thalassemia intermedia syndromes, when blood supply to the expanded marrow may be insufficient, even with increased plasma transferrin saturation, to satisfy the demands of the erythoblasts.[112] When erythropoietin therapy for the anemia of chronic renal disease was introduced, it was noted that even in patients with adequate or increased amounts of storage iron, the stimulation of erythropoiesis was typically accompanied by a drop in transferrin saturation,[85] and the appearance of hypochromic red cells.[99] In some transfusion-dependent iron-loaded patients, an initial drop in serum ferritin concentration after starting erythropoietin therapy (Fig. 11.7) was followed by a recovery to previous levels once a new steady state at a high hemoglobin concentration was reached.[113] The evidence of impaired iron supply was accompanied by a poor response to the erythropoietin

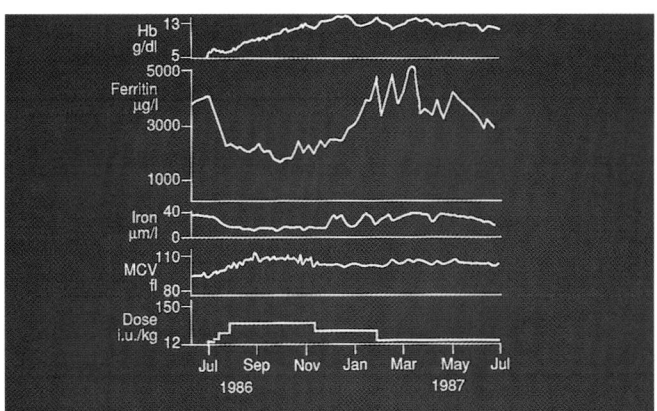

Fig. 11.7 Serial measures of iron status in a patient with chronic renal failure starting treatment with recombinant human erythropoietin. Despite high pretreatment iron stores, related to multiple previous red cell transfusions, serum iron and serum ferritin fell during the phase of hemoglobin regeneration, but recovered at the new steady state at a higher hemoglobin concentration.

which could be reversed by iron therapy (usually small amounts of intravenous iron). This functional (rather than absolute) iron deficiency also provided further evidence that the serum ferritin concentration was dependent on the flux of iron through the macrophages, rather than being directly related to the amount of iron stores. During the initial phase of erythropoietin treatment, the need for blood transfusions was replaced by the production of young red cells: the macrophages were required to supply additional iron for erythropoiesis at a time when their uptake of iron from senescent red cells had fallen. This net drain of iron from the macrophage could be expected to reduce the amount of labile iron available within the cell, and thus reduce the stimulus for translation of ferritin mRNA, despite the relatively inert hemosiderin iron stores remaining almost unchanged.

Treatment

With the introduction of erythropoietin therapy for the anemia of renal disease, the emphasis has moved away from avoiding iron therapy and its associated risk of iatrogenic iron overload.[114] The aim now is to maintain the iron supply (assessed by transferrin saturation or the percentage of hypochromic red cells), and thus the response to erythropoietin, through regular small doses of intravenous iron (e.g. 100 mg iron sucrose each month), provided the serum ferritin does not exceed 500–1000 µg/l.[113,115]

The pathophysiology of the anemia of renal failure has much in common with the 'anemia of chronic disorders', considered in the following section.

Anemia of chronic disorders

A normochromic normocytic anemia develops in patients with a variety of inflammatory disorders provided these last more than a few days. Where the inflammatory stimulus is prolonged the anemia may become more microcytic. The severity of the anemia is proportional to that of the underlying disorder, which may be infection, malignancy or an autoimmune disease such as rheumatoid arthritis. Inflammatory stimulation of the synthesis of acute-phase proteins is reflected in an increase in plasma viscosity or erythrocyte sedimentation rate, and may be obvious on a blood film by the presence of increased formation of red cell rouleaux. The pathogenesis of the anemia is multifactorial, involves the activation of cellular immunity and the production of a range of inflammatory cytokines, and is accompanied by an alteration in the handling of iron by macrophages (and other iron-donating cells) that results in characteristic changes in measures of iron status.

Pathogenesis

Impaired production of erythropoietin

Patients with the anemia of chronic disorders generally have reduced amounts of erythropoietin in the urine,[116] and lower serum concentrations of erythropoietin compared with patients with other causes for anemia.[117,118] However, this is not a universal finding, and patients with juvenile chronic arthritis may retain a normal erythopoietin drive to the marrow:[119] this may account for the more profound red cell microcytosis often encountered in these patients, where limitations on the iron supply to the erythron appear to play a more dominant role (see below). Pro-inflammatory cytokines interleukin-1 (IL-1) and tumor necrosis factor-α (TNF-α) are likely to mediate reduced erythropoietin production by the kidney in response to anemic hypoxia.[120]

Inhibition of erythropoiesis

IL-1 and TNF-α, as well as interferon-γ (IFN-γ), directly inhibit the growth of erythroid progenitors (BFU-E and CFU-E)[120,121] through promotion of apoptosis.[122] In part, this apoptosis may be mediated through the increased production of nitric oxide.[123] The latter may also inhibit heme synthesis since it activates IRP which is then able to bind to IRE stem loop structures[124] and may thus reduce the translation of the mRNA for ALAS. A greater amount of erythropoietin is required to restore CFU-E growth *in vitro* in the presence of high concentrations of TNF-α or

IFN-γ.[125] The effects of reduced erythropoietin production and direct cytokine inhibition of erythropoiesis are thus likely to combine to suppress erythropoiesis in inflammatory disorders.

Decreased red cell survival

Activation of macrophages and enhanced erythophago-cytosis is responsible for a modest reduction in red cell survival in inflammatory conditions.[126,127] Although the reduction in red cell survival would not, on its own, be sufficient to produce significant anemia, it compounds the impaired erythroid response (see above) mediated via inflammatory cytokines.

Reduction in iron supply to the erythroid marrow

Inflammation, and the anemia of chronic disorders, is associated with reduced serum iron concentrations, and retention of iron within macrophages. The circulating transferrin concentration also tends to be reduced, and the reduction of transferrin saturation is thus often less severe than in iron-deficiency anemias. The end result is that iron is redistributed from circulating red cells to macrophage iron stores. Despite increased marrow iron staining and raised serum ferritin values, there is a modestly reduced iron supply to the erythroblasts and red cells may become progressively more microcytic (Fig. 11.8). The finding that serum concentrations of trans-ferrin receptor are not generally increased in the anemia of chronic disorders (unlike iron deficiency)[72] may relate to cytokine-induced inhibition of receptor synthesis. Alternatively, a balanced decrease in both erythropoiesis and iron supply, so that the iron requirements of individual erythroblasts continue to be met, could mean that there is no activation of transferrin receptor synthesis through the IRP/IRE regulatory mechanism. In patients with inflammatory disorders who develop more marked red cell microcytosis there may be either more severe impairment of iron supply to the erythron,[128] or the suppression of erythropoiesis may be less marked (as appears to be the case in juvenile chronic arthritis).[119] In both these circumstances the expectation is that the serum transferrin receptor concentration will be raised, though the ratio of serum transferrin receptor to log ferritin may not be increased unless there is a coincidental absolute iron deficiency (Fig. 11.9).[80,129]

The changes in iron metabolism can be related to altered production of pro- and anti-inflammatory cytokines and/or their downstream products.[130] Inflammation, and

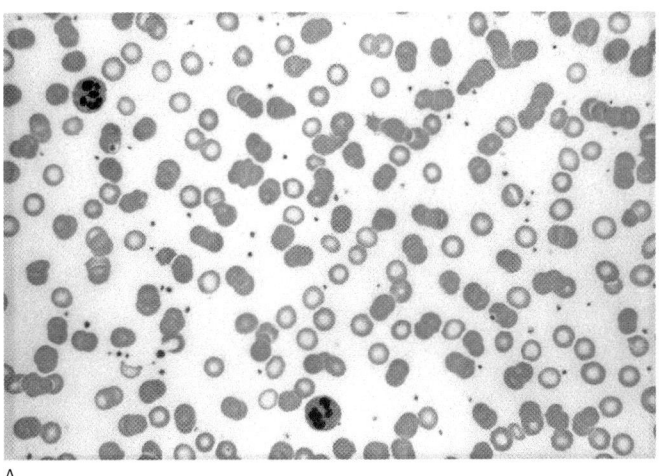
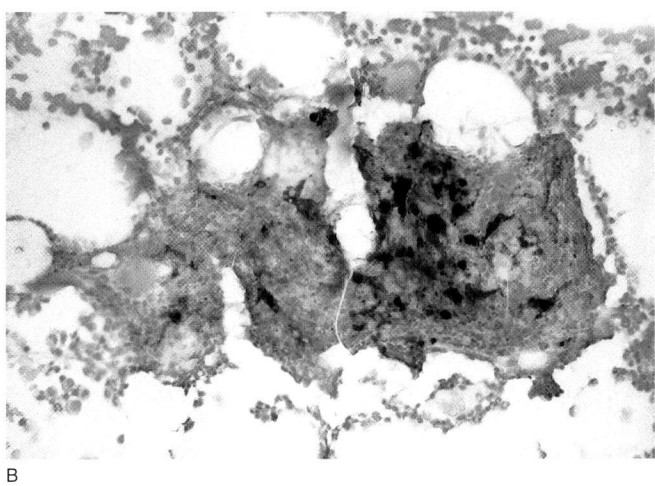

A   B

Fig. 11.8 Peripheral blood film (A) and bone marrow aspirate stained for iron (B) from a 63-year-old woman with active rheumatoid arthritis (Hb 7.2 g/dl, MCV 66 fl). Marked hypochromia and rouleaux of the red cells (ESR 110 mm/h) was accompanied by plentiful marrow iron stores. These are the features of macrophage 'iron block' in a severe case of the anemia of chronic disorders. From Postgraduate Haematology 4/e by Hoffbrand, Lewis and Tuddenham.[171] Reprinted by permission of Elsevier Science Ltd.

the pro-inflammatory cytokines IL-1 and TNF-α, stimulate ferritin synthesis within macrophages and hepatocytes,[131,132] through an effect on transcription and translation of the mRNA which is independent of the IRP/IRE regulatory mechanism. By contrast, γ-IFN activates IRP, an effect that is blocked by the anti-inflammatory cytokines IL-4, IL10 and IL-13, thus allowing increased ferritin translation.[133] Ferritin thus behaves as an acute-phase protein, with synthesis being increased by a variety of pathways in inflammation, contributing to the classic 'RE block' in iron release from macrophages. Differences in the proportions or types of cytokine expression may account for variation in the degree of erythroid suppression and red cell microcytosis in different inflammatory disorders.

Recent studies suggest that the antimicrobial protein, hepcidin, produced by the liver in response to inflammation, may play a major role in controlling the release of iron to plasma not only from macrophages, but also from duodenal mucosal cells.[68] Increased amounts of circulating hepcidin might account for the reduced iron absorption seen in inflammatory disorders,[134] as well as iron retention by macrophages (see discussion on page 210 of the molecular regulation of iron absorption).

Diagnosis

The finding of a mild to moderate normochromic anemia in association with an obvious underlying disorder usually makes the clinical diagnosis of the anemia of chronic disorders, and the pattern of disturbance of the measures of iron status usually helps to confirm the diagnosis (see Table 11.1). Difficulty may arise when there is a possi-

bility of iron deficiency coexisting with the anemia of chronic disorders. Here the increased intracellular ferritin synthesis by macrophages and hepatocytes (see above) can lead to serum ferritin values which are within the normal reference range, even where iron stores are absent. Values even as high as 100 μg/l may still be associated with absent iron stores where there is an acute-phase response. Furthermore these values must be considered in relation to the accompanying anemia, since there may still be inadequate iron stores to permit full regeneration of the hemoglobin once the inflammatory stimulus is removed. The serum transferrin receptor concentration, or the transferrin receptor/log ferritin index (see Fig. 11.9), may yield a better distinction between anemia of chronic disorders alone (low index) and combined with iron deficiency (raised index).[80] However, bone marrow examination, and Perls' stain for hemosiderin iron, may still be the quickest way to be certain whether there are iron stores present.

Treatment

The main approach is to treat the underlying inflammatory disorder. In many cases it is the underlying disease rather than the accompanying anemia that gives rise to the main symptoms. However, where the anemia is impairing quality of life (e.g. in association with cancer), red cell transfusion may help. A more sustained rise in hemoglobin may be obtained with recombinant erythropoietin therapy, but the response is variable and usually not clinically significant: again this is likely to reflect differences in the range of cytokines produced, and larger doses of erythropoietin may be needed where

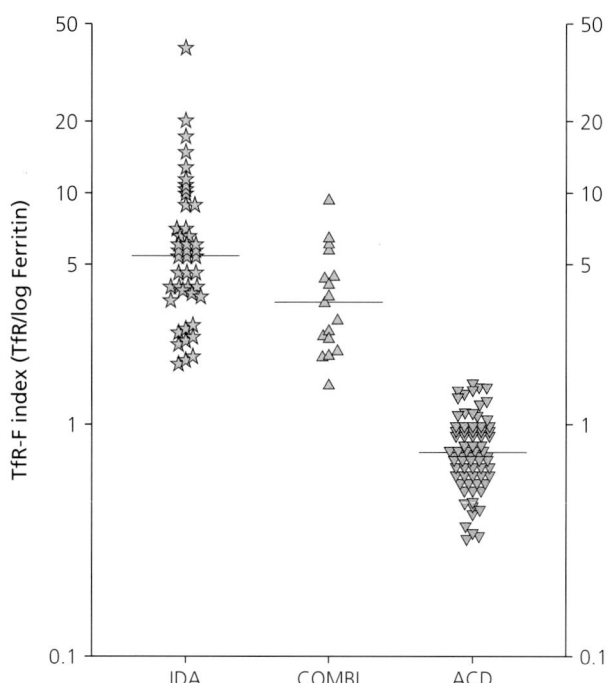

Fig. 11.9 The serum transferrin receptor/log ferritin index in patients with iron-deficiency anemia (IDA), anemia of chronic disorders (ACD), or a combination of the two (COMBI). The index produces a good separation of those patients with iron deficiency, whether or not they have an accompanying inflammatory disorder. From: Punnonen K, Irjala K, Rajanaki A. Serum transferrin receptor and its ratio to serum ferritin in the diagnosis of iron deficiency. *Blood* 1997; 89: 1052–1057. Copyright American Society of Hematology, used by permission.

erythroid suppression is most marked. Iron supplementation is likely to be ineffective, and carries the theoretical objection that it may impair immune function where the underlying disease is infective or malignant in origin. The possibility that iron chelators might be used to treat the anemia by 'shuttling' iron out of macrophage iron stores has been raised.[135] However, this remains speculative.

Iron overload

Iron overload may be primarily the result of a genetically determined increase in iron absorption, as in hereditary hemochromatosis, or secondary to disturbance of erythropoiesis, other diseases, or environmental factor(s) (Table 11.3). The distinction is not always clear-cut. For example, coinheritance of the C282Y mutation of the *HFE* gene (see below) may contribute to iron loading in diseases such as porphyria cutanea tarda,[136] and a non-HFE-related genetic component may be required to allow the dietary iron loading in sub-Saharan iron overload.[137] However, the severe secondary iron overload that

accompanies some genetic or acquired anemias is either the result of regular red cell transfusions or a marked increase in iron absorption mediated by the 'erythroid regulator'. An additional contribution from a hemochromatosis gene is not required for the development of iron overload, but in occasional patients might make this more severe.[138]

Iron-overload disorders (Table 11.3)

Severe iron overload, whether primary or secondary, is arbitrarily defined as greater than 5 g excess iron,[139] and hemochromatosis as the combination of such iron overload with iron-induced tissue damage. Hereditary hemochromatosis now encompasses several genetic abnormalities that result in excessive iron absorption and eventual parenchymal iron overload. By contrast, excess iron in macrophages appears relatively non-toxic. In patients receiving multiple red cell transfusions, or parenteral iron, the iron is first released within macrophages, but subsequently undergoes redistribution via transferrin to parenchymal tissues.

Primary iron overload

HFE-related hereditary hemochromatosis

Genetics

The disorder is inherited as an autosomal recessive, and is one of the most common of the single-gene disorders found in populations of North-European origin. The *HFE* gene is located on the short arm of chromosome 6, very close to the HLA-A locus, and codes for an HLA-class-1-like protein.[25] In the UK over 90% of patients with hereditary hemochromatosis are homozygous for a point mutation responsible for a cysteine to tyrosine substitution at amino acid 282 (C282Y). The frequency of the C282Y mutation is around 9% in the UK, but only 0.5% in Italy.[140] A second mutation, substituting a histidine with aspartic acid at amino acid 63 (H63D), is more common in the general population, and has a less-defined role in predisposing towards iron loading. A further 4% of patients were found to be compound heterozygotes (C282Y/H63D), though most individuals with this genotype are not iron loaded. The proportion of patients with one or other of these genotypes declines on moving south through Europe, and is lowest in Italy (70%). A third, much rarer, mutation (S65C) is over-represented among patients with hemochromatosis who have at least

Table 11.3 Causes of iron overload. Conditions in the upper part of the table may potentially give rise to severe iron overload (> 5 g excess in adults) and consequent risk of tissue damage. In those conditions below the line any increase in total iron burden is small: redistribution of body iron may play a major role, and a localized increase in tissue iron may then have more specific clinical effects than those of generalized iron overload

Condition	Features of iron overload	Prevalence of iron overload
Primary iron overload		
HFE-related		
• Hereditary hemochromatosis, type 1	Autosomal recessive. Chromosome 6p. *HFE* mutations, especially C282Y Increased iron absorption	Common in those of North-European origin
Non-HFE-related		
• Hereditary hemochromatosis, type 2	Juvenile hemochromatosis. Severe. Chromosome 1q. Gene unknown	Rare
• Hereditary hemochromatosis, type 3	Autosomal recessive. More severe than type 1. Chromosome 7q. TfR2 mutations	Small proportion of adult hemochromatosis
Ferroportin mutations	Increased absorption or decreased iron release from macrophages. Autosomal dominant. Chromosome 2q	Unknown, but probably uncommon
Aceruloplasminemia	Impaired release of iron from macrophages. Autosomal recessive. Chromosome 3q	Very rare
Congenital atransferrinemia	Increased iron absorption. Impaired utilization by erythron. Autosomal recessive	Very rare
Neonatal hemochromatosis	Mechanisms unknown. Some related to maternal illness, others autosomal recessive	Rare
Secondary iron overload		
Iron-loading anemias		
• Massive ineffective erythropoiesis (severe β-thalassemia syndromes, sideroblastic anemias, congenital dyserythropoietic anemias)	Increased iron absorption and/or blood transfusion	Common, as a result of thalassemia, in those of Mediterranean, Middle-Eastern, and Asian origin. Other causes rare
• Refractory hypoplastic anemias (e.g. chronic renal failure, pure red cell aplasia, aplastic and myelodysplastic syndromes)	Blood transfusion	Relatively common where adequate transfusion services available
• Severe chronic hemolytic anemias (e.g. pyruvate kinase deficiency, congenital spherocytosis, sickle cell disease)	Blood transfusion (increased absorption in some cases?)	Rare as causes of severe iron overload
Sub-Saharan dietary iron overload	Increase in both dietary iron and iron absorption. Gene unknown	Common in sub-Saharan Africa
Causes of modest iron overload		
• Chronic liver disease (alcoholic cirrhosis, portocaval anastamosis)	Increased iron absorption	Common
• Porphyria cutanea tarda	Increased iron absorption. Increased frequency of HFE mutations	Relatively uncommon
Local iron overload		
• Lung (idiopathic pulmonary hemosiderosis)	Pulmonary hemorrhage	Rare
• Renal (e.g. paroxysmal nocturnal hemoglobinuria, sickle cell disease)	Hemoglobinuria with renal tubular hemosiderosis	Rare

one chromosome without one of the other identified mutations, and is probably associated with a mild form of the disease.[141] Less than a quarter of heterozygotes for the C282Y mutation show mild increases in iron status, but clinical complications of iron overload are not a feature.[142] The mechanism by which the impaired cell membrane expression of the mutant HFE protein may enhance iron absorption is discussed elsewhere.

Clinical features

A sustained positive iron balance leads to progressive accumulation of iron, and presentation, usually in middle age, with evidence of iron-induced organ damage. A variety of clinical presentations mean that a high degree of clinical suspicion is necessary. Weakness and fatigue are prominent, while arthralgia, and impotence in males are common.[143,144] The arthritis particularly affects the second and third metacarpal–phalangeal joints, and a destructive arthropathy of the hip and knee joints may also occur. Late-onset diabetes, abnormal liver function tests, or skin pigmentation may all trigger a suspicion of hemochromatosis. In younger patients cardiac failure and arrhythmias are more common at presentation, most likely reflecting a more rapid accumulation of iron. Abdominal pain may result from hepatic enlargement or hepatocellular carcinoma.

Diagnosis

An increase in transferrin saturation is the first biochemical abnormality in the development of iron overload, and signifies an increased risk of parenchymal tissues taking up excess iron. A fasting saturation of greater than 55% (men and postmenopausal women) or 50% (premenopausal women) suggests a risk of iron accumulation:[64] a parallel measurement of serum ferritin allows an estimate of the current accumulation of excess iron stores. The guidelines published by the British Committee for Standards in Haematology[64] indicate how testing for *HFE* mutations may now allow confirmatory liver biopsy to be restricted to: (1) those patients with a raised ferritin as well as transferrin saturation but who lack *HFE* mutations (where the question is whether there is an alternative explanation, e.g. hepatitis C, alcoholic or fatty liver disease, or whether an increased hepatic iron index (Table 11.1) shows iron overload consistent with non-HFE hemochromatosis); and (2) patients with homozygous C282Y or C282Y/H63D, but who have a serum ferritin $> 1000\,\mu g/l$, or abnormal liver function tests (where the question is whether fibrosis has progressed to cirrhosis, with the consequent need to monitor for the development of hepatocellular carcinoma during follow-up). The guidelines further suggest that in patients with a raised fasting transferrin saturation, but no evidence of increased iron stores (i.e. normal serum ferritin), the measures of iron status should be repeated at annual intervals whether or not *HFE* genotyping confirms HFE-related hemochromatosis: regular phlebotomy or liver biopsy, respectively, can then be carried out if the serum ferritin becomes elevated.

Patients with *HFE* mutations and a raised serum ferritin, but to a level of $< 1000\,\mu g/l$ and with no evidence of liver damage, do not require a diagnostic liver biopsy. Quantitative phlebotomy – estimating the total amount of iron removed (at approximately 200 mg per unit of blood) before iron stores are exhausted, provides both treatment and confirmation of the diagnosis of iron overload.

Treatment

Removal of the excess iron by regular phlebotomy cannot reverse established cirrhosis and does not help the arthropathy, but even in those with established disease there is a reduction in mortality from cardiac and hepatic failure. Hepatocellular carcinoma is now a major cause of death in those with cirrhosis, and regular monitoring with serum α-fetoprotein and liver ultrasound imaging may allow prompt treatment.

Patients diagnosed and treated before cirrhosis has developed have a normal life expectancy.[143] Phlebotomy at a rate of 450 ml/week is usually well tolerated, and should continue until iron stores are exhausted (serum ferritin $< 20\,\mu g/l$). This may need to be continued for over 2 years since the excess iron is usually greater than 10 g in those with established tissue damage, and may exceed 30 g in total. The rate of phlebotomy may need to be reduced if the hemoglobin drops below 12 g/l. Thereafter phlebotomy from 2 to 6 times each year should be carried out to maintain the serum ferritin below $50\,\mu g/l$ and transferrin saturation at $< 50\%$.

Screening

Counselling and testing (phenotypic and genotypic) should be offered to siblings and parents, and considered for partners and children, of probands. Siblings in particular are at high (1 in 4) risk of having also inherited the hemochromatosis genes.

Population screening remains more controversial, since although there are clear benefits in early identification of those at risk, with an effective treatment available, the penetrance of the disease remains uncertain. A population-based study in Busselton, Australia, identified 1 in 200 adults (16 subjects) as being homozygous for C282Y, of which nearly all had increased transferrin saturations, and half had clinical features consistent with hemochromatosis.[145] However, in a large number of healthy blood donors,[146] none of the C282Y homozygotes had any symptoms or family history of iron overload, and only 20% had elevated transferrin saturations and serum ferritin. A similar low penetrance was seen among individuals attending a US health appraisal clinic, where

C282Y homozygotes had a normal age distribution, and less than 1% had symptoms that could have been related to hemochromatosis.[147] Both these studies could be biased in favor of healthy members of the population, but a study showing a high penetrance of iron overload and disease-related conditions in homozygous relatives of probands[148] is potentially biased in the opposite direction. Penetrance is likely to be dependent on an interaction of genetic with physiologic and environmental factors (e.g. symptomatic iron overload is less frequent in women before the menopause, while a high alcohol intake, enhancing the bioavailability of dietary iron,[149] is common in men with symptomatic disease). However, a systematic search for polymorphisms in genes coding or transferrin receptor 1, ferroportin, ceruloplasmin, ferritin, IRP-1, IRP-2 and hepcidin, has revealed no potentially explanatory associations in patients with HFE-related hemochromatosis.[150]

Non HFE-related hereditary hemochromatosis

This is defined by the presence of genetically determined iron overload with the clinical features of hereditary hemochromatosis, but a wild-type *HFE* genotype. Two disorders are so far characterized:

- *Hereditary hemochromatosis type 2 (juvenile hemochromatosis)* is a rare severe form of iron overload which presents before the age of 30 years with cardiomyopathy and gonadal failure.[151] It maps to chromosome 1q, but the gene has not yet been identified. The severity of the iron loading has led to the hypothesis that it may hold a clue to the identity of the 'erythroid' regulator of iron absorption.
- *Hereditary hemochromatosis type 3* results from homozygous mutations in the gene coding transferrin receptor 2 on chromosome 7q22.[37,152] Since inactivation of TfR2 causes iron overload, it seems likely that it is part of the mechanism controlling iron absorption. One suggestion is that by impairing hepatocyte iron uptake it may lead to a reduction in the liver's production of hepcidin, and a loss of this proposed brake on iron absorption.[68]

Ferroportin mutations

Two families have been described with an autosomal dominant form of iron overload associated with ferroportin mutations. The first was characterized by early iron accumulation in macrophages, a high serum ferritin, and a low tolerance of phlebotomy.[153,154] The main effect was on reticuloendothelial iron release, and the partial loss of function clearly did not extend to impairment of iron absorption. By contrast, the mutation present in the other family is thought to give enhanced ferroportin-mediated iron transport to account for the iron-overload phenotype.[155]

Neonatal hemochromatosis

This is a rare severe form of hemochromatosis, characterized by congenital cirrhosis or hepatitis and widespread tissue iron loading.[156] In some cases it may be related to maternal infection, but others show features consistent with autosomal recessive inheritance: the genetic basis is unknown.

Congenital atransferrinemia

This very rare disorder is characterized by severe microcytic anemia and parenchymal liver iron overload.[157] It illustrates the essential role for transferrin in delivering iron to the erythron, and the transferrin-independent pathways for iron release to plasma and uptake by the liver.

Aceruloplasminemia

This is an autosomal recessive disorder caused by mutations in the ceruloplasmin gene,[158,159] and characterized by diabetes, retinal degeneration and neurologic disease (extrapyramidal signs, cerebellar ataxia and dementia). Hepatic iron loading may be resistant to phlebotomy[49] consistent with the ferroxidase role of ceruloplasmin in promoting cellular iron efflux.

Secondary iron overload
Parenteral iron loading

In transfusion-dependent anemias, each unit of red cells delivers approximately 200 mg iron. In congenital anemias such as β-thalassemia major this can add up to 100 g iron by the end of the second decade of life, by which time most patients will have died from the toxic effects of the excess iron.[160] These include cardiac arrhythmias and heart failure, diabetes and failure of puberty, and cirrhosis. The rate of iron loading through regular transfusion is considerably greater than the maximum possible through increased iron absorption, and pathologic changes may therefore occur somewhat later where the latter route predominates.[139]

Increased iron absorption

Increased oral intake of iron does not normally result in significant iron loading[59] unless there is some additional contributing factor. In sub-Saharan iron overload a combination of unusually high dietary iron bioavailability with an underlying (unknown) genetic defect is required to produce the disorders.[137] In patients with iron-loading anemias associated with massive erythroid expansion, for example the β-thalassemia intermedia syndromes and congenital sideroblastic anemias shown in Figure 11.10,[52] and congenital dyserythropoietic anemias,[161] the rate of iron loading is directly related to the degree of erythroid expansion.[162] For a given degree of erythroid expansion, as assessed by ferrokinetic studies of plasma iron turnover, the 'erythroid' regulator appears more active in association with dyserythropoiesis than hemolysis.[53] However, even in HbH disease, where the defect is primarily hemolytic, iron overload from excessive iron absorption can be a problem.[163] It may be expected that the heightened iron absorption related to the 'erythroid' regulator will have an even greater effect if the diet contains readily available iron. The risk of iron loading via the gastrointestinal route may be concealed in some patients in whom a mild and asymptomatic anemia coexists with a marked expansion of dyserythropoietic marrow. Such patients may be at particular risk of misguided oral iron therapy[164] and liver biopsy may be needed to determine the true extent of iron loading.

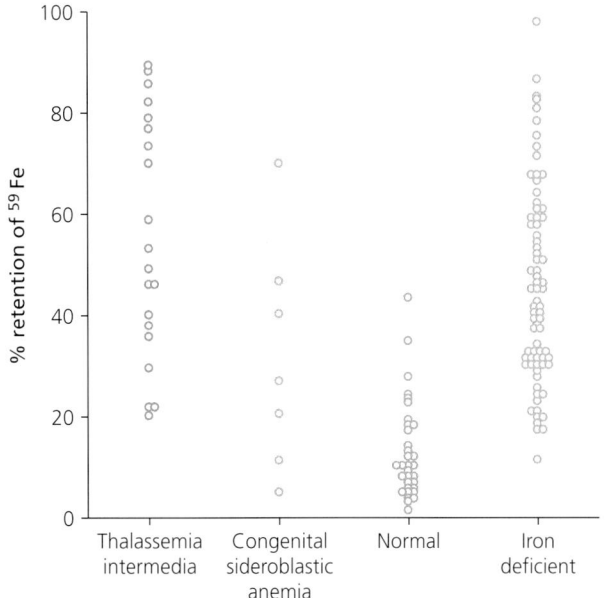

Fig. 11.10 Iron absorption from a test dose of 5 mg ^{59}Fe ferrous sulfate measured by whole body counting. Patients with massive ineffective erythropoiesis had iron retention similar to that of patients with iron deficiency, despite the fact that they had already accumulated substantial amounts of excess iron. From Pippard and Weatherall, 1984,[162] with permission.

Pathogenesis of iron-induced damage

Changes of liver fibrosis are seen very early in the development of iron overload in transfusion-dependent thalassemia.[165] In the liver, lipid peroxidation by iron-catalyzed hydroxyl radicals[166] results in impairment of membrane-dependent functions of mitochondria, including mitochondrial respiration, and damage to lysosomes resulting in their increased fragility. In iron overload, the lysosomal uptake of ferritin results in partial ferritin degradation to insoluble hemosiderin, and this may also increase the lysosomal fragility. Pathologic fibrogenesis is mediated by the activation and proliferation of hepatic stellate cells, probably as the result of iron-induced oxidative stress. The degree of damage in various organs is not always clearly correlated with their iron content. In particular, the heart may show functional impairment despite relatively low and patchy iron deposition.

Treatment

Management of secondary iron overload is mainly dependent on the use of iron chelation therapy. It is the metabolically active iron within cells which is both the main catalyst for free radical formation and the major source of chelatable iron.[167] Desferrioxamine is the main iron chelating agent in clinical use, and has to be given as a continuous infusion on a regular daily basis to produce effective iron removal. Nevertheless, when used conscientiously in this way, maintainance of serum ferritin below 2500 µg/l prevents cardiac complications of iron overload,[168] and is associated with improved pubertal growth and prolongation of survival. Its main disadvantage is the need for parenteral administration, and numerous potential orally active alternative chelators have been investigated in the last 20 years. Only one, deferiprone, has had any significant clinical exposure, and there remain some concerns about both its efficacy and safety.[169] The approach to management of secondary iron overload has recently been comprehensively reviewed by Porter.[170]

REFERENCES

1. Dallman PR, Beutler E, Finch CA 1978 Annotation: Effects of iron deficiency exclusive of anaemia. British Journal of Haematology 40: 179–184
2. Aisen P 1994 Iron metabolism: an evolutionary perspective. In: Brock JH, Halliday JW, Pippard MJ, Powell LW (eds), Iron metabolism in health and disease. Saunders, London, 1–30
3. DeMaeyer E, Adiels-Tegman M 1985 The prevalence of anaemia in the world. Rapport Trimestriel de Statistiques Sanitaires Mondiales 38: 302–316
4. Cook JD, Finch CA, Smith NJ 1976 Evaluation of the iron status of a population. Blood 48: 449–455
5. Expert Scientific Working Group 1985 Summary of a report on

assessment of the iron nutritional status of the United States population. American Journal of Clinical Nutrition 42: 1318–1330

6. McCance RA, Widdowson EM 1937 Absorption and excretion of iron. Lancet ii: 680–684

7. Finch CA, Duebelbeiss K, Cook JD et al 1970 Ferrokinetics in man. Medicine 49: 17–53

8. Ponka P 1997 Tissue-specific regulation of iron metabolism and heme synthesis: distinct control mechanisms in erythroid cells. Blood 89: 1–25

9. Levy JE, Montross LK, Andrews NC 2000 Genes that modify the hemochromatosis phenotype in mice. Journal of Clinical Investigation 105: 1209–1216

10. Andrews NC 2000 Iron homeostasis: insights from genetics and animal models. Nature Reviews Genetics 1: 208–217

11. Huebers H, Josephson B, Huebers E et al 1981 Uptake and release of iron from human transferrin. Proceedings of the National Academy of Sciences, USA 78: 2572–2576

12. Huebers H, Csiba E, Huebers E, Finch CA 1985 Molecular advantage of diferric transferrin in delivering iron to reticulocytes: a comparative study. Proceedings of the Society of Experimental Biology and Medicine 179: 222–226

13. Edwards CQ, Kushner JP 1993 Screening for hemochromatosis. New England Journal of Medicine 328: 1616–1620

14. Bainton DF, Finch CA 1964 The diagnosis of iron deficiency anemia. American Journal of Medicine 37: 62–70

15. Morgan EH, Baker E 1988 Role of transferrin receptors and endocytosis in iron uptake by hepatic and erythroid cells. Annals of the New York Academy of Sciences 256: 65–82

16. Fleming MD, Romano MA, Su MA et al 1998 Nramp2 is mutated in the anemic Belgrade (b) rat: evidence of a role for Nramp2 in endosomal iron transport. Proceedings of the National Academy of Sciences, USA 95: 1148–1153

17. Andrews NC 1999 The iron transporter DMT1. International Journal of Biochemistry and Cell Biology 31: 991–994

18. Kuhn LC 1994 Molecular regulation of iron proteins. Baillière's Clinical Haematology 7: 763–785

19. Cairo G, Peitrangelo A 2000 Iron regulatory proteins in pathobiology. Biochemistry Journal 352: 241–250

20. May A, Bishop DF 1998 The molecular biology and pyridoxine responsiveness of X-linked sideroblastic anaemia. Haematologica 83: 56–70

21. Bekri S, Kispal G, Lange H et al 2000 Human ABC7 transporter: gene structure and mutation causing X-linked sideroblastic anemia with ataxia with disruption of cystosolic iron-sulfur protein maturation. Blood 96: 3256–3264

22. Maguire A, Hellier K, Hammans S, May A 2001 X-linked cerebellar ataxia and sideroblastic anaemia associated with a missense mutation in the ABC7 gene predicting V411L. British Journal of Haematology 115: 910–917

23. Becker E, Richardson DR 2001 Frataxin: its role in iron metabolism and the pathogenesis of Friedreich's ataxia. International Journal of Biochemistry and Cell Biology 33: 1–10

24. Gordon N 2000 Friedreich's ataxia and iron metabolism. Brain Development 22: 465–468

25. Feder JN, Gnirke A, Thomas W et al 1996 A novel MHC class I-like gene is mutated in patients with hereditary haemochromatosis. Nature Genetics 13: 399–408

26. West AP, Jr, Giannetti AM, Herr AB et al 2001 Mutational analysis of the transferrin receptor reveals overlapping HFE and transferrin binding sites. Journal of Molecular Biology 313: 385–397

27. Riedel HD, Muckenthaler MU, Gehrke SG et al 1999 HFE downregulates iron uptake from transferrin and induces iron-regulatory protein activity in stably transfected cells. Blood 94: 3915–3921

28. Waheed A, Parkkila S, Zhou XY et al 1997 Hereditary hemochromatosis: effects of C282Y and H63D mutations on association with beta2-microglobulin, intracellular processing, and cell surface expression of the HFE protein in COS-7 cells. Proceedings of the National Academy of Sciences, USA 94: 12384–12389

29. Waheed A, Parkkila S, Saarnio J et al 1999 Association of HFE protein with transferrin receptor in crypt enterocytes of human duodenum. Proceedings of the National Academy of Sciences USA 96: 1579–1584

30. Parkkila S, Parkkila AK, Waheed A et al 2000 Cell surface expression of HFE protein in epithelial cells, macrophages, and monocytes. Haematologica 85: 340–345

31. Fleming RE, Sly WS 2002 Mechanisms of iron accumulation in hereditary hemochromatosis. Annual Reviews in Physiology 64: 663–680

32. Weiss G, Houston T, Kastner S et al 1997 Regulation of cellular iron metabolism by erythropoietin: activation of iron-regulatory protein and upregulation of transferrin receptor expression in erythroid cells. Blood 89: 680–687

33. Brittenham GM 1994 The red cell cycle. In: Brock JH, Halliday JW, Pippard MJ, Powell LW (eds), Iron metabolism in health and disease. Saunders, London, 31–62

34. Kawabata H, Yang R, Hirama T et al 1999 Molecular cloning of transferrin receptor 2. A new member of the transferrin receptor-like family. Journal of Biological Chemistry 274: 20826–20832

35. West AP, Jr, Bennett MJ, Sellers VM et al 2000 Comparison of the interactions of transferrin receptor and transferrin receptor 2 with transferrin and the hereditary hemochromatosis protein HFE. Journal of Biological Chemistry 275: 38135–38138

36. Fleming RE, Migas MC, Holden CC et al 2000 Transferrin receptor 2: continued expression in mouse liver in the face of iron overload and in hereditary hemochromatosis. Proceedings of the National Academy of Sciences, USA 97: 2214–2219

37. Camaschella C, Roetto A, Cali A et al 2000 The gene TFR2 is mutated in a new type of haemochromatosis mapping to 7q22. Nature Genetics 25: 14–15

38. Gutierrez JA, Yu J, Wessling-Resnick M 1998 Characterization and chromosomal mapping of the human gene for SFT, a stimulator of Fe transport. Biochemistry and Biophysics Research Communications 253: 739–742

39. Brock JH 1994 Iron in infection, immunity, inflammation and neoplasia. In: Brock JH, Halliday JW, Pippard MJ, Powell LW (eds) Iron metabolism in health and disease. Saunders, 353–389

40. Raja KB, Simpson RJ, Peters TJ 1992 Investigation of a role for reduction in ferric iron uptake by mouse duodenum. Biochimica et Biophysica Acta 1135: 141–146

41. McKie AT, Barrow D, Latunde-Dada GO et al 2001 An iron-regulated ferric reductase associated with the absorption of dietary iron. Science 291: 1755–1759

42. Gunshin H, Mackenzie B, Berger UV et al 1997 Cloning and characterization of a mammalian proton-coupled metal-ion transporter. Nature 388: 482–488

43. Fleming RE, Migas MC, Zhou X et al 1999 Mechanism of increased iron absorption in murine model of hereditary hemochromatosis: increased duodenal expression of the iron transporter DMT1. Proceedings of the National Academy of Sciences, USA 96: 3143–3148

44. Uzel C, Conrad ME 1998 Absorption of heme iron. Seminars in Hematology 35: 27–34

45. McKie AT, Marciani P, Rolfs A, et al 2000 A novel duodenal iron-regulated transporter, IREG1, implicated in the basolateral transfer of iron to the circulation. Molecular Cell 5: 299–309

46. Brittenham GM, Weiss G, Brissot P et al 2000 Clinical consequences of new insights in the pathophysiology of disorders of iron and heme metabolism. Hematology. American Society of Hematology Education Program 39–50

47. Vulpe CD, Kuo YM, Murphy TL et al 1999 Hephaestin, a ceruloplasmin homologue implicated in intestinal iron transport, is defective in the sla mouse. Nature Genetics 21: 195–199

48. Harris ZL, Durley AP, Man TK, Gitlin JD 1999 Targeted gene disruption reveals an essential role for ceruloplasmin in cellular iron efflux. Proceedings of the National Academy of Sciences, USA 96: 10812–10817

49. Hellman NE, Schaefer M, Gehrke S et al 2000 Hepatic iron overload in aceruloplasminaemia. Gut 47: 858–860

50. Goya N, Miyazaki S, Kodate S, Ushio B 1972 A family of congenital atransferrinemia. Blood 40: 239–245

51. Lynch SR, Skikne BS, Cook JD 1989 Food iron absorption in idiopathic hemochromatosis. Blood 74: 2187–2193

52. Pippard MJ, Callender ST, Warner GT, Weatherall DJ 1979 Iron absorption and loading in beta-thalassaemia intermedia. Lancet 2: 819–821

53. Pootrakul P, Kitcharoen K, Yansukon et al 1988 The effect of erythroid hyperplasia on iron balance. Blood 71: 1124–1129

54. Cavill I, Woorwood M, Jacobs A 1975 Internal regulation of iron absorption. Nature 256: 328–329

55. Finch CA 1994 Regulators of iron balance in humans. Blood 84: 1697–1702

56. Raja KB, Simpson RJ, Pippard MJ, Peters TJ 1988 *In vivo* studies on the relationship between intestinal iron (Fe^{3+}) absorption, hypoxia and erythropoiesis in the mouse. British Journal of Haematology 68:373–378

57. Skikne BS, Cook JD 1992 Effect of enhanced erythropoiesis on iron absorption. Journal of Laboratory and Clinical Medicine 120: 746–751

58. Hughes RT, Smith T, Hesp R et al 1992 Regulation of iron absorption in iron loaded subjects with end stage renal disease: effects of treatment with recombinant human erythropoietin and reduction of iron stores. British Journal of Haematology 82: 445–454

59. Sayers MH, English G, Finch C 1994 Capacity of the store-regulator in maintaining iron balance. American Journal of Hematology 47: 194–197

60. Tchernitchko D, Bourgeois M, Martin ME, Beaumont C 2002 Expression of the two mRNA isoforms of the iron transporter Nramp2/DMT1 in mice and function of the iron responsive element. Biochemical Journal 363: 449–455

61. Zoller H, Kock RO, Theurl I et al 2001 Expression of the duodenal iron transporters divalent-metal transporter 1 and ferroportin 1 in iron deficiency and iron overload. Gastroenterology 120: 1412–1419

62. Griffiths WJ, Sly WS, Cox TM 2001 Intestinal iron uptake determined by divalent metal transporter is enhanced in HFE-deficient mice with hemochromatosis. Gastroenterology 120: 1420–1429

63. Zoller H, Pietrangelo A, Vogel W, Weiss G 1999 Duodenal metal-transporter (DMT-1, NRAMP-2) expression in patients with hereditary haemochromatosis. Lancet 353: 2120–2123

64. Dooley J, Worwood M 2000 Genetic haemochromatosis. Guidelines on diagnosis and therapy compiled on behalf of the British Committee for Standards in Haematology. Darwin Medical Communications, Abingdon

65. Andrews NC 1999 Disorders of iron metabolism. New England Journal of Medicine 34: 1986–1995

66. Fillet G, Beguin Y, Baldelli L 1989 Model of reticuloendothelial iron metabolism in humans: abnormal behaviour in idiopathic hemochromatosis and in inflammation. Blood 74: 844-851

67. Pigeon C, Ilyin G, Courselaud B et al 2001 A new mouse liver-specific gene, encoding a protein homologous to human antimicrobial peptide hepcidin, is overexpressed during iron overload. Journal of Biological Chemistry 276: 7811–7819

68. Nicolas G, Bennoun M, Devaux I et al 2001 Lack of hepcidin gene expression and severe tissue iron overload in upstream stimulatory factor 2 (USF2) knockout mice. Proceedings of the National Academy of Sciences, USA 98: 8780–8785

69. Worwood M 1994 Laboratory determination of iron status. In: Brock JH, Halliday JW, Pippard MJ, Powell LW (eds), Iron metabolism in health and disease. Saunders, London, 449–476

70. Cook JD 1999 The measurement of serum transferrin receptor. American Journal of Medical Sciences 318: 269–276

71. Cazzola M, Beguin Y 1992 New tools for clinical evaluation of erythron function in man. British Journal of Haematology 80: 278–284

72. Ferguson BJ, Skikne BS, Simpson KM et al 1992 Serum transferrin receptor distinguishes the anemia of chronic disease from iron deficiency anemia. Journal of Laboratory and Clinical Medicine 19: 385–390

73. Cazzola M, Beguin Y, Bergamaschi G et al 1999 Soluble transferrin receptor as a potential determinant of iron loading in congenital anemias due to ineffective erythropoiesis. British Journal of Haematology 106: 752–755

74. Worwood M 1986 Serum ferritin. Clinical Science 70: 215–220

75. Worwood M, Cragg SJ, Jacobs A et al 1980 Binding of serum ferritin to concanavalin A: patients with homozygous B thalassaemia and transfusional iron overload. British Journal of Haematology 46: 409–416

76. Brittenham GM, Cohen AR, McLaren CE et al 1993 Hepatic iron stores and plasma ferritin concentration in patients with sickle cell anemia and thalassemia major. American Journal of Hematology 42: 81–85

77. Beaumont C, Leneuve P, Devaux I et al 1995 Mutation in the iron responsive element of the L ferritin mRNA in a family with dominant hyperferritinaemia and cataract. Nature Genetics 11: 444–446

78. Cazzola M, Bergamaschi G, Tonon L et al 1997 Hereditary hyperferritinemia-cataract syndrome: relationship between phenotypes and specific mutations in the iron-responsive element of ferritin light-chain mRNA. Blood 90: 814–821

79. Skikne BS, Flowers CH, Cook JD 1990 Serum transferrin receptor: a quantitative measure of tissue iron deficiency. Blood 75: 1870–1876

80. Punnonen K, Irjala K, Rajamaki A 1997. Serum transferrin receptor and its ratio to serum ferritin in the diagnosis of iron deficiency. Blood 89: 1052–1057

81. Pasquale D, Chikkappa G 1995. Bone marrow biopsy imprints (touch preparations) for assessment of iron stores. American Journal of Hematology 48: 201–202

82. Barron BA, Hoyer JD, Tefferi A 2001 A bone marrow report of absent stainable iron is not diagnostic of iron deficiency. Annals of Hematology 80: 166–169

83. Bassett ML, Halliday JW, Powell LW 1986 Value of hepatic iron measurements in early haemochromatosis and determination of the critical iron level associated with fibrosis. Hepatology 6: 24–29

84. Angelucci E, brittenham GM, McLaren CE et al 2000 Hepatic iron concentration and total body iron stores in thalassemia major. New England Journal of Medicine 343: 327–331

85. Eschbach JW, Egrie JC, Downing MR et al 1987 Correction of the anemia of end-stage renal disease with recombinant human erythropoietin: results of a combined Phase I and II clinical trial. New England Journal of Medicine 316: 73–78

86. Buss DH 1995 Dietary sources and intakes of iron. In: Iron. Nutritional and physiological significance. Report of the British Nutrition Foundation Task Force. Chapman Hall, London, 13–16

87. Gregory J, Foster K, Tyler H, Wiseman M 1990 The dietary and nutritional survey of British adults. HMSO, London

88. Department of Health 1989 Dietary reference values for food energy and nutrients for the United Kingdom. HMSO, London

89. Rockey DC, Cello JP 1993 Evaluation of the gastrointestinal tract in patients with iron-deficiency anemia. New England Journal of Medicine 329: 1691–1695

90. Carmel R, Weiner JM, Johnson CS 1987 Iron deficiency occurs frequently in patients with pernicious anemia. Journal of the American Medical Association 257: 1081–1083

91. Gross SJ, Stuart MJ, Swender PT et al 1976 Malabsorption of iron in children with iron deficiency. Journal of Pediatrics 88: 795–799

92. Lee PL, Halloran C, Trevino R et al 2001. Human transferrin G277S mutation: a risk factor for iron deficiency anaemia. British Journal of Haematology 115: 329–333

93. Larrick JW, Hyman ES 1984. Acquired iron-deficiency anemia caused by an antibody against the transferrin receptor. New England Journal of Medicine 311: 214–218

94. Hartman KR, Barker JA 1996 Microcytic anemia with iron malabsorption: an inherited disorder of iron metabolism. American Journal of Hematology 51: 269–275

95. Pearson HA, Lukens JN 1999. Ferrokinetics in the syndrome of familial hypoferremic microcytic anemia with iron malabsorption. Journal of Pediatric Hematology and Oncology 21: 412–417

96. Charlton RW, Bothwell TH 1982 Definition, prevalence and prevention of iron deficiency. Clinics in Haematology 11: 309–325

97. Garrett S, Worwood M 1994 Zinc protoporphyrin and iron-deficient erythropoiesis. Acta Haematologica 91: 21–25

98. Brugnara C 2000 Reticulocyte cellular indices: a new approach in the diagnosis of anemias and monitoring of erythropoietic function. Critical Reviews in Clinical Laboratory Sciences 37: 93–130

99. MacDougall IC, Cavill I, Hulme B et al 1992 Detection of functional iron deficiency during erythropoietin treatment: a new approach. British Medical Journal 304: 225–226

100. Berger M, Brass LF 1987 Severe thrombocytopenia in iron deficiency anemia. American Journal of Hematology 24: 425–428

101. Soff GA, Levin J 1988 Thrombocytopenia associated with repletion of iron in iron-deficiency anemia. American Journal of Medical Sciencess 295: 35

102. McKnight GS, Lee DC, Hemmaplardh D et al 1983 Transferrin gene expression. Effects of nutritional iron deficiency. Journal of Biological Chemistry 255: 144–147

103. Hallberg L, Bengtsson C, Lapidus et al 1993 Screening for iron deficiency: an analysis based on bone marrow examinations and serum ferritin determinations in a population sample of women. British Journal of Haematology 85: 787–798

104. Kimura H, Finch CA, Adamson JW 1986 Hematopoiesis in the rat: quantitation of hematopoietic progenitors and the response to iron deficiency anemia. Journal of Cell Physiology 126: 298–306

105. Jacobs A 1961 Iron-containing enzymes in the buccal epithelium. Lancet ii: 1331–1333

106. Jacobs A, Kilpatrick GS 1964 The Paterson–Kelly syndrome. British Medical Journal 2: 79–82

107. Dallman PR 1987 Iron deficiency and the immune response. American Journal of Clinical Nutrition 46: 329–334

108. Edgerton VR, Gardner GW, Ohira Y et al 1979 Iron-deficiency anaemia and its effect on worker productivity and activity patterns. British Medical Journal 2: 1546–1549

109. Basta SS, Soekirman MS, Karyadi D, Scrimshaw MS 1979 Iron deficiency anemia and the productivity of adult males in Indonesia. American Journal of Clinical Nutrition 32: 916–925

110. Finch CA, Gollnick PD, Hlastala MP et al 1979 Lactic acidosis as a result of iron deficiency. Journal of Clinical Investigation 64: 129–137

111. Lansdown R, Wharton BA 1995 Iron and mental and motor behaviour in children. In: Iron. Nutritional and physiological significance. Report of a British Nutrition Foundation Task Force. Chapman and Hall, London, 65–78

112. Pootrakul P, Wattanasaree J, Anuwatanakulchai M, Wasi P 1984 Increased red blood cell protoporphyrin in thalassemia: a result of relative iron deficiency. American Journal of Clinical Pathology 82: 289–293

113. Drueke TB, Barany P, Cazzola M et al 1997 Management of iron deficiency in renal anemia: guidelines for the optimal therapeutic approach in erythropoietin-treated patients. Clinical Nephrology, 48: 1–8

114. Gokal R, Millard PR, Weatherall DJ et al 1979 Iron metabolism in haemodialysis patients. Quarterly Journal of Medicine 48: 369–91

115. MacDougall IC 1999 Strategies for iron supplementation: oral versus intravenous. Kidney International 69: S61–S66

116. Douglas SW, Adamson JW 1975 The anemia of chronic disorders: studies of marrow regulation and iron metabolism. Blood 45: 55–65

117. Baer AN, Dessypris EN, Goldwasser E, Krantz SB 1987 Blunted erythropoietin response to anaemia in rheumatoid arthritis. British Journal of Haematology 66: 559–564

118. Miller CB, Jones RJ, Piantadosi S et al 1990 Decreased erythropoietin response in patients with the anemia of cancer. New England Journal of Medicine 322: 1689–1692

119. Cazzola M, Ponchio L, de Benedetti F et al 1996 Defective iron supply for erythropoiesis and adequate endogenous erythropoietin production in the anemia associated with systemic-onset juvenile chronic arthritis. Blood 87: 4824–4830

120. Kranz SB 1994 Pathogenesis and treatment of the anemia of chronic disease. American Journal of Medical Sciences 307: 353–359

121. Wang CQ, Udupa KB, Lipschitz DA 2002 Interferon-gamma exerts its negative regulatory effect primarily on the earliest stages of murine erythroid progenitor cell development. Journal of Cell Physiology 162: 134–138

122. Selleri C, Sato T, Anderson S et al 1995 Interferon-gamma and tumor necrosis factor-alpha suppress both early and late stages of hematopoiesis and induce programmed cell death. Journal of Cell Physiology 165: 538–546

123. Maciejewski JP, Selleri C, Sato T et al 1995 Nitric oxide suppression of human hematopoiesis *in vitro*. Contribution to inhibitory action of interferon-gamma and tumor necrosis factor-alpha. Journal of Clinical Investigation 96: 1085–1092

124. Weiss G, Goossen B, Doppler W et al 1993 Translational regulation via iron-responsive elements by the nitric oxide/NO-synthase pathway. Embo Journal 12: 3651–3657

125. Means RT, Krantz SB 1991 Inhibition of human erythroid colony formation by IFN-gamma can be corrected by human recombinant erythropoietin. Blood 78: 2564–2570

126. Dinant HJ, De Maat CEM 1992 Erythropoiesis and mean red cell lifespan in normal subjects and in patients with the anaemia of active rheumatoid arthritis. British Journal of Haematology 39: 437–444

127. Means RT, Krantz SB 1992 Progress in understanding the pathogenesis of the anemia of chronic disease. Blood 80: 1639–1647

128. Kivivuori SM, Pelkonen P, Ylijoki H et al 2000 Elevated serum transferrin receptor concentration in children with juvenile chronic arthritis as evidence of iron deficiency. Rheumatology 39: 193–197

129. Punnonen K, Kaipiainen-Seppanen O, Riittinen L et al 2000 Evaluation of iron status in anemic patients with rheumatoid arthritis using an automated immunoturbidimetric assay for transferrin receptor. Clinical Chemistry and Laboratory Medicine 38: 1297–1300

130. Brittenham GM, Weiss G, Brissot P et al 2000 Clinical consequences of new insights in the pathophysiology of disorders of iron and heme metabolism. Hematology. American Society of Hematology Education Program 39–50

131. Konijn AM, Carmel N, Levy R, Hershko C 1981 Ferritin synthesis in inflammation II. Mechanism of increased ferritin synthesis. British Journal of Haematology 49: 361–370

132. Rogers JT, Bridges KR, Durmowicz GP et al 1990 Translational control during the acute phase response. Ferritin synthesis in response to interleukin-1. Journal of Biological Chemistry 265: 14572–14578

133. Weiss G, Bogdan C, Hentze MW 1997. Pathways for the regulation of macrophage iron metabolism by the anti-inflammatory cytokines IL-4 and IL-13. Journal of Immunology 158: 420–425

134. Weber J, Werre JM, Julius HW, Marx JJM 1988 Decreased iron absorption in patients with active rheumatoid arthritis, with and without iron deficiency. Annals of the Rheumatic Diseases 47: 404–409

135. Vreugdenhill G, Swaak AJG, De Jeu-Jaspars C, van Eijk HG 1990 Correlation of iron exchange between the oral iron chelator 1,2-dimethyl-3-hydroxypyrid-4-one(L1) and transferrin and possible antianaemic effects of L1 in rheumatoid arthritis. Annals of the Rheumatic Diseases 49: 956–957

136. Roberts AG, Whatley SD, Morgan RR et al 1997 Increased frequency of the haemochromatosis Cys282Tyr mutation in sporadic porphyria cutanea tarda. Lancet 349: 321–323

137. Gordeuk V, Mukiibi J, Hasstedt SJ et al 1992 Iron overload in Africa. Interaction between a gene and dietary iron content. New England Journal of Medicine 326: 95–100

138. Rees DC, Singh BM, Luo LY et al 1998 Nontransfusional iron overload in thalassemia. Association with hereditary hemochromatosis. Annals of the New York Academy of Sciences 850: 490–494

139. Pippard MJ 1994 Secondary iron overload. In: Brock JH, Halliday JW, Pippard MJ, Powell LW (eds), Iron metabolism in health and disease. Saunders, London, 271–309

140. Merryweather-Clarke AT, Pointon JJ, Shearman JD, Robson KJ 1997 Global prevalence of putative haemochromatosis mutations. Journal of Medical Genetics 34: 275–278

141. Mura C, Raguenes O, Ferec C. HFE mutations analysis in 711 hemochromatosis probands: evidence for S65C implication in mild form of hemochromatosis. Blood 93: 2502–2505

142. Bulaj ZJ, Griffen LM, Jorde LB et al 1996 Clinical and biochemical abnormalities in people heterozygous for hemochromatosis. 335: 1799–1805

143. Niederau C, Fischer R, Purschel A et al 1991 Long-term survival and causes of death in patients with hereditary hemochromatosis. Gastroenterology 110: 1107–1119

144. Adams PC, Deugnier Y, Moirand R, Brissot P 1997 The relationship between iron overload, clinical symptoms, and age in 410 patients with genetic hemochromatosis. Hepatology 25: 162–166

145. Olynyk JK, Cullen DJ, Aquilia S et al 1999 A population-based study of the clinical expression of the hemochromatosis gene. New England Journal of Medicine 341: 718–724

146. Jackson HA, Carter K, Darke C et al 2001 HFE mutations, iron deficiency and overload in 10,500 blood donors. British Journal of Haematology 114: 474–484

147. Beutler E, Felitti VJ, Koziol JA et al 2002 Penetrance of 845G – > A (C282Y) HFE hereditary haemochromatosis mutation in the USA. Lancet 359: 211–218

148. Bulaj ZJ, Ajioka RS, Phillips JD et al 2000 Disease-related conditions in relatives of patients with hemochromatosis. New England Journal of Medicine 343: 1529–1535

149. Charlton RW, Jacobs P, Seftel H, Bothwell TH 1964 Effect of alcohol on iron absorption. British Medical Journal 2: 1427–1429

150. Lee PL, Gelbart T, West C et al 2001 A study of genes that may modulate the expression of hereditary hemochromatosis: transferrin receptor-1, ferroportin, ceruloplasmin, ferritin light and heavy chains, iron regulatory proteins (IRP)-1 and -2, and hepcidin. Blood Cells Molecules and Diseases 27: 783–802

151. Kelly AL, Rhodes DA, Roland JM et al 1998 Hereditary juvenile haemochromatosis: a genetically heterogenous life-threatening iron-storage disease. Quarterly Journal of Medicine 91: 607–618

152. Roetto A, Totaro A, Piperno A et al 2001 New mutations inactivating transferrin receptor 2 in hemochromatosis type 3. Blood 97: 2555–2560

153. Pietrangelo A, Montosi G, Totaro A et al 1999 Hereditary hemochromatosis in adults without pathogenic mutations in the hemochromatosis gene. New England Journal of Medicine 341: 725–732

154. Montosi G, Donovan A, Totaro A et al 2001 Autosomal-dominant hemochromatosis is associated with a mutation in the ferroportin (SLC 11A3) gene. Journal of Clinical Investigation 108: 619–623

155. Njajou OT, Vaessen N, Joosse M et al 2001 A mutation in SLC 11A3 is associated with autosomal dominant hemochromatosis. Nature Genetics, 28: 213–214

156. Kelly AL, Lunt PW, Rodrigues F et al 2001 Classification and genetic features of neonatal haemochromatosis: a study of 27 affected pedigrees and molecular analysis of genes implicated in iron metabolism. Journal of Medical Genetics 38: 599–610

157. Goya N, Miyazaki S, Kodate S, Oshio B 1972 A family of congenital atransferrinemia. Blood 40: 239–245

158. Yoshida K, Furihata K, Takeda S et al 1995 A mutation in the ceruloplasmin gene is associated with systemic hemosiderosis in humans. Nature Genetics 9: 267–272

159. Harris ZL, Takahashi Y, Miyajima H et al 1995 Aceruloplasminemia: molecular characterization of this disorder of iron metabolism. Proceedings of the National Academy of Sciences, USA 92: 2539–2543

160. Modell B 1979 Advances in the use of iron-chelating agents for the treatment of iron overload. Progress in Hematology 11: 267–312

161. Wickramasinghe SN, Thein SL, Srichairatanakool S, Porter JB 1999 Determinants of iron status and bilirubin levels in congenital dyserythropoietic anaemia type I. British Journal of Haematology 107: 522–525

162. Pippard MJ, Weatherall DJ 1984 Iron absorption in non-transfused iron loading anaemias: prediction of risk for iron loading and response to iron chelation treatment, in β thalassaemia

163. Chen FE, Ooi C, Ha SY et al 2000 Genetic and clinical features of hemoglobin H disease in Chinese patients. New England Journal of Medicine 343: 544–550

164. Peto TEA, Pippard MJ, Weatherall DJ 1983 Iron overload in mild sideroblastic anaemias. Lancet i: 375–378

165. Iancu TC, Neustein HB, Landing BH 1977 The liver in thalassaemia major: ultrastructural observation. In: Iron Metabolism. Ciba Foundation Symposium 51. North Holland: Elsevier; p. 293–309

166. McCord JM 1998 Iron, free radicals, and oxidative injury. Seminars in Hematology 35: 5–12

167. Pippard MJ, Callender ST, Finch CA 1982 Ferrioxamine excretion in iron-loaded man. Blood 60: 288–294

168. Olivieri NF, Nathan DG, MacMillan JH et al 1994 Survival in medically treated patients with homozygous β-thalassemia. New England Journal of Medicine 331: 574–578

169. Pippard MJ, Weatherall DJ 2000 Oral iron chelation therapy for thalassaemia: an uncertain scene. British Journal of Haematology 111: 2–5

170. Porter JB 2001 Practical management of iron overload. British Journal of Haematology 115: 239–252

171. Pippard MJ, Hoffbrand AV 1999 Iron. In: Hoffbrand AV, Lewis SM, Tuddenham EGD, editors. Postgraduate Haematology. 4th ed. Oxford: Butterworth Heinemann; p. 23–46

intermedia and congenital sideroblastic anaemias. Haematologia 17: 407–414

Macrocytic anemia

12

SN Wickramasinghe

Megaloblastic hemopoiesis

Vitamin B$_{12}$-related and folate-related causes of megaloblastic anemia
Vitamin B$_{12}$
Folates

Vitamin B$_{12}$-independent and folate-independent causes of megaloblastic erythropoiesis
Abnormalities of nucleic acid synthesis
Uncertain etiology

Macrocytosis with normoblastic erythropoiesis

There are two groups of macrocytic anemias: those associated with megaloblastic hemopoiesis and those associated with normoblastic hemopoiesis. The most common causes of megaloblastic hemopoiesis are vitamin B_{12} or folate deficiency. Disturbances of vitamin B_{12} or folate metabolism may also cause this type of hemopoiesis as may vitamin B_{12} or folate-independent mechanisms.

Megaloblastic hemopoiesis[1-3]

Paul Ehrlich first used the term megaloblast in 1880 to describe a type of morphologically abnormal erythroblast seen in the bone marrow of patients with untreated pernicious anemia. It was subsequently found that megaloblasts occur in many other conditions (see Tables 12.1 and 12.2). Megaloblastic erythropoiesis is characterized by three features: (1) erythroblasts that are larger than normal at all stages of maturation; (2) a dissociation between cytoplasmic and nuclear maturity leading to early and late polychromatic erythroblasts with well-hemoglobinized (i.e. polychromatic) cytoplasm having nuclei with considerably smaller quantities of condensed chromatin than their normal counterparts (Figs 12.1 and 12.2); and (3) the generation of macrocytes (Fig. 12.3). In megaloblastic erythropoiesis there is also an increased prevalence of early and late polychromatic erythroblasts with dysplastic features (see Chapter 5), an increased

number of basophilic erythropoietic cells relative to more mature erythroblasts (Fig. 12.4) and erythroid hyperplasia. The severity of each of these morphologic abnormalities increases with increasing severity of the anemia.

Megaloblastic erythropoiesis is considerably more ineffective than normoblastic erythropoiesis and the extent of ineffectiveness is proportional to the extent of the anemia. The ineffectiveness of megaloblastic erythropoiesis results from an abnormality of the red cell

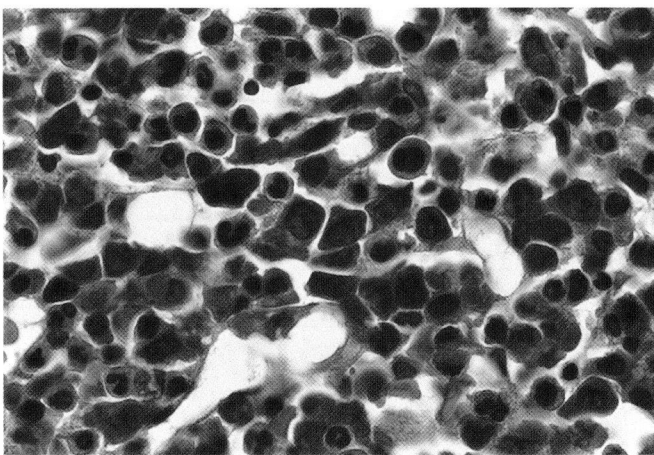

Fig. 12.2 Clot section of aspirated marrow showing several megaloblasts. These have relatively little condensed chromatin and contain several nucleoli some of which abut on the nuclear membrane.

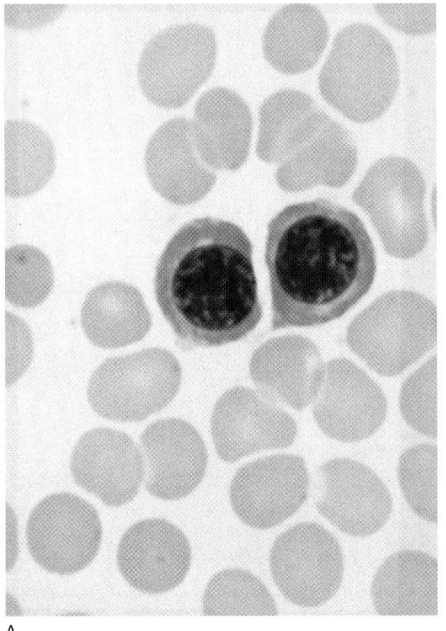
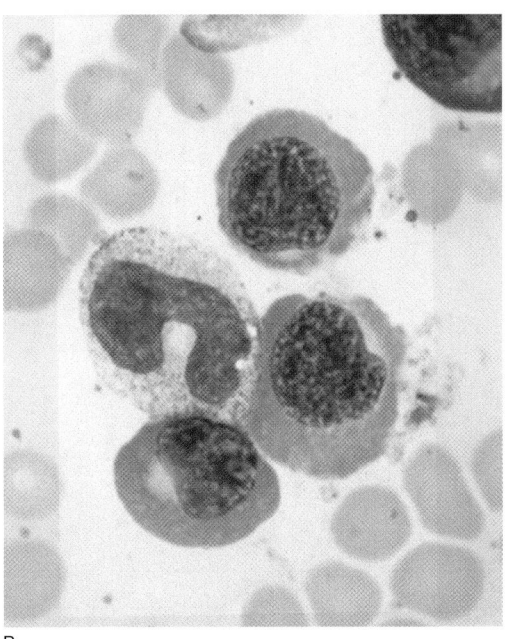

A   B

Fig. 12.1 (A,B) Differences between megaloblastic and normoblastic erythropoiesis as seen in bone marrow smears. (A) Two early polychromatic normoblasts from a healthy adult. (B) Three early polychromatic megaloblasts (and one neutrophil metamyelocyte) from a patient with severe pernicious anemia. May–Grünwald–Giemsa stain.

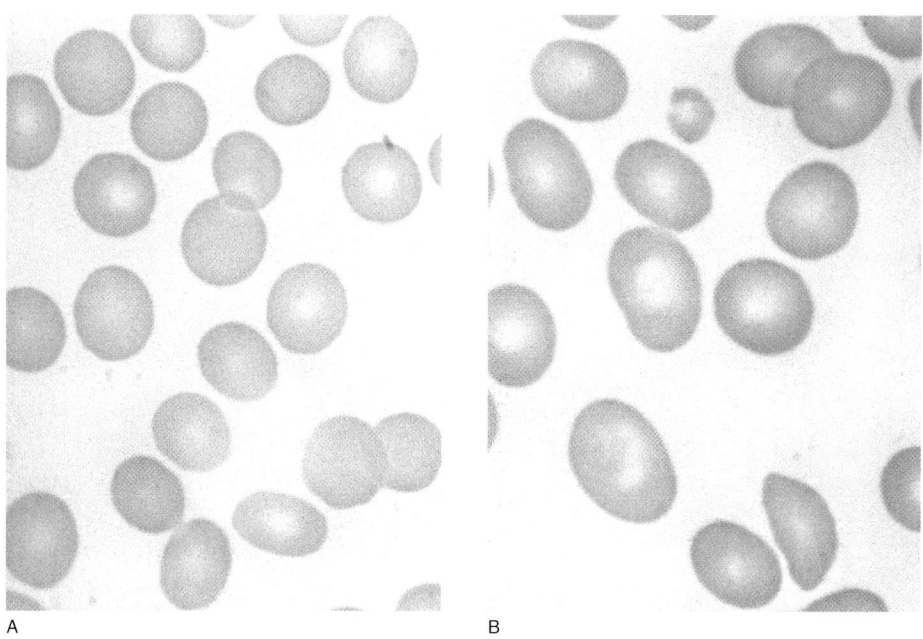

Fig. 12.3 (A,B) Red cells from a healthy adult (A) and from a case of severe pernicious anemia (B). The patient's red cells are macrocytic and oval in shape. May–Grünwald–Giemsa stain.

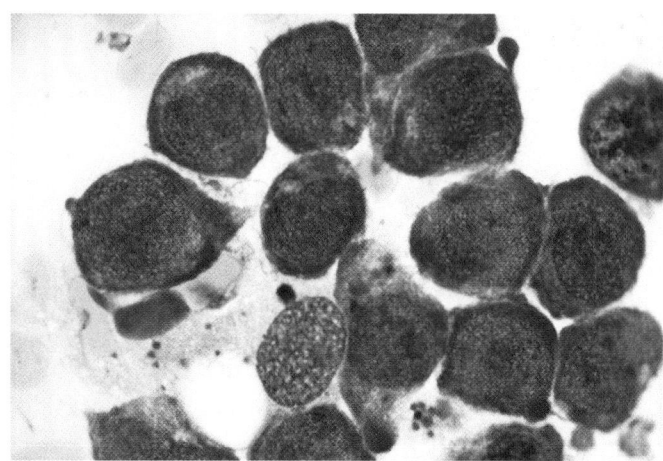

Fig. 12.4 Bone marrow smear from a patient with severe pernicious anemia showing a marked increase in the proportion of basophilic erythropoietic cells. May–Grünwald–Giemsa stain.

precursors which leads to the phagocytosis by bone marrow macrophages of a substantial proportion of the early and late polychromatic megaloblasts. Some vitamin B₁₂-deficient or folate-deficient early polychromatic megaloblasts seem to become arrested at all stages of the cell cycle.

Usually, patients with megaloblastic erythropoiesis also show morphologic abnormalities ('megaloblastic changes') in cells of the granulocyte series. The two most striking abnormalities are the formation of giant metamyelocytes in the marrow (Fig. 12.5) and the presence of hypersegmented neutrophil granulocytes in the blood

(Fig. 12.6). The giant metamyelocytes are 17–30 μm or more in diameter and usually have long horseshoe-shaped nuclei, sometimes with one or more bud-like protuberances. In addition, these cells may contain cytoplasmic vacuoles, nuclear perforations or poorly staining chromatin. Giant metamyelocytes have DNA contents in the entire range between the diploid (2c) and tetraploid (4c) values and seem to result from an abnormal type of development in promyelocytes and myelocytes that have been arrested or retarded during their progress through the cell cycle. Most of these giant cells appear to be phagocytosed by bone marrow macrophages but a few undergo nuclear segmentation and develop into giant polymorphonuclear leukocytes known as macropolycytes (Fig. 12.7). Such macropolycytes have hyperdiploid DNA contents. By contrast, hypersegmented neutrophils have diploid DNA contents and appear to be derived from normal-looking metamyelocytes with diploid DNA contents.

Megakaryocytes are usually normal or increased in number and occasionally display markedly hypersegmented nuclei.

Vitamin B₁₂-related and folate-related causes of megaloblastic anemia

The vitamin B₁₂- and folate-related causes of macrocytosis with megaloblastic erythropoiesis are given in Table 12.1.

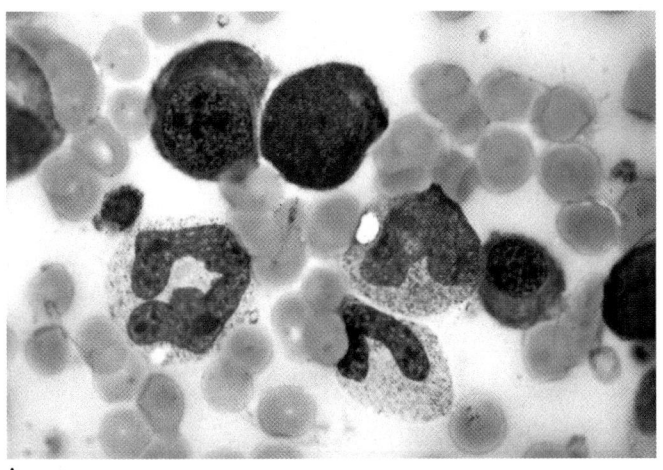
A

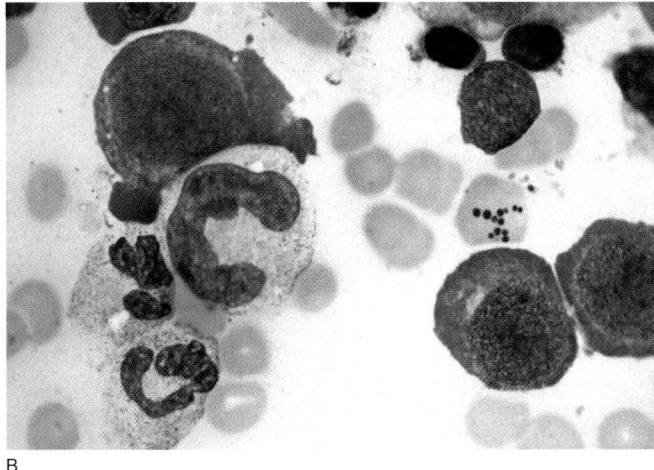
B

Fig. 12.5 (A,B) Marrow smear from a patient with pernicious anemia. (A) Giant metamyelocyte, normal-sized neutrophil band form and neutrophil myelocyte with a slightly indented nucleus. The nucleus of the giant metamyelocyte has a bud-like protrusion along its length. (B) Giant metamyelocyte adjacent to two normal-sized neutrophil granulocytes. May–Grünwald–Giemsa stain.

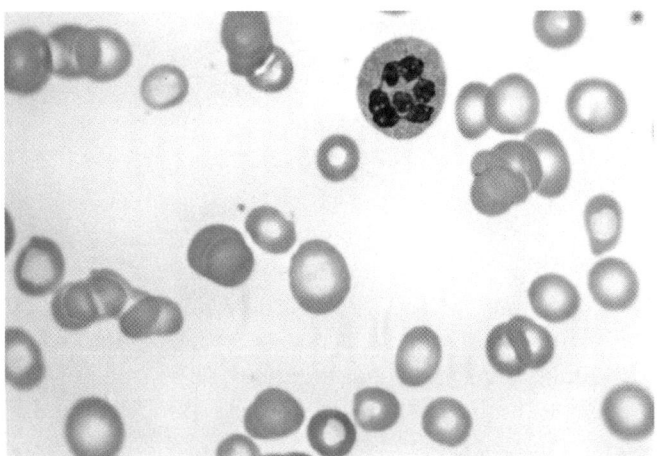

Fig. 12.6 Hypersegmented neutrophil and macrocytes in the blood smear of a patient with pernicious anemia. May–Grünwald–Giemsa stain.

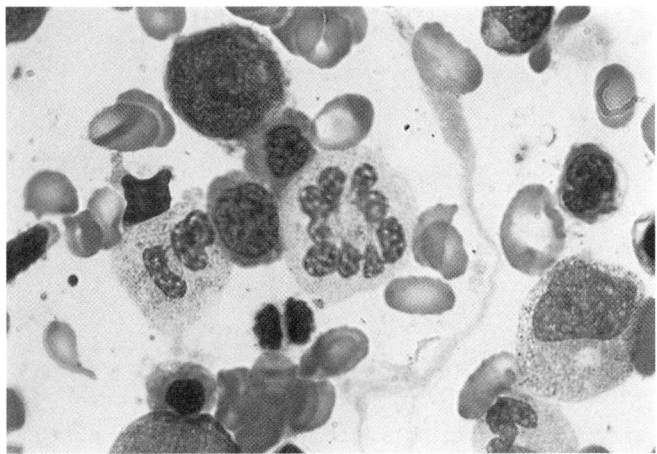

Fig. 12.7 Hypersegmented macropolycyte and a normal-sized neutrophil with two nuclear segments from the bone marrow smear of a patient with pernicious anemia. The nuclear and cytoplasmic areas of the macropolycyte are similar to those of the giant metamyelocytes in Figure 12.5. May–Grünwald–Giemsa stain.

Vitamin B_{12}

The vitamin B_{12} molecule consists of two parts aligned at right angles to each other: (1) a planar corrin nucleus (containing four pyrrole rings); and (2) the ribonucleotide of 5,6-dimethylbenzimidazole. A cobalt atom is located at the center of the corrin nucleus and is coordinately bonded to the four pyrrole rings and to one of the nitrogen atoms of the ribonucleotide as well as to an organic group such as methyl, deoxyadenosyl, cyano or hydroxo. The two naturally occurring B_{12} coenzymes have the methyl or deoxyadenosyl group and are known as methylcobalamin and deoxyadenosylcobalamin, respectively. In nature, vitamin B_{12} is synthesized exclusively by microorganisms. Synthesis by bacteria in the rumen serves as the main source of B_{12} in herbivores. Other animals and man obtain B_{12} by consuming foods of animal origin, including dairy products. Vegetables and fruits are devoid of vitamin B_{12} except by virtue of contamination by bacteria. A mixed diet contains about 5–30 μg vitamin B_{12} per day and 1–3 μg of this are absorbed. The vitamin in food is largely protein-bound and is released from its bound state within the stomach by the action of the proteolytic enzyme pepsin. Most of the released B_{12} rapidly attaches to a B_{12}-binding protein found in saliva and gastric juice known as R-binder. Subsequently, B_{12} is released from the R-binder in the jejunum as a result of its degradation by pancreatic trypsin. The released B_{12} then combines with intrinsic factor, a glycoprotein secreted by the parietal cells of the fundus and body of the stomach. The vitamin B_{12}–intrinsic factor complex, which is resistant to digestion, passes down to the distal half of the ileum where absorption takes place via specific receptor sites on the brush border of the mucosal cells. There is a mucosal delay of a few hours before the absorbed vitamin B_{12} enters the portal blood. Most of the newly-absorbed vitamin B_{12} in portal blood is attached to transcobalamin II (TC II) and most of the vitamin B_{12} in systemic blood to transcobalamin I (TC I).

Vitamin B_{12} is mainly found in the liver, the hepatic stores being 2–5 mg. The absorption of 1–3 µg vitamin B_{12} per day balances an inevitable daily loss of the same magnitude. Loss occurs largely in the urine and feces via desquamation of epithelial cells and in the bile. There is an enterohepatic circulation of vitamin B_{12}: about 3–6 µg is excreted daily into the intestinal tract, mainly in the bile, of which all but about 1 µg is reabsorbed in the terminal ileum. If intrinsic factor is absent or ileal absorption is defective there is failure to conserve vitamin B_{12} secreted in the bile.

The biochemical mechanisms by which vitamin B_{12} deficiency leads to its main clinical consequences of anemia, peripheral neuropathy and subacute combined degeneration of the spinal cord remain uncertain.[2] Only two reactions are known to require vitamin B_{12} in man. These are: (1) the isomerization of methylmalonyl coenzyme A to succinyl coenzyme A, which is dependent on deoxyadenosylcobalamin; and (2) the methylation of homocysteine to methionine, which requires the enzyme

homocysteine-methionine methyl transferase, the methyl donor 5-methyltetrahydrofolate (methyl-THF) and the coenzyme methylcobalamin. During the latter reaction the methyl-THF is converted to THF and impairment of this reaction in bone marrow cells results in defective methylation of deoxyuridylate to thymidylate due to a decreased availability of 5,10-methylenetetrahydrofolate (5,10-methylene-THF) (Fig. 12.8). Defective thymidylate synthesis is thought to lead to defective DNA synthesis, including misincorporation of uracil into DNA and, consequently, to the development of megaloblastic hemopoiesis and anemia.[2] The mechanism by which impairment of the transferase reaction results in decreased levels of 5,10-methylene-THF is still controversial. Some have suggested that this impairment results in trapping of intracellular folates in the form of 5-methyl-THF which cannot be converted to 5,10-methylene-THF.[4,5] Others have considered that the important consequence of the impairment of the transferase reaction is the failure of methionine synthesis which in turn results in a reduced availability of formate and inadequate formylation of tetrahydrofolate, formyltetrahydrofolate being the precursor of 5,10-methylene-THF-polyglutamate (Fig. 12.8).[6]

The biochemical mechanisms underlying the neurologic damage induced by vitamin B_{12} deficiency also

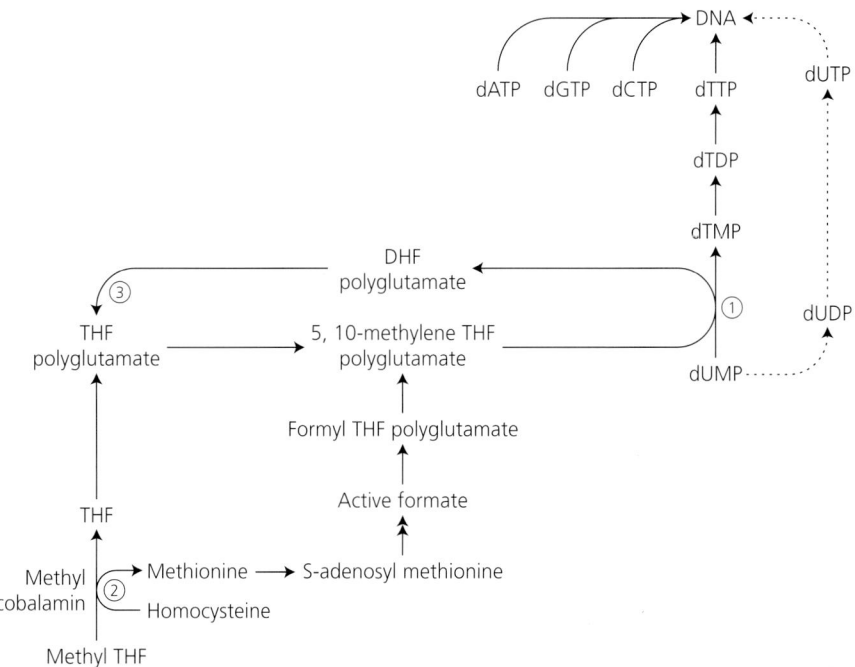

Fig. 12.8 Biochemical pathways involved in vitamin B_{12} and folate deficiency. The interrupted lines show how uracil is misincorporated into DNA as a consequence of impaired methylation of deoxyuridine monophosphate (dUMP) to deoxythymidine monophosphate (dTMP). dUDP, deoxyuridine diphosphate; dUTP, deoxyuridine triphosphate; dTDP, deoxythymidine diphosphate; dTTP, deoxythymidine triphosphate; THF, tetrahydrofolate; DHF, dihydrofolate; 1, thymidylate synthase; 2, homocysteine methyltransferase (methionine synthase); 3, dihydrofolate reductase.

remains uncertain.[2,7,8] The balance of evidence suggests that the neurologic damage may result from a failure to methylate basic proteins in myelin sheaths secondary to a failure of the synthesis of S-adenosylmethionine from methionine as a consequence of the decreased methylcobalamin-dependent conversion of homocysteine to methionine (Fig. 12.8).

The clinicopathologic features of subacute combined degeneration of the cord and the peripheral neuropathy caused by vitamin B_{12} deficiency are described in the section on pernicious anemia. These neurologic abnormalities have also developed in patients with vitamin B_{12} deficiency due to veganism, partial or total gastrectomy, abnormal small intestinal bacterial flora, ileal resection and the Imerslund–Gräsbeck syndrome. A severe peripheral neuropathy has been reported in inadequately-treated patients with congenital transcobalamin II deficiency.

Causes of vitamin B_{12} deficiency (Table 12.1)

Inadequate dietary intake

Veganism.[9,10] As vitamin B_{12} is not found in vegetables or fruit, strict vegetarians (vegans – i.e. those who do not eat meat or fish and do not take appreciable amounts of milk, milk products or eggs) must have a very low dietary intake of this vitamin. The largest group of vegans is found amongst the Hindus. Although the majority of vegans have low serum vitamin B_{12} levels, most vegans have normal hematological values, including mean cell volumes (MCVs), and appear to be in good health. Apparently an intact enterohepatic circulation of vitamin B_{12} together with the very small quantities of vitamin B_{12} absorbed from the diet ensure adequate supplies of the vitamin to marrow and other cells despite the reduced vitamin B_{12} stores. However, some vegans with a low serum B_{12} level develop a megaloblastic anemia which responds to treatment with either oral or parenteral vitamin B_{12} and a few suffer from vitamin B_{12} neuropathy. Breast-fed infants of vegan mothers may develop vitamin B_{12} deficiency during the first year of life.[11] People on a predominantly vegetarian diet who consume some dairy products may also develop low serum B_{12} levels and it is possible that some of them have an additional acquired defect in the ability to release B_{12} from food (see below).

Gastric lesions

Pernicious anemia[3] In this condition impaired vitamin B_{12} absorption and vitamin B_{12} deficiency result from a marked reduction in the secretion of intrinsic factor

Table 12.1 Vitamin-B_{12}-related and folate-related causes of macrocytosis with megaloblastic erythropoiesis

Vitamin-B_{12}-related
(a) Inadequate dietary intake: veganism
(b) Gastric lesions: pernicious anemia, total or partial gastrectomy, congenital intrinsic factor deficiency, congenitally abnormal intrinsic factor
(c) Intestinal lesions: stagnant loop syndrome, ileal resection, Crohn's disease, chronic tropical sprue, fish tapeworm, selective malabsorption with proteinuria (Imerslund–Gräsbeck syndrome)
(d) Other causes of malabsorption of vitamin B_{12}: food cobalamin malabsorption, some drugs, chronic pancreatitis, Zollinger–Ellison syndrome, HIV infection, irradiation, graft versus host disease, etc.
(e) Acquired abnormality of cobalamin metabolism: nitrous oxide toxicity
(f) Inherited abnormalities of cobalamin transport and metabolism

Folate-related
(a) Inadequate dietary intake
(b) Malabsorption: coeliac disease, jejunal resection, tropical sprue
(c) Increased requirement or loss: pregnancy, prematurity, hemolytic anemia, malignant disease, chronic inflammatory disease, long-term dialysis, congestive heart failure, liver disease
(d) Acquired abnormality of folate metabolism: dihydrofolate reductase inhibitors
(e) Complex mechanism: anticonvulsant therapy, ethanol abuse, oral contraceptive drugs
(f) Congenital disorders of folate absorption and metabolism

secondary to gastric atrophy. The vitamin B_{12} deficiency may lead to anemia, neurologic damage or both. The disease is common in people of Northern European extraction but also occurs in Africans, Asians, Chinese and other races. Pernicious anemia is uncommon before the age of 30 years and the incidence increases with advancing age, most patients being 50–70 years old. According to the old literature, the overall prevalence in the UK is about 1 per 1000 of the population, and approaches 1% after the age of 60 years. A recent study showed that the prevalence of mild cobalamin deficiency due to undiagnosed pernicious anemia amongst the multiethnic population of Los Angeles, California, aged 60 years or over was at least 2.7% in women and 1.4% in men; the prevalence was 4.3% in black women and 4.0% in white women.[12] The male:female ratio in pernicious anemia is about 1:1.5. A family history of pernicious anemia is present in about 20% of patients. Autoimmune diseases (thyroid diseases, vitiligo, hypoparathyroidism and hypofunction of the adrenal glands) are more common in patients with pernicious anemia and their relatives than in the general population, and patients show a slightly higher than normal incidence of the blood group A. Male patients have a slightly increased incidence of gastric carcinoma. There is a more substantial increase in gastric carcinoid tumors but these are mostly relatively benign.[13]

The above data indicate that there is a genetic predisposition to the development of gastric atrophy and that autoimmune mechanisms are involved. However, the absence of intrinsic factor and parietal cell antibodies in some cases of pernicious anemia suggests that these antibodies are a consequence rather than the cause of the damage to the gastric mucosa. Instead, it appears from studies of a murine model of autoimmune chronic atrophic gastritis that cell-mediated immunity may be involved.[14] Indeed, the gastric mucosa in pernicious anemia shows infiltration with plasma cells and lymphocytes, with an excess of CD4[+] cells. In addition, its histology improves and both acid and intrinsic factor (IF) secretion increases during a period of steroid administration.

As is the case in some developing countries now, when pernicious anemia was first recognized in the developed world over a century ago, the disease was diagnosed at an advanced stage, usually with severe megaloblastic anemia, other cytopenias and progressive neurologic abnormalities. Today, with the availability of automated full blood counts (including MCVs) and automated serum B_{12} and folate and red cell folate assays, B_{12} deficiency is usually diagnosed at an early stage. In one study, 44% of B_{12}-responsive patients had hematocrit values within the normal range and 36% had MCVs within the normal range.[15] For the same reasons, the prevalence and severity of B_{12} neuropathy is now less than in the past.

Symptoms and signs. Symptoms are of slow onset and may include tiredness, weakness, dyspnea, a sore tongue and gastrointestinal disturbances (anorexia, nausea, vomiting, dyspepsia, constipation, diarrhea) and loss of weight. There may be slight jaundice, a low-grade pyrexia and slight enlargement of the spleen.

Neurologic symptoms, which affect only some patients, usually begin in the lower limbs and are symmetrical. The most frequent of these are paresthesiae in the extremities, difficulty in walking and muscle weakness. Others include poor vision, stiffness of the limbs, impotence and impairment of bladder and rectal control. Neurologic signs include sensory loss (particularly loss of position and vibration sense), ataxia, positive Romberg sign, impairment of memory and, less commonly, the features of spastic paraplegia. The severity of neurologic impairment correlates inversely with the hematocrit;[16] about a quarter of cases with B_{12} neuropathy are not anemic and a slightly lower proportion do not have a high MCV.[17]

Laboratory investigations and treatment. Patients diagnosed very early have a hemoglobin level and MCV within the reference range. Those diagnosed early have a high MCV (macrocytosis) and high mean cell hemoglobin (MCH) associated with a hemoglobin level within the reference range. Later, there is both macrocytosis and mild to severe anemia. In anemic patients, the reduction of the red cell count is more marked than that of the hemoglobin level. Usually some of the macrocytes are oval in shape (see Fig. 12.3). With increasing anemia, the red cells also show an increasing degree of anisocytosis and poikilocytosis. The poikilocytes include tear-drop-shaped and irregularly-shaped cells as well as small red cell fragments. There is a rough inverse correlation between the degree of anemia and the MCV; unusually mild degrees of macrocytosis for the extent of anemia are found when there are many small red cell fragments (usually in patients with Hb less than 7 g/dl) and in patients with coexistent iron deficiency, chronic disorder, or thalassemia syndrome. The circulating neutrophil granulocytes of most cases show a tendency towards hypersegmentation of their nuclei, more than 3% of the neutrophils containing five or more nuclear segments. There may be mild neutropenia or thrombocytopenia, particularly in severely anemic patients.

The bone marrow is hypercellular and in severely anemic patients there may be an almost complete replacement of fat cells by hemopoietic cells. Hemopoiesis is megaloblastic in type. The myeloid/erythroid (M/E) ratio is usually reduced but may be increased. The quantity of stainable iron in the marrow fragments is usually normal or increased. There are abnormal sideroblasts but few, if any, ringed sideroblasts.

The serum bilirubin level may be slightly elevated and the serum lactate dehydrogenase is frequently increased. The serum iron is high but falls within 48 h of a single injection of vitamin B_{12}. The serum vitamin B_{12} level is below the normal range in 95–97% of cases. However, a low serum vitamin B_{12} level should be considered as presumptive rather than definitive evidence of vitamin B_{12} deficiency as low levels are also seen in about one-third of patients with folate deficiency. Furthermore, low vitamin B_{12} levels may be found in pregnant women or in the elderly, sometimes without any hematologic, neurologic or biochemical disturbances attributable to a deficiency of this vitamin. Red cell folate levels are low in 60% of patients with pernicious anemia and normal in the remainder. The serum folate level is low in 10% of cases and high in 20%. Parietal cell antibodies, directed against the α and β subunits of the proton pump (H[+], K[+] ATPase) of the gastric parietal cell,[14] are found in the serum in about 85% of patients and IgG intrinsic factor antibodies in 55%. The gastric juice contains an IgA antibody against intrinsic factor in about 60% of cases; there is no correlation between the presence of this IgA antibody and of the IgG antibody.

Because of the impairment of the adenosylcobalamin-dependent conversion of methylmalonyl CoA to succinyl CoA, plasma methylmalonic acid (MMA) levels are increased in vitamin B_{12} deficiency (but not in folate deficiency). In addition, the impairment of the methylation of homocysteine, which is dependent both on methylcobalamin and methyl-THF, leads to an increase in plasma homocysteine (HCYS) levels in either vitamin B_{12} or folate deficiency. Nearly all clinically confirmed cases of vitamin B_{12} deficiency have increased levels of plasma MMA or HCYS or both and less than 2% of confirmed cases of folate deficiency (without renal failure) have increased plasma MMA levels.[18] Whereas increased MMA levels are highly specific for vitamin B_{12} deficiency, increased HCYS levels are less specific, being found in patients with impaired renal function, alcoholism and some inborn errors of homocysteine metabolism.

There is a histamine-fast or pentagastrin-fast achlorhydria. The pH of gastric juice is usually alkaline, but may vary between 6 and 8; after the injection of pentagastrin, the pH usually becomes more alkaline and in any case does not fall by more than 0.5 units. The intrinsic factor content of pentagastrin-stimulated gastric juice is very low, being in the range 0–250 U/h (normal, > 2000 U/h). Vitamin B_{12} absorption tests, such as the Schilling test, show impaired absorption of an orally-administered physiologic dose of ^{57}Co- or ^{58}Co-labeled vitamin B_{12}; this impaired absorption is improved by the simultaneous oral administration of intrinsic factor.

The diagnosis of pernicious anemia requires the demonstration of a gross impairment of intrinsic factor secretion. This is usually achieved indirectly by performing a Schilling test, with and without intrinsic factor.[3,19] The majority of patients have megaloblastic hemopoiesis and a low serum vitamin B_{12} level, but this combination of abnormalities occurs in other conditions. Furthermore, some patients with a vitamin B_{12} neuropathy may show no morphologic abnormalities in either the blood or the bone marrow. The diagnosis of pernicious anemia cannot be maintained in the absence of a histamine-fast or pentagastrin-fast achlorhydria but this type of severe achlorhydria is not uncommon in elderly subjects with adequate intrinsic factor secretion. Parietal cell antibodies are not specific for pernicious anemia, being found in a small percentage of healthy individuals (2% of those less than 30 years of age and 16% of those greater than 60 years) and in a higher proportion of individuals with various disorders such as myxedema, Graves' disease,

iron deficiency anemia and gastritis without pernicious anemia. By contrast, intrinsic factor antibodies are virtually confined to pernicious anemia.

Patients with pernicious anemia may be initially treated with six intramuscular injections, each of 1 mg hydroxocobalamin, over 2–12 weeks to replenish body stores. This should be followed by 1 mg hydroxocobalamin intramuscularly every 3 months, throughout life. Hematologic abnormalities are rapidly and completely reversed by vitamin B_{12} therapy. Neurologic symptoms of recent onset may improve considerably over 6–12 months.

Histopathology. At necropsy, untreated cases of advanced pernicious anemia show pallor and fatty change in most organs. In the heart, the fatty change causes a 'tabby-cat striation' of the myocardium. The liver and spleen are slightly enlarged and contain heavy deposits of hemosiderin as well as foci of extramedullary hemopoiesis. There is replacement of the yellow fatty marrow of long bones by hyperplastic hemopoietic marrow which is deep red in color. The expansion of the marrow causes a thinning of the bone cortex and loss of trabeculae. There is severe atrophy of the mucosa and muscle coat of the upper two-thirds of the stomach. Histologic examination of the mucosa reveals only a few scattered glands and these are lined by mucus-secreting cells (Fig. 12.9). There is a lack of oxyntic and peptic cells with a variable degree of infiltration by lymphocytes and plasma cells. The epithelium of the tongue, esophagus and intestine is also thinned. Cytologic and histologic studies show that the epitheial cells lining the buccal cavity, tongue, stomach, jejunum, bronchial tree, urinary tract, vagina and cervix uteri display 'megaloblastic changes' – particularly an increase in cell and nuclear size.

In some patients, the features of subacute combined degeneration of the spinal cord may be seen (Fig. 12.10).[20] There is patchy degeneration of the dorsal columns and pyramidal and spinocerebellar tracts causing a grayish discoloration of the white matter. Usually, the foci of degeneration initially affect (and are most extensive in) the lower cervical and upper thoracic segments of the cord and gradually spread upwards into the upper cervical segments and downwards into the lumbar segments. The dorsal columns and spinocerebellar tracts are most affected in the upper part of the spinal cord and the pyramidal tracts in the lower part. Microscopically, there is marked swelling of the myelin sheaths (giving the affected areas a vacuolated appearance) followed by degeneration of the axons; the degenerating myelin sheaths and axons are removed by phagocytic cells which become laden with lipid. Extensive damage is eventually followed by substantial gliosis. Similar degenerative changes may be present in the posterior nerve roots. Foci of demyelination may also occur in the white matter of the cerebral hemispheres and the medulla oblongata. In long-standing cases, there is secondary degeneration of the long tracts in areas of the spinal cord not directly involved by the disease. The cerebrospinal fluid shows an increase of protein (usually less than 100 mg/dl) in

about half the patients with subacute combined degeneration of the cord.

There may be evidence of a peripheral neuropathy with loss of nerve fibers and the muscles may show denervation atrophy.[3,20] Bilateral optic atrophy has been reported occasionally.

Juvenile pernicious anemia. This disorder affects older children and is similar to pernicious anemia in adults except that a higher proportion of cases (about 50%) have an associated autoimmune endocrinopathy, some cases suffer from mucocutaneous candidiasis and parietal cell antibodies are usually not present.

Pernicious anemia and hypogammaglobuninemia. A number of cases have been reported in which pernicious anemia was associated with hypogammaglobulinemia and occasionally with a selective deficiency of IgA. Differences from classical pernicious anemia have included onset between the third and fourth decade, atrophy of the mucosa in the entire stomach including the pyloric antrum and absence of plasma cells in the mucosal infiltrate.

Total or partial gastrectomy.[21,22] Total gastrectomy results in the removal of the intrinsic-factor-secreting cells and therefore inevitably leads to a megaloblastic anemia due to vitamin B_{12} deficiency. This anemia appears 2–10 years after the operation; the long delay represents the time taken for normal vitamin B_{12} stores to run out after the abrupt cessation of vitamin B_{12} absorption. It is best to commence regular B_{12} therapy soon after the gastrectomy.

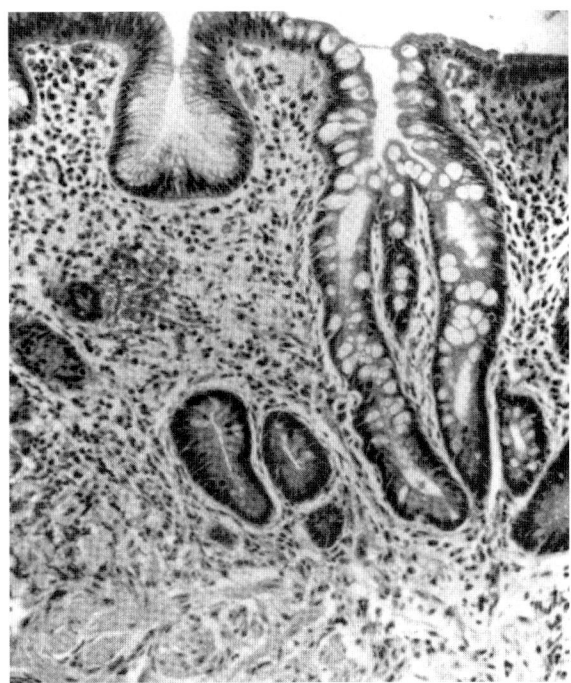

Fig. 12.9 Biopsy of the gastric mucosa in pernicious anemia showing a paucity of gastric glands. The few glandular elements seen contain mucous-secreting cells. The mucosal layer contains increased numbers of lymphocytes and plasma cells. Hematoxylin–eosin. Courtesy of Dr I Chanarin.

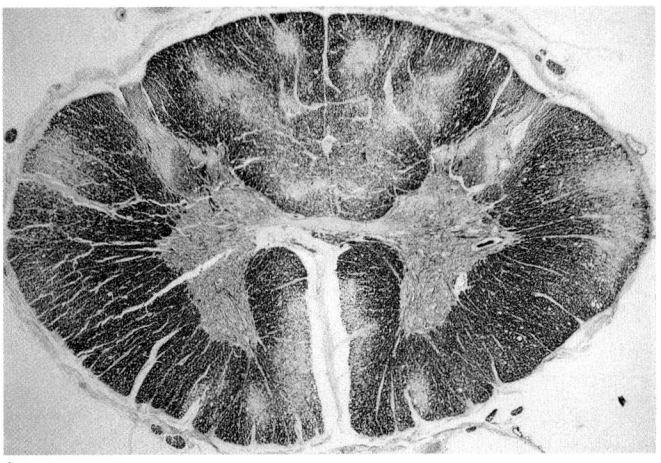

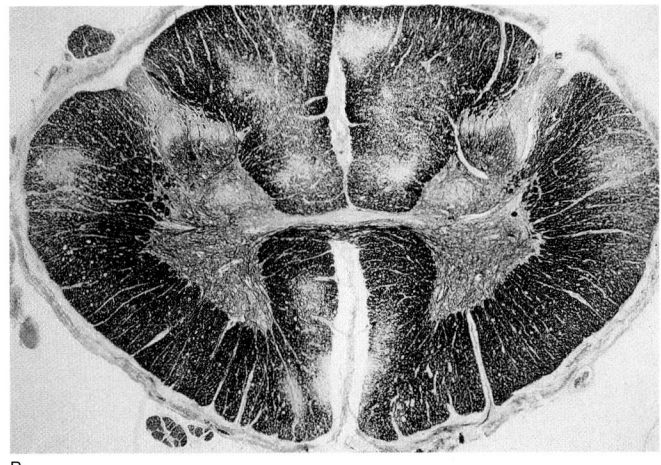

A

B

Fig. 12.10 (A,B) The cervical (A) and thoracic (B) spinal cord showing advanced subacute combined degeneration. Particularly the posterior and lateral columns but also the anterior columns show pale areas, indicating demyelination. Weigert–Pal method for myelin. Courtesy of Professor F Scaravilli, Department of Neuropathology, Institute of Neurology, University College London, UK.

Anemia due to iron deficiency develops in about half the cases subjected to partial gastrectomy, and anemia or neuropathy due to vitamin B_{12} deficiency in about 5% of the cases. The iron-deficiency anemia usually appears during, and the vitamin B_{12}-deficiency anemia after the first five postoperative years. The probability of developing vitamin B_{12} deficiency is a function of the amount of stomach resected. In most cases, the vitamin B_{12} deficiency appears to result from a combination of the loss of intrisnic-factor-secreting mucosa at operation and the subsequent atrophy of the remainder of the gastric mucosa. Sometimes, the deficiency may result from a failure to release vitamin B_{12} from food due to a deficiency of acid and gastric pepsin (see below). In a few cases, and particularly when blind loops have been created (as happens during a Polya gastrectomy), the vitamin B_{12} deficiency is a consequence of the development of an abnormal intestinal bacterial flora.

Congenital intrinsic factor deficiency.[23,24] Patients with this rare syndrome present with megaloblastic anemia, usually during the first 3 years of life. The syndrome is characterized by the absence of intrinsic factor but the presence of hydrochloric acid and pepsin in gastric juice, a normal-looking gastric mucosa, the absence of parietal cell and intrinsic factor antibodies and an autosomal recessive inheritance. Heterozygotes are clinically normal.

Congenitally abnormal intrinsic factor.[24,25] A single case has been described in which a severe megaloblastic anemia was due to homozygosity for the production of a mutant intrinsic factor molecule. This abnormal intrinsic factor bound vitamin B_{12} but failed to promote vitamin B_{12} absorption.

Intestinal lesions

Abnormal intestinal bacterial flora.[26] Vitamin B_{12} deficiency may develop in conditions in which there is small-intestinal stasis. Such conditions include multiple jejunal diverticula, small-intestinal strictures, intestinal involvement in systemic sclerosis, and stagnant intestinal loops resulting either from gastrointestinal surgery or from fistulae complicating regional iletis or tuberculosis. The intestinal stasis results in the presence of an increased number of bacteria (e.g. enterobacteria, bacteroides, streptococci, lactobacilli and Gram-positive anaerobes) within the proximal part of the small gut. These bacteria convert vitamin B_{12} from ingested food into inactive cobamides and thus decrease the availability of vitamin B_{12} for absorption at the terminal ileum.[27] Patients with vitamin B_{12} deficiency due to the presence of an abnormal

intestinal bacterial flora show a decreased absorption of an oral dose of radiolabeled vitamin B_{12} which is not improved when the vitamin is given with intrinsic factor. However, they show a substantial improvement in absorption soon after a course of a broad-spectrum antibiotic such as tetracycline.

Ileal resection,[28] **Crohn's disease and chronic tropical sprue.** As mentioned, vitamin B_{12} is absorbed in the terminal ileum. A deficiency of this vitamin due to impairment of its absorption may, therefore, develop in diseases affecting the lower part of the ileum (e.g. Crohn's disease, chronic tropical sprue) or after resections of more than about 60 cm of the terminal ileum. The extent of impairment of B_{12} absorption is proportional to the extent of resection.

Megaloblastic anemia is present in 60–90% of patients with tropical sprue. About 90% of patients with this disease malabsorb vitamin B_{12} and many also malabsorb folate. The absorption of vitamin B_{12} frequently returns to normal after a course of broad-spectrum antibiotics and in the early stages of the disease may improve following therapy with folic acid.

Infestation with the fish tapeworm (*Diphyllobothrium latum***).**[29,30] Infestation with this tapeworm is seen in people living around the freshwater lakes of Finland, the Baltic States, northern Italy, Switzerland, Germany, Romania, the Soviet Union, Japan and North America. However, megaloblastic anemia caused by this tapeworm is more or less confined to Finland, the Baltic States and the Soviet Union. Infestation occurs by eating raw or partly cooked fish containing a larval form. The adult tapeworm may grow to a length of 10 m and is found attached by its head to the mucosa of the ileum. Only a few per cent of infested humans develop megaloblastic hemopoiesis or neurologic abnormalities due to vitamin B_{12} deficiency. The tapeworm causes these effects by extracting vitamin B_{12} from food. Although most fish tapeworms are attached to the distal half of the small intestine, the worms of anemic individuals are attached much higher up and it appears that parasites with a high attachment may extract more vitamin B_{12} than others. Vitamin B_{12} deficiency due to infestation with the fish tapeworm is becoming less common because of pollution of the lakes and a consequent reduction in the population of potentially infective fish. Whereas in the past about 20% of Finns harbored the fish tapeworm this figure had come down to about 2% in 1977.[31]

Selective malabsorption of vitamin B_{12} with proteinuria (Imerslund–Gräsbeck syndrome).[32,33] This rare congenital disorder is inherited as an autosomal recessive character and patients present with megaloblastic anemia between the ages of 1 and 15 years. The anemia results from a failure of the terminal ileum to absorb vitamin B_{12} from the vitamin B_{12}–intrinsic-factor complex. The defect of absorption only affects vitamin B_{12}, the absorption of other substances being entirely normal. The gastric juice contains normal quantities of intrinsic factor and the histology of the stomach and terminal ileum is normal. In some cases there is decreased intrinsic factor–cobalamin receptor activity in the ileal mucosa but in one case there appeared to be over-expression of an active but unstable receptor.[34] Over 90% of cases have proteinuria (0.2–1 g protein/1 urine) but there are usually no other defects of renal function. Renal biopsy has shown no consistent pattern of abnormality. The anemia is corrected by parenteral vitamin B_{12} but the mild proteinuria persists.

Other causes of malabsorption of vitamin B_{12}, usually without megaloblastic anemia. In several of the situations discussed in this section, the malabsorption has usually not been sufficiently severe or has not been allowed to continue for a sufficiently long period to cause the development of megaloblastic anemia.

Malabsorption of food cobalamin.[35–37] There is now growing evidence that many patients with a low serum vitamin B_{12} level fail to adequately release this vitamin from its protein-bound state in food as a consequence of impaired secretion of acid and pepsin by the stomach. Such patients usually have no hematologic or obvious neurologic abnormality. However, some cases have abnormal homocysteine and methylmalonic acid levels, give abnormal deoxyuridine suppressed values or show neuro-electrophysiologic abnormalities. A few patients display hematologic abnormalities or neurologic dysfunction. In an occasional case the gastric dysfunction has progressed to involve intrinsic factor secretion and pernicious anemia has developed. In food cobalamin malabsorption, the conventional Schilling test gives a normal result but a modification of the test employing protein-bound instead of free radiolabeled vitamin B_{12} gives an abnormal result: the vitamin is usually bound *in vitro* to egg or chicken serum. Conditions associated with food cobalamin malabsorption are non-specific gastritis, *Helicobacter pylori* gastritis, partial gastrectomy, vagotomy, gastric bypass surgery for treatment of obesity, bacterial overgrowth in the stomach, alcohol abuse and the use of acid suppressing drugs. The latter incude cimetidine, omeprazole, ranitidine and gelusil. About 45% of unexplained low serum vitamin B_{12} levels,

in patients who have not been subjected to gastric surgery, may be caused by malabsorption of food cobalamin. Patients with food cobalamin malabsorption respond to vitamin B_{12} given orally.

Some drugs. Malabsorption of vitamin B_{12} has been demonstrated in patients receiving aminosalicylates, neomycin, colchicine, slow-release potassium chloride, metformin, phenformin, cholestyramine and large doses of vitamin C. Rarely, megaloblastic anemia has developed following prolonged treatment with aminosalicylates or metformin.

Chronic pancreatitis. Vitamin B_{12} malabsorption, rarely with megaloblastic anemia, has also been described in severe pancreatic disease. Here, the impaired secretion of trypsin by the diseased pancreas causes reduced degradation of vitamin B_{12}–R-binder complexes and, consequently, reduced availability of the vitamin for binding to intrinsic factor.

Zollinger–Ellison syndrome. The vitamin B_{12} malabsorption that occurs in this syndrome may be caused by inactivation of pancreatic trypsin leading to impaired release of the vitamin from salivary and gastric R binder.

HIV infection. Low serum vitamin B_{12} levels and abnormal Schilling test results are frequently seen in the later stages of HIV infection but only a few patients show evidence of tissue B_{12} deficiency such as abnormal deoxyuridine-suppressed values and elevated plasma methylmalonic acid or homocysteine levels. Rarely is there a hematologic response to parenteral vitamin B_{12} therapy. The low serum vitamin B_{12} levels appear to be frequently due to reduced levels of transcobalamin I.[38]

Other causes. Impaired absorption of vitamin B_{12} has been reported in about 30% of cases of gluten-sensitive enteropathy, after total body irradiation, after ileal irradiation (e.g. during radiotherapy to the cervix), in graft versus host disease, in giardiasis and in folate, protein, riboflavin or pyridoxine deficiency.

Acquired abnormality of cobalamin metabolism

Inactivation of vitamin B_{12} by nitrous oxide.[39,40] The continuous exposure of patients to a mixture of 50% N_2O and 50% O_2 for 5–6 days or more (once used in the management of severe tetanus) may cause bone marrow aplasia with severe megaloblastic changes in the residual hemopoietic cells.[41] Continuous exposure for 5–24 h (e.g. during the postoperative ventilation of patients who have undergone cardiac bypass surgery) often induced mildly megaloblastic erythropoiesis.[42] It is also possible that the intermittent use of nitrous oxide over long periods (e.g. Entonox – a mixture of equal parts of N_2O and O_2 – inhaled for 15–20 min two or three times a day to facilitate physiotherapy) may induce megaloblastic changes.[43] Furthermore, neuropathy resembling that seen in vitamin B_{12} deficiency has been described in dentists repeatedly exposed to N_2O over a long period.[44] These effects seem to result from the oxidation of methyl cobalamin by N_2O and its consequent inactivation.

Inherited abnormalities of cobalamin transport and metabolism

Congenital transcobalamin II deficiency.[45–47] A few children have been reported in whom a megaloblastic anemia resulted from the complete absence of transcobalamin II (TC II). This transcobalamin is concerned with the active transport of vitamin B_{12} into all cell types and away from the epithelial cells of the terminal ileum (following absorption from the vitamin-B_{12}–intrinsic-factor complex). Most patients present with severe megaloblastic anemia, leukopenia, thrombocytopenia and failure to thrive within a few weeks of birth. Neurologic damage is usually seen only when vitamin B_{12} therapy is delayed. The inheritance is as an autosomal recessive character. Some patients have additional features such as marked hypogammaglobulinemia, granulocyte dysfunction, bizarre red cell morphology or erythroid hypoplasia. Since most of the vitamin B_{12} in serum is bound to transcobalamin I, the serum vitamin B_{12} level is normal. By contrast, the unsaturated vitamin B_{12}-binding capacity of the serum, which is normally largely dependent on the presence of apotranscobalamin II, is greatly reduced (normal range, 1000 ± 200 pg/ml). There is also an impairment of the absorption of vitamin B_{12} which is not corrected by the administration of intrinsic factor. The anemia responds to the regular injection of 1000 μg vitamin B_{12} twice or thrice a week. These massive doses probably work, despite the absence of the specific transport protein, by causing free vitamin B_{12} to enter cells by passive diffusion.

Congenitally abnormal transcobalamin II. Megaloblastic anemia responsive to parenteral vitamin B_{12} in a patient with high serum cobalamin levels has been described which was caused by homozygosity for a congenitally abnormal TCII molecule: the abnormal TC II binds vitamin B_{12} but the TC II–B_{12} complex does not bind to the TC II receptor.[48] In another patient, pancytopenia at the age of 6 weeks appeared to be due to double heterozygosity for the absence of TC II and for the abnormal TC II molecule.[49]

Methylmalonic acidurias.[24,50] These rare congenital disorders result from an impairment of the conversion of methylmalonyl CoA to succinyl CoA, a reaction which is dependent both on adenosylcobalamin and on the apoenzyme methylmalonyl CoA mutase. Affected children have severe metabolic acidosis with high concentrations of methylmalonic acid in the urine, blood and CSF. The primary defect lies in various mutations in the methylmalonyl CoA mutase apoenzyme, in which case the disorder is unresponsive to vitamin B_{12}, or a deficiency of adenosylcobalamin, in which case the disorder is vitamin B_{12} responsive. Two groups of patients with adenosylcobalamin deficiency exist, CblA in which there is a failure to reduce vitamin B_{12} from the cob(III)-alamin to the cob(I)alamin form and CblB in which there is a failure to convert cob(I)alamin to adenosylcobalamin. Cases with a mutation in methylmalonyl CoA mutase are treated by restricting the intake of amino acids that use the proprionate pathway but several develop complications such as infarction of the basal ganglia, pancreatitis, nephritis and cardiomyopathy and do not survive long.

Combined deficiency of adenosylcobalamin and methylcobalamin.[24,50] Affected patients have both methylmalonic aciduria due to a failure to synthesize adenosylcobalamin, and homocystinuria and hypomethioninemia due to a failure to synthesize methyl-cobalamin. Three groups of cases with different primary defects are recognized, namely CblC, CblD and CblF disease, and of these CblC disease is the most common. The majority of CblC cases present in infancy with lethargy, feeding difficulties and failure to thrive. Others present in childhood or adolescence with neurologic symptoms such as spasticity, psychosis or a retinopathy with perimacular pigmentation. In most cases, there is megaloblastic anemia and there may be macrocytosis, hypersegmented polymorphs or thrombocytopenia. Impaired methylation of deoxyuridylate in marrow cells has been demonstrated both in patients with megaloblastic and in those with normoblastic erythropoiesis.

Methylcobalamin deficiency. In this deficiency, defective methylcobalamin synthesis leads to homocystinuria and hypomethioninemia in the absence of methylmalonic aciduria. Two groups of disorders exist, CblE disease and CblG disease. CblG disease is caused by impaired methylation of cob(I)alamin on its aponenzyme methionine synthase due to mutations in methionine synthase. CblE disease is caused by mutations in a reductase which is required for the reduction of cobalamin to cob(I)alamin prior to its methylation. The diagnosis is often made before the age of 2 years but has sometimes been made in adults. Clinical features include megaloblastic anemia, and various neurologic disturbances. The hematologic and biochemical abnormalities are reversed by parenteral hydroxocobalamin administered frequently but the neurologic deficits tend to show only a partial correction.

Folates

The folates are a family of compounds derived from the biologically inactive parent compound pteroyl monoglutamic acid (folic acid). Most intracellular folates are pteroyl polyglutamates with a total of 3–7 (usually 4, 5 or 6) glutamic acid residues linked together by γ-carboxy peptide bonds. By contrast most of the extracellular folates are monoglutamates. Naturally occurring intracellular and extracellular folates are also in the reduced di- or tetrahydrofolate form and, in addition, contain a single carbon unit in various states of reduction (e.g. methyl, formyl, methylene).

Folates are present in all types of animal and vegetable foods; particularly high concentrations are found in yeast, spinach, Brussels sprouts and liver. The folate content of an average diet is about 680 μg/day, and is greatly influenced by the method of preparation of food. Folates are rapidly destroyed by heat and 30–90% may be lost during cooking. About 80% of a 200 μg dose of ^{3}H-pteroylglutamic acid is absorbed; less folate is absorbed from dietary polyglutamates than monglutamates. The amount of folate absorbed by an adult is 100–200 μg per day. Prior to absorption, dietary pteroyl polyglutamates are first hydrolysed into monoglutamates, probably in the lumen of the gut, by the enzyme folate conjugase. The enterocyte converts the folate monoglutamates into 5-methyltetrahydrofolate before transfer to portal blood. The jejunum and upper part of the ileum absorb folate more actively than the remainder of the small intestine.

The total folate content of the human body is about 6–10 mg; most of this is found in the liver. The daily absorption of 100–200 μg folate is balanced by an equal loss of folate in sweat, desquamated cells (e.g. skin cells) and urine. Because of the relatively large daily requirement, folate stores may become depleted and folate deficiency develop within 3–4 months of taking a folate-depleted diet.

Folate coenzymes are involved in the transfer of single carbon units in a number of reactions. 5,10-methylenetetrahydrofolate is required for the methylation of deoxyuridylate to thymidylate. 10-formyltetrahydrofolate and 5,10-methenyltetrahydrofolate are involved in the supply of carbons 2 and 8 of the purine ring, respectively. 5-methyltetrahyrdrofolate participates in methionine synthesis. Other folate-dependent reactions in humans include the conversion of serine to glycine and the degradation of histidine through formiminoglutamic acid to glutamic acid.

Folate deficiency causes megaloblastic hemopoiesis but rarely leads to neurologic damage. Some workers have attributed the hematological changes to impaired DNA synthesis secondary to defective methylation of deoxyuridylate to thymidylate. However, studies of DNA synthesis have suggested that most folate- (or vitamin B$_{12}$-) deficient human marrow cells elongate daughter DNA strands at a normal rate and incorporate nucleic acid precursors (other than deoxyuridine) into DNA at normal or even enhanced rates. It now appears that the defective methylation of deoxyuridylate in folate deficiency results in an increase in the intracellular pool of deoxyuridine triphosphate and, consequently, to misincorporation of uracil into DNA[51] and this may well be the biochemical basis of the megaloblastic change. A very few folate-responsive patients with subacute combined degeneration of the cord have been reported in whom cobalamin deficiency seemed to have been excluded.

Folate and neural tube defects

There is an important but incompletely understood association between folate and neural tube defects. When folic acid (4 mg/day orally) is given before conception and during the first trimester of pregnancy to women with a previous infant with a neural tube defect, the probability of producing another baby with such a defect is markedly reduced.[52] A lower dose of folate (400 μg/day) has been recommended to reduce the risk of the first occurrence of a neural tube defect.[53] In addition, there is an increased incidence of neural tube defects and other congenital malformations in the babies of women receiving anticonvulsant drugs such as sodium valproate, carbamazepine, phenytoin and primidone.[54]

Causes of folate deficiency (Table 12.1)

Inadequate dietary intake Megaloblastic anemia due to a dietary folate deficiency tends to occur in the poor, the neglected elderly, the mentally disturbed, chronic alcoholics, and infants fed almost exclusively on goat's milk (which only contains 12% of the folate in cow's milk). 'Goat's milk anemia' has been reported in various countries including Germany, Italy, New Zealand and the USA. Inadequate folate intake contributes to the development of folate deficiency after gastric surgery, in patients with prolonged severe illnesses and in patients with epilepsy receiving anticonvulsant drugs.

Malabsorption Diseases such as gluten-sensitive enteropathy and tropical sprue, which affect the upper part of the small intestine, often cause anemia due to malabsorption of folate. Reduced absorption of folate is also seen after partial gastrectomy or jejunal resection and when Crohn's disease affects the upper small intestine. In addition, it has been reported in patients taking salazopyrine.

Increased requirement or loss An increased requirement of folate due to increased nucleic acid turnover may lead to folate deficiency, particularly in those taking suboptimal quantities of folate in their diet. An increased requirement occurs in pregnancy because of the needs of the growing fetus,[55] in chronic hemolytic anemias and chronic idiopathic myelofibrosis because of increased proliferation of erythropoietic cells and marrow cells (including fibroblasts), respectively, and in premature infants because of the rapid growth during the first 2–3 months. There is also an increased folate requirement in various malignant diseases (leukemia, lymphoma, myeloma, carcinoma), presumably due to increased proliferation of neoplastic cells.

Before the use of folate supplements during pregnancy, megaloblastic anemia was found in the latter part of pregnancy in 2.8% of women in the UK.[56] However, examination of the bone marrow revealed that megaloblastic hemopoiesis was much more common, being found in 25% and in over 50%, respectively, of women in the UK and in South India. With the increasing awareness of the importance of adequate folate intake preconceptually and during pregnancy, the incidence of megaloblastic anemia of pregnancy in the developed world is now quite low. Megaloblastic anemia is particularly common in twin pregnancies and is most likely to present after the 36th week of gestation, around the time of delivery or early in the postpartum period.

The folate requirement of the newborn per unit weight is 10-fold that of an adult and premature babies may develop megaloblastic anemia at 4–6 weeks of age.

Patients with chronic inflammation such as those with tuberculosis or severe rheumatoid arthritis tend to become folate-deficient, probably because of a combination of: (1) inadequate intake (as the result of a poor appetite); (2) increased urinary loss; and (3) an increased requirement to support the increased formation of chronic inflammatory cells. In psoriasis and exfoliative dermatitis there may also be inceased loss of folate via desquamation of skin cells. It has been postulated that fever itself may interfere with folate metabolism by inhibiting temperature-sensitive folate coenzymes.

Some folate is lost during long-term hemodialysis or peritoneal dialysis as folates are only loosely bound to plasma proteins. This loss is modest but may aggravate negative folate balance caused by other mechanisms. There is a substantial increase in the urinary loss of folate (to $> 100\,\mu g/day$) in some patients with congestive heart failure or liver disease that has been attributed to hepatocellular damage.

Acquired abnormality of folate metabolism

Therapy with dihydrofolate reductase inhibitors.[57,58] The enzyme dihydrofolate reductase, which is present in most mammalian cells, catalyses the reduction of dihydrofolate to tetrahydrofolate. The dihydrofolate which is reduced in this way is derived both from the diet and from the 5,10-methylenetetrahydrofolate-dependent methylation of deoxyuridylate to thymidylate. In the latter reaction the folate coenzyme is oxidized to dihydrofolate. The administration of dihydrofolate reductase inhibitors (such as methotrexate, pyrimethamine and triamterene) appears to cause megaloblastic hemopoiesis by impairing the regeneration of 5,10-methylenetetrahydrofolate from dihydrofolate and thus reducing the rate of methylation of deoxyuridylate. Trimethoprim, which is present in co-trimoxazole (Septrin), is a weak inhibitor of mammalian dihydrofolate reductase: when used in conventional dosage it causes megaloblastic hemopoiesis only in patients with a preexisting impairment of the methylation of deoxyuridylate due, for example, to a mild degree of vitamin B_{12} or folate deficiency. When necessary, the hematologic effects of dihydrofolate reductase inhibitors may be reversed using folinic acid (5-formyl tetrahydrofolate).

Complex or unknown mechanism

Anticonvulsant therapy and ethanol abuse. Most patients with macrocytosis associated with anticonvulsant therapy[58,59] or chronic alcoholism[3,58,60–62] do not suffer from folate deficiency (see below). In those who do, the deficiency seems to be mainly caused by an inadequate diet. However, malabsorption of folate has been described both in treated epileptics (conflicting data) and chronic alcoholics, and may contribute to the development of folate deficiency. There is also some evidence that anticonvulsant drugs and, possibly, ethanol may induce enzymes involved in folate catabolism.

Oral contraceptive drugs. Folate-responsive megaloblastic anemia has been reported in only a few women on the contraceptive pill in whom other causes of folate deficiency appeared to have been excluded. The evidence that the pill has a significant effect on folate status is weak and controversial. Some data suggest that the pill may cause impaired folate absorption and increased urinary folate loss.

Congenital disorders of folate absorption and metabolism[24,63] Eighteen patients with *hereditary folate malabsorption* have been reported so far, in whom there appears to be an abnormality in a transport system specific for folic acid. The condition presents in the first few months of life with megaloblastic anemia (and other hematologic abnormalities such as macrocytosis, leukopenia and, occasionally, thrombocytopenia), vomiting, diarrhea, mouth ulcers, recurrent infections, failure to thrive and neurologic abnormalities. The latter include hypotonia, seizures, mental retardation and ataxia. Folate levels in serum, red cells and CSF are very low. The hematologic abnormalities and gastrointestinal symptoms respond to high doses of folic acid given orally or smaller doses parenterally, and in some cases seizures improve.

The most frequent inherited disorder of folate metabolism is *methylene tetrahydrofolate reductase (MTHFR) deficiency*. Patients may present at any time from infancy to childhood. Symptoms vary markedly in different cases and some infants are severely ill with seizures, abnormalities of gait, breathing disorders and coma. Megaloblastic anemia or other hematologic abnormalities are usually absent. Serum, red cell and CSF folate levels are reduced, plasma homocysteine levels are increased, plasma methionine levels are normal or reduced and there is homocysteinuria. Arterial and venous thombosis may occur and the histopathologic features of subacute combined degeneration of the cord have been found at autopsy.

Table 12.2 Vitamin-B_{12}-independent and folate-independent causes of macrocytosis with megaloblastic erythropoiesis

Abnormalities of nucleic acid synthesis
(a) Therapy with antipurines (e.g. mercaptopurine, thioguanine, azathioprine), antipyrimidines (e.g. fluorouracil, azauridine, cytarabine), hydroxyurea, cyclophosphamide, procarbazine, acyclovir. Arsenic poisoning.
(b) Orotic aciduria, Lesch–Nyhan syndrome

Uncertain etiology
(a) Anticonvulsant therapy,[a] chronic alcoholism[a]
(b) Myelodysplastic syndromes, erythroleukemia
(c) Congenital dyserythropoietic anemia, types I and III
(d) Thiamine-responsive anemia

[a] See also Table 12.1.

Rare cases of megaloblastic hemopoiesis with normal or high serum folate levels have been caused by *glutamate formiminotransferase deficiency* or *cyclodeaminase deficiency* (in which there is increased formiminoglutamic acid in blood and urine after histidine loading), *dihydrofolate reductase deficiency, methionine synthase deficiency* or deficiency of other (unidentified) enzymes involved in folate metabolism. Mental retardation has developed in some cases.

Vitamin B_{12}-independent and folate-independent causes of megaloblastic erythropoiesis

(Table 12.2)

Abnormalities of nucleic acid synthesis

Drug-induced impairment of DNA synthesis[57,58]

A number of drugs interfering with DNA synthesis cause macrocytosis with megaloblastic erythropoiesis. These include mercaptopurine, thioguanine and azathioprine (which interfere with purine synthesis), fluorouracil (which inhibits thymidylate synthase), cytarabine (which inhibits DNA polymerase), and hydroxyurea (which inhibits ribonucleotide reductase). Other drugs which cause megaloblastic changes by vitamin B_{12}-independent or folate-independent mechanisms include zidovudine, cyclophosphamide, procarbazine and acyclovir. Arsenic poisoning also causes megaloblastic changes.

Orotic aciduria[64,65]

This is a rare inherited disorder of pyrimidine synthesis characterized by severe megaloblastic anemia, failure to thrive, the excretion of large quantities (0.5–1.5 g/d) of orotic acid in the urine and impaired cellular (but not humoral) immunity. The disorder is caused by a greatly reduced activity of two enzymes, orotidylic pyrophosphorylase and orotidylic decarboxylase, which are involved in the conversion of orotic acid to uridine monophosphate, a precursor of the pyrimidine bases of DNA. Affected patients appear to be homozygotes for an autosomal recessive gene and present between the ages of 3 months and 7 years. The serum vitamin B_{12} and red cell folate levels are normal and there is no response to vitamin B_{12} or folate therapy. Both the anemia and the failure of growth and development respond well to the daily administration of 1–1.5 g uridine.

Lesch-Nyhan syndrome[66]

This syndrome is characterized by mental retardation, choreoathetosis, self-mutilation (especially biting of the lips and fingers), gout, and a sex-linked recessive inheritance. It is caused by a deficiency of the enzyme hypoxanthine phosphoribosyltransferase, which is involved in purine synthesis. Some cases have a megaloblastic anemia that is responsive to adenine.

Children with the Lesch–Nyhan syndrome may also have an increased susceptibility to infection due to defective function of B-lymphocytes. Evidence of B-cell dysfunction includes a reduced number of B-cells, decreased IgG levels, reduced isoagglutinin titers and an impaired response to pokeweed mitogen.

Uncertain etiology

Anticonvulsant therapy[3,58]

Some patients who develop megaloblastic erythropoiesis as a consequence of treatment with phenytoin (either on its own or in combination with other anticonvulsant drugs) do not suffer from a folate deficiency or an impairment of the methylation of deoxyuridylate due to any other cause. In these cases, the megaloblastic changes appear to be the result of a folate-independent drug-induced impairment of DNA synthesis and erythroblast proliferation.

Chronic alcoholism[3,58]

A proportion of chronic alcoholics display megaloblastic erythropoiesis, usually of a mild degree, in the absence of evidence of folate deficiency such as a low serum, red cell or hepatic folate level or an abnormality in the methylation of deoxyuridylate as judged by the deoxyuridine suppression test. In addition to megaloblasts, the bone marrow often shows vacuolation of proerythroblasts and ringed sideroblasts. All these abnormalities are rapidly reversed on stopping alcohol consumption and presumably result from a direct effect of ethanol or its metabolites on erythropoietic cells. There is some evidence to support the hypothesis that the bone marrow damage is at least partly caused by acetaldehyde generated locally by the metabolism of ethanol by bone marrow macrophages.[67]

Myelodysplastic syndromes and erythroleukemia[58]

The megaloblastic erythropoiesis seen in these disorders is not primarily caused by vitamin B_{12} or folate deficiency

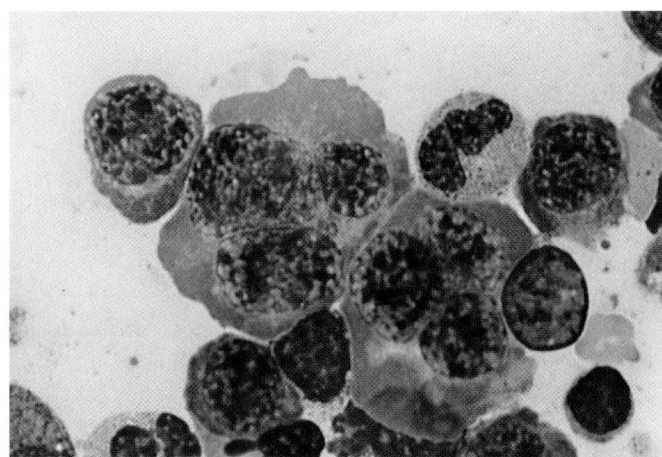

Fig. 12.11 Marrow smear from a child with thiamine-responsive anemia showing megaloblastic change and two multinucleate megaloblasts. May–Grünwald–Giemsa stain.

but may occasionally be complicated by folate deficiency as a result of an increased requirement for folate.

Thiamine-responsive anemia[68,69]

This rare autosomal recessive disorder is characterized by megaloblastic anemia (Fig. 12.11), mild thrombocytopenia and leukopenia, sensorineural deafness and diabetes mellitus; the megaloblastic anemia is refractory to vitamin B_{12}, folate or pyridoxine therapy. Some cases also have sideroblastic erythropoiesis. The anemia, but not the progressive deafness, responds to the oral administration of large doses (20–100 mg/day) of thiamine. In some cases, thiamine also improves the diabetes. Patients do not show any of the clinical features of the syndrome (beriberi) produced by dietary deficiency of thiamine and appear not to be deficient in this vitamin. The disease gene has been localized to chromosome 1q23.2–23.3 and the gene product may be a thiamine transporter.[69,70]

Macrocytosis with normoblastic erythropoiesis[3,58]

The conditions in which at least a proportion of the patients with macrocytosis have normoblastic erythropoiesis are listed in Table 12.3. Chronic alcohol abuse is a very common cause of macrocytosis (usually without anemia). The extent of alcohol consumption that induces macrocytosis varies considerably in different individuals; only about 35% of subjects who consume 100–800 g (mean 380 g) alcohol per day (equivalent to an average of a bottle of spirits per day) develop MCVs above the

Table 12.3 Causes of macrocytosis with normoblastic erythropoiesis

Normal neonates (physiologic)
Chronic alcoholism[a]
Chronic liver disease[a]
Hemolytic anemia[a]
Hypothyroidism
Therapy with anticonvulsant drugs[a]
Normal pregnancy
Chronic pulmonary disease (with hypoxia)
Heavy smoking
Myelodysplastic syndromes[a]
Hypoplastic and aplastic anemia

[a] Some cases show megaloblastic erythropoiesis.

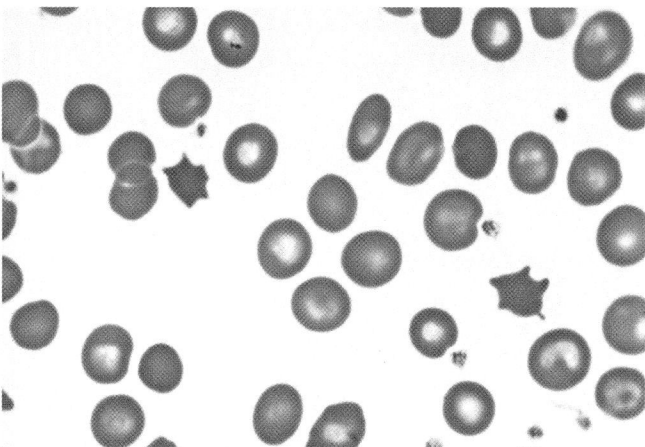

Fig. 12.12 Photomicrograph of a blood film of a 70-year-old man with severe hypothyroidism (Hb 9.1 g/dl; MCV 95 fl). Two acanthocytes are seen. May–Grünwald–Giemsa stain.

normal range.[71] Alcohol-induced macrocytosis is associated with normoblastic erythropoiesis in about 70% of the cases and in these the macrocytosis is independent of folate deficiency or an impairment of the 5,10-methylenetetrahydrofolate-dependent methylation of deoxyuridylate. Similarly, phenytoin-induced macrocytosis is occasionally associated with normoblastic erythropoiesis, usually with no evidence of impairment of the methylation of deoxyuridylate. The mechanism underlying the macrocytosis in both these conditions is uncertain but may be an impairment of cell proliferation by a direct effect of alcohol or the drug or their metabolites on erythroblasts. The macrocytosis seen in non-folate-deficient patients with hemolytic anemia results from various erythropoietin-induced alterations in the kinetics of erythropoiesis; the reticulocytes produced by patients with stimulated erythropoiesis are considerably larger than normal reticulocytes and mature into rounded macrocytes. About 25% of cases of hypothyroidism (without associated pernicious anemia) have macrocytic red cells and in these the macrocytosis seems to be a

manifestation of a deficiency of thyroid hormones. Patients with hypothyroidism may also have acanthocytes in their blood films (Fig. 12.12). Even those patients with hypothyroidism whose MCVs are within the normal range show some fall in the MCV when they become euthyroid.[72] In women who are not iron- or folate-deficient there is a slight but progressive increase in the MCV throughout pregnancy and occasionally the MCV may rise above the reference range for adults.[73] Another cause of macrocytosis with normoblastic erythropoiesis is chronic pulmonary disease.[74] Here, the macrocytosis is sometimes associated with true polycythemia secondary to a reduced PO_2 in arterial blood and has been attributed to a swelling of red cells.

REFERENCES

1. Wickramasinghe SN 1995 Morphology, biology and biochemistry of cobalamin- and folate-deficient bone marrow cells. Baillière's Clinical Haematology 8(3): 441–459
2. Wickramasinghe SN 1999 The wide spectrum and unresolved issues of megaloblastic anemia. Seminars in Hematology 36: 3–18
3. Chanarin I 1990 The megaloblastic anaemias, 3rd edn. Blackwell Scientific Publications, Oxford
4. Herbert V, Zalusky R 1962 Interrelation of vitamin B_{12} and folic acid metabolism: folic acid clearance studies. Journal of Clinical Investigation 41: 1263–1276
5. Noronha JM, Silverman M 1962 On folic acid, vitamin B_{12}, methionine and formiminoglutamic acid metabolism. In: Heinrich HC (ed), Vitamin B_{12} and intrinsic factor. Enke, Stuttgart, 728–736
6. Chanarin I, Deacon R, Lumb M, Perry J 1980 Vitamin B_{12} regulates folate metabolism by the supply of formate. Lancet ii: 505–507
7. Scott JM, Dinn JJ, Wilson P, Weir DG 1981 The pathogenesis of subacute combined degeneration: a result of methyl group deficiency. Lancet 2: 334–337
8. Weir DG, Scott JM 1995 The biochemical basis of the neuropathy in cobalamin deficiency. Baillière's Clinical Haematology 8(3): 479–497
9. Matthews JH, Wood JK 1984 Megaloblastic anaemia in vegetarian Asians. Clinical and Laboratory Haematology 6: 1–7
10. Campbell M, Lofters WS, Gibbs WN 1982 Rastafarianism and the vegans syndrome. British Medical Journal 285: 1617–1618
11. Monagle PT, Tauro GP 1997 Infantile megalobastosis secondary to maternal vitamin B_{12} deficiency. Clinical and Laboratory Haematology 19: 23–25
12. Carmel R 1996 Prevalence of undiagnosed pernicious anemia in the elderly. Archives of Internal Medicine 156: 1097–1100
13. Kokkola A, Sjoblom SM, Haapiainen R et al 1998 The risk of gastric carcinoma and carcinoid tumours in patients with pernicious anaemia. Scandinavian Journal of Gastroenterology 33: 88–92
14. Glesson PA, Toh BH 1991 Molecular targets in pernicious anaemia. Immunology Today 12: 233–238
15. Stabler SP, Allen RH, Savage DG, Lindenbaum J 1990 Clinical spectrum and diagnosis of cobalamin deficiency. Blood 76: 871–881
16. Healton EB, Savage DG, Brust JCM et al 1991 Neurologic aspects of cobalamin deficiency. Medicine 70: 229–245
17. Lindenbaum J, Healton EB, Savage DG et al 1988 Neropsychiatric disorders caused by cobalamin deficiency in the absence of anemia or macrocytosis. New England Journal of Medicine 318: 1720–1728
18. Savage DG, Lindenbaum J, Stabler SP, Allen RH 1994 Sensitivity of serum methylmalonic acid and total homocysteine determinations for diagnosing cobalamin and folate deficiencies. American Journal of Medicine 96: 239–246
19. Schilling RF 1953 A new test for intrinsic factor activity. Journal of Laboratory and Clinical Medicine 42: 946
20. Pant SH, Ashbury AK, Richardson EP 1968 The myelopathy of pernicious anaemia. A neuropathological reappraisal. Acta Neurologica Scandinavica 44 (suppl 35): 1–36

21. Deller DJ, Witts LJ 1962 Changes in the blood after partial gastrectomy with special reference to vitamin B$_{12}$. I. Serum vitamin B$_{12}$, haemoglobin, serum iron, and bone marrow. Quarterly Journal of Medicine 31: 71–88

22. Johnson HD, Hoffbrand AV 1970 The influence of extent of resection, type of anastamosis, and ulcer site on the haematological side effects of gastrectomy. British Journal of Surgery 57: 33–37

23. McIntyre OR, Sullivan LW, Jeffries GH, Silver RH 1965 Pernicious anemia in childhood. New England Journal of Medicine 272: 981–986

24. Rosenblatt DS, Whitehead VM 1999 Cobalamin and folate deficiency: acquired and hereditary disorders in children. Seminars in Hematology 36: 19–34

25. Katz M, Mehlman CS, Allen RH 1974 Isolation and characterization of an abnormal human intrinsic factor. Journal of Clinical Investigation 53: 1274–1283

26. Donaldson RM 1970 Small bowel bacterial overgrowth. Advances in Internal Medicine 16: 191–212

27. Brandt LJ, Bernstein LH, Wagle A 1977 Production of vitamin B$_{12}$ analogues in patients with small bowel bacterial overgrowth. Annals of Internal Medicine 87: 546–551

28. Thompson WG, Wrathell E 1977 The relation between ileal resection and vitamin B$_{12}$ absorption. Canadian Journal of Surgery 20: 461–464

29. Von Bondsdorff B 1977 Diphyllobothriasis in man. Academic Press, London.

30. Anonymous 1977 Anaemia and the fish tapeworm. Lancet i: 292

31. Saarni M, Palva I, Ahrenberg P 1977 Finns and the fish tapeworm. Lancet i: 806

32. Gräsbeck R 1972 Familial selective vitamin B$_{12}$ malabsorption. New England Journal of Medicine 287: 358

33. Altay C, Cetin M, Gumruk F et al 1995 Familal selective vitamin B$_{12}$ malabsorption (Imerslund–Gräsbeck syndrome) in a pool of Turkish patients. Pediatric Hematology and Oncology 12: 19–28

34. Eaton DM, Livingston JH, Seetharam B, Puntis JWL 1998 Overexpression of an unstable intrinsic factor–cobalamin receptor in Imerslund–Gräsbeck syndrome. Gastroenterology 115: 173–176

35. Carmel R, Sinow RM, Karnaze DS 1987 Atypical cobalamin deficiency. Subtle biochemical evidence of deficiency is commonly demonstrable in patients without megaloblastic anemia and is often associated with protein-bound cobalamin malabsorption. Journal of Laboratory and Clinical Medicine 109: 454–463

36. Carmel R, Sinow RM, Siegel ME, Samloff IM 1988 Food cobalamin malabsorption occurs frequently in patients with unexplained low serum cobalamin levels. Archives of Internal Medicine 148: 1715–1719

37. Carmel R 1995 Malabsorption of food cobalamin. Baillière's Clinical Haematology 8(3): 639–655

38. Remacha A, Cadafalch J 1999 Cobalamin deficiency in patients infected with the human immunodeficiency virus. Seminars in Hematology 36: 75–87

39. Chanarin I 1980 Cobalamins and nitrous oxide: a review. Journal of Clinical Pathology 33: 909–916

40. Chanarin I 1982 The effects of nitrous oxide on cobalamins, folates and on related events. In: Golberg L (ed), CRC critical reviews on toxicology, vol 10. CRC Press, Florida, 179–213

41. Lassen HCA, Henriksen E, Neukirch F, Kristensen HS 1956 Treatment of tetanus. Severe bone marrow depression after prolonged nitrous oxide anaesthesia. Lancet i: 527–530

42. Amess JAL, Burman JF, Rees GM et al 1978 Megaloblastic haemopoiesis in patients receiving nitrous oxide. Lancet ii: 339–342

43. Nunn JF, Sharer NM, Gorchein A et al 1982 Megaloblastic haemopoiesis after multiple short-term exposure to nitrous oxide. Lancet i: 1379–1381

44. Layzer RB 1978 Myeloneuropathy after prolonged exposure to nitrous oxide. Lancet ii: 1227–1230

45. Burman JF, Mollin DL, Sourial NA, Sladden RA 1979 Inherited lack of transcobalamin II in serum and megaloblastic anaemia: a further patient. British Journal of Haematology 43: 27–38

46. Hall CA 1992 The neurologic aspects of transcobalamin II deficiency. British Journal of Haematology 80: 117–120

47. Kaikov Y, Wadsworth, LD, Hall CA, Rogers PC 1991 Transcobalamin II deficiency: case report and review of the literature. European Journal of Pediatrics 150: 841–843

48. Haurani FI, Hall CA, Rubin R 1979 Megaloblastic anemia as a result of an abnormal transcobalamin II (Cardoza). Journal of Clinical Investigation 64: 1253–1259

49. Seligman PA, Steiner LL, Allen RH 1980 Studies of a patient with megaloblastic anemia and an abnormal transcobalamin II. New England Journal of Medicine 303: 1209–1212

50. Linnell JC, Bhatt HR 1995 Inherited errors of cobalamin metabolism and their management. Baillière's Clinical Haematology 8(3): 567–601

51. Blount BC, Mack MM, Wehr CM et al 1997 Folate deficiency causes uracil misincorporation into human DNA and chromosome breakage: implications for cancer and neuronal damage. Proceedings of the National Academy of Sciences USA 94: 3290–3295

52. MRC Vitamin Study Research Group 1991 Prevention of neural tube defects: results of the Medical Research Council vitamin study. Lancet ii: 131–137

53. Department of Health, Scottish Office Home and Health Department, Welsh Office, Department of Health and Social Services Northern Ireland 1992 Folic acid and the prevention of neural tube defects: report from an expert advisory group. Department of Health, London

54. Christensen B, Rosenblatt DS 1995 Effects of folate deficiency on embryonic development. Baillière's Clinical Haematology 8(3): 617–637

55. Chanarin I, Rothman D, Ward A, Perry J 1968 Folate status and requirement in pregnancy. British Medical Journal 2: 390–394

56. Giles C 1966 An account of 335 cases of megaloblastic anaemia of pregnancy and the puerperium. Journal of Clinical Pathology 19: 1–11

57. Scott JM, Weir, DG 1980 Drug-induced megaloblastic change. Clinics in Haematology 9: 587–606

58. Wickramasinghe SN 1981 The deoxyuridine suppression test: a review of its clinical and research applications. Clinical and Laboratory Haematology 3: 1–18

59. Reynolds EH, Laundy M 1978 Haematological effects of anticonvulsant treatment. Lancet ii: 682

60. Wu A, Chanarin I, Levy AJ 1974 Macrocytosis of chronic alcoholism. Lancet i: 829–831

61. Unger KW, Johnson D, Jr 1974 Red blood cell mean corpuscular volume: a potential indicator of alcohol usage in a working population. American Journal of the Medical Sciences 267: 281–289

62. Wickramasinghe SN, Corridan B, Hasan R, Marjot DH 1994 Correlations between acetaldehyde-modified haemoglobin, carbohydrate-deficient transferrin (CDT) and haematological abnormalities in chronic alcoholism. Alcohol and Alcoholism 29: 415–423

63. Zittoun J 1995 Congenital errors of folate metabolism. Baillière's Clinical Haematology 8(3): 603–616

64. Smith LH Jr 1973 Pyrimidine metabolism in man. New England Journal of Medicine 288: 764–771

65. Rajantie J 1981 Orotic aciduria in lysinuric protein intolerance: dependence on the urea cycle intermediates. Pediatric Research 15: 115–119

66. Van der Zee SPM, Lommen EJP, Trijbels JMF, Shretlen EDAM 1970 The influence of adenine on the clinical features and purine metabolism in the Lesch–Nyhan syndrome. Acta Paediatrica Scandinavica 59: 259–264

67. Wickramasinghe SN, Hasan R 1993 Possible role of macrophages in the pathogenesis of ethanol-induced bone marrow damage. British Journal of Haematology 83: 574–579

68. Haworth C, Evans DIK, Mitra J, Wickramasinghe SN 1982 Thiamine responsive anaemia: a study of two further cases. British Journal of Haematology 50: 549–561

69. Fleming JC, Tartaglini E, Steinkamp MP et al 1999 The gene mutated in thiamine-responsive anaemia with diabetes and deafness (TRMA) encodes a functional thiamine transporter. Nature Genetics 22: 305–308

70. Diaz GA, Banikazemi M, Oishi K et al 1999 Mutations in a new gene encoding a thiamine transporter cause thiamine-responsive megaloblastic anaemia syndrome. Nature Genetics 22: 309–312

71. Wickramasinghe SN, Corridan B, Hasan R, Marjot DH 1994 Correlations between acetaldehyde-modified haemoglobin, carbohydrate-deficient transferrin (CDT) and haematological abnormalities in chronic alcoholism. Alcohol and Alcoholism 29: 415–423

72. Horton L, Coburn RJ, England JM, Himsworth RL 1976 The haematology of hypothyroidism. Quarterly Journal of Medicine 45: 101–123

73. Chanarin I, McFadyen IR, Kyle R 1974 The physiological macrocytosis of pregnancy. British Journal of Obstetrics and Gynaecology 84: 504–508

74. Freedman BJ, Pennington DG 1963 Erythrocytosis in emphysema. British Journal of Haematology 9: 425–430

Recommended Reading

Bhatt HR, James VHT, Besser GM et al 1994 Advances in Thomas Addison's diseases, Vols 1 and 2. Journal of Endocrinology, Bristol

Wickramasinghe SN (ed) 1995 Megaloblastic anaemia. Bailliere's clinical haematology, Vol 8/No 3. Baillière Tindall, London

Carmel R (ed) 1999 Beyond megaloblastic anemia: new paradigms of cobalamin and folate deficiency. Seminars in hematology, Vol 36/No 1. WB Saunders, Philadelphia

Aplastic anemia: acquired and inherited

13

EC Gordon-Smith

Acquired aplastic anemia

Definition and differential diagnosis

Etiology
Drugs
Industrial domestic chemicals
Viruses

Criteria for severity

Pathophysiology
The stem cell in aplastic anemia
The microenvironment in aplastic anemia
The immune process in pathogenesis

Hematology

Clinical presentation

Clinical course

Clonal evolution in aplastic anemia

Treatment
Immunosuppressive treatment
Growth factors in aplastic anemia
Stem cell transplantation
Volunteer unrelated and mismatched transplants

Conclusion

Inherited aplastic anemias

Fanconi anemia
Cytogenetic findings
Genetic basis of Fanconi anemia
Hematologic features
Clinical course
Treatment
Conclusion

Acquired aplastic anemia

Acquired aplastic anemia is an uncommon disorder which in Europe and the United States affects about 2 per million of the population per annum, with a higher incidence in other parts of the world, including Southeast Asia, where the incidence may be 2–3 times higher.[1] The difference in incidence seems to be environmental rather than ethnic since people from those areas who settle in the United States have a similar incidence to Caucasians. Any age may be affected but there are two peaks, one occurring in adolescents and young adults, a second rise occurring after the age of 60 years, this bimodal distribution being most marked in white males.[2-4] Overall the male:female ratio of cases is about equal but there may be a preponderance of males in the younger or adolescent age group.[4]

Definition and differential diagnosis

Acquired aplastic anemia is defined by peripheral blood pancytopenia with a hypocellular bone marrow in which normal hemopoiesis is replaced to a greater or lesser extent by fat cells in the absence of genetic, malignant or predictable myelosuppressive causes. Remaining hemopoietic precursors and circulating blood cells are morphologically normal or show only minor abnormalities. The exclusions in the definition emphasize that other diseases may produce a similar morphologic picture to acquired aplastic anemia and these need to be ruled out in coming to a diagnosis (Table 13.1). One of the difficulties in early studies of aplastic anemia was the lack of rigor in defining cases. Undoubtedly in earlier

reports of a high incidence of aplastic anemia (AA), particularly in elderly patients, cases of myelodysplastic anemia, sometimes with a cellular marrow, were included and the incidence of the disease over-estimated.[5,6]

In addition to the conditions listed in Table 13.1, hairy cell leukemia (HCL) may be misdiagnosed as AA. The bone marrow aspirate in HCL is often aparticulate and dilute, hairy cells may be scanty and the marrow trephine appears to show hypocellularity, but the reticulin is increased and the hemopoietic tissue is not replaced by fat cells but by the abundant cytoplasm of hairy cells. Immunophenotyping will detect the HCL.

Etiology

In about one-quarter to one-third of the patients with acquired AA, suspicion may be directed to a particular agent, usually a drug or virus as the precipitating cause. Thus, in the great majority of patients no etiological agent can be identified.

Drugs

The list of drugs which have been recorded as precipitating AA is long,[7-10] but mostly only single or a few cases have been reported for each drug and the evidence against many of the drugs is slim. Some of the more commonly implicated drugs are listed in Table 13.2. A difficulty in determining the role of drug exposure to the development of AA is the delay between exposure to the drug and the identification of marrow damage. Typically there is a delay of 2–3 months between first exposure and the onset of pancytopenia. This delay may be longer though an exposure which took place for a short period

Table 13.1 Differential diagnosis of acquired aplastic anemia

Pathophysiology	Examples	Differential features
Inherited AA	FA	Chromosome fragility Dysmorphism Family history
	Dyskeratosis congenita	Nail/skin changes Leukoplakia X-linked, family history
Malignant AA	Hypoplastic MDS	Blood cell morphology Cytogenetics
	Acute leukemia (presenting as AA)	Spontaneous remission followed by leukemic relapse
Toxic AA	Irradiation Chemotherapy	History of exposure
Antibody-mediated	Autoimmune pancytopenia	Multiple autoantibodies

AA, aplastic anemia; FA, Fanconi anemia; MDS, myelodysplastic syndrome.

Table 13.2 Drugs which are strongly associated with an increased risk of aplastic anemia

Drug	Examples	Selected references

Antibiotics	Chloramphenicol
	Sulfonamides
	  Sulfasalazine
	  Co-trimoxazole
		See text
		18

Anti-inflammatory agents	Phenylbutazone Oxyphenbutazone Indomethacin Sulindac Diclofenac Piroxicam Penicillamine Gold salts Mesalazine	10,19,20 10,20
Thyrostatic	Carbimazole Thiouracils Potassium perchlorate	

Anticonvulsant	Hydantoins
	  Phenytoin
	  Mephenytoin
	Carbamazepine
	Ethosuximide
		10

Psychotropic	Phenothiazines	10
Antimalarial	Quinacrine (Mepacrine) Maloprim	
Antidiabetic	Chlorpropamide Carbutamide Tolbutamide	10

Note: Many of these drugs have also been associated with a variety of other blood dyscrasias, particularly neutropenia or agranulocytosis.

6 months to 1 year before weakens the association and exposure which ended more than 1 year earlier makes the association unlikely.

Chloramphenicol

Chloramphenicol was introduced into clinical practice in 1949 and it was predicted that it would cause blood dyscrasias on the basis of its structural relationship to amidopyrine.[11] The first case of AA was reported in 1950.[12] It has been estimated that somewhere between 1:25 000 and 1:60 000 people exposed to oral chloramphenicol develop AA.[13,14] The evidence is purely epidemiologic, there being no tests to demonstrate that chloramphenicol is responsible for AA in any particular case. The difficulty of the epidemiologic approach to these rare events is illustrated by the debate over the possible association of chloramphenicol ophthalmic preparations with AA.[15] Case analysis suggests that there is no greater incidence with these preparations than the background.[16] Chloramphenicol also causes a dose-dependent suppression of hemopoiesis,

particularly affecting erythropoiesis, through its action on mitochondrial DNA. There is reticulocytopenia with vacuolation of erythroid and granulocytic progenitor cells.[17] This suppression is not related to the development of prolonged AA. Other anti-infective agents, particularly sulfonomides have been implicated in AA.[18]

Non-steroidal anti-inflammatory drugs

Non-steroidal anti-inflammatory drugs (NSAIDs) have been incriminated in AA. Phenylbutazone and oxyphenbutazone have the highest incidence of aplasia in this group.[19] The indole derivatives indomethacin and sulindac have both been reported in association with AA.[20] It seems possible that the development of AA in response to NSAIDs is, at least in some respects, a class effect in that there have been cases of relapse of AA which followed exposure to one NSAID when the patient was subsequently given another, chemically unrelated NSAID.[21]

Gold salts

Gold salts have a high incidence of hematologic adverse reactions. Neutropenia and eosinophilia are common.[22,23] Persistence with gold injections in the face of a falling neutrophil count may lead to aplasia or aplasia may appear without warning. Gold salts are one of the few drugs for which careful monitoring of blood counts may prevent the development of aplasia.

Anti-thyroid drugs

Anti-thyroid drugs, methimazole, propylthiourcil and carbimazole, have a significantly increased risk of AA as well as agranulocytosis. The agranulocytosis appears to have drug-dependent immune pathogenesis[24] but the pathogenesis of the rarer aplasia is unknown.

Industrial domestic chemicals

Benzene is a myelotoxin. Exposure to sufficient levels leads inevitably to marrow damage but there seems to be wide variation in the dose required between individuals and it is doubtful whether it produces aplasia of the idiosyncratic variety although cases have been described.[10] Nevertheless, the perception that benzene solvents might cause AA led to the production of Stoddard's solvent, an aliphatic organic solvent. Unfortunately this too has been associated with aplasia.[25] Insecticides,[26] DDT,[27] lindane (γ-hexachlorocyclohexane)[28,29] pentachlorophenols[30] and aniline hair dyes[31] have each been linked to the development of idiosyncratic AA though epidemiologic evidence is often weak.[10] Considering the very widespread use of DDT and the paucity of reported cases it seems that this compound has little or no haematologic toxicity and that reports may well be confounded by the solvents, including benzene, in the preparation of DDT for spraying.

Viruses

Hepatitis

Hepatitis, presumably of viral origin, is a precursor of AA in about 5–10% of cases in the West, perhaps double this in the Far East.[32] In the majority of cases no specific hepatitis virus can be identified and the association is based on clinical grounds and the presence of abnormal liver function tests. The delay between the clinical hepatitis and the onset of pancytopenia is of the order of 6–12 weeks, a similar period to that between drug exposure and aplasia. There is some suggestion that chloramphenicol administration followed by hepatitis is particularly likely to be associated with AA.[33] Further evidence to support the association is the finding that in one series over a quarter of patients who underwent orthotopic liver transplant for fulminant liver failure following viral hepatitis developed AA whereas patients transplanted for other reasons had no marrow failure.[34] The prognosis in these patients has been poor, though this relates to the severity of the marrow depression and not the supposed viral agent. The patients respond equally well to immunosuppressive therapy or stem cell transplantation[35] as others with the same degree of marrow failure.

Parvovirus

Parvovirus B19 infection in non-immune individuals may lead to a transient pure red cell aplasia of clinical importance to people with hemolytic anemia (see Chapter 14). The virus specifically infects the erythroid burst-forming units (BFU-E) and does not normally produce true AA.

Epstein–Barr virus (EBV)

EBV infection is commonly accompanied by neutropenia or thrombocytopenia probably of an immune origin. Rarely, there may be true marrow aplasia which behaves like other cases of acquired disease,[36] though within this group there are some patients who develop pancytopenia with marrow aplasia in whom there is spontaneous recovery in 4–6 weeks.

Criteria for severity

A classification of the severity of the marrow damage in AA was devised in the 1970s to allow the comparison of the effectiveness of different treatment in this disease without a gross imbalance in the severity of the different groups.[37] The original classification was based on observations of survival curves of collective series of drug-induced AA which showed that there appeared to be two populations, one with a median survival of a few months and a 1-year survival of < 10%, another which had a more prolonged survival, even though the patients remained with a degree of pancytopenia.[7] Studies of these patients' peripheral blood and bone marrow allowed prognostic features to be devised which identified the severe aplastic anemia (SAA) and the non-severe aplastic anemia (NSAA). It is clear that the degree of marrow damage is not a double population but a spectrum and improving support and treatments has led to modification of the classification into three groups, very severe aplastic anaemia (VSAA) having been added[38] (Table 13.3). The classification includes an assessment of the degree of hypocellularity of the marrow based on the trephine biopsy findings. This is the most subjective of the measurements, particularly as the cellularity may vary quite considerably in different samples and indeed in the same sample, the so called 'hot pockets'.[39]

Pathophysiology

Normal hemopoiesis takes place in the specialized environment of the bone marrow with pleuripotent hemopoietic stem cells giving rise to a variety of committed progenitors which produce the mature cells for the circulation. The production is controlled by many factors, stimulatory, inhibitory and differentiating, some within the stroma in which hemopoiesis takes place, others derived from the circulation.[40] In normal hemopoiesis there is a balance between the rate of cell production and cell loss, both through maturation and escape into the circulation and through apoptosis of progenitor cells which provide redundant capacity. The process is controlled in part through the action of cytokines such as granulocyte-colony stimulating factor (G-CSF), erythropoietin (Epo), thrombopoietin (Tpo), stem cell factor (SCF) and many others, and inhibitors such as tissue growth factor-β (TGF-β). It has been considered that AA might be the result of damage of the hemopoietic stem cells directly, to the microenvironment in which they proliferate or to a failure of the control factors or to combinations of these aberrations.

Table 13.3 Gradation of severity of acquired aplastic anemia

Grade of severity	Definition	
	Peripheral blood	**Bone marrow**[a]
VSAA	Neutrophils < 0.2 × 10^9/l Platelets < 20 × 10^9/l Reticulocytes < 20 × 10^9/l Transfusion dependent	< 25% normal cellularity Moderately hypocellular < 30% Remaining cells hemopoietic
SAA	Neutrophils < 0.5 > 0.2 × 10^9/l Otherwise as for VSAA	As for VSAA
NSAA	Neutrophils < 1.5 > 0.5 × 10^9/l Platelets < 100 > 20 × 10^9/l Reticulocytes < 60 > 20 × 10^9/l	Hypocellular

[a] The bone marrow in aplastic anemia is often patchy in cellularity and the assessment of cellularity, even with a good trephine, may be difficult.
NSAA, non-severe aplastic anemia; SAA, severe aplastic anemia, VSAA, very severe aplastic anemia.

The stem cell in aplastic anemia

There are qualitative and quantitative abnormalities of hemopoietic stem cells in AA.[41] Short-term colony assays of committed progenitor cells – colony-forming units (CFU-C, CFU-E), burst-forming units (BFU-E) – are markedly reduced in AA and remain low even after recovery.[41–43] Committed progenitors, identified by long-term culture initiating cells (LTCIC) are also reduced and have a poorer proliferative potential than normal stem cells, with poorer survival of colony-forming cells in long-term bone marrow culture.[41–47]

The microenvironment in aplastic anemia

Long-term cultures depend upon a viable and confluent stroma for proper growth. Cross-over experiments have shown that stroma grown from AA marrow can support colony-forming cells from normal marrow but that colony forming cells (CD34$^+$) from aplastic marrow will not grow on normal nor aplastic marrow suggesting that the stroma is not at fault in the pathogenesis of AA.[41,47] However, it should be remembered that it is not always possible to grow stroma from AA and there may be a degree of heterogeneity in the pathophysiology.

There might also be a deficiency of growth factors or growth factor binding in the failure of hemopoiesis but measurement has failed to find any evidence for this. Epo,[48–50] (Tpo)[51,52] and G-CSF levels are increased in AA[53] though the concentration of circulating G-CSF is low in both normals and patients with AA. SCF level in soluble form in the plasma appears to be in the normal range[54] though others have found reduced levels of circulating SCF.[55,56] These observations might explain why Epo is

ineffective in the treatment of AA whereas G-CSF may have a part to play in direct stimulation of bone marrow stem cells.[43,57] The marrow stroma consists of four main cell types: fibroblasts, endothelial cells, adipocytes and macrophages. Further evidence that the stroma is not primarily involved in the pathogenesis of AA is the observation that following a successful stem cell transplant the stroma, with the exception of macrophages, remains of host origin and is able to support the new hemopoiesis adequately.

The immune process in pathogenesis

Since the introduction of immunosuppressive treatment for AA, particularly of antilymphocyte globulin (ALG),[58,59] the prognosis of AA has been greatly improved. ALG was originally prepared using human peripheral blood lymphocytes. Refinement occurred with the use of thoracic duct lymphocytes as immunogen and more recently with lymphocytes from excised thymus or cell lines derived from T-lymphocytes. These preparations are usually designated antithymocyte globulin (ATG). In this chapter 'ALG' is used to encompass all preparations including ATG. It should be emphasized that ALG/ATG preparations are biological products which contain a variety of antibodies directed against many T-cell antigens (and some non T-cell) and that different commercial preparations are by no means bioequivalent.[60,61] It has been generally assumed that immune processes play a role at least in maintaining the aplasia[62] even if the initial damage, perhaps brought about by exposure to drug or virus, may not be immune mediated. It is also evident that antibody-mediated inhibition of the hemopoiesis, whilst it may occur, is very rare and is not the pathway by which immune suppression of hemopoiesis usually occurs. It was recognized early on that certain -cell subsets could inhibit hemopoiesis in normal marrow[63,64] and that, at least in some aplastic patients, removal of T-cells from aspirated marrow would enhance the *in vitro* colony-forming activity.[63] Activated T-cells (Thy-1) will produce inhibitors of hemopoiesis including interferon-γ (IFN-γ) and IFN-γ may be elevated in the blood and bone marrow of patients with AA.[65] IFN-γ is produced normally in response to virus infections and certainly some virus infections will inhibit hemopoiesis, but the precise role, if any, of the activated T-lymphocytes and production of IFN-γ in the pathogenesis of idosyncratic AA is not yet known. The subject has been reviewed by Nakao.[66] The strongest evidence remains the response to immunosuppressive therapy.

Hematology

The peripheral blood film shows pancytopenia without gross morphologic abnormalities in the remaining cells. There may be some macrocytosis of remaining red cells usually with an absolute reticulocytopenia. A relative reticulocytosis should always raise the possibility of

associated paroxysmal nocturnal hemoglobinuria (PNH). Granulocytes often show increased staining of granules, the so-called toxic granulation of neutropenia. The neutrophil alkaline phosphatase score is increased (it falls if PNH develops). Monocytes may be reduced in proportion to the granulocytes. Platelets are reduced and of small and uniform size. There is usually a variable reduction in the lymphocyte count, but sometimes the count is normal or even increased so that the total white cell count may be normal. A reduction in the CD4:CD8 ratio of T-cells may occur[67-69] but this is by no means universal and seems to be non-specifically related to infections or multiple transfusions. Abnormal cells are not seen. The bone marrow aspirate is normally easily obtained, typically with many fragments which have a lacy, empty appearance (Fig. 13.1A). The cell trails are hypocellular with a relative increase in lymphocytes and plasma cells and other non-hemopoietic forms. There may be a minor degree of dyserythropoiesis but in general remaining hemopoietic precursors are normal in appearance. Lymphocytes and plasma cells may appear to be increased but this is because of the lack of hemopoietic cells and there is no consistent increase in

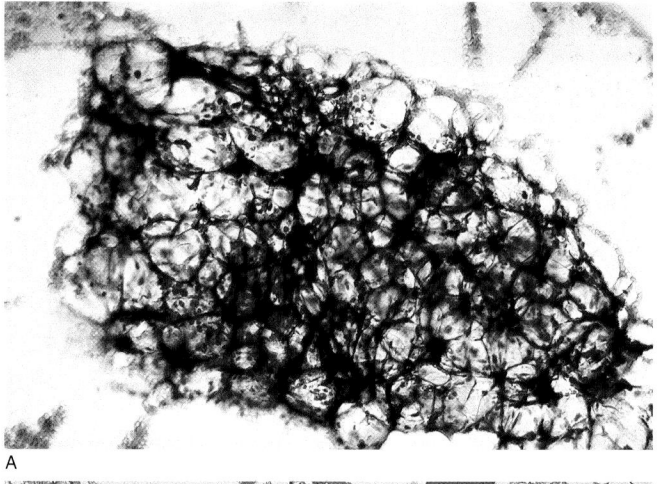

A

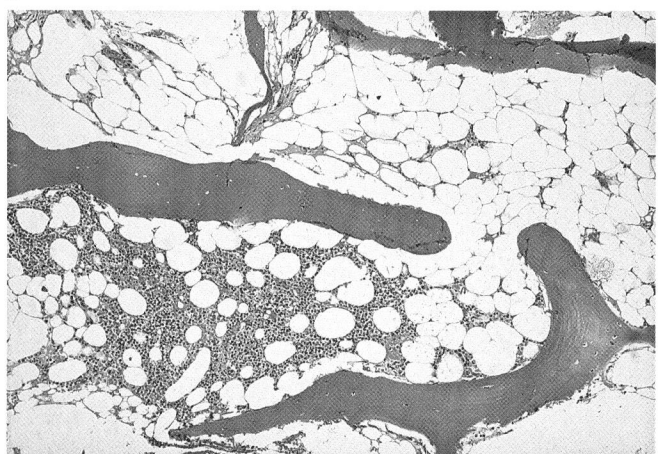

C

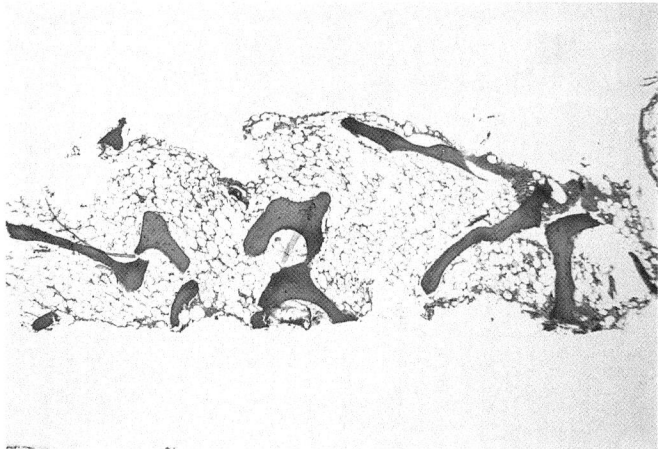

B

Fig. 13.1 (A) Fragment from a bone marrow aspirate of a patient with severe aplastic anemia showing typical 'lacy' appearance of the fragment which contains a little or no hemopoietic cells. (B) Trephine biopsy from a patient with severe aplastic anemia showing the disappearance of hemopoietic cells between the trabeculae and displacement by fat cells. (C) Trephine biopsy from a patient with severe aplastic anemia showing a residual island of apparently normal hemopoiesis in an otherwise fatty marrow.

lymphocytes or in any subset in the marrow taken from patients with AA. In the early stages of AA, macrophages appear active with increased intracellular iron and erythrophagocytsis may be prominent. In a proportion of cases the hypocellularity of the marrow is patchy with areas of cellular marrow remaining. The bone marrow aspirate under these circumstances may be misleadingly cellular. A trephine biopsy (sometimes more than one) is necessary to assess cellularity properly.

The trephine shows the fat replacement of marrow with or without the remaining islands of cellularity (Fig. 13.1B,C). The presence or absence of cellular 'hot pockets'[39] does not correlate with the severity of the peripheral blood pancytopenia and the apparent cellularity of a trephine specimen may not be reflected in the blood count. Non-hematopoietic cells remain, sometimes giving the impression of a chronic inflammatory infiltrate. Reticulin fibers are scanty, commensurate with the degree of hypocellularity. The most common misdiagnosis of AA is to make it on the basis of a blood tap for an aspirate in the presence of pancytopenia without obtaining adequate trephine specimens.

Special tests may be of interest but little use in the diagnosis and prognosis of AA. Ferrokinetic studies using ^{59}Fe usually shows a prolonged iron clearance. Iron utilization is always decreased and the failure of utilization reflects the severity of the aplasia. ^{52}Fe studies confirm the poor iron clearance, most of the iron being taken up by the liver, and the ^{52}Fe scan may demonstrate well the patchy nature of the marrow failure, with islands of active erythropoiesis being seen in an otherwise non-erythropoietic marrow.

Cytogenetic studies on bone marrow are required at presentation of patients with AA, mainly to exclude hypoplastic myelodysplastic syndrome (MDS). Typically, chromosome configuration and number are normal in AA but it is now clear that in a number of cases there may be evidence for a clone of cytogenetically abnormal cells to be present at presentation which may be stable or transient but does not seem to affect response to treatment.[70]

Clinical presentation

The clinical features derive from the decrease in peripheral blood cells and are non-specific. The patient may be feeling completely well at the time when easy bruising or petechiae appear or may have a more of less prolonged period of feeling tired from anemia. Sometimes infection is the presenting feature but this seems to be less common in idiosyncratic AA than bleeding manifestations. The spleen, liver and lymph nodes are not enlarged and jaundice is only a feature in those patients with post-

hepatitic aplasia who have a prolonged cholestatic phase after the infection.

At presentation it is necessary to take a detailed drug, occupational and symptomatic history to try to establish an etiologic agent so that this may be avoided in the future. Unfortunately, even if such an occupational or other exposure is suspected there is no way of proving the suspicion.

Clinical course

The clinical course is modified by the transfusion support and antibiotic therapy which the patient receives. There are some events which may interrupt the clinical course apart from the catastrophies associated with the low platelet count and neutropenia. The proliferative capacity of the marrow is greatly reduced but the marrow also appears to be unstable in that abnormal clones of cells, PNH, myelodysplastic or leukemic, may appear during the disease, sometimes all three in the same individual. In patients who have a remission or partial response about 25–40% will develop a clonal disorder or relapse within 5–10 years, though this is not necessarily associated with a poor prognosis.[71,72] The degree of aplasia may vary and the course of the disease is not always predictable.

Some, perhaps most, patients present with a degree of pancytopenia which stabilizes over a long period of time (months or years). In general, the greater the degree of pancytopenia the worse the prognosis as indicated in the grading of severity in Table 13.1. Patients with lesser degrees of pancytopenia, particularly those with a relative preservation of granulocytes, have a better prognosis, but clearly this is not a stepwise progression but a continuous spectrum.

A minority of patients present with minor degrees of pancytopenia or deficiency in only one cell line, but over the succeeding months or years the aplasia gradually becomes more profound. This is most usually observed in patients who present with amegakaryocytic thrombocytopenia which progresses over a period of years to true AA.

Clonal evolution in aplastic anemia

The pathophysiology of AA needs to take into account the observation of the frequent emergence of abnormal clones of cells in the aplastic hemopoiesis.[71,72] The most common event is for PNH clones to emerge, sometimes more than one clone in a single individual.[73,74] The frequency and diversity of the somatic mutations which lead to PNH suggest that such clones occur in normal marrow but are not expressed because normal hemopoiesis swamps the progeny of the clone. When the marrow is damaged in AA the PNH clone may have a growth advantage and may come to dominate hemopoiesis or at least provide a substantial part of it. There is evidence that PNH clones do arise in normal marrow which supports the above hypothesis.[75] Since the PNH phenotype lacks a range of surface proteins normally attached by the phosphatidyl inositol glycan (PIG) anchor, it is tempting to surmise that the target for immune attack lies within these proteins and that absence of the proteins in the PNH clone allows the PNH precursor cell to escape the immune destruction. The same may be true of other cytogenetic abnormalities which are common in MDS or acute leukemia. Whilst progression to MDS, or less commonly acute myeloid leukemia (AML), may occur, hemopoiesis in some AA patients produces clones with abnormal cytogenetics which are commonly seen in MDS, but in the aplastic setting may be transient or stable without progressing to a more malignant phase.[70]

Treatment

The choice of treatment for AA depends upon a number of factors, the age of the patient, the severity of the bone marrow damage, the availability of suitable donor and the general health of the patient. Whichever mode of treatment is eventually advanced the most important aspect is to be able to provide comprehensive support for the patient with blood products and infection control. The two main treatment modalities are immunosuppression and stem cell transplantation, each of which has its own advantages and disadvantages.

Immunosuppressive treatment

The suggestion that antilymphocyte globulin could be used to treat AA first came in 1970 from George Mathé and colleagues in Paris[58] though formal clinical trials did not take place until 1977.[59] In that European trial half the patients with SAA achieved remission whereas previous experience had suggested an approximate 10% 1-year survival. Subsequent control trials confirmed the effectiveness of this form of treatment.[76,77] Approximately two out of three of the patients achieved remission defined as freedom from transfusion, following a first course of treatment with ALG.

A variety of treatment schedules have been tried for ALG but there has been no clear advantage shown for any over the 5-day course usually given which was originally determined by the amount of ALG available for trials.

The actual dosage used may vary from one preparation to another depending upon the biological standardization of that product and producers will usually indicate the recommended dose in terms of mg/kg or vials/10 kg for their particular produce. ALG is given through a central venous line to avoid problems with phlebitis over 16 h daily for 5 days. Fever, rigors and general lethargy are common in the first 2 days of treatment, the subsequent days usually remaining trouble-free. Some 7–10 days post-infusion serum sickness, with rash, joint pain and fever, may occur, modified by giving corticosteroids 1 mg/kg/day increasing if necessary if serum sickness occurs. Problems with fluid balance, liver-function abnormalities and occasional more prolonged joint pains may occur. The use of ALG on its own produces a response in up to 65% of patients by about 6 months[78] though relapse may be as high as 40% over the subsequent 10 years.[71,72] By relapse is meant a return to transfusion dependence and may be brought about by a true reversion to aplasia, the emergence of a PNH clone or the development of myelodysplasia. As support improved, so the survival rates improved, for those who did not show a response to the first course of ALG. Subsequent courses also produce remission as defined by freedom from transfusion and some patients have received multiple courses. The main causes of failure of support measures are refractoriness to platelet transfusions and antibiotic-resistant infections, especially fungal.

ALG therapy requires hospital admission, ideally in an isolation facility, for up to 3 weeks, so attempts have been made to find alternative forms of immunosuppression. Early attempts with monoclonal antibodies proved unsatisfactory. Cyclosporin used alone is effective in some patients[79] but a smaller proportion responded first time, perhaps 50%, the combination of ALG and cyclosporin being more effective in NSAA than cyclosporin alone.[80] When given together with ALG the addition of cyclosporin seems to improve the remission rate, particularly in SAA and perhaps shortens the time for remission.[80,81] When used in combination the schedule is to start cyclosporin after the ALG at 5 mg/kg/day in divided doses, adjusting the dose to achieve steady state whole blood values around 100–200 mg/1. Cyclosporin is continued for a minimum of 6 months. If there is a response the drug is continued until a plateau is obtained and then cautiously reduced. A proportion of patients' responses are cyclosporin dependent.

Growth factors in aplastic anemia

The effect of G-CSF on neutrophil production in AA has been extensively investigated. Five to ten mg/kg daily by subcutaneous injection raises the neutrophil count in most patients except those with VSAA,[82] but the effect lasts only as long as G-CSF is given. A pilot study of ALG, cyclosporin and G-CSF in Europe has given encouraging results[38] so that a randomized trial is in progress. A study of G-CSF given to children with AA in Japan also suggested a beneficial effect on outcome, though these were concerns about the induction of AA,[83] so far not confirmed.

Cyclophosphamide

Interest was raised in the use of high-dose cyclophosphamide as immunosuppression for patients who failed to respond to ALG.[84] Responses were seen in seven out of 10 patients and there was no evidence of clonal evolution in a 10-year follow-up. The time to response and the period of severe pancytopenia were prolonged. However, a randomized controlled trial of cyclophosphamide compared with ALG showed that the toxicity of the cyclophosphamide far outweighed the potential benefit[85] and its use without stem cell transplant is not recommended.

Anabolic steroids

Anabolic steroids[86] were the only form of bone marrow stimulation before the introduction of immunosuppression and cytokines. Responses are undoubtedly achieved in NSAA though control trials have failed to demonstrate a benefit in SAA. Nevertheless, anabolic steroids do have a place in the management of AA, though side-effects, virilization and hepatotoxicity make them difficult to manage.

In summary, immunosuppression with ALG and cyclosporin is the first treatment option for patients with all degrees of severity of AA who do not have an HLA-matched sibling donor, for patients with NSAA irrespective of donor availability, for patients over 30 years with a donor who have SAA or NSAA (but not VSAA) and for patients with systemic disease which makes stem cell transplantation high risk. The response should be assessed at 4 months. If there is no response or partial response, a second course of ALG, either with ALG sourced from another animal or even the same source,[87] should be given to patients without a sibling donor. For those with a donor, a decision may have to be made to proceed with a stem cell transplantation.

Stem cell transplantation

Transplant for AA using bone marrow from HLA-matched sibling donors was introduced by E. Donnell

Thomas and colleagues in 1969.[88] An early trial demonstrated superiority of this treatment over support and anabolic steroids,[89] the only non-transplant treatment then available. Subsequent experience worldwide recorded by the European Bone Marrow Transplant (EBMT) Group and the International Bone Marrow Transplant Registry (IBMTR), as well as the continuing reports from Seattle, indicated that some 70–80% of patients transplanted using cyclophosphamide (50 mg/kg/day × 4) conditioning and cyclosporin to reduce rejection and graft-versus-host disease (GVHD), survive with grafts. These results are overall similar to treatment with ALG in terms of survival but transplantation has an advantage in children and young adults and in patients with VSAA. A proportion of surviving patients (about 15%) have chronic GVHD and late relapse may occur but the risk of clonal evolution is small compared with the 40% post-ALG.

Volunteer unrelated and mismatched transplants

The very long time it may take to achieve remission with immunosuppression as well as the risk of clonal evolution have led to the use of unrelated volunteers as a source of stem cells for transplantation. Early results were encouraging,[90] but subsequent experience is more disappointing[91,92] with a high risk of graft failure unless the conditioning regime was increased to greatly toxic levels. Failure of grafts under these circumstances meant inevitable death. There may be a place for such transplants in children with VSAA providing a full-matched donor is found. An alternative approach is the use of relatively mild conditioning with ALG and cyclophosphamide with post-graft immunosuppression with cyclosporin in the expectation that if the graft fails autologous reconstitution may yet occur. This approach is similar in concept to the 'low-dose' transplants which aim to achieve mixed chimerism. In the meantime, unrelated transplants for AA should only be carried out in experienced centers so that assessment of results can be meaningful.

Conclusion

The treatment of AA has improved greatly over the last 30 years. The platform from which successful treatment may develop is the provision of adequate support services. Allogeneic stem cell transplantation from an HLA-matched sibling is the treatment of choice for severe AA in children and young adults. If a sibling donor is available stem cell transplantation may be used as a first treatment for older adults with very severe AA. Other patients would be treated with immunosuppression using antilymphocyte globulin and cyclosporin, and the results of trials including growth factors are still awaited.

Inherited aplastic anemias

A number of inherited disorders lead on to bone marrow failure with features of AA. The most important ones are listed in Table 13.4. Far and away the most common of these is Fanconi anemia which is discussed in detail below.

Fanconi anemia

Fanconi anemia (FA) is inherited as an autosomal recessive disease and is associated with multiple developmental abnormalities, particularly of the skin and skeleton (Fig. 13.2A–C).[93] There is wide genetic and phenotypic heterogeneity. Cases have been described in all populations, with a higher incidence in populations where there is a founder effect,[94] or a stable population with little ethnic variability.[95]

Cytogenetic findings

FA is characterized by the appearance of multiple breaks and aberrations in the chromosomes of peripheral blood lymphocytes when stimulated into metaphase by phytohemagglutinin[96] and this increased fragility is further enhanced by exposure to clastogenic agents such as diepoxybutane (DEB) or mitomycin C (MMC) (Fig. 13.3).[97,98] These observations are the basis of the specific diagnostic test for FA which is performed on peripheral blood lymphocytes.[99] FA may present in adult life with AA or acute leukemia. The FA screen should be performed on all children or young adults presenting with AA or acute myeloid leukemia.

Genetic basis of Fanconi anemia

There are at least seven distinct genes which may lead to the phenotype of FA (*fanc A-G*), of which five genes have been cloned, *A*,[100,101] *C*,[102] *D2*,[103] *F*[104] and *G*.[105] Multiple mutations have been described in many of these genes[106,107] which lead mostly to null mutations or less commonly to predicted altered protein. Except when there is a founder effect, most patients seem to be compound heterozygotes. *Fanc-G* is identical to a gene *xrcc-9*[105] involved in the cell cycle regulation or possibly post-replication repair, but the function of the other genes is unknown. An important step in understanding the function of Fanconi genes has been the observation that one gene, *fanc-D2*, interacts with *brca-1*, the susceptibility gene in most familial breast and ovarian cancers. It is thought that the gene products of *fanc-A, C, F* and *G* form a complex which activates *fanc-D2* by mono-ubiquitination[108] which in turn affects *brca-1*. However, there is no excess of breast or ovarian cancer in patients with FA and the exact relationship is by no means clear.[109] It is presumed that the pathways are

Table 13.4 Congenital bone marrow failure syndromes

Disease	Clinical features	Hematology	Inheritance	Genetics
Fanconi anemia	See text	AA develops age 5–10 in majority. Some delayed	Autosomal recessive	At least 7 genes involved in pathway (see text)
Dyskeratosis congenita	Reticulated hyper-pigmentation of skin of face, neck, shoulders Dystrophic nails Leukoplakia and oral cancer	AA develops 10–30 years	(1) x-linked recessive (2) Autosomal dominant (3) Autosomal recessive	xq28 dyskerin gene[123] (DKC1)
Shwachman–Diamond syndrome	Exocrine pancreatic insufficiency Metaphyseal dysostosis	Neutropenia About 20–25% develop pancytopenia Increased MDS and leukemia[124]	Autosomal recessive	Chromosome 7[125] (antromeric)
Pearson's syndrome	Exocrine pancreatic insufficiency	Ringed sideroblasts vacuolated precursors Pancytopenia present early	Sporadic	Mitochondrial[126] DNA deletions

AA, aplastic anemia; MDS, myelodysplastic syndrome.

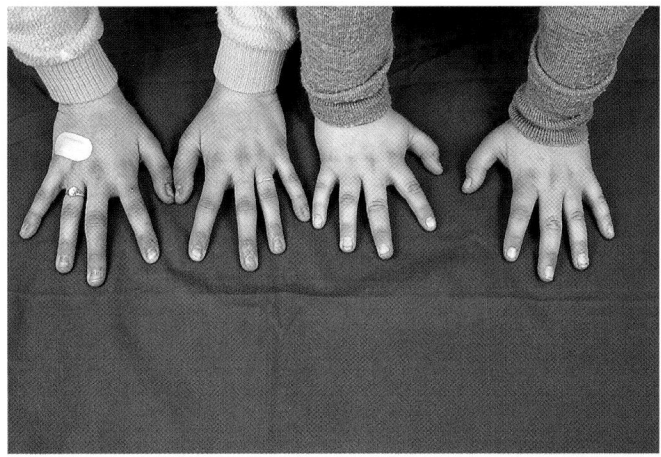

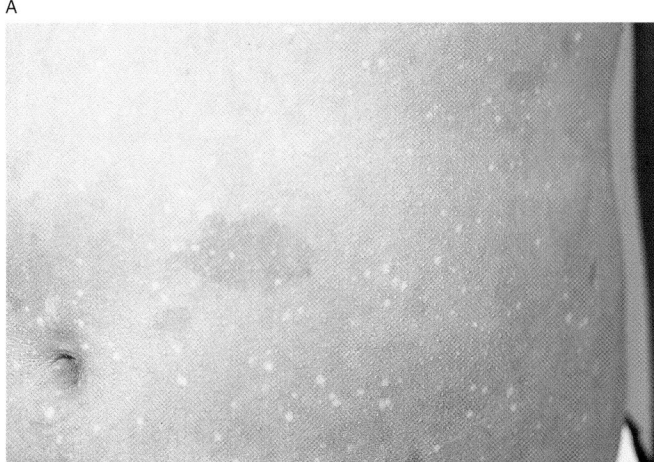

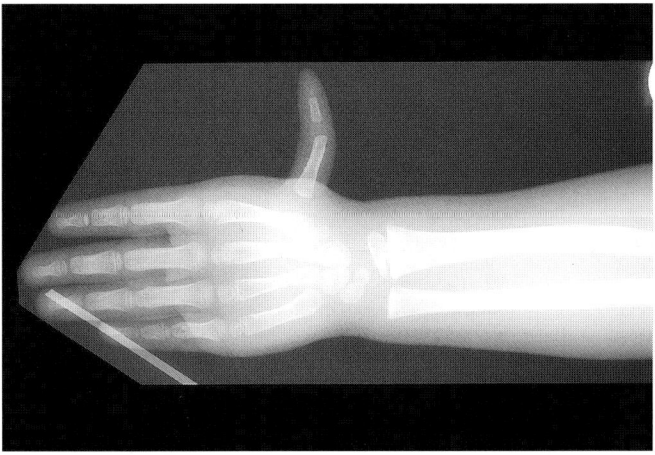

Fig. 13.2 (A) Hands from two siblings with Fanconi anemia showing abnormalities of the thumbs and little fingers. (B) Skin on the trunk of a patient with Fanconi anemia showing café au lait patches and depigmented spots. (C) X-ray of a child with Fanconi anemia showing abnormalities of the thumb.

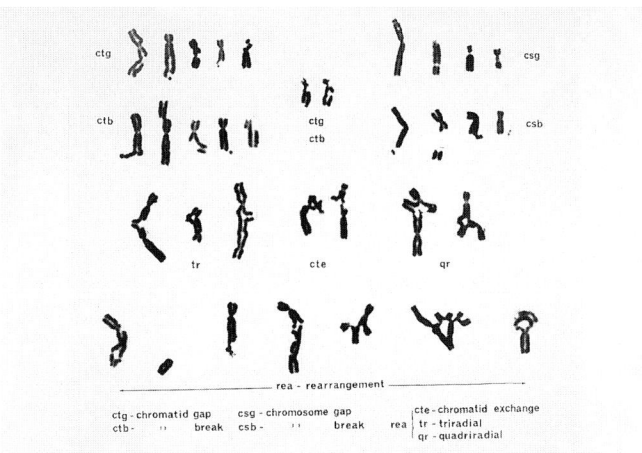

Fig. 13.3 Karyotype from peripheral blood lymphocytes stimulated with phytohemoglobin and clastogens from a case of Fanconi anemia. Numerous breaks, anomalies and reduplications are present.

Hematologic features

The blood count at birth is usually normal or nearly normal and remains so during infancy. Bone marrow failure develops slowly though there is considerable variation at the age at which the failure becomes apparent.[110] Some mutations, for example the IVS 4+4 A→T mutation common in Ashkenazi Jews of the *fanc-C* gene, are associated with a high incidence of morphologic disorders, early presentations and a high incidence of transformation to AA.[111] Overall, 85–90% of patients with FA develop bone marrow failure with a median age at presentation of 7–8 years and an overall risk of developing acute leukemia of about 1%. The disorder may present in adult life, sometimes with the onset of acute leukemia. As intimated, there is some correlation with genetic subtype both for dysmorphisms and for hematological presentation.[112,113]

Clinical course

Once bone marrow failure sets in the outlook is poor with the majority of patients going on to irreversible bone marrow failure and death from infection or hemorrhage. Acute leukemia, usually myeloid, may also develop. Solid tumors, particularly squamous tumors involving the tongue, oropharynx or genital tract are also more common than in the general population, and may cause death in patients who survive to adult life. With good supportive care patients may survive for several years, though again there is considerable heterogeneity. In adults fertility is decreased, particularly in males, but there are many examples of successful pregnancies in women with FA.[114]

involved in chromosome repair, possibly specifically of the damage caused by DNA cross-linking agents. The commonest genes involved in FA are *fanc-A, fanc-C* and *fanc-G*.[107]

Treatment

Anabolic steroids

Most patients with incipient bone marrow failure due to FA will respond to anabolic steroids,[86,114] but the effect is temporary. Anabolic steroids will delay the onset of transfusion dependency by up to 2 years and may prolong median life span by about the same amount. The problems of prolonged treatment relate to abnormalities of liver function, including peliosis hepatis and the emergence of hepatocellular carcinoma (Fig. 13.4), which are the consequence of the high doses of these agents which are required to stimulate bone marrow function. A typical dose of oxymethalone would be 2.5 mg/kg/day. Parenteral anabolic steroids do not damage the liver. Other major problems are the virilization including aggressive behavior in children, and hypercholesterolemia with an increased risk of coronary artery disease. Prolonged therapy may also result in hypogonadal function and aspermia. Even in patients who do not develop severe hepatocellular damage the effectiveness of anabolic steroids tends to wear off after about 2 years.

Hemopoietic stem cell transplantation (HSCT)

HSCT is the only way of curing the bone marrow failure of FA but it will neither influence the development of solid tumors nor of course affect problems associated with somatic anomalies. Patients with FA have an increased susceptibility to the effects of cytotoxic agents and radiotherapy[115] and the conditioning regime should be suitably modified to account for this.[116] Various schedules have been proposed using reduced doses of cyclophosphamide compared with those used for acquired AA (25–100 mg/kg over 4 days) combined with low-dose total body irradiation (200–500 c).[114] In figures gathered from the International Bone Marrow Transplant Registry, a 2-year probability of survival was 66% (58–73%) after HLA identical sibling transplant, but only 29% (18–43%) after alternative donor transplant.[117] Whilst the results of HLA-matched sibling transplants improve, those with volunteer donors remain disappointing. An exception to this is in Japan where perhaps the genetic diversity in the HLA system is less than in the rest of the world.[118] As already mentioned, there is a higher incidence of squamous carcinomas in FA even without transplantation and this risk may be enhanced by the procedure.[114,119]

Gene therapy

FA should be a suitable disease for treatment with gene therapy since the transfected stem cell ought to have a growth advantage over the remaining FA cells.[120] Such an approach has been attempted for *fanc-c* patients, so far without evidence of sustained engraftment.[121,122]

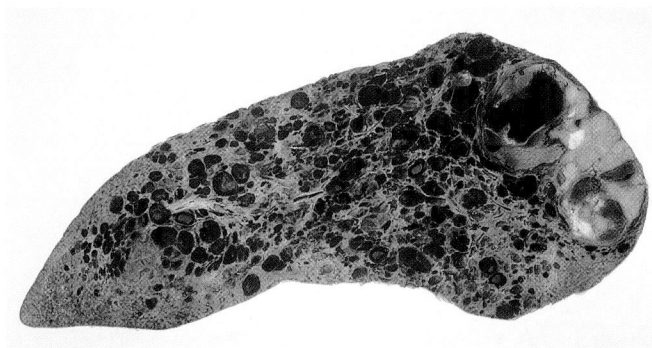

A

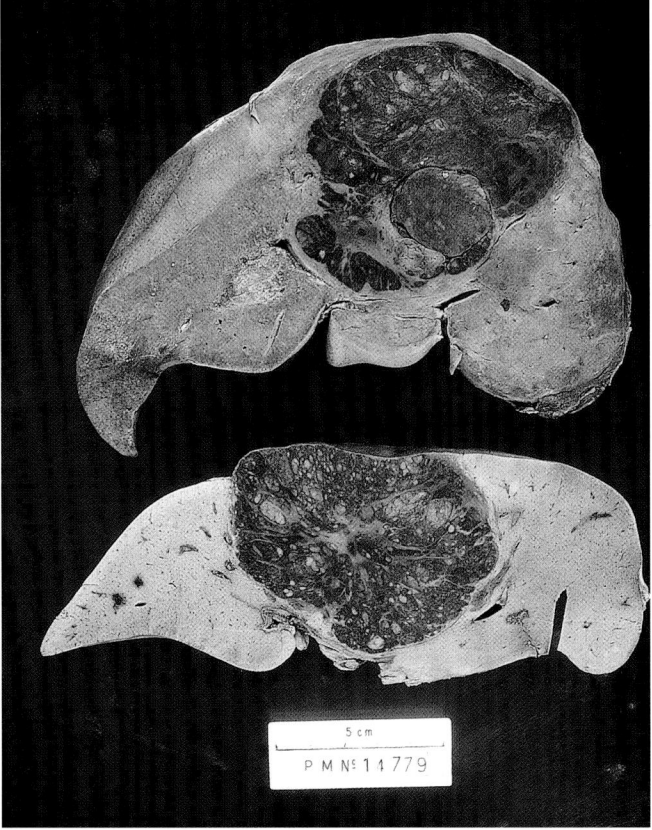

B

Fig. 13.4 (A) Section of liver showing extensive peliosis hepatis (venous lakes) with an area of hepatocellular carcinoma with necrosis and calcification in the right lobe. (B) Hepatocellular carcinoma developing in a liver from a Fanconi patient without prior peliosis hepatis.

Conclusion

The underlying biological/biochemical defects in FA are slowly emerging but the basic defect, whether a failure to repair DNA cross-link damage to chromosomes or some other pathway, remains elusive. So far the genetic knowledge has not transplanted into improved therapeutic measures though knowledge of the specific gene defect may help with prognosis. Changes in HSCT may yet hold further hope for sufferers from FA and gene therapy remains a possibility.

REFERENCES

1. Gordon-Smith EC, Issaragrisil S 1992 Epidemiology of aplastic anaemia. Baillière's Clinical Haematology 5: 475–491
2. Szklo M, Sensenbrenner L, Markowitz J et al 1985 Incidence of aplastic anemia in metropolitan Baltimore: a population based study. Blood 66: 115–119
3. Linet MS, McCaffrey LD, Morgan WF et al 1986 Incidence of aplastic anemia in a three county area of South Carolina. Cancer Research 46: 426–429
4. Mary JY, Baumelou E, Guiguet M & the French Cooperative Group for Epidemiological Study of Aplastic Anemia in France 1990 A prospective multicentre study. Blood 75: 1646–1653
5. Bottiger LE, Westerholme B 1972 Aplastic anaemia I: incidence and aetiology. Acta Medica Scandinavica 192: 315–318
6. Anonymous 1987 Incidence of aplastic anemia; relevance of diagnostic criteria. By the international agranulocytosis and aplastic anemia study. Blood 70: 1718–1721
7. Williams DM, Lynch RE, Cartwright GE 1973 Drug induced aplastic anemia. Seminars in Hematology 10: 195–223
8. Heimpel H, Heit W 1980 Drug induced aplastic anemia: clinical aspects. Clinical Hematology 9: 641–662
9. Gordon-Smith EC 1989 Aplastic anaemia – aetiology and clinical features. Bailliere's Clinical Haematology 2: 1–18
10. Young NS, Alter BP 1994 Drugs and chemicals. In: Young NS, Alter BP (eds), Aplastic anemia acquired and inherited. WB Saunders, Philadelphia, 100–132
11. Smadel JE 1949 Chloramphenicol (chloromycetin) in the treatment of infectious diseases. American Journal of Medicine 7: 671–685
12. Rich ML, Ritterhof RJ, Hoffmann RJ 1950 A fatal case of aplastic anemia following chloramphenicol (chloromycetin) therapy. Annals of Internal Medicine 33: 1459–1467
13. Smick KM, Condit PK, Procter RL et al 1964 Fatal aplastic anemia. An epidemiological study of its relationship to the drug chloramphenicol. Journal of Chronic Diseases 17: 899–914
14. Wallerstein RO, Condit PK, Kasper CK et al 1969 A statewide study of chloramphenicol and fatal aplastic anemia. Journal of the American Medical Association 208: 2045–2050
15. Doona M, Walsh JB 1995 Use of chloramphenicol as topical eye medication: time to cry halt? (Editorial). British Medical Journal 310: 1217–1218
16. Gordon-Smith EC, Marsh JC, Geary CG 1995 Is it time to stop using chloramphenicol on the eye? Prospective study of aplastic anaemia should give the answer (letter). British Medical Journal 311: 451
17. Scott JL, Finegold SM, Belkin GA et al 1965 A controlled double-blind study of the hematological toxicity of chloramphenicol. New England Journal of Medicine 272: 1137–1142
18. Kaufman DW, Kelly JP, Levy M, Shapiro S 1991 The drug etiology of agranulocytosis and aplastic anemia. In: Monographs in epidemiology and biostatistics, vol 18. Oxford University Press, New York 204–216
19. Inman WHW 1977 Study of fatal bone marrow suppression with special reference to phenylbutazone and oxyphenbutazone. British Medical Journal i: 1500–1505
20. (Anonymous) The International Agranulocytosis and Aplastic Anemia Study 1986 Risks of agranulocytosis and aplastic anemia. A first report of their relation to drug use with special reference to analgesics. Journal of the American Medical Association 256: 1749–1757
21. Andrews R, Russel N 1990 Aplastic anaemia associated with a non-steroidal anti-inflammatory drug; relapse after exposure to another such drug. British Medical Journal 301: 38
22. Kean WF, Annastassiades TP 1979 Long term chrysotherapy: incidence and efficacy during sequential time periods. Arthritis and Rheumatism 22: 495–501
23. Kay AGL 1976 Myelotoxicity of gold. British Medical Journal i: 1266–1268
24. Fibbe WE, Claas FH, van der Star-Dijkstra W et al 1986 Agranulocytosis induced by propylthiouracil: evidence of a drug dependent antibody reacting with granulocytes, monocytes and hematopoietic progenitor cells. British Journal of Haematology 64: 363–373
25. Prager D, Peters C 1970 Development of aplastic anaemia and the exposure to Stoddard solvent. Blood 35: 286–287
26. Sanchez-Medal L, Castenedo JP, Garcia-Rojas F 1963 Insecticides and aplastic anemia. New England Journal of Medicine 269: 1365–1367
27. Stormant RT 1955 The present status of chlordane. Journal of the American Medical Association 158: 1364–1367
28. Brahams D 1994 Lindane exposure and aplastic anemia. Medicine and the law. Lancet 343: 1092
29. Rugman FP, Cosstick R 1990 Aplastic anaemia associated with organochlorine pesticide: case reports and review of evidence. Journal of Clinical Pathology 43: 98–101
30. Roberts HJ 1990 Pentachlorophenol-associated aplastic anemia and red cell aplasia, leukemia and other blood disorders. Journal of the Florida Medical Association 77: 86–90
31. Hopkins JE, Manoharan A 1985 Severe aplastic anaemia following the use of hair dye: report of two cases and review of the literature. Postgraduate Medical Journal 61: 1003–1005
32. Young NS, Issaragrisil S, Ch'en WC et al 1986 Aplastic anaemia in the Orient. British Journal of Haematology 62: 1–6
33. Hagler L, Pastore RA, Bergin JJ et al 1975 Aplastic anemia following viral hepatitis: Report of two fatal cases and review of the literature. Medicine (Baltimore) 54: 139–164
34. Tzakis AG, Arditi M, Whitington PF et al 1988 Aplastic anemia complicating orthotopic liver transplantation for non-A, non-B hepatitis. New England Journal of Medicine 319: 393–396
35. Camitta BM, Nathan DG, Forman EN et al 1974 Posthepatitic severe aplastic anemia – an indication for early bone marrow transplantation. Blood 43: 473–483
36. Lazarus KH, Baehner RL 1981 Aplastic anemia complicating infectious mononucleosis: a case report and review of the literature. Pediatrics 67: 907–910
37. Camitta BM, Rappeport JM, Parkman R et al 1975 Selection of patients for bone marrow transplantation in severe aplastic anemia. Blood 45: 355–363
38. Bacigalupo A, Bruno B, Sarocco P et al 2000 Antithymocyte globulin, cyclosporin, prednisolone and granulocyte-colony stimulating factor for severe aplastic anemia: an update of the GITMO/EBMT study on 100 patients. Blood 95: 1931–1934
39. Kansu E, Erslev AJ 1976 Aplastic anaemia with 'hot pockets'. Scandinavian Journal of Haematology 17: 326–334
40. Broxmeyer HE 1999 The hematopoietic system: principles of therapy with hematopoietically active cytokines. In: Ganser A, Hoelzer D (eds), Cytokines in the treatment of hematopoietic failure. Marcel Dekker, New York, 1–37
41. Marsh JCW, Chang J, Testa NG et al 1991 *In vitro* assessment of marrow 'stem cell' and stromal function in aplastic anaemia. British Journal of Haematology 78: 258–267
42. Maciewski JP, Anderson S, Katevas P et al 1994 Phenotypic and functional analysis of bone marrow progenitor cell compartment in bone marrow failure. British Journal of Haematology 87: 227–234
43. Scopes J, Daly S, Atkinson R et al 1996 Aplastic anemia: evidence for dysfunctional bone marrow progenitor cells and the corrective effect of granulocyte colony stimulating factor. Blood 87: 3179–3185
44. Lord BI, Heyworth CM, Testa NG 1997 An introduction to primitive haematopoietic cells. In: Testa NG, Lord BI, Dexter TM (eds), Haematopoietic lineages in health and disease. Marcel Dekker, New York, 1–27
45. Bacigalupo A, Figari O, Tong J et al 1995 Long-term marrow culture in patients with aplastic anemia compared with marrow transplant recipients and normal controls. Experimental Hematology 23: 1472–1477
46. Maciejewski JP, Selleri C, Sata T et al 1996 A severe and consistent deficit in marrow and circulating primitive hematopoietic cells (long-term culture-initiating cells) in acquired aplastic anemia. Blood 88: 1983–1991
47. Marsh JCW, Testa NG 2000 Stem cell defect in aplastic anemia. In: Schrezenmeier H, Bacigalupo A (eds), Aplastic anemia. Pathophysiology and treatment. Cambridge University Press, Cambridge, 1–20

48. Gaines Das RE, Milne A, Rowley M et al 1992 Serum immunoreactive erythropoietin in patients with idiopathic aplastic and Fanconi's anaemias. British Journal of Haematology 82: 601–607

49. Schrezenmeier H, Noe G, Raghavachar A et al 1994 Serum erythropoietin and serum transferrin receptor levels in aplastic anaemia. British Journal of Haematology 88: 286–294

50. Kojima S, Matsuyama T, Kodera Y 1995 Circulating erythropoietin in patients with acquired aplastic anaemia. Acta Haematologica 94: 117–122

51. Marsh JCW, Gibson FM, Prue RL et al 1996 Serum thrombopoietin levels in patients with aplastic anaemia. British Journal of Haematology 95: 605–610

52. Kojima S, Matsuyama T, Kodera Y et al 1997 Measurement of endogenous plasma thrombopoietin in patients with acquired aplastic anaemia by a sensitive enzyme-linked immuno-sorbent assay. British Journal of Haematology 97: 538–543

53. Kojima S, Matsuyama T, Kodera Y et al 1996 Measurement of endogenous plasma granulocyte colony-stimulating factor in patients with acquired aplastic anemia by a sensitive chemiluminescent immunoassy. Blood 87: 1303–1308

54. Kojima S, Matsuyama T, Kodera Y 1997 Plasma levels and production of soluble stem cell factor by marrow stromal cells in patients with aplastic anaemia. British Journal of Haematology 99: 440–446

55. Nimer SD, Leung DHY, Wolin MJ et al 1994 Serum stem cell factor in patients with aplastic anemia. International Journal of Hematology 60: 499–512

56. Wodnar-Filipowicz A, Lyman SD, Gratwohl, A et al 1993 Levels of soluble stem cell factor in serum of patients with aplastic anemia. Blood 81: 3259–3264

57. Bacigalupo A, Brochia G, Corda G et al 1995 Antilymphocyte globulin, cyclosporin and granulocyte colony-stimulating factor in acquired severe aplastic anemia (SAA). A pilot study by the EBMT SAA Working Party. Blood 85: 1348–1353

58. Mathe G, Amiel JL, Schwarzenberg L, Choay J et al 1970 Bone marrow graft in man after conditioning by antilymphocytic serum. British Medical Journal 2: 131–136

59. Speck B, Gluckman E, Haak HL, van Rood JJ 1977 Treatment of aplastic anaemia by antilymphocyte globulin with and without allogeneic bone marrow infusions. Lancet 2: 1145–1148

60. Rebellato LM, Gross U, Verbanac KM, Thomas JM 1994 A comprehensive definition of the major antibody specificities in polyclonal rabbit antithymocyte globulin. Transplantation 57: 685–694

61. Bonnefoy-Berard N, Vincent C, Revillard JP 1991 Antibodies against functional leukocyte surface molecules in polyclonal antilymphocyte and antithymocyte globulins. Transplantation 51: 669–673

62. Young NS 2000 Hemopoietic cell destruction by immune mechanisms in acquired aplastic anaemia. Seminar of Hematology 37: 3–14

63. Bacigalupo A, Podesta M, Mingari MC et al 1981 Immune suppression of hematopoiesis in aplastic anemia: activity of T-γ lymphocytes. Journal of Immunology 125: 1449–1453

64. Bacigalupo A, Podesta M, Frassoni F et al 1982 Generation of CFU-C suppressor cells *in vitro*. A multistep process. British Journal of Haematology 52: 421–427

65. Zoumbos N, Djeu J, Young N 1985 Interferon is the suppressor of hematopoiesis generated by stimulated lymphocytes in vitro. Proceedings of the National Academy of Sciences of the United States of America 82: 188–192

66. Nakao S 2000 Role of T-lymphocytes in the pathophysiology of aplastic anemia. In: Schrezenmeier H, Bacigalupo A (eds), Aplastic anemia: pathophysiology and treatment. Cambridge University Press, Cambridge, 41–57

67. Kuriyama K, Tomonager M, Jinnai I et al 1984 Reduced helper (OKT4+): suppressor (OKTT8+) ratios in aplastic anaemia: relation to immunosuppressive therapy. British Journal of Haematology 57: 329–336

68. Ruiz-Arguelles GJ, Katzman JA, Cano-Castellanos R 1984 Lymphocyte subsets in patients with aplastic anaemia. American Journal of Hematology 16: 267–275

69. Kojima S, Matsuyama K, Kodera Y, Okada J 1989 Circulating activated suppressor T lymphocytes in hepatitis-associated aplastic anaemia. British Journal of Haematology 71: 147–151

70. Geary CG, Harrison CJ, Philpott NJ et al 1999 Abnormal erythrocyte clones in patients with aplastic anaemia: response to immunosuppressive therapy. British Journal of Haematology 104: 271–274

71. Tichelli A, Gratwohl A, Würsch A et al 1988 Late haematological complications in severe aplastic anaemia. British Journal of Haematology 69: 413–418

72. De Planque MM, Bacigulupo A, Würsch A et al 1989 Long term follow-up of severe aplastic anaemia patients treated with antilymphocyte globulin. British Journal of Haematology 73: 1121–1126

73. Bessler M, Mason P, Hillmen P, Luzzatto L 1994 Somatic mutations and cellular selection in paroxysmal nocturnal haemoglobinuria. Lancet 343: 951–953

74. Hillmen P, Hows JM, Luzzatto L 1992 Two distinct patterns of glycophosphatidylinositol linked protein deficiency in the red cells of patients with paroxysmal nocturnal haemoglobinuria. British Journal of Haematology 80: 399–405

75. Araten DJ, Nafa K, Pakdeeswuan K, Luzzatto L 1999 Clonal populations of haematopoietic cells with paroxysmal nocturnal haemoglobinuria genotype and phenotype are present in normal individuals. Proceedings of the National Academy of Sciences of the United States of America 96: 5209–5214

76. Camitta B, O'Reilly RJ, Sensenbrenner L et al 1983 Antithoracic duct lymphocyte globulin therapy of severe aplastic anemia. Blood 62: 883–885

77. Champlin R, Ho W, Gale RP 1983 Antithymocyte globulin treatment of patients with aplastic anemia. New England Journal of Medicine 308: 113–118

78. Bacigalupo A, Hows J, Gluckman E et al 1988 Bone marrow transplantation (BMT) versus immunosuppression for the treatment of severe aplastic anaemia (SAA): a report of the EBMT SAA Working Party. British Journal of Haematology 70: 177–182

79. Gluckman E, Esperon-Bourdeau H, Baruchel A et al 1992 Multicentre randomized study comparing cyclosporin A alone and antithymocyte globulin with prednisolone for treatment of severe aplastic anemia. Blood 79: 2540–2546

80. Marsh JC, Schrezenmeier H, Marin P et al 1999 Prospective randomised multicentre study comparing cyclosporin alone with the combination of antithymocyte globulin and cyclosporin for the treatment of patients with non-severe aplastic anaemia: a report from the EBMT Severe Aplastic Anaemia Working Party. Blood 2191–2195

81. Frickhofen N, Kaltwasser JP, Schrezenmeier H et al 1991 Treatment of aplastic anemia with antilymphocyte globulin and methyl prednisolone, with and without cyclosporin. New England Journal of Medicine 324: 1297–1304

82. Schrezenmeier H 2000 Role of cytokines in the treatment of aplastic anemia. In: Schrezenmeier H, Bacigalupo A (eds), Aplastic anemia: pathophysiology and treatment. Cambridge University Press, Cambridge, 197–229

83. Kojima S, Fukuda M, Miyajima T, Horibe K 1991 Treatment of aplastic anemia in children with recombinant human granulocyte colony-stimulating factor. Blood 77: 937–941

84. Brodsky RA, Sensenbrenner LI, Rapperport JM et al 1996 Complete remission in severe aplastic anemia after high-dose cyclophosphamide without bone marrow transplantation. Blood 87: 491–494

85. Tisdale JF, Dunn DE, Geller N et al 2000 High-dose cyclophosphamide in severe aplastic anaemia: a randomised trial. Lancet 356: 1554–1559

86. Shahidi NT, Diamond LK 1959 Testosterone-induced remission in aplastic anemia. J Dis Childhood 98: 293–303

87. Tichelli A, Passweg JR, Nissen C et al 1998 Repeated treatment with horse antilymphocyte globulin for severe aplastic anaemia. British Journal of Haematology 100: 393–400

88. Storb R, Thomas ED, Buckner CD et al 1974 Allogenic marrow grafting for treatment of aplastic anemia. Blood 43: 157–180

89. Camitta BM, Thomas ED, Nathan EG et al 1979 A prospective study of autologous and bone marrow transplantation for treatment of severe aplastic anemia. Blood 53: 504–514

90. Gordon-Smith EC, Fairhead SM, Chipping PM et al 1982 Bone marrow transplantation for severe aplastic anemia using histocompatible unrelated volunteer donors. British Medical Journal 285: 835–837

91. Bacigalupo A, Hows J, Gordon-Smith EC et al 1988 Bone marrow transplantation for severe aplastic anaemia from donors other than HLA identical siblings: A report of the BMT Working Party. Bone Marrow Transplant 3: 531–535

92. Hows J, Stone JV, Camitta BM 2000 Alternative donor bone marrow transplantation for severe acquired aplastic anemia. In: Schrezenmeier H, Bacigalupo A, (eds). Aplastic Anemia: Pathophysiology and Treatment. Cambridge University Press, Cambridge, 258–274

93. Fanconi G 1967 Familial constitutional panmyelocytopathy, Fanconi's anaemia (FA). 1. Clinical aspects. Seminars in Hematology 4: 233–240

94. Rossendorff J, Bernstein R, MacDougall L, Jenkins T 1987 Fanconi anaemia: another disease of unusually high prevalence in the Africaans population of South Africa. American Journal of Medical Genetics 27: 793–797

95. Savria A, Zatterale A, del Principle D, Joenje H 1996 Fanconi anemia for Italy: high prevalence for complementation group A in two geographic clusters. Human Genetics 97: 599–603

96. Schroeder TM, Kurth R 1971 Spontaneous chromosomal breakage and high incidence of leukaemia in inherited disease. Blood 37: 96–112

97. Sasaki MS, Tonomura A 1973 A high susceptibility of Fanconi's anemia to chromosome breakage by DNA cross-linking agents. Cancer Research 35: 1829–1836

98. Auerbach AD, Rogatko A, Schroeder-Kurth TM 1989 International Fanconi anemia registry: relation of clinical symptoms to diepoxybutane sensibility. Blood 73: 391–396

99. Auerbach AD, Ghash R, Pollio PC, Zhang M 1989 Diepoxybutane test for prenatal and postnatal diagnosis of Fanconi anemia. In: Schroeder-Kurth TM, Auerbach AD, Obe G (eds), Fanconi anemia. Clinical cytogenetic and experimental aspects. Springer, Berlin, 71–104(F)

100. Lo Ten Foe JR, Rooimans MA, Bosnoyan-Collins L et al 1996 Expression cloning of a cDNA for the major Fanconi anemia gene, FAA. Nature Genetics 14: 320–323

101. The Fanconi Anemia/Breast Cancer Consortium 1996 Proportional cloning of the Fanconi anemia group A gene. Nature Genetics 14: 324–328

102. Strathdee CA, Gavish H, Shannon WR, Buchwald M 1992 Cloning of cDNAs for Fanconi's anemia by functional complementation. Nature 356: 763–767

103. Timmers C, Taniguchi T, Hejna J et al 2001 Positional cloning of novel Fanconi anaemia gene, FANCD2. Molecular Cell 7: 241–248

104. de Winter JP, Rooimans MA, van der Weel L et al 2000 The Fanconi anemia gene *FANCF* encodes a novel protein with homology to ROM. Nature Genetics 24: 15–16

105. de Winter JP, Waisfisz Q, Rooimans MA et al 1998 The Fanconi anemia groups G gene is identical with XRCC9. Nature Genetics 20: 281–283

106. Carreau M, Buchwald M 1998 The Fanconi anaemia genes. Pediatrics 10: 65–69

107. D'Apolito M, Zelante L, Sarola A 1998 Molecular basis of Fanconi anaemia. Hematologia 83: 533–542

108. Garcia-Higuera I, Taniguchi T, Ganesan S et al 2001 Interaction of the Fanconi anemia proteins and BRCA1 in a common pathway. Molecular Cell 7: 249–262

109. Youssoufian H 2001 Fanconi anaemia and breast cancer: what's the connection? Nature Genetics 27: 352–353

110. Butterini A, Gale R, Veilander PC et al 1994 Hematologic abnormalities in Fanconi anemia: an International Fanconi Anemia Registry Study. Blood 84: 1600–1655

111. Gillio AP, Valander PC, Batish SD et al 1997 Phenotypic consequences of mutations in the Fanconi anaemia FAC gene: an international Fanconi anemia registry study. Blood 90: 105–110

112. Alter BP 1993 Fanconi's anaemia and its variability. British Journal of Haematology 85: 9–14

113. Faivre L, Guardiola P, Lewis C et al 2000 Association of complementation group and mutation type with clinical outcome in Fanconi anemia. Blood 96: 4064–4069

114. Young NS, Alter BP 1994 Clinical features of Fanconi's anaemia. In: Aplastic anemia, acquired and inherited. WB Saunders, Philadelphia, 275–309

115. Berger R, Bernheim A, Gluckman E, Gisselbrecht C 1980 *In vitro* effect of cyclophosphamide metabolities on chromosomes of Fanconi anaemia patients. British Journal of Haematology 45: 565–568

116. Gluckman E, Devergie A, Dutreix J 1983 Radiosensitivity in Fanconi anaemia: application to the conditioning regimen for bone marrow transplantation. British Journal of Haematology 54: 431–440

117. Gluckman E, Auerbach AD, Horowitz MM et al 1995 Bone marrow transplantation for Fanconi anemia. Blood 86: 2856–2862

118. Yamada T, Tachibana A, Shimizu T et al 2000 Novel mutations of the FANCG gene causing alternative splicing in Japanese Fanconi anemia. Journal of Human Genetics 45: 159–166

119. Flowers MED, Doney KC, Storb R et al 1992 Marrow transplantation for Fanconi anemia with or without leukaemic transformation: an update on the Seattle experience. Bone Marrow Transplant 9: 167–173

120. Fu K-L, Lo Ten Foe JR, Joenje H et al 1997 Functional correlation of Fanconi group A hematopoietic cells by retroviral gene transfer. Blood 90: 3296–3303

121. Liu JM, Kim S, Read EJ et al 1999 Engraftment of hematopoietic progenitor cells transduced with the Fanconi anemia group C gene (FANCC). Human Gene Therapy 10: 2337–2346

122. Lui JM 2000 Genetic correction of Fanconi anemia. In: Schrezenmeier H, Bacigalupo A (eds), Aplastic anemia: pathophysiology and treatment. Cambridge University Press, Cambridge, 368–379

123. Knight SW, Heiss NS, Vulliamy TJ et al 1999 X-linked dyskeratosis congenita is predominantly caused by missense mutations in the DKC1 gene. American Journal of Human Genetics 65: 50–58

124. Smith OP, Hann IM, Chessells JM et al 1996 Haematological abnormalities in Shwachman–Diamond syndrome. British Journal of Haematology 94: 279–284

125. Goobie S, Popovic M, Morrison J et al 2001 Shwachman-Diamond syndrome with exocrine-pancreatic dysfunction and bone marrow failure maps to the centromeric region of chromosome 7. American Journal of Human Genetics 68: 1048–1054

126. Muraki K, Nishimura S, Goto Y et al 1997 The association between haematological manifestation and mtDNA deletions in Pearson syndrome. Journal of Inherited Metabolic Diseases 20: 697–703

Pure red cell aplasia and sideroblastic anemias

14

SN Wickramasinghe

Pure red cell aplasia

Diamond-Blackfan anemia (constitutional erythroid hypoplasia, congenital erythroblastopenia, erythrogenesis imperfecta)

Acquired pure red cell aplasia (PRCA)

Hereditary sideroblastic anemias

X-linked inheritance

Autosomal recessive inheritance

Maternal inheritance

Thiamine-responsive anemia

Acquired sideroblastic anemias

Sideroblastic anemia secondary to drugs and chemicals

Idiopathic or primary acquired sideroblastic anemia (refractory anemia with ringed sideroblasts)

Bone marrow in sideroblastic anemias

Pure red cell aplasia

In some patients anemia develops due to a selective hypoplasia or aplasia of erythropoietic cells. The other cell lines in the marrow are usually unaffected and both the leukocyte and platelet counts in the blood are generally normal. The bone marrow normally shows a marked deficiency of erythropoietic cells at all stages of maturation or a total absence of erythroblasts. Occasionally, there are increased numbers of pronormoblasts (sometimes with giant forms) and basophilic normoblasts and an absence of more mature cells. The absolute reticulocyte count in the blood is very low. Pure red cell aplasia occurs both as a congenital defect (Diamond-Blackfan anemia) and as an acquired defect.[1-3]

Diamond–Blackfan anemia (constitutional erythroid hypoplasia, congenital erythroblastopenia, erythrogenesis imperfecta)[4-6]

This syndrome is characterized by the onset, usually during the first four months of life, of anemia due to selective hypoplasia of the red cell precursors. 10% of cases are familial and others sporadic. In familial cases, both autosomal recessive and autosomal dominant inheritance have been proposed. There are also other variations in the clinical and biologic characteristics of the disease in different patients, suggesting the possibility of more than one primary defect. The anemia, which is macrocytic at diagnosis in two-thirds of the cases, becomes progressively worse and is eventually severe. Most patients have increased levels of HbF and erythrocyte adenosine deaminase (a purine salvage pathway enzyme). About 25% of patients have congenital abnormalities; these include skeletal anomalies affecting the lateral aspects of the limbs (e.g. triphalangeal thumbs), webbing of the neck and short stature. There is an increased risk of developing hematologic and other malignancies including osteogenic sarcoma.[7] The marrow shows few or no erythroblasts but is normal in other respects. The plasma erythropoietin concentration is increased but the BFU-E are reduced. The latter may show erythropoietin dose-dependence but are relatively erythropoietin-insensitive.[6] Long-term bone marrow cultures have revealed no defect in the bone marrow stroma and confirmed a defect in erythroid progenitors; some cases also had a defect in CFU-GM.[8] About 80% of the patients respond to treatment with corticosteroids, erythroblasts reappearing in the bone marrow. Occasional steroid-responsive and non-responsive patients remit spontaneously, sometimes at puberty. Steroid non-responsive cases require regular transfusions. Some patients with Diamond-Blackfan anemia have been treated, usually successfully, by bone marrow transplantation.[6] Various mutations (nonsence, missence, splice sites and frameshift) of the ribosomal protein S19 (RPS19) gene have been found in 24% of cases[9] but the mechanism by which this mutation causes anemia remains uncertain.

Acquired pure red cell aplasia (PRCA)

The causes of acquired PRCA may be grouped under four headings: (1) viral infections, (2) immunologic disturbances, (3) myelodysplasia, and (4) chemicals and drugs.

Viral infections. PRCA develops following infection with parvovirus B19,[10] which causes a mild febrile disorder (erythema infectiosum) in children and may cause arthropathy in adults. Individuals with a normal red cell life-span have a transient arrest of erythropoiesis with an absence of reticulocytes but do not drop their hemoglobin to any appreciable extent: recovery of erythropoiesis occurs when anti-B19 IgM and IgG antibodies develop 10–12 d after infection. In various chronic hemolytic anemias (e.g. hereditary spherocytosis and sickle cell anemia), the abrupt cessation of erythropoiesis in the face of a markedly shortened red cell life-span leads to a rapid and life-threatening fall in the hemoglobin level. With supportive therapy with red cell transfusions when necessary, recovery occurs spontaneously in 1–2 weeks. The receptor for B19 is a globoside expressed mainly on some CFU-E and on pronormoblasts and more mature erythroblasts; on erythroid cells this globoside is the P antigen. Infection of erythroid cells causes apoptosis. The marrow may contain giant pronormoblasts with cytoplasmic vacuolation and, occasionally, eosinophilic nuclear inclusions. In addition to the anemia, there may sometimes be a variable reduction of the neutrophil and platelet counts by uncertain mechanisms. In conditions associated with immunosuppression (e.g. congenital immunodeficiency and immunodeficiency secondary to immunosuppressive drugs, HIV infection and T-large granular lymphocyte leukemia[11]) and in some patients without evident immunosuppression,[12] parvovirus B19 infection persists and causes chronic PRCA. Chronic PRCA secondary to B19 infection responds to high-dose intravenous immunoglobulin therapy.

Rarely, pure red cell aplasia may complicate the course of primary atypical pneumonia, infectious mononucleosis (Epstein-Barr [EB] virus infection) or mumps. Immunologic mechanisms may be involved in the pathogenesis of the PRCA in patients with chronic EB virus infection as *in vitro* studies have shown that their T-cells inhibit erythropoiesis.

Immunologic PRCA. No associated disorder can be found in some cases of chronic acquired pure red cell aplasia. However about 30% of cases are associated with the presence of a thymic tumour. A number of cases are associated with rheumatoid arthritis, systemic lupus erythematosus,[13,14] myasthenia gravis, Felty's syndrome,[15] antiphospholipid syndrome,[16] non-Hodgkin's and Hodgkin's lymphoma,[17] B cell chronic lymphocytic leukemia (CLL), T cell CLL, large granular lymphocyte (LGL) leukemia,[18] angioimmunoblastic lymphadenopathy, carcinoma of the bronchus, breast or stomach, acute viral hepatitis during pregnancy,[19] renal insufficiency, therapy with immunosuppressive drugs such as azathioprine and protein-energy malnutrition. PRCA may precede the diagnosis of carcinoma by several months or the development of frank leukemia by several years. Some patients treated with recombinant human erythropoietin have also developed PRCA; such patients have anti-erythropoietin antibodies and their serum blocks erythroid colony formation by normal bone marrow cells.[20] The association of pure red cell aplasia with thymoma, autoimmune disorders, anti-erythropoietin antibodies and the above-mentioned malignant diseases, and the response of some cases to immunosuppressive therapy (corticosteroids, anti-thymocyte globulin, cyclophosphamide, cyclosporin A) suggest that immunologic mechanisms may underly the aplasia in at least some patients. This view is supported by studies in a few cases that have shown the presence of antibodies directed against erythroblasts, morphologically unrecognized erythroid progenitor cells or erythropoietin (in cases not treated with erythropoietin). Furthermore, the possibility that alterations in T-lymphocyte sub-populations may underly the red cell aplasia in some patients has been raised by the observation that patients with PRCA associated with thymoma, lymphoma, CLL and LGL leukemia have T-cells that suppress the growth of erythroid cells *in vitro*.

Antibody- or cell-mediated suppression of erythroid progenitors has also been demonstrated[21] in some cases of *transient erythroblastopenia of childhood*.[3] This condition usually affects children aged 1 yr or older, is unrelated to parvovirus B19 infection, and often resolves spontaneously within 4–8 weeks. In addition to the reticulocytopenia, some patients have neutropenia. Viral infections and hereditary factors have also been implicated in the pathogenesis.

Myelodysplasia. Rarely, PRCA occurs and may be an early manifestation, in the myelodysplastic syndromes[22] (Chapter 19).

Chemicals and Drugs. Pure red cell aplasia has followed exposure to benzene and treatment with drugs such as phenytoin sodium, chloramphenicol, azathioprine, procainamide, sulphonamides and sodium valproate.[23,24] Some of these drugs may act by immunologic mechanisms.

Sideroblastic anemia

The sideroblastic anemias are diagnosed on the basis of a characteristic appearance of the bone marrow after staining by Perls' acid ferrocyanide method; their defining feature is the presence of a complete or partial perinuclear ring of abnormally coarse siderotic granules in a substantial proportion of the erythroblasts (Fig. 14.1).

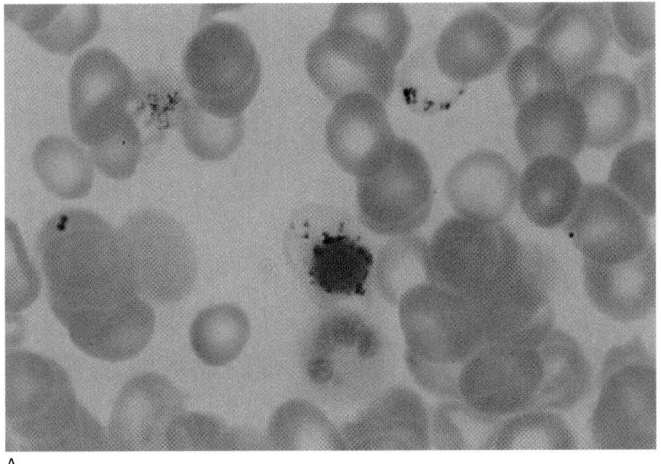
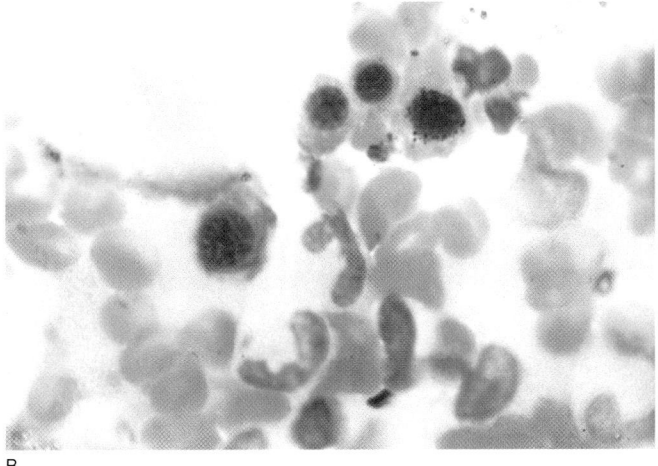

A   B

Fig. 14.1 (A, B) Marrow smear from a patient with hereditary sideroblastic anemia (A) and primary acquired sideroblastic anemia (B). Each of the photomicrographs shows a ringed sideroblast and (A) also contains siderocytes. Perls' acid ferrocyanide stain.

Electron microscope studies have revealed that the majority of the siderotic granules consist of iron-laden mitochondria. The iron-containing material is found between the mitochondrial cristae (Fig. 14.2). The affected mitochondria sometimes display degenerative changes such as the loss of some or all of the cristae and the presence of abnormally electron-lucent areas in the mitochondrial matrix. Studies of heme synthesis have shown different defects in various patients, the two most commonly observed being reduced activity of the enzymes aminolevulinic acid (ALA) synthase and ferrochelatase. The sideroblastic anemias occur as inherited or acquired conditions.

Hereditary sideroblastic anemias

The hereditary sideroblastic anemias (HSAs) are rare; the inheritance is usually X-linked but may also be autosomal recessive or maternal. There may be mild or moderate splenomegaly. The severity of these disorders varies markedly. Some patients die in infancy or childhood; others have a normal or near-normal life span.

X-linked inheritance

The common form of X-linked sideroblastic anemia is caused by mutations in the erythroid-specific 5-aminolevulinate synthase gene (*ALAS2* gene) located at Xp11.21.[25–27] So far, 18 different mutations in this gene have been reported to cause sideroblastic anemia and the activity of the enzyme ALAS is usually reduced to 3–40% of normal. Pyridoxal phosphate is required both for enzyme activity and enzyme stability. Xp11.21-linked HSA is often detected in childhood or adolescence but may sometimes be diagnosed late in life.[28] Anemia is usually confined to males; female carriers generally show only minor changes in the blood and marrow. Rarely, anemia may be encountered in heterozygous females due to skewed Lyonization. Most patients respond to pharmacologic doses (i.e. 5–500 mg per day) of pyridoxine orally. In a patient with pyridoxine-refractory sideroblastic anemia, a point mutation in the ALAS2 gene caused abnormal proteolytic processing of the enzyme precursor and instability of the enzyme.[29] If a secondary folate deficiency develops, there may also be some response to folate therapy. The anemia is sometimes severe and then requires treatment with regular blood transfusion. Even untransfused patients may develop iron overload leading to cirrhosis of the liver, diabetes mellitus and cardiac dysfunction.

Both the mean cell volume (MCV) and mean cell hemoglobin (MCH) are low, and may be as low as 58 fl and 18 pg respectively. The white cell and platelet counts are usually normal but may be slightly decreased. The blood film shows many hypochromic, microcytic red cells.

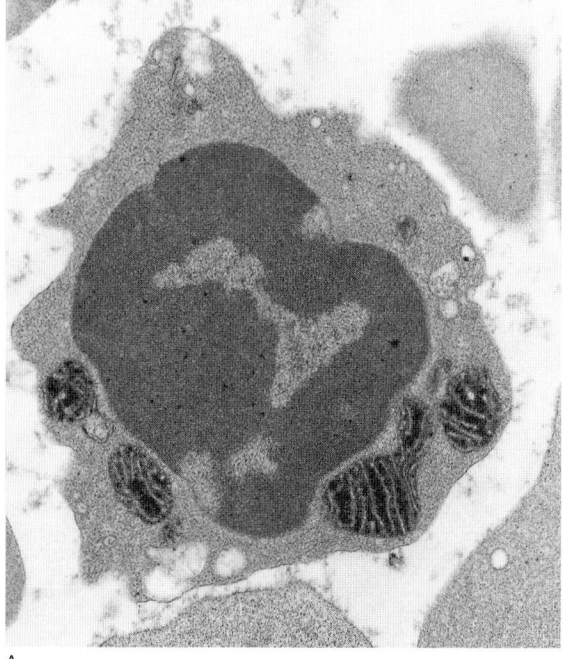 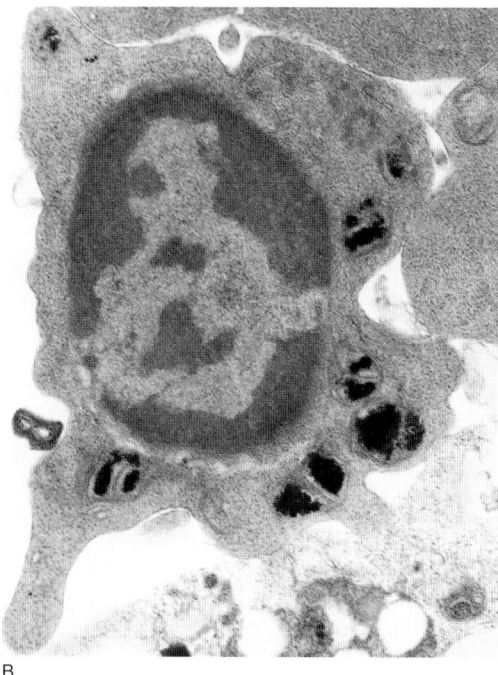

A   B

Fig. 14.2 (A, B) Electron micrographs of ringed sideroblasts from a case of hereditary sideroblastic anemia (A) and a case of primary acquired sideroblastic anemia (B). Note the presence of very electron-dense iron-containing material between the cristae of the mitochondria. Uranyl acetate and lead citrate. (A) × 20 000; (B) × 17 800.

Some cases have a variable number (up to 50%) of normochromic normocytic red cells (Fig. 14.3). Apart from the microcytosis, there is anisocytosis and poikilocytosis and there may be some target cells. The blood film may also contain an occasional cell with basophilic stippling or Pappenheimer bodies and a very occasional late erythroblast; the number of such cells increases after splenectomy.

A mutation affecting another gene on the X-chromosome located at Xq13 causes a recessive disorder in infants and young children characterized by non-progressive cerebellar ataxia, a mild hypochromic microcytic anemia and sideroblastic erythropoiesis.[30] This condition is known as X-linked sideroblastic anemia with ataxia (XLSA/A) and the mutant gene, *ABC7*, codes for a putative mitochondrial iron transporter.

Autosomal recessive inheritance

In one English family with severe HSA (MCV 65 fl), linkage to *ALAS2* was excluded by linkage analysis and the disease seemed to be inherited as an autosomal recessive character.[31]

Maternal inheritance

In HSAs due to mutations in mitochondrial DNA, the MCV is increased and the blood film shows macrocytes as well as some hypochromic microcytes. Pearson's syndrome is a rare and often fatal maternally-inherited disorder of infancy caused by mutations in mitochondrial DNA.[32] It is characterized by sideroblastic anemia, a high MCV, neutropenia and impaired pancreatic, hepatic and renal function. Recently, a pedigree with maternally-inherited sideroblastic anemia, a raised MCV and a dimorphic red cell population has been described in which a mutation in mitochondrial DNA was postulated.[33] The patients did not have the other features of Pearson's syndrome.

Thiamine-responsive anemia

Some cases of thiamine-responsive anemia are associated with sideroblastic erythropoiesis.[34] This autosomal recessive disorder is characterized by megaloblastic anemia, mild thrombocytopenia and leukopenia, progressive sensorineural deafness and diabetes mellitus. The disease is caused by a mutation in a gene on 1q 23.2–23.3, named *SLC19A2*, coding for a thiamine carrier.[35–37] Pharmacologic doses of thiamine correct the anemia and may improve the diabetes.

Acquired sideroblastic anemias

The acquired sideroblastic anemias can be subdivided into: (1) those secondary to the ingestion of certain drugs and toxic substances; and (2) primary or idiopathic acquired sideroblastic anemia (a myelodysplastic syndrome; also see Chapter 19).

Sideroblastic anemia secondary to drugs and chemicals

The drugs and toxic agents reported to cause sideroblastic erythropoiesis are listed in Table 14.1;[38,39] the commonest is undoubtedly alcohol. The red cells of cases of secondary sideroblastic anemia resemble those of the primary acquired type in being dimorphic with a small population of hypochromic microcytes.

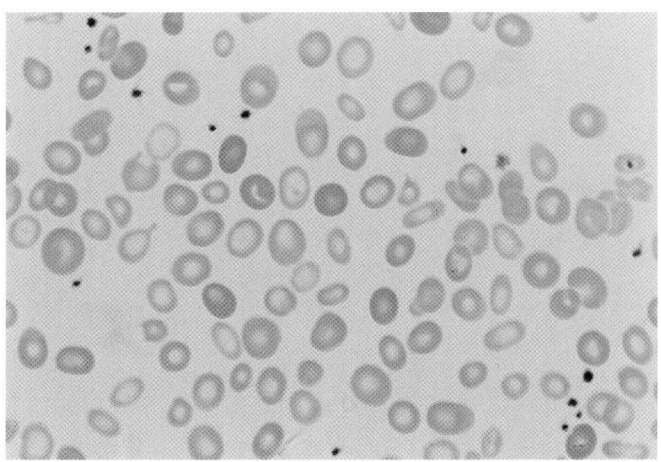

Fig. 14.3 Peripheral blood smear from an untransfused patient with hereditary sideroblastic anemia showing some normochromic and many markedly hypochromic red cells. May–Grünwald–Giemsa stain.

Table 14.1 Classification of sideroblastic anemias

Hereditary sideroblastic anemias
1. Xp11.21-linked (mutation in *ALAS2* gene)
2. Xq13.1–13.3-linked, with ataxia
3. Autosomal recessive inheritance
4. Maternal inheritance (primary mitochondrial DNA mutations, e.g. Pearson's syndrome)
5. Thiamine-responsive anemia

Acquired sideroblastic anemias
1. Drugs and toxic substances (chloramphenicol, isoniazid, cycloserine, pyrazinamide, progesterone, azathioprine, alcohol, lead, arsenic, zinc)
2. Idiopathic or primary acquired sideroblastic anemias (refractory anemia with ringed sideroblasts)

Idiopathic or primary acquired sideroblastic anemia (refractory anemia with ringed sideroblasts)

This disorder accounts for about one-third of the cases of acquired sideroblastic anemia and usually affects the elderly. The average age at diagnosis is about 70 years (range, 37–86 years). Some patients have heteroplastic mutations in mitochondrial DNA which may impair the function of the mitochondrial respiratory chain and thereby interfere with mitochondrial iron metabolism and heme synthesis and cause iron-loading of mitochondria.[40] Similarly, mutations in mitochondral DNA have been reported in childhood myelodysplasia with ringed sideroblasts.[41] In some other patients, the mutation responsible for the sideroblastic change may affect nuclear DNA and indirectly cause mitochondrial damage.

Mild splenomegaly may be found. Some cases show a partial hematologic response to pyridoxine administered orally. Those patients who develop a secondary folate deficiency may show some response to folate therapy.

In primary acquired sideroblastic anemia, the hemoglobin is usually between about 6 and 10 g/dl and the MCV is frequently raised. The reticulocyte percentage is normal or slightly increased. The leukocyte and platelet counts are usually normal but may be slightly reduced and very occasionally, thrombocytosis may be seen. The blood film is characteristically dimorphic with a major population of well-hemoglobinized, normocytic or macrocytic cells and a second population of hypochromic microcytes that are often misshapen (Fig. 14.4). The percentage of microcytes varies widely from less than 1 to 30. The well-hemoglobinized cell population may also show poikilocytosis and there may be a few target cells. A very few cells displaying basophilic stippling or Pappenheimer bodies and a very occasional circulating erythroblast may be present.

Primary acquired sideroblastic anemia usually runs a relatively benign course with a median survival of 10 years; these patients often die of conditions unrelated to the anemia. According to the early literature, in about 10% of patients the disease evolves into acute myeloid leukemia.[42] The neutrophils of such patients may show hypogranular cytoplasm, Auer rods, the acquired Pelger–Huët anomaly or a low neutrophil alkaline phosphatase (NAP) score for a considerable period prior to the development of overt leukemia. However, more recent studies indicate that when the dysplastic changes are confined to the erythroid series, there is no increase in the risk of transformation to acute myeloid leukemia.[43] Oncogenic *N Ras* mutations are rare in primary acquired

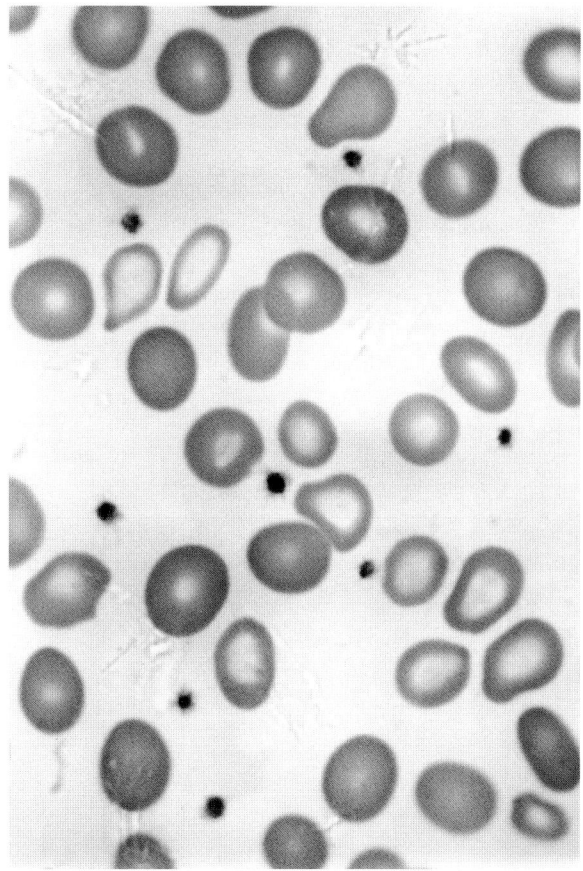

Fig. 14.4 Peripheral blood smear from an untransfused patient with primary acquired sideroblastic anemia showing both normochromic and markedly hypochromic cells. May–Grünwald–Giemsa stain.

sideroblastic anemia and this may be related to the good prognosis in this condition.[44] As in the hereditary sideroblastic anemias, primary acquired sideroblastic anemias may be complicated by hemosiderosis with hepatic, myocardial and pancreatic damage. The iron overload is not related to the presence of the hemochromatosis mutations Cys282Tyr and His63Asp.[45]

Bone marrow in sideroblastic anemias

The marrow usually shows erythroid hyperplasia with some increase in the proportion of basophilic erythropoietic cells. These changes are often more frequent and more marked in primary acquired sideroblastic anemia than in the hereditary or other acquired types. Erythropoiesis is usually micronormoblastic with poor hemoglobinization of the cytoplasm in the inherited type and either macronormoblastic or megaloblastic in the primary acquired type. The megaloblastic change is sometimes partly or wholly caused by a secondary folate deficiency but is more often unrelated to folate status. A characteristic finding in all types of sideroblastic anemia is the presence of some polychromatic erythroblasts with areas of feebly-staining ('transparent' or 'vacuolated') cytoplasm (Fig. 14.5). Such cells may also contain several coarse basophilic granules and pyknotic nuclei which are often irregularly shaped. Some of these polychromatic erythroblasts have very scanty cytoplasm with indistinct or ragged edges.

The defining feature of sideroblastic erythropoiesis is the presence of many ringed sideroblasts in the marrow (usually ≥15% of the erythroblasts). It should be noted that ringed sideroblasts may be present at a very low frequency in normal marrow and that the proportion of such cells is slightly increased in many disorders of erythropoiesis. Therefore, the diagnosis of sideroblastic erythropoiesis requires the presence of substantial numbers of ringed sideroblasts. Ringed sideroblasts are seen at all stages of erythroblast maturation in primary acquired sideroblastic anemia and many cases of alcohol-induced sideroblastic anemia. By contrast, they are more or less confined to the late polychromatic erythroblast compartment in hereditary sideroblastic anemia due to mutations in the ALAS2 gene and in most other types of acquired sideroblastic anemia.

In primary acquired sideroblastic anemia, the accumulation of large quantities of iron within the mitochondria is associated with and possibly causes: (1) an impairment of proliferation in the early polychromatic erythroblast compartment;[46] and (2) a gross suppression of protein biosynthesis in some early and late polychromatic erythroblasts.[47] The anemia in this disorder is largely the consequence of a high death rate amongst both the early and late polychromatic erythroblasts (i.e. due to a gross degree of ineffective erythropoiesis). By contrast, there is usually a lesser degree of ineffective erythropoiesis in the hereditary sideroblastic anemias, presumably because in this disorder, marked iron loading of the mitochondria and consequent cell death is more or less confined to the non-dividing late polychromatic erythroblasts.[48] Impaired hemoglobin synthesis and the production of poorly-hemoglobinized microcytes also play a significant role in the pathogenesis of the anemia in the hereditary disorder.

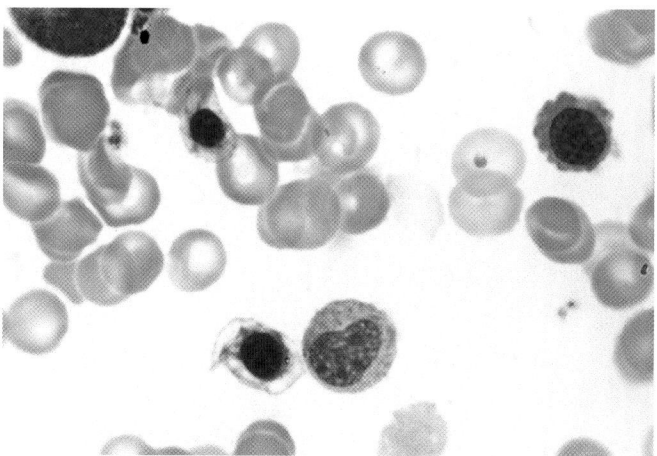

Fig. 14.5 Marrow smear from a patient with primary acquired sideroblastic anemia showing two late polychromatic erythroblasts with feebly-staining ('vacuolated') areas in the cytoplasm and one early polychromatic erythroblast with well-stained cytoplasm. May–Grünwald–Giemsa stain.

REFERENCES

1. Krantz SB 1974 Pure red cell aplasia. New England Journal of Medicine, 291: 345–350
2. Young NS, Abkowitz JL, Luzzatto L 2000 New insights into the pathophysiology of acquired cytopenias. Hematology – American Society of Hematology Education Program 18–38
3. Fisch P, Handgretinger R, Schaefer HE 2000 Pure red cell aplasia. British Journal of Haematology 111: 1010–1022
4. Diamond LK, Wang WC, Alter BP 1976 Congenital hypoplastic anemia. Advances in Pediatrics 22: 349–378
5. Hardisty RM 1976 Diamond-Blackfan anemia. In: Porter R, Fitzsimons DW (eds) Ciba Foundation Symposium 37 (new series) on congenital disorders of erythropoiesis. Elsevier, Amsterdam, 89–101
6. Dianzani I, Garelli E, Ramenghi U 1996 Diamond–Blackfan anemia: a congenital defect in erythropoiesis. Haematologica 81: 560–572
7. Lipton JM, Federman N, Khabbaze Y et al 2001 Osteogenic sarcoma associated with Diamond–Blackfan anemia: a report from the Diamond–Blackfan Anemia Registry. Journal of Pediatric Hematology and Oncology 23:39–44
8. Santucci MA, Bagnara GP, Strippoli P et al 1999 Long-term bone marrow cultures in Diamond–Blackfan anemia reveal a defect of both granulomacrophage and erythroid progenitors. Experimental Hematology 27: 9–18
9. Willig T-N, Draptchinskaia N, Dianzani I et al 1999 Mutations in ribosomal protein S19 gene and Diamond–Blackfan anemia: wide variations in phenotypic expression. Blood 94: 4294–4306
10. Brown KE 2000 Haematological consequences of parvovirus B19 infection. Bailliere's Clinical Haematology 13: 245–259
11. Kondo H, Mori A, Watanabe J et al 2001 Pure red cell aplasia associated with parvovirus B19 infection in T-large granular lymphocyte leukemia. Leukemia and Lymphoma 42: 1439–1443
12. de Las Nieves Lopez MA, Medina Perez Mf, Gonzalez Hermoso C 2000 Erythroblastopenia and parvovirus B19 infection in a healthy child. Haematologica 85(E-letters): E07
13. Jimeno Sainz A, Blazquez Encinar JC, Conesa V 2001 Pure red aplasia as the first manifestation of systemic lupus erythematosus. American Journal of Medicine 111: 78–79
14. Habib GS, Saliba WR, Froom P 2002 Pure red cell aplasia and lupus. Seminars in Arthritis and Rheumatism 31: 279–283
15. La Montagna G, Baruffo A, Abbadessa A, Felaco T 1999 Pure red cell aplasia in Felty's syndrome: a case report of successful reversal after cyclosporin A treatment. Clinical Rheumatology 18: 244–247
16. Walton T, Karim Y, Wright D et al 2001 The association of pure red cell aplasia with the antiphospholipid syndrome. Lupus 10: 899–901
17. Cobcroft R 2001 Pure red cell aplasia associated with small lymphocytic lymphoma. British Journal of Haematology 113: 260
18. Go RS, Li CY, Tefferi A, Phyliky RL 2001 Acquired pure red cell aplasia associated with lymphoproliferative disease of granular T lymphocytes. Blood 98: 483–485
19. Ohno Y, Itakura A, Sano M, Mizutani S 2002 Pure red cell aplasia and acute hepatitis during pregnancy. Gynecologic and Obstetric Investigation 53: 112–113

20. Casadevall N, Nataf J, Viron B et al 2002 Pure red cell aplasia and antierythropoietin antibodies in patients treated with recombinant erythropoietin. New England Journal of Medicine 346: 469–475

21. Freedman MH, Saunders EF 1983 Transient erythroblastopenia of childhood: varied pathogenesis. American Journal of Hematology 14: 247–254

22. Park S, Merlat A, Guesnu M et al 2000 Pure red cell aplasia associated with myelodysplastic syndromes. Leukemia 14: 1709–1710

23. Bunn HF 2002 Drug-induced autoimmune red cell aplasia. New England Journal of Medicine 346: 522–523

24. Farkas V, Szabo M, Renyi I et al 2000 Temporary pure red cell aplasia during valproate monotherapy: clinical observations and spectral electroencephalographic aspects. Journal of Child Neurology 15: 485–487

25. Bottomley SS, May BK, Cox TC et al 1995 Molecular defects of erythroid 5-aminolevulinate synthase in X-linked sideroblastic anemia. Journal of Bioenergetics and Biomembranes 27: 161–167

26. Edgar AJ, Wickramasinghe SN 1998 Hereditary sideroblastic anaemia due to a mutation in exon 10 of the erythroid 5-aminolaevulinate synthase gene. British Journal of Haematology 100: 389–392

27. Edgar AJ, Vidyatilake HMS, Wickramasinghe SN 1998 X-linked sideroblastic anaemia due to a mutation in the erythroid 5-aminolaevulinate synthase gene leading to an arginine[170] to leucine substitution. European Journal of Haematology 61: 55–58

28. Cotter PD, May A, Fitzsimons EJ et al 1995 Late-onset X-linked sideroblastic anemia. Missense mutations in the erythroid δ-aminolevulinate synthase (*ALAS2*) gene in two pyridoxine-responsive patients initially diagnosed with acquired refractory anemia and ringed sideroblasts. Journal of Clinical Investigation 96: 2090–2096

29. Furuyama K, Fujita H, Nagai T et al 1997 Pyridoxine refractory X-linked sideroblastic anemia caused by a point mutation in the erythroid 5-aninolevulinate synthase gene. Blood 90: 822–830

30. Allikmets R, Raskind WH, Hutchinson A et al 1999 Mutation of a putative mitochondrial iron transporter gene (ABC7) in X-linked sideroblastic anemia and ataxia (XLSA/A). Human Molecular Genetics 8: 743–749

31. Jardine PE, Cotter PD, Johnson SA et al 1994 Pyridoxine-refractory congenital sideroblastic anemia with evidence for autosomal inheritance: exclusion of linkage to ALAS2 at Xp11.21 by polymorphism analysis. Journal of Medical Genetics 31: 213–218

32. Smith OP, Hann IM, Woodward CE, Brockington M 1995 Pearson's marrow/pancreas syndrome: haematological features associated with deletion and duplication of mitochondrial DNA. British Journal of Haematology 90: 469–472

33. Tuckfield A, Ratnaike S, Hussein S, Metz J 1997 A novel form of hereditary sideroblastic anemia with macrocytosis. British Journal of Haematology 97: 279–285

34. Bazarbachi A, Muakkit S, Ayas M et al 1998 Thiamine-responsive myelodysplasia. British Journal of Haematology 102: 1098–1100

35. Labay V, Raz T, Baron D et al 1999 Mutations in SLC19A2 cause thiamine-responsive megaloblastic anaemia associated with diabetes mellitus and deafness. Nature Genetics 22: 300–304

36. Fleming JC, Tartaglini E, Steinkamp MP et al 1999 The gene mutated in thiamine-responsive anaemia with diabetes and deafness (TRMA) encodes a functional thiamine transporter. Nature Genetics 22: 305–308

37. Diaz G A, Banikazemi M, Oishi K et al 1999 Mutations in a new gene encoding a thiamine transporter cause thiamine-responsive megaloblastic anaemia syndrome. Nature Genetics 22: 309–312

38. Brodsky RA, Hasegawa S, Fibach E et al 1994 Acquired sideroblastic anaemia following progesterone therapy. British Journal of Haematology 87: 859–862

39. Fiske DN, McCoy HE, Kitchens CS 1994 Zinc-induced sideroblastic anemia: report of a case, review of the literature and description of the hematologic syndrome. American Journal of Hematology 46: 147–150

40. Gattermann N 2000 From sideroblastic anemia to the role of mitochondrial DNA mutations in myelodysplastic syndromes. Leukaemia Research 24: 141–151

41. Bader-Meunier B, Rötig A, Mielot F et al 1994 Refractory anemia and mitochondrial cytopathy in childhood. British Journal of Haematology 87: 381–385

42. Cheng DS, Kushner JP, Wintrobe MM 1979 Idiopathic refractory sideroblastic anemia: incidence and risk factors for leukemic transformation. Cancer 44: 724–731

43. Germing U, Gattermann N, Aivado M et al 2000 Two types of acquired idiopathic sideroblastic anaemia (AISA): a time-tested distinction. British Journal of Haematology 108: 724–728

44. Beris Ph, Samii K, Matthes T et al 1998 Study of the N Ras (codons 12, 13 and 61) in 42 patients with acquired sideroblastic anemia (ASA). Schweizerische Medizinische Wochenschrift 128 (suppl 96): 64S

45. Beris Ph, Samii K, Darbellay R et al 1999 Iron overload in patients with sideroblastic anaemia is not related to the presence of the haemochromatosis Cys282Tyr and His63Asp mutations. British Journal of Haematology 104: 97–99

46. Wicramasinghe SN, Chalmers DG, Cooper EH 1968 A study of ineffective erythropoiesis in sideroblastic anaemia and erythraemic myelosis. Cell and Tissue Kinetics 1: 43–50

47. Wickramasinghe SN, Hughes M 1978 Capacity of ringed sideroblasts to synthesize nucleic acids and protein in patients with primary acquired sideroblastic anaemia. British Journal of Haematology 38: 345–352

48. Wickramasinghe SN, Fulker MJ, Losowsky MS, Hall R 1971 Microspectrophotometric and electron microscopic studies of bone marrow in hereditary sideroblastic anaemia. Acta Haematologica 45: 236–244

Congenital dyserythropoietic anemias

15

SN Wickramasinghe

Congenital dyserythropoietic anemia, type I

Congenital dyserythropoietic anemia, type II
(hereditary erythroblastic multinuclearity with
positive acidified serum lysis test, HEMPAS)

Congenital dyserythropoietic anemia, type III

Other types of congenital dyserythropoietic anemia

Diagnosis of congenital dyserythropoietic anemia

These are a mixed group of uncommon inherited anemias.[1-4] The anemia is predominantly caused by a considerable increase in ineffective erythropoiesis and a proportion of the erythroblasts usually show morphologic abnormalities indicative of dyserythropoiesis (dysplastic changes). The ineffectiveness of erythropoiesis is suggested by a suboptimal reticulocyte response for the degree of anemia despite erythroid hyperplasia. Mainly on the basis of the nature of the dysplastic changes seen by light and electron microscopy, the congenital dyserythropoietic anemias (CDAs) have been divided into three classical types designated CDA types I, II and III (Table 15.1) and four other groups designated CDA groups IV–VII.

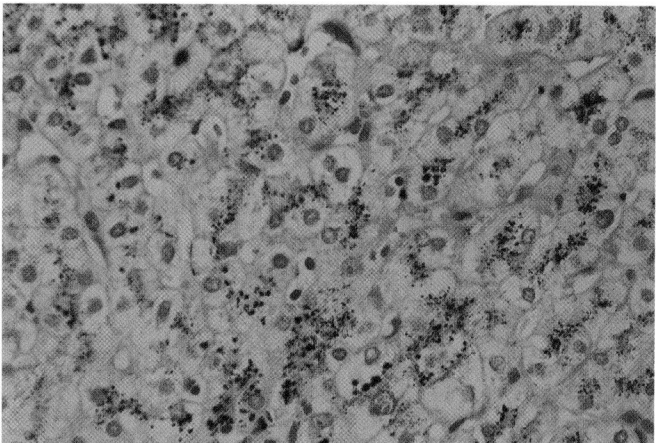

Fig. 15.1 Needle biopsy of the liver of a 40-year-old patient with CDA type I who had received few transfusions, showing grade 4/4 iron overload. Perls' stain.

Congenital dyserythropoietic anemia, type I[4-8]

This disorder may be diagnosed at birth, during the neonatal period or at any time during the first five decades of life. It may also present *in utero,* with manifestations of fetal anemia requiring antenatal transfusions. Patients usually have a mild to moderate anemia and may show mild jaundice, hepatosplenomegaly and cholelithiasis. A few cases are severely anemic and transfusion-dependent. There is a tendency for some patients who have received few or no transfusions to develop marked iron overload (Fig. 15.1). Some cases have congenital abnormalities such as syndactyly, aberrations of the bones of the hands and feet (absence or hypoplasia of some phalanges, additional phalanges), dysplastic nails, short stature and abnormal pigmentation of areas of the skin (Fig. 15.2). The disorder is inherited as an autosomal recessive character. In a highly inbred group of Israeli

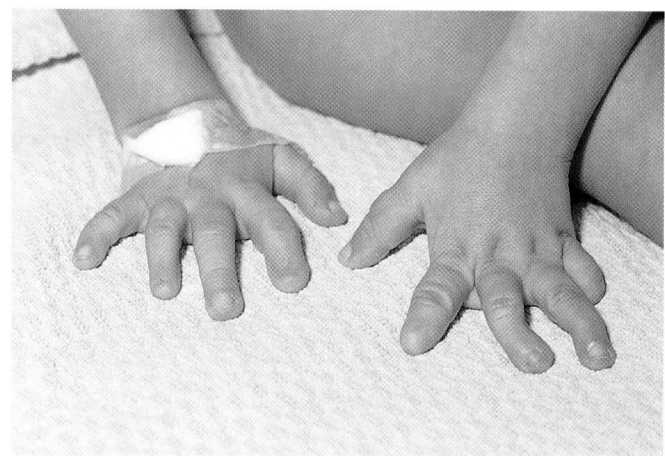

Fig. 15.2 Dysmorphic features in the hands of a child with CDA type I. In the left hand, the middle finger has an additional phalanx, the index finger lacks a distal phalanx and the little finger lacks two phalanges. Nails are missing or very small and dysplastic in two fingers of each hand. Courtesy of Professor T Pearson.

Table 15.1 Characteristics of CDA types I, II and III

	Type I	Type II	Type III
Inheritance	Autosomal recessive	Autosomal recessive	*Familial form:* autosomal dominant *Sporadic form:?* autosomal recessive or new dominant mutation
Localization of disease gene	15q15.1–15.3	20q11.2 (in ~ 90% of cases)	Swedish family: 15q22
Red cells	Macrocytes	Normocytes	Macrocytes
Erythroblasts (a) Light microscopy	Internuclear chromatin bridges	Binucleate polychromatic eythroblasts	Giant erythroblasts with up to 12 nuclei per cell
(b) Electron microscopy	'Swiss-cheese' appearance of heterochromatin	Peripheral cisternae	—
Ham test	Negative	Positive	Negative
Biochemistry	—	Underglycosylation of band 3	—

Bedouin, the disease gene *(CDAN1)* has been localized to chromosome 15q15.1–15.3. Identical haplotypes were found within the region containing *CDAN1* in the Bedouin patients but different haplotypes were found in six English cases.[8]

The average hemoglobin (Hb) is 9.0 g/dl (range 6.0–12.6 g/dl), the mean cell volume (MCV) is increased in 75% of cases, the blood film shows macrocytes and stippled red cells (Fig. 15.3) and the reticulocyte count is normal or only slightly raised. There is intense erythroid hyperplasia in the marrow (Fig. 15.4) and erythropoiesis shows megaloblastic features. Some of the more mature basophilic erythroblasts and many of the early and late polychromatic erythroblasts show dyserythropoietic features. The characteristic morphologic abnormality is an internuclear chromatin strand connecting pairs of

almost completely separated polychromatic erythroblasts (0.6–2.8 strands per 100 erythroblasts) (Fig.15.5A, B). There is also an increase in the percentage of binucleate polychromatic erythroblasts, which account for 3.5–7.0% of all erythroblasts. The latter may contain nuclei of different size and show partial fusion of the two nuclear masses; the two nuclei within the same cell may display different staining characteristics (Fig. 15.6). The most striking ultrastructural abnormality is the presence of nuclei with a spongy or 'Swiss-cheese' appearance in a high proportion (up to 60%) of the mononucleate early and late polychromatic erythroblasts; these nuclei have multiple rounded electron-lucent areas within abnormally electron-dense heterochromatin (Fig. 15.7). Nuclei having the 'Swiss-cheese' appearance may also contain nuclear-membrane-lined cytoplasmic intrusions, some-

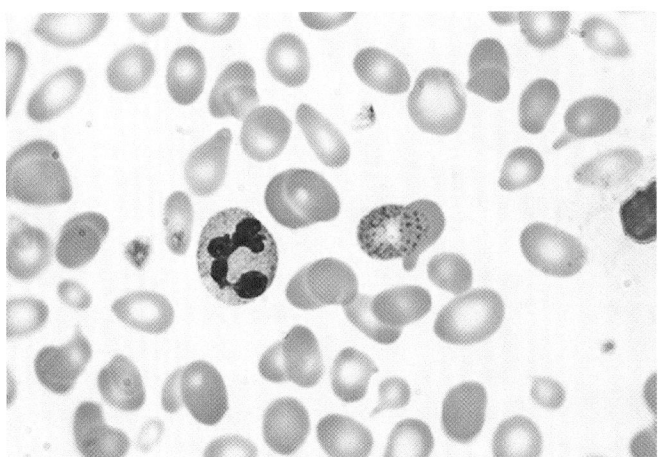

Fig. 15.3 Blood film of a case of CDA type I, showing oval macrocytes, moderate anisopoikilocytosis including tear-drop-shaped cells and a coarsely-stippled red cell. May–Grünwald–Giemsa stain.

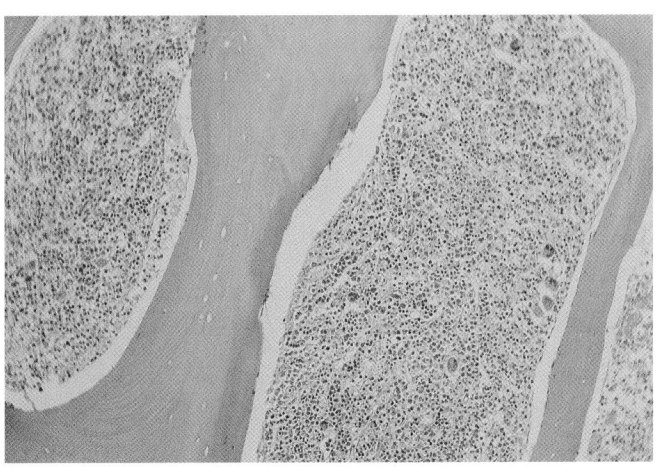

Fig. 15.4 Trephine biopsy of bone marrow from a patient with CDA type I, showing an intensely hypercellular marrow with complete replacement of fat cells by hemopoietic (largely erythropoietic) cells. Hematoxylin and eosin.

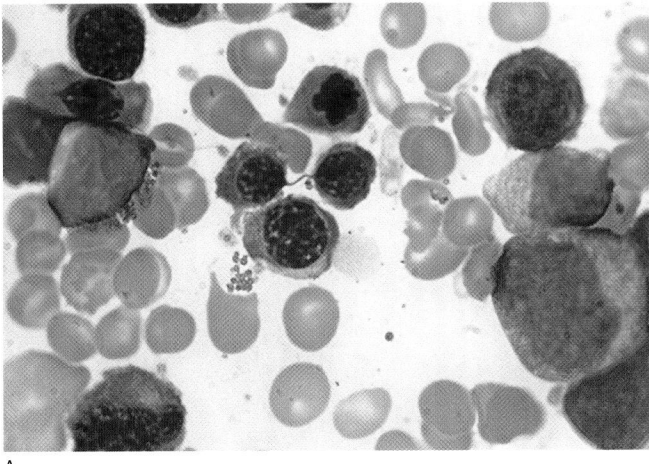

A

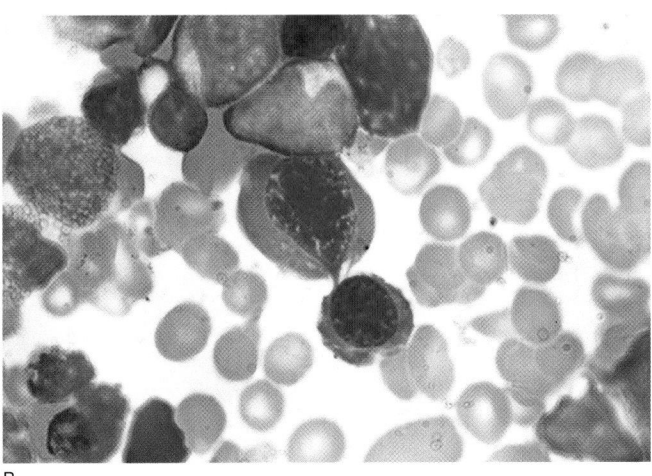

B

Fig. 15.5 (A, B) Internuclear chromatin strands joining incompletely separated erythroblasts in a marrow smear from a case of CDA type I. In (A) the chromatin strand connects two nuclei of equal size and in (B) the joined nuclei are unequal. May–Grünwald–Giemsa stain.

times with cytoplasmic organelles (Fig. 15.7b). An abnormally low percentage of mononucleate early polychromatic erythroblasts synthesize DNA; the non-DNA-synthesizing cells have DNA contents between the 2c and 8c values (1c = the haploid DNA content, i.e. the DNA content of a spermatozoon) and appear to be derived from the maturation of cells which have become arrested during their progress through the cell cycle. There is a marked increase in ineffective erythropoiesis as the result of a high rate of intramedullary destruction of the morphologically abnormal cells.

Some patients show a hematological response to splenectomy. Several cases have responded to interferon-α, with an increase in Hb, a decrease in MCV, a decrease in the proportion of erythroblasts with the 'Swiss-cheese' ultrastructural abnormality and a decrease in ineffective erythropoiesis.[1,9]

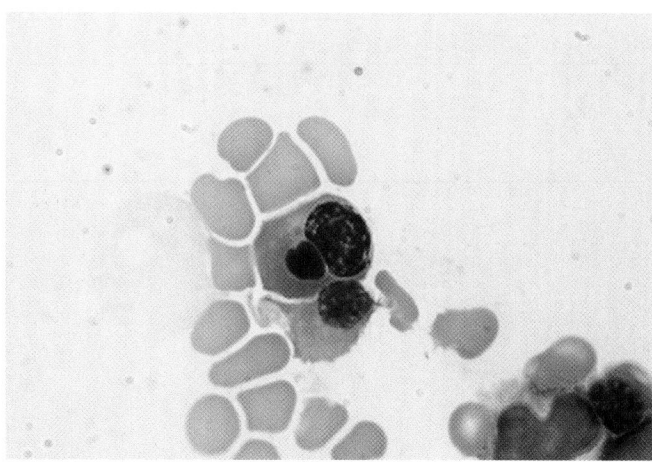

Fig. 15.6 Marrow smear from a case of CDA type I showing a binucleate erythroblast in which the two nuclei have stained differently. The other two erythroblasts in the photomicrograph are joined by an internuclear chromatin strand that has been stretched during the preparation of the smear. May–Grünwald–Giemsa stain.

Congenital dyserythropoietic anemia, type II (hereditary erythroblastic multinuclearity with positive acidified serum lysis test, HEMPAS)[10–12]

This is the commonest type of CDA. Many of the reported cases have had southern Italian ancestry but cases have also been reported from northwest Europe and north Africa. Clinical features include mild to moderate anemia, mild jaundice, splenomegaly in 65% of cases, cholelithiasis and a tendency to develop iron-overload. Patients usually present between 1 month and 25 years but there is frequently a delay in establishing the diagnosis. The disorder is inherited as an autosomal recessive character and in about 90% of cases the disease gene (*CDAN2*) is on chromosome 20q11.2.

The average Hb is about 8 g/dl. The red cells are normochromic and normocytic and show moderate anisocytosis, poikilocytosis and basophilic stippling. The reticulocyte count is either normal or only slightly raised.

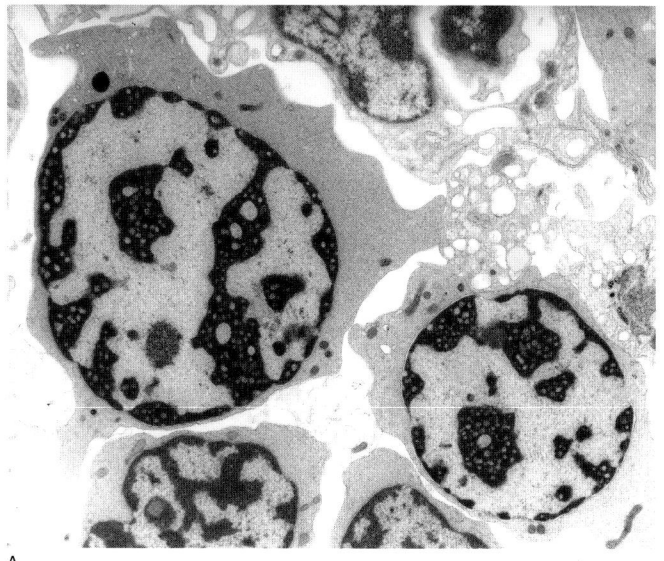

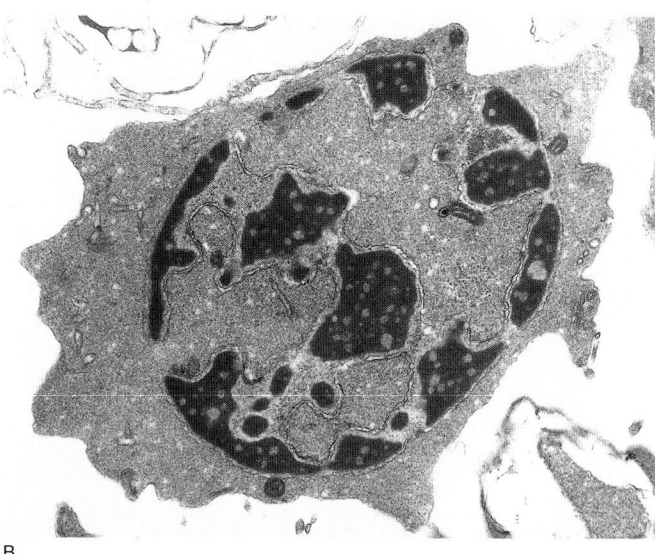

A

B

Fig. 15.7 (A, B) Electron micrographs of erythroblasts from a case of CDA type I, showing the 'Swiss-cheese' abnormality of the heterochromatin. (A) Two erythroblasts with abnormally electron-dense, spongy heterochromatin adjacent to two cells with normal-looking heterochromatin. (B) Erythroblast displaying invaginations of the nuclear membrane. There are nuclear-membrane-bound areas enclosing cytoplasm and cytoplasmic organelles within the nucleus. Uranyl acetate and lead citrate.

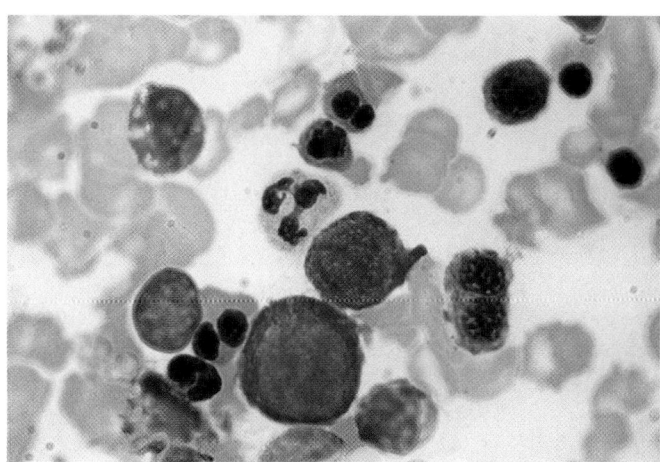

Fig. 15.8 Bone marrow smear of a patient with CDA type II, showing three binucleate late polychromatic erythroblasts and one binucleate early polychromatic erythroblast. The two nuclei of one of the late erythroblasts are stuck together and each shows a bud-like protrusion. May–Grünwald–Giemsa stain.

Some cases are only mildly anemic or not anemic and occasional patients are transfusion-dependent, even without coinheritance of β-thalassemia trait. The bone marrow shows normoblastic erythroid hyperplasia. A few of the basophilic erythropoietic cells and early polychromatic erythroblasts and 10–35% of the late erythroblasts are binucleate; the nuclei are usually of equal size (Fig. 15.8). In addition, a small proportion of the erythroblasts are trinucleate or multinucleate. Many of the mononucleate and binucleate late erythroblasts have orthochromatic cytoplasm and highly-condensed, apparently structureless nuclei. The anemia results from ineffectiveness of erythropoiesis, there being a high rate of phagocytosis of mononucleate and binucleate late erythroblasts by bone marrow macrophages. Electron microscope studies reveal a characteristic double membrane (consisting of smooth endoplasmic reticulum) aligned parallel to and at a distance of 40–60 nm from the cell membrane in a substantial proportion of the late erythroblasts (Fig. 15.9A,B). These double membranes are referred to as peripheral cisternae. Bone marrow macrophages are often laden with lipid and appear as pseudo-Gaucher cells (Fig. 15.9C).

The red cells give a positive acidified serum lysis test with about 30% of fresh ABO-compatible normal sera but not with the patient's own serum. The reactive sera contain an IgM antibody that combines specifically with an antigen on HEMPAS red cells. This antibody can be removed by absorption with red cells of cases of HEMPAS but not of patients with paroxysmal nocturnal hemoglobinuria.

The anion transport protein (band 3) of the red cell membrane is underglycosylated and, consequently, is thinner and moves faster than normal on SDS polyacrylamide gel electrophoresis (SDS-PAGE). Different glycosylation enzymes have been found to be reduced in activity in different patients and linkage analyses have excluded N-acetylglucosaminyltransferase II and α-mannosidase II as the disease genes.

Splenectomy results in a substantial increase in Hb in some cases.

Congenital dyserythropoietic anemia, type III[1,13–15]

This is the rarest of the three classical types of CDA. Two forms of CDA type III exist, one which is inherited as an autosomal dominant characteristic and a sporadic form which could either be due to a new dominant mutation or possibly be inherited as an autosomal recessive character. The family with the autosomal dominant form of CDA type III that has been most investigated is from northern Sweden and contains 34 affected individuals in five generations. In this family, the disease gene (*CDAN3*) has been localized to chromosome 15q22.

The clinical features of the Swedish cases of CDA type III include mild or moderate anemia, mild jaundice, cholelithiasis, increased prevalence of monoclonal gammopathy of uncertain significance and myeloma and, in older patients, visual symptoms associated with macular degeneration and angioid streaks. The spleen is not palpable and iron overload does not develop, at least partly because of increased iron loss from hemosiderinuria secondary to some intravascular hemolysis. The disorder runs a relatively benign course. Most cases are diagnosed in older children or adults.

The features of the sporadic form of CDA type III vary from case to case and include hepatosplenomegaly (in most cases), a mongoloid face, mental retardation, hemosiderinuria, severe iron overload (one case), and the development of Hodgkin's disease and T-cell lymphoma (two cases).

In CDA type III, the Hb is usually between 7 and 14 g/dl, the MCV is usually high or normal and the granulocyte and platelet counts are normal. The blood film shows macrocytes (and, sometimes, occasional giant erythrocytes), poikilocytosis, fragmented red cells and basophilic stippling. The reticulocyte count is normal or slightly raised. The acidified serum lysis test is negative. The bone marrow shows marked erythroid hyperplasia, megaloblastic erythropoiesis in the absence of vitamin B_{12} or folate deficiency and the presence of some large uninucleate erythroblasts with big lobulated nuclei and

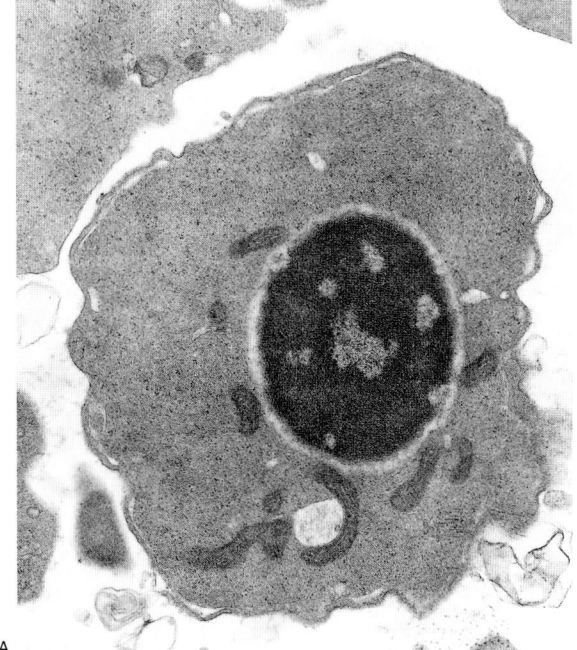

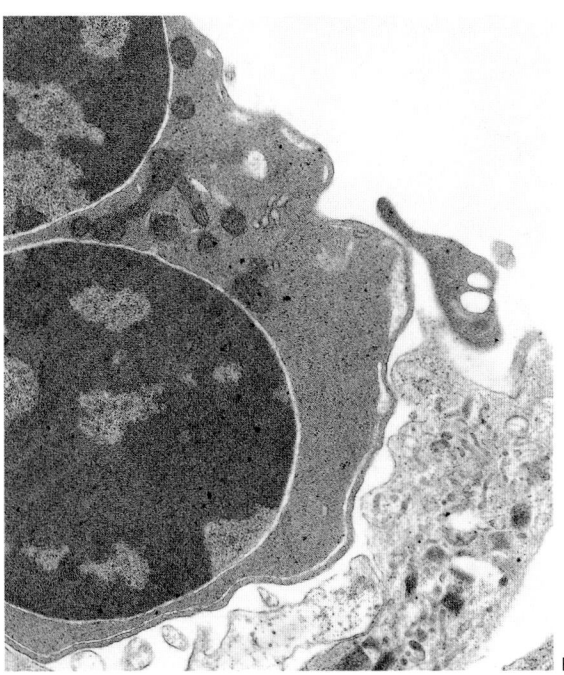

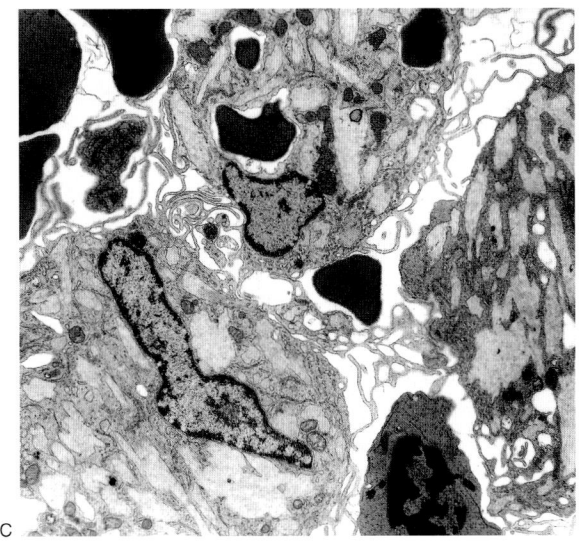

Fig. 15.9 (A–C) Electron micrographs of bone marrow cells from a case of CDA type II. (A) (B) A mononucleate and a binucleate late polychromatic erythroblast showing the characteristic double membrane running parallel to the cell membrane. (C) Cluster of three pseudo-Gaucher cells, each with several large electron-lucent secondary lysosomes containing lipid. Uranyl acetate and lead citrate. (A) × 14 500; (B) × 17 700; (C) × 4800. (C) From Wickramasinghe.[4]

many giant multinucleate erythroblasts with up to 12 nuclei per cell. The tendency to multinuclearity begins in the basophilic erythropoietic cells but is most marked in the early and late polychromatic erythroblasts. Over 35% of all erythroblasts may be binucleate or multinucleate (Fig. 15.10) and the latter may have total DNA contents up to 40c. Sometimes the two nuclei of a binucleate cell or two or more of the nuclei within a multinucleate cell are joined together either by a narrow strand of chromatin or over a wide area of contact. The nuclear masses within multinucleate erythroblasts are rounded in outline and equal in size and staining characteristics in some cells but irregular in shape, unequal in size or different in their staining characteristics in others. The giant mononucleate

erythroblasts have DNA contents up to 20c. Other abnormalities affecting erythroblasts include coarse basophilic stippling of the cytoplasm and karyorrhexis. Electron microscope studies show a variety of non-specific abnormalities including differences in the ultrastructural appearances of different nuclei within the same multinucleate cell (Fig. 15.11). In addition, in some patients occasional erythroblast sections contain stellate or branching intracytoplasmic inclusions composed of precipitated β-globin chains (Fig. 15.12).[16,17] The anemia results largely from ineffective erythropoiesis; both mononucleate and multinucleate cells may be seen within bone marrow macrophages.

Other types of congenital dyserythropoietic anemia[1,3]

About 40% of the cases of CDA diagnosed in the UK are of types other than types I–III and the most frequent of these has been designated CDA group IV. A tentative classification of other forms of CDA is given in Table 15.2.

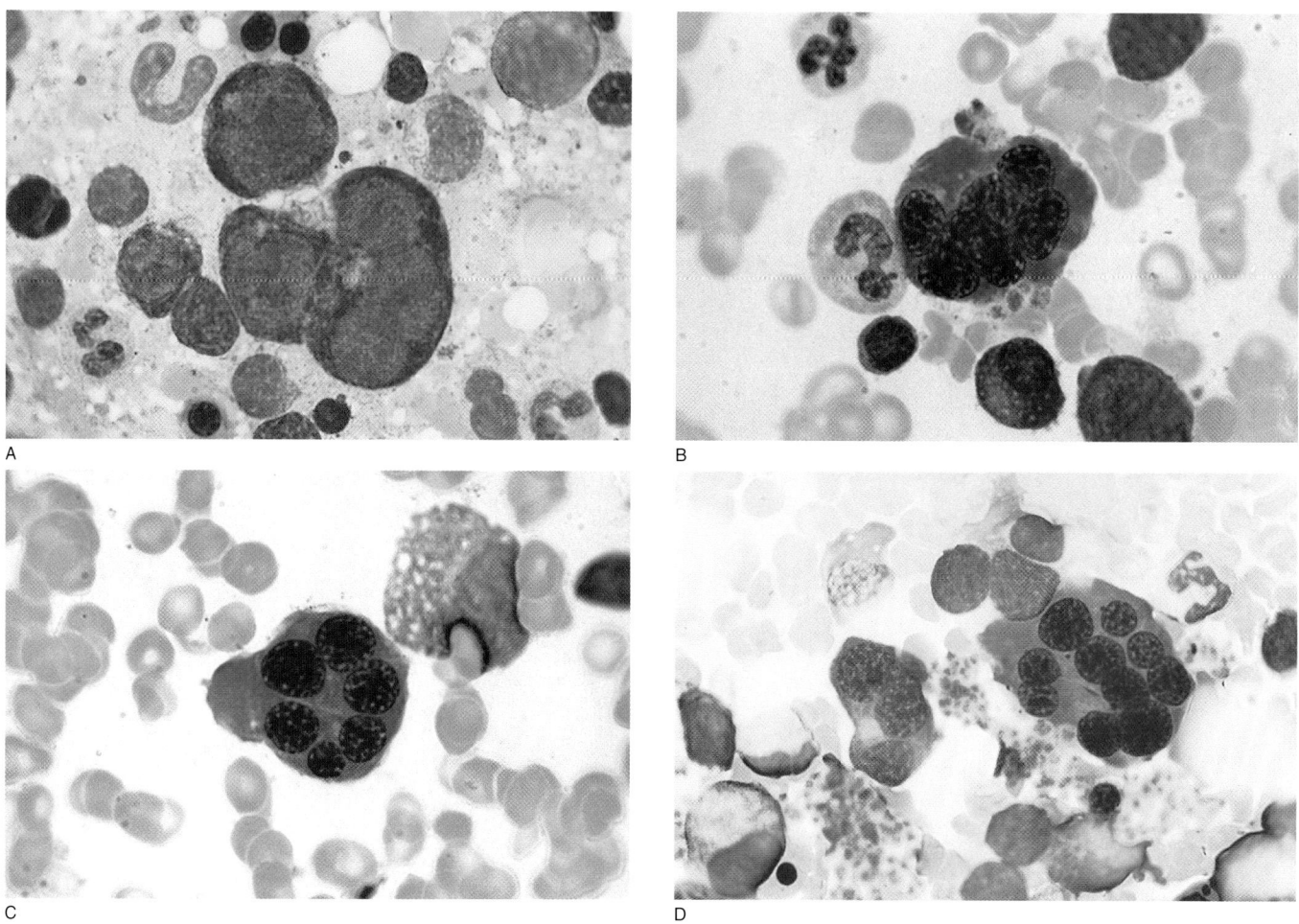

Fig. 15.10 (A–D) Bone marrow cells of a patient from the Swedish family with CDA type III. (A) Tetranucleate basophilic erythropoietic cell near two mononucleate basophilic erythropoietic cells. (B)–(D) Giant multinucleate polychromatic erythroblasts. The cell in (D) contains 10 nuclei. May–Grünwald–Giemsa stain.

Table 15.2 Defining features of CDA groups IV–VII

Group	Essential features
IV	Severe transfusion-dependent anemia Marked normoblastic erythroid hyperplasia with a slight to moderate increase in the percentage of erythroblasts with very irregular or karyorrhectic nuclei (Fig. 15.13) Absence of precipitated protein within erythroblasts
V	Normal or near-normal Hb with normal or slightly increased MCV Predominantly unconjugated hyperbilirubinemia Marked normoblastic/slightly megaloblastic erythroid hyperplasia Little or no erythroid dysplasia
VI	Normal or near-normal Hb with marked macrocytosis (MCV 119–125 fl) Erythroid hyperplasia with cobalamin- and folate-independent florid megaloblastic erythropoiesis (Fig. 15.14)
VII[17]	Severe transfusion-dependent anemia Severe normoblastic erythroid hyperplasia with irregular nuclear shapes in many erythroblasts (Fig. 15.15) Intraerythroblastic inclusions resembling precipitated globin that fail to react with antibodies to α- or β-globin chains (Fig. 15.16)

In most cases, inheritance is likely to have been as an autosomal recessive character or there may have been a new dominant mutation. However, in CDA group V, both autosomal recessive and dominant patterns of inherit-ance have been suggested. Homozygosity for pyruvate kinase deficiency should be excluded before the diagnosis of CDA group IV is considered. Splenectomy has been beneficial in some cases of CDA group IV.

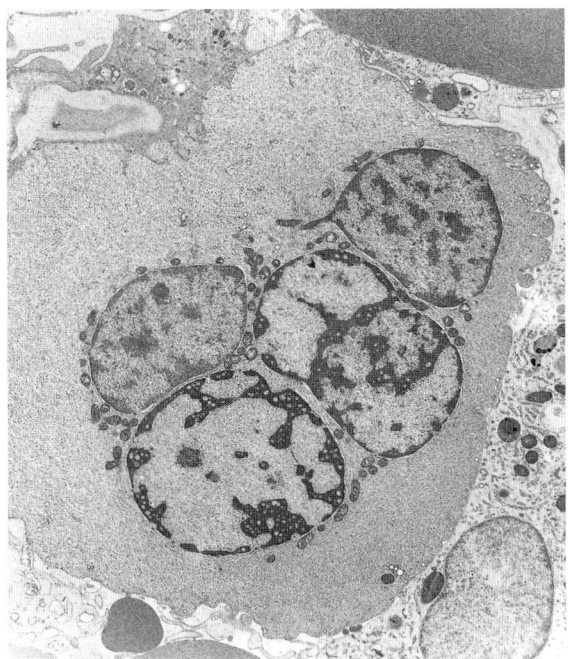

Fig. 15.11 Electron micrograph of a giant multinucleate erythroblast from a case with the sporadic form of CDA type III. Note the different ultrastructural appearances of the different nuclei within the same cell. Uranyl acetate and lead citrate. × 3500.

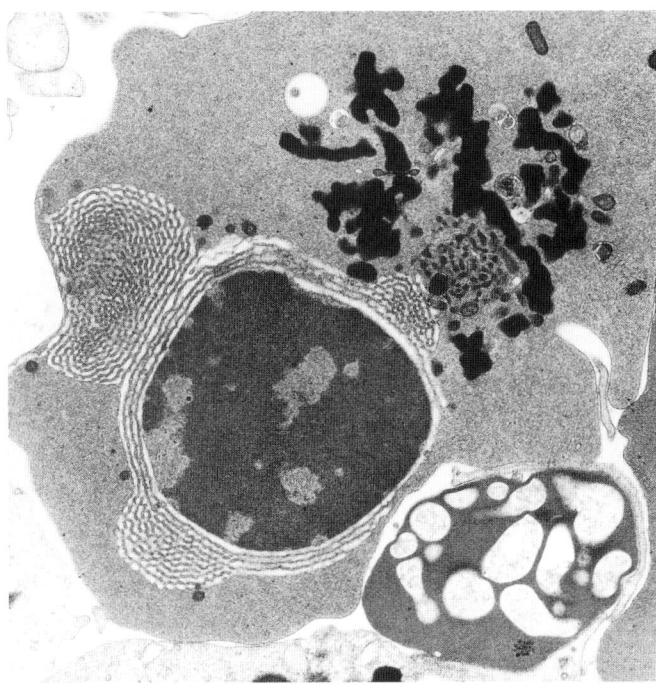

Fig. 15.12 Electron micrograph of an eythroblast from a patient with the sporadic form of CDA type III, showing branching intracytoplasmic inclusions and extensive reduplication of the nuclear membrane. From Wickramasinghe and Goudsmit.[16]

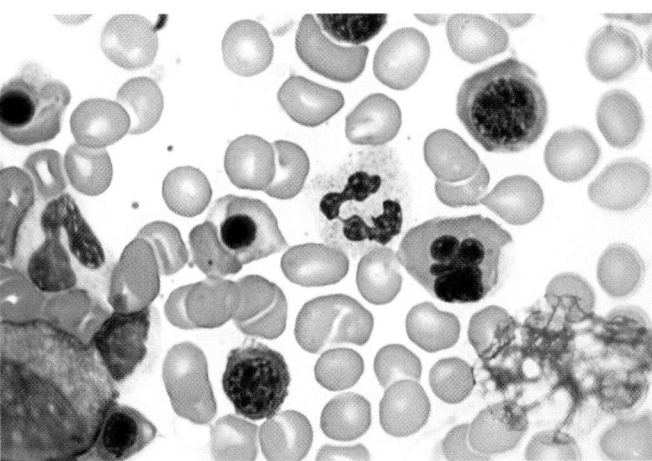

Fig. 15.13 Erythroblasts from a marrow smear from a case of CDA group IV. One of the erythroblasts has a lobulated nucleus. May–Grünwald–Giemsa stain.

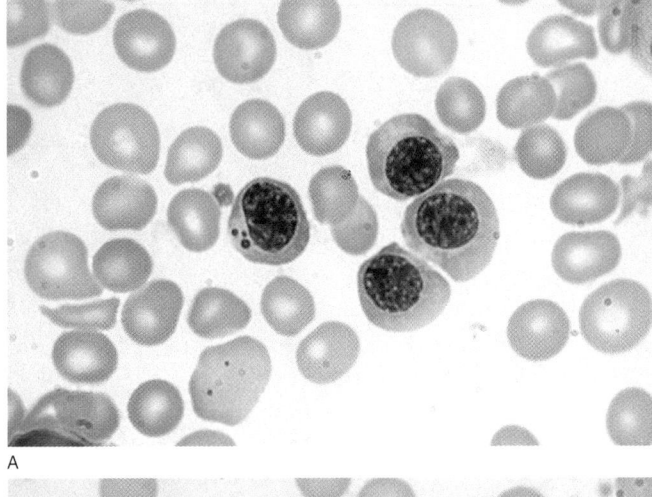

A

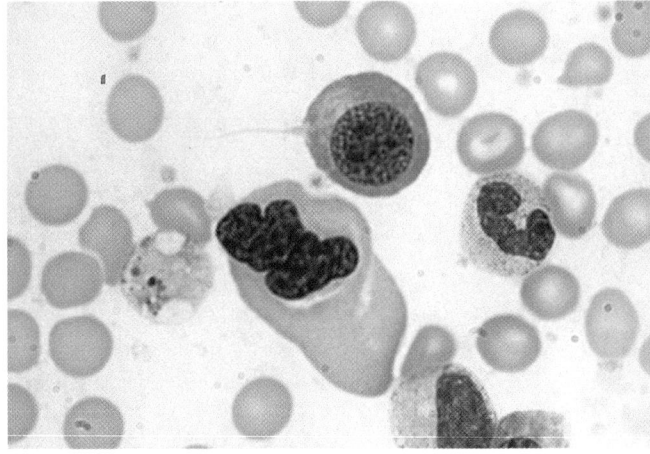

B

Fig. 15.14 (A, B)Megaloblasts from a case of CDA group VI. The megaloblastic change is florid despite an Hb of 14.5 g/dl (MCV 125 fl). One of the megaloblasts and a polychromatic macrocyte in (A) contain Howell–Jolly bodies and the binucleate megaloblast in (B) has irregular nuclear outlines. May–Grünwald–Giemsa stain.

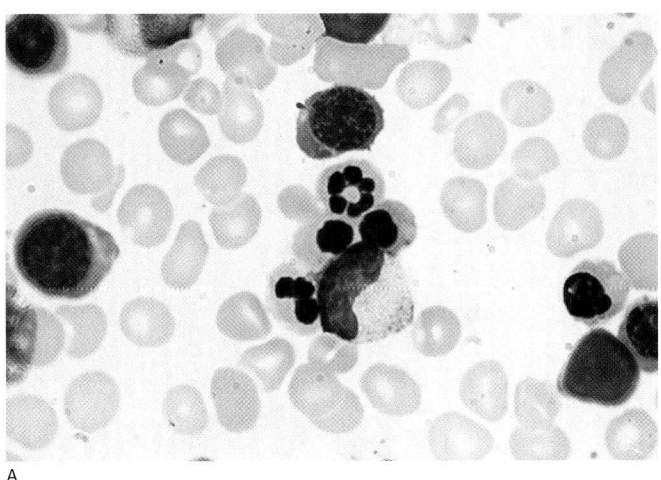

A

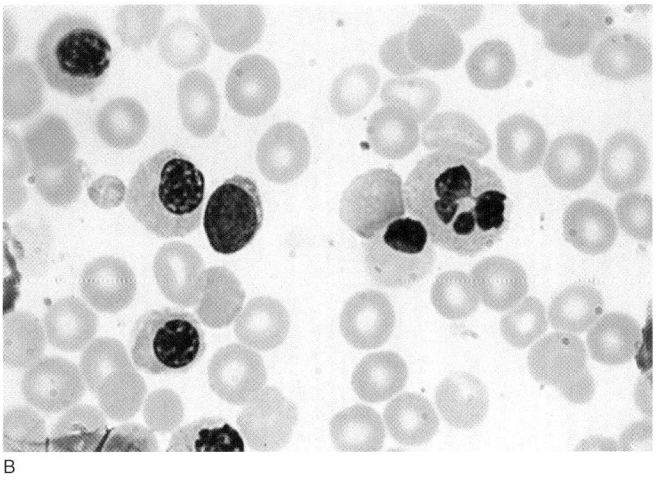

B

Fig. 15.15 (A, B) Cells from marrow smears of two patients with CDA group VII. (A) One of the late erythroblasts has a ring-shaped nucleus with six nuclear segments and another has a nucleus with three segments. (B) One of the erythroblasts has four nuclear masses joined by fine chromatin strands.

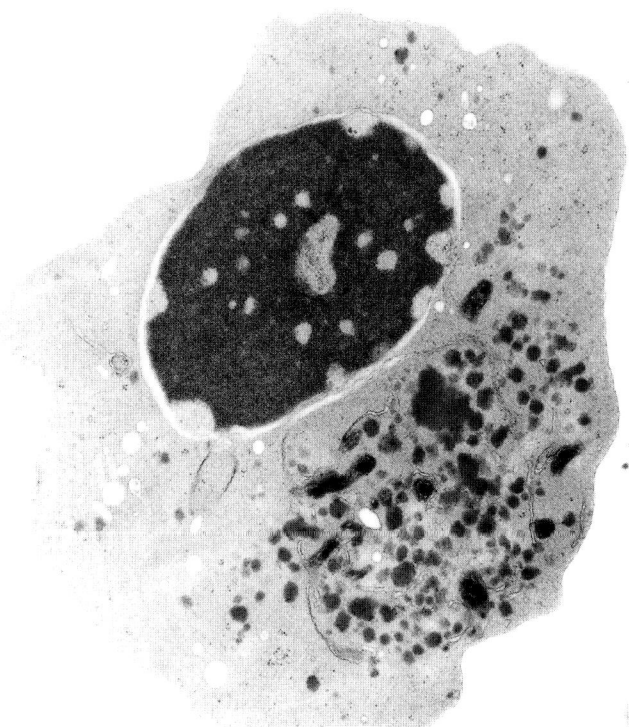

Fig. 15.16 Electron micrograph of an erythroblast from a patient with CDA group VII, showing multiple electron-dense foci of precipitated non-globin protein. Much of this material appears to be enclosed within a double membrane. From Wickramasinghe et al.[17] Uranyl acetate and lead citrate.

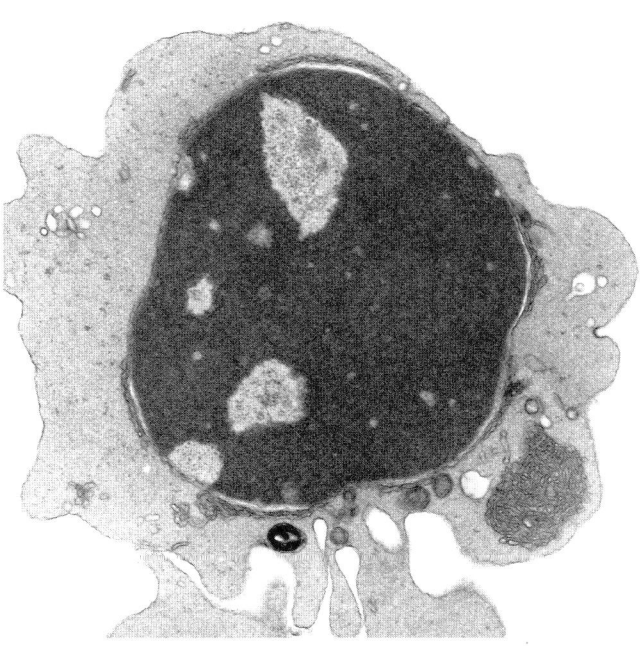

Fig. 15.17 Electron micrograph of an erythroblast from a child with a deficiency of erythroid CD44, showing a compact mass of double membranes within the cytoplasm. Intertwining double membranes are also apposed to large areas of the nuclear membrane. Uranyl acetate and lead citrate.

In addition to CDA groups IV–VII, single cases or families of CDA with unique features have been reported. For example, a Danish patient with CDA had a deficiency of erythroid but not leukocyte CD44, the Colton blood group phenotype Co(a- b-), 50% HbF, small amounts of embryonic globin chains in some red cells, a marked reduction of aquaporin I (the channel-forming integral protein or CHIP) but no mutation in the gene encoding CHIP and novel intraerythroblastic inclusions.[18] The inclusions consisted of large compact masses of double membranes (Fig. 15.17). In another family, the blood films of a non-anemic father and daughter showed oval macrocytes and basophilic stippling of red cells and bone marrow smears from the father showed dysplastic changes in erythroblasts including internuclear chromatin strands joining nearly-completely separated erythroblasts. However, unlike in CDA type I, the ultrastructure of erythroblast heterochromatin was normal.[19]

Diagnosis of congenital dyserythropoietic anemia

The possibility of CDA should be considered whenever there is a suboptimal absolute reticulocyte count for the degree of anemia, unexplained hyperbilirubinemia or unexplained iron overload. Acquired dyserythropoiesis and causes of congenital dyserythropoiesis of known etiology (conventionally not included under the heading CDA) must be excluded. Causes of acquired and congenital dyserythropoiesis[4] are given in Chapter 5. The diagnosis of specific types or groups of CDA depends on the demonstration of their characteristic features and especially on the light and electron microscope appearances of the bone marrow erythroblasts.

REFERENCES

1. Wickramasinghe SN 2000 Congenital dyserythropoietic anemias. Current Opinion in Hematology 7: 71–78
2. Delaunay J, Iolascon A 1999 The congenital dyserythropoietic anaemias. Baillière's Clinical Haematology 12(4): 691–705
3. Wickramasinghe SN 1998 Congenital dyserythropoietic anaemias: clinical features, haematological morphology and new biochemical data. Blood Reviews 12: 178–200
4. Wickramasinghe SN 1997 Dyserythropoiesis and congenital dyserythropoietic anaemias. British Journal of Haematology 98: 785–797
5. Tamary H, Shalev H, Luria D et al 1996 Clinical features and studies of erythropoiesis in Israeli Bedouins with congenital dyserythropoietic anemia type I. Blood 87: 1763–1770
6. Shalev H, Tamary H, Shaft D et al 1997 Neonatal manifestations of congenital dyserythropoietic anemia type I. Journal of Pediatrics 131: 95–97
7. Tamary H, Shalmon L, Shalev H et al 1998 Localization of the gene for congenital dyserythropoietic anemia type I to a < 1-cM interval on chromosome 15q15.1–15.3. American Journal of Human Genetics 62: 1062–1069
8. Hodges VM, Molloy GY, Wickramasinghe SN 1999 Genetic heterogeneity of congenital dyserythropoietic anemia type I. Blood 94: 1139–1140
9. Lavabre-Bertrand T, Blanc P, Navarro R et al 1995 Alpha-interferon therapy for congenital dyserythropoiesis type I. British Journal of Haematology 89: 929–932
10. Iolascon A, D'Agostaro G, Perrotta S et al 1996 Congenital dyserythropoietic anemia type II. Molecular basis and clinical aspects. Haematologica 81: 542–558
11. Gasparini P, del Giudice EM, Delaunay J et al 1997 Localization of the congenital dyserythropoietic anemia II locus to chromosome 20q11.2 by genomewide search. American Journal of Human Genetics 61: 1112–1116
12. Iolascon A, De Mattia D, Perrotta S et al 1998 Genetic heterogeneity of congenital dyserythropoietic anemia type II. Blood 92: 2593–2594
13. Sandstrom H, Wahlin A 2000 Congenital dyserythropoietic anaemia type III. Haematologica 85: 753–757
14. Sandström H, Wahlin A, Eriksson M et al 1994 Intravascular haemolysis and increased prevalence of myeloma and monoclonal gammopathy in congenital dyserythropoietic anaemia, type III. European Journal of Haematology 52: 42–46
15. Lind L, Sandström H, Wahlin A et al 1995 Localization of the gene for congenital dyserythropoietic anemia type III, CDAN3, to chromosome 15q21–q25. Human Molecular Genetics 4: 109–112
16. Wickramasinghe SN, Goudsmit R 1987 Precipitation of β-globin chains within the erythropoietic cells of a patient with congenital dyserythropoietic anaemia, type III. British Journal of Haematology 65: 250–251
17. Wickramasinghe SN, Lee MJ, Furukawa T et al 1996 Composition of the intra-erythroblastic precipitates in thalassaemia and congenital dyserythropoietic anaemia (CDA): identification of a new type of CDA with intra-erythroblastic precipitates not reacting with monoclonal antibodies to α- and β-globin chains. British Journal of Haematology 93: 576–585
18. Parsons SF, Jones J, Anstee DJ et al 1994 A novel form of congenital dyserythropoietic anemia (CDA) associated with deficiency of erythroid CD44 and a unique blood group phenotype [In (a-b-), Co(a-b-)]. Blood 83: 860–868
19. Wickramasinghe SN, Spearing RL, Hill GR 1998 Congenital dyserythropoiesis with intererythroblastic chromatin bridges and ultrastructurally-normal erythroblast heterochromatin: a new disorder. British Journal of Haematology 103: 831–834

Polycythemia (the erythrocytoses)

M Messinezy   JD van der Walt   TC Pearson

16

Introduction

Hematocrit (PCV) and red cell mass (RCM)

Polycythemia vera (PV)

Clinical features

Investigations for the diagnosis of PV

Exclusion of causes of secondary erythrocytosis

Examination of karyotype and demonstration of clonality

Minor degrees of splenomegaly

Serum erythropoietin (Epo)

Culture studies of BFU-E (burst-forming units – erythroid)

Bone marrow appearances and disease progression

Differential diagnosis of bone marrow appearances

Spleen histology

Treatment of PV

Secondary erythrocytosis

Management of secondary erythrocytosis

Idiopathic erythrocytosis

Management of idiopathic erythrocytosis

Apparent erythrocytosis

Management of apparent erythrocytosis

Introduction

'Polycythemia' is derived from Greek words meaning 'too many cells in the blood'. The name in itself does not suggest which type(s) of cells are being referred to, and therefore the term 'erythrocytoses' is to be preferred. This makes it clear that these diseases relate to too many red cells. There are a number of types of erythrocytosis each of which is considered in this chapter. First and clearly distinct from the rest is *polycythemia vera* (PV). This differs from the other erythrocytoses in being a clonal disorder[1] originating from a single neoplastic stem cell in the bone marrow. PV is also a member of the group of interrelated myeloproliferative disorders[2] (primary thrombocythemia, chronic idiopathic myelofibrosis, chronic myeloid leukemia) sharing many of their features. The term polycythemia is still appropriate for this clonal disorder because PV is the only erythrocytosis in which not only red cells but often also white cells and platelets are increased. The older name was polycythemia rubra vera but this is both cumbersome and slightly misleading as it is usually not only the red cells that are involved. Another name for PV was primary polycythemia which usefully indicates that the abnormality originates in the bone marrow rather than being secondary to a pathologic process outside it. However, the recent recognition of a primary congenital erythrocytosis, namely truncation of the erythropoietin receptor (see below), means that confusion could arise. Therefore, PV is now the preferred name and links satisfactorily with the historically established older name. There are three additional erythrocytoses to be considered: *secondary, idiopathic* and *apparent erythrocytosis*.

Hematocrit (PCV) and red cell mass (RCM)

Though packed cell volume (PCV) and hemoglobin (Hb) values both depend on the number of red cells present, PCV is the more reliable indicator on which the definition of erythrocytosis is based.[3] This is because the not uncommon association with iron deficiency will lower the Hb rather more than the PCV value, thereby resulting in some patients with borderline erythrocytosis being missed. *Erythrocytosis is present when the PCV is > 0.51 in males and > 0.48 in females* though as with all 'normal' values, each laboratory should ideally generate its own reference range. However, a normal PCV may be misleading in situations where there could be an increased RCM as in splenomegaly, or if the plasma volume is expanded. In iron deficiency (microcytosis) some elec-

Table 16.1 Traditional classification of the erythrocytoses

Erythrocytosis (PCV males > 0.51 females > 0.48)	
Absolute erythrocytosis (increased RCM)	Apparent erythrocytosis (normal RCM)
• Polycythemia vera • Secondary erythrocytosis • Idiopathic erythrocytosis	

PCV, packed cell volume; RCM, red cell mass.

tronic red cell counters underestimate the real PCV value. The true PCV when there is microcytosis is obtained by the microhematocrit method or by applying a correction to the electronic counter result.

Once PCV estimation has established the presence of an erythrocytosis, the next stage in its elucidation is measurement of RCM traditionally by a chromium isotope red cell labeling dilution method or by technetium labeling. There has been considerable controversy about how best to standardize and express the results of this time-consuming estimation. Though ml/kg body weight is still widely used, it can underestimate the RCM in obesity because fat tissue is relatively avascular. The preferred expression of a result is by comparison of the measured value of RCM with that predicted to be normal for the patient's gender, height and weight.[4] Since 98–99% of normal individuals have a measured RCM value falling within ± 25% of the predicted value for their height and weight, this is defined as a 'normal' RCM. *Values of RCM ≥ 25% above the predicted value are called an 'absolute erythrocytosis'.* Since the RCM measurement itself has an error of ± 5%, results may be misinterpreted, especially when close to the upper limit for the 'normal' RCM. If the PCV is 0.60 or greater in males, and greater than 0.56 in females, it is not essential to measure the RCM, as there will almost certainly be an absolute erythrocytosis. Three types of erythrocytosis (primary erythrocytosis which includes congenital erythrocytosis and PV, secondary erythrocytosis, idiopathic erythrocytosis) have an absolute increase in RCM (absolute erythrocytosis) while erythrocytosis associated with a normal RCM is known as apparent erythrocytosis (Tables 16.1 and 16.2). Unfortunately, it is possible for two causes of erythrocytosis to coexist in a single patient, especially when elderly.

Polycythemia vera (PV)

PV is so far the only known example of erythrocytosis due to an intrinsic or primary bone marrow defect which is acquired rather than congenital (Table 16.2), though there are occasional familial cases. It is now well

Table 16.2 Extended subclassification of absolute erythrocytosis

		Absolute erythrocytosis		
Primary		Secondary		Idiopathic
Congenital	Acquired	Congenital	Acquired	
• Truncation Epo receptor	• Polycythemia vera	• High-oxygen-affinity Hb • Autonomous high Epo production	• Hypoxemia • Renal tumors, etc.	

Epo, erythropoietin.

established that the red cells, granulocytes and platelets in PV are all derived from a single aberrant bone marrow stem cell resulting from one or more somatic mutations. The abnormal clone differentiates into red and white cells with normal morphology. The basic abnormality is in the clone's apparently autonomous proliferation and lack of response to normal controlling mechanisms. The molecular aberrations present in PV are currently being defined but the abnormality is unlikely to be identical in all patients.

Clinical features

Like most clonal disorders, PV is a disease of older age groups (though not exclusively), the median age at presentation being 55–60 years, with slight male preponderance. Presentation as an incidental blood count finding is common but a large proportion of patients present with vascular complications (30–50%).[5] These may be arterial (particularly cerebral thrombosis) or venous and include microvascular digital occlusion (Fig. 16.1). The occlusive tendency is due partly to the increased PCV

and Hb with resultant reduction in peripheral blood flow but also to the platelets which may be increased in number, abnormal in size and function and marginalized towards the endothelial surface by the increased volume of red cells. Concurrently, there may also be an increased hemorrhagic risk, which can result, for example, in dramatic hematomas after surgical procedures. Aquagenic pruritus and gout are classical features occurring in a minority of patients. Palpable splenomegaly when present (in about one-third of patients with PV) is a very important finding because, being a hallmark of myeloproliferative disorders, it distinguishes PV from the other erythrocytoses. The splenomegaly could of course occasionally be due to the incidental presence of other diseases.

Investigations for the diagnosis of PV

A modern scheme of major and minor criteria for the diagnosis of PV[6] is shown in Table 16.3. The criteria act as a reminder of relevant investigations in patients who have an absolute erythrocytosis. A raised RCM (absolute erythrocytosis) is the defining feature that distinguishes PV from the other myeloproliferative disorders (primary thrombocythemia, chronic idiopathic myelofibrosis,

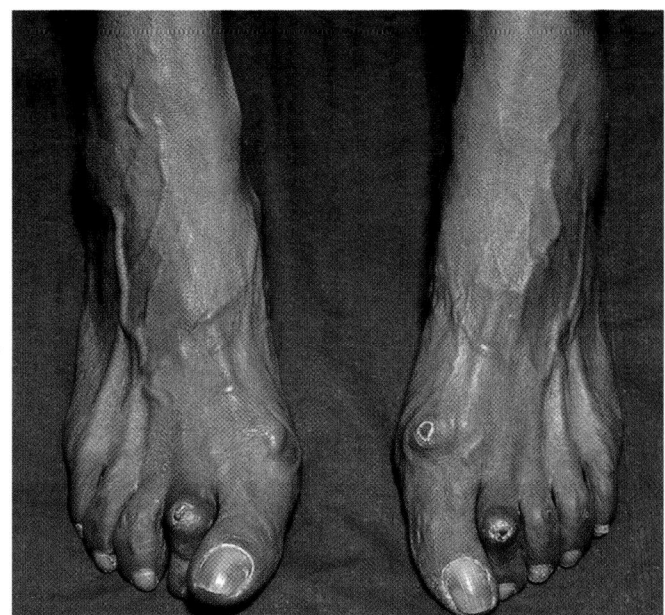

Fig. 16.1 Gangrenous toes in PV.

Table 16.3 Criteria for diagnosis of PV

	MAJOR criteria	
in all	• Raised RCM	
in all	• Absence of secondary erythrocytosis	
	AND $\rightarrow$	OR
either *or*	• Palpable splenomegaly • Acquired abnormal karyotype	TWO MINOR criteria • Platelets > 400 × 10⁹/l • Neutrophils > 10 × 10⁹/l > 12.5 × 10⁹/l in smokers • Very low serum Epo *or* characteristic BFU-E growth • mild splenomegaly by imaging

BFU-E, Erythroid burst-forming units; Epo, erythropoietin; RCM, red cell mass.

chronic myeloid leukemia). Absolute erythrocytosis is also, of course, a feature of secondary erythrocytosis which needs to be excluded in all patients suspected of having PV (see below). However there are a number of factors that may confuse the issue. In the first place, iron deficiency is not unusual in PV mainly because of hemorrhage and may be unsuspected unless routinely considered. If iron deficiency is found, it is often difficult to be certain whether the RCM would have been raised in its absence and preliminary iron therapy is not usually an option. Secondly, splenomegaly with associated red cell pooling and plasma volume expansion may lower the PCV sometimes into the normal range so that the need to measure the RCM may not be considered. Finally, common sense suggests that PV at its earliest stage may not yet have achieved an absolute erythrocytosis at the time the RCM is measured.

Once a raised RCM has been established and secondary erythrocytosis has been excluded, either palpable splenomegaly or an acquired abnormal karyotype are major criteria which will establish the diagnosis of PV in the small number of patients in whom they are present.

The majority of patients with PV also have a neutrophil leukocytosis ($> 10.0 \times 10^9$/l) or thrombocytosis ($> 400 \times 10^9$/l) or both, though there can be reasons other than PV for these findings which are only minor criteria. Further minor criteria (only two minor criteria are necessary for the diagnosis of PV in patients without either palpable splenomegaly or abnormal karyotype) are a reduced serum erythropoietin (Epo) level (or characteristic erythroid burst-forming units [BFU-E] growth) or mild splenomegaly by imaging. These are discussed below.

Exclusion of causes of secondary erythrocytosis

Table 16.4 shows some of the large number of conditions that may be associated with acquired secondary erythrocytosis, predominantly via increased Epo secretion. These, as well as congenital causes of secondary erythrocytosis (Table 16.2), are discussed in greater detail in the secondary erythrocytosis section below. However, exclusion of causes of secondary erythrocytosis is essential in order to make the diagnosis of PV. Not unexpectedly, this may not always be possible, either because the cause is unusual and has not been recognized or looked for, or because the condition is at an early stage that is not detectable by the methods used. In addition, some of the more common causes could by chance coexist with PV in the same patient. Routine screening for hypoxemia by pulse oximetry is usual, but the value of 92% oxygen

Table 16.4 Causes of acquired secondary erythrocytosis

Stimulation of Epo secretion *by arterial hypoxemia:*
• Chronic lung disease (± smoking)
• Cyanotic congenital heart disease
• Sleep apnea syndrome
• High altitude

Presumed stimulation of Epo secretion *without arterial hypoxemia:*
• Renal lesions (adenocarcinoma, cysts, diffuse disease, hydronephrosis, renal transplant, artery stenosis)
• Hepatoma, liver cirrhosis, hepatitis
• Tumors (adrenal, bronchial carcinoma, fibroids, cerebellar hemangioblastoma)
• Androgen therapy

Epo, erythropoietin.

saturation traditionally taken as the dividing line is insecure (see below). Abdominal ultrasound for renal and hepatic conditions (as well as spleen sizing), carbon-monoxy hemoglobin level, p50 estimation to demonstrate the presence of a high-oxygen-affinity hemoglobin, and serum Epo estimation are all deemed essential screening tests in a patient with absolute erythrocytosis.

Examination of karyotype and demonstration of clonality

It soon became clear even in the early days of chromosome analysis, that unlike in chronic myeloid leukemia (CML), there was not going to be a single chromosome abnormality that defined all patients with PV. Nevertheless, karyotypic analysis has been revealing in these patients[7] and deeper understanding at gene and molecular level may explain pathogenetic mechanisms or at least have prognostic implications for patients in whom the abnormalities are found. Only about 10–15% of patients with PV are currently found to have a karyotypic abnormality at diagnosis, the commonest being 20q and 13q deletions, followed by trisomies of 1, 8 and 9 (Fig. 16.2).[8] Such findings are good evidence of a clonal abnormality and therefore diagnostically helpful in PV. In the future, many other abnormalities are likely to be found at gene level which are not currently evident by routine methods of karyotypic analysis. A link between some such abnormalities and the pathologic process is suggested by the fact that translocations seem to occur at sites of tumor suppressor genes, which may lead not only to dominantly-acting fusion oncogenes but also to gene loss which may disturb normal hematopoiesis. A need for diagnostic caution is suggested by the fact that similar karyotypic abnormalities are found in myelodysplastic syndromes. These syndromes form a spectrum overlap-

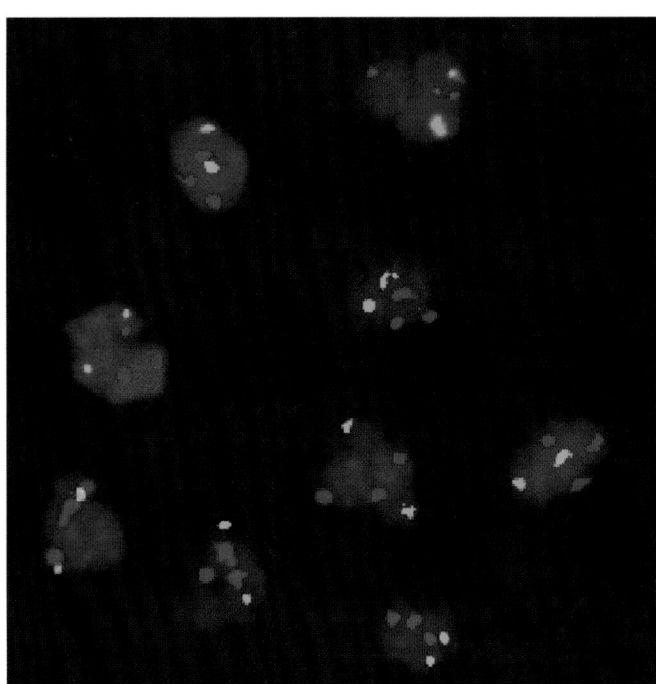

Fig. 16.2 Trisomy 8 in PV revealed by FISH. Interphase fluorescence *in situ* hybridization (I-FISH) was applied to blood neutrophils from a PV patient. Red dots identify chromosome 8 centromeres, green dots identify chromosome 9 centromeres (by kind permission of NB Westwood and AM Gruszka–Westwood).

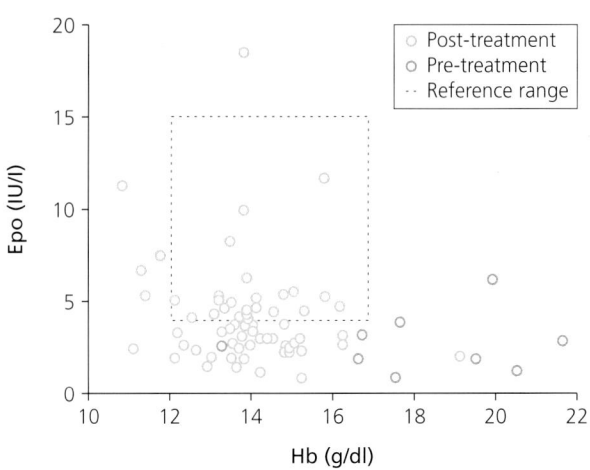

Fig. 16.3 Relationship between serum Epo and Hb in PV. From Messinezy,[13] with permission.

ping in some cases with the features of myeloproliferative disorders.

Attempts made to demonstrate disease clonality in a more direct fashion than by karyotypic analysis have been less successful than hoped.[9] One method using X-linked probes, such as the HUMARA gene, apart from being only applicable to females, has major drawbacks in that apparent clonality is frequently demonstrated in normal older women.[10] A reliable and universally applicable way of demonstrating clonality could provide the single marker needed for the easy diagnosis of PV but it is not yet available.

Minor degrees of splenomegaly

While palpable splenomegaly is a major diagnostic criterion of PV, the significance to be attached to lesser degrees of splenomegaly, where the spleen is not yet palpable, are still uncertain. Moreover the imaging methods used are poorly standardized. Radioisotope volume measurements of the spleen are possible[11] but cumbersome. Ultrasound volume measurements are being developed. Currently, measurement of maximum spleen length on abdominal ultrasound is at least easy and a convenient alternative. Its use can largely but not entirely separate patients with PV from those with other

erythrocytoses. A maximum length of 12 cm can be taken as the upper limit of normal but this is not a precise value because of variability due to age and body size (a complicated formula is available that takes these factors into account).[12] Moreover, lack of precision in the ultrasound technique and sometimes an inability to exclude other causes of mild splenomegaly, makes this measurement only a minor criterion in the diagnosis of PV.

Serum erythropoietin (Epo)

Values well below the normal range are found in the majority of patients with PV even after treatment has returned the PCV to normal (Fig. 16.3).[13] Some centers attach major significance to this finding in the diagnosis of PV. However, a need for caution is indicated by the fact that low levels can also be found in some patients with apparent or with idiopathic erythrocytosis especially at pretreatment raised Hb values and also in many patients with the myeloproliferative disorder primary thrombocythemia. Moreover, low values are seen in those rare familial erythrocytoses[14,15] due to mutation of the Epo receptor gene causing truncation of the cytoplasmic portion of the Epo receptor and consequent inability to switch off the signal following Epo binding (hypersensitivity to Epo). This condition resembles PV in being a primary erythrocytosis (abnormality intrinsic to the bone marrow) but is congenital rather than acquired (Table 16.2). Recent ELISA kit methods for measuring serum Epo are more reliable than past methods but there is still considerable variability and the reference range should ideally be determined by each laboratory. The use of serum Epo estimation as only a minor diagnostic criterion of PV seems realistic at present.

Culture studies of BFU-E (burst-forming units – erythroid)

Culture of red cell progenitors *in vitro* has been seen as a promising way of attempting to reveal differences between PV and the other erythrocytoses. BFU-E in PV patients are hypersensitive to a number of different growth factors including Epo, IL-3 and insulin-like growth factor. Endogenous erythroid colonies (EEC) which grow in serum-containing media without any addition of Epo are believed to be a marker of PV.[16,17] They probably grow because of hypersensitivity to the small amount of Epo in the serum contained in the culture medium. The reliability of such observations may be suspect and technical improvements in terms of Epo response curves or the effect of other growth factors (Interferon and IL-3) on growth in serum-free media in the presence of Epo have been used at the expense of sensitivity, cost and convenience.[18] Moreover, BFU-E hypersensitivity to Epo is also found in the rare erythrocytoses resulting from cytoplasmic Epo receptor truncation mentioned above and is not therefore specific to PV. Though certain observations are still regarded as a minor criterion in the diagnosis of PV, tests involving culture of red cell progenitors are costly, difficult to standardize, and unlikely to become routine.

Bone marrow appearances and disease progression

The histopathology of the bone marrow in PV shares features in common with other members of the group of chronic myeloproliferative disorders (CMPD). The differ-ential diagnosis is considered below. The appearance of the bone marrow in PV depends on the phase of the disease. Three phases are recognized, referred to here as proliferative phase, spent phase and acute transformation.

In the proliferative phase, the marrow is usually markedly hypercellular, but cellularity is variable and may be normocellular in 5% of cases[19] (Figs. 16.4 and 16.5). The proliferation is a panmyelosis – erythropoiesis, megakaryopoiesis and granulopoiesis are all increased in PV. Erythropoiesis and granulopoiesis are morphologically unremarkable[20] but megakaryopoiesis shows significant morphological abnormalities (Fig. 16.6) that may be of value in distinguishing PV from the other CMPD.[21] The megakaryocytes appear in clusters and have a pleomorphic appearance[22] – there is a wide range in megakaryocyte size, ranging from micromegakaryocytes with simple nuclei to giant forms with multiple nuclear segments.[21–23] The sinusoids may be dilated and branching with intrasinusoidal hemopoiesis.[20] Eosinophilia and basophilia may be noted.[20]

Iron stores are either markedly reduced or completely absent.[19,22] This may be noted on hematoxylin and eosin staining and confirmed by Perls' stain for iron. There is increased reticulin staining in the initial diagnostic biopsy in a minority of cases of PV, advanced collagen sclerosis with or without osteosclerosis being seen in approximately 5% of cases.[24]

After 5–20 years from diagnosis, the proliferative phase is followed in 10–20% of patients by the usually gradual evolution of the spent phase.[25,26] After 20 years, as many as 30% of surviving patients may progress to a spent phase with so-called post-polycythemic myelofibrosis. This coincides with a falling Hb level, increasing splenomegaly and a leukoerythroblastic blood picture with the appearance of tear-drop poikilocytes.[25] The bone

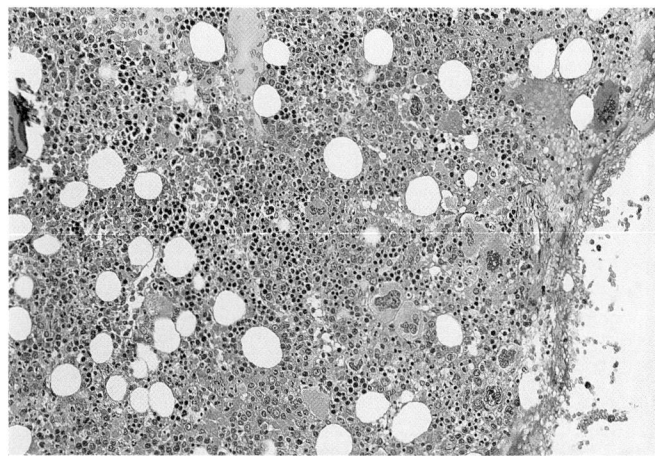

Fig. 16.4 PV showing panmyelosis and a moderately hypercellular marrow.

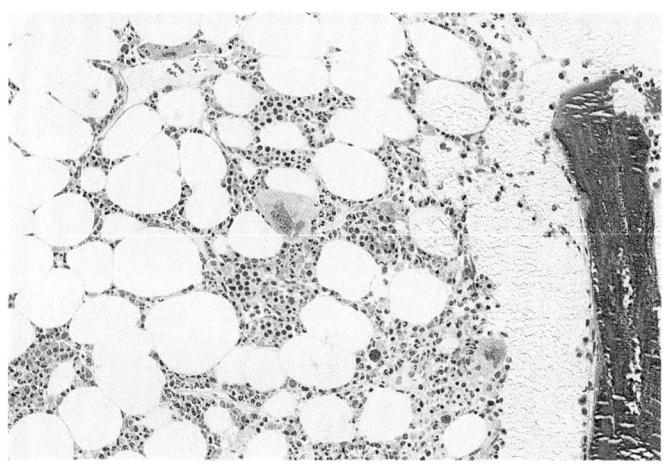

Fig. 16.5 A case of PV showing a normocellular marrow. Characteristic megakaryocytes are seen.

marrow, which may at first be cellular, shows increasing reticulin fibers (Figs 16.7–16.9) and, in some cases, collagenous fibrosis[25] (Figs 16.10–16.14) which may be demonstrated by the elastic-van Gieson stain. The spent phase is associated with a poor prognosis and higher incidence of progression to acute leukemia.[20]

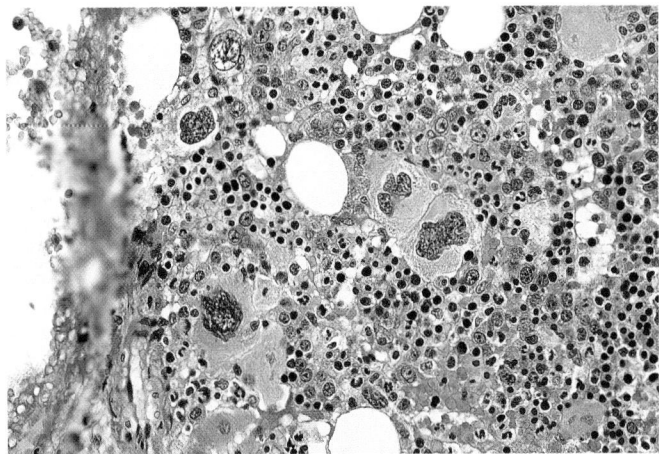

Fig. 16.6 Detail showing megakaryocyte morphology and erythroid proliferation.

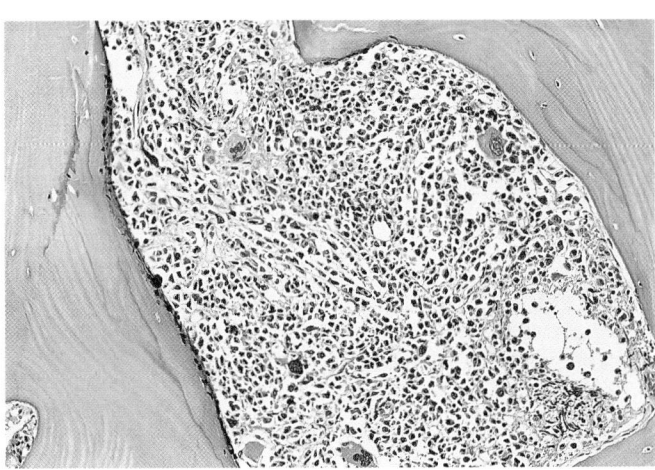

Fig. 16.7 A case of PV showing a markedly hypercellular marrow and early myelofibrosis.

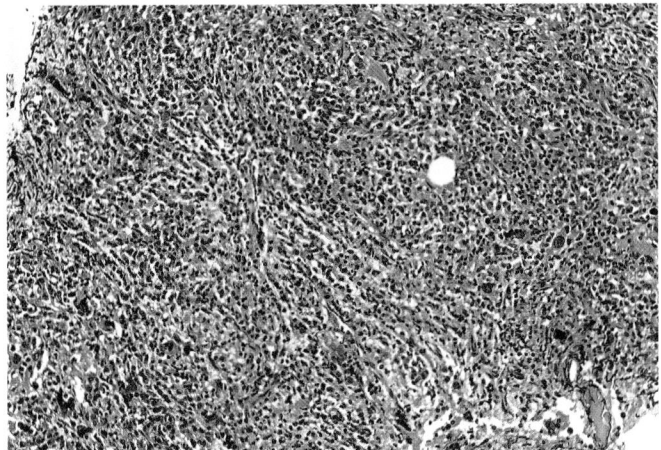

Fig. 16.8 A case of PV showing a markedly hypercellular marrow and established myelofibrosis.

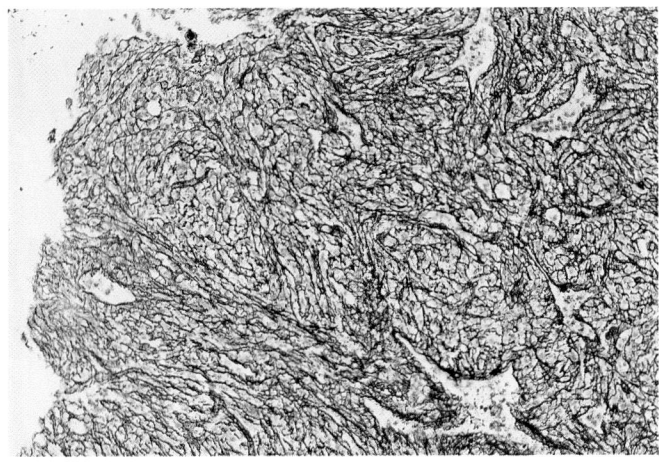

Fig. 16.9 Reticulin stain on Fig. 16.8 showing dense reticulin.

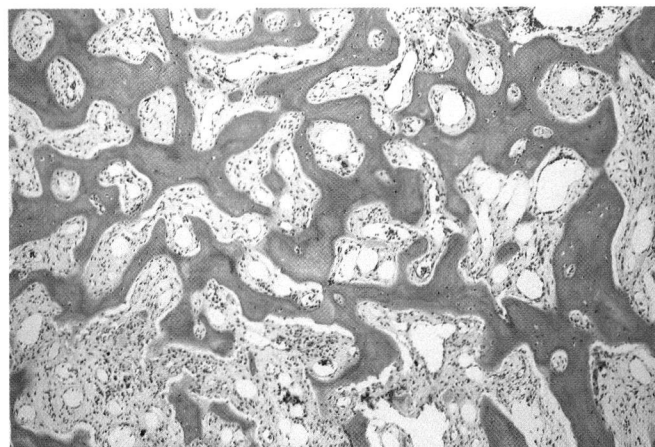

Fig. 16.10 Spent phase showing osteomyelofibrosis and a hypocellular marrow.

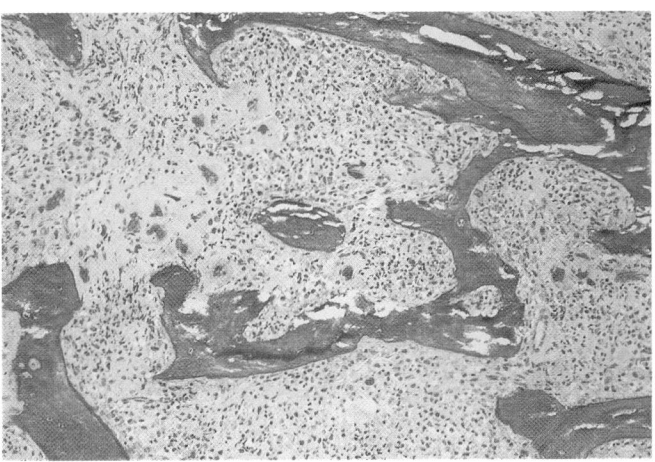

Fig. 16.11 Spent phase showing osteomyelofibrosis and a hypercellular marrow.

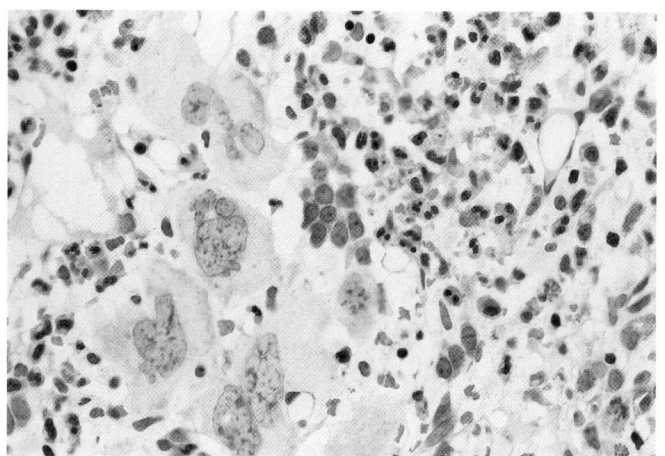

Fig. 16.12 Detail of Fig. 16.11 showing megakaryocyte morphology and erythroid proliferation.

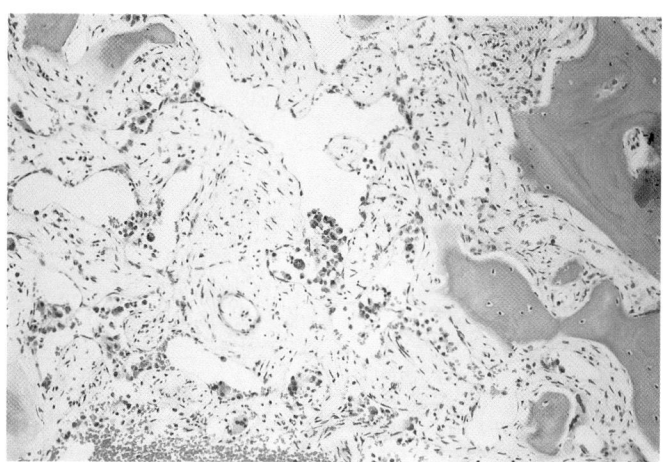

Fig. 16.13 Detail of Fig. 16.11 showing dilated sinusoids.

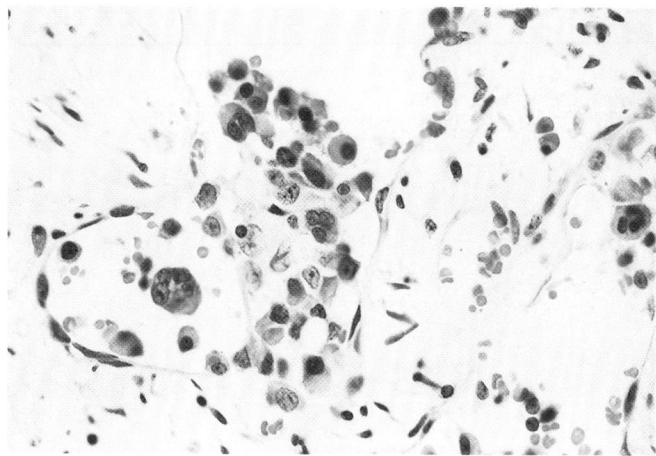

Fig. 16.14 Detail of Fig. 16.11 showing intrasinusoidal hemopoiesis.

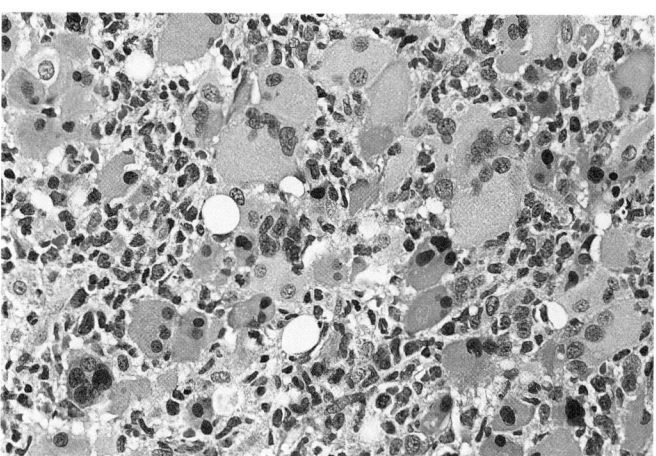

Fig. 16.15 A case of acute transformation of PV showing marked megakaryocyte proliferation in a background of myeloid blasts.

Between 5 and 10% of PV patients progress to acute transformation (Fig. 16.15).[20,27] The incidence is higher in patients who have been treated with ^{32}P or alkylating agents.[20,25,27] Any type of acute myeloid leukemia may occur,[27] while acute lymphoblastic leukemia[28,29] is very rare.

Megakaryoblastic transformation is distinctly uncommon.[30] Other malignancies have also been found to occur in PV and include chronic lymphocytic leukemia and other non-Hodgkin's lymphomas.[27,31] The development of lymphoid neoplasia has led to the suggestion that expansion of a pluripotential hemopoietic stem is involved in both PV and the lymphoid neoplasia.[29,31] In ^{32}P treated patients who survive 20 years, the combined risk of myelodysplasia, leukemia and lymphoma reaches 30%.[26] Myelodysplasia may precede the development of acute leukemia[32,33] and may present without the prior development of myelofibrosis.[32] Progression to other chronic myeloproliferative disorders is very rare but Ph[1]-positive chronic myeloid leukemia[34,35] and chronic neutrophilic leukemia have been described.[36]

The assessment of transformation in the marrow does not differ from that of *de novo* disease. The trephine biopsy should be always assessed in conjunction with the peripheral blood findings and the bone marrow aspirate. Nevertheless, immunocytochemical techniques are particularly useful in cases of peripheral pancytopenia and 'dry taps' associated with myelofibrosis. Commonly available antibodies that are particularly suitable for paraffin sections of bone marrow include:[20] CD3 (T-cells), CD10 (various B-cell neoplasms including lymphoblastic leukemia), CD20 (B-cells excluding plasma cells), CD79a (B-cells), CD34 (hemopoietic stem cells and early myeloid and lymphoid precursors), CD61 (megakaryocytes and precursors), CD68-DAKO PG-M1 (macrophages and monocytes), Glycophorin A (erythroid series from erythroblasts onwards), neutrophil elastase (neutrophil granulocytes and their precursors) and myeloperoxidase (granulocyte precursors).

Differential diagnosis of bone marrow appearances

The differential diagnosis depends on whether the biopsy has been taken as part of the investigation of erythrocytosis or on whether the pathologist is confronted with a hypercellular marrow in which there is a prominent erythroid component. In all cases, clinical and hematologic data should be taken into account,[37] but there are important morphologic differences that should allow a diagnosis in most cases, particularly when considering the early proliferative phase of PV.

Secondary erythrocytosis (see below), being in fact hyperplasia rather than a true myeloproliferative disorder, may show a hypercellular marrow with a prominent erythroid component,[20,25] but lacks the characteristic panmyelosis, megakaryocyte abnormalities[21,22,25] and iron depletion[19,22] typical of PV (Fig. 16.16 and 16.17). The same criteria apply to reactive hyperplasia following such conditions as hemolysis (Fig. 16.18).

Distinction of PV from the other CMPD is an occasional problem, particularly when clinical and laboratory findings are atypical. Primary thrombocythemia does not exhibit trilineage proliferation and the megakaryocytes are very large and do not show the variation in sizes from large to small seen in PV.[22,23] Chronic idiopathic myelofibrosis may cause difficulty, particularly in the so-called prefibrotic stage. However, erythropoiesis is not increased and the megakaryocytes exhibit marked morphologic atypicality not seen in the early proliferative phase of PV.[23] Chronic granulocytic leukemia does not show an increase in erythropoiesis and megakaryocytes are small with hypolobated nuclei.[23] The presence of visible iron in CMPD other than PV is useful additional evidence against a diagnosis of PV in which iron is usually absent.[19,22]

In the late stages of PV, the development of fibrosis or acute transformation may render the distinction from other CMPD difficult or impossible. However, a previous clinical history or preceding biopsies should allow an informative assessment to be made.[25]

Spleen histology

In common with other CMPD, the spleen may be involved in PV.[38] In the early proliferative phase, there is congestion with mature erythrocytes but no extramedullary hemopoiesis.[38] Later in the evolution of the disease, in the spent phase, there is prominent trilineage extramedullary hemopoiesis (Fig. 16.19).[38] The development of extramedullary hemopoiesis correlates with increasing reticulin in the bone marrow and the development of a leuko-erythroblastic blood picture.

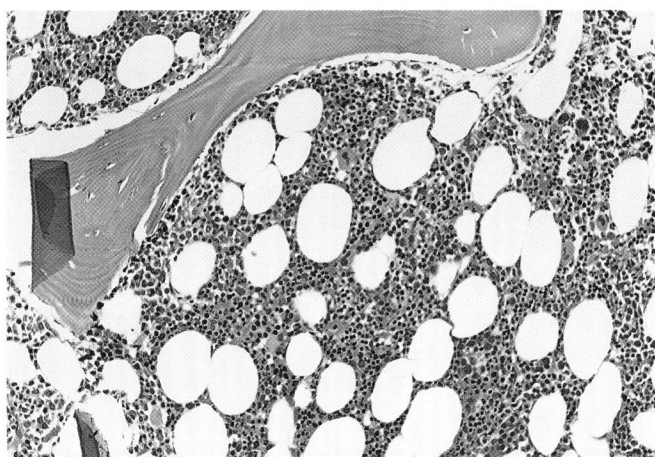

Fig. 16.16 A case of secondary erythrocytosis. Cellularity is mildly increased due to erythroid hyperplasia but megakaryocyte morphology is normal.

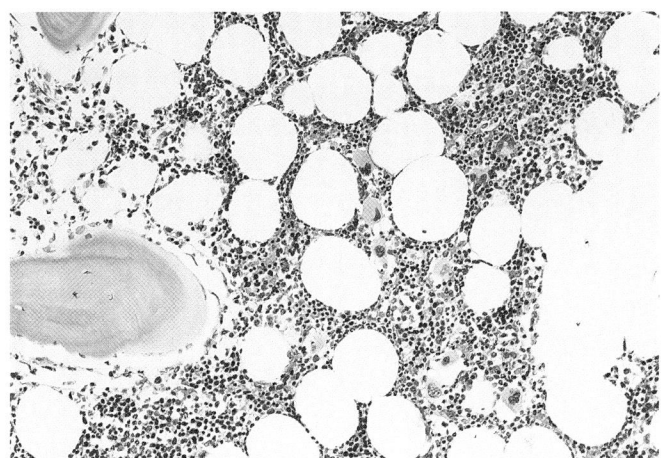

Fig. 16.17 Perls' stain for iron in Fig. 16.16 confirms normal iron stores.

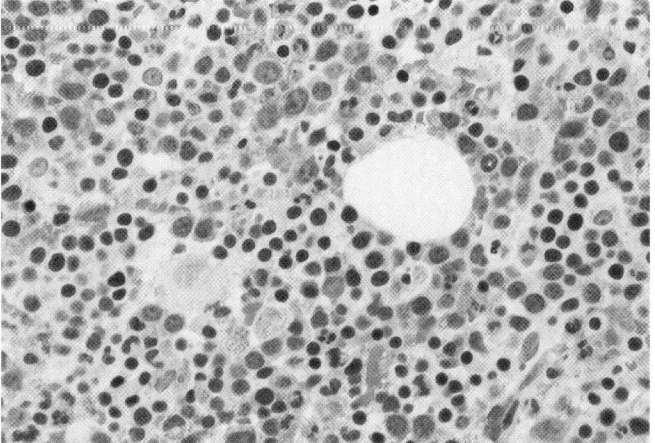

Fig. 16.18 Erythroid hyperplasia in a case of hemolysis. Iron stores are conspicuously visible as golden brown pigment.

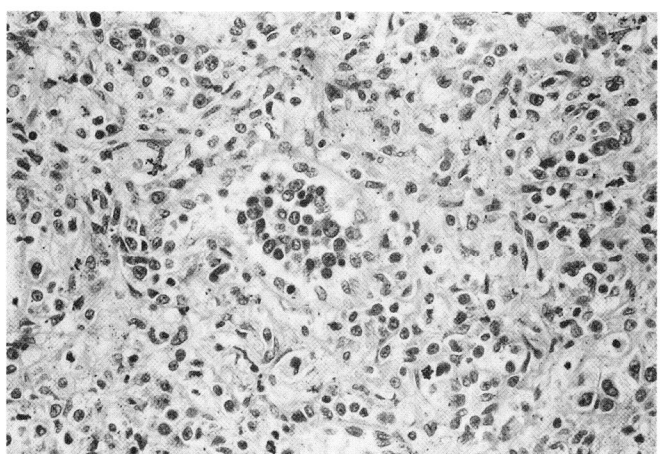

Fig. 16.19 The spleen in PV showing extramedullary hemopoiesis and intrasinusoidal erythropoiesis.

Treatment of PV

While not curative, the treatment currently available for PV restores the expected life span from only about 18 months in the untreated patient[39] to almost normal, at least in the elderly. Vascular occlusion is the commonest cause of death in the untreated patient. Regular venesection to maintain the PCV below 0.45 is recommended[3] in order to reduce this risk and should be accompanied by a cytoreductive agent if the platelet count is raised, or if there is increasing splenomegaly. Hydroxyurea is the preferred agent at present,[40] the aim being to maintain the platelet count below 400×10^9/l. This drug, which inhibits the synthesis of DNA by acting on ribonucleotide reductase, also reduces the amount of venesection required. The possibility that it may have a small leukemogenic potential (5% at 10 years) has not yet been clearly established. Anagrelide[41] is a relatively new drug whose antiproliferative action is confined to the platelet series. This may prove to be a drawback in PV where an action against all cell lines is desirable. Alpha-interferon[42] has the attraction of a non-mutagenic agent and can successfully control both PCV and platelet count. The need for injections and occurrence of troublesome side-effects mean that few patients succeed in using interferon long term. However, the potential of entirely suppressing the abnormal clone with this agent is attractive. The use of ^{32}P or low-dose busulfan as myelosuppressants is now largely confined to the elderly because of the leukemogenic risk of these drugs over and above that inherent in PV itself. Ideal treatment for PV should also reduce the risk of disease progression to myelofibrosis and more rarely to acute leukemia.[26,43] While it appears that the former can probably be achieved by myelosuppression, the search for a drug to achieve the latter will be more elusive since suppression of the abnormal clone will be required.

Secondary erythrocytosis

All patients with an increased RCM (absolute erythrocytosis) need to be examined for the possibility that this is secondary to pathology outside the bone marrow (see Table 16.4). Secondary erythrocytosis is often difficult to prove conclusively and the situation can be further confused because the stimulus to erythropoiesis may not yet, at the time of testing, be sufficient to increase the RCM to the value defined as an absolute erythrocytosis. Moreover, while these disorders stimulate erythropoiesis via the Epo mechanism (sometimes increased appropriately due to hypoxic stimulation of the oxygen sensor in the kidney, and sometimes increased inappropriately) a raised serum Epo value is not always found in these patients. Conditions associated with secondary erythrocytosis, such as tumors, may also cause leukocytosis and thrombocytosis resulting in a mistaken diagnosis of PV.

Of the congenital (see Table 16.2) causes of secondary erythrocytosis, a mutant high-oxygen-affinity hemoglobin should routinely be excluded by p50 estimation. If a left-shifted oxygen dissociation curve is demonstrated without being able to identify an abnormal hemoglobin, congenital low 2,3-diphosphoglycerate (2,3DPG) is a rare possibility. Individuals (and sometimes families) with autonomous high Epo production[44] also fall into the congenital category.

The acquired (see Table 16.2) causes of secondary erythrocytosis are numerous,[45] the two commonest groups being those associated with arterial hypoxemia (lung disease and cyanotic congenital heart disease) and those with renal lesions (Fig. 16.20). Unfortunately, common conditions such as moderate chronic lung disease or renal cysts are not necessarily the cause of erythrocytosis when present. Moreover, the miscellaneous tumors that have sometimes been associated with erythrocytosis are either very common (fibroids, bronchial carcinoma) or very rare (cerebellar hemangioblastoma [Fig. 16.21]), which makes them easy to miss as a cause. Nevertheless, routine testing of renal function and liver function as well as abdominal ultrasound to visualize these organs (as well as to estimate spleen size) should always be performed.

Estimation of arterial oxygen saturation by pulse oximeter conveniently avoids arterial puncture, but when the hypoxemia is not severe, interpretation can be difficult. First, though an oxygen saturation of 92% is the traditional dividing line below which erythrocytosis is expected, this is not based on secure scientific evidence;

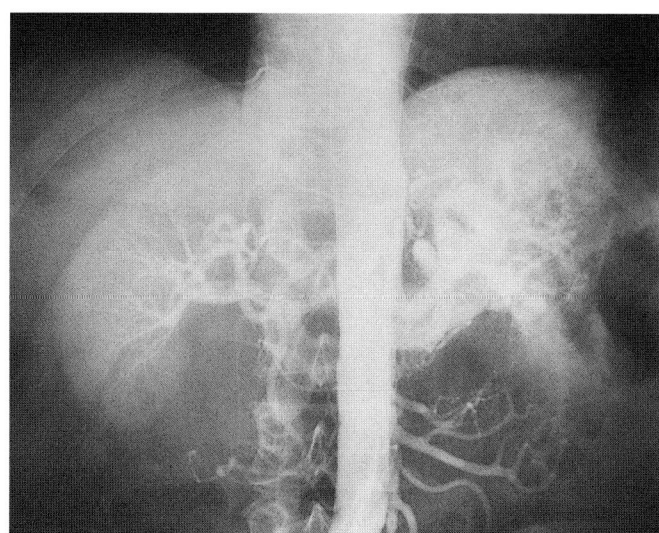

Fig. 16.20 Angiogram of hypernephroma.

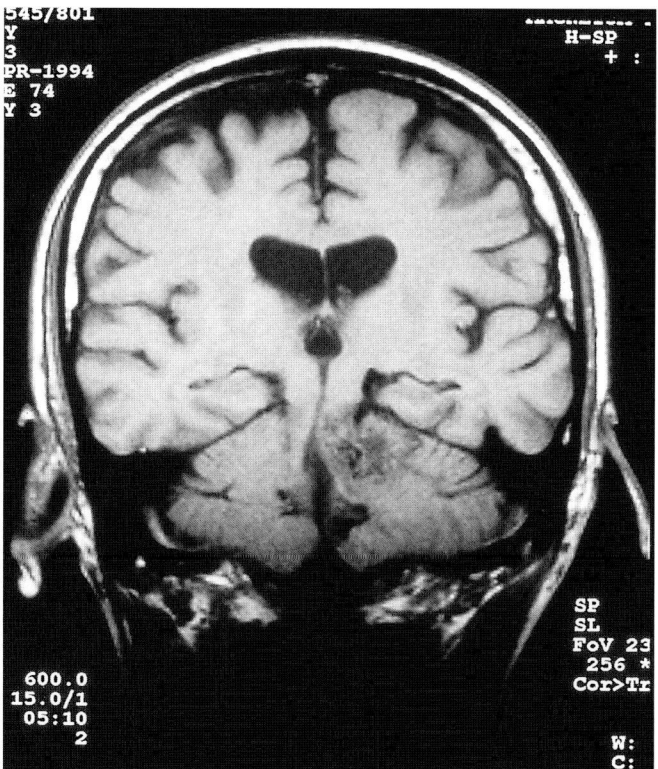

Fig. 16.21 MRI scan of cerebellar hemangioblastoma.

second, most oximeters include COHb values in their oxygen saturation reading which reduces the true oxygen saturation in many smokers to values < 92%; third, the oxygen saturation at night (and even in repose) may be considerably lower from a clinic reading. Ideally, a formula that sums the time spent at different degrees of arterial hypoxemia through 24 h could be useful as an indication of the total hypoxemic stimulus. Certainly, a low threshold for diagnosing both sleep apnea

syndrome[46] and nocturnal hypoxemia in those with chronic obstructive airways disease (COAD) is needed.

Management of secondary erythrocytosis

Excessive erythrocytosis and the resulting raised viscosity must increase cardiac workload. It is also likely to promote thrombosis, though less so than in PV with its additional platelet abnormalities. However, mild erythrocytosis is also a useful compensatory response in hypoxemia. Without having prospective long-term studies on the value of venesection in secondary erythrocytosis, a sensible compromise is to maintain the PCV at around 0.51–0.53 by venesection when there is arterial hypoxemia, and at lower values (< 0.45) in patients with renal causes or a history of thrombosis or ischemia. There is no place for the use of cytotoxic drugs.

Idiopathic erythrocytosis

This self-explanatory term includes all patients who have an absolute erythrocytosis but no evidence that this is due either to a primary or secondary cause. Alternative names such as benign or pure erythrocytosis[47] have been used but may be misleading. It is clearly a heterogenous condition, and as ways of diagnosing PV and secondary erythrocytosis are refined, fewer patients will fall into this category. Already certain patients who were previously part of this group now have a specific diagnosis such as those with Epo receptor abnormalities (primary congenital erythrocytosis) or familial autonomous raised Epo secretion (secondary erythrocytosis) and more such subgroups are likely to be defined. Meanwhile some of the patients currently in the idiopathic erythrocytosis group may have the following explanations or alternative pathologies:

- They are among 1–2% of normal people with RCM above the reference range.
- They are at an early stage of PV with as yet insufficient features to meet the diagnostic criteria of PV.
- They (theoretically) may have clonal proliferation only involving the erythroid series.
- There may be an underlying unrecognized or previously unknown cause of secondary erythrocytosis.

To avoid wrong inclusion in the idiopathic erythrocytosis group, stringent investigation of patients for features of PV and of secondary erythrocytosis, not only at presentation but also at follow-up, is necessary. Continuing close observation makes it more likely that an underlying pathology may be revealed in time. Careful studies of patients in this group are likely to be a fruitful source for elucidation of new, detailed pathogenetic mechanisms causing erythrocytosis. As always, the possibility of more than one coexisting factor needs to be borne in mind.

Management of idiopathic erythrocytosis

While diagnostic elucidation is the main aim in patients whose erythrocytosis appears to be idiopathic, management may also include reducing the risk of thrombosis by venesection (but not cytotoxic agents). In the absence of clear scientific evidence, a practical compromise is to reduce the PCV to < 0.45 if it is persistently ≥ 0.54. Lower PCV values ≥ 0.51) may suggest the need for venesection in patients with other thrombotic risk factors (hypertension, hyperlipidemia, diabetes, strong family history) or in those having past or present ischemic events.

Apparent erythrocytosis

A variety of names have been used in the past (Geisböck's syndrome, stress, pseudo, relative and spurious polycythemia) for conditions which do not have clear features distinguishing them from each other and can conveniently be brought together under the diagnostic category of apparent erythrocytosis.[48] This term applies to patients with a persistently raised PCV but whose RCM is in the normal range (not 25% or more above the predicted RCM for an individual of that height and weight). Unlike the other categories of erythrocytosis discussed in this chapter, patients with apparent erythrocytosis do not therefore have an absolute erythrocytosis.

Many investigators have observed that apparent erythrocytosis tends to occur in individuals who are obese, hypertensive, on diuretics, or cigarette/alcohol users. Such correlations are not necessarily an indication of cause and effect, but there is no doubt that correction of these factors often coincides with a reduction in PCV, and is the first line in the management of these patients. There are a number of possible explanations for the raised PCV in apparent erythrocytosis:

- individuals representing one extreme of the normal physiologic range of PCV (RCM in higher part of normal range and plasma volume in lower part of normal range);

- plasma volume reduction (as in dehydration);
- small increase in red cell mass triggering compensatory plasma volume reduction for control of blood volume; and
- early stage of conditions leading to absolute erythrocytosis.

The different interacting factors associated with plasma-volume control are difficult to measure and elucidate, but relevant observations include finding that arterial hypoxemia can reduce plasma volume, perhaps partly by altering capillary permeability. In milder cases of hypoxemia, this process may predominate over the expected stimulation of erythropoiesis.

Management of apparent erythrocytosis

In the absence of a prospective study to see whether PCV reduction reduces the incidence of vascular occlusion in these patients, venesection tends in practice to be confined, as in idiopathic erythrocytosis, to those patients with the higher PCV values (e.g. ≥ 0.54) or where there are other thrombotic risk factors. Once a venesection regime has started (aim PCV < 0.45) it is no longer possible to be sure which patients (perhaps one-third of the total) would spontaneously return to a normal PCV and which might go on to develop an absolute erythrocytosis. Consequently, elucidation of the different pathogenetic mechanisms can become more difficult but should nevertheless be considered during follow-up.

Acknowledgment

We are most grateful to Monica Nestor for preparation of the manuscript.

REFERENCES

1. Adamson JW, Fialkow PJ, Murphy S et al 1976 Polycythemia vera: stem cell and probable clonal origin of the disease. New England Journal of Medicine 295: 913–916
2. Dameshek W 1951 Some speculations on the myeloproliferative syndromes. Blood 6: 372–375
3. Guthrie DL, Pearson TC 1982 PCV measurement in the management of polycythaemic patients. Clinical and Laboratory Haematology 4: 257–265
4. Pearson TC, Guthrie DL, Simpson J et al 1995 Red cell mass and plasma volume interpretation in normal adults. British Journal of Haematology 89: 748–756
5. Berlin NI 1995 Classification of the polycythemias and the initial clinical features in polycythemia vera. In: Wasserman LR, Berk PD, Berlin NI (eds), Polycythemia vera and the myeloproliferative disorders. WB Saunders, Philadelphia, 22–30
6. Pearson TC, Messinezy M 1996 The diagnostic criteria of polycythaemia rubra vera Leukemia and Lymphoma 22 (suppl 1): 87–93
7. Diez Martin JL, Graham DL, Petitt RM et al 1991 Chromosome studies in 104 patients with polycythemia vera. Mayo Clinic Proceedings 66: 287–299

8. Bench AJ, Nacheva EP, Champion KM et al 1998 Molecular genetics and cytogenetics of myeloproliferative disorders. Baillières Clinical Haematology 11: 819–848

9. Briere J, El-Kassar N 1998 Clonality markers in polycythaemia and primary thrombocythaemia. Baillières Clinical Haematology 11: 787–801

10. Champion KM, Gilbert JGR, Asimakopoulos FA et al 1997 Clonal haemopoiesis in normal elderly women: implications for the myeloproliferative disorders and myelodysplastic syndromes. British Journal of Haematology 97: 920–926

11. Carneskog J, Wadenvik H, Fjälling M et al 1996 Assessment of spleen size using gamma camera scintigraphy in newly diagnosed patients with essential thrombocythaemia and polycythaemia vera. European Journal of Haematology 56: 158–162

12. Messinezy M, MacDonald LM, Nunan TO et al 1997 Spleen sizing by ultrasound in polycythaemia and thrombocythaemia: comparison with SPECT. British Journal of Haematology 98: 103–107

13. Messinezy M, Westwood NB, Woodcock SP et al 1995 Low serum erythropoietin – a strong diagnostic criterion of primary polycythemia even at normal haemoglobin levels. Clinical and Laboratory Haematology 17: 217–220

14. De la Chapelle A, Träskelin A-L, Juvonen E et al 1993 Truncated erythropoietin receptor causes dominantly inherited benign human erythrocytosis. Proceedings of the National Academy of Sciences USA 90: 4495–4499

15. Kralovics R, Indrak K, Stopka T et al 1997 Two new epo receptor mutations: truncated epo receptors are most frequently associated with primary familial and congenital polycythemias. Blood 90: 2057–2061

16. Reid CDL 1987 The significance of endogenous erythroid colonies (EEC) in haematological disorders. Blood Reviews 1: 133–140

17. Partanen S, Huvonen E, Ikkala E et al 1989 Spontaneous erythroid colony formation in the differential diagnosis of erythrocytosis. European Journal of Haematology 42: 327–330

18. Westwood NB, Pearson TC 1996 Diagnostic applications of haemopoietic progenitor culture techniques in polycythaemias and thrombocythaemias. Leukemia and Lymphoma 22 (suppl 1): 95–103

19. Ellis JT, Peterson P, Geller SA, et al 1986 Studies of the bone marrow in polycythemia vera and the evolution of myelofibrosis and second hematologic malignancies. Seminars in Hematology 23: 144–155

20. Naeim F 1998 Chronic myeloproliferative disorders. In: Naeim F, Pathology of bone marrow, 2nd edn Williams & Wilkins, Baltimore, 166–188

21. Thiele J, Kvasnicka HM, Fischer R 1999 Histochemistry and morphometry on bone marrow biopsies in chronic myeloproliferative disorders – aids to diagnosis and classification. Annals of Hematology 78: 495–506

22. Thiele J, Zankovich R, Schneider G et al 1988 Primary (essential) thrombocythemia versus polycythemia vera rubra. A histomorphometric analysis of bone marrow features in trephine biopsies. Analytical and Quantitative Cytology and Histology 10: 375–382

23. Thiele J, Kvasnicka HM, Volker D et al 1999 Clinicopathological diagnosis and differential criteria of thrombocythemias in various myeloproliferative disorders by histopathology, histochemistry and immunostaining from bone marrow biopsies. Leukemia and Lymphoma 33: 207–218

24. Georgii A, Vykoupil KF, Buhr T et al 1990 Chronic myeloproliferative disorders in bone marrow biopsies. Pathology, Research and Practice 186: 2–27

25. Brunning RD, McKenna RW 1994 Tumors of the bone marrow. In: Rosai J, Sobin LH (eds) Atlas of tumor pathology, third series, fascicle 9. Armed forces Institute of Pathology, Washington 195–254

26. Najean Y, Rain JD, Dresch C et al 1996 Risk of leukaemia, carcinoma and myelofibrosis in 32P- or chemotherapy-treated patients with polycythaemia vera: a prospective analysis of 682 cases. The 'French Cooperative Group for the Study of Polycythaemias. Leukemia and Lymphoma 22 (suppl 1): 111–119

27. Georgii A, Buhr T, Buesche G et al 1996 Classification and staging of Ph-negative myeloproliferative disorders by histopathology from bone marrow biopsies. Leukaemia and Lymphoma 22: 15–29

28. Neilson D, Patton WN, Williams MD et al 1994 Polycythaemia rubra vera transforming to acute lymphoblastic leukaemia with a common immunophenotype. Journal of Clinical Pathology 47: 471–472

29. Braich TA, Grogan TM, Hicks MJ et al 1986 Terminal lymphoblastic transformation in polycythaemia vera. American Journal of Medicine 80: 304–306

30. Wong KF, Chan JK, Ma SK et al 1993 Megakaryoblastic transformation of polycythemia vera associated with hypercalcemia. American Journal of Hematology 43: 240–242

31. Steinberg E, Ben-Dor D, Lugassy G et al 1995 Anaplastic B-cell (Ki-1) lymphoma developing in a patient with polycythaemia vera. Leukaemia and Lymphoma 19: 507–509

32. Holcombe RF, Treseler PA, Rosenthal DS 1991 Chronic myelomonocytic leukemia transformation in polycythaemia vera. Leukemia 5: 606–610

33. Sanchez Fayos J, Prieto E, Roman A et al 1996 Polycythaemia vera as a multiphasic clonal myelopathy: diagnostic profile, chronic pathological progression and effect of therapy on the survival of 74 cases. Sangre 41: 447–457

34. Hoppins EC, Lewis JP 1975 Polycythaemia rubra vera progressing Ph^{1-} positive chronic myelogenous leukaemia. Annals of Internal Medicine 83: 820–823

35. Haq AU 1990 Transformation of polycythemia vera to Ph-positive chronic myelogenous leukemia. American Journal of Hematology 35: 110–113

36. Higuchi T, Oba R, Endo M et al 1999 Transition of polycythemia vera to chronic neutrophilic leukemia. Leukaemia and Lymphoma 33: 203–206

37. Wolf BC, Neiman RS 1988 The bone marrow in myeloproliferative and dysmyelopoietic syndromes. Hematology/Oncology Clinics of North America 2: 669–694

38. Wolf BC, Banks PM, Mann RB et al 1988 Splenic hematopoiesis in polycythaemia vera. A morphologic and immunohistologic study. American Journal of Clinical Pathology 89: 69–75

39. Chievitz E, Thiede, T 1962 Complications and causes of death in polycythaemia vera. Acta Medica Scandinavica 172: 513–523

40. Fruchtman SM, Mack K, Kaplan ME et al 1997 From efficacy to safety: a Polycythemia Vera Study group report on hydroxyurea in patients with polycythemia vera. Seminars in Hematology 34: 17–23

41. Anagrelide Study Group 1992 Anagrelide, a therapy for thrombocythemic states: experience in 577 patients. American Journal of Medicine 92: 69–76

42. Silver RT 1997 Interferon alfa: effects of long-term treatment for polycythemia vera. Seminars in Hematology 34: 40–50

43. Landaw SA 1995 Acute leukemia in polycythemia vera. In: Wasserman LR, Berk PD, Berlin NI (eds), Polycythemia vera and the myeloproliferative disorders. WB Saunders, Philadelphia, 154–165

44. Distelhorst CW, Wagner DS, Goldwasser E et al 1981 Autosomal dominant familial erythrocytosis due to autonomous erythropoietin production. Blood 58: 1155–1158

45. Pearson TC, Lewis SM 1998 Non-leukaemic myeloproliferative disorders. In: Hoffbrand AV, Lewis SM, Tuddenham EGD (eds.), Postgraduate haematology. Butterworth Heinemann, Oxford 505–529

46. Moore-Gillon JC, Treacher DF, Gaminara EJ et al 1986 Intermittent hypoxia in patients with unexplained polycythaemia. British Medical Journal 293: 588–590

47. Prchal JT, Sokol L 1996 'Benign erythrocytosis' and other familial and congenital polycythemias. European Journal of Haematology 57: 263–268

48. Pearson TC 1991 Apparent polycythaemia. Blood Reviews 5: 205–213

Disorders affecting leucocyte lineages

Abnormalities in leucocyte morphology and number 299

Disorders of phagocyte function 321

Myelodysplastic disorders 331

Acute leukemias 351

The chronic lymphoid and myeloid leukemias and systemic mastocytosis 381

Lymphoma 405

Abnormalities in immunoglobulin synthesizing cells 437

Abnormalities in leukocyte morphology and number

17

SN Wickramasinghe

Inherited abnormalities of granulocyte morphology
Pelger–Huët anomaly
Hereditary hypersegmentation of neutrophil nuclei
May–Hegglin anomaly
Chediak–Higashi syndrome
Myeloperoxidase deficiency
Alder–Reilly anomaly
Jordans' anomaly (familial vacuolization of leukocytes)
Lactoferrin deficiency ('specific granule' deficiency)

Acquired abnormalities of granulocyte morphology
Shifts to the left or right
Toxic granulation of neutrophils
Döhle bodies
Macropolycytes
Acquired Pelger–Huët anomaly
Acquired myeloperoxidase deficiency
Botryoid nuclei
Other abnormalities

Leukopenia

Neutropenia
Drugs, chemicals and ionizing radiation

Immune neutropenia
Dialysis neutropenia
Chronic idiopathic neutropenia
Cyclical neutropenia
Familial benign chronic neutropenia
Neutropenia in healthy black population
Severe congenital neutropenia (infantile genetic agranulocytosis, Kostmann's syndrome)
Congenital aleukia (reticular dysgenesis)
Other rare neutropenic syndromes

Eosinopenia

Basopenia

Monocytopenia

Lymphocytopenia

Leukocytosis

Neutrophil leukocytosis

Eosinophil leukocytosis
Idiopathic hypereosinophilic syndrome

Basophil leukocytosis

Lymphocytosis and monocytosis
Infectious mononucleosis
Atypical manifestations of EBV infections

Blood leukocytes may show abnormalities of their morphology, number or function or combinations of such abnormalities. Many diseases are associated with changes in the concentration of one or more types of circulating leukocytes. Although such changes are often non-specific they may provide diagnostic clues. Alterations in the concentration of circulating leukocytes usually represent a response of the body to diseases of various tissues other than the blood and bone marrow but may also result from diseases of the hemopoietic system. The leukemias may cause an increase or a decrease in the concentrations of mature leukocytes in the blood as well as an impairment of leukocyte function. They are discussed separately in Chapters 20 and 21.

Inherited abnormalities of granulocyte morphology

Pelger–Huët anomaly[1,2]

This disorder is inherited as an autosomal dominant trait and affects 1 in 5000 people. It is characterized by a marked reduction in the number of nuclear segments in neutrophil granulocytes. Heterozygotes have bilobed spectacle-like nuclei in 50–70% of their neutrophil granulocytes (Fig. 17.1A) and round or oval unsegmented nuclei in 20–40%. The affected nuclei have abnormally coarse chromatin. There are no abnormalities in the number or, usually, function[3] of neutrophils. The condition should not be confused with the left-shift seen in a reactive neutrophil leukocytosis. Homozygotes for the Pelger–Huët anomaly are rare and show round or oval nuclei in all neutrophil granulocytes. An acquired abnormality resembling the Pelger–Huët anomaly may be seen in myelodysplastic states and some other conditions.

Hereditary hypersegmentation of neutrophil nuclei[4]

This rare condition is inherited as an autosomal dominant character. The proportion of neutrophils with five or more lobes is normally 2–3% but in these cases is usually greater than 10%. The neutrophils appear to have adequate function.

May–Hegglin anomaly[1,5,6]

This is a rare disorder that is inherited as an autosomal dominant trait. It is characterized by intracytoplasmic inclusions in all types of granulocytes and in monocytes.

Other features are giant hypogranular platelets, thrombocytopenia (in one-third of the cases), a moderate reduction in platelet life span and, occasionally, a mild to severe hemorrhagic tendency. The cytoplasmic inclusions are 2–5 µm in diameter, appear grayish-blue when stained by a Romanowsky method, and are composed of stacks of rough endoplasmic reticulum. They are similar to Döhle bodies both in appearance and composition but tend to be larger, more rounded and discrete, and to affect a much higher percentage of the granulocytes. Despite the morphologic abnormality in neutrophils, there is no increased susceptibility to infections. Platelet function is abnormal, accounting for the mild bleeding diathesis in some cases without thrombocytopenia. The gene for this disorder has been localized to chromosome 22q12.3–13.1.[7]

Chediak–Higashi syndrome[1,8,9]

This autosomal recessive condition is characterized by the presence of a reduced number of granules and the formation of some abnormally large granules (by progressive fusion of normally-formed granules) in most granule-containing cells. The affected cells include the neutrophils, eosinophils, lymphocytes, monocytes, melanocytes, Schwann cells of peripheral nerves, fibroblasts, vascular endothelial cells, renal tubular cells and the parenchymal cells of the adrenal and pituitary glands. There is a deficiency of platelet dense-granules, leading to easy bruising and bleeding. The large granules in leukocytes vary from a pale slate-gray to a dark reddish color (Romanowsky stain) (Figs 17.1 B,C,D). Despite the presence of some giant melanin granules, the reduction of the total number of melanin granules in the skin, iris and retina gives rise to partial oculocutaneous albinism with silvery hair, photophobia and nystagmus. There is a marked reduction in circulating natural killer cells (NK cells).[10] The leukocyte abnormalities are associated with recurrent infections, particularly of the respiratory tract and skin, that cause death during infancy or early childhood; however, the use of prophylactic antibiotics and the effective treatment of infections has resulted in longer survival. The infecting organism is usually *Staphylococcus aureus* but may be *Streptococcus pyogenes*, *Haemophilus influenzae* or *Streptococcus pneumoniae*. Some affected children and particularly those who live beyond early childhood, develop a terminal accelerated phase. This is characterized by a lymphoma-like picture with lymphadenopathy, hepatosplenomegaly, neuropathy, widespread infiltration of tissues by non-malignant lymphohistiocytic cells, and pancytopenia. Death results from the complications of pancytopenia. The giant granules present in neutrophils (Fig. 17.1B) are peroxidase-positive and

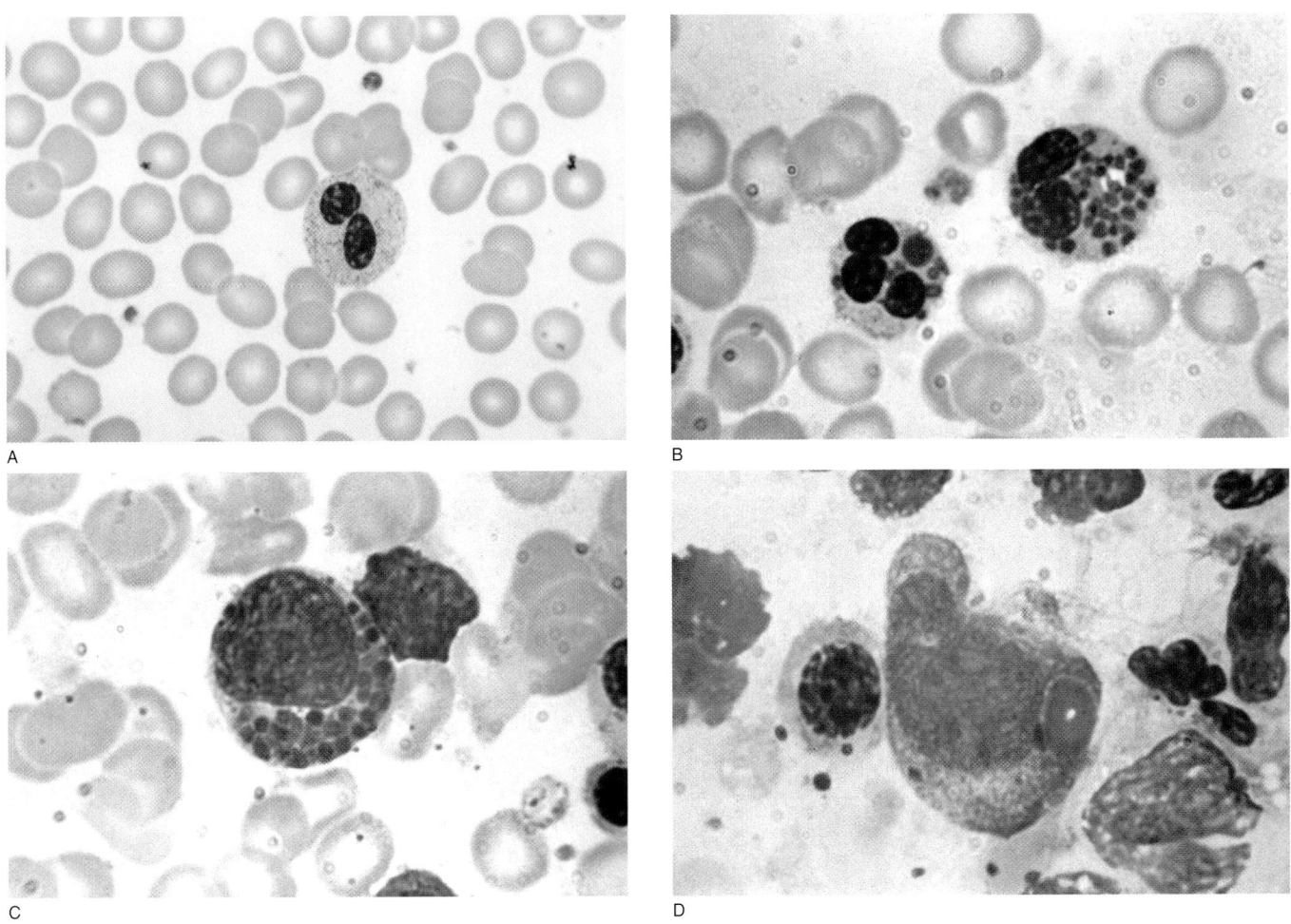

Fig. 17.1 (A–D) Two inherited abnormalities of the morphology of neutrophils. (A) Peripheral blood neutrophil showing the inherited Pelger–Huët anomaly. (B–D) Cells from a marrow smear of a patient with the Chediak–Higashi syndrome showing the presence of giant granules within the neutrophil series. (B) Two neutrophils with giant granules. (C) Neutrophil myelocyte with giant granules. (D) Neutrophil promyelocyte with two giant granules. May–Grünwald–Giemsa stain. (B–D) Courtesy of Professor J W Stewart.

represent primary granules that have fused together. Specific and gelatinase granules are not involved in the formation of giant granules.[11] The neutrophils have morphologically normal specific granules and increased numbers of autophagic vacuoles. They display normal phagocytic activity, defective chemotaxis, defective degranulation and delayed killing of some bacteria. The primary defect in the Chediak–Higashi syndrome is unknown but may involve the formation, fusion or trafficking of vesicles. It has been postulated that the defects in neutrophil function may result from an increased rate of depolymerization of tubulin,[12] the major structural protein of microtubules.

Myeloperoxidase deficiency[13,14]

The introduction of automated differential counting based on cytochemical reactions for myeloperoxidase to detect neutrophils has revealed that a deficiency of myeloperoxidase in neutrophils (but not of the peroxidase in eosinophils) is relatively common (1:2000). In Romanowsky-stained blood smears the neutrophils are morphologically normal. Most individuals with myeloperoxidase deficiency do not have an increased susceptibility to infections, indicating that enzymes other than myeloperoxidase play a role in the killing of bacteria by neutrophils. However, occasional myeloperoxidase-deficient patients suffer from recurrent infections. Neutrophils of myeloperoxidase-deficient patients show normal phagocytosis, an altered respiratory burst, an initial delay in killing bacteria and markedly impaired killing of fungi.

Myeloperoxidase levels are undetectable or reduced and a number of different mutations in the myeloperoxidase gene have been reported. Myeloperoxidase deficiency is inherited as an autosomal recessive character; most affected individuals are compound heterozygotes.[15]

Alder–Reilly anomaly[1,16]

This anomaly consists of the presence of abnormally coarse azurophilic or deeply basophilic cytoplasmic granules in neutrophils and, sometimes, in blood lymphocytes and monocytes. In lymphocytes the individual granules may occur within vacuoles and are occasionally comma-shaped. The Alder–Reilly anomaly is found in various types of mucopolysaccharidoses including Hunter–Hurler syndrome, and Maroteaux–Lamy polydystrophic dwarfism. These syndromes, which are inherited as autosomal recessive traits, are caused by deficiencies of enzymes involved in the degradation of the carbohydrate components of mucopolysaccharides; the anomalous granules consist of the uncatabolized carbohydrate components. Only a proportion of patients with these syndromes display the anomaly in blood cells. The Alder–Reilly anomaly is easily confused with toxic granulation of the neutrophils but differs from the latter in that it may also affect lymphocytes and monocytes.

Jordans' anomaly (familial vacuolization of leukocytes)

Vacuolation of neutrophil promyelocytes and more mature cells of the neutrophil series and of monocytes and occasional lymphocytes has been reported in a few families. The cases include two brothers with progressive muscular dystrophy and two sisters with ichthyosis.[17] Up to 10 lipid-containing vacuoles, 2–5 μm in diameter, may be present per cell.

Lactoferrin deficiency ('specific granule' deficiency)[18,19]

In this condition, recurrent infection from birth is associated with a deficiency in neutrophils of lactoferrin, vitamin B_{12}-binding protein, gelatinase and alkaline phosphatase, and impairment of neutrophil chemotaxis and adherence. The neutrophils of affected patients have bilobed nuclei and possess few or no specific granules or abnormal specific granules (empty, elongated vesicular sacs). Peroxidase-positive primary granules are decreased in size and are deficient in the antimicrobial peptides termed defensins.[20] There is a marked reduction of lactoferrin mRNA in marrow cells and it has been suggested that the deficiency of several granule proteins may result from an abnormality affecting a transcription factor.[19] A mutation in the *C/EBPE* gene, coding for a transcription factor involved in granulocytopoiesis, has been found in some but not all cases (see Chapter 18).

Acquired abnormalities of granulocyte morphology

Shifts to the left or right

In some conditions (e.g. infections) the proportion of band forms and neutrophils with only two nuclear segments may increase, and some metamyelocytes and myelocytes and a very occasional myeloblast may be seen in the blood. When this happens the neutrophil series is described as showing a shift to the left. In other conditions there is an increased proportion of neutrophils with four or five or more nuclear segments. This occurs in vitamin B_{12} or folate deficiency (see Chapter 12) and may also be seen in renal disease and iron-deficiency anemia.

Toxic granulation of neutrophils

(Figs 17.2B,C)

'Toxic granules' are fine or coarse reddish-violet granules (Romanowsky stain) that are found scattered throughout the cytoplasm of neutrophils. They frequently occur in severe infections but are also seen in non-infective inflammatory states and in normal pregnancy. The primary granules of neutrophil promyelocytes and myelocytes are azurophilic but those of normal mature neutrophils lose this property. Toxic granules seem to result from an abnormality in the maturation of the primary granules with a consequent retention of their azurophilic property.[21] Neutrophils with toxic granulation may also show increased cytoplasmic basophilia, vacuolation or Döhle bodies.

Döhle bodies[22,23]

These are rounded, oval or rod-shaped pale grayish-blue inclusions found within the cytoplasm of neutrophils, usually at the periphery and protruding beyond the normal contour of the cell (Figs 17.2D and 17.3). They are 1–2 μm long and consist of stacks of rough endoplasmic reticulum. Döhle bodies are found in normal pregnancy, various infections, in patients with various neoplasms and after severe burns.

Macropolycytes

These are very large polymorphonuclear leukocytes (diameter >16 μm) which often have hypersegmented nuclei with 6–14 nuclear segments. They may be found

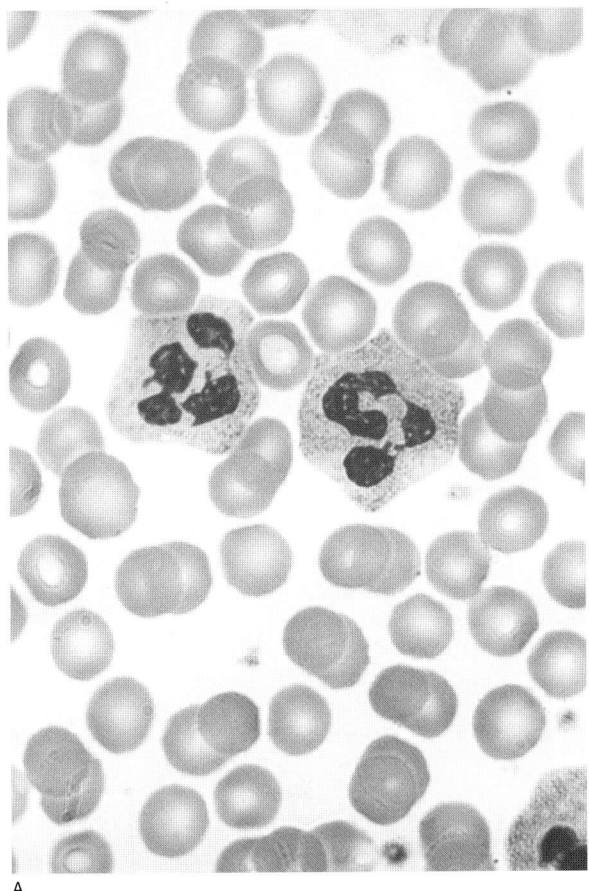

A

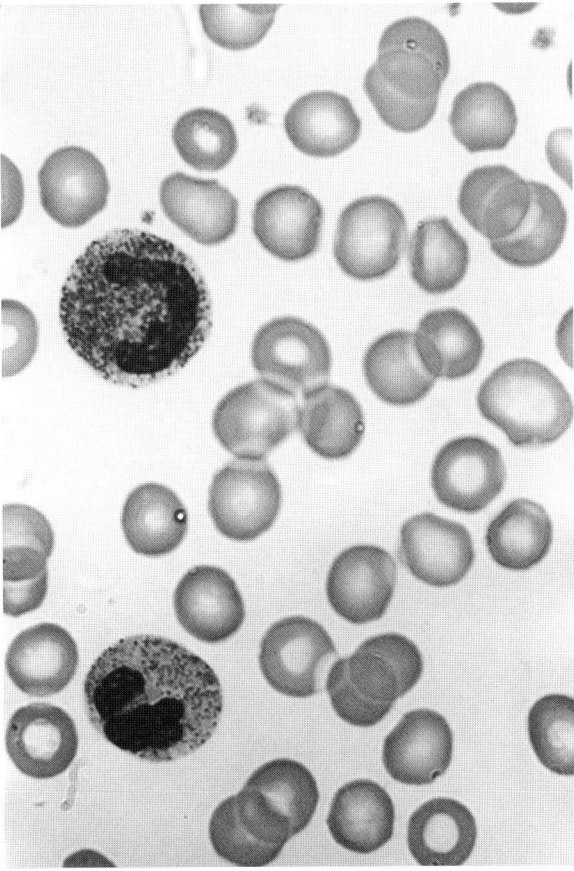

B

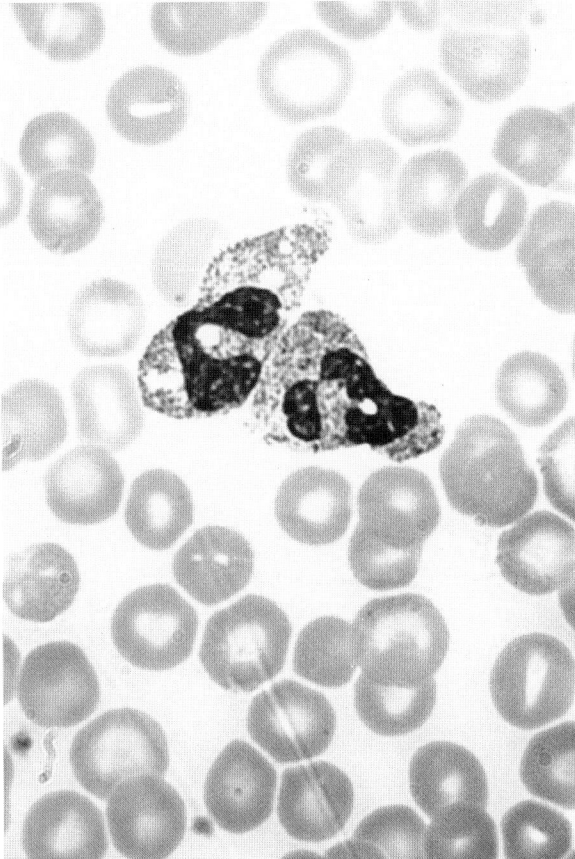

C

Fig. 17.2 (A–E) Some acquired abnormalities of the morphology of peripheral blood neutrophils. (A) Two normal neutrophils (for comparison). (B) Toxic granulation in a patient with a left-shift due to an infection. One of the cells is a band form (juvenile neutrophil). (C) Vacuolation and toxic granulation in a patient with an acute infection.

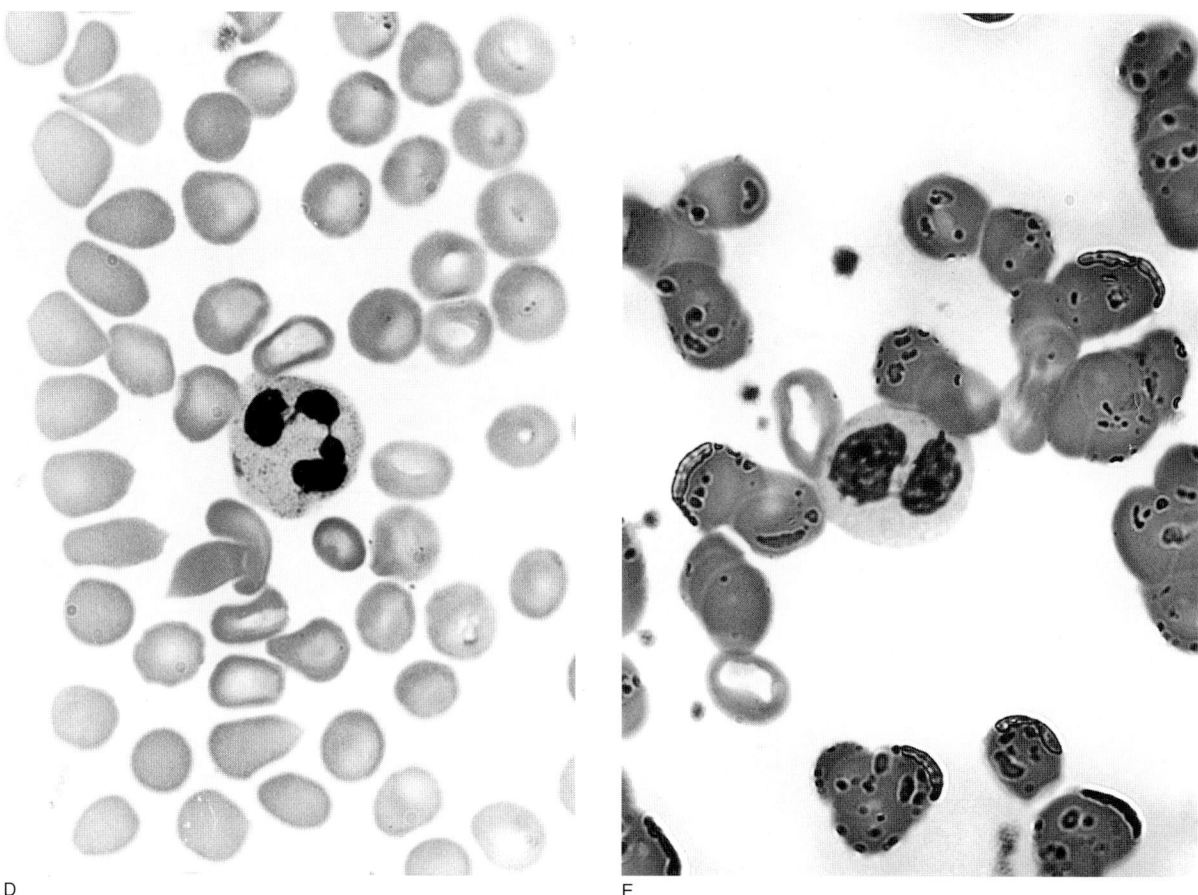

D   E

Fig. 17.2 *(Cont'd)* (D) Neutrophil from a patient with an acute infection showing an elongated Döhle body at its periphery. (E) Hypogranular neutrophil with the acquired Pelger–Huët anomaly from a patient with a myelodysplastic syndrome. May–Grünwald–Giemsa stain.

in the blood in vitamin B$_{12}$ or folate deficiency and in infections, myeloproliferative disorders and drug-induced marrow damage.

The macropolycytes seen in vitamin B$_{12}$ deficiency have tetraploid or hypotetraploid DNA contents and appear to result from nuclear segmentation in those giant metamyelocytes that are not phagocytosed by bone marrow macrophages (see Chapter 12).

The occurrence of macropolycytes has been reported as an inherited condition in a single family.

Acquired Pelger–Huët anomaly

Neutrophils resembling those in the inherited Pelger-Huët anomaly are frequently seen in the myelodysplastic syndromes (Fig. 17.2E, also see Fig. 19.7) and in acute leukemia, and rarely in chronic granulocytic leukemia and myelofibrosis. The acquired Pelger–Huët anomaly develops transiently in patients treated with paclitaxel and docetaxel[24] and the anomaly has also been found in patients with severe hematological toxicity caused by valproic acid.[25]

Acquired myeloperoxidase deficiency

An acquired myeloperoxidase deficiency may occur in acute myeloid leukemia, myelodysplastic syndromes and myeloproliferative disorders as well as in Hodgkin's disease, lead poisoning and pregnancy.

Botryoid nuclei[26,27]

In patients with heat stroke, over 50% of the neutrophils contain increased numbers of small, moderately pyknotic nuclear segments which are clustered like grapes on a stem.

Other abnormalities

Hypogranular neutrophils (acquired 'specific granule' deficiency) are found especially in myelodysplastic syndromes (Fig. 17.2E, also see Fig. 19.5) but may also be seen in other conditions such as Ph-negative chronic myeloid leukemia, chronic myelomonocytic leukemia and acute myeloid leukemia. In addition, they may be found in neonates and in patients with burns. Rarely,

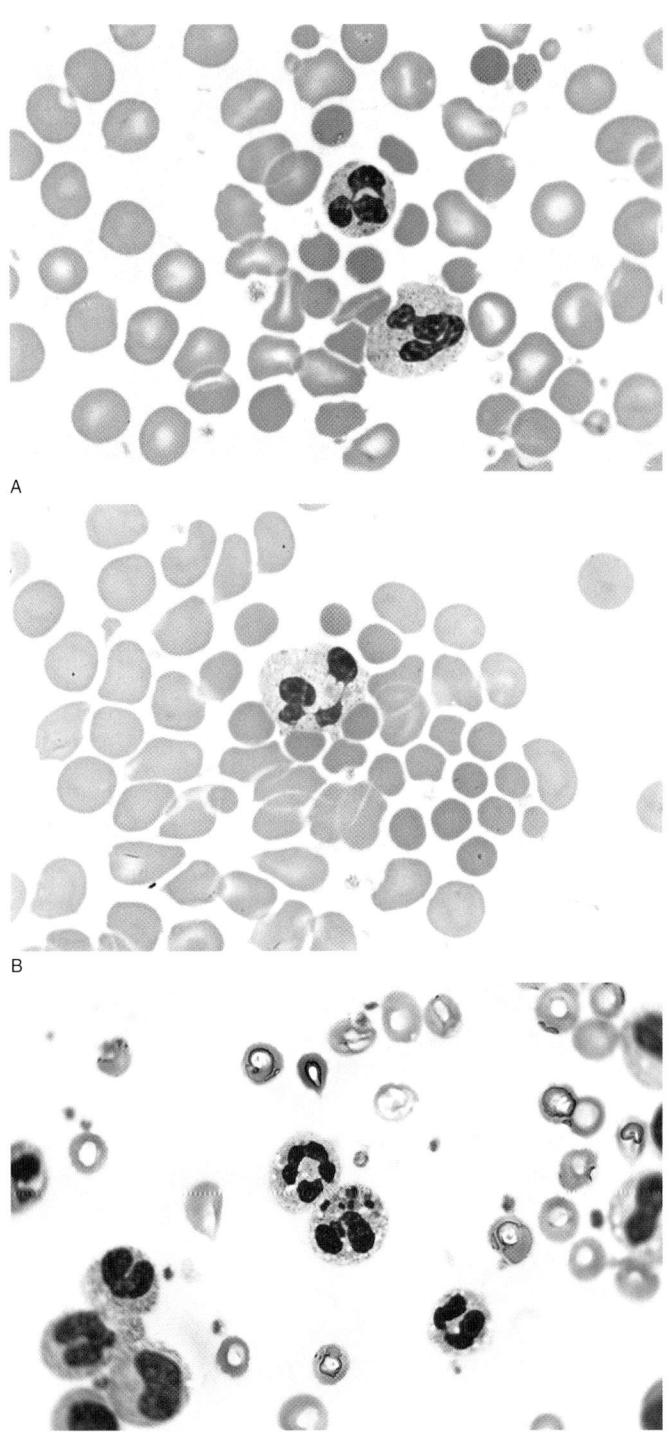

A

B

C

Fig. 17.3 (A–C) Some acquired abnormalities of the morphology of peripheral blood neutrophils. (A) and (B) Neutrophils from a patient with extensive burns. One of the cells in (A) has an elongated peripheral Döhle body and the cell in (B) contains three rounded Döhle bodies. (C) Buffy coat cells from a case of meningococcal meningitis showing a granulocyte containing phagocytosed diplococci. May–Grünwald–Giemsa stain.

ingested microorganisms may be seen within circulating neutrophils, for example in meningococcal meningitis (Fig. 17.3C).

Leukopenia

The term leukopenia is applied to a decrease in the concentration of circulating white blood cells below the reference range. The terms granulocytopenia, neutropenia, eosinopenia, basopenia, lymphocytopenia and monocytopenia are used to describe reductions in the concentrations of circulating granulocytes, neutrophils, eosinophils, basophils, lymphocytes and monocytes correspondingly.

Neutropenia

Neutropenia may arise from: (1) various disorders of bone marrow function resulting in a decreased rate of release of neutrophils from the marrow into the circulation; (2) a shift of neutrophils from the circulating to the marginated cell pools (see Chapter 1); (3) a reduction of the $T_{1/2}$ of circulating neutrophils; and (4) combinations of the above. A decrease in the rate of release of neutrophils from the marrow (i.e. a decrease of effective neutrophil granulocytopoiesis) may be caused by a reduction in the rate of production of neutrophil precursors (i.e. decreased total neutrophil granulocytopoiesis), an increased intramedullary destruction of neutrophil precursors (i.e. increased ineffective neutrophil granulocytopoiesis), or an impairment of the release of bone marrow neutrophils into the blood. A reduction of the $T_{1/2}$ of circulating neutrophils may be due to destruction of circulating cells (e.g. by antibodies or a hyperactive spleen) or an accelerated rate of egress of neutrophils from the blood into tissues. Because of the difficulties involved in the quantitative assessment of total, effective and ineffective neutrophil granulocytopoiesis in humans, the mechanisms underlying the neutropenia in many clinical situations and especially in any individual patient are frequently a matter of uncertainty. When neutropenia is caused by ineffective neutrophil granulocytopoiesis due to intramedullary destruction of the most mature neutrophil precursors, or by an increased loss of circulating cells, there is a compensatory increase of total neutrophil granulocytopoiesis. In many neutropenic states the marrow contains few cells beyond the neutrophil myelocyte stage because of an accelerated release of neutrophil metamyelocytes and marrow neutrophils into the circulation.

The conditions that may be associated with a neutropenia are listed in Table 17.1. Many of these are discussed elsewhere in this volume. A neutropenia may be seen in certain phases of diseases caused by a number of infectious agents. The mechanisms underlying this

Table 17.1 Causes of neutropenia

Infections
   Viral: measles, mumps, rubella, influenza, infectious
     mononucleosis, infectious hepatitis, HIV, parvovirus,
     dengue, yellow fever
   Bacterial: brucellosis, typhoid, paratyphoid, overwhelming
     pyogenic infections (septicemia), miliary tuberculosis
   Rickettsial: typhus
   Protozoal: malaria, kala-azar, trypanosomiasis
   Fungal: histoplasmosis, blastomycosis

Drugs (see Table 17.2), alcohol and other chemicals

Ionizing radiation

Hypersplenism

Leukemia, including CD3$^+$ large granular lymphocyte leukemia

Myelodysplastic syndromes

Aplastic anemia and paroxysmal nocturnal hemoglobinuria

Bone marrow infiltration

Myelofibrosis

Megaloblastic anemia

Anaphylactic shock

Immune neutropenia
   Amidopyrine-induced agranulocytosis
   Systemic lupus erythematosus (SLE)
   Rheumatoid arthritis, scleroderma
   Autoimmune neutropenia
   Neonatal alloimmune neutropenia

Hemophagocytic syndromes

Dialysis neutropenia

Chronic idiopathic neutropenia

Cyclical neutropenia

Familial benign chronic neutropenia

Neutropenia in blacks (physiologic)

Severe congenital neutropenia

Congenital aleukia

Other rare neutropenic syndromes

Miscellaneous: hyperthyroidism, hypopituitarism, Addison's
   disease, Kawasaki disease, copper deficiency, starvation,
   anorexia nervosa

neutropenia, which only affects a proportion of infected patients (e.g. about 50% of patients with typhoid), are uncertain. They may include an endotoxin-induced shift of neutrophils from the circulating to the marginated cell pools, a reduced $T_{1/2}$ of circulating granulocytes (due either to destruction of cells within the circulation or to an accelerated rate of egress of cells from the blood) and a failure of the bone marrow to adequately increase the rate of effective granulocytopoiesis. In certain circumstances infection may be associated both with a failure to adequately increase effective granulocytopoiesis and

with an exhaustion of the marrow granulocyte pool so that neutropenia is seen together with a left shift. This is particularly common in very severe bacterial infections and in bacterial infections in neonates and alcoholics (who normally have a reduced marrow granulocyte pool). The neutropenia induced by certain drugs (e.g. chlorpromazine) or found in aplastic anemia and cyclical neutropenia is caused by decreased total granulocytopoiesis. The neutropenia found in megaloblastic anemias and in individuals receiving some drugs (e.g. methotrexate) is caused by increased ineffective granulocytopoiesis, usually with some reduction in the $T_{1/2}$ of the circulating granulocytes. Finally, the low neutrophil counts found in hypersplenism, amidopyrine-induced agranulocytosis, autoimmune neutropenia (including systemic lupus erythematosus [SLE]) and neonatal alloimmune neutropenia are caused by a reduction of the $T_{1/2}$ of these cells in the blood.

Drugs, chemicals and ionizing radiation[28]

The commonest drug-induced blood dyscrasia is a neutropenia.[29] Some drugs (e.g. alkylating agents or antifolate drugs), certain chemicals (e.g. benzene) and irradiation induce a neutropenia in all individuals in a dose-dependent manner. Other drugs produce neutropenia only in occasional individuals and this phenomenon is usually at least partly based on a genetic polymorphism of drug metabolism. Drugs of the latter category may either cause neutropenia as part of an aplastic anemia or induce a selective neutropenia. Furthermore, several of the drugs causing aplastic anemia in susceptible individuals initially cause a neutropenia that subsequently progresses to aplastic anemia. Drugs that may occasionally cause selective neutropenia are listed in Table 17.2. The relatively high-risk drugs amongst these include amidopyrine and the antithyroid drugs. Some of the drugs listed in Table 17.2 usually induce a mild to moderate neutropenia that is asymptomatic and does not progress despite continuation of the drug; others usually cause a complete or virtually complete absence of neutrophils (agranulocytosis). Agranulocytosis[30–32] results in a life-threatening clinical syndrome characterized by fever, sweating, vomiting, sore throat, dysphagia due to necrotic ulceration of the mouth and pharynx, extreme prostration and, frequently, death from overwhelming infection. At necropsy, necrotic ulcers are found in the mucous membrane of the entire alimentary tract as well as in the vagina. The prognosis is considerably improved if the offending drug is stopped and infection is adequately controlled by antibiotic therapy. Drugs or

Table 17.2 Some drugs which may cause a selective neutropenia in occasional patients

Analgesic drugs
  Amidopyrine, dipyrone

Antibacterial drugs
  Cephalosporins, chloramphenicol, clindamycin, co-trimoxazole (sulphamethoxazole-trimethoprim), other sulphonamides, doxycycline, dapsone, gentamicin, isoniazid, lincomycin, metronidazole, nitrofurantoin, penicillins, rifampicin, streptomycin, tetracycline, vancomycin

Anticoagulant drugs
  Dicoumarol, phenindione

Anticonvulsant drugs
  Carbamazepine, ethosuximide, phenytoin, primidone, sodium valproate, troxidone (trimethadione)

Antidiabetic drugs
  Chlorpropamide, tolbutamide

Antihistamines
  Brompheniramine, chlorpheniramine, mepyramine, promethazine, trimeprazine

Anti-inflammatory drugs
  Celecoxib, fenoprofen, ibuprofen, indomethacin, oxyphenbutazone, penicillamine, phenylbutazone, sodium aurothiomalate

Antimalarial drugs
  Amodiaquine, dapsone, hydroxychloroquine, pamaquin pyrimethamine, quinine

Antithyroid drugs
  Carbimazole, methimazole, methylthiouracil, potassium perchlorate, propylthiouracil

Anxiolytic, antipsychotic and antidepressant drugs
  Amitriptyline, chlordiazepoxide, chlorpromazine, clozapine, diazepam, imipramine, meprobamate, mianserin, prochlorperazine, promazine, thioridazine, trifluoperazine, trimeprazine

Cardiovascular drugs
  Captopril, diazoxide, hydralazine, methyldopa, pindolol, procainamide, propranalol, quinidine

Diuretics
  Bendrofluazide, bumetanide, chlorothiazide, chlorthalidone, hydrochlorothiazide, spironolactone

Miscellaneous
  Allopurinol, arsenicals, cimetidine, colchicine, griseofulvin, levamisole, levodopa

their metabolites might induce neutropenia by one or both of two mechanisms: (1) impairment of bone marrow function; and (2) destruction of circulating neutrophils.[33]

The classical example of a drug that causes agranulocytosis by a toxic effect on the marrow is chlorpromazine. This drug causes a transient and moderate neutropenia in one-third of individuals receiving it. It causes agranulocytosis in about 1 in 1200 individuals, usually after a cumulative dose of 10–20 g over 20–30 days. Chlorpromazine appears to cause agranulocytosis by

inhibiting DNA synthesis and cell proliferation in the granulocyte precursors of susceptible individuals. At the time of the agranulocytosis, the marrow shows few or no neutrophil granulocytopoietic cells. The susceptibility of occasional individuals to develop agranulocytosis following therapy with chlorpromazine or other sulphur-containing drugs such as carbimazole or metiamide may depend on their genetically determined ability to oxidize the drug to highly-reactive myelotoxic metabolites (sulphoxides) more rapidly than most individuals.[34] It is likely that many other drugs that cause neutropenia do so by directly or indirectly impairing biochemical processes within granulocytopoietic cells or by causing some form of immune destruction of these cells.

The best understood example of a drug that causes agranulocytosis by destroying circulating neutrophils is amidopyrine. Individuals with amidopyrine-induced agranulocytosis give a history of previous exposure to the drug and may, after recovery from the initial agranulocytosis, show a recurrence of agranulocytosis within 12 h of a test dose. The serum of such individuals contains an antibody that causes agglutination of neutrophils and an acute neutropenia in the presence of the drug. It has been suggested that the antibody may be directed against complexes between drug metabolites and cellular components. The marrow shows increased granulocytopoietic activity and a depletion of the more mature precursors.

Immune neutropenia[35]

As has already been mentioned, the agranulocytosis induced by amidopyrine, and possibly also by other drugs, is often attributed to the destruction of circulating neutrophils and, possibly, also of neutrophil precursors by drug-related immune mechanisms. There is also evidence that some drug metabolites may directly damage neutrophils and their precursors through the myeloperoxidase system.[36]

Excluding the drug-related neutropenias, immune neutropenia may be divided into autoimmune neutropenia and alloimmune neonatal neutropenia.

Autoimmune neutropenia may be seen in various collagen vascular disorders, including rheumatoid arthritis (especially Felty's syndrome), SLE, Sjögrens syndrome, scleroderma, polymyositis and polymyalgia rheumatica. A number of mechanisms seem to be involved in the pathogenesis of the neutropenia, including a clonal increase in large granular T-lymphocytes (which may inhibit neutrophil granulocytopoiesis), antibodies against neutrophils, circulating immune complexes and cell-mediated immunity. Autoimmune neutropenia may also be found in association with autoimmune hemolytic anemia, immune thrombocytopenic purpura or both. It may also occur in patients with large granular lymphocyte syndrome and Hodgkin's and non-Hodgkin's lymphoma. Chronic autoimmune neutropenia[37,38] is usually a relatively mild disease unassociated with other autoimmune disorders, characterized by recurrent infections, particularly of the oropharynx and skin; in some cases the antineutrophil antibody has the specificity anti-NA2 or pan-Fcγ RIII (CD16, NA1/NA2). Some cases requiring treatment have responded to granulocyte colony stimulating factor (G-CSF).

In the syndrome called neonatal alloimmune neutropenia (also see Chapter 30),[39,40] the neutrophils and neutrophil precursors of the fetus are destroyed by the transplacental passage of maternal IgG alloantibodies formed against HLA or neutrophil-specific antigens (NA1 and NA2) present on fetal but not on maternal neutrophils. Most cases recover spontaneously. The neutropenia is occasionally severe and may cause life-threatening neonatal infections: such cases respond to G-CSF.

Dialysis neutropenia[41,42]

Shortly after commencing a hemodialysis 'run', contact of plasma with dialysis membranes causes activation of complement via the alternative pathway. Activated complement components lead to increased neutrophil adhesiveness and aggregation, with consequent sequestration in the lungs and to a lesser extent in vessels elsewhere, and thus to a marked neutropenia. Acute cardiopulmonary failure may occur. After some hours, neutropenia is reversed and a rebound neutrophilia occurs.

Chronic idiopathic neutropenia[35,43,44]

This disorder of unknown etiology, affects children as well as adults. Neutropenia develops (without splenomegaly) and lasts for 1 or more years. The condition resembles chronic autoimmune neutropenia except for the lack of clear evidence for an immune basis. In chronic idiopathic neutropenia, there may also be a monocytosis. In addition, both CD8+ and CD4+ T-lymphocytes and to a lesser extent NK cells are reduced.[45] Recovery occurs spontaneously. Both affected children and adults usually have moderate neutropenia and only suffer from an increased susceptibility to minor infections. Some are more severely affected.

The $T_{1/2}$ of circulating neutrophils is normal in most but not all cases, as is the size of the marginated blood granulocyte pool. However, both the neutropenia and the T-lymphocytopenia may be at least partly due to increased extravasation of these cells[46,47] as there is a marked elevation of serum levels of endothelial cell-derived soluble cell adhesion molecules (sELAM, sICAM, sVCAM) indicating endothelial cell activation. Patients also have elevated levels of two potent endothelial cell activators, IL1-β and TNF-α, in their serum.

The number of proliferating neutrophil precursors in the marrow is usually normal or subnormal indicating a failure to increase granulocytopoietic activity in response to the neutropenia. The number of non-dividing precursors, particularly the juvenile neutrophils and segmented neutrophils, is reduced in about a third of the cases. However, a proportion of cases show different cytokinetic disturbances (e.g. increased numbers of proliferating precursors, shortened $T_{1/2}$ of blood granulocytes, or an increase in the marginated granulocyte pool), suggesting that chronic idiopathic neutropenia may include a number of pathogenetically-different conditions. Although the bone marrow usually contains normal or increased numbers of granulocyte-macrophage colony-forming units (CFU-GM), the formation of colony-stimulating factor by marrow macrophages is defective.[48] In other studies, bone marrow stromal cells of some cases have shown reduced expression of G-CSF mRNA.[49] In contrast to the above findings, there are reduced numbers of CFU-GM in long-term marrow cultures and the culture supernatants contain increased or normal levels of G-CSF. However, the supernatants contain increased levels of the inhibitory cytokine TGF-β1, raising the possibility that granulocytopoiesis may be impaired due to an imbalance between stimulatory and inhibitory cytokines.[50] *In vitro* studies have shown that some cases of acquired idiopathic neutropenia have T-cells (sometimes with the phenotype of cytotoxic/suppressor cells) which inhibit the growth of autologous CFU-GM.[51]

Symptomatic patients have responded to treatment with low doses of recombinant human G-CSF.[52]

Cyclical neutropenia[53–55]

This is a rare disorder in which neutropenia occurs for 4–10 days at intervals of 15–35 days (average, 21 days). Most cases present in infancy or childhood with periodic bouts of fever, malaise, headache, sore throat, oral ulceration, skin infections or, occasionally, infections of the lungs and other organs. Such bouts occur during the neutropenic phases, last for a few days and recur over many years. They are sometimes accompanied by arthralgia or abdominal pain. About half the cases show a monocytosis during the neutropenic phase and some show an eosinophilia. The neutrophil count becomes nearly normal between the symptomatic periods but there is usually an increased proportion (50–80%) of juvenile (unsegmented) neutrophils. The cyclical neutropenia results from cyclical changes in neutrophil granulocytopoiesis; a severe hypoplasia of the neutrophil series precedes the onset of neutropenia. Cyclical neutropenia has been transferred by bone marrow transplantation to a histocompatible sibling with acute lymphoblastic leukemia.[56] In some cases the condition is inherited as a dominant trait with high penetrance and variable expression. In such cases there are mutations involving the neutrophil elastase gene (see Chapter 18). Individual patients have benefitted from therapy with testosterone, prednisolone or lithium or from plasmapheresis and most patients respond to treatment with G-CSF.

Familial benign chronic neutropenia[57,58]

This disorder, which is inherited as an autosomal dominant trait, is characterized by chronic neutropenia, sometimes associated with monocytosis and hypergammaglobulinemia and, occasionally, with moderate eosinophilia. Some cases have only a mild or moderate neutropenia and are asymptomatic. Others have a more severe neutropenia and suffer from repeated attacks of severe stomatitis and recurrent boils from infancy and from periodontal disease. However, even these cases run a relatively benign course. The bone marrow is normocellular and usually shows few neutrophil precursors beyond the myelocyte stage.

Neutropenia in healthy black population

Ethnic variations in the normal neutrophil count are mentioned in Chapter 1.

Severe congenital neutropenia (infantile genetic agranulocytosis, Kostmann's syndrome)[59]

This condition is usually inherited as an autosomal dominant trait. Affected patients suffer from very severe neutropenia (bordering on complete agranulocytosis) and recurrent infections (e.g. boils and carbuncles). Prior to the availability of recombinant human G-CSF, they usually died from overwhelming sepsis during infancy but with antibiotic therapy occasionally survived to the second decade. Some cases have an absolute monocytosis and eosinophilia and may develop hypergammaglobulinemia. The bone marrow shows normal, increased or decreased cellularity of the neutrophil series, with an

absence of cells beyond the promyelocyte/myelocyte stage. The neutrophils and their precursors show prominent vacuolation. Only rare neutrophil colonies are formed when marrow is cultured on soft agar and electron-microscopic studies of such colonies show gross abnormalities of maturation (asynchronous nucleocytoplasmic maturation, convoluted nuclei, paucity of granules). Cells in monocyte and eosinophil colonies mature normally.[60] The neutropenia appears to result from an intrinsic defect in an early progenitor cell which causes ineffectiveness of neutrophil granulocytopoiesis. Some cases develop acute myeloid leukemia.

Most patients respond rapidly to treatment with G-CSF, with an increase of the neutrophil count to within the normal range. No abnormalities have been found in G-CSF production or in the G-CSF receptor.[61] There is a marked increase within neutrophils of the SH2-containing protein tyrosine phosphatases SHP-1 and SHP-2, suggesting that in Kostmann's syndrome there may be an abnormality of dephosphorylation of proteins involved in intracellular signaling pathways.[62] Recently, it has been shown that a high proportion of cases of dominantly-inherited severe congenital neutropenia have mutations in the gene for neutrophil elastase (see Chapter 18).

Congenital aleukia (reticular dysgenesis)[63]

In this rare disorder, no granulocytes, monocytes or lymphocytes are present in the blood and there are no lymphocytes in the thymus. There are also no peripheral lymphoid tissues. The bone marrow shows erythropoiesis and megakaryocytopoiesis but no lymphopoiesis, monocytopoiesis or granulocytopoiesis. Affected individuals die of infection shortly after birth.

Other rare neutropenic syndromes

Neutropenia has been described as a feature of a number of other rare syndromes usually affecting one or very few cases. In Schwachman's syndrome,[64,65] which is inherited as an autosomal recessive trait, neutropenia is associated with frequent infections, malabsorption due to congenital pancreatic hypoplasia, metaphyseal chondrodysplasia, thrombocytopenia and defective neutrophil motility.

In the syndrome of 'cartilage-hair hypoplasia',[66] the neutropenia is associated with dwarfism, abnormally fine and sparse hair, hyperextensible joints and lymphopenia.

Neutropenia has occasionally been associated with hypogammaglobulinemia[67] (sometimes with elevated IgM levels) as a familial or non-familial characteristic and, in the rare disorder known as myelokathexis, there is in addition neutrophil degeneration and hypersegmentation (see Chapter 18).

Neutropenia is also a feature of two disorders of neutrophil function, the 'lazy leukocyte syndrome'[68] (in which recurrent mouth and ear infections are associated with an impairment of the release of neutrophils from the marrow, normal neutrophil morphology, and an impaired response to chemotactic stimuli) and the Chediak–Higashi syndrome.

The term congenital dysgranulopoietic neutropenia has been used to describe a disorder affecting six unrelated children who had recurrent severe bacterial infections since birth, marked neutropenia, impaired neutrophil migration, normal numbers of colony-forming cells in the bone marrow, normal or slightly increased colony-stimulating activity in the serum, and prominent morphologic and ultrastructural abnormalities in cells at and after the neutrophil promyelocyte/myelocyte stage.[69] The abnormalities of the cells included numerous autophagic vacuoles, abnormally electron-lucent primary granules, myelinization of primary granules, granule fusion, absence or marked decrease of secondary granules, and maturation of the cytoplasm ahead of the nucleus.[69]

Eosinopenia[70]

A transient eosinopenia develops after the administration of corticotrophin, corticosteroids, adrenaline or histamine or in response to severe exercise, emotional stress, trauma, surgery and most acute viral and bacterial infections. In the case of corticosteroid therapy, the eosinopenia appears to result both from an impairment of the release of eosinophils from the marrow and the increased margination (or sequestration) of blood eosinophils. An eosinopenia may also be seen in normal pregnancy and during labor and in Cushing's syndrome, acromegaly, SLE and aplastic anemia.

Basopenia[71]

A basophil granulocytopenia (basopenia) may be found in acute hypersensitivity reactions, acute stress, hyperthyroidism, Cushing's syndrome and pregnancy as well as in response to the administration of progesterone, corticosteroids or corticotrophin. The blood basophil count falls on the day of ovulation.

Monocytopenia

A monocytopenia is seen in cases of aplastic anemia, particularly when there is a marked neutropenia[72] and

in AIDS. It is characteristic of 'hairy cell' leukemia (see Chapter 22). Monocytopenia also occurs after the administration of corticosteroids.[73]

Lymphocytopenia[74]

Temporary lymphocytopenia (lymphopenia) develops after the administration of corticosteroids. In addition, lymphocytopenia, probably due to elevated plasma cortisol levels, is seen following surgery or trauma and in many acute illnesses, such as most infections (including malaria), burns and heart failure. Other causes of lymphocytopenia include Cushing's syndrome, uremia, SLE, advanced carcinoma and Hodgkin's disease, aplastic anemia, agranulocytosis, myelodysplastic syndromes, alcohol abuse, anorexia nervosa and graft-versus-host disease. Lymphocytopenia is also found in some congenital and acquired immune deficiency syndromes including AIDS and immune deficiency secondary to radiotherapy or treatment with immunosuppressive drugs (e.g. after organ transplantation or cytotoxic chemotherapy).

Leukocytosis

An increase in the concentration of circulating leukocytes above the reference range for the age of an individual is termed leukocytosis. This can be due to an increase in one or more of the five types of leukocytes normally present in blood or to the appearance of immature leukocytes in the circulation, or both. Increases in the neutrophils, eosinophils, basophils, monocytes or lymphocytes are described as neutrophil leukocytosis (neutrophilia), eosinophil leukocytosis (eosinophilia), basophil leukocytosis (basophilia), monocytosis and lymphocytosis, respectively.

Neutrophil leukocytosis

Neutrophil leukocytosis may be generated by one or more of the following mechanisms: (1) a shift of cells from the marginated to the circulating blood neutrophil pools; (2) an increased rate of entry of neutrophils into the blood; (3) a prolonged $T_{1/2}$ of neutrophils in the circulation; and (4) a decreased rate of egress of neutrophils from the blood into the tissues.

Some of the causes of a neutrophil leukocytosis are listed in Table 17.3. The high neutrophil counts seen after exercise and electric shocks, in emotional states, and in patients with vomiting, convulsions or paroxysmal tachycardia, are caused by a shift of cells from the marginated to the circulating pool. The neutrophil leukocytosis seen in most other conditions results from an increased rate of release of neutrophils from the marrow into the blood. This occurs acutely as a result of the emptying of the marrow granulocyte pool into the blood and more chronically in association with an increased rate of production of marrow granulocytes. The first of these mechanisms is responsible for the initial acute neutrophilia in response to bacterial endotoxins, corticosteroids and etiocholanolone. The second operates when there is a sustained neutrophil leukocytosis as in conditions such as infections, inflammation and malignant disease. In some patients with carcinoma or sarcoma the increased neutrophil granulocytopoiesis appears to result from the production by the tumor cells of proteins which stimulate the growth of CFU-GM.[75,76] The high

neutrophil leukocyte counts in the chronic myeloproliferative disorders result partly from increased production of leukocytes in the marrow and partly from an abnormally long survival time ($T_{1/2}$) of these cells in the blood. The neutrophil leukocytosis seen in patients on long-term corticosteroid therapy is associated with a normal rate of release of neutrophils from the marrow into the blood and a decreased rate of egress from the blood into the tissues. The commonest cause of neutrophil leukocytosis is an acute infection with a pyogenic organism. However, neutrophil leukocytosis also occurs in infections with certain non-pyogenic organisms (e.g. in poliomyelitis, herpes zoster, typhus). Tuberculosis does not usually cause a neutrophil leukocytosis but may do so when there is rapid local spread of tubercle bacilli, as for example in tuberculous meningitis. In acute infections involving the organisms listed in Table 17.3, the neutrophil counts are usually in the range $10–30 \times 10^9/l$ (but may be $> 80 \times 10^9/l$) and the eosinophil and basophil counts are reduced. Severe infections may be accompanied by a shift to the left and the development of toxic granulation and Döhle bodies within neutrophils. Young children may respond to acute infections with a lymphocytosis rather than a neutrophil leukocytosis.

Eosinophil leukocytosis[70]

An eosinophilia may occur in many conditions, several of which are listed in Table 17.4. It is most commonly caused by allergic disorders in non-tropical areas and by parasitic infestations (Figs 17.4 and 17.5) in tropical areas. In the case of parasitic infestations the highest eosinophil counts are found with metazoan parasites which invade tissues or the blood. A tropical syndrome characterized by

Table 17.3 Causes of neutrophil leukocytosis

Physiologic
  Neonates (Chapter 1)
  Exercise, emotion
  Pregnancy
  Parturition
  Lactation

Pathologic
  Certain acute infections
    Bacterial: various pyogenic cocci, *Escherichia coli*,
      Pseudomonas aeruginosa, Corynebacterium diphtheriae,
      Francisella tularensis
    Spirochaetal: syphilis, Weil's disease
    Rickettsial: typhus, Rocky Mountain spotted fever
    Chlamydial: psittacosis
    Viral: rabies, poliomyelitis, smallpox, herpes simplex
      infection, herpes zoster, chickenpox
    Protozoal: *Pneumocystis carinii* infection
    Mycotic: actinomycosis, coccidioidomycosis
    Helminthic: liver fluke, filariasis
  Acute inflammation not caused by infections
    Surgical operations, burns, infarcts, hepatic necrosis, crush
      injuries, rheumatoid arthritis, rheumatic fever, vasculitis,
      myositis, pancreatitis, hypersensitivity reactions, etc.
  Endocrine/metabolic
    Cushing's syndrome, acute thyrotoxicosis, uremia, diabetic
      acidosis, gout
  Acute hemorrhage
  Acute hemolysis
  Chronic myeloproliferative disorders
    Chronic granulocytic leukemia, polycythemia rubra vera,
      myelofibrosis
  Malignant disease
    Carcinoma, lymphoma, etc.
  Drugs
    Adrenaline, corticosteroids, lithium
  Hereditary neutrophilia
  Miscellaneous
    Convulsions, paroxysmal tachycardia, electric shock,
      vomiting, after splenectomy, postneutropenic rebound
      neutrophilia, cigarette smoking

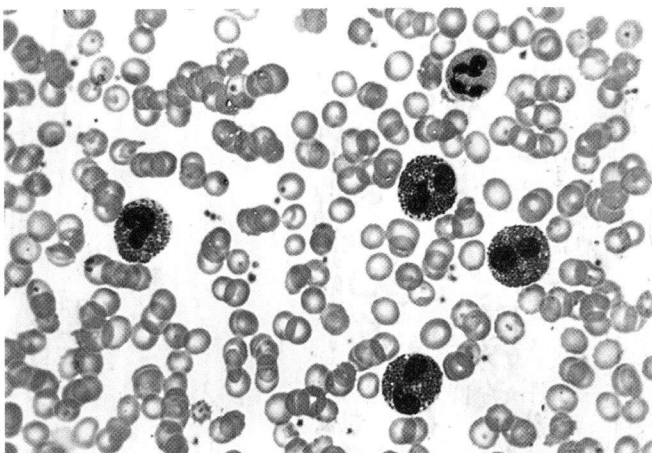

Fig. 17.4 Peripheral blood film of a patient with a reactive eosinophilia secondary to a parasitic infection. May–Grünwald–Giemsa stain.

Table 17.4 Causes of eosinophil leukocytosis

Parasitic infestations
  Metazoan infestations:[77] ancylostomiasis (hookworm infestation), angiostrogyliasis, ascariasis, clonorchiasis, cysticercosis, echinococcosis (hydatid cyst), fascioliasis, fasciolopsiasis, filariasis (Fig. 17.5), gnathostomiasis, loiasis, onchocerciasis, paragonimiasis, schistosomiasis, strongyloidiasis, toxocariasis, trichinellosis, visceral larva migrans (toxocariasis)
  Arthropod infestations: scabies

Certain fungal and bacterial infections
  Allergic pulmonary aspergillosis, chronic tuberculosis (occasionally), coccidioidomycosis, disseminated histoplasmosis, *Pneumocystis pneumoniae* infection, scarlet fever

Allergic disorders
  Bronchial asthma, atopic eczema, hay fever, allergic vasculitis, Stevens–Johnson syndrome, drug sensitivity (gold, sulphonamides, penicillin)

Graft-versus-host reaction

Skin diseases
  Pemphigus, bullous pemphigoid, eczema, psoriasis, herpes gestationis, subcutaneous eosinophilic angiolymphoid hyperplasia with eosinophilia, eosinophilic lymphofolliculosis (Kimura's disease), granulomatous dermatitis with eosinophilia (Well's disease), diffuse fasciitis with eosinophilia (Schulman's syndrome)

Postinfection rebound eosinophilia

Reactive 'pulmonary' eosinophilia
  Löffler's syndrome (pulmonary infiltration with eosinophilia), tropical pulmonary eosinophilia

Idiopathic hypereosinophilic syndrome

Leukemias and chronic myeloproliferative disorders
  Chronic granulocytic leukemia, polycythemia rubra vera, acute lymphoblastic leukemia (cALL and T-ALL),[78] eosinophilic leukemia

Other malignant diseases
  Mycosis fungoides, Sézary syndrome, Hodgkin's disease, other lymphomas (T-cell), angioimmunoblastic lymphadenopathy, carcinoma (usually with metastasis), multiple myeloma, heavy chain disease

Systemic mastocytosis

Connective tissue disorders
  Churg–Strauss syndrome (variant of polyarteritis nodosa), systemic necrotizing vasculitis (variant of polyarteritis nodosa), systemic sclerosis, rheumatoid arthritis

Thrombocytopenia with absent radii

Certain disorders of neutrophils
  Job's syndrome, severe congenital neutropenia, familial benign chronic neutropenia, cyclical neutropenia

Wiskott–Aldrich syndrome

Cyclical eosinophilia with angioedema

Hereditary eosinophilia

Miscellaneous
  Ulcerative colitis, Crohn's disease, eosinophilic gastroenteritis, Goodpasture's syndrome, pancreatitis, chronic active hepatitis, after splenectomy, after irradiation of intra-abdominal tumors

Idiopathic

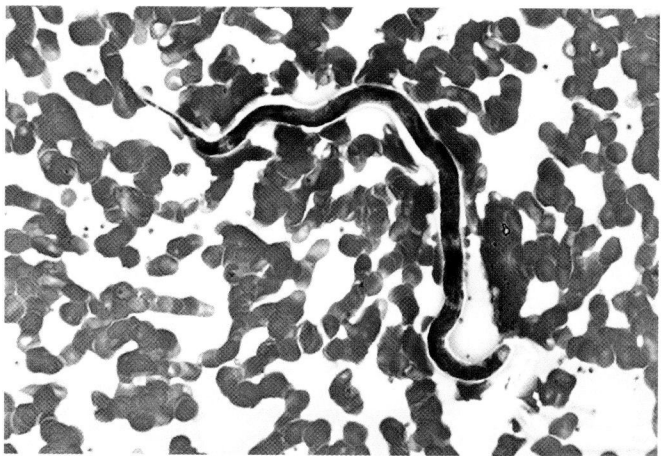

Fig. 17.5 Microfilaria in the blood of a patient with loiasis. May–Grünwald–Giemsa stain.

eosinophilia, lymph node enlargement and pulmonary symptoms has been described under the name tropical eosinophilia: although microfilariae are absent from the blood, this syndrome is caused by occult filariasis, the microfilariae being destroyed in the tissues by an immune mechanism.

Very high eosinophil counts are also seen in the hypereosinophilic syndrome (see below). The eosinophilia associated with malignant tumors may be caused by a tumor-derived glycoprotein which stimulates eosinophil granulocytopoiesis.[79] Tumors may also elaborate a factor chemotactic for eosinophils which resembles eosinophil chemotactic factor for anaphylaxis (ECF-A).

Idiopathic hypereosinophilic syndrome[80–82]

The idiopathic hypereosinophilic syndrome (IHES) is an acquired disorder of unknown etiology. It is characterized by hypereosinophilia (eosinophil count $> 1.5 \times 10^9/l$) of more than 6 months duration and pulmonary and other organ dysfunction secondary to infiltration by eosinophils. The tissue damage is caused by specific secretory products of eosinophils. The majority of patients are males. The absolute eosinophil count ranges from $1.5 \times 10^9/l$ up to $100–300 \times 10^9/l$. Eosinophils are frequently vacuolated and extensively degranulated (Fig. 17.6A, B). Both hypersegmented and non-segmented forms are seen and some cells may have doughnut-shaped nuclei (Fig. 17.6B). Eosinophil IgG Fc receptors may be increased. Neutrophils of patients with IHES may show aberrant staining, the granules being larger and often more basophilic than those of normal neutrophils (Fig. 17.6C). Anemia and thrombocytopenia may occur. The bone

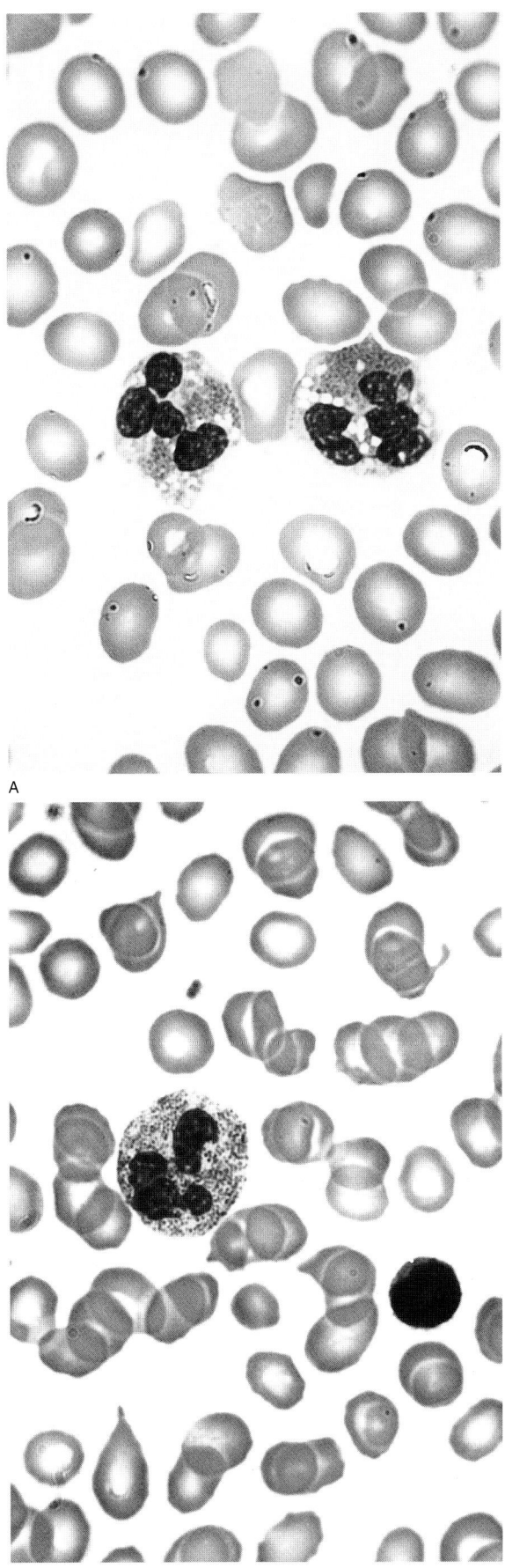

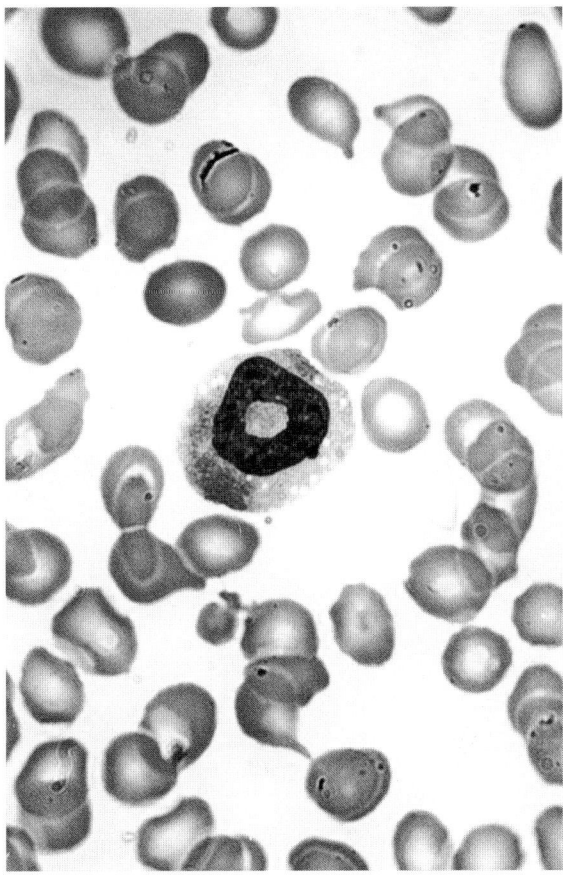

Fig. 17.6 (A–C) Blood film from a patient with the hypereosinophilic syndrome. (A) Two abnormal eosinophil granulocytes which are vacuolated and partially degranulated and which show increased nuclear segmentation. (B) Partially degranulated eosinophil granulocyte with a ring-shaped nucleus. (C) Neutrophil granulocyte with abnormally large, basophilic granules (the granules are smaller than those of a basophil granulocyte). May–Grünwald–Giemsa stain.

marrow shows an increase of eosinophils and eosinophil myelocytes; bone marrow cells show less degranulation and vacuolation than peripheral blood cells.

Cardiac damage (Löffler's endocarditis) may develop in IHES but may also occur in patients with sustained reactive hypereosinophila, including that due to filariasis and toxocariasis.[83–85] In the acute phase there is necrosis of myocardium, particularly subendocardial myocardium, with infiltration by eosinophils and other leukocytes. Other cardiac lesions include mural thrombosis with underlying eosinophil infiltration, pericarditis and arteritis. Valves may show fibrosis or formation of vegetations. The mural thrombi may give rise to single or multiple emboli. In the chronic phase subendocardial fibrosis occurs, initially with a surrounding zone of inflammation; chordae become shortened, valves, particularly the mitral and tricuspid, become incompetent and a restrictive cardiomyopathy and arrhythmias develop. Endomyocardial biopsy may be used to confirm the diagnosis.

Other features found in some cases of IHES include anorexia, weight loss, fever, night sweats, hepatomegaly, splenomegaly and lymphadenopathy (with eosinophil infiltration), vasculitis (including retinal and choroidal vasculitis), pulmonary fibrosis, and damage to the central and peripheral nervous system. Vasculitic lesions are often associated with thrombosis and increased plasma levels of β-thromboglobulin and platelet factor 4, which suggest activation of platelets. Levels of fibrinogen and factor-VIII-related-antigen are increased, probably as a reaction to tissue damage. Choroidal and retinal vasculitis may be demonstrated by fluorescein angiography, which shows hemorrhage, microaneurysms, attenuation of vessels and areas of avascularity. Neurologic lesions (mononeuritis multiplex, peripheral neuritis) are common; they may be a consequence of embolism, vasculitis, thrombosis, hemorrhage, or damage by eosinophil-derived neurotoxin (Rnase 2). Diarrhea due to eosinophilic gastroenteritis may occur.

The diagnosis of IHES involves the exclusion both of known causes of eosinophilia and of eosinophilic leukemia. The diagnosis of eosinophilic leukemia can be made when there is a clonal cytogenetic abnormality in bone marrow cells (see Chapter 21) or presumptive evidence of clonality in females from analysis of X-chromosome inactivation patterns in purified eosinophils.[86] Some patients diagnosed as having IHES subsequently develop a clonal cytogenetic abnormality, undergo a blastic transformation or develop tumors composed of myeloblasts and eosinophils (granulocytic sarcoma). Evidently, such patients initially had eosinophilic leukemia rather than IHES, with disease progression occurring subsequently.

Tissue damage similar to that seen in IHES also occurs when eosinophilia is secondary to a malignant disorder such as Hodgkin's disease, non-Hodgkin's lymphoma or acute lymphoblastic leukemia.[87]

Basophil leukocytosis[71]

A reactive basophil leukocytosis may occur in hypersensitivity reactions, hypothyroidism, ulcerative colitis, smallpox, chickenpox and the idiopathic hypereosinophilic syndrome. Basophil leukocytosis also occurs in chronic granulocytic leukemia, polycythemia rubra vera, essential thrombocythemia, myelofibrosis, basophilic leukemia, eosinophilic leukemia and Ph-positive acute leukemia. In the case of chronic granulocytic leukemia, a further and considerable increase in both immature and mature basophils may precede transformation of the disease to a more malignant phase.

Lymphocytosis and monocytosis

The various causes of lymphocytosis and monocytosis are listed in Tables 17.5 and 17.6. The two chronic infections, tuberculosis and brucellosis, may be associated with an increase in either or both cell types. The only acute bacterial infection that is frequently associated with a lymphocytosis is whooping cough (pertussis); in some children with this disorder the lymphocyte count may exceed $50 \times 10^9/l$. A lymphocytosis may be found in several viral infections. In infectious mononucleosis the high lymphocyte count is accompanied by large, atypical lymphocytes. Changes very similar to those of infectious mononucleosis may be seen in cytomegalovirus infection,

Table 17.5 Causes of lymphocytosis

Physiologic
  Infants and young children (Chapter 1)

Certain viral infections
  Infectious mononucleosis, cytomegalovirus infection, infectious hepatitis, chickenpox, smallpox, measles, rubella, mumps, influenza, primary HIV infection

Certain bacterial infections
  Pertussis, brucellosis, tuberculosis, secondary and congenital syphilis

Bacterial infections in infants and young children

Chronic lymphocytic leukemia

Lymphomas, Waldenström's macroglobulinemia and heavy chain disease

Post-splenectomy

Table 17.6 Causes of monocytosis[88]

Physiologic
  Infants

Certain bacterial infections
  Tuberculosis, brucellosis, secondary syphilis, subacute bacterial endocarditis, typhoid, recovery from many acute infections

Certain protozoal infections
  Leishmaniasis (visceral and cutaneous), malaria, trypanosomiasis (Fig. 17.7)

Certain rickettsial infections
  Typhus, Rocky Mountain spotted fever

Myelodysplastic syndromes

Acute monocytic and acute and chronic myelomonocytic leukemias

Chronic granulocytic leukemia, atypical Ph-negative chronic myeloid leukemia, juvenile chronic myelomonocytic leukemia, polycythemia rubra vera, myelofibrosis

Other malignant diseases
  Hodgkin's disease, other lymphomas, carcinoma, multiple myeloma, malignant histiocytosis

Miscellaneous
  Cyclical neutropenia, chronic idiopathic neutropenia, recovery from drug-induced neutropenia, ulcerative colitis, regional enteritis, sarcoidosis, connective tissue disease, post-splenectomy, lipid storage diseases

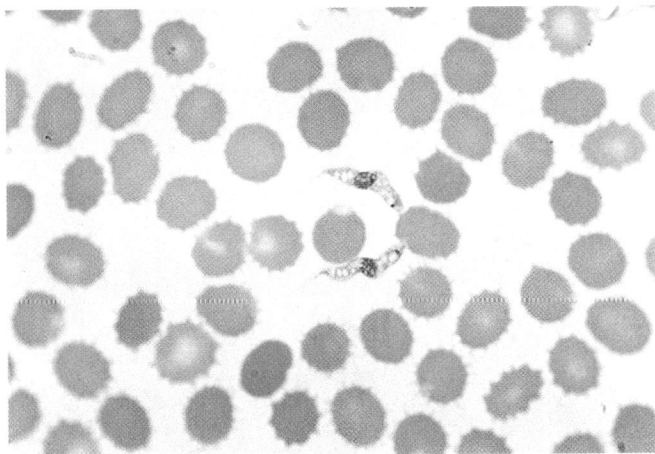

Fig. 17.7 Two trypanosomes in the blood smear of a patient with African trypanosomiasis. May–Grünwald–Giemsa stain.

and similar but lesser changes may be seen in toxoplasmosis, malaria, infectious hepatitis, primary infection with HIV (Chapter 5), other viral infections, as a sequel of immunization, and as part of a reaction to drugs.

Infectious mononucleosis[89]

Infectious mononucleosis is a clinical syndrome resulting from an acute self-limiting primary infection by the Epstein–Barr virus (EBV). This syndrome is characterized by fever, pharyngitis, the presence of increased numbers of highly atypical lymphocytes ('mononuclear cells') in the peripheral blood, and the production of heterophile antibodies (see below). EBV infects and replicates in the B-lymphocytes and epithelial cells of the pharynx and also in a small proportion of T-cells. All three cell types have the specific receptor for EBV, namely CD21 (C3d receptor). Primary infection is followed by the establishment of a long-term carrier state.

Clinical features

In children, primary infections are often asymptomatic or clinically mild. Typical infectious mononucleosis usually develops when primary infections occur in adolescents and young adults; however, small numbers of typical cases are seen in younger and older persons. Fever and malaise are usual. Acute tonsillitis and pharyngitis may be severe, sometimes with the formation of a pseudomembrane resembling that of diphtheria. Cervical lymph nodes are commonly enlarged and lymphadenopathy may be generalized (hence the synonym 'glandular fever'). Splenomegaly is common, with spontaneous splenic rupture a rare complication. Hepatic enlargement and jaundice occur in a minority. Other clinical features are multiple but less common. They include edema of the eye-lids, rash and arthritis and the clinical manifestations of pericarditis, meningitis, encephalitis, nephritis, pneumonitis, retinitis, uveitis, myocarditis, parotiditis, mononeuritis and transverse myelitis.

Peripheral blood

The lymphocytes are increased in number and many have atypical morphology (hence 'atypical mononucleosis') (Fig. 17.8). Atypical features include large size, irregular shape, increased cytoplasmic basophilia, diffuse chromatin pattern, prominent nucleoli and a scalloped margin at points of contact with other cells. The atypical lymphocytes are not the virus-infected B-lymphocytes, but are T-lymphocytes. These T-lymphocytes may contain tartrate-resistant acid phosphatase (the same isoenzyme as is found in hairy cell leukemia) and may show block-positivity when stained by the periodic acid-Schiff (PAS) method. The majority of atypical cells have the phenotype of CD8+ cytotoxic/suppressor T-cells. The proliferation of EBV-infected B-cells is limited by EBV-specific cytotoxic T-cells that recognize various EBV antigens. There is also a reduction in the number of CD4+ T-cells, secondary to viral gp350-related Fas-mediated apoptosis.[90] The eosinophil count is reduced. Neutrophil alkaline

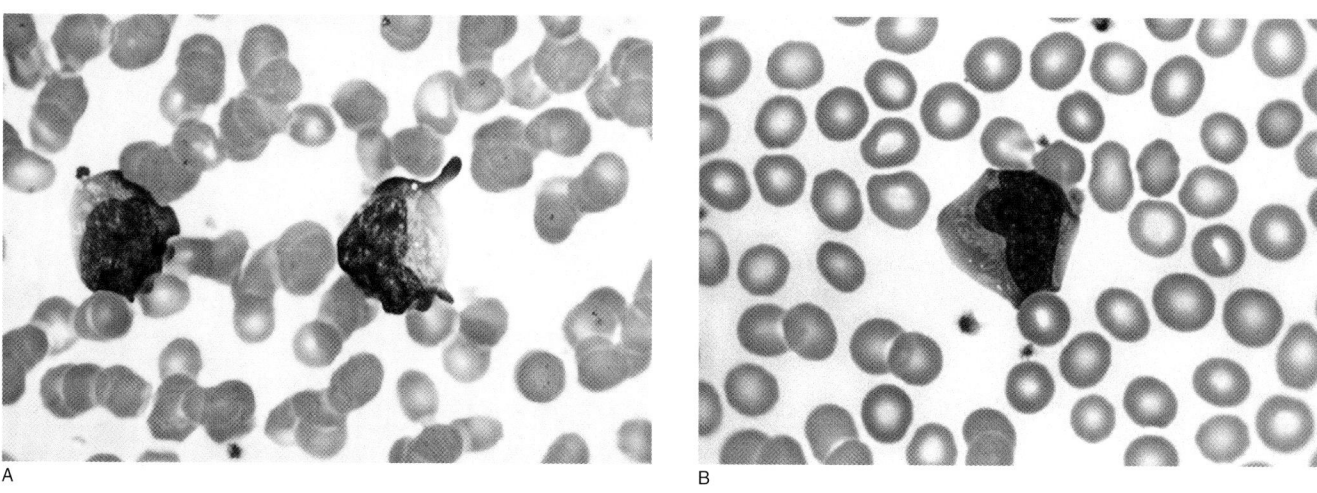

Fig. 17.8 (A,B) Atypical lymphocytes in the blood films of two patients with infectious mononucleosis. In addition to the features mentioned in the text, the cell in (A) showed increased basophilia at the periphery of the cytoplasm, another commonly found atypical feature. May–Grünwald–Giemsa stain.

phosphatase tends to be low. Hematological complications include autoimmune hemolytic anemia due to a cold antibody with anti-i specificity, thrombocytopenia due to peripheral destruction of platelets, and rarely granulocytopenia or aplastic anemia, the latter occuring several weeks after infectious mononucleosis. Another rare complication is severe pancytopenia secondary to hemophagocytosis.[91] Disseminated intravascular coagulation has been observed in association with the hemophagocytic syndrome.

Serological features. Infectious mononucleosis is accompanied by the development of multiple antibodies that may be categorized as: (1) virus-specific antibodies; (2) heterophile antibodies; and (3) autoantibodies. Heterophile antibodies are antibodies formed in response to antigens of one species that cross-react with antigens on the cells of other species.

The most characteristic heterophile antibody (which is the basis of the Paul Bunnell test and other simpler screening tests for infectious mononucleosis) is an agglutinin of sheep or horse red blood cells which is adsorbed by ox red cells but not by guinea-pig kidney. Agglutinins of rhesus monkey, goat and camel erythrocytes and hemolysins of ox red cells may also occur. Antibodies may also develop against bacteria, and against viruses other than EBV.

Autoantibodies that may develop in infectious mononucleosis include anti-i and less often anti-I, anti-IgG (rheumatoid factor), antinuclear factor and the antibodies responsible for a positive Wassermann reaction.

A presumptive diagnosis of infectious mononucleosis may be made when typical clinical and hematological features are associated with the presence of a heterophile antibody. A definitive diagnosis requires serologic evidence of a recent primary EBV infection, namely the demonstration of IgM antibody to VCA (viral capsid antigen). Individuals with a past infection have IgG but not IgM antibodies to VCA and have antibodies to EBNA (EBV-determined nuclear antigen). Measurement of virus-specific antibodies is of no value in severely immunocompromised patients; in such cases the diagnosis of EBV infection is difficult and requires the demonstration of the EBV genome or related proteins in tissues.

Bone marrow

The marrow aspirate is infiltrated with atypical pleomorphic lymphocytes. There are focal accumulations of lymphocytes, and granulomas composed of lymphocytes, histiocytes (macrophages) and epithelioid cells. The granulomas tend to be smaller than those in tuberculosis and sarcoidosis and giant cells are infrequent.[92]

When infectious mononucleosis is associated with a hemophagocytic syndrome (Chapter 5), the bone marrow shows increased numbers of promonocytes and phagocytic histiocytes that are cytologically more mature than the cells of malignant histiocytosis. Bone marrow aplasia is a rare complication.[93]

Atypical manifestations of EBV infection

Patients with defective immunity may have an atypical outcome following primary EBV infection.

X-linked lymphoproliferative disease (Duncan's syndrome)

This is an X-linked recessive condition in which there is a more-or-less specific inability to deal with the EB virus, usually due to mutations in the gene encoding SLAM (signaling-lymphocyte activation molecule)-associated protein, located on Xq25. In affected boys, primary EBV infection causes a life-threatening illness, with fulminant hepatitis, hemophagocytic syndrome and a 50% mortality. Some patients subsequently develop aplastic anemia, acquired hypogammaglobulinemia, or lymphoproliferative disorders including B-cell lymphoma (diffuse large B-cell lymphoma or small non-cleaved cell lymphoma).[94] The aplastic anemia may respond to corticosteroids, antithymocyte globulin or immunosuppression followed by syngeneic stem cell transplantation and appears to have an immunologic basis.

Chronic active EBV infection

Primary EBV infection may sometimes run a prolonged course of more than 6 months (even years), and this presumably occurs in individuals with a lesser degree of immunologic inadequacy than in Duncan's syndrome. The features of chronic active EBV infection are severe malaise, persistent or intermittent fever, enlargement of lymph nodes, hepatosplenomegaly and an unusual antibody response pattern to EBV. Rarely, chronic active EBV infection may be severe with persistent high fever, extreme lymphadenopathy, interstitial pneumonitis, anemia, neutropenia, thrombocytopenia, polyclonal gammopathy and unusually high IgG antibody titers to EBV-related antigens such as VCA and EA (early antigen).

Lymphoproliferative disorders in immunocompromised subjects

Occasional cases of ataxia-telangiectasia[95] or Wiskott–Aldrich syndrome have developed EBV-genome-positive lymphoma. Patients who are immunosuppressed following renal or other transplantation and who are carriers of EBV may develop polyclonal proliferations of B-lymphocytes carrying the viral genome as a consequence of the inhibition of EBV-specific cytotoxic T-lymphocytes; in some cases evolution to a monoclonal lymphoma occurs.[96,97] An immunosuppressed recipient of a bone marrow transplant also developed a monoclonal immunoblastic sarcoma of donor cell origin which carried EBV DNA.[98] Although EBV does not cause Burkitt's lymphoma-type lymphoproliferative disorders in primary immunodeficiency states or after transplantation, about half the Burkitt's lymphoma-type lymphoproliferative disorders developing in AIDS are EBV-genome-positive.

REFERENCES

1. Brunning RD 1970 Morphological alterations in nucleated blood and marrow cells in genetic disorders. Human Pathology 1: 99–124
2. Skendzel LP, Hoffman GC 1962 The Pelger anomaly of leukocytes: forty cases in seven families. American Journal of Clinical Pathology 37: 294–301
3. Johnson CA, Bass DA, Trillo AA et al 1980 Functional and metabolic studies of polymorphonuclear leukocytes in the congenital Pelger–Huet anomaly. Blood 55: 466–469
4. Undritz VE 1964 Eine neue Sippe mit erblich-konstitutionellen Hochsegmentierung der Neutrophilenkerne Undritz. Schweizerische Medizinische Wochenschrift 94: 1365
5. Oski FA, Naiman JL, Allen DM, Diamond LK 1962 Leukocyte inclusions – Döhle bodies – associated with platelet abnormality (The May–Hegglin Anomaly). Report of a family and review of the literature. Blood 20: 657–667
6. Noris P, Spedini P, Belletti S et al 1998 Thrombocytopenia, giant platelets, and leukocyte inclusion bodies (May–Hegglin anomaly): clinical and laboratory findings. American Journal of Medicine 104: 355–360
7. Martignetti JA, Heath KE, Harris J, Bizzaro N et al 2000 The gene for May–Hegglin anomaly localizes to a < 1-Mb region on chromosome 22q12.3–13.1. American Journal of Human Genetics 66: 1449–1454
8. Blume RS, Wolff SM 1972 The Chediak–Higashi syndrome: studies in four patients and a review of the literature. Medicine (Baltimore) 51: 247–280
9. Introne W, Boissy RE, Gahl WA 1999 Clinical, molecular, and cell biological aspects of Chediak–Higashi syndrome. Molecular Genetics and Metabolism 68: 283–303
10. Virelizier J-L, Lagrue A, Durandy A et al 1982 Reversal of natural killer defect in a patient with Chediak–Higashi syndrome after bone marrow transplantation. New England Journal of Medicine 306: 1055–1056
11. Kjeldsen L, Calafat J, Borregaard N 1998 Giant granules of neutrophils in Chediak–Higashi syndrome are derived from azurophil granules but not from specific and gelatinase granules. Journal of Leukocyte Biology 64: 72–77
12. Oliver JM 1978 Cell biology of leukocyte abnormalities – membrane and cytoskeletal function in normal and defective cells. A review. American Journal of Pathology 93: 221–270
13. Kitahara M, Eyre HJ, Simonian Y et al 1981 Hereditary myeloperoxidase deficiency. Blood 57: 888–893
14. Larrocha C, Fernandez de Castro M, Fontan G et al 1982 Hereditary myeloperoxidase deficiency: study of 12 cases. Scandinavian Journal of Haematology 29: 389–397
15. Petrides PE 1998 Molecular genetics of peroxidase deficiency. Journal of Molecular Medicine 76: 688–698
16. Groover RV, Burke EC, Gordon H, Berdon WE 1972 The genetic mucopolysaccharidoses. Seminars in Hematology 9: 371–402
17. Rozensajn L, Klajman A, Yaffe D, Efrati P 1966 Jordans' anomaly in white blood cells. Blood 28: 258
18. Parmley RT, Tzeng DY, Baehner RL, Boxer LA 1983 Abnormal distribution of complex carbohydrates in neutrophils of a patient with lactoferrin deficiency. Blood 62: 538–548
19. Lomax KJ, Gallin JI, Rotrosen D et al 1989 Selective defect in myeloid cell lactoferrin gene expression in neutrophil specific granule deficiency. Journal of Clinical Investigation 83: 514–519
20. Parmley RT, Gilbert CS, Boxer LA 1989 Abnormal peroxidase-positive granules in 'specific granule' deficiency. Blood 73: 838–844
21. Schofield KP, Stone PC, Beddall AC, Stuart J 1983 Quantitative cytochemistry of the toxic granulation blood neutrophil. British Journal of Haematology 53: 15–22
22. Itoga T, Laszlo J 1962 Döhle bodies and other granulocytic alterations during chemotherapy with cyclophosphamide. Blood 20: 668–674
23. Abernathy MR 1966 Döhle bodies associated with uncomplicated pregnancy. Blood 27: 380–385

24. Juneja SK, Matthews JP, Luzinat R et al 1996 Association of acquired Pelger–Huët anomaly with taxoid therapy. British Journal of Haematology 93: 139–141

25. Ganick DJ, Sunder T, Finley JL 1990 Severe hematologic toxicity of valproic acid. A report of four patients. American Journal of Pediatric Hematology and Oncology 12: 80–85

26. Hernandez JA, Aldred SW, Bruce JR et al 1980 'Botryoid' nuclei in neutrophils of patients with heatstroke. Lancet ii: 642–643

27. Boutilier MB, Hardy NM, Saffos RO 1981 Botryoid nuclei in neutrophils of patients with heatstroke. Lancet i: 53

28. de Gruchy GC 1975 Drug-induced blood disorders. Blackwell Scientific Publications, Oxford

29. Arneborn P, Palmblad J 1982 Drug-induced neutropenia – a survey for Stockholm 1973–1978. Acta Medica Scandinavica 212: 289–292

30. Dameshek W, Colmes A 1936 The effect of drugs in the production of agranulocytosis with particular reference to amidopyrine hypersensitivity. Journal of Clinical Investigation 15: 85

31. Hartl W 1965 Drug allergic agranulocytosis (Schultz's disease). Seminars in Hematology 2: 313–337

32. Pisciotta AV 1971 Drug-induced leukopenia and aplastic anemia. Clinical Pharmacology and Therapeutics 12: 13–43

33. Pisciotta AV 1973 Immune and toxic mechanisms in drug-induced agranulocytosis. Seminars in Hematology 10: 279–310

34. Ritchie JC, Sloan TP, Idle JR, Smith RL 1980 Ciba Foundation Symposium 76 on environmental chemicals, enzyme function and human disease. Elsevier, Amsterdam, 219

35. Dale DC 1998 Immune and idiopathic neutropenia. Current Opinion in Hematology 5: 33–36

36. Uetrecht JP 1996 Reactive metabolites and agranulocytosis. European Journal of Haematology 57 (suppl): 83–88

37. Boxer LA, Greenberg MS, Boxer GJ, Stossel TP 1975 Autoimmune neutropenia. New England Journal of Medicine 293: 748–753

38. Verheugt FWA, von dem Borne AEG Kr, van Noord-Bokhorst JC, Engelfriet CP 1978 Autoimmune granulocytopenia: the detection of granulocyte antibodies with the immunofluorescence test. British Journal of Haematology 39: 339–350

39. Verheugt FW, van Noord-Bokhorst JC, von dem Borne AEG, Engelfriet CP 1979 A family with allo-immune neonatal neutropenia: group-specific pathogenicity of maternal antibodies. Vox Sanguinis 36: 1–8

40. Halvorsen K 1965 Neonatal leucopenia due to fetomaternal leucocyte incompatibility. Acta Paediatrica Scandinavica 54: 86–90

41. Agar JW, Hull JD, Kaplan M, Pletka PG 1979 Acute cardiopulmonary decompensation and complement activation during hemodialysis. Annals of Internal Medicine 90: 792–793

42. Jacob HS, Craddock PR, Hammerschmidt DE, Moldow CF 1980 Complement-induced granulocyte aggregation: an unsuspected mechanism of disease. New England Journal of Medicine 302: 789–794

43. Price TH, Lee MY, Dale DC, Finch CA 1979 Neutrophil kinetics in chronic neutropenia. Blood 54: 581–594

44. Kyle RA 1980 Natural history of chronic idiopathic neutropenia. New England Journal of Medicine 302: 908–909

45. Kyriakou D, Papadaki HA, Sakellariou D et al 1997 Flow-cytometric analysis of peripheral blood lymphocytes in patients with chronic idiopathic neutropenia of adults. Annals of Hematology 75: 103–110

46. Papadaki HA, Eliopoulos GD 1998 Selective loss of peripheral blood CD45RO+ T lymphocytes correlates with increased levels of serum cytokines and endothelial cell-derived soluble cell adhesion molecules in patients with chronic idiopathic neutropenia of adults. Annals of Hematology 77: 153–159

47. Papadaki HA, Eliopoulos GD 1998 Enhanced neutrophil extravasation may be a contributing factor in the determination of neutropenia in patients with chronic idiopathic neutropenia of adults. European Journal of Haematology 61: 272–277

48. Greenberg PL, Mara B, Steed S, Boxer L 1980 The chronic idiopathic neutropenia syndrome: correlation of clinical features with *in vitro* parameters of granulocytopoiesis. Blood 55: 915–921

49. Kohgo Y, Hirayama Y, Matsunaga T et al 1994 Chronic idiopathic neutropenia associated with abnormal expression of granulocyte colony-stimulating factor mRNA of bone marrow stromal cells. International Journal of Hematology 59: 177–180

50. Papadaki HA, Giouremou K, Eliopoulos GD 1999 Low frequency of myeloid progenitor cells in chronic idiopathic neutropenia of adults may be related to increased production of TGF-β by bone marrow stromal cells. European Journal of Haematology 63: 154–162

51. Bagby GC Jr, Lawrence H J, Neerhout RC 1983 T-lymphocyte-mediated granulopoietic failure. *In vitro* identification of prednisone-responsive patients. New England Journal of Medicine 309: 1073–1078

52. Bernini JC, Wooley R, Buchanan GR 1996 Low-dose recombinant human granulocyte colony-stimulating factor therapy in children with symptomatic chronic idiopathic neutropenia. Journal of Pediatrics 129: 551–558

53. Reimann HA, De Berardinis CT 1949 Periodic (cyclic) neutropenia, an entity. Blood 4: 1109

54. von Schulthess GK, Fehr J, Dahinden C 1983 Cyclic neutropenia: amplification of granulocyte oscillations by lithium and long-term suppression of cycling by plasmapheresis. Blood 62: 320–326

55. Dale DC, Hammond WP IV 1988 Cyclic neutropenia: a clinical review. Blood Reviews 2: 178

56. Krance RA, Spruce WE, Forman SJ et al 1982 Human cyclic neutropenia transferred by allogeneic bone marrow grafting. Blood 60: 1263–1266

57. Cutting HO, Lang JE 1964 Familial benign chronic neutropenia. Annals of Internal Medicine 61: 876

58. Busch FH 1990 Familial benign chronic neutropenia in a Danish family. Ugeskrift for Laeger 152: 2565–2566

59. Kostmann R 1956 Infantile genetic agranulocytosis. Acta Paediatrica Scandinavica 45 (suppl 105): 1

60. Zucker-Franklin D, L'Esperance P, Good RA 1977 Congenital neutropenia: an intrinsic cell defect demonstrated by electron microscopy of soft agar colonies. Blood 49: 425–436

61. Guba SC, Sartor CA, Hutchinson R et al 1994 Granulocyte colony-stimulating factor (G-CSF) production and G-CSF receptor structure in patients with congenital neutropenia. Blood 83: 1486–1492

62. Tidow N, Kasper B, Welte K 1999 SH2-containing protein tyrosine phosphatases SHP-1 and SHP-2 are dramatically increased at the protein level in neutrophils from patients with severe congenital neutropenia (Kostmann's syndrome). Experimental Haematology 27: 1038–1045

63. De Vaal OM, Seynhaeve V 1959 Reticular dysgenesis. Lancet ii: 1123

64. Schwachman H, Diamond LK, Oski FA, Khaw KT 1964 The syndrome of pancreatic insufficiency and bone marrow dysfunction. Journal of Pediatrics 65: 645

65. Aggett PJ, Harries JT, Harvey BA, Soothill JF 1979 An inherited defect of neutrophil mobility in Schwachman syndrome. Journal of Pediatrics 94: 391–394

66. Lux SE, Johnston RB Jr, August CS et al 1970 Chronic neutropenia and abnormal cellular immunity in cartilage-hair hypoplasia. New England Journal of Medicine 282: 231–236

67. Lonsdale D, Deodhar SD, Mercer RD 1967 Familial granulocytopenia and associated immunoglobulin abnormality. Report of three cases in young brothers. Journal of Pediatrics 71: 790–801

68. Miller ME, Oski FA, Harris MB 1971 Lazy-leucocyte syndrome. A new disorder of neutrophil function. Lancet i: 665–669

69. Parmley RT, Crist WM, Ragab AH et al 1980 Congenital dysgranulopoietic neutropenia: clinical, serologic, ultrastructural, and in vitro proliferative characteristics. Blood 56: 465–475

70. Beeson PB, Bass DA 1977 The eosinophil. Saunders, Philadelphia

71. Dvorak HF, Dvorak AM 1975 Basophil leukocytes: structure, function and role in disease. Clinics in Haematology 4: 651–683

72. Twomey JJ, Douglass CC, Sharkey O Jr 1973 The monocytopenia of aplastic anemia. Blood 41: 187–195

73. Rinehart JJ, Sagone AL, Balcerzak SP et al 1975 Effects of corticosteroid therapy on human monocyte function. New England Journal of Medicine 292: 236–241

74. Zacharski LR, Linman JW 1971 Lymphocytopenia: its causes and significance. Mayo Clinic Proceedings 46: 168–173

75. Kimura N, Niho Y, Yanase T 1982 A high level of colony-stimulating activity in a lung cancer patient with extensive leucocytosis, and the establishment of a CSA producing cell line (KONT). Scandinavian Journal of Haematology 28: 417–424

76. Hocking W, Goodman J, Golde D 1983 Granulocytosis associated with tumor cell production of colony-stimulating activity. Blood 61: 600–603

77. Leder K, Weller PF 2000 Eosinophilia and helminthic infections. Baillière's Clinical Haematology 13(2): 301–317

78. Narayanan G, Hussain BM, Chandralekha B et al 2000 Hypereosinophilic syndrome in acute lymphoblastic leukaemia – case report and literature review. Acta Oncologica 39: 241–243

79. Slungaard A, Ascensao J, Zanjani E, Jacob HS 1983 Pulmonary

carcinoma with eosinophilia. Demonstration of a tumor-derived eosinophilopoietic factor. New England Journal of Medicine 309: 778–781

80. Anonymous 1983 The hypereosinophilic syndrome. Lancet i: 1417–1418

81. Spry CJ, Tai PC 1976 Studies on blood eosinophils. II. Patients with Löffler's cardiomyopathy. Clinical and Experimental Immunology 24: 423–434

82. Bain BJ 2000 Hypereosinophilia. Current Opinion in Hematology 7: 21–25

83. Brockington IF, Olsen EG 1972 Eosinophilia and endomyocardial fibrosis. Postgraduate Medical Journal 48: 740–741

84. Corssmit EP, Trip MD, Durrer JD 1999 Loffler's endomyocarditis in the idiopathic hypereosinophilic syndrome. Cardiology 91: 272–276

85. Thomas K, Nixdorff U, Manger B et al 2000 Hypereosinophilia with myocardial involvement due to toxocariasis. Diagnosis of regional myocardial perfusion abnormalities by pulsed tissue Doppler echocardiography. Medizinische Klinik 95: 163–167

86. Chang HW, Leong KH, Koh DR, Lee SH 1999 Clonality of isolated eosinophils in the hypereosinophilic syndrome. Blood 93: 1651–1657

87. Yakulis R, Bedetti CD 1983 Löffler's endocarditis. Occurrence with malignant lymphoma with a high content of epithelioid histiocytes ('Lennert's lymphoma'). Archives of Pathology and Laboratory Medicine 107: 531–534

88. Maldonado JE, Hanlon DG 1965 Monocytosis: a current appraisal. Mayo Clinic Proceedings 40: 248

89. Okano M 2000 Haematological associations of Epstein–Barr virus infection. Bailliére's Clinical Haematology 13(2): 199–214

90. Tanner JE, Alfieri C 1999 Epstein–Barr virus induces Fas (CD95) in T cells and Fas ligand in B cells leading to T-cell apoptosis. Blood 94: 3439–3447

91. Okano M, Gross TG 1996 Epstein–Barr virus-associated hemophagocytic syndrome and fatal infectious mononucleosis. American Journal of Hematology 53: 111–115

92. Krause JR, Kaplan SS 1981 Bone marrow findings in infectious mononucleosis and mononucleosis-like diseases in the older adult. Scandinavian Journal of Haematology 28: 15–22

93. Ahronheim GA, Auger F, Joncas JH et al 1983 Primary infection by Epstein–Barr virus presenting as aplastic anemia. New England Journal of Medicine 309: 313–314

94. Purtilo DT 1980 Epstein–Barr-virus-induced oncogenesis in immune-deficient individuals. Lancet i: 300–303

95. Saemundsen AK, Berkel AI, Henle W et al 1981 Epstein–Barr-virus-carrying lymphoma in a patient with ataxia-telangiectasia. British Medical Journal 282: 425–427

96. Hanto DW, Frizzera G, Gajl-Peczalska KJ et al 1982 Epstein–Barr virus-induced B-cell lymphoma after renal transplantation: acyclovir therapy and transition from polyclonal to monoclonal B-cell proliferation. New England Journal of Medicine 306: 913–918

97. Hopwood P, Crawford DH 2000 The role of EBV in post-transplant malignancies: a review. Journal of Clinical Pathology 53: 248–254

98. Schubach WH, Hackman R, Neiman PE et al 1982 A monoclonal immunoblastic sarcoma in donor cells bearing Epstein–Barr virus genomes following allogeneic marrow grafting for acute lymphoblastic leukemia. Blood 60: 180–187

Disorders of phagocyte function

JR Brown   AJ Thrasher

18

Introduction

Disorders of phagocyte maturation

Leukocyte adhesion molecule deficiencies

Phagocyte signaling abnormalities

Deficiencies of the phagocyte respiratory burst

Extrinsic disorders of phagocytosis

Introduction

Metchnikoff in the 19th century identified phagocytes as an essential and primary component in the elimination of a harmful agent, and predicted that defects in phagocyte function would predispose the host to microbial invasion.[1] Subsequently, patients with decreased phagocyte counts or compromised phagocytic function (for either inherited or acquired reasons) have been shown to suffer recurrent and often fatal infections. The cells implicated in these disorders arise primarily from the myeloid lineage, namely eosinophils, neutrophils, monocytes, macrophages and dendritic cells. During an infection and the subsequent inflammatory reaction, phagocyte production and activation is initiated by enhanced proliferation and maturation of phagocyte precursors in the bone marrow, which are then released into the circulation at an accelerated rate (Fig. 18.1A). Competent phagocytic cells (Fig. 18.1B) activate specific adhesive receptors which aid in rolling and firm adhesion to the endothelium. In response to gradients of chemokinetic and chemotactic molecules, the phagocytes traverse the endothelial wall and migrate towards the site of infection. Interactions between the phagocyte and microbe precede engulfment, degranulation and activation of the respiratory burst, which in combination result in killing primarily within the phagocytic vacuole. Defects in any part of this complex process manifest as immunodeficiency of phagocyte function, highlighted in Figure 18.1. Primary defects of phagocytes are the result of genetic mutations (Table 18.1), many of which have been identified very recently, and the result of which affect adhesion, migration, respiratory burst activity and degranulation.

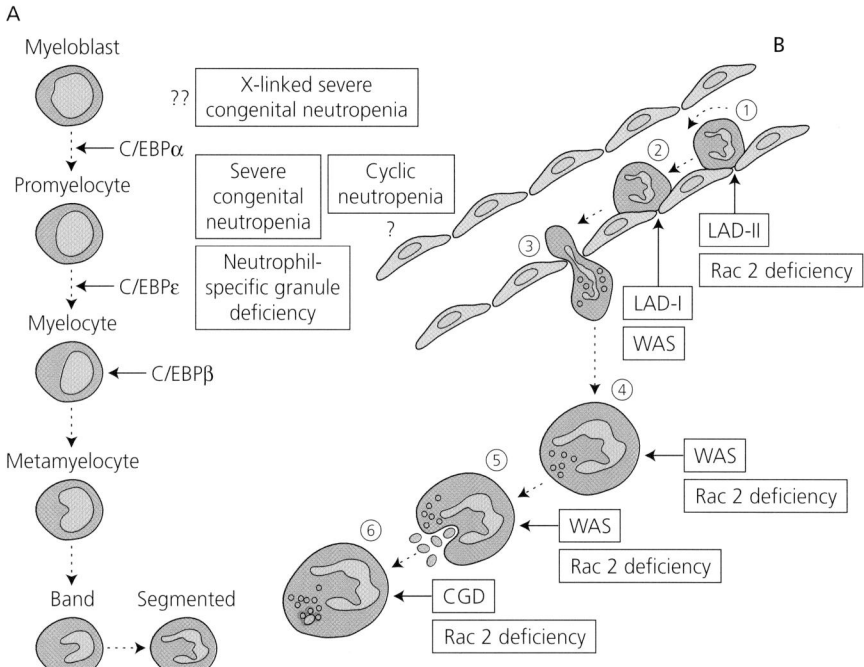

Fig. 18.1 Schematic drawings of myelopoiesis (A) and phagocyte functions (B). Myelopoiesis (A) proceeds by commitment of myeloid precursors and subsequent differentiation into granulocytes and monocytes (dotted arrows). Various transcription factors have been shown to be involved in key stages of myeloid development, including members of the CCAAT/enhancer binding protein (C/EBP) including α, β and ε (solid arrows). Recently, two patients with neutrophil specific granule deficiency have been shown to have mutations in C/EBPε. Severe congenital neutropenia is thought to result from maturational arrest at the promyelocytic stage and in many cases is due to mutations in the gene encoding neutrophil elastase. The mechanism for neutropenia and monocyopenia in X-linked congenital neutropenia is at present unknown. The initiation of inflammation (B; dotted arrows) begins with phagocyte activation by rolling (1), adhesion (2), and transmigration (3) of the endothelium; chemotactic migration to the site of infection (4), followed by bacterial phagocytosis (5) degranulation and intracellular killing (6). Phagocyte deficiencies can affect any part of this process as indicated by solid arrows. CGD – chronic granulomatous disease; LAD – leukocyte adhesion deficiency; WAS – Wiskott-Aldrich syndrome.

Table 18.1 Phagocyte immunodeficiency diseases

Disease	Genetic defect	Phenotypic defect
Disorders of phagocyte maturation		
Severe congenital neutropenia	AD and sporadic; *ELA2* mutation	Developmental arrest of myeloid precursors. Maturational arrest at promyelocytic stage
Cyclic neutropenia	AD and sporadic; *ELA2* mutation	Fluctuations between normal granulocyte counts and severe neutropenia with 21-day periodicity. Increased apoptosis in myeloid precursors
X-linked severe congenital neutropenia	X-linked Activating *WAS* mutation	Neutropenia and monocytopenia
Neutrophil-specific granule deficiency	AR *C/EBP ε* mutation	Absent secondary and tertiary granules. Primary granules lack defensins
Myelokathexis	AD	Myeloid hyperplasia in bone marrow with cytoplasmic vacuolation of neutrophils, nuclear hypersegmentation, and pyknotic nuclear lobes connected by thin filaments
Leukocyte adhesion molecule deficiencies		
LAD-I	AR *ITB2* mutation	High peripheral neutrophil counts, and inability to make pus
LAD-II (CDG-IIc)	AR GDP-fucose transporter mutation	Granulocytes unable to bind to selectins on endothelium. Congenital disorder of fucosylation
Phagocyte signaling abnormalities		
WAS	X-linked *WAS* mutation	Dysfunctional actin polymerization in hematopoietic cells. Defects of adhesion, migration and phagocytosis
Rac 2 deficiency	AD *RAC 2* mutation	Abnormal granulocyte chemotaxis, respiratory burst, degranulation. High peripheral neutrophil counts
Deficiencies of the phagocyte respiratory burst		
CGD	X-linked *CYBB* mutation AR *CYBA, NCF1 NCF2* mutation	Phagocytes unable to produce superoxide

AD, autosomal dominant; AR, autosomal recessive; C/EBP, CCAAT/enhancer binding protein; *ELA2*, elastase2 gene; CDG, congenital disorder of glycosylation; CGD, chronic granulomatous disease; WAS, Wiskott–Aldrich syndrome.

Disorders of phagocyte maturation

Severe congenital neutropenia (SCN), otherwise known as Kostmann syndrome, is characterized by circulating neutrophil counts of less than 200/µl, and is usually diagnosed at birth or soon thereafter.[2] Bone marrow studies in these patients indicate a relatively selective defect of neutrophil formation, and a maturational arrest at the promyelocytic stage (Fig. 18A). Approximately 10% of patients with SCN develop acute myeloid leukemia or myelodysplasia, often accompanied by monosomy 7 and trisomy 21 cytogenetic abnormalities.[3,4] Cyclic neutropenia, in contrast, is characterized by regular and consistent oscillations of neutrophil count, usually with a periodicity of 21 days which clinically manifests as fever, mouth ulcers and infection at the nadir (which lasts from 3 to 6 days) of the neutrophil count.[5,6] Most patients with either disorder respond to granulocyte-colony stimulating factor (G-CSF) therapy, although refractory cases, and those complicated by hematologic malignancy may be rescued by hematopoietic stem cell transplantation.

Most frequently, SCN follows an autosomal dominant inheritance, or arises sporadically. Occasionally, SCN may arise as an autosomal recessive disorder, suggesting that there may at least be some genetic heterogeneity. Similarly, cyclic neutropenia usually follows an autosomal dominant or sporadic pattern of inheritance. The underlying genetic lesions that account for the majority of cases of SCN or cyclic neutropenia have recently been identified. Initially, it was postulated that constitutional mutations of the gene encoding the G-CSF receptor were responsible for SCN, but it is now clear that these mutations occur somatically, and in association with the development of myeloid malignancy.[7] Detailed studies of families with autosomal dominant cyclic neutropenia identified a genetic lesion mapping to a region on chromosome 19p13.3 containing the genes for three neutrophil serine proteases, azurcidin, proteinase 3 and neutrophil elastase (*ELA2*). It was subsequently determined that mutations in and around the sequence coding for the active site of *ELA2* (which is synthesized at the promyelocytic stage of neutrophil development; Fig. 18.1A), were responsible for this form of cyclic neutropenia.[8] Furthermore, because many of the hematological features of cyclic neutropenia are shared with SCN, it was later determined that heterozygous mutations in the same gene account for about 75% of autosomal dominant SCN.[9] The diversity of mutations in SCN has been shown to be much wider than in cyclic neutropenia, in which most are clustered around the active site. There may therefore be some correlation between genotype and clinical phenotype.

Neutrophil elastase is a monomeric, 218-amino acid (25 kDa), chymotryptic serine protease synthesized by promyelocytes and promonocytes during the early stages of primary granule production, and is formed as a proenzyme during differentiation before final storage in cytoplasmic granules in its active state.[10] It has activity against many proteins including matrix components and clotting factors, and is effectively neutralized by a number of endogenous inhibitors including the serpins α1-antitrypsin and monocyte/neutrophil elastase inhibitor (MNEI; gene symbol *ELANH2*) and the non-serpin, elfin. The mechanism by which defective elastase function results in neutropenia remains uncertain, although it has previously been shown to have cell-stimulating activity.[11,12] Accelerated apoptosis of myeloid progenitors has also been observed in patients with cyclic neutropenia.[13] One possibility is that haploinsufficiency of enzymatic activity causes reduced survival or increased apoptosis of myeloid precursors because of disturbances in the hematopoietic microenvironment. Evidence against this is provided by the observation of wide variability that known mutations have on enzymatic activity, and the fact that null mutant mice generated by gene targeting are not neutropenic. It is also possible that the mutant protein interferes in a dominant negative way with sub-cellular trafficking or post-translational processing of the normal enzyme, or by gain of function toxicity.

Most recently, a family with X-linked congenital neutropenia and monocytopenia have been shown to have a mutation in the gene encoding the Wiskott–Aldrich syndrome (WAS) protein (WASp, see later).[14] These patients are quite distinct from those with WAS phenotypically, with normal or near normal platelet counts and platelet volumes, and none of the typical immunologic abnormalities. In this family, it appears that WASp is rendered constitutively active by a genetic mutation in the conserved GTPase-binding domain (based on the ability of mutant protein to enhance Arp2/3-mediated actin polymerization), and within the autoinhibitory hydrophobic core. The mechanisms by which this leads to neutropenia and monocytopenia remain obscure. Mutations resulting in typical or attenuated WASp almost invariably occur outside this region. One clear possibility is that constitutively active WASp is myelotoxic, and although this remains speculative, over-expression of normal WASp can certainly compromise cellular viability (AT, unpublished observations).

During hematopoiesis, cellular proliferation, differentiation and survival are largely dependent on the regulation of gene expression by the actions of transcription factors. Members of the CCAAT/enhancer binding protein (C/EBP) family of transcription factors are key regulators of cellular differentiation and function in many tissues. Six homologous members of this family have been identified (C/EBPα, β, γ, δ, ε and ξ), each existing as distinct isoforms.[15] All members have been shown to possess an activation domain, a DNA-binding basic region and are able to homodimerize and heterodimerize with each other through a leucine-rich dimerization domain, termed the leucine zipper, which determines specificity of dimer formation. C/EBPα, β, δ and ε are all expressed during hematopoiesis (Fig. 18.1A); however, C/EBPε, the newest member of the family, is expressed exclusively in cells of myeloid and T-cell lineages.[16] Targeted disruption of the *C/EBPε* gene in mice results in defects of granulopoiesis, neutrophil phagocytosis and bacterial killing, migration, and impaired cytokine production after an inflammatory challenge.[17,18] In addition, there is accelerated apoptosis in maturing granulocytic cells.[19]

Neutrophil specific granule deficiency (SGD) is a very rare congenital disorder characterized by a lack of specific (secondary) granule proteins such as lactoferrin, transcobalamin, collagenase, gelatinase B (tertiary granules), abnormalities of migration, disaggregation and bactericidal activity, and atypical bilobed nuclei. Primary granules are markedly depleted of defensins although expression of myeloperoxidase and lysozyme is unaffected. Eosinophils also lack eosinophilic-specific granules and are undetectable by Giemsa–Wright staining. Despite the lack of lactoferrin in neutrophils, saliva from patients contains normal levels suggesting a specific defect of myeloid granulopoiesis. Given the striking similarity between SGD and mutant mice generated by targeting of the *C/EBPε* gene it is unsurprising that mutations have now been found in at least two patients.[20,21] However other patients with SGD do not appear to have defects in this gene suggesting that it may be genetically heterogeneous.[22]

Myelokathexis is a rare cause of severe chronic neutropenia and is characterized by degenerative changes and hypersegmentation in mature neutrophils which are also functionally abnormal.[23] In the bone marrow, there is relative granulocytic hyperplasia with cytoplasmic vacuolation, nuclear hypersegmentation, and pyknotic nuclear lobes connected by thin filaments. Some evidence points to an intrinsic acceleration of apoptosis in neutrophil precursors.[13] The molecular basis for this condition has not yet been determined. In association with *w*arts, *h*ypogammaglobulinemia, and recurrent respiratory tract *i*nfections, *m*yelokathexis forms part of the WHIM syndrome, which is inherited in an autosomal dominant fashion.[24]

Leukocyte adhesion molecule deficiencies

Leukocyte adhesion disorders arise from defects in cell aggregation and adhesion to extracellular matrix and vascular endothelium. Integrins are a large family of molecules involved in intercellular and cell-substratum adhesion. Each is a heterodimer of non-covalently linked α and β chains. The members of a particular family share a common β chain, but each possess a unique α chain. The best known of the integrins are from the $β_2$ family, and expression of these are confined primarily to monocytes, neutrophils, and activated lymphocytes. These are known as lymphocyte-function-associated antigen (LFA-1 or CD11a/CD18), complement receptor-3 (CR3, Mac-1 or CD11b/CD18), p150,95 (or CD11c/CD18), and $αvβ_2$ or (CD11d/CD18). All $β_2$ integrins are constitutively represented on the plasma membrane of the leukocyte, and are both quantitatively and functionally upregulated by activation of the cell. The counter-receptors for leukocyte integrin molecules are members of the immunoglobulin gene superfamily, intercellular adhesion molecule-1 (ICAM-1) and ICAM-2, which are expressed on endothelial cells. Resting leukocytes (particularly B lymphocytes and cells of the monocyte–macrophage lineage) themselves express a third ligand for LFA-1, ICAM-3, which is constitutively expressed, and which may be important for interleukocyte signaling.

Two distinct human disorders of leukocyte adhesion have been recognized (leukocyte adhesion deficiency type 1 [LAD 1], and LAD type 2 [LAD II]) (Fig. 18.1B). LAD I is a rare inherited disease characterized in its severe form by delayed separation of the umbilical cord, recurrent life-threatening bacterial (usually with *Staphylococcus aureus* and Gram-negative enteric organisms) and fungal infections, gingivitis, impaired pus formation, delayed wound healing, and chronic leukocytosis.[25] Lymphocytes, monocytes and granulocytes show defects of adhesion to endothelial cells, cell migration, cell-mediated cytolysis and antigen presentation. Surprisingly, patients are not overtly susceptible to viral infection. LAD 1 is an autosomal recessive disorder caused by mutations in the *ITB2* gene encoding CD18 which is located on chromosome 21.[26,27] Patients with LAD I are therefore deficient in their cell-surface expression of the glycoprotein $β_2$-integrin

subunit (CD18). Most mutations in the *ITB2* gene are heterogeneous and found in a highly conserved ~ 240-residue domain.[27] The degree of deficiency of the molecule usually correlates well with the severity of the clinical condition. Patients suffering from the severe form of the disease (less than 1% normal cell surface expression of CD18) die in childhood unless treated by hematopoietic stem cell transplantation, whereas those with moderate disease (2–5% expression) can survive into adulthood. Recently, a patient with phenotypically severe LAD I was shown to express between 40 and 60% of normal levels of CD18.[28] In this patient, one of the mutant alleles was expressed normally, but could not be activated. Both Mac-1 on neutrophils and LFA-1 on T-cells failed to bind ligands such as fibrinogen and ICAM-1, respectively, or to display a $β_2$-integrin activation epitope. In contrast, the patient's T-cells showed some binding activity to ICAM-2 and ICAM-3 when treated with divalent cations, suggesting that the most significant abnormality was of interaction between LFA-1 and ICAM-1. Similarly, another variant patient has been described with absent CD11/CD18 activation but normal levels of expression.[29] This patient presented with myelodysplastic syndrome and infectious complications typical of severe LAD 1 and has been shown to have markedly impaired $β_2$-and $β_3$-integrin cell adhesion, yet normal levels of expression. For this patient it is proposed that the phenotype is due to abnormalities of inside-out signaling mechanisms that regulate the activity of integrins of these classes, rather than an intrinsic molecular defect.[29]

LAD II has been described in only a few patients.[30,31] It results from a general defect in fucose metabolism leading to an absence of sialyl-Lewis X (SLeX) and other fucosylated ligands for selectins, which are a group of cell-adhesion molecules expressed on endothelial cells, and mediate rolling along the endothelium before firm attachment is achieved. The phenotype of the immunodeficiency is similar to that of LAD I, but less severe. Additional features include severe mental retardation and short stature suggesting that these molecules are also important in development. LAD II is now known to belong to a growing group of congenital disorders of glycosylation (CDG), in which glycosylation of proteins is defective due to molecular lesions in genes required for the assembly of lipid-linked oligosaccharides, their transfer to nascent proteins (CDG-I), or the processing of protein-bound glycans (CDG-II). Missense genetic mutations in patients with LAD II (also know known as CDG-IIc) have been identified in a highly conserved GDP-fucose transporter, which explains the observed defect of GDP-fucose import into the Golgi apparatus where fucosylation takes place.[32–34] Fucosylation of fibroblasts from LAD-II patients grown *in vitro* can be corrected by fucose addition to culture medium.[36] Similarly, oral fucose treatment of LAD-II patients can restore selectin ligands and improve the immuno-deficiency, suggesting that the defective transporter has partial activity, or that less-efficient independent pathways exist.[33,36]

Phagocyte signaling abnormalities

Many aspects of phagocyte function depend on the ability to modulate shape and therefore dynamically organize the actin cytoskeleton. Two inherited disorders are now known to produce abnormalities of these processes. The Wiskott–Aldrich syndrome (WAS) is a rare inherited X-linked recessive disease characterized by immune dys-regulation (deficiency and autoimmunity) and micro-thrombocytopenia.[37] In its less severe form, known as X-linked thrombocytopenia (XLT), mutations in the same gene produce the characteristic platelet abnormality but minimal immunologic disturbance. In the absence of hematopoietic stem cell transplantation, many patients with WAS die in childhood and early adulthood from hemorrhage, infection or lymphoreticular malignancy.

The *WAS* gene encodes a 502 amino acid proline-rich intracellular protein (WASp) expressed exclusively in hematopoietic cells, which belongs to a recently defined family of more widely expressed proteins involved in transduction of signals from receptors on the cell surface to the actin cytoskeleton. The Rho family GTPases (Cdc42, Rac and Rho) regulate many aspects of cell function including cytoskeletal rearrangement, progression through cell cycle, and vesicle trafficking.[38] WASp binds to the GTP-bound form of Cdc42 *in vitro*, less well to GTP-bound Rac, but not to Rho, and clusters physically with polymerized actin. These findings and others have led to the suggestion that WASp is a direct effector for Cdc42, although its multidomain structure undoubtedly supports a multifunctional role in the regulated assembly of cytoskeletal complexes. Cdc42 induces the formation of distinct actin-filament-containing protrusions known as filopodia in fibroblast and monocytic cell lines. In contrast, growth-factor-induced activation of the related GTP-binding protein Rac leads to accumulation of an actin network at the cell periphery producing lamellipodia and membrane ruffling. Cdc42 and Rac have also been shown to participate in the establishment of cell-substratum focal adhesion complexes distinct from Rho-induced focal adhesions. For WASp, the interaction with Cdc42/Rac

has been shown to be mediated through a Cdc42/Rac interactive binding (CRIB) motif (or GTPase-binding domain, GBD), which is found in many downstream effectors of Cdc42 and Rac. In addition, the C-terminal portion of WASp has been shown to interact directly with the actin-related protein (Arp)2/3 complex, indicating the critical regulatory role for WASp in the nucleation and branching of actin filaments.[39] In its inactive state, WASp is thought to block the Arp2/3-binding site by intramolecular interactions between the C-terminus and the GBD.[40] WASp therefore acts as a regulated scaffold for the organized recruitment of signaling molecules and effector proteins at sites of new actin polymerization. In the absence of WASp, macrophages and dendritic cells have now been shown to have marked abnormalities of chemotaxis, chemokinesis, adhesion and phagocytosis of both opsonized particles and apoptotic cells.[41–48]

In neutrophils, the GTPase Rac has been shown to be critical for activity of the NADPH oxidase, through inter-action with p67[phox] (see below).[49] Both Rac 1 and Rac 2 are highly homologous although Rac2 accounts for > 96% of the Rac protein expressed in neutrophils. A single male infant has now been described with a point mutation in one allele of the *Rac2* gene.[50,51] This results in an inability of the mutant protein to bind GTP, and dominant inhibition of the normal protein. Clinically, this patient suffered from recurrent infections, poor wound healing, and absence of pus in infected areas. His peripheral neutrophil count was also high, and when tested *in vitro* neutrophils exhibited decreased chemotaxis, polarization, azurophilic granule secretion, and superoxide anion production.

Deficiencies of the phagocyte respiratory burst

Chronic granulomatous disease (CGD) is a rare genetic disorder caused by defects in the enzyme responsible for the oxidative or 'respiratory' burst in all phagocytes.[49,52] Failure to produce a respiratory burst results in characteristic susceptibility to severe and recurrent infections by catalase-positive organisms, *S. aureus*, *Burkholderia cepacia*, *Aspergillus* sp. and *Serratia marcescens*, and also a tendency to develop granulomatous inflammation, particulary affecting hollow organs.

The NADPH-oxidase catalyses the formation of superoxide, which is a precursor for the generation of potent oxidant compounds, by transmembrane passage of electrons from NADPH to molecular O_2. It is most abundant in phagocytic cells, particularly neutrophils, eosinophils and cells of the monocyte/macrophage lineage, consisting of a membrane-bound flavocytochrome b_{558} and four cytosolic factors, p47^{phox}, p67^{phox}, p40^{phox} and p21rac, which translocate to the membrane on activation of the cell (the suffix *phox* represents *phagocyte oxidase*).[53] Activation is initiated classically by opsonized particles, but also by many soluble inflammatory mediators. The redox center of the oxidase is the flavocytochrome b_{558}, which consists of two proteins with apparent molecular weights of 23 kDa (p22^{phox}, α subunit) and 76–92 kDa (gp91^{phox}, β subunit) respectively, and are arranged as a 1:1 heterodimer. Both p22^{phox} and gp91^{phox} are missing in cells derived from most CGD patients with a molecular lesion of either subunit, indicating that mutual interaction is necessary for assembly of the mature complex. Biosynthesis of gp91^{phox} glycoprotein is also dependent on the incorporation of two non-identical heme groups for each heterodimer within membrane-spanning α helices, one predicted to lie near the inner face, and the other towards the outer face of the cell. The locations of the binding sites for the substrate NADPH, and for the electron carrier flavin adenine dinucleotide (FAD) are now known to lie within the C-terminal region of gp91^{phox} itself (although an additional NADPH-binding site may exist on p67^{phox}). Final transfer of electrons across the cell membrane is probably mediated by the two, associated heme groups. The membrane-spanning N-terminal region of the flavocytochrome has recently been identified as the site of a charge-compensating H$^+$ conductance during activation of the respiratory burst, and may also therefore be responsible for maintaining intracellular (preventing deleterious acidification) and phagosomal pH (for optimal activity of proteolytic enzymes).

The flavocytochrome b_{558} almost certainly comprises the complete electron transporting system and forms the membrane docking site for the cytosolic components. In resting neutrophils, the plasma membrane is devoid of flavocytochrome b_{558}, which resides almost exclusively in specialized light density intracellular vesicles and within the membranes of specific granules. When the cell is activated the plasma membrane invaginates to form the phagocytic vacuole with which vesicles containing flavocytochrome b_{558} fuse. The cytosolic components form an activation complex which translocates to the membrane to associate with the flavocytochrome b_{558}. Assembly of the complete NADPH-oxidase complex may induce conformational changes in flavocytochrome b_{558} which permit binding of the substrate NADPH, and which are energetically favorable for electron transport.

The majority of CGD patients follow an X-linked recessive inheritance (67%; X91^0 CGD) and are genetically heterogeneous, whilst the remaining cases are autosomal recessive and are equally distributed among females and males.[54] The second most common cause of CGD is A47^{0}CGD. In contrast to other forms of CGD, a GT dinucleotide deletion at a GTGT repeat at the boundary between the first intron and second exon is found in the majority of mutant alleles, resulting in a chain terminator at amino acid residue 51.[55] This has now been found to arise from recombination events (probably partial) between the p47^{phox} gene and highly homologous pseudogenes, which contain the GT deletion.[56–58] Treatment for CGD is dependent on prophylaxis against both bacterial and fungal infection with antibiotics. Stem cell transplantation may also be curative, and is a reasonable option particularly if an HLA-matched sibling donor is available.

Extrinsic disorders of phagocytosis

Once localized to the area of inflammation, phagocytic cells directly attack invading microorganisms. They do this by internalization of particles into phagocytic vacuoles, or phagosomes. On the cell surface, leukocytes express carbohydrate mannosyl–fucosyl receptors that can bind non-encapsulated microbes carrying these surface sugars in the absence of opsonization, in addition to high-affinity receptors for IgG and complement, FcR and CR1/CR3, respectively, which co-operate with each other to bind to their corresponding ligands. Opsonization of particles with IgG and fragments of complement, in particular C3 breakdown products such as C3bi, renders them much more susceptible to phagocytosis. Deficiency of these components (e.g. IgG in X-linked agammaglobulinemia (XLA), X-linked hyper IgM syndrome, and common variable immunodeficiency (CVID)) results in susceptibility to infection by organisms whose main route of destruction is by phagocytosis, in particular, pyogenic bacteria. Mannose-binding lectin (MBL) is a soluble defense collagen (related to C1q, and pulmonary surfactant protein (SP-A)) which can activate complement independently of the classical and alternative pathways.[59] In addition, it acts as an opsonin of mannose-rich pathogens, and has been shown to directly enhance FcR-mediated phagocytosis by both monocytes and macrophages. These ligands are elements of innate immunity which may be particularly important as a first line of defense before the generation of cellular immunity and high-affinity specific antibodies, and may be functionally most important in children between the ages of 6 months (at a time when maternal antibody levels have waned) and 2 years (before which time the generation of anti-carbohydrate IgG is inefficient). Genetically determined MBL deficiency is associated with increased susceptibility and severity of infection.

REFERENCES

1. Yang KD, Quie PG, Hill HR 1999 Phagocytic system. In: Ochs HD, Smith CIE, Puck JM, (eds), Primary immunodeficiency diseases. A molecular and genetic approach. Oxford University Press, New York, 82–96
2. Kostmann R 1956 Infantile genetic agranulocytopenia: new recessive lethal disease in man. Acta Paediatrica Scandinavia 45(suppl 105): 1–78
3. Freedman MH, Bonilla MA, Fier C et al 2000 Myelodysplasia syndrome and acute myeloid leukemia in patients with congenital neutropenia receiving G-CSF therapy. Blood 96(2): 429–436
4. Tschan CA, Pilz C, Zeidler C et al 2001 Time course of increasing numbers of mutations in the granulocyte colony-stimulating factor receptor gene in a patient with congenital neutropenia who developed leukemia. Blood 97(6): 1882–1884
5. Dale DC, Hammond WP 4th 1988 Cyclic neutropenia: a clinical review. Blood Reviews 2(3): 178–185
6. Haurie C, Dale DC, Mackey MC 1998 Cyclical neutropenia and other periodic hematological disorders: a review of mechanisms and mathematical models. Blood 92(8): 2629–2640
7. Tidow N, Pilz C, Teichmann B et al 1997 Clinical relevance of point mutations in the cytoplasmic domain of the granulocyte colony-stimulating factor receptor gene in patients with severe congenital neutropenia. Blood 89(7): 2369–2375
8. Horwitz M, Benson KF, Person RE et al 1999 Mutations in ELA2, encoding neutrophil elastase, define a 21-day biological clock in cyclic haematopoiesis. Nature Genetics 23(4): 433–436
9. Dale DC, Person RE, Bolyard AA et al 2000 Mutations in the gene encoding neutrophil elastase in congenital and cyclic neutropenia. Blood 96(7): 2317–2322
10. Bode W, Meyer E Jr, Powers JC 1989 Human leukocyte and porcine pancreatic elastase: X-ray crystal structures, mechanism, substrate specificity, and mechanism-based inhibitors. Biochemistry 28(5): 1951–1963
11. Wakasugi K, Schimmel P 1999 Two distinct cytokines released from a human aminoacyl-tRNA synthetase. Science 284(5411): 147–151
12. Champagne B, Tremblay P, Cantin A et al 1998 Proteolytic cleavage of ICAM-1 by human neutrophil elastase. Journal of Immunology 161(11): 6398–6405
13. Aprikyan AA, Liles WC, Rodger E et al 2001 Impaired survival of bone marrow hematopoietic progenitor cells in cyclic neutropenia. Blood 97(1): 147–153
14. Devriendt K, Kim AS, Mathijs G et al 2001 Constitutively activating mutation in WASP causes X-linked severe congenital neutropenia. Nature Genetics 27(3): 313–217
15. Lekstrom-Himes J, Xanthopoulos KG 1998 Biological role of the CCAAT/enhancer-binding protein family of transcription factors. Journal of Biological Chemistry 273(44): 28545–28548
16. Antonson P, Stellan B, Yamanaka R et al 1996 A novel humanCCAAT/enhancer binding protein gene, C/EBPepsilon, is expressed in cells of lymphoid and myeloid lineages and is localized on chromosome 14q11.2 close to the T-cell receptor alpha/delta locus. Genomics 35(1): 30–38
17. Yamanaka R, Barlow C, Lekstrom-Himes J et al 1997 Impaired granulopoiesis, myelodysplasia, and early lethality in CCAAT/enhancer binding protein epsilon-deficient mice. Proceedings of the National Academy of Sciences USA 94(24): 13187–13192
18. Lekstrom-Himes J Xanthopoulos KG 1999 CCAAT/enhancer binding protein epsilon is critical for effective neutrophil-mediated response to inflammatory challenge. Blood 93(9): 3096–3105
19. Verbeek W, Wachter M, Lekstrom-Himes J et al 2001 C/EBPepsilon −/− mice: increased rate of myeloid proliferation and apoptosis. Leukemia 15(1): 103–111
20. Lekstrom-Himes JA, Dorman SE, Kopar P et al 1999 Neutrophil-specific granule deficiency results from a novel mutation with loss of function of the transcription factor CCAAT/enhancer binding protein epsilon. Journal of Experimental Medicine 189(11): 1847–1852
21. Gombart AF, Shiohara M, Kwok SH et al 2001 Neutrophil-specific granule deficiency: homozygous recessive inheritance of a frameshift mutation in the gene encoding transcription factor CCAAT/enhancer binding protein–epsilon. Blood 97(9): 2561–2567
22. Lekstrom-Himes JA 2001 The role of C/EBP(epsilon) in the terminal stages of granulocyte differentiation. Stem Cells 19(2): 125–133
23. Bassan R, Viero P, Minetti B et al 1984 Myelokathexis: a rare form of chronic benign granulocytopenia. British Journal of Haematology 58(1): 115–117
24. Gorlin RJ, Gelb B, Diaz GA et al 2000 WHIM syndrome, an autosomal dominant disorder: clinical, hematological, and molecular studies. American Journal of Medical Genetics 91(5): 368–376
25. Etzioni A, Doerschuk CM, Harlan JM 1999 Of man and mouse: leukocyte and endothelial adhesion molecule deficiencies. Blood 94(10): 3281–3288
26. Anderson DC, Springer TA 1987 Leukocyte adhesion deficiency: an inherited defect in the Mac-1, LFA-1, and p150,95 glycoproteins. Annual Review of Medicine 38: 175–194
27. Hogg N, Bates PA 2000 Genetic analysis of integrin function in man: LAD-1 and other syndromes. Matrix Biology 19(3): 211–222
28. Hogg N, Stewart MP, Scarth SL et al 1999 A novel leukocyte adhesion deficiency caused by expressed but nonfunctional beta2 integrins Mac-1 and LFA-1. Journal of Clinical Investigation 103(1): 97–106
29. Kuijpers TW, Van Lier RA, Hamann D et al 1997 Leukocyte adhesion deficiency type 1 (LAD-1)/variant. A novel immunodeficiency syndrome characterized by dysfunctional beta2 integrins. Journal of Clinical Investigation 100(7): 1725–1733
30. Etzioni A, Frydman M, Pollack S et al 1992 Brief report: recurrent severe infections caused by a novel leukocyte adhesion deficiency. New England Journal of Medicine 327(25): 1789–1792
31. Marquardt T, Brune T, Luhn K et al 1999 Leukocyte adhesion deficiency II syndrome, a generalized defect in fucose metabolism. Journal of Pediatrics 134(6): 681–688
32. Lubke T, Marquardt T, von Figura K et al 1999 A new type of carbohydrate-deficient glycoprotein syndrome due to a decreased import of GDP-fucose into the golgi. Journal of Biological Chemistry 274(37): 25986–25989
33. Luhn K, Wild MK, Eckhardt M et al 2001 The gene defective in leukocyte adhesion deficiency II encodes a putative GDP-fucose transporter. Nature Genetics 28(1): 69–72
34. Lubke T, Marquardt T, Etzioni A et al 2001 Complementation cloning identifies CDG-IIc, a new type of congenital disorders of glycosylation, as a GDP-fucose transporter deficiency. Nature Genetics 28(1): 73–76
35. Karsan A, Cornejo CJ, Winn RK et al 1998 Leukocyte Adhesion Deficiency Type II is a generalized defect of de novo GDP-fucose biosynthesis. Endothelial cell fucosylation is not required for neutrophil rolling on human nonlymphoid endothelium. Journal of Clinical Investigation 101(11): 2438–2445
36. Marquardt T, Luhn K, Srikrishna G et al 1999 Correction of leukocyte adhesion deficiency type II with oral fucose. Blood 94(12): 3976–3985
37. Thrasher AJ, Burns S, Lorenzi R et al 2000 The Wiskott–Aldrich syndrome: disordered actin dynamics in haematopoietic cells. Immunological Reviews 178: 118–128
38. Mackay DJ, Hall A 1998 Rho GTPases. Journal of Biological Chemistry 273(33): 20685–20688
39. Machesky LM, Insall RH 1998 Scar1 and the related Wiskott–Aldrich syndrome protein, WASP, regulate the actin cytoskeleton through the Arp2/3 complex. Current Biology 8(25): 1347–1356
40. Kim AS, Kakalis LT, Abdul-Manan N et al 2000 Auto-inhibition and activation mechanisms of the Wiskott–Aldrich syndrome protein. Nature 404(6774): 151–158
41. Binks M, Jones GE, Brickell PM et al 1998 Intrinsic dendritic cell abnormalities in Wiskott–Aldrich syndrome. European Journal of Immunology 28(10): 3259–3267
42. Thrasher AJ, Jones GE, Kinnon C et al 1998 Is Wiskott–Aldrich syndrome a cell trafficking disorder? Immunology Today 19(12): 537–539
43. Zicha D, Allen WE, Brickell PM et al 1998 Chemotaxis of macrophages is abolished in the Wiskott–Aldrich syndrome. British Journal of Haematology 101(4): 659–665
44. Badolato R, Sozzani S, Malacarne F et al 1998 Monocytes from Wiskott–Aldrich patients display reduced chemotaxis and lack of cell polarization in response to monocyte chemoattractant protein-1 and formyl-methionyl-leucyl-phenylalanine. Journal of Immunology 161(2): 1026–1033

45. Linder S, Nelson D, Weiss M et al 1999 Wiskott–Aldrich syndrome protein regulates podosomes in primary human macrophages. Proceedings of the National Academy of Sciences USA 96(17): 9648–9653
46. Lerenzi R, Brickell PM, Katz DR et al 2000 Wiskott–Aldrich syndrome protein is necessary for efficient IgG-mediated phagocytosis. Blood 95(9): 2943–2946
47. Leverrier Y, Lorenzi R, Blundell MP et al 2001 Cutting edge: the Wiskott–Aldrich syndrome protein is required for efficient phagocytosis of apoptotic cells. Journal of Immunology 166(8): 4831–4834
48. Burns S, Thrasher AJ, Blundell MP et al 2001 Configuration of human dendritic cell cytoskeleton by Rho GTPases, the WAS protein, and differentiation. Blood 98(4), 1142–1149
49. Segal AW, Abo A 1993 The biochemical basis of the NADPH oxidase of phagocytes. Trends in Biochemical Sciences 18(2): 43–47
50. Ambruso DR, Knall C, Abell AN et al 2000 Human neutrophil immunodeficiency syndrome is associated with an inhibitory Rac2 mutation. Proceedings of the National Academy of Sciences USA 97(9): 4654–4659
51. Williams DA, Tao W, Yang F et al 2000 Dominant negative mutation of the hematopoietic-specific Rho GTPase, Rac2, is associated with a human phagocyte immunodeficiency. Blood 96(5): 1646–1654
52. Goldblatt D, Thrasher AJ 2000 Chronic granulomatous disease. Clinical and Experimental Immunology 122(1): 1–9
53. Babior BM 1999 NADPH oxidase: an update. Blood 93: 1464–1476
54. Roos D, de Boer M, Kuribayashi F et al 1996 Mutations in the X-linked and autosomal recessive forms of chronic granulomatous disease. Blood 87(5): 1663–1681
55. Casimir CM, Bu-Ghanim HN, Rodaway AR et al 1991 Autosomal recessive chronic granulomatous disease caused by deletion at a dinucleotide repeat. Proceedings of the National Academy of Sciences USA 88(7): 2753–2757
56. Gorlach A, Lee PL, Roesler J et al 1997 A p47-phox pseudogene carries the most common mutation causing p47-phox-deficient chronic granulomatous disease. Journal of Clinical Investigation 100(8): 1907–1918
57. Roesler J, Curnutte JT, Rae J, et al 2000 Recombination events between the p47-phox gene and its highly homologous pseudogenes are the main cause of autosomal recessive chronic granulomatous disease. Blood 95(6): 2150–2156
58. Vazquez N, Lehrnbecher T, Chen R et al 2001 Mutational analysis of patients with p47-phox-deficient chronic granulomatous disease: The significance of recombination events between the p47-phox gene (NCF1) and its highly homologous pseudogenes. Experimental Hematology 29(2): 234–243
59. Jack DL, Klein NJ, Turner MW 2001 Mannose-binding lectin: targeting the microbial world for complement attack and opsonophagocytosis. Immunological Reviews 180: 86–99

Myelodysplastic disorders

19

TJ Hamblin   BS Wilkins

Definition

Epidemiology

Classification

Diagnosis

Blood-film examination
Red cells
White cells
Platelets

Bone marrow aspirate
Erythropoiesis
Granulopoiesis
Thrombopoiesis

The role of trephine biopsy in the assessment of myelodysplastic syndromes

General histologic features of myelodysplastic syndromes

Assessment of spatial distribution of hemopoiesis in MDS

Assessment of cytologic features in trephine biopsy sections in MDS

Histologic assessment of myelodysplasia in hypoplastic bone marrow

Histiologic features of secondary myelodysplasia

Use of immunochemistry and fluorescent *in situ* hybridization in trephine biopsy sections in myelodysplasia

Karyotype

Genetic abnormalities

Cell biology

Other abnormalities

Pathogenesis

Natural history

Management

It has been known for many years that some leukemias smoulder for a long time before catching fire. The terms, smouldering leukemia, oligoblastic leukemia and pre-leukemia were applied. It had also been recognized that some obscure anemias were unresponsive to the usual hematinics. They were variously known as refractory anemia, sideroachrestic anemia and sideroblastic anemia. It was also known that some of these anemias accumulated blasts in the bone marrow and eventually transformed to acute leukemia. However, it needed an international classification from the French–American–British (FAB) Group[1] (Table 19.1) to prompt hematologists regularly to diagnose the syndrome and then to realize that it is relatively common.

Definition

Myelodysplastic syndrome (MDS) may be defined as a clonal disorder of hematopoietic stem cells that retain the ability to differentiate into end-stage cells, but do so in a disordered and ineffective manner. Consequently, the bone marrow is usually hypercellular in the face of peripheral blood cytopenias. The hallmarks of MDS are morphologic abnormalities of red cells, white cells and platelets and of their precursors, some of which may be quite subtle (Table 19.2). As time progresses there is a tendency for cells to lose the ability to differentiate so that blast cells build up. The syndrome may culminate in acute leukemia.

Epidemiology

MDS is usually idiopathic, occuring predominately in those over 60 years. A Leukemia Research Fund (LRF) study put the annual incidence at 3.6 per 100 000 but this masks the fact that many cases remain undiagnosed.[2] One group has suggested a prevalence of 1 in 500 in those over 60 years.[3] In those over 85 years it represents about a quarter of all hematologic malignancies. Although some think it is getting commoner, this apparent increase in incidence simply reflects a greater willingness to perform bone marrow investigations in the elderly.[4]

Secondary MDS, which tends to occur in younger people, develops after exposure to certain chemicals, particularly benzene and its derivatives, and to cytotoxic drugs, especially alkylating agents. The younger age at

Table 19.1 FAB group classification of MDS

Type	Peripheral blood	Bone marrow
RA	< 1% blasts	Dyshemopoiesis in one, two or all three lineages; < 5% blasts
RARS	< 1% blasts	As RA with ring sideroblasts comprising > 14% erythroblasts
RAEB	< 5% blasts	As RA with 5–20% blasts
RAEBt	< 5% blasts	As RA with 20–30% blasts or as RAB with Auer rods
CMML	As any of above with > 10⁹/l monocytes	As any of the above plus promonocytes

RA, refractory anemia; RARS, RA with ring sideroblasts; RAEB, RA with excess of blasts; RAEBt, RAEB in transformation; CMML, chronic myelomonocytic leukemia.
Variants that do not fit well into this classification include hypoplastic MDS, fibrotic MDS and juvenile myelomonocytic leukemia.

Table 19.2 Morphologic abnormalities of blood and bone marrow cells in MDS

Lineage	Blood	Bone marrow
Red cells	Macrocytes Aniso-poikilocytosis Dimorphic picture Polychromasia Punctate basophilia Normoblasts Reticulocytopenia	Erythroid hyperplasia Multinuclearity Dyskaryorrhexis Megaloblasts Cytoplasmic vacuoles Howell–Jolly bodies Ringed sideroblasts
White cells	Hypogranular neutrophils Unilobed or bilobed neutrophils (Pelger cells) Hypersegmented neutrophils Monocytosis (often with multiple, elongated nuclear lobes) Promonocytes (with fine azurophil granules) Degranulated eosinophils	Hypogranularity of myeloid precursors Increased promonocytes Increased blast cells (type I with scanty agranular cytoplasm and type II with sparse granules
Platelets	Agranular platelets Giant platelets Megakaryocyte fragments	Micromegakaryocytes Large megakaryocytes with single round or oval nucleus Large megakaryocytes with multiple small round nuclei Megakaryoblasts

presentation of idiopathic MDS in developing countries suggests a less rigorous control of noxious chemicals in these communities. Familial MDS is rare, but also occurs at a young age. Childhood MDS is very rare, but unusual diseases such as juvenile myelomonocytic leukemia (JMML) are often included within the classification.

Classification

The FAB group recognized that those patients with more than 5% blast cells in their bone marrows had shorter survivals and were more likely to transform to acute leukemia. This formed the basis for their classification of the syndrome. Two other factors, the presence of mono-cytes and the presence of ringed sideroblasts, further defined the syndrome. Finally, a demarcation had to be made between MDS and acute leukemia. An arbitrary 30% of blast cells in the marrow became the threshold for acute myeloblastic leukemia. A category, refractory anemia with excess of blasts in transformation, for those patients with between 20 and 30% marrow blast cells became the transition category. The final classification (Table 19.1) also had prognostic value.

Because, only a third of patients die from leukemia, a third die from irrelevant causes and a third from their cytopenias, several prognostic scoring systems[5–9] have been introduced to take account of the prognostic import-ance of cytopenias. Others recognized that age, serum lactate dehydrogenase (LDH) and chromosomal aber-rations also influenced survival, and that the effect of the blast count was subtler than the FAB group had appreciated, with patients with 5–10% blast cells doing better than those with 11–20%. A coming-together of all those who had designed scoring systems produced the International Prognostic Scoring System (IPSS)[10] (Table 19.3). This system has been independently validated in clinical practice.[11]

In 1997 the WHO group[12] reclassified MDS (Table 19.4). The refractory anemia with excess of blasts in transform-ation (RAEBt) group was eliminated and patients with > 20% blast cells were designated as acute myeloblastic leukemia. Refractory anemia and refractory anemia with sideroblasts should henceforth refer only to cases with unilineage dysplasia. There is little disagreement that 'pure sideroblastic anemia' is an entity that seldom, if ever, transforms to acute leukemia,[13] but 'pure refractory anemia' is less well defined. Stand-alone dyserythropoiesis is often found in both normal marrows and in inflam-matory conditions. Without karyotypic abnormalities or another clonal marker this subtype will be very difficult

Table 19.3 International Prognostic Scoring System for MDS

Prognostic variable	Score value				
	0	0.5	1	1.5	2
% bone-marrow blasts	< 5	5–10	—	11–20	21–30
Karyotype	Good	Intermediate	Poor		
Cytopenias	0/1	2/3			

Good karyotype = –Y, del(5q) or del(20q)
Poor karyotype = 3 or more abnormalities (complex) or chromosome 7 abnormalities
Intermediate = all other abnormalities.
Risk groups: Low scores 0, Intermediate 1 scores 0.5–1, Intermediate 2 scores 1.5–2, High scores > 2.
Median survivals are age related:
For low-risk group, 11.8 years for patients < 60 years and 4.8 years for patients > 60 years.
For intermediate 1 group: 5.2 years for patients < 60 years and 2.7 years for patients > 60 years.
For intermediate 2 group, 1.8 years for patients < 60 years and 1.1 years for patients > 60 years.
For high risk group: 0.3 years for patients < 60 years and 0.5 years for patients > 60 years.

Table 19.4 WHO classification of MDS

Myelodysplastic syndromes
1. Refractory anemia:
   (a) with ringed sideroblasts (RARS)
   (b) without ringed sideroblasts
2. Refractory cytopenia with multilineage dysplasia
3. Refractory anemia with excess blasts
   (a) Type I with 5–9% blasts
   (b) Type II with 10–19% blasts
4. 5q- syndrome
5. Myelodysplastic syndrome, unclassifiable

Myelodysplastic/myeloproliferative diseases
1. Chronic myelomonocytic leukemia
2. Atypical chronic myeloid leukemia
3. Juvenile myelomonocytic leukemia

Acute myeloblastic leukemia
1. Acute myeloid leukemia with multilineage dysplasia
2. Acute myeloid leukemia and myelodysplastic syndromes, therapy related

to diagnose. Cases with dysplastic features in two or more lineages should be known as refractory cytopenias with multilineage dysplasia. There was disagreement about chronic myelomonocytic leukemia (CMML). The pathologists in the group proposed a new category of MDS with myeloproliferative features (alternatively myelodysplastic, myeloproliferative disease, MDS/MPD) to include CMML, JMML and atypical chronic myeloid leukemia (aCML).

Particular types of acute myeloblastic leukemia (AML) pass through an oligoblastic phase, often showing dys-plastic features in granulocytic line. They have character-istic chromosomal translocations: t(8;21), t(15;17), and inv

16 abnormalities. These should not be categorized as MDS, but as distinct entities: varieties of AML. The 5q-syndrome is also a distinct entity and is so categorized as a variant of MDS. Refractory anemia with excess of blasts (RAEB) was separated into RAEB I with 5–9% blast cells and RAEB II with 10–19% blast cells. Some cases of AML may be recognized as having derived from MDS and this should be stated. Some of these cases will be what had been previously diagnosed as RAEB in transformation (RAEBt) and some will have been called AML. It is probable that a large proportion of cases of AML in the elderly will fall into this category.

Finally, it was recognized that some cases do not fit into this or any classification and should be categorized as MDS unclassifiable. Although the WHO classification encountered some opposition[14] it has been retrospectively evaluated by the Dusseldorf group and found to have prognostic value.[15]

Diagnosis

The majority of patients with MDS are asymptomatic and are diagnosed because a blood test has been performed for an irrelevant reason. Some will present with the symptoms of anemia (tiredness, breathlessness and lassitude), thrombocytopenia (bruising or bleeding), or neutropenia (recurrent infections, mouth ulcers). CMML may have some features of a myeloproliferative syndrome with moderate degrees of hepatosplenomegaly. In patients with high monocyte counts the abnormal monocytes become tissue macrophages and may produce pathology remote from the bone marrow. Gum hypertrophy, pleural and pericardial effusion, painful swollen joints and skin deposits have all been reported on rare occasions.

A full blood count may show anemia, neutropenia or thrombocytopenia. A raised mean cell volume (MCV) is frequently found and may be the only abnormality in the blood count. The differential diagnosis includes other causes of macrocytic anemia: B12 or folate deficiency, alcohol, liver disease, hypothyroidism and hemolytic anemia; and other causes of cytopenias: acute leukemia, aplastic anemia, drug-induced cytopenias, immune thrombocytopenia and marrow infiltration with various tumors. The morphologic abnormalities seen in AIDS have some similarities to those of MDS. Diagnosis of MDS will almost certainly depend on bone marrow examination although this may be legitimately resisted in the very elderly. Sometimes there are sufficient abnormalities on the blood film to make the diagnosis, and sometimes there are changes that make bone marrow aspirate and trephine biopsy imperative.

Blood film examination

The ability to diagnose MDS crucially depends on the optimum staining of blood and bone marrow films. We prefer Jenner–Giemsa staining, but the stain used is a matter of personal preference. Staining varies enormously from laboratory to laboratory, so each observer should become familiar with his or her own laboratory's stain. Films sent for a second opinion should be sent unstained. It is important that the stain used picks up granularity in neutrophils well and also reveals basophilic stippling in red cells. Tired, end-of-the-day stains are treacherous.

Red cells

Anemia is the most common feature of MDS but it is not necessarily present. Sometimes the only feature on the blood count suggestive of MDS is a raised MCV. Usually the red cells are large, but they may be of normal size and very occasionally small. Many textbooks list sideroblastic anemia among the causes of a low MCV. This is very misleading and only applies to the rare hereditary form. Refractory anemia with ring sideroblasts (RARS) is associated with a raised or normal MCV.

Frequently the red cells in MDS vary in size and shape (anisopoikilocytosis). Oval macrocytes are common. When these are accompanied by small hypochromic cells, so as to give a dimorphic picture, RARS should be suspected (Fig. 19.1). However, small hypochromic red cell fragments may be seen in all forms of MDS. A preponderance of small hypochromic red cells is rarely seen and should

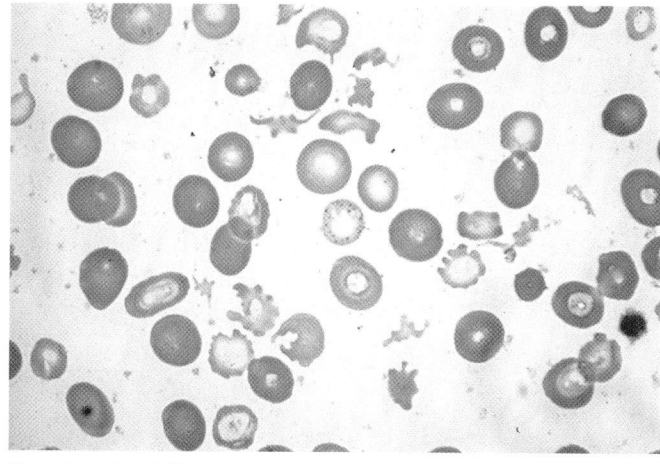

Fig. 19.1 Blood film from patient with RARS showing anisocytosis, poikilocytosis, anisochromasia, basophilic stippling and irregularly shaped red cells.

suggest acquired haemoglobin H (HbH) disease (Fig. 19.2). This is a very rare finding in MDS, usually in elderly men, but may be revealed in the usual way with supravital staining (Fig. 19.3).

Variation is cell shape is common. Poikilocytosis with tear-drop cells, acanthocytes and cell fragments are all frequently seen. MDS is a rare cause of elliptocytosis. However, red cell size and shape may be normal. Howell–Jolly bodies are occasionally seen. Rather more common is basophilic stippling which may be fine or coarse (Fig. 19.4). Fine basophilic stippling confined to large misshapen hypochromic cells usually indicates RARS.

White cells

Neutropenia is the rule in MDS. Although it may be severe, it is frequently mild. In CMML, the reverse is often true. In addition to the absolute monocytosis that defines the condition, there is usually a neutrophil leukocytosis. The neutrophil count is often $> 10 \times 10^9/l$ and we have seen cases with neutrophil counts $> 50 \times 10^9/l$.

The granularity of neutrophils is an important feature. Classically, there are few if any neutrophil granules (Fig. 19.5), but sometimes hypergranularity is seen (Fig. 19.6). Rarely, giant granules typical of those seen in Chediak–Higashi syndrome have been identified. Auer rods are sometimes seen, but they have no prognostic significance.

Neutrophil lobulation is the other feature to observe. Pseudo Pelger–Huët cells are neutrophils with unilobular or bilobed neutrophils with normal condensation of the nucleus (Fig. 19.7). It is important to distinguish these cells from myelocytes and metamyelocytes where the nucleus remains relatively uncondensed. Frequently, pseudo Pelger cells are seen together with hypogranularity.

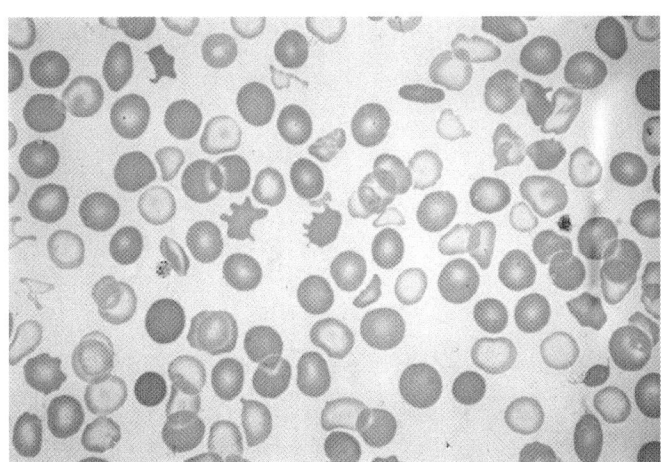

Fig. 19.2 Blood film from a patient with acquired HbH disease showing very hypochromic population together with anisocytosis and poikilocytosis and irregularly shaped red cells.

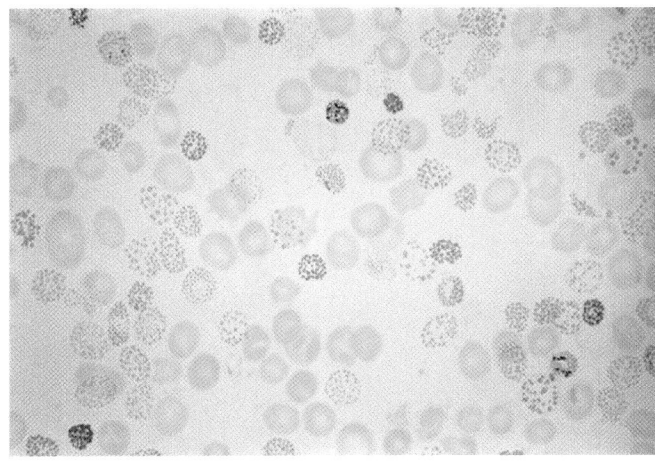

Fig. 19.3 Blood film from a patient with acquired HbH disease showing 'golf ball' inclusions when stained with brilliant cresyl blue.

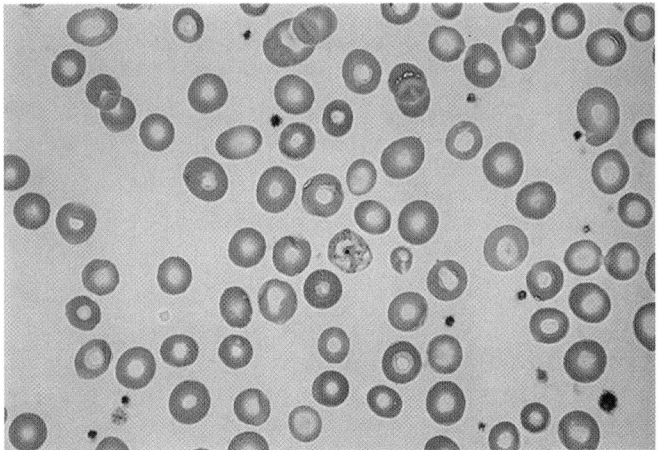

Fig. 19.4 Blood film from a patient with RARS showing a Howell–Jolly body in a cell with coarse basophilic stippling.

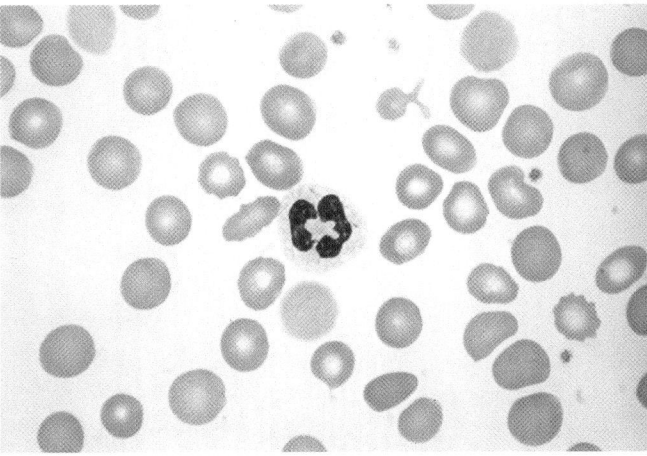

Fig. 19.5 Blood film from a patient with RA showing a hypogranular neutrophil.

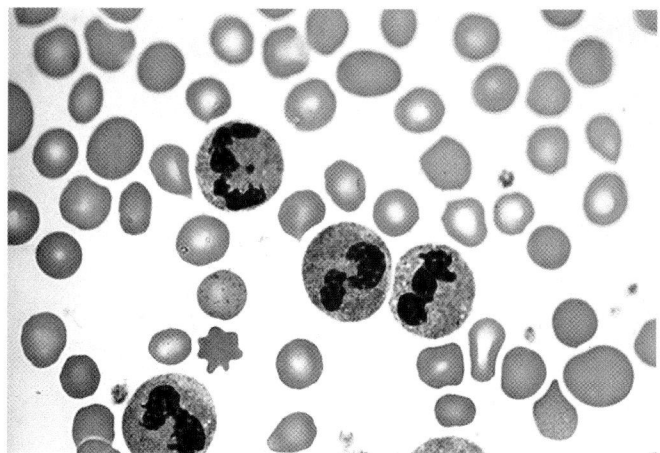

Fig. 19.6 Blood film from a patient with RA showing hypergranular neutrophils.

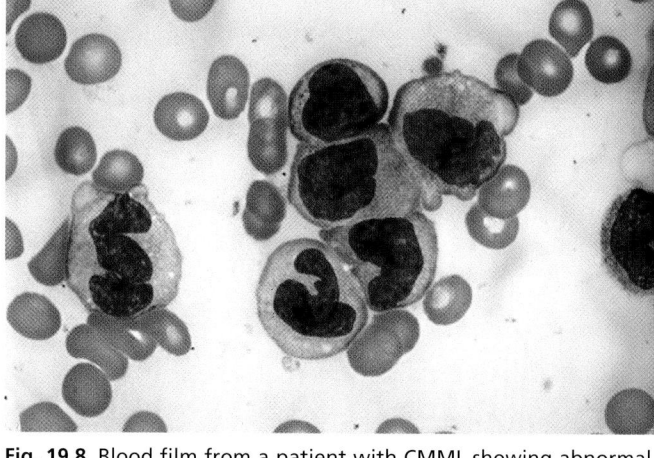

Fig. 19.8 Blood film from a patient with CMML showing abnormal monocytes.

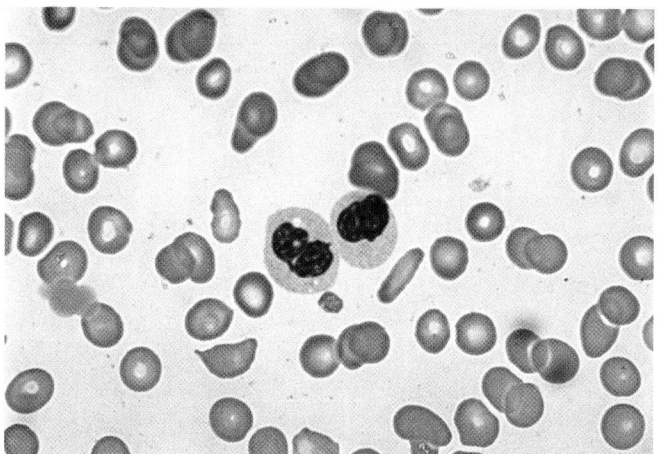

Fig. 19.7 Blood film from a patient with RA showing pseudo-Pelger–Huët cells.

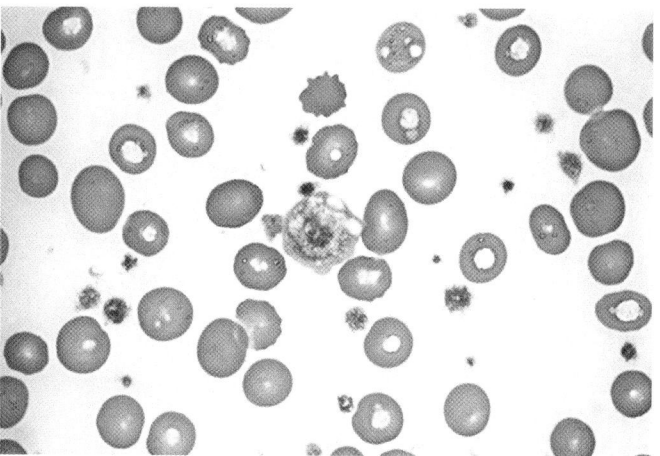

Fig. 19.9 Blood film from a patient with RA showing a giant platelet.

Occasionally, hyperlobulated polymorphs are seen. An unusual feature is arachnoid lobulation, where the nuclear lobules look like the segments of a spider's leg.

Monocytes are increased in CMML (Fig. 19.8). One of the difficulties with the FAB classification is the magic number of $10^9/l$ monocytes. Some cases skip between refractory anemia (RA) and CMML from week to week as their monocyte count hovers either side of this number. Monocytes often have multiple, elongated nuclear lobes. Promonocytes, with fine azurophil granules, may also be seen. The diagnosis of CMML may be difficult to make because the monocytosis may be slight, and the predominant feature of the blood film is a granulocytosis. These granulocytes may have minimal dysplastic features. The differentiation between CMML and chronic myeloid leukemia is discussed below.

Degranulated eosinophils are sometimes a feature. Eosinophils with basophilic granules and vice versa are sometimes seen.

Platelets

Thrombocytopenia is common. Thrombocytosis is rare, but occurs in the 5q– syndrome. It is important to distinguish myeloproliferative thrombocythemia from the thrombocytosis of MDS. The former should not have dysplastic features. Sometimes thrombocytosis accompanies the finding of ring sideroblasts.

Giant platelets or megakaryocte fragments may circulate in MDS (Fig. 19.9). Agranular platelets may also be seen.

Bone marrow aspirate

A well-prepared, freshly stained bone marrow aspirate is the key to the diagnosis of MDS. Which is the best Romanowsky stain continues to be a matter of argument. For most of us the answer is – the one you are used to. Interpreting bone marrow aspirates in MDS can be difficult. Nothing replaces practice. Some of the morphologic abnormalities are very subtle and referral of the slides for expert opinion is sometimes necessary. However, even experts disagree. Most disagreements arise from the recognition of mild degrees of RA.

Typically, the marrow is hypercellular, but cellularity is better appreciated from trephine biopsy than from the aspirate films. This is one of the reasons that the two investigations should be seen as complementary.

Erythropoiesis

All the features seen in the blood may be present, but the bone marrow aspirate gives the opportunity of examining the whole of erythropoiesis. In many cases there is erythroid hyperplasia, but pure red cell aplasia is a rare finding. Frequently, the red cell precursors appear megaloblastic. Multinuclear forms are common (Fig. 19.10), and megaloblastic anemia forms one of the chief differential diagnoses. Mitotic figures are common (Fig. 19.11) and there is frequently dyskaryorrhexis (literally, abnormal bursting of a cell nucleus). Pyknosis, nuclear budding and intranuclear bridging are frequently seen. There is often asynchrony between the maturation of nucleus and cytoplasm, with fully hemoglobinized cells with uncondensed nuclei.

Ringed sideroblasts are red cell precursors with an accumulation of iron in the mitochondria, which stains blue with Perls' stain. Older classifications, which counted the number of granules, have been superseded by a definition of a ring as one that extends at least a third of the way around the nucleus. Over half of cases of MDS have some sideroblasts. Arbitrarily, when ringed sideroblasts comprise > 15% of the total erythroblast population the disease is designated RARS (Figs 19.12 and 19.13).

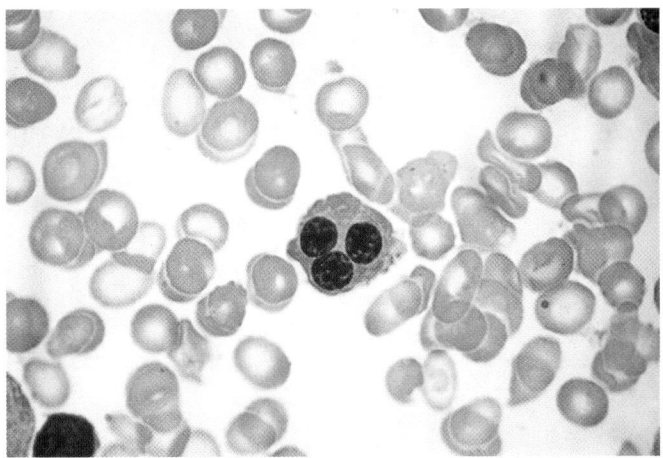

Fig. 19.10 Bone marrow film from a patient with RA showing a trinucleate normoblast.

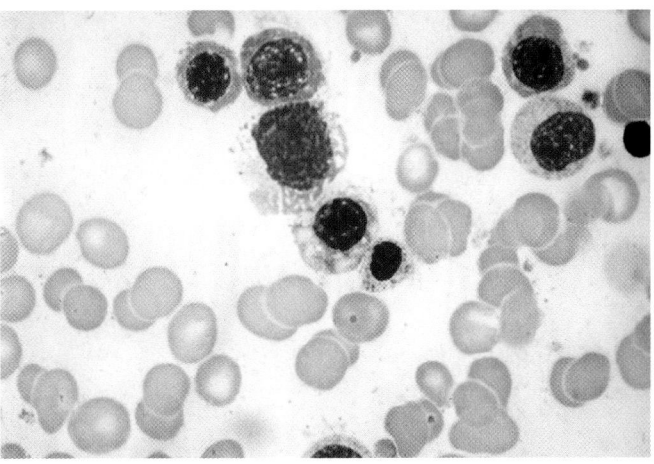

Fig. 19.12 Bone marrow film from a patient with RARS showing vacuolated and stippled normoblasts.

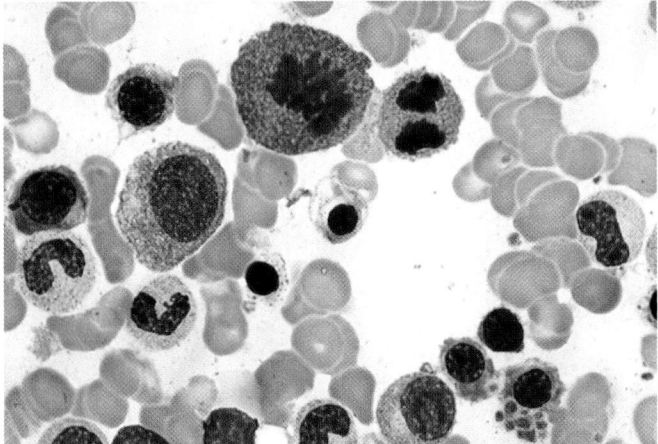

Fig. 19.11 Bone marrow film from a patient with RARS showing mitotic figures, and vacuolated and stippled normoblasts.

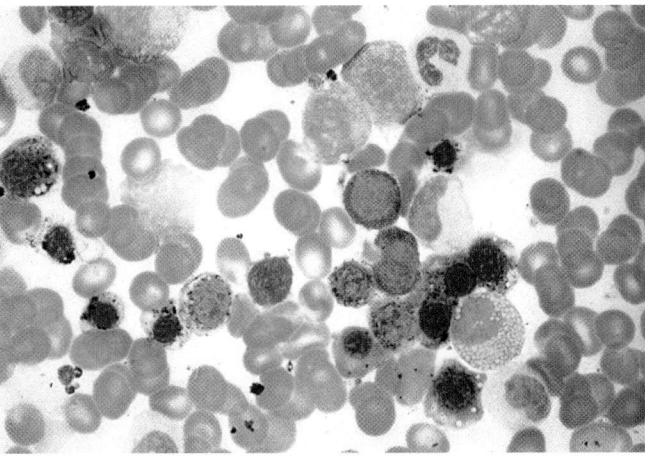

Fig. 19.13 Bone marrow film from a patient with RARS stained with Perls' stain showing ringed sideroblasts.

Granulopoiesis

Again, all the features seen in the blood may be present. Absence of secondary granules may be a feature of all myeloid precursor cells (Fig. 19.14), but primary azurophil granules are usually present in promyelocytes and some myeloblasts. Interestingly, it is very unusual for the myeloid cells in MDS not to stain with myeloperoxidase albeit less densely than in normals. On the other hand the cells are usually negative for leukocyte alkaline phophatase. Especially in CMML, an apparently hybrid cell with both myeloid and monocytic characteristics is seen. These paramyeloblasts stain positively for both chloro-acetate esterase (granulocyte specific) and α-naphthyl acetate esterase (monocyte specific).

An accurate blast cell count is important prognostically. It may be difficult to distinguish myeloblasts from promyelocytes. The FAB group recognized two types of blast cells. Type I blast cells are myeloblasts of variable size without granules or Auer rods (Fig. 19.15). The nuclear chromatin is uncondensed and there are usually one or two nucleoli. A type II blast cell is usually larger with rather more cytoplasm, and contains a few azurophil granules. They are distinguishable from promyelocytes, which have a slightly eccentric nucleus, which is rather more condensed with less distinct nucleoli, and an obvious Golgi zone (Fig. 19.16). Abnormal promyelocytes may also have excessive granules (more than six) resembling those seen in M3 AML though without the bilobed or monocytoid nucleus. Goasguen and colleagues[16] later described a type III blast cell with more than 20 azurophil granules but without a Golgi zone (Fig. 19.17).

Thrombopoiesis

Both very few and very many megakaryocytes are sometimes seen in MDS, but usually the numbers are normal.

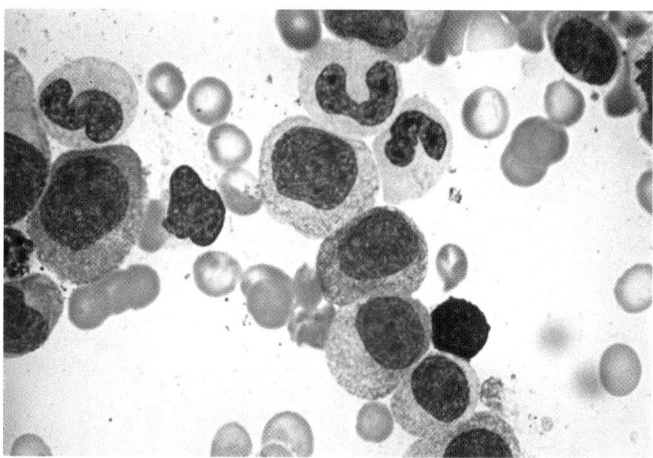

Fig. 19.14 Bone marrow film from a patient with RA showing hypogranular myeloid cells at different stages of maturation.

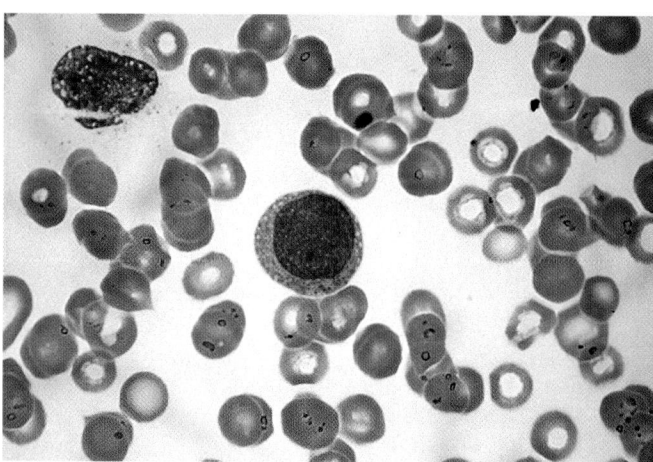

Fig. 19.16 Bone marrow film from a patient with RAEB showing a type II myeloblast.

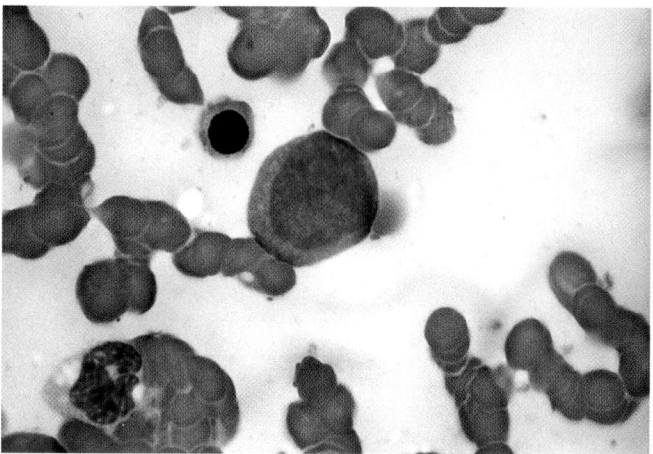

Fig. 19.15 Bone marrow film from a patient with RAEB showing a type I myeloblast.

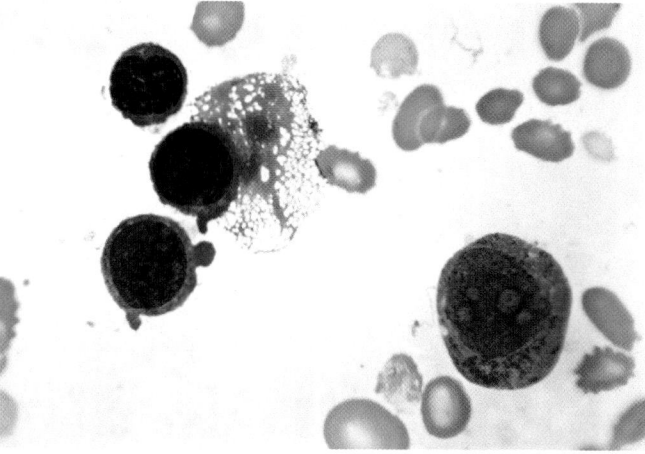

Fig. 19.17 Bone marrow film from a patient with RAEB showing a type III myeloblast.

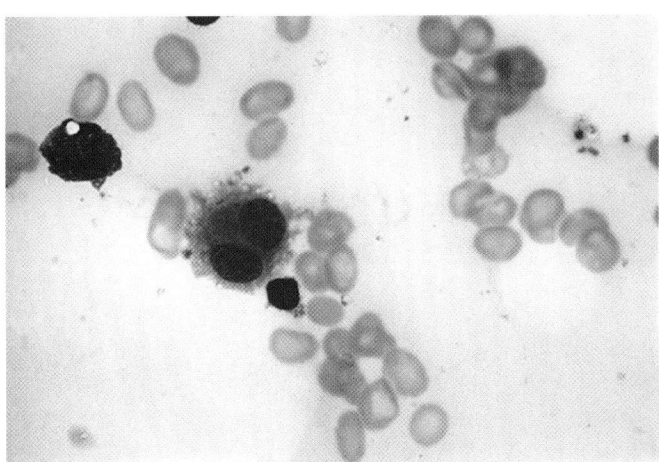

Fig. 19.18 Bone marrow film from a patient with RA showing micromegakaryocytes.

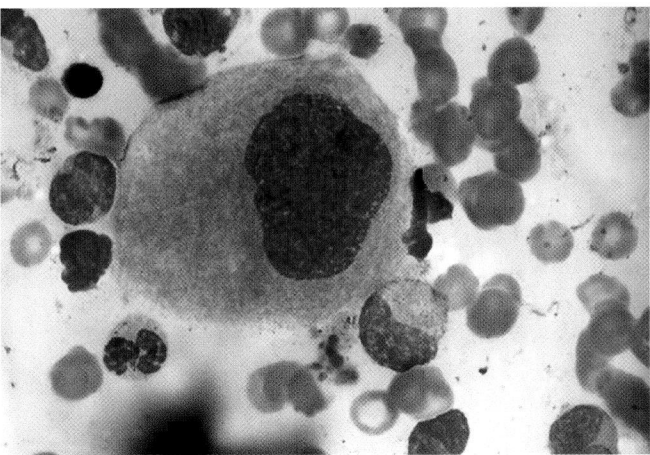

Fig. 19.20 Bone marrow film from a patient with 5q-syndrome showing a mononuclear megakaryocyte.

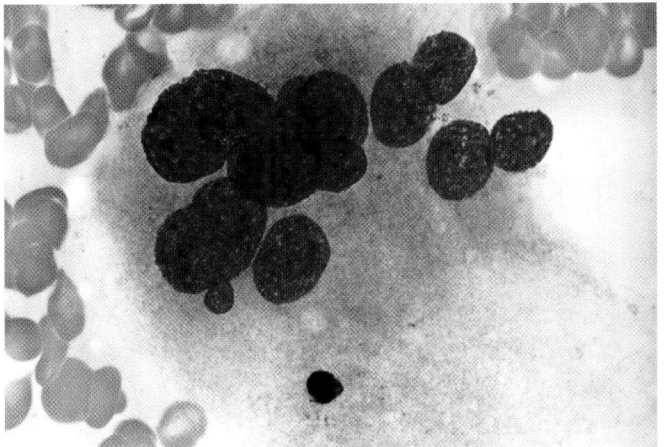

Fig. 19.19 Bone marrow film from a patient with RA showing a giant megakaryocyte with multiple dispersed nuclei.

There are characteristically three types of abnormal megakaryocyte seen: micromegakaryocytes (Fig. 19.18), giant megakaryocytes with multiple dispersed nuclei (Fig. 19.19), and moderate-sized megakaryocytes with a single round eccentric nucleus (Fig. 19.20). This last type is characteristic of the 5q⁻ syndrome, but is not confined to it.

The role of trephine biopsy in the assessment of myelodysplastic syndrome

Trephine biopsy is rarely essential for the diagnosis of MDS but offers useful information in addition to that obtained from cytologic assessment of peripheral blood and aspirated bone marrow.[17–19] The particular value of trephine biopsy in this context is for the demonstration of spatial disturbance of hemopoietic tissue within the marrow, which cannot be appreciated in samples obtained by aspiration. Cytologic abnormalities in the various hemopoietic cell lineages can also be seen in histologic sections of bone marrow, although aspirate films show these features in more subtle detail and are the preferred preparation in which to make assessment of cytologic features of dysplasia. In any patient in whom aspiration proves difficult, trephine biopsy is recommended as it can supply much of the information that may be lacking from suboptimal aspirate films.

General histologic features of myelodysplastic syndrome

Histologic sections in most patients with MDS will show hypercellularity of hemopoietic tissue but, in some cases, will appear normocellular or hypocellular. It is important to remember the expected range of cellularity is wide in the older age group within which most cases of MDS arise, but is generally lower as age increases. When relatively young patients present with suspected MDS, what might appear to be increased cellularity should not be overestimated.

Stromal components of the bone marrow usually appear relatively normal in MDS; there may be a mild increase in reticulin but collagen fibrosis is uncommon[20] and disturbances of trabecular bone remodeling, including new bone formation, are rare. Marked stromal abnormalities such as edema or fibrosis should raise suspicion of secondary myelodysplasia or an overlap myeloproliferative/myelodysplastic syndrome.

Histologic features seen in trephine biopsy sections in MDS do not correlate well with individual subtypes as defined by the FAB or WHO classification systems. In general, it is possible to determine that an individual example of MDS has 'low-grade' features, consistent with FAB categories myelodysplastic syndrome – refractory anemia (MDS-RA), RARS, other refractory cytopenias or the 5q-syndrome, or 'high-grade' features in keeping with MDS-RAEB or RAEBt.[21,22] This distinction can be made on the basis of prevalence of early myelomonocytic cells (myeloblasts, promyelocytes and promonocytes) within sections (Figs 19.21 and 19.22). Recognition of myeloblasts may be difficult but increased numbers of promyelocytes, usually accompanied by disproportionately reduced numbers of metamyelocytes and neutrophil polymorphs, are generally easy to recognize. It should be noted that in chronic myelomonocytic leukemia (discussed in Chapter 21), the presence of large numbers of immature myelomonocytic cells does not correlate well with the biologic aggressiveness of the disease in individual patients.

Assessment of spatial distribution of hemopoiesis in MDS

As mentioned above, trephine biopsy sections have the particular value in MDS of allowing assessment of the spatial distribution of hemopoietic cells. In normal bone marrow, promyelocytes and myelocytes are localized preferentially at the margins of bone trabeculae and around the adventitial aspects of arterioles and venules coursing through intertrabecular spaces.[23] Metamyelocytes and neutrophil polymorphs are found in increasing numbers with progression towards the centers of intertrabecular marrow spaces. Developing monocytes are more randomly distributed and are difficult to distinguish from early granulocytic cells in histologic sections.[24] Erythroid cells form orderly clusters in non-paratrabecular areas of the marrow spaces, with mid- and late normoblasts predominating. Megakaryocytes are usually found singly, in the central parts of intertrabecular spaces, and sometimes the plane of section allows their location at the edge of sinusoids to be seen.

In the MDS, and in secondary forms of myelodysplasia, this topographic arrangement is disturbed to a greater or lesser extent. Displacement of early granulocyte precursors from trabecular margins is a frequent finding and, accompanying this, scattered metamyelocytes and neutrophil polymorphs may be found immediately adjacent to trabecular margins. The presence of myeloblasts and promyelocytes in groups in the central parts of intertrabecular spaces is seen less commonly (Fig. 19.23).[25] The latter phenomenon has been a source of debate for many years, since some authors have claimed that such abnormal localization of immature precursors (ALIP) is of adverse prognostic significance in patients whose blast cell counts in blood and aspirated marrow are low. However, it has proved difficult to define objective criteria for the recognition and quantification of ALIP. In most cases where ALIP is seen in daily practice, it is present in the context of a blood or bone marrow blast cell count consistent with FAB categories of MDS-RAEB, RAEBt or even AML; in this context it has no independent prognostic value. It should also be noted that ALIP is not a phenomenon specific to MDS; it can be seen in reactive conditions and myeloproliferative disorders, in which it is of no known significance.

Spatial disorganization of erythropoiesis is represented by erythroid cell clusters occupying paratrabecular areas

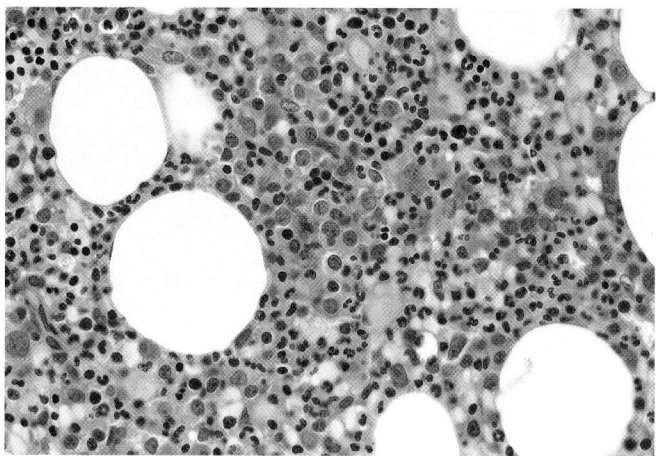

Fig. 19.21 Histology of 'low-grade' myelodysplasia in MDS-RA. Hematoxylin and eosin-stained section of decalcified, paraffin-embedded bone marrow trephine biopsy core; original magnification × 40.

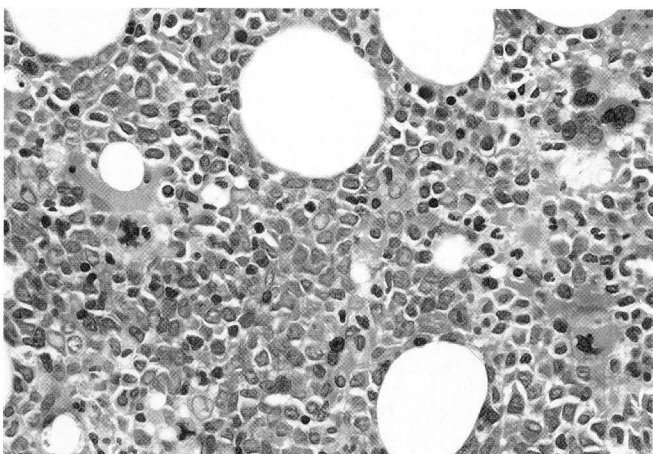

Fig. 19.22 Histology of 'high-grade' myelodysplasia in MDS-RAEB. Hematoxylin and eosin-stained section of decalcified, paraffin-embedded bone marrow trephine biopsy core; original magnification × 40.

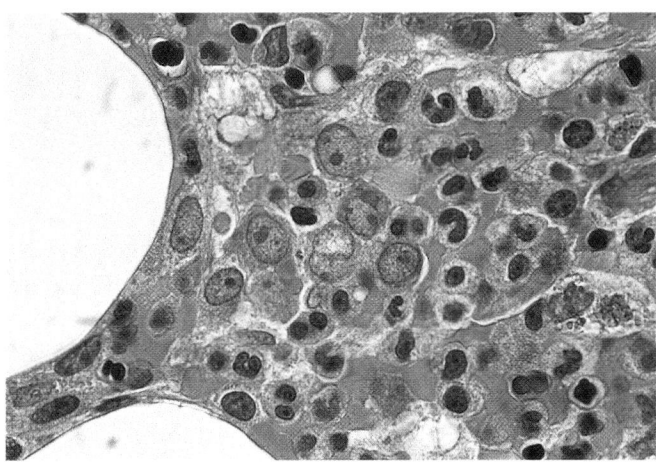

Fig. 19.23 Immature myelomonocytic cells in the center of an intertrabecular space; so-called 'ALIP'. Hematoxylin and eosin-stained section of decalcified, paraffin-embedded bone marrow trephine biopsy core; original magnification × 100.

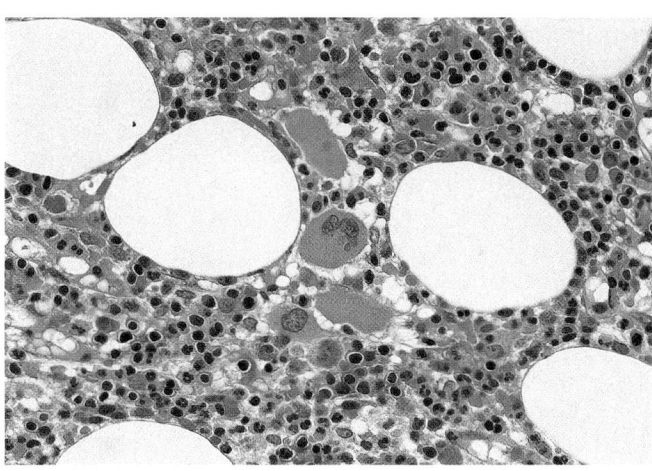

Fig. 19.25 Cluster of atypical, small megakaryocytes in MDS. Hematoxylin and eosin-stained section of decalcified, paraffin-embedded bone marrow trephine biopsy core; original magnification × 40.

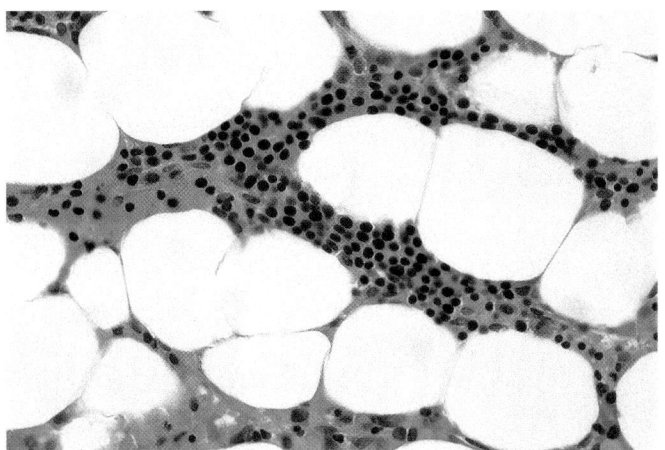

Fig. 19.24 Dyplastic erythropoiesis with irregular clustering of erythroid precursor cells, each cell at a similar (in this example, relatively late) stage of maturation to its neighbors; in normal erythroid cell clusters, a mixture of maturational stages would be present. Hematoxylin and eosin-stained section of decalcified, paraffin-embedded bone marrow trephine biopsy core; original magnification × 40.

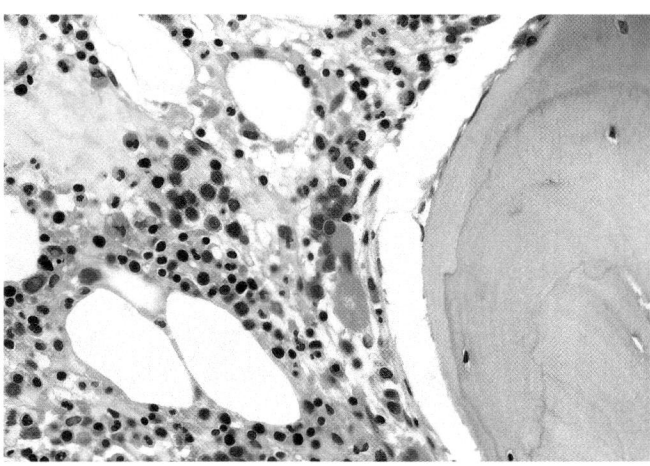

Fig. 19.26 Displacement of atypical megakaryocytes to the paratrabecular region in MDS. Hematoxylin and eosin-stained section of decalcified, paraffin-embedded bone marrow trephine biopsy core; original magnification × 40.

of the marrow and also by loss of the normal organization of individual clusters. The clusters are frequently enlarged, with increased numbers of proerythroblasts and early normoblasts. The cells in some clusters may appear synchronous, rather than reflecting a spectrum of maturational stages of erythropoiesis (Fig. 19.24). In some patients, erythropoiesis may appear dispersed, with absent or infrequent formation of cell clusters. It is curious that, despite striking cytologic findings in aspirated bone marrow, erythropoiesis is frequently hyperplastic but otherwise apparently normal in many patients with MDS-RARS, in whom trephine biopsy histology may be remarkable for its lack of dysplastic features.

Assessment of megakaryocyte morphology and distribution is critical to the interpretation of bone marrow trephine biopsy histology in MDS.[26–29] Cytologic features are discussed below but spatial distribution of megakaryocytes, as for other hemopoietic lineages, is often highly abnormal. Because of their relatively large size and distinctive morphology, it is usually easy to detect clustering of megakaryocytes (Fig. 19.25) and their displacement from perisinusoidal to paratrabecular locations (Fig. 19.26). Occasional clusters of 2–3 megakaryocytes may be found in normal or reactive bone marrow but larger groupings are highly atypical and indicate pathology such as myelodysplasia or a chronic myeloproliferative disorder. Paratrabecular location of megakaryocytes has similar significance and is extremely rare in other contexts, unless the bone marrow is severely hypoplastic for other reasons. Even in the latter situation, the possibility of hypoplastic MDS should be considered carefully.

Assessment of cytologic features in trephine biopsy sections in MDS

Cytologic features of myelodysplasia in developing hemopoietic cells are best seen in bone marrow aspirate films. In decalcified trephine biopsy sections it is usually not possible to detect hypogranularity in granulocytic cells and nuclear abnormalities such as pseudo-Pelger changes can be seen only with difficulty. Failure of nuclear condensation and lobulation in terminally differentiated neutrophil polymorphs can be seen in occasional cases. Abnormalities of granulation may be visible in high-quality sections of plastic-embedded trephine biopsies. Since these are generally thinner than those cut from paraffin-embedded specimens (1–2 mm compared with 4–5 mm), familiarity with the normal degree of granularity visible in thin sections is essential. More readily appreciable are abnormalities in the proportions of developing granulocytes present representing different stages of maturation; there are frequently increased promyelocytes and myelocytes accompanied by reduced numbers of metamyelocytes and neutrophils. It is even more difficult in trephine biopsy sections than aspirate films to determine precisely which cells among the immature granulocytes are truly myeloblasts.

In the erythroid series, dysplastic cytology is frequently represented by a megaloblast-like appearance of individual nucleated red cell precursors. As with granulopoiesis, however, it is usually easier to appreciate the imbalance in relative numbers of cells at different stages of maturation. Increased numbers of dysplastic proerythroblasts and reduced numbers of later cells alter the composition of erythroid nests; absence of the familiar late normoblasts, abundant in normal bone marrow, is an important clue to the presence of erythroid dysplasia in trephine biopsy sections. The megaloblast-like proerythroblasts may be confused with early myelomonocytic precursors, and may even suggest ALIP, but staining reveals their basophilic cytoplasm, often with a perinuclear halo, allowing their distinction from other immature hemopoietic cells.

Cells of megakaryocytic lineage demonstrate the most readily appreciable dysplastic cytologic features in bone marrow trephine biopsy sections. Because megakaryocytes tend to remain adherent to particles in aspirate films,

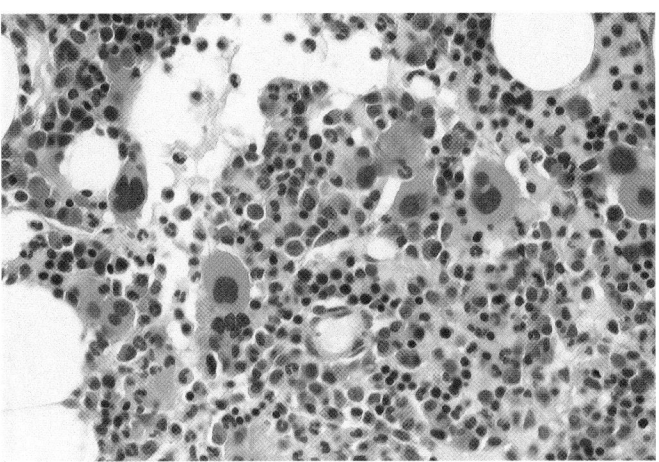

Fig. 19.27 Small, monolobular megakaryocytes typical of the 5q-syndrome. Hematoxylin and eosin-stained section of decalcified, paraffin-embedded bone marrow trephine biopsy core; original magnification × 40.

trephine biopsy is often superior for their assessment. Megakaryocyte numbers are frequently increased, with striking spatial abnormalities as described above, and their size is often variable but generally smaller than normal. True micromegakaryocytes, similar in size to promyelocytes, are difficult to see without specific immunohistochemical staining, but small megakaryocytes are usually easy to recognize. In addition to their reduced size, these cells typically have reduced numbers of nuclear lobules; the mean number of nuclear lobules per megakaryocyte in normal bone marrow is between 6 and 10. Monolobular small megakaryocytes are particularly associated with the 5q-syndrome (Fig. 19.27) but are also present, together with a heterogeneous population of less-distinctive dysplastic megakaryocytes, in other forms of myelodysplasia.

One aspect of cytology in myelodysplasia is often only appreciable in bone marrow trephine biopsy sections and not in aspirate films. This is the increased apoptotic activity that contributes to ineffective hemopoiesis in patients with MDS.[30,31] Apoptotic nuclei, recognizable by their characteristic patterns of nucleic acid condensation, can be seen scattered throughout the hemopoietic tissue and, sometimes, clustered inside the cytoplasm of stromal macrophages. However, increased apoptotic activity also occurs in other conditions involving increased cell turnover in the bone marrow, including hyperplastic states (e.g. associated with septicemia or in response to malignant disease elsewhere in the body), chronic myeloproliferative disorders and acute leukemias. Undue significance should not be attributed to finding increased apoptotic activity in bone marrow trephine biopsy sections if other features of dysplasia are absent.

Histologic assessment of myelodysplasia in hypoplastic bone marrow

Assessment of myelodysplasia in hypocellular bone marrow specimens poses particular difficulties due to the paucity of hemopoietic tissue available for assessment.[32,33] Aspiration may have been unsuccessful or may have yielded a suboptimal sample, so that trephine biopsy has an important role to play. The differential diagnosis includes primary MDS, secondary myelodysplasia (see below) and disorders such as hypoplastic/aplastic anemia, paroxysmal nocturnal hemoglobinuria and hypoplastic acute myeloid leukemia. The same criteria should be applied in assessing hemopoietic cell distribution and cytologic features as in normocellular or hypercellular trephine biopsy sections. Even with very little hemopoietic tissue to evaluate, it should be possible to determine whether the biopsy shows: (1) hypoplastic normal hemopoiesis; (2) hypoplastic dysplastic hemopoiesis with evidence of at least partial maturation within each hemopoietic lineage; or (3) hypoplastic acute leukemia with blast cells and minimal or no evidence of maturation.

Histologic features of secondary myelodysplasia

Dysplastic hemopoiesis may occur in response to a variety of, often poorly characterized, systemic diseases and toxic insults to the bone marrow. A familiar example is the myelodysplasia associated with infection by the human immunodeficiency virus (HIV).[34] Hemopoietic recovery following cytotoxic chemotherapy is also often transiently dysplastic,[35] in addition to the predictable megaloblastosis caused by use of folate antagonists.

It is not always possible to determine by bone marrow examination whether dysplasia is primary or secondary but trephine biopsy histology provides important clues to indicate the likelihood of one versus the other. The main features that indicate a secondary origin for myelodysplasia are abnormalities of the bone marrow stroma, reflecting toxic or inflammatory injury of stromal cells, occurring in addition to hemopoietic cell damage. At the least, increased stromal reticulin (grade 2–3) is usually present. In addition, there is often stromal edema, indicated by separation of hemopoietic cells in the interstitium and widening of sinusoidal lumens (Figs 19.28 and 19.29). In more severe injury, gelatinous change occurs; evidence for this may be found in aspirate films as well as in histologic preparations, with irregular

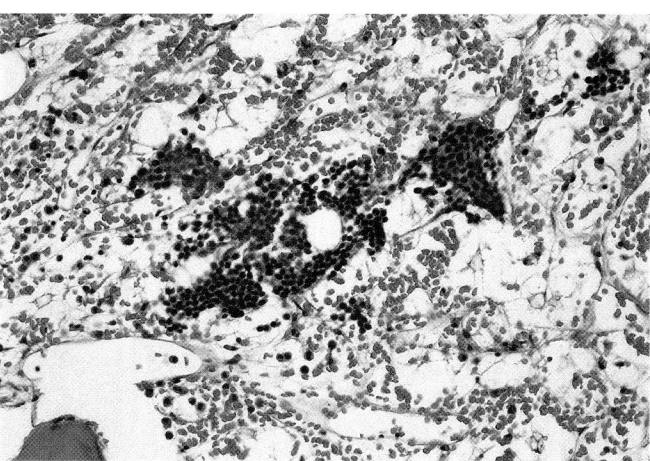

Fig. 19.28 Stromal edema and red cell extravasation, presumed to represent stromal responses to inflammatory or toxic injury. Atypical, cohesive-appearing, 'synchronous' clusters of erythropoietic cells are prominent and other hemopoietic cells are widely separated in the background. Non-nucleated red cells are present throughout the edematous interstitium and a distended sinusoidal lumen can be seen (bottom left) adjacent to the end of a bony trabecula. Hematoxylin and eosin-stained section of decalcified, paraffin-embedded bone marrow trephine biopsy core; original magnification × 20.

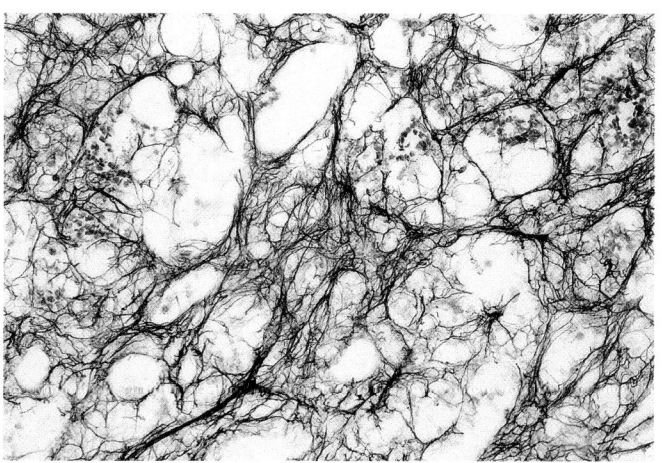

Figure 19.29 Reticulin staining of the same case shows diffuse, grade 3 increase in interstitial reticulin fibers. Silver-stained section of decalcified, paraffin-embedded bone marrow trephine biopsy core; original magnification × 20.

masses eosinophilic, periodic acid–schiff (PAS)-positive material in particles and trails. In histologic sections, distinction between severe edema and gelatinous change can be confirmed by alcian blue staining; edema fluid remains unstained but, in gelatinous change, the stroma stains turquoise/blue. Stromal injury is occasionally sufficiently severe to cause collagen fibrosis, particularly if necrosis has occurred. Evidence of previous necrosis may be found in the form of dead bone trabeculae or fragments of amorphous debris in the fibrotic stroma showing dystrophic calcification. Recent severe systemic illness or exposure to cytotoxic agents may leave a distinct cement line around many bone trabeculae, reflecting transient inhibition of normal bone remodeling (Fig. 19.30). Stromal injury may also lead to new bone formation; this is usually only focal and minor in extent but rare patients, for unknown reasons, respond to toxic bone marrow injury with florid neo-osteogenesis.

Other features suggestive of a secondary origin for dysplasia are the presence of inflammatory cells, particularly plasma cells, in increased numbers in the stroma and the finding of reactive lymphoid nodules or granulomas.

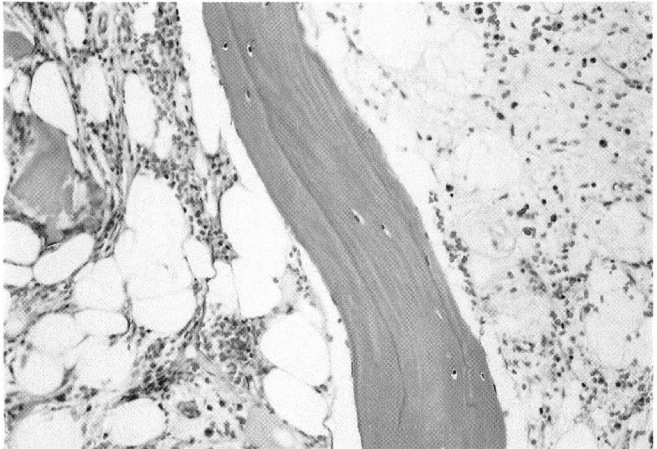

Figure 19.30 Distinct cement line around a bone trabecula representing a recent period of decreased bone remodeling, as a response to cytotoxic therapy, followed by recovery. Hematoxylin and eosin-stained section of decalcified, paraffin-embedded bone marrow trephine biopsy core; original magnification × 10.

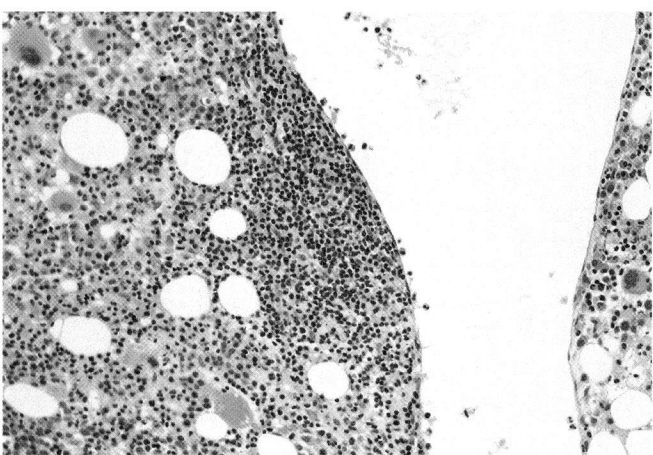

Fig. 19.31 Poorly defined aggregate of small lymphoid cells abutting the margin of a dilated sinusoid in a case of MDS-RA; the site and organization of this infiltrate are atypical and, considered in isolation, would raise suspicion of a low-grade lymphoid neoplasm. Hematoxylin and eosin-stained section of decalcified, paraffin-embedded bone marrow trephine biopsy core; original magnification × 20.

If lymphoid nodules are seen, it should be remembered that such aggregates, sometimes with atypical features, might also occur in association with primary MDS (Fig. 19.31). The differential diagnosis must include, in addition, bone marrow involvement by lymphoma provoking secondary myelodysplasia (see Chapter 22). Distinguishing between these alternatives can be extremely difficult and requires integration of all clinical, hematologic, cytogenetic and molecular genetic information available for the individual patient under consideration. Even with such information, it may be necessary to follow the patient's subsequent progress, including re-biopsy of their bone marrow, to establish the nature and clinical significance of such abnormalities.

Use of immunohistochemistry and fluorescent *in situ* hybridization in trephine biopsy sections in myelodysplasia

Immunohistochemistry can be very helpful in interpreting trephine biopsy histology in myelodysplastic conditions when cytologic abnormalities cause difficulty in the recognition of cells belonging to the various hemopoietic lineages.[36] Cells of the granulocytic series, at all stages of maturation, can be demonstrated by immunostaining for muramidase (lysozyme) or the CD68 variant recognized by monoclonal antibody KP1. Use of neutrophil elastase as a target antigen for immunohistochemistry may be unreliable in MDS if hypogranularity of granulocytes is a feature; otherwise, it can be useful to demonstrate the distribution of promyelocytes and myelocytes. Later granulocytes (metamyelocytes and neutrophil polymorphs) express CD15 and the calprotectin molecule recognized by monoclonal antibody Mac387. Numbers of eosinophil, basophil and monocyte precursors are not usually sufficient to cause problems in interpreting the results of these immunostains. However, caution is needed in any patient who does have a significant increase in any of these cell types in their blood or aspirated bone marrow, since the expression by such cells of the antigens described above is incompletely characterized at present.

The identity and distribution of dysplastic erythroid cells can be confirmed by immunohistochemistry to demonstrate glycophorin A or C; glycophorin C is expressed slightly earlier in erythropoiesis than is glycophorin A. Megakaryocytes are usually easily recognizable from their cytologic features but atypical forms, micromegakaryocytes and megakaryoblasts can be highlighted by immunostaining for CD61 (platelet glycoprotein IIIa) or CD42b (platelet glycoprotein Ib).

An interesting recent application of immunohisto-chemistry in MDS has been for the enumeration of CD34[+] hemopoietic stem cells in bone marrow trephine biopsy sections. It has been reported that the CD34[+] count assessed in this way has prognostic value, with higher counts predicting increased likelihood of leukemic trans-formation.[37,38] To date, CD34 immunohistochemistry has not been put into widespread use, at least in the UK, but it may become more widely practiced if the predictive value is confirmed in larger studies. Evaluation of CD34 positivity in bone marrow trephine biopsy sections must be undertaken with care to exclude capillary endothelial cells. Endothelial cells express this antigen strongly and, particularly when cut in cross-section, cannot always be seen to be associated with a vascular lumen. With experience, hemopoietic cells can be recognized by their characteristic granular immunohistochemical staining pattern with monoclonal antibody QBEnd10, reactive with class I CD34 (Fig. 19.32).

As understanding of the genetic basis of hemopoietic disorders, including primary MDS, increases, interest in demonstrating cytogenetic abnormalities *in situ* in bone marrow trephine biopsy sections is growing. Despite the limitations of visualizing signals in sectioned nuclei, in which only part of the chromosomal complement of any cell is represented, methodology has been developed for successful demonstration of numerical chromosomal abnormalities and translocations by fluorescent DNA *in situ* hybridization (FISH) in trephine biopsy sections.[39,40] Applications of FISH to histologic preparations repre-senting MDS have, as yet, been very limited but the prospect of further studies in this area is exciting.

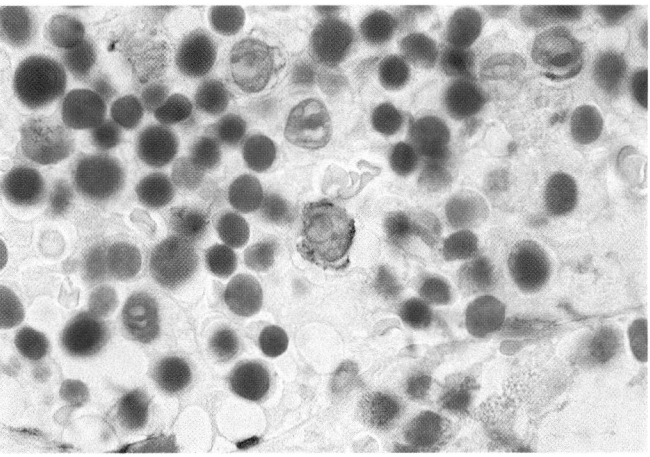

Fig. 19.32 Primitive hemopoietic cell expressing CD34 with a characteristic granular distribution, as shown by immunohistochemistry using monoclonal antibody QBEnd10 (Novocastra Laboratories Ltd, Newcastle upon Tyne, UK). Streptavidin-biotin immunoperoxidase method using section of decalcified, paraffin-embedded bone marrow trephine biopsy core; original magnification × 100.

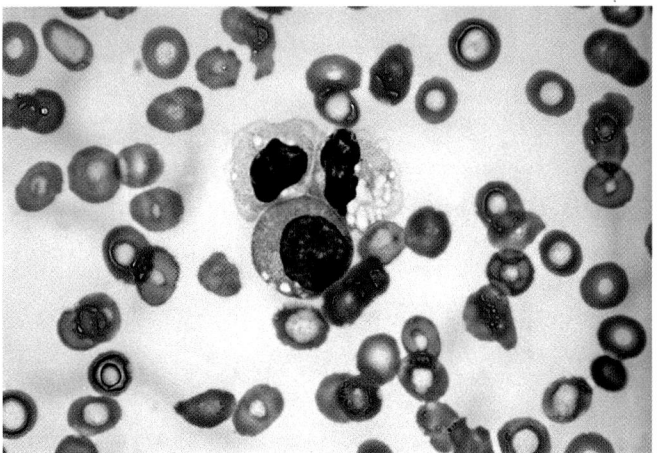

Fig. 19.33 Blood film from a patient with RA showing vacuolated pseudo-Pelger cells characteristically seen in association with abnormalities of chromosome 17p.

Karyotype

If possible, direct chromosomal analysis of the bone marrow should be performed in MDS. Clonal cytogenetic abnormalities are found in approximately 50% of cases of primary MDS[41,42] and more than 90% of cases of secondary MDS.[43,44] The more advanced the disease, the greater the incidence of karyotypic abnormality. Even when a normal karyotype is found, monosomies and tri-somies are sometimes detected by FISH.[45] An abnormal karyotype gives important prognostic information. Common chromosomal abnormalities include del (5q), −7, +8, del (20q) and −Y. Some specific associations are recognized: for example, isolated del (5q)[46,47] commonly occurs in older women with a macrocytic anemia, normal or raised platelet count, monolobated megakaryocytes and a good prognosis. Del (5q) is not confined to this group; it may be found in other forms of MDS that do not

have such a benign prognosis, but then the breakpoint on chromosome 5 is different (being telomeric to 5q31).

Deletions of 17p are characterized by small vacuolated pseudo-Pelger cells;[48,49] rearrangements of 3q26 are asso-ciated with raised platelet counts and micromega-karyocytes;[50] and a rare t(5:12) translocation is found in some cases of CMML.[51]

Genetic abnormalities

In general it is not known what genetic effects of the commonest chromosomal abnormalities produce. Abnor-malities at 3q23 cause activation of the *EVI-1* gene[52] while those of 17p affect *p53*. However, gene mappers have yet to isolate the responsible genes on 5q and 7q despite many years of effort.

The t(5:12) translocation dysregulates the ras signaling pathway,[53] and mutations of the *ras* gene have been a regular finding. Various authors have found mutations, mostly involving *N-ras*, in between 9 and 40% of cases of MDS,[54,55] especially CMML. Most mutations involve a G to A transition at codon 12 or 13. A rare association between juvenile myelomonocytic leukemia and neurofibromatosis is caused by a mutation of the *NF1* gene.[56] This gene product is a GTPase-activating protein that also interacts with *ras,* converting it from an active to an inactive form.

Other genetic abnormalities encountered in MDS include hypermethylation of the cyclin-dependent kinase inhibitor p15,[57] mutations in the gene coding for receptor for macrophage colony stimulating factor (*c-fms*)[58] and mutations of *p53*. In some cases of RARS mutations of the mitochondrial gene encoding mitochondrial cytochrome C oxidase have been seen.[59]

Cell biology

The growth of marrow progenitor cells in short-term culture is abnormal in MDS.[60] In some cases there is no growth, but more commonly there is a reduction of myeloid colony-forming units (CFU-GM), erythroid burst-forming units (BFU-E) and mixed granulocyte-erythroid-macrophage-megakaryocytic colony units (CGU-GEMM), with an increase in clusters and defective maturation of cells within individual colonies. In general, the defects are worse in patients with greater numbers of blasts in the marrow. In CMML and JMML, CFU-GM growth is increased, due to over production of granulocyte-macrophage colony-stimulating factor (GM-CSF).

In dissecting the causes of these abnormalities, it appears that there is a defect of colony-forming cells in responding to growth factors by proliferation and differentiation. Increasing concentrations of these factors improves response, laying a basis for treatment of MDS with growth factors.[61] Growth in long-term marrow

culture is poor in MDS and seldom sustained for longer than 2 weeks.[62]

Of great recent interest is the discovery of increased apoptosis in MDS,[63,64] which has been demonstrated by a variety of techniques. When CD34+ cells are studied, it is most apparent in early MDS. Increased bone marrow blast cell counts are associated with a significant reduction of apoptosis.

Immune function is impaired in MDS.[65-68] A wide range of supposedly auto-immune diseases has been found in association with MDS. It is likely that these represent disorders of macrophage rather than lymphoid function. Although the susceptibility to infection is caused by defects in granulocyte or macrophage number and function there is considerable evidence that lymphocytes are affected by the disease (Table 19.5). One possible cause for this is that lymphocytes are involved in the dysplastic clone via a common progenitor. There is conflicting evidence for this (Table 19.6), but recent opinion favors the immune system being affected by abnormal activities of monocytes and dendritic cells, which certainly are part of the clone.

Other abnormalities

A wide range of laboratory abnormalities may be found in MDS. These are largely epiphenomena that give little insight into the pathogenesis of MDS. They are detailed in Table 19.7.

Pathogenesis

Most workers view MDS as the result of the cumulative acquisition of multiple genetic errors occurring over a long period. Some of these abnormalities may be congenital, but most are acquired. The acquired genetic abnormalities may be random errors, but some environmental insults increase the risk. Chief among these have been exposure to X-irradiation, alkylating agents and benzene and its derivatives. Some individuals may be more prone to this process because they lack effective detoxifying enzymes.[86-88]

Table 19.5 Immunologic abnormalities associated with MDS

Immunoglobulins	B-cells	T-cells	NK cells
Polyclonal hypergammaglobulinemia	Normal in number	T-cell lymphopenia	Reduced in number
Hypogammaglobulinemia	Functionally immature	Reduced CD4+ cells	Functionally immature
Monoclonal gammopathy		Impaired T-cell function	
Anti-red cell antibodies			

Table 19.6 Evidence of lymphoid involvement in myelodysplastic syndrome

Transformation of MDS to acute lymphoblastic leukemia
Occurs but very rare

Co-existent MDS and lymphoid malignancies
Commoner than would be expected by chance, but mainly involves myeloma and chronic lymphocytic leukemia (CLL)

Inactivation of same X chromosome in lymphoid and myeloid cells
Most frequently not found but well reported index cases

Same cytogenetic abnormality in lymphoid and myeloid cells
Occurs but very rare

Same oncogene mutations in lymphoid and myeloid cells
Few case reports only

Table 19.7 Other abnormal pathologic findings in MDS

Investigation	Abnormality
Serum B12[69]	Often high, but coincident pernicious anemia has been reported
Serum LDH[70]	High levels carry poor prognosis
Ferrokinetics[71]	Shortened red cell survival; ineffective erythropoiesis
HbF[72]	Often raised in JMML
Ham's test[73]	Positive rarely
Red cell enzymes[74]	Raised levels of several enzymes on glycolytic pathway
Direct antiglobulin test[75]	Positive in 8%
Serum lysozme[76]	Raised in CMML
Granulocyte function[77]	Reduced motility, adherence, phagocytosis and bacterial killing
NAP score[78]	Often low
Platelet function[79]	Prolonged bleeding time, reduced aggregation with adrenaline and collagen
Monocyte function[80–85]	Increased cytokine production and receptors for immunoglobulin and complement; decreased cytoplasmic enzymes and phagocytosis

CMML, chronic myelomonocytic leukemia; JMML, juvenile myelomonocytic leukemia; NAP, neutrophil alkaline phosphatase.

Natural history

Although some individuals may follow an indolent course, in most the condition will progress. Cytopenias will become worse and bone marrow blast cell counts will increase. In this elderly group, around a third will develop acute leukemia, a third will die of the consequence of cytopenias and a third will die from an unrelated cause.[5]

Management

Treatment for MDS is unsatisfactory. The keystone is good supportive care. Even in patients who develop acute myeloblastic leukemia, the course is often indolent and no attempt at aggressive therapy should be initiated until the pace of the disease is established. Many patients require no treatment beyond the psychological support of a concerned physician. However, cytopenias lead to infections bleeding and bruising and the symptoms of anemia. Judicious use of red cell transfusions and appropriate antibiotics is essential. Some patients will require platelet transfusions. Those patients expected to live for a considerable time on red cell transfusion will need to consider iron chelation therapy with desferrioxamine.

Some authorities recommend the use of hemopoietic growth factors. Both granulocyte colony stimulating factor (G-CSF) and GM-CSF raise the neutrophil count, but neither has been shown to improve survival in MDS.[89] In patients with a low transfusion requirement and a serum eythropoietin level lower than 200 μg/l, recombinant eythropoietin therapy will raise the hemoglobin in between 30 and 50% of patients with RA or RAEB.[90] In RARS the addition of G-CSF to the eythropoietin is synergistic and necessary to raise the hemoglobin.[91]

Low-dose chemotherapy with cytarabine produces responses in 16% of patients,[92] but cytopenias are often prolonged and this treatment has fallen out of favor. Other agents being used in low doses experimentally include 5-azacytidine,[93] aclarubicin,[94] melphalan[95,96] and decitabine.[97] There is no clear evidence that any of these is better than cytarabine, although melphalan has the advantage of being an oral drug.

High-dose chemotherapy has a dismal record. Over 80% of patients are > 60 years of age and many are too frail to withstand the side-effects of this form of therapy. Many trials have reported complete response rates of over 50% of those patients treated, but these responses seldom last longer than a year, and there are very few long-term survivors.[98]

Some patients are cured by bone marrow allograft. Unfortunately, only about 3% of MDS patients are suitable for this extreme form of therapy (personal communication – Jeanne E Anderson). Non-myelo-ablative transplant is currently being investigated as a potential treatment for MDS patients up to the age of 70 years.[99]

Other experimental treatments include immuno-suppression with either anti-thymocyte globulin[100] or cyclosporin,[101] thalidomide,[102] which is believed to exert its effect via the bone marrow stroma, and farnesyl transferase inhibitors,[102] which exert their effect by interfering with the *ras* signaling pathway. Finally, newer approaches to ablative therapy include the use of radiolabeled monoclonal antibodies.[103]

REFERENCES

1. Bennett JM, Catovsky D, Daniel MT et al 1992 Proposals for the classification of the myelodysplastic syndrome. British Journal of Haematology 51: 189–199
2. Cartwright RA, Alexander FE, McKinney PA, Ricketts TJ 1990 Leukaemia and Lymphoma: An atlas of distribution within areas of England and Wales 1984–1988. LRF, London.
3. Williamson PJ, Kruger A, Reynolds PJ et al 1994 Establishing the incidence of myelodysplastic syndromes. British Journal of Haematology 87: 743–745
4. Aul C, Gattermann M, Schneider W et al 1992 Age related incidence and other epidemiological aspects of myelodysplastic syndromes. British Journal of Haematology 82: 358–367
5. Mufti GJ, Stevens J, Oscier DG et al 1985 Myelodysplastic syndromes: a scoring system with prognostic importance. British Journal of Haematology 59: 425–433
6. Sanz GF, Sanz MA, Vallespi T et al 1989 Two regression models and a scoring system for predicting survival and planning treatment in myelodysplastic syndrome: a multivariate analysis of prognostic factors in 370 patients. Blood 74: 395–408
7. Goasguen JE, Gerand R Bizet M et al 1990 Prognostic factors of myelodysplastic syndromes – a simplified 3D scoring system. Leukemia Research 14: 255–262
8. Mora E, Lazzarino M Castello A et al 1990 Risk assessment in myelodysplastic syndromes: value of clinical, haematological and bone marrow histologic findings at presentation. European Journal of Haematology 45: 94–100
9. Aul C, Gattermann N, Heyll A et al 1992 Primary myelodysplastic syndromes: analysis of prognostic factors in 235 patients and proposals for an improved scoring system. Leukemia 6: 52–59
10. Greenberg P, Cox C, LeBeau M M et al 1997 International scoring system for evaluating prognosis in myelodysplastic syndromes. Blood 89: 2079–2088
11. Estey E, Keating M, Pierce S et al 1997 Application for international scoring system for myelodysplasia to MD Anderson patients. Blood 90: 2843–2846
12. Harris NL, Jaffe ES, Diebold J et al 1999 WHO classification of neoplastic diseases of the hematopoietic and lymphoid tissues: Report of the clinical advisory committee meeting – Airlie House, Virginia, November 1997. Journal of Clinical Oncology 17: 3835–3849
13. Germing U, Gattermann N, Aivado M et al 2000 Two types of acquired idiopathic sideroblastic anaemia (AISA): a time-tested distinction. British Journal of Haematology 108: 724–728
14. Greenberg P, Anderson J, de Witte T et al 2000 Problematic WHO reclassification of myelodysplastic syndromes. Members of the International MDS Study Group. Journal of Clinical Oncology 18: 3447–3452
15. Germing U, Gattermann N, Strupp C et al 2000 Validation of the WHO proposals for a new classification of primary myelodysplastic syndromes: a retrospective analysis of 1600 patients. Leukemia Research 24: 983–992
16. Goasguen JE, Bennett JM, Cox C et al 1991 Prognostic implication and characterization of the blast cell population in the myelodysplastic syndrome. Leukemia Research 15: 1159–1165
17. Tricot G, de Wolf Peeters C, Hendrickx B, Verwilghen RL 1984 Bone marrow histology in myelodysplastic syndromes. British Journal of Haematology 56: 423–430
18. Delacrétaz F, Schmidt P-M, Piguet D et al 1987 Histopathology of myelodysplastic syndromes: the FAB classification. American Journal of Clinical Pathology 87: 180–186
19. Bartl R, Frisch B, Baumgart R 1992 Morphologic classification of the myelodysplastic syndromes (MDS): combined utilization of bone marrow aspirates and trephine biopsies. Leukemia Research 16: 15–33
20. Maschek H, Georgii A, Kaloutsi V et al 1992 Myelofibrosis in primary myelodysplastic syndromes: a retrospective study of 352 patients. European Journal of Haematology, 48: 208–214
21. Rios A, Cañizo C, Sanz MA et al 1990 Bone marrow biopsy in myelodysplastic syndromes: morphological characteristics and contribution to the study of prognostic factors. British Journal of Haematology 75: 26–33
22. Maschek H, Gutzmer R, Choritz H, Georgii A 1994 Life expectancy in primary myelodysplastic syndromes: a prognostic score based upon histopathology from bone marrow biopsies of 569 patients. European Journal of Haematology 53: 280–287
23. Wilkins BS 1992 Occasional Article: The histology of normal haemopoiesis. Journal of Clinical Pathology 245: 645–649
24. Wilkins BS, Jones DB 1992 Cell-stroma interactions in monocytopoiesis. FEMS Microbiology and Immunology 105: 347–354
25. Tricot G, de Wolf-Peeters C, Vlietnck R, Verwilghen RL 1984 Bone marrow histology in the myelodysplastic syndromes II. Prognostic value of abnormal localization of immature precursors in MDS. British Journal of Haematology 58: 217–225
26. Fox SB, Lorenzen J, Heryet A et al 1990 Megakaryocytes in myelodysplasia: an immunohistochemical study on bone marrow trephines. Histopathology, 17: 69–74
27. Thiele J, Fischer R 1991 Megakaryocytopoiesis in haematological disorders: diagnostic feature of bone marrow biopsies. Virchows Archives (A), 418: 87–97
28. Thiele J, Quitmann H, Wagner S, Fischer R 1991 Dysmegakaryopoiesis in myelodysplastic syndromes (MDS): an immunomorphometric study of bone marrow trephine biopsy specimens. Journal of Clinical Pathology 44: 300–305
29. Wong K, Chan JKC 1991 Are 'dysplastic' and hypogranular megakaryocytes specific markers for myelodysplastic syndrome? British Journal of Haematology 77: 509–514
30. Clark DM, Lampert IA 1990 Apoptosis is a common histopathological finding in myelodysplasia: the correlate of ineffective haematopoiesis. Leukemia and Lymphoma 2: 415–418
31. Thiele J, Zirbes TK, Wiemers P et al 1997 Incidence of apoptosis in HIV-myelopathy, myelodysplastic syndromes and non-specific inflammatory lesions of the bone marrow. Histopathology 30: 307–311
32. Yoshida Y, Oguma S, Uchjino H, Maekawa T 1988 Refractory myelodysplastic syndromes with hypocellular bone marrow. Journal of Clinical Pathology 41: 763–767

33. Orazi A, Albitar M, Heerema NA et al 1997 Hypoplastic myelodysplastic syndromes can be distinguished from acquired aplastic anemia by CD34 and PCNA immunostaining of bone marrow biopsy specimens. American Journal of Clinical Pathology 107: 268–274

34. Thiele J, Zirbes TK, Bertsch HP et al 1996 AIDS-related bone marrow lesions – myelodysplastic features or predominant inflammatory-reactive changes (HIV myelopathy)? A comparative morphometric study by immunohistochemistry with special emphasis on apoptosis and PCNA-labelling. Annals of Cell Pathology 11: 141–157

35. Wilkins BS, Bostanci AG, Ryan MF, Jones DB 1993 Haemopoietic regrowth after chemotherapy: an immunohistochemical study of bone marrow trephine biopsy specimens. Journal of Clinical Pathology 46: 915–921

36. Mangi MH, Mufti GJ 1992 Primary myelodysplastic syndromes: diagnostic and prognostic significance of immunohistochemical assessment of bone marrow biopsies. Blood 79: 98–205

37. Soligo DA, Oriani A, Annaloro C et al 1994 CD34 immunohistochemistry of bone marrow biopsies: prognostic significance in primary myelodysplastic syndromes. American Journal of Hematology 46: 9–17

38. Horny H-P, Wehrmann M, Schlicker HUH et al 1995 QBENDIO for the diagnosis of myelodysplastic syndromes in routinely processed bone marrow biopsy specimens. Journal of Clinical Pathology 48: 291–294

39. Green AJ, Wilkins BS, Ross F et al 1997 Fluorescence in situ hybridisation in fixed, decalcified bone marrow trephine biopsies. Journal of Pathology 182 (suppl): 4A.

40. Thiele J, Schmitz B, Fuchs R et al 1998 Detection of the bcr/abl gene in bone marrow macrophages in CML and alterations during interferon therapy – a fluorescence *in situ* hybridization study on trephine biopsies. Journal of Pathology 186: 331–335

41. Mufti GJ 1992 Chromosomal deletions in the myelodysplastic syndrome. Leukemia Research 16: 35–41

42. Morel P, Hebbar M, Lai J-L et al 1993 Cytogenetic analysis has strong independent prognostic value in *de novo* myelodysplastic syndromes and can be incorporated in a new scoring system: a report on 408 cases. Leukemia 7: 1315–1323

43. Kantarjian HM, Keating MJ, Walters RS et al 1986 Therapy-related leukemia and myelodysplastic syndrome: clinical, cytogenetic, and prognostic features. Journal of Clinical Oncology 4: 1748–1757

44. Levine EG, Bloomfield CD 1992 Leukemias and myelodysplastic syndromes secondary to drug, radiation, and environmental exposure. Seminars in Oncology 19: 47–84

45. Lessard M, Herry A, Berthou C et al 1998 FISH investigation of 5q and 7q deletions in MDS/AML reveals hidden translocations, insertions and fragmentations of the same chromosomes. Leukemia Research 22: 303–312

46. Van den Berghe H, Cassiman JJ, David G et al 1974 Distinct haematological disorder with deletion of long arm of No. 5 chromosome. Nature 251: 437–438

47. Van den Berghe H, Michaux L 1997 5q-, twenty-five years later: a synopsis. Cancer Genetics and Cytogenetics 94: 1–7

48. Lai JL, Zandecki M, Fenaux P et al 1990 Translocations (5;17) and (7;17) in patients with *de novo* or therapy-related myelodysplastic syndromes or acute nonlymphocytic leukemia. A possible association with acquired pseudo-Pelger–Huet anomaly and small vacuolated granulocytes. Cancer Genetics and Cytogenetics 46: 173–183

49. Jary L, Mossafa H, Fourcade C et al 1997 The 17p-syndrome: a distinct myelodysplastic syndrome entity? Leukemia and Lymphoma 25: 163–168

50. Ohyashiki K, Ohyashiki JH, Hojo H et al 1990 Cytogenetic findings in adult acute leukemia and myeloproliferative disorders with an involvement of megakaryocyte lineage. Cancer 65: 940–948

51. Berkowicz M, Rosner E, Rechavi G et al 1991 Atypical chronic myelomonocytic leukemia with eosinophilia and translocation (5;12). A new association. Cancer Genetics and Cytogenetics 51: 277–278

52. Ohyashiki JH, Ohyashiki K, Shimamoto T et al 1995 Ecotropic virus integration site-1 gene preferentially expressed in post-myelodysplasia acute myeloid leukemia: possible association with GATA-1, GATA-2, and stem cell leukemia gene expression. Blood 85: 3713–3718

53. Srivastava A, Boswell HS, Heerema NA et al 1988 K-ras2 oncogene overexpression in myelodysplastic syndrome with translocation 5;12. Cancer Genetics and Cytogenetics 35: 61–71

54. Lyons J, Janssen JW, Bartram C et al 1988 Mutation of Ki-ras and N-ras oncogenes in myelodysplastic syndromes. Blood 71: 1707–1712

55. Padua RA, Carter G, Hughes D 1988 RAS mutations in myelodysplasia detected by amplification, oligonucleotide hybridization, and transformation. Leukemia 2: 503–510

56. Ludwig L, Janssen JW, Schulz AS, Bartram CR 1993 Mutations within the FLR exon of NF1 are rare in myelodysplastic syndromes and acute myelocytic leukemias. Leukemia 7: 1058–1060

57. Quesnel B, Guillerm G, Vereecque R et al 1998 Methylation of the p15(INK4b) gene in myelodysplastic syndromes is frequent and acquired during disease progression. Blood 91: 2985–2990

58. Padua RA, Guinn BA, Al-Sabah AI et al 1998 RAS, FMS and p53 mutations and poor clinical outcome in myelodysplasias: a 10-year follow-up. Leukemia 12: 887–892

59. Broker S, Meunier B, Rich P et al 1998 MtDNA mutations associated with sideroblastic anaemia cause a defect of mitochondrial cytochrome c oxidase. European Journal of Biochemistrey 258: 132–138

60. Oscier DG 1987 Myelodysplastic syndromes. Ballière's Clinical Haematology 1: 389–426

61. Thomas X, Guyotat D, Campos L et al 1991 *In vitro* effects of recombinant hemopoietic growth factors on progenitor cells from patients with myelodysplastic syndromes. Leukemia Research 5: 29–36

62. McMullin MF, Buckley O, Magill MK Irvine AE 1998 Long-term bone marrow culture profiles in patients with myelodysplastic syndromes are not explicable by defective apoptosis. Leukemia Research 22: 735–740

63. Greenberg PL 1998 Apoptosis and its role in the myelodysplastic syndromes: implications for disease natural history and treatment. Leukemia Research 22: 1123–1136

64. Parker JE, Mufti GJ 2000 Excessive apoptosis in low risk myelodysplastic syndromes (MDS). Leukemia and Lymphoma 40: 1–24

65. Hamblin TJ 1996 Immunological abnormalities in myelodysplastic syndrome. Seminars in Hematology 33: 150–162

66. Hamblin TJ 1992 Immunological abnormalities in myelodysplastic syndromes. Hematology and Oncology Clinics of North America 6: 571–586

67. Hamblin TJ 1994 Immunological abnormalities in myelodysplastic syndromes. In: Galton DAG, Mufti GJ (eds), The myelodysplastic syndromes. Churchill Livingstone, Edinburgh, 97–114

68. Hamblin TJ 2002 Immunology of myelodysplastic syndromes. In: Bennett JMB (ed), Myelodysplastic symdromes: pathobiology and treatment. Marcel Dekker, New York, in press

69. Jacobs A 1985 Myelodysplastic syndromes: pathogenesis, functional abnormalities, and clinical implications. Journal of Clinical Pathology 38: 1201–1217

70. Wimazal F, Sperr WR, Kundi M et al 2001 Prognostic value of lactate dehydrogenase activity in myelodysplastic syndromes. Leukemia Research 25: 287–294

71. May SJ, Smith SA, Jacobs A et al 1985 The myelodysplastic syndrome: analysis of laboratory characteristics in relation to the FAB classification. British Journal of Haematology 59: 311–319

72. Newman DR, Pierre RV, Linman JW 1973 Studies in the diagnostic significance of haemoglobin F levels. Mayo Clinic Proceedings 48: 199–202

73. Hauptman GM, Sondag D, Lang JM, Oberling F 1978 False positive acidified serum lysis test in a preleukaemic dyserythropoiesis. Acta Haematologica 59: 73–79

74. Lintula R 1986 Red cell enzymes in myelodysplastic syndromes: a review. Scandinavian Journal of Haematology 36 (suppl 45): 56–59

75. Mufti GJ, Figes AN, Hamblin TJ et al 1986 Immunological abnormalities in myelodysplastic syndromes. I serum immunoglobulins and autoantibodies. British Journal of Haematology 63: 143–147

76. Solal-Celigny P, Desaint B, Herrera A et al 1984 Chronic myelomoncytic leukaemia according to the FAB classification analysis of 35 cases. Blood 63: 634–638

77. Ruutu T 1986 Granulocyte function in the myelodysplastic syndromes. Scandinavian Journal of Haematology 36 (suppl 45): 66–70

78. Bendix-Hansen K, Bergmann OJ 1985 Evaluation of neutrophil alkaline phosphatase (NAP) activity in untreated myeloproliferative syndromes and in leukaemoid reactions. Scandinavian Journal of Haematology 35: 219–224

79. Rasi V, Lintula R 1986 Platelet function in the myelodysplastic syndromes. Scandinavian Journal of Haematology 36 (suppl 45): 71–73

80. Kitigawa M, Saito I, Yoshida S 1997 Overexpression of tumor necrosis factor alpha and interferon gamma by bone marrow cells from patients with myelodysplastic syndromes. Leukemia 11: 2049–2056

81. Shetty V, Mundle S, Alvi S et al 1996 Measurement of apoptosis proliferation and three cytokines in 46 patients with myelodysplastic syndromes. Leukemia Research 20: 891–900

82. Verhoef GEG, DeScouwer P, Ceuppens JL et al 1992 Measurement of serum cytokine levels in patients with myelodysplastic syndromes. Leukemia 6: 1268–1272

83. Menconboni M, Castello G, Lerza R et al 1996 Production of tumor necrosis factor and granulocyte colony stimulating factor by bone marrow accessory cells in myelodysplastic patients. European Journal of Haematology 56: 148–152

84. Rigolin GM, Howard J, Buggins A et al 1999 Phenotypic and functional characteristics of monocyte derived dendritic cells from patients with myelodysplastic syndromes. British Journal of Haematology 107: 844–850

85. Kyriakou D, Liapi D, Kyriakou E et al 2000 Aberrant expression of the major sialoglycoprotein (CD43) on the monocytes of patients with myelodysplastic syndromes. Annals of Hematology 79: 198–205

86. Davies SM, Robison LL, Buckley JD et al 2000 Glutathione S-transferase polymorphisms in children with myeloid leukemia: a Children's Cancer Group study. Cancer Epidemiology Biomarkers and Prevention 9: 563–566

87. Chen H, Sandler DP, Taylor JA et al 1996 Increased risk for myelodysplastic syndrome in individuals with glutathione transferase theta (*GSTT1*) gene defect. Lancet 347: 295–297

88. Shpilberg O, Dorman JS, Shahar A Kuller LH 1997 Molecular epidemiology of hematological neoplasms – present status and future directions. Leukemia Research 21: 265–284

89. Seipelt G, Ottmann OG, Hoelzer D 2000 Cytokine therapy for the myelodysplastic syndrome. Current Opinion in Hematology 7: 156–160

90. Kurzrock R, Talpaz M, Estey E et al 1991 Erythropoietin treatment in patients with myelodysplastic syndromes and anemia. Leukemia 5: 985–990

91. Hellstrom-Lindberg E, Negrin R, Stein R et al 1997 Erythroid response to treatment with G-CSF plus erythropoietin for the anaemia of patients with myelodysplastic syndrome: proposal for a predictive model. British Journal of Haematology 99: 344–351

92. Cheson BD 1998 Standard and low-dose chemotherapy for the treatment of myelodysplastic syndromes. Leukemia Research 22 (suppl 1): S17–21

93. Chitambar CR, Libnoch JA, Matthaeus WG et al 1991 Evaluation of continuous infusion low-dose 5-azacytidine in the treatment of myelodysplastic syndromes. American Journal of Hematology 37: 100–104

94. Shibuya T, Teshima T, Harada M et al 1990 Treatment of myelodysplastic syndrome and atypical leukemia with low-dose aclarubicin. Leukemia Research 14: 161–167

95. Omoto E, Deguchi S, Takaba S et al 1996 Low-dose melphalan for treatment of high-risk myelodysplastic syndromes. Leukemia 10: 609–614

96. Denzlinger C, Bowen D, Benz D et al 2000 Low-dose melphalan induces favourable responses in elderly patients with high-risk myelodysplastic syndromes or secondary acute myeloid leukaemia. British Journal of Haematology 108: 93–95

97. Pinto A, Zagonel V 1993 5-Aza-2'-deoxycytidine (Decitabine) and 5-azacytidine in the treatment of acute myeloid leukemias and myelodysplastic syndromes: past, present and future trends. Leukemia 7 (suppl 1): 51–60

98. Hamblin TJ 1992 Intensive chemotherapy in myelodysplastic syndromes. Blood Reviews 6: 215–219

99. Giralt S, Khouri I, Champlin R 1999 Non myeloablative 'mini transplants'. Cancer Treatment and Research 101: 97–108

100. Molldrem JJ, Jiang YZ, Stetler-Stevenson M et al 1998 Haematological response of patients with myelodysplastic syndrome to antithymocyte globulin is associated with a loss of lymphocyte-mediated inhibition of CFU-GM and alterations in T-cell receptor Vbeta profiles. British Journal of Haematology 102: 1314–1322

101. Jonasova A, Neuwirtova R, Cermak J et al 1998 Cyclosporin A therapy in hypoplastic MDS patients and certain refractory anaemias without hypoplastic bone marrow. British Journal of Haematology 100: 304–309

102. Cheson BD, Zwiebel JA, Dancey J Murgo A 2000 Novel therapeutic agents for the treatment of myelodysplastic syndromes. Seminars in Oncology 27: 560–577

103. Bunjes D, Buchmann I, Duncker C et al 2001 Rhenium 188-labeled anti-CD66 (a, b, c, e) monoclonal antibody to intensify the conditioning regimen prior to stem cell transplantation for patients with high-risk acute myeloid leukemia or myelodysplastic syndrome: results of a phase I-II study. Blood 98: 565–572

Acute leukemias

20

DM Swirsky   SJ Richards   PAS Evans

Introduction

Classification systems

Acute lymphoblastic leukemia

Clinical presentation

Classification

Cytology, cytochemistry and histopathology

Immunophenotypic diagnosis of ALL

Precursor B-cell ALL

Precursor T-cell ALL

Detection of residual disease in ALL
Cytogenetic abnormalities in ALL

Molecular genetics and disease monitoring in ALL

Residual disease monitoring in ALL

Acute myeloid leukemia

Blast cell morphology in AML

Cytochemical reactions in AML

AML with recurrent translocations
AML with t(8;21)
AML with t(15;17)
AML with inv(16) and t(16;16)
AML with t(v;11)(v;q23)

AML with multilineage dysplasia

AML therapy related

AML not otherwise categorized
Acute myeloblastic leukemia minimally differentiated (FAB M0)

Acute myeloblastic leukemia with maturation (FAB M1)
Acute myeloblastic leukemia with maturation (FAB M2)
Acute myelomonocytic leukemia (FAB M4)
Acute monocytic leukemia (FAB M5A and M5B)
Acute erythroid leukemia (FAB M6)
Acute megakaryocytic leukemia (FAB M7)
Acute basophilic leukemia
Acute panmyelosis with marrow fibrosis

Hypocellular forms of AML

Extramedullary AML (chloromas, granulocytic sarcomas)

CNS leukemia in AML

Immunophenotypic diagnosis of AML
Poorly differentiated AML
AML with evidence of maturation (AML-M2)
Acute promyelocytic leukemia (AML-M3)
Acute myelomonocytic leukemia (AML-M4)
Acute monocytic leukemia (AML-M5)
Acute myeloid leukemia M6 and M7

Detection of residual disease

Cytogenetics in AML

Molecular diagnosis in AML

Residual disease monitoring in AML

Acute biphenotypic leukemia

Introduction

The acute leukemias are divided broadly into two major categories, acute lymphoblastic leukemia (ALL) and acute myeloid leukemia (AML). Biphenotypic acute leukemias have features of both major types, and the acute leukemias of infancy have specific features. The acute leukemias are clonal malignant diseases of early hemopoietic progenitor cells. The lymphoblastic forms are characterized by homogeneous blast cell populations and both diagnosis and classification are based on the blast cell immunophenotype and cytogenetics. In the myeloid forms, which always have some increase in myeloid blasts, considerable maturation of multiple myeloid lineage cell types may be present. Diagnosis and classification are based on morphology and cytochemistry as well as the blast cell immunophenotype and cytogenetic abnormalities. The recently proposed World Health Organization (WHO) classification also takes account of chromosomal abnormalities of known prognostic significance and preceding events such as myelodysplasia or chemo/radiotherapy. The accurate diagnosis and classification of the acute leukemias requires multiple diagnostic techniques; microscopy (morphology, cytochemistry and histology), immunophenotyping (flow cytometry and immunohistochemistry) and genetics (metaphase karyotyping, fluorescence *in situ* hybridization [FISH] and molecular genetics). All of these are complementary in arriving at an accurate and informative diagnosis. There are significant differences in the acute leukemias encountered at different ages. Approximately 80% of patients with AML are over the age of 15 years, whereas 85% of patients with ALL are under the age of 15 years. Both types of acute leukemia can occur at any age. Within each major type of acute leukemia there are significant biological differences at different ages. Diagnosis is primarily based on examination of blood and bone marrow, but the presenting pathology may involve lymph nodes, CSF, skin, testes and other soft tissues.

Classification systems

Since 1976 the French–American–British (FAB) classification of acute leukemias, and its subsequent revisions, has been generally accepted.[1–4] The FAB system is based almost entirely on morphologic and cytochemical criteria, and was conceived prior to the introduction of immunophenotyping, and before the impact of cytogenetic abnormalities on prognosis was known. In ALL the morphologic assessment of the disease has no useful role in classification, which is entirely based on immunophenotyping and

cytogenetic abnormalities, and in which the leukemic blast population is generally homogeneous. Acute myeloid leukemia is different; morphologic assessment remains important as multiple myeloid lineages may be involved, maturation of leukemic cells is common and dysplastic changes may be present. Morphologic and cytochemical assessment remain central to diagnosis. Undifferentiated AML requires immunophenotypic diagnosis. AML may be secondary to a preceding myelodysplastic syndrome, myeloproliferative disorder or chemo/radiotherapy. There are important prognostic subgroups defined by cytogenetic abnormalities.

Recently, a Clinical Advisory Committee of the WHO has outlined a new classification of neoplastic diseases of the hematopoietic system including acute leukemia which draws together morphologic, immunophenotypic, cytogenetic and clinical features in a classification system that reflects relevant biological and clinical disease entities.[5,6]

Acute lymphoblastic leukemia

Clinical presentation

Symptoms may be of abrupt onset, or more insidiously occurring over a period of weeks or even months. Patients usually present with the clinical signs of marrow failure, namely tiredness and pallor (anemia), infections (neutropenia) and purpura, bruising or gum bleeding (thrombocytopenia). Fever may be present, and half of children with the disease have bony pain. Less commonly, lymphadenopathy, the signs associated with a mediastinal mass or CNS disease may be the presenting features. Rarely, testicular or other soft-tissue disease may be the first sign of the disease. Minor hepatosplenomegaly is common. Approximately 25% of patients have a leukocyte count of $< 5 \times 10^9/l$, 50% between 5 and $50 \times 10^9/l$, and 25% $> 50 \times 10^9/l$. Leukocyte counts $> 500 \times 10^9/l$ are occasionally seen. At the time of diagnosis the marrow is usually hypercellular, with replacement of normal hemopoiesis by the blast cells. Rare patients present with marrow hypoplasia, before developing a typical leukemic picture.[7,8] Such patients may improve spontaneously or respond transiently to aplasia-directed immunosuppressive treatment before the leukemia becomes apparent. Patients with T-lineage ALL may present with signs associated with a mediastinal mass. The marrow is usually heavily infiltrated and the circulating circulating blast cell count may be high ($> 100 \times 10^9/l$). Occasionally, patients may have minimal or absent bone marrow disease. The WHO system recognizes 'T-lymphoblastic lymphoma' of the mediastinum and T-lineage ALL as a single biological entity with different clinical presentations.

Classification

The FAB classification of acute lymphoblastic leukemia is based on morphology alone and recognizes three types of cell, namely: small homogeneous blasts with round nuclei and scanty cytoplasm (L1); larger blasts with irregular nuclei, prominent nucleoli and more abundant cytoplasm (L2); and basophilic cells with prominent cytoplasmic vacuoles (L3). The L3 type include the majority of cases previously termed B-ALL (now excluded in the WHO classification), which express surface-membrane immunoglobulin (SMIg), but also includes other types of ALL, particularly those with t(1;19).[9]

The WHO classification largely adopts the 1994 REAL (Revised European–American classification of Lymphoid Neoplasms) classification of lymphoid neoplasms.[10] The principle underlying the WHO classification (for both lymphoid and myeloid neoplasms) is that distinct disease entities of clinical utility should be recognized. This requires the integration of relevant information previously excluded from classification systems. The factors contributing to diagnostic entities variously include morphology, immunophenotype, genetics and clinical features, depending on the specific disease. Thus for ALL the WHO classification recognizes precursor T- and B-cell neoplasms corresponding to acute lymphoblastic leukemia, but excludes cases with the t(8;14)(q24;q32), (and the rarer variants with t(2;8)(p12;q24) and t(8;22)(q24;q11)), which are classed as mature B-cell neoplasms, having undergone immunoglobulin gene rearrangement and expressing surface immunoglobulin. They correspond to the cells of Burkitt's lymphoma, which in the WHO system is classified with the mature B-cell neoplasms. Cases which present with peripheral blood involvement are termed Burkitt cell leukemia.

Precursor B-cell neoplasms are further subdivided by the presence or absence of specific recurring cytogenetic abnormalities, namely: t(9;22)(q34;q11); t(1;19)(q23;p13); t(12;21)(p12;q22); and t(various;11q23). However, it seems likely that B-lineage ALL will continue to be subdivided into pre-pre-B, Common, and pre-B types, based on the expression of CD10 and cytoplasmic μ chain. Similarly T-lineage ALL will continue to be subdivided into pre-T and T-ALL on the basis of cytoplasmic or membrane CD3 expression (see below).

Cytology, cytochemistry and histopathology

The morphology of lymphoid blasts on well-prepared Romanowsky-stained smears of blood or marrow is variable (Fig. 20.1). The FAB system recognizes three types of blast cell, designated L1, L2 and L3.[1] In L1 cases (the majority) the blasts are small or medium-sized with round nuclei and fine but densely packed homogeneous chromatin. Nucleoli are small and usually single or absent. Cytoplasm is scanty and weakly basophilic. Cytoplasmic vacuoles may be present. L2 blasts are larger, with irregular nuclei showing clefting or indentation. Nucleoli are more prominent, often large and occasionally multiple. Cytoplasm is relatively abundant and may be finely reticulated. Basophilia is variable. Scanty azurophil granules are rarely present in both L1 and L2 blasts. L3 blasts are medium/large cells with round or slightly irregular nuclei and coarse chromatin. Nucleoli are usually prominent but single. Moderate amounts of deeply basophilic cytoplasm are present and the majority of cases show prominent cytoplasmic vacuolation. Mitoses may be frequent. Rarely, ALL may present with an associated hypereosinophilia.[11] The hypereosinophilia may precede the diagnosis of ALL and there is a possible association with the translocation t(5;14)(q31.1;q32.3).[12,13]

There are no positive diagnostic cytochemical stains that distinguish ALL. Lymphoblasts are negative when stained for myeloperoxidase. Very rarely, coarse granular or globular positivity with Sudan Black B may be present.[14,15] T-lineage ALL frequently shows localized or polar staining with acid phosphatase, but these appear-

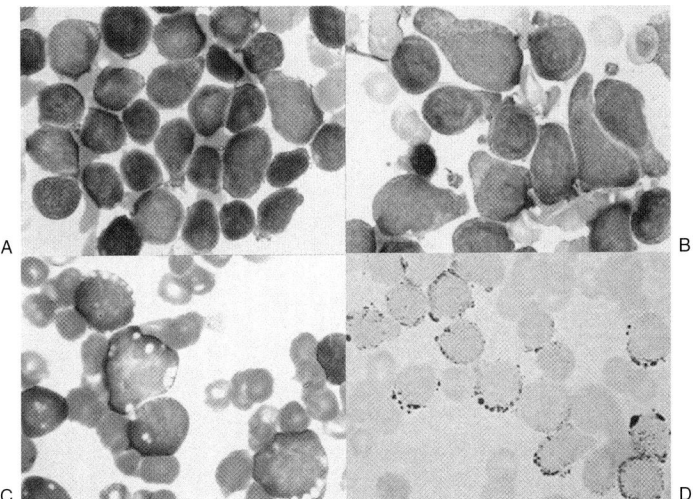

Fig. 20.1 (A–C) May–Grünwald–Giemsa stain showing lymphoblasts with variable morphology. (D) Periodic acid-Schiff reaction showing typical blocks and granules on a clear cytoplasmic background.

ances are not specific.[16] Esterase stains are largely unhelpful.[17] The periodic acid–Schiff (PAS) reaction is useful in identifying lymphoblasts, which usually show fine granules or blocks of positivity (Fig. 20.1). These are found in up to 95% of cases, although they may be very rare, occurring in less than 1% of blasts. The distinctive feature of positivity in lymphoblasts is the absence of any diffuse cytoplasmic staining, which is invariably present in myeloid lineage cells (discussed below). Lymphoblasts show a glass-clear cytoplasm in which positive granules and blocks are sharply defined. Neutrophils stain strongly and serve as an internal control for the quality of the PAS stain.[17]

The marrow trephine biopsy usually shows maximal hypercellularity due to diffuse replacement by blast cells. The lymphoblast population is usually homogeneous. In the majority of cases the cells are small with scanty cytoplasm. Nuclei show finely stippled chromatin, often with peripheral condensation. Nucleoli are small and seldom multiple. A minority of cases (10–15%), corresponding to the L2 type morphologically, show larger cells with irregular nuclei and increased cytoplasm. T-lineage ALL may show some degree of nuclear irregularity, and the nuclei may be small and hyperchromatic.[18] Varying degrees of reticulin fibrosis (reversible on successful treatment) may be present in approximately half the cases.[19] This is of no clinical consequence, but may be severe enough to make the marrow inaspirable. It may be commoner in B-lineage than T-lineage ALL.[20] Areas of marrow necrosis, usually patchy, but occasionally

extensive, may be present, and can delay diagnosis if no circulating blasts are present.[21] Cases presenting as aplastic anemia may show a degree of reticulin fibrosis not generally seen in true aplasia, and are usually of common-ALL phenotype (Fig. 20.2).[7,8]

At both presentation or relapse almost any organ system can be infiltrated by leukemia. The CNS (Fig. 20.2), and in boys, the testis (Fig. 20.3), are favored sites of relapse (sanctuary sites). Blast cells may be clustered if involvement is limited. Diagnosis is by immunohistochemistry. The hemopoietic nature of the cells is best

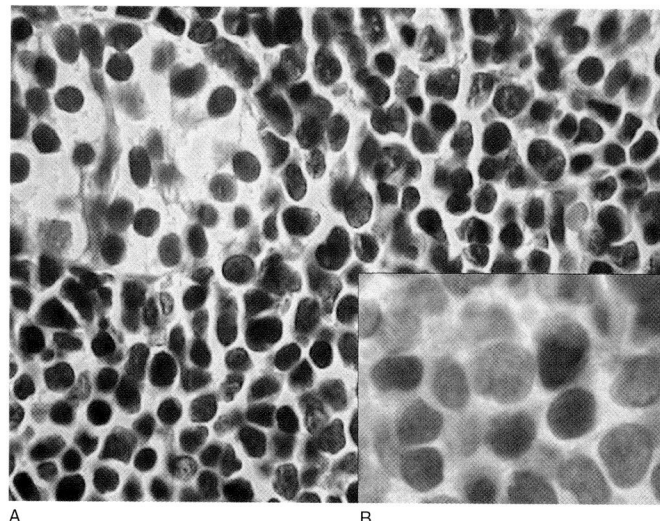

Fig. 20.3 (A) Hematoxylin and eosin stain. Testis invaded by common ALL. Blast cells are homogeneous. A seminifierous tubule is at top left. (B) TdT-positive blasts.

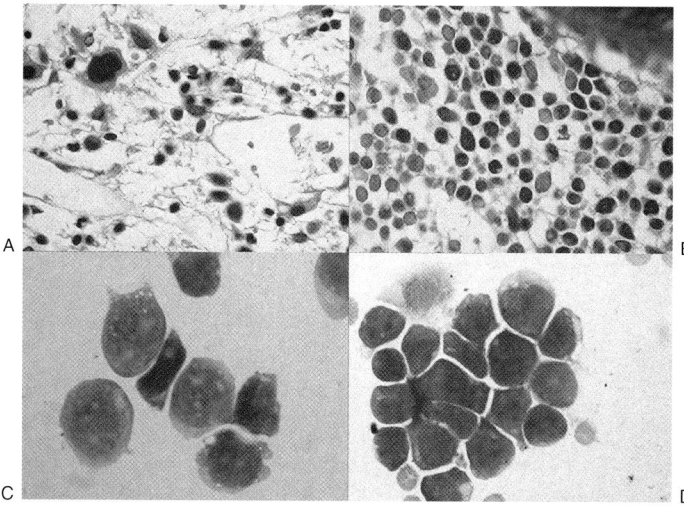

Fig. 20.2 (A) Hematoxylin and eosin stain. Marrow biopsy from a 14-year-old girl with pancytopenia showing hypocellularity, stromal edema and mild fibrosis. (B) Same patient 11 weeks later showing marrow replacement by common ALL. (C) CSF cytospin from a patient with CNS relapse of T-ALL. (D) Cytospin of vitreous fluid showing lymphoblasts from a child with ALL and a deposit involving the iris.

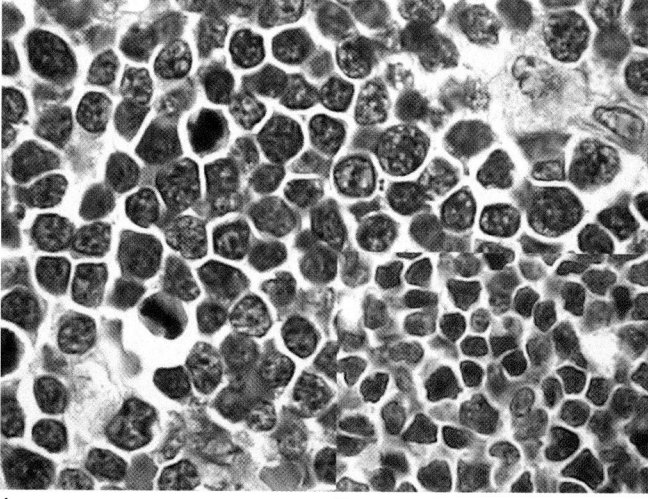

Fig. 20.4 T-cell acute lymphoblastic leukemia. (A) Hematoxylin and eosin stain. Mediastinal lymph node from an 8-year-old girl replaced by large blasts with vesicular chromatin and prominent nucleoli. Mitotic figures are present. (B) TdT-positive blasts. Immunophenotype cCD3[+], CD1a[+], CD5[+],CD4[−], CD8[+], CD38[+] CD45[+], TdT[+].

Table 20.1 Immunophenotypic features of acute lymphoblastic leukemia

Type of leukemia	Antigen expression													
	CD 45	CD 19[a]	CD 34	CD 10	TdT	CD 20	CD 22[b]	CD 79	clgM	cCD 3	CD 1a	CD 7	CD 4[c]	CD 8
Pre-pre-B	+	+	+	–	+	–	+	–	–	–	–	–	–	–
Common	(+)/–	+	+/(–)	+	+	–	+	–	–	–	–	–	–	–
Pre-B	(+)/–	+	+/(–)	+	+	–	+	–	+	–	–	–	–	–
Burkitt	+	+	–	+	–	+	+	+	+	–	–	–	–	–
Pre-T	+	–	+	(+)	+	–	–	–	–	+	–	+	(+)	(+)
T	+	–	–	–	+	–	–	–	–	+	+	+	(+)	(+)

[a] Unreactive in fixed tissues.
[b] Unreliable in fixed tissues.
[c] Unreliable on resin sections.

demonstrated by the presence of CD45 (leukocyte common antigen), although 25% of B-lineage ALL may be negative, and the correct diagnosis and lineage (T or B) established by immunostaining with a panel of antibodies directed against TdT, CD1a, CD3, CD4, CD7, CD8, CD10, CD19, CD20, CD22, CD34, CD79α and cytoplasmic IgM (Table 20.1). A particular problem is the diagnosis of T-ALL from fine-needle aspirates of a mediastinal mass, where normal T-cell precursors may be present in thymomas.

Immunophenotypic diagnosis of ALL

Immunophenotyping of blast cells by flow cytometry in suspected cases of ALL is an essential component of multiparameter approach to diagnosis. In the majority of cases of ALL, it is immunophenotyping that provides the objective information for definitive diagnosis. Comprehensive multicolor flow cytometry studies at presentation are essential for accurate diagnosis and detection of aberrant phenotypes which can be used for monitoring responses to therapy and detecting residual disease at the end of treatment episodes.

The ability to detect intracellular antigens by flow cytometry has considerably improved the diagnostic accuracy of immunophenotyping.[22] Nuclear terminal deoxynucleotidyl transferase (TdT), cytoplasmic CD79α (B-lineage), CD3 (T-lineage) and myeloperoxidase (myeloid lineage) are reliably detectable.[23] Simultaneous assessment of the three cytoplasmic antigens by multicolor flow cytometry together with membrane markers such as CD34 or CD45 to identify the blast cells, is a powerful technique which virtually eliminates the possibility of a misdiagnosis. In the rare instances where coexpression of two of these lineage specific cytoplasmic antigens occurs, a diagnosis of biphenotypic leukemia can be made, though this needs to be taken in the context of the membrane immunophenotype.

Precursor B-cell ALL

Diagnosis of B-lineage ALL requires demonstration of expression of B-lineage associated antigens expressed either in the cytoplasm (CD79α or IgM) or on the surface membrane (CD19 or CD22). The precursor nature of the cells is established by expression of the nuclear enzyme TdT or the membrane markers CD10 and CD34. Failure to express the surface immunoglobulin light chains kappa or lambda, membrane CD79β or high levels of CD45 are also features of precursor B-cells. Subclassification of precursor B-ALL based on patterns of antigen expression is detailed in Table 20.1, and although these phenotypic diagnostic groups are distinct, the important differential diagnosis is between pre-pre (pro) B-ALL (CD10⁻) and the CD10⁺ (common/pre-B-ALL), as the former have a significantly poorer prognosis.[24] The aberrant expression of myeloid antigens in these disorders not only provides an opportunity for monitoring residual disease, but also can predict cases with prognostic cytogenetic abnormalities with a high degree of accuracy. Childhood precursor B-ALL with the t(12;21) shows a characteristic immunophenotype with high-intensity CD10 and HLA-DR expression, low CD45 and CD20, heterogeneous CD34 expression and increased levels of the myeloid antigens CD13 and CD33.[25] CD9 negativity is also frequently seen amongst this genotypic subgroup of ALL.[26] The t(12;21) is found in 25–30% of pediatric ALL cases and confers a good prognosis despite lack of hyperdiploidy. The presence of a t(1;19) found in approximately 5% of precursor B-ALL is associated with a pre-B phenotype of CD19⁺CD10⁺CD22⁺CD34⁻CD20⁺/⁻.[27,28] In ALL the presence of a t(4;11) or t(11;19), disrupting the MLL gene on 11q23 is associated with a poor prognosis, a pre-pre-B phenotype of CD19⁺CD10⁻ and coexpression of the myeloid antigens CD15 and CD65.[29] The monoclonal antibody 7.1 appears to identify cases with MLL gene rearrangements though its use in routine diagnosis is not widespread.[29] In a recently published study, a clear correlation has been established between the poor prognosis translation t(9;22) (or molecular BCR/ABL fusion) in *de novo* adult precursor B-ALL and a unique phenotype of homogeneous CD10 and CD34 expression together with low and heterogeneous expression of CD38 and aberrant CD13 expression.[30] The careful analysis of immunophenotype in ALL provides an effective prescreening process for requesting specific molecular or cytogenetic testing for the known prognostic translocations and provides information that can be used for immediate treatment stratification of patients.

Precursor T-cell ALL

Acute lymphoblastic leukemia of T-lineage is defined by expression of cytoplasmic or membrane CD3. The precursor nature of the cells is demonstrated by expression of TdT (Fig. 20.4) or the thymocyte marker CD1a. The expression of CD2, CD5, CD7, CD4 and CD8 can also be used to demonstrate a precursor cell phenotype as levels of expression differ between mature (post-thymic) T-cells and prethymic/thymic cells. The most frequent phenotype seen in T-cell ALL is thymic CD1a+ with CD7, CD2, CD5 and cytoplasmic or weak membrane CD3 positivity. There is frequent coexpression of CD4 and CD8. More primitive forms (pre-T) are CD1a−, CD7+, cCD3+ and negative for CD2, CD5, CD4 and CD8. This subtype can be CD34+, and show weak expression of CD10 and myeloid antigens.[31] These patients may show a poorer prognosis than the thymic types.[32] For pediatric cases expression of membrane T-cell receptor (TCR)γδ was associated with better event-free survival at 4 years than TCRαβ cases, though expression of these TCR molecules is not an independent prognostic marker.[33]

Detection of residual disease in ALL

Multicolor flow cytometry, can detect low levels of residual leukemic cells with an aberrant phenotype. These methods rely upon differentiating leukemic cells from a background of normal lymphoid cells based on aberrant or abnormal blast cell phenotypes identified at presentation.[34–37] These aberrant features include: (1) inappropriate absence, reduction or increase in antigen expression; (2) expression of antigens associated with a different lineage; (3) asynchronous antigen expression; and (4) abnormal light-scatter characteristics. A different approach that can be applied to all precursor B-cell ALL cases, relies on the detection of abnormalities in the normal B-cell differentiation pathway and has been shown to be effective in predicting relapse.[38] This method

can be applied to patients in whom there is no detailed presentation immunophenotype. Moreover, it can be applied systematically as it uses combinations of antibodies that delineate specific predictable stages of B-cell ontogeny.

Cytogenetic abnormalities in ALL

Cytogenetic abnormalities can be detected in up to 90% of cases of ALL. In large clinical trials a significant number of cases fail to yield metaphases, and a further large proportion yield only normal metaphases.[39] The significance of normal metaphases in acute leukemia is uncertain. There is good evidence that prognostically significant translocations (e.g. t(9;22)) can be present, identified by reverse transcription-polymerase chain reaction (RT-PCR) or FISH, where metaphase cytogenetics is normal.[40] One of the most important recurring abnormalities in childhood ALL is the t(12;21), which is only identifiable by molecular techniques. The diagnosis of ALL is incomplete if all these cytogenetic techniques are not routinely employed. Despite these difficulties, many of the abnormalities identified are of prognostic significance independent of other useful prognostic indicators which include age, leukocyte count and CNS disease at diagnosis.[41–47] There are significant differences between the incidence of specific abnormalities in children (hyperdiploidy common, t(9;22) rare) and adults (hyperdiploidy rare, t(9;22) common). The clinical significance of some recurring translocations or ploidy changes is controversial or neutral, but there is general agreement about others. The majority of prognostically important abnormalities are associated with B-lineage ALL. The t(9;22) in ALL carries a poor prognosis in both children and adults.[39,48] The t(4;11) carries a poor prognosis, particularly in infants, and overall all 11q23 abnormalities involving disruption of the MLL gene are adverse.[49] The t(1;19), initially thought to be adverse, is probably of neutral significance.[50,51] Ploidy changes are important, with hypodiploid and near-haploid karyotypes carrying an adverse prognosis.[41,43,52] Conversely, hyperdiploidy carries a favorable prognosis. The t(12;21), which is the commonest recurrent abnormality in childhood B-lineage disease, is a favorable finding.[53]

T-lineage ALL has fewer clinically significant chromosomal groups. The t(10;14) has been identified as a favorable finding in children. Cases with normal karyotypes fare better than those with any chromosomal abnormality.[54,55] Table 20.2, which is not exhaustive, summarizes the significance and approximate frequencies of the main chromosomal abnormalities in ALL.

Table 20.2 Chromosomal abnormalities in acute lymphoblastic leukemia

Chromosomal abnormality	Genes involved	Methods of Detection	Prognostic significance	Frequency	
				Children	Adults
B-lineage disease					
t(12;21)(p12;q22)	TEL-AML1	PCR FISH	Favorable	20–30%	~3%
t(9;22)(q34;q11)	BCR–ABL	Metaphase PCR FISH	Adverse	3–5%*	25–40%[a]
t(1;19)(q23;p13)	PBX-E2A	Metaphase PCR	Doubtful	5%	3%
t(4;11)(q21;q23)	MLL-AF4	Metaphase PCR FISH	Adverse in children Neutral in adults	3% (37% in infants < 1 year)	3%
All MLL translocations including t(4;11)(q21;q23)	MLL	Metaphase PCR FISH	Adverse overall	6% (70% in infants < 1 year)	7%
Del (6q)	Unknown	Metaphase	Neutral	9%	< 1%
Near-haploid	Not applicable	Metaphase	Adverse	< 1%	< 1%
Hypodiploid < 45 chromosomes	Not applicable	Metaphase	Adverse	1%	4%
Hyperdiploid > 50 chromosomes	Not applicable	Metaphase	Favorable	25%	1–2%
T-lineage disease					
del (6q)	Not applicable	Metaphase	Neutral	19%	Unknown
del(9p), including i(9q)	Not Applicable	Metaphase	Neutral	9–10%	Unknown
t(11;14)(p13;q11)	LM02-TCR8	Metaphase	Neutral	7%	Unknown
t(10;14)(q24;q11)		Metaphase	Favorable	6%	Unknown

[a] Depends on age limits separating pediatric group from adults.
FISH, fluorescent *in situ* hybridization; PCR, polymerase chain reaction.

Molecular genetics and disease monitoring in ALL

The majority of the translocations associated with ALL result in the formation of chimeric fusion genes. Breakpoints frequently occur over very large molecular distances within intronic gene sequences and are not readily amplifiable. However, following mRNA synthesis and subsequent reverse transcription to a stable cDNA template, these translocations become accessible to polymerase chain reaction (PCR) amplification using exon specific primers (RT-PCR).

The t(9;22) in ALL usually creates a chimeric fusion gene which gives rise to a 190 kD protein. The breakpoints in the ABL gene on chromosome 9 are consistently between exons 1 and 2, with multiple breakpoints in the minor breakpoint region involving the 5′E1A exon of the BCR gene on chromosome 22.[56,57] Less frequently, breakpoints usually associated with chronic myeloid leukemia (CML), giving rise to a 210 kD fusion protein are detected in ALL.[58] It has been postulated that Ph[1] positive ALL may possibly be two separate diseases, the majority presenting as *de novo* ALL, and rare cases derived from chronic myeloid leukemia presenting clinically in lymphoid blast transformation.[59] The ability to detect these different breakpoints is only possible using an RT-PCR strategy.

ALL with the t(1;19) is invariably of Pre-B-ALL subtype.[60,61] The abnormality is detectable in 25% of cases of Pre-B-ALL expressing cytoplasmic Igµ. Overall, 6% of pediatric patients carry this translocation.[60] Breakpoints on both chromosomes are conserved allowing a single assay to be designed capable of detecting all cases.[62] Disruption of the MLL gene at 11q23 is frequently observed in ALL. The gene involved has sequence homology with the drosophila trithorax gene and is termed HRX.[63] Although breaks are tightly clustered within an 8.5 Kb region, between exons 5 and 11, detection of this abnormality using RT-PCR is complicated by the variety of different translocation partners associated with this gene. Interpretation is further hampered by the diverse pattern of breakpoints within both MLL and the partner gene.[64] A multiplex strategy capable of detecting the majority of breakpoints has been described which uses eight parallel PCR reactions to identify 29 chromosomal aberrations.[65] However, FISH-based detection of MLL gene disruption is a more appropriate alternative.[66]

RT-PCR provides the most suitable means to detect the cytogenetically cryptic t(12;21), which gives rise to the TEL/AML1 fusion gene.[67,68] This abnormality has a frequency of between 20 and 30% in childhood ALL cases.[69] It is said to confer a favorable prognosis in patients and is commonly seen in children between 2 and 10 years of age.

Abnormalities involving the TAL-1 gene at 1p32 are found in approximately 15% of T-ALL cases. The most common of these involves a 95kb 5′ deletion resulting in disruption of the SCL gene, while a third of the abnormalities show a t(1;14)(p32;q11).[70]

Lineage assignment using antigen receptor gene rearrangements would conceptually provide useful diagnostic information in ALL. However, promiscuous, cross-lineage rearrangements are frequently encountered. Although unsuitable for lineage assignment these rearrangements have been extensively used to identify clonal specific markers with which to monitor the effects of therapy in patients with ALL (discussed below).

Residual disease monitoring in ALL

Present treatment protocols for ALL achieve clinical remission in around 95% of children and 70% of adults.[71] Thirty per cent of children and 70% of adult patients will still relapse on these intensive regimens.[72] The clone detectable at relapse is identical to that identified at presentation in the majority of cases. The immunophenotypic detection of residual disease has been discussed earlier in this chapter. RT-PCR-based techniques looking for translocations and DNA PCR for the detection of somatic gene rearrangements are conventionally employed for the analysis of residual disease in acute leukemia.

Monitoring for the presence of the t(9;22) during treatment and after allogeneic bone marrow transplantation is clinically useful in chronic myeloid leukemia, and its use in ALL has also been reported, where positivity post-bone marrow transplantation is predictive of relapse.[73–76] Persistent detection of the t(4;11) by RT-PCR during treatment is associated with a poor outcome.[77] However, the presence of a t(1;19) following consolidation therapy did not predict relapse.[78] Increasingly, the t(12;21) has also been used to monitor residual disease in childhood ALL.[79]

Clone-specific IgH or TCR gene rearrangements are in many cases of ALL the only marker available to monitor residual disease. Data derived from Southern hybridization analysis have shown that lineage-independent rearrangements of the TCR genes occur frequently in cases of precursor B-ALL, most frequently seen are rearrangements of the gamma and delta loci, conversely, IgH rearrangements are also seen in a small number of T-ALL cases. The gold standard for residual disease monitoring involves the creation of allele-specific oligonucleotides (ASO) that are subsequently used to identify clonally related cells in follow-up material.

Cross-lineage rearrangements of both the TCR gamma and delta genes have been utilized to monitor residual disease in ALL.[80–82] The immunoglobulin heavy chain gene (IgH) offers the most appropriate target for residual disease detection, detectable by PCR in over 94% of cases of precursor B-ALL.[83] Amplification with consensus IgH primers using presentation material, which contains predominantly leukemic cells, will produce a product that is both size and sequence specific. The unique size of each patient's clonal DNA PCR product can also be used to identify and monitor residual disease.[84]

Residual disease detection above a level of 10^{-3} at either the end of induction or prior to late intensification is associated with a poor prognosis.[84–86]

Serial quantification of residual disease in ALL provides the most accurate means of interpreting the cytoreductive effects of chemotherapy and may be the only means of predicting relapse. Initially, quantification was performed using a limiting dilution assay in combination with conventional ASO PCR.[87,88] Modified PCR amplification to include a competitor molecule has also been used to assess the level of residual leukemia. Both techniques have been largely superseded by real-time quantitative (RQ)-PCR (Taqman) techniques that utilise the 5′ exonuclease activity of Taq polymerase to accurately quantify residual ALL.[89,90]

Acute myeloid leukemia

Acute myeloid leukaemia (AML) is the single term which embraces a diverse group of diseases. The common strand is a proliferation of early myeloid progenitors, with or without maturation. The disease may be expressed in only one of the myeloid lineages (predominantly granulocyte, monocyte, erythroid and megakaryocyte, less commonly eosinophil or basophil) or several. Morphological dysplasia of maturing cells may be absent or prominent. It generally arises *de novo*, but may be a secondary event following a previous preleukemic state (myelodysplasia and myeloproliferative disorders), or known leukemogenic stresses such as chemotherapy (particularly with alkylating agents and topoisomerase II inhibitors) or radiation treatment. There are specific subtypes defined by linked morphology, cytogenetic abnormalities and clinical features. The pattern of disease types varies with age. This diversity of morphologic, clinical and genetic components has presented difficulties with the definition of AML, notably the separation from myelodysplastic syndromes with increased blast cell percentages in the marrow, and its classification. The FAB classification (Table 20.3), proposed in 1976[1] and subsequently modified[2] is based on blast percentage in the marrow, predominant cell type present and the presence or absence of maturation. It includes specific categories

Table 20.3 French–American–British (FAB) classification of acute myeloid leukemia (AML)

FAB category	Criteria for FAB typing	Cytochemistry
M0 (AML with minimal evidence of myeloid maturation)	• Morphologically undifferentiated blasts • Myeloid phenotype • Lymphoid markers negative	• < 3% blasts positive for SBB or MPO • No Auer rods present on SBB or MPO • Esterases negative in the blast cells
M1 (AML without maturation)	• Blasts > 90% of BM NEC • Maturing monocytic cells < 10% • Maturing granulocytes < 10%	• 3–100% blasts positive for SBB or MPO • Usually localized pattern of positivity • SBB or MPO positive Auer rods frequently present • Chloroacetate positive cells < 10% • NSE or BE positive cells scanty or absent
M2 (AML with maturation)	• Blasts 30–89% of NEC • Maturing granulocytes > 10% of NEC • Monocytic component < 20%	• 3–100% blasts positive for SBB or MPO • SBB or MPO positive Auer rods frequently present • SBB or MPO negative neutrophils may be present if dysplastic • Chloroacetate positive cells > 10% (maturing granulocytes) • NSE or BE positive cells scanty or absent
M3 (Hypergranular promyelocytic leukemia) M3variant (Hypogranular promyelocytic leukemia)	• M3 shows marrow replacement by granular and hypergranular promyelocytes • M3variant shows mainly agranular basophilic cells, bilobed nuclei	• SBB and MPO show characteristic heavy staining filling the cytoplasm • Multiple SBB or MPO positive Auer rods present, often obscured by heavy cytoplasmic staining • Majority of cells are chloroacetate esterase positive • Auer rods are chloroacetate positive • Leukemic promyelocyes show a deep pink cytoplasmic blush with PAS stain • t(15;17) demonstrable by cytogenetics, RT-PCR or FISH • Microparticulate nuclear PML protein pattern
M4 (Acute myelomonocytic leukemia)	• Blasts > 30% of NEC • Granulocyte component > 20% of BM NEC • Monocytic component > 20% of BM NEC	• Esterase stains show a mixture of chloroacetate and NSE or BE positive cells, usually > 20% of each • Some cells may show both types of esterase • 3–100% blasts positive for SBB or MPO, localized pattern in the myeloblasts, scattered pattern in monoblasts/monocytes • SBB or MPO positive Auer rods common • SBB or MPO negative neutrophils if dysplasia present
M4Eo	• Typical large 'eosinobasophils' present which define presence of inv/del/t(16)	• Usually conforms to M4 by conventional criteria, but may occasionally by M2 by FAB criteria • Inv/del/t(16) demonstrable by cytogenetics, RT-PCR or FISH
M5a and M5b (Acute monoblastic leukemia without maturation [M5a] and with maturation [M5b])	• Blasts > 30% of BM NEC • > 80% monocytic component of BM NEC • M5a when monoblasts > 80% of BM NEC • M5b when monoblasts < 80% of BM NEC	• Usually > 80% of BM cells show NSE or BE positivity • Chloroacetate positive cells usually rare, but always < 20% • SBB and MPO may be negative in the blasts/monocytes • SBB or MPO positive Auer rods rare
M6 (Erythroleukemia)	• Erythroid cells (all stages) > 50% of BM cells • Myeloid blasts > 30% of BM NEC	• Some/many erythroid precursors positive on PAS stain, rarely all negative • Some myeloid blasts SBB or MPO positive • SBB or MPO positive Auer rods occasionally present
M7 (Acute megakaryoblastic leukemia)	• Blasts mainly megakaryoblasts shown by immunologic methods	• Immunologic confirmation of megakaryocytic blasts required (> 30%) • Trephine biopsy may be helpful • Megakaryoblasts may show platelet like granules on PAS stain • Focal NSE (but not BE) positivity may be present • Myeloid blasts may show SBB or MPO positivity and rarely Auer rods

BE, butyrate esterase; BM, bone marrow; FISH, fluorescent *in situ* hybridization; MPO, myeloperoxidase; NEC, non-erythroid cells; NSE, non-specific esterase; PAS, periodic acid–Schiff; PML, promyelocytic leukemia; RT-PCR, reverse transcription-polymerase chain reaction; SBB, Sudan black B.

for acute promyelocytic leukemia, which was described 20 years prior to the discovery of the t(15;17),[91,92] and myelomonocytic leukemia with specifically abnormal eosinophil precursors (M4Eo) which includes most of the cases with inv(16)(p13;q22), t(16;16)(p13;q22) and del(16)(q22). Immunophenotyping plays no part in classifying the majority of cases in the FAB system, being necessary only for the identification of acute megakaryoblastic leukemia (M7) and minimally differentiated AML (M0) which is myeloperoxidase and esterase negative, identifiable only by immunophenotyping, including identification of immunoreactive cytoplasmic myeloperoxidase.[3,4]

The accumulated evidence of clinically relevant preceding events, cytogenetic abnormalities and multilineage dysplasia has led to the proposal of a new classification system by a clinical advisory committee of the WHO.[5,6] The principle follows that for lymphoid neoplasms; to define as far as possible clinically distinct disease entities, with the remainder classified by morphology and immunophenotype along the lines of the FAB classification with the addition of two new categories, acute basophilic leukemia and panmyelosis with myelofibrosis.

The WHO system redefines the marrow blast percentage required to diagnose AML downwards from 30 to 20% of marrow cells. This is based on the clinical behavior of the FAB category refractory anemia with excess blasts in transformation (RAEB-T), which tends to run a short acute clinical course much like AML.[93] The WHO classification divides AML into four groups: (1) AML with recurrent cytogenetic abnormalities; (2) AML with multilineage dysplasia; (3) AML, therapy related; and (4) AML not otherwise categorized (defined by morphology and immunophenotype) (Table 20.4). It assumes the availability of, and incorporates, metaphase cytogenetics, RT-PCR and FISH technologies as part of the diagnostic process. The pathology of AML is discussed below using the WHO framework.

Blast cell morphology in AML

Myeloblasts are variably sized. The nucleus is often eccentrically placed and characteristically appears partly attached to the cytoplasmic membrane. Chromatin is fine, and nucleoli multiple. There may be notching or internal folding of the chromatin. The N:C ratio is variable, but generally lower than in lymphoblasts. Type I myeloblasts are agranular, type II blasts have up to 20 fine azurophil granules. Type III blasts have been described which have more abundant granules, and need to be distinguished from promyelocytes, which are larger, show some

Table 20.4 WHO classification of acute myeloid leukemia (AML)

1. AML with recurrent translocations
   AML with t(8;21)(q22;q22)
   AML with t(15;17)(q22;q21) and variants (promyelocytic leukemia)
   AML with inv(16)(p13;q22), t(16;16)(p13;q22) or del(16)(q22) [M4Eo]
   AML with (v;11q23)

2. AML with multilineage dysplasia
   AML with prior myelodysplastic syndrome
   AML without prior myelodysplastic syndrome

3. AML therapy related
   Alkylating agent-related
   Epipodophyllotoxin-related
   Other

4. AML not otherwise categorized (FAB equivalent in parentheses)
   AML minimally differentiated (M0)
   AML without maturation (M1)
   AML with maturation (M2)
   Acute myelomonocytic (M4)
   Acute monocytic (M5)
   Acute erythroid leukemia (M6)
   Acute megakaryocytic leukemia (M7)
   Acute basophilic leukemia
   Acute panmyelosis with myelofibrosis
   Myeloid sarcoma

chromatin condensation and more abundant cytoplasm. Auer rods may be rare or frequent. Up to 70% of myeloblastic leukemias show Auer rods on myeloperoxidase or Sudan black B stains, with somewhat fewer cases showing them on Romanowsky stains. Occasionally, they are present in more mature granulocytes. Auer rods are definitive proof of a myeloid origin in acute leukemia. Monoblasts are larger than myeloblasts and have a low N:C ratio. The nucleus is surrounded by abundant basophilic or gray/blue cytoplasm. Fine azurophil granules may be numerous and cytoplasmic vacuolation may be present. Maturation to promonocytes and monocytes is marked by lobulation or folding of the nucleus and lessening of cytoplasmic basophilia.

Erythroblasts are large cells with round, central nuclei and deeply basophilic cytoplasm. Leukemic erythroblasts may show multiple vacuoles arranged concentrically, usually at the cytoplasmic margin. Nuclear rosetting or multinuclearity can occur at all stages of maturation. Megakaryoblasts are difficult to identify with certainty on a Romanowsky stain. Their size is variable, often small, and the only clue may be cytoplasmic blebs or a tail of cytoplasm. They are not synonymous with micromegakaryocytes, which may also be very small, but show deeply staining condensed chromatin, irregular cytoplasmic projections or blebs, and often exhibit recognizable platelet granules.

Cytochemical reactions in AML

Cytoplasmic cytochemical reactions complement the Romanowsky stain and immunophenotype, principally in confirming the myeloid nature of blasts, giving information on lineage involvement. The findings in AML usually reflect the staining patterns of normal counterparts, but abnormal patterns may be seen in dysplastic cells. Myeloperoxidase (MPO) and Sudan black B (SBB) are equivalent stains and define agranular blasts as myeloid. Auer rods are positive with both stains and are seen more frequently than on Romanowsky stains. In myeloblasts the positivity is usually localized. Monoblasts are frequently negative, but if positive, show a fine scattered granular pattern. Eosinophil granules are strongly positive with MPO, but show a negative core with SBB. Leukemic (and normal) promyelocytes stain heavily, with positive granules filling the cytoplasm. Hypogranular leukemic promyelocytes show the same pattern. Dysplastic metamyelocytes and neutrophils frequently show scanty or no granular positivity due to failure of specific granule formation. This does not always correlate directly with hypogranularity on the Romanowsky stain.

The carboxylic esterases are essential in defining monocyte and granulocyte components. Chloroacetate esterase (CAE) is specific for granulocytes and mast cells. Blasts are usually negative, cytoplasmic positivity appears at the blast/promyelocyte transition stage. Promyelocytes stain strongly, a helpful feature in hypogranular promyelocytic leukemia, where the Auer rods are also CAE positive. Unlike MPO and SBB, dysplastic granulocytes stain well with CAE. Monoblasts and monocytes generally stain strongly with α-naphthyl butyrate or α-naphthyl acetate esterase (non-specific esterase, NSE). NSE also stains megakaryocytes and some megakaryoblasts. Rarely, in promyelocytic leukemia the dominant esterase may be NSE, or the cells may show mixed positivity with CAE positive Auer rods and diffuse NSE cytoplasmic positivity. Double staining of cells is also seen in acute myelomonocytic leukemia and, to a varying degree, in dysplastic myelocytes and neutrophils.

The PAS stain for glycogen and acid glycoproteins is helpful, but does not give lineage-specific information. Myeloblasts are negative or show a faint diffuse cytoplasmic blush. Strong positivity does not appear until the neutrophil stage is reached. Promyelocytic leukemia cells show a distinctive strong diffuse positivity. Monoblasts frequently display fine granules, often at the cell periphery. Normal erythroid precursors are negative at all stages, but dysplastic erythroblasts at all stages may be positive. When present, the positivity is coarsely granular

in proerythroblasts and diffuse in later normoblasts. Megakaryocytes show mixed block, granular and diffuse positivity, a pattern seen in micromegakaryocytes, where the granules may be concentrated in cytoplasmic blebs. Basophils may show large irregular blocks of positivity.

Perls' stain for free iron is useful for demonstrating ringed sideroblasts in occasional cases with multilineage dysplasia. If abnormal basophils or mast cells are suspected, toluidine blue staining confirms the presence of these specific granules, including cases where the basophils are agranular on the Romanowsky stain.

AML with recurrent translocations

AML with t(8;21)

Cases of AML with t(8;21) are seen predominantly in younger patients (median age around 30 years), constituting at least 12% of cases in children, and 8% of all patients under the age of 55 years.[94,95] This incidence is an underestimate as there is good evidence that metaphase cytogenetics misses some cases detected by RT-PCR.[96] The t(8;21) is predictive of a high remission rate and improved overall survival.[94]

The t(8;21) is characterized by recognizable morphology and cytochemistry (Fig. 20.5), but the blast

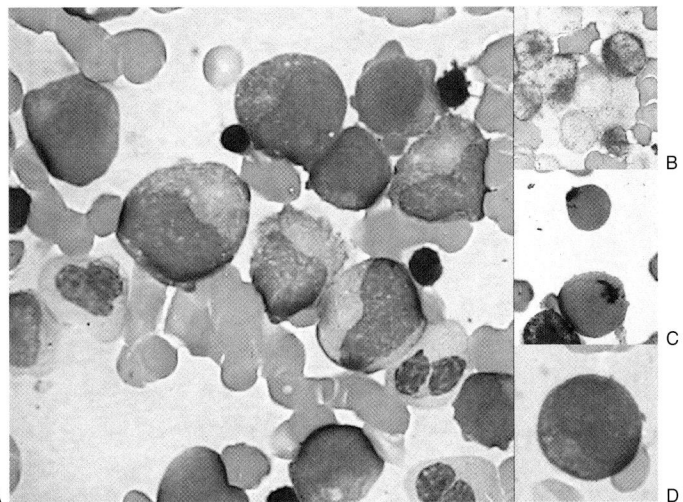

Fig. 20.5 AML with t(8;21), differentiated (FAB M2) type. (A) May–Grünwald–Giemsa stain. Blasts are basophilic. The promyelocyte shows granules over the Golgi region but all the maturing forms are agranular with the characteristic flat featureless cytoplasm. (B) Chloroacetate esterase (CAE) showing blue granules in the maturing granulocytes. (C) Sudan black B showing typical localized positivity with one Auer rod visible. (D) May–Grünwald–Giemsa stain showing a classical t(8;21) blast with slightly indented nucleus and a slender Auer rod overlying the pale Golgi region in the nuclear indentation.

percentage in the marrow is highly variable.[97] The t(8;21) defines the disease, irrespective of blast count. Although most cases are acute myeloblastic leukemia with maturation (FAB M2), 20–30% show little maturation (FAB M1), and rare cases show less than 20% blasts. Such cases are defined as AML despite a blast count that would normally define a myelodysplastic syndrome. The morphology is almost always of myeloblastic/granulocytic type, with one-third of cases showing abnormal eosinophils.[97] The abnormal eosinophils have been shown to carry the translocation, and rarely may be the predominant presenting feature in the blood and marrow.[98,99]

The blast cells are basophilic, and variable in size. Nuclei are usually eccentrically placed and frequently show an indentation containing a pale Golgi region. Chromatin is fine with two or more prominent nucleoli. Auer rods, often notably long and slender, are invariably present but may be rare. Blasts may be type I or type II, blending into type III blasts and promyelocytes. The blasts and promyelocytes may show large globular (pseudo-Chediak) granules. Dysplastic granulocyte maturation is always present. Myelocytes are often agranular, and beyond this stage the cytoplasm is usually an abnormal peach color. Auer rods may be present in granulocytes at all stages including neutrophils. Classically dysplastic agranular pseudo-Pelger neutrophils are usually present, and occasionally mononuclear neutrophils with round nuclei showing mature clumped chromatin are seen.

Eosinophils, if present show variable granule size and staining. Nuclear maturation may be defective with hypolobation. Rarely, Auer rods are demonstrable in eosinophils by MPO and SBB staining. Megakaryocytes and erythroid precursors show minor, if any, dysplastic changes. There is indirect and direct evidence that erythroid precursors do not carry the translocation.[100,101] Rarely, there may be a substantial increase in mast cells. This is of unknown significance and may persist when remission has been obtained.

The cytochemical appearances in t(8;21) are characteristic. Virtually all the blasts show MPO or SBB positivity, typically tightly localized in the nuclear indentation. Auer rods are seen more frequently than on Romanowsky stains. The pseudo-Chediak granules stain as large globules, particularly with MPO. Myelocytes stain normally, with strong positivity filling the cytoplasm, but metamyelocytes and neutrophils may be negative. The blasts may show localized chloroacetate positivity and positive Auer rods. CAE-positive Auer rods are not generally seen in AML except in cases of t(8;21) and promyelocytic leukemia. Later maturing granulocytes show normal patterns of CAE positivity.

Although no single feature is pathognomonic of t(8;21), the blast cell morphology and cytochemistry and the pattern of dysplastic maturation of neutrophils and eosinophils taken together are moderately predictive of the presence of the translocation.[102]

AML with t(15;17)

Acute promyelocytic leukemia is a distinct clinicopathologic syndrome within AML. The characteristic proliferation of abnormal (hyper)granular promyelocytes in association with a defibrination syndrome was recognized in 1957.[91] The associated t(15;17) was fully described by Rowley et al in 1977.[92] In 1980, Golomb et al described the 'microgranular' (hypogranular) morphologic variant that comprises approximately 20–30% of cases.[103] The FAB group incorporated this as the M3variant subtype (M3v). More recently, some confusion has arisen due to the use of the term variant to describe the rare cases with t(11;17)(q3;q21) and even rarer t(5;17)(q23;q12) as 'variant' promyelocytic leukemia.[104,105] The t(15;17) involves the fusion of the PML (promyelocytic leukemia) gene on chromosome 15 to the RARA (retinoic acid receptor alpha) gene on chromosome 17. This PML/RARA fusion gene and its product are the target for the successful differentiation therapy of the disease using All-*trans*-retinoic acid (ATRA) first reported by Huang et al in 1988, which also rapidly corrects the coagulopathy present in most cases.[106] The cytogenetic variants with t(11;17) and t(5;17) do not respond to ATRA, do not show the classical 'faggot' cells with multiple Auer rods and can be distinguished morphologically from true promyelocytic leukemia.[107] Combined therapy with ATRA and conventional chemotherapy has resulted in high remission rates and improved survival in promyelocytic leukemia with t(15;17) detected by metaphase cytogenetics, RT-PCR or FISH.

Hypergranular promyelocytic leukemia usually presents as a pancytopenia. There may be few circulating abnormal promyelocytes. The marrow is hypercellular, and may clot quickly on aspiration. The specific morphologic features of hypergranular promyelocytic leukemia (Fig. 20.6) may only be present in a minority of cells in the marrow. Typical nuclei are bilobed with overlap of the two lobes (also described as reniform or figure-of-eight). Nucleoli may be preserved. The cytoplasm is granular, with accentuated azurophilic staining that gives a red or deep reddish-purple hue to the granules. Hypergranularity is often so extensive that the nuclear borders are obscured. The granule content of the promyelocytes varies widely within and between cases. The pathognomonic cell contains multiple Auer rods (faggots or

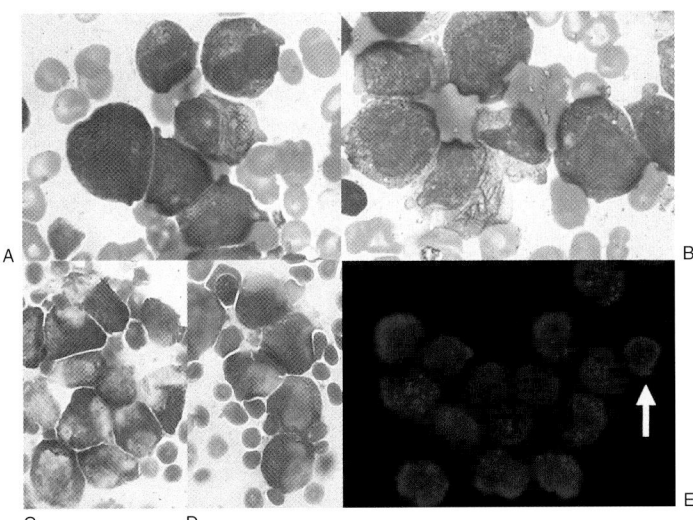

Fig. 20.6 Hypergranular acute promyelocytic leukemia. (A and B) May–Grünwald–Giemsa stain. Each picture shows one cell with typical multiple Auer rods. The remaining promyelocytes illustrate the variability of granule content in APML. (C) Myeloperoxidase stain (diaminobenzidine). Typical heavy staining filling the cytoplasm. (D) Chloroacetate esterase (CAE) showing typical intense staining. (E) Nuclear PML protein immunofluorescence showing abnormal microparticulate pattern. One cell (arrow) shows the normal wild-type pattern of discrete bodies (courtesy of Dr S. O'Connor).

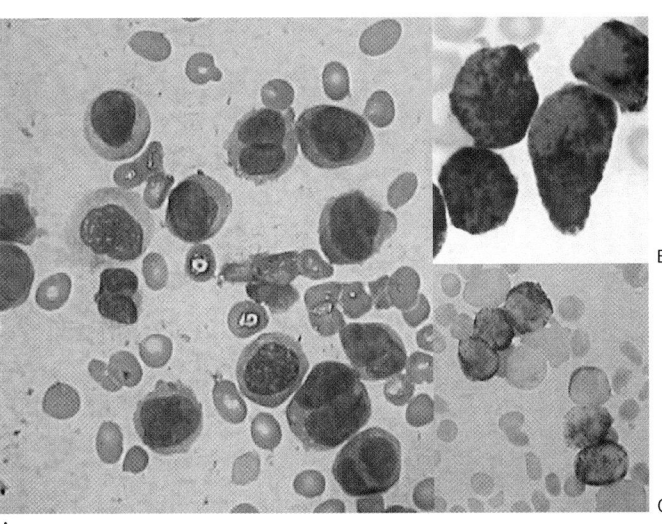

Fig. 20.7 Hypogranular acute promyelocytic leukemia. (A) Peripheral blood May–Grünwald–Giemsa stain. Note the bilobed nuclei and basophilic cytoplasm. The cell at bottom right has 'dusty' cytoplasm but granules are absent. (B) Sudan black B stain showing typical heavy cytoplasmic positivity. (C) Strong cytoplasmic chloracetate esterase (CAE) positivity in the majority of cells.

bundles), with or without accompanying granules. These may be apparent on trephine biopsy sections, particularly on Giemsa-stained sections. Agranular blast cells may be present, but seldom account for more than 5–10% of cells. Neutrophil maturation shows variable dysplasia. Residual erythropoiesis may be megaloblastic, but there are generally no other signs of dyserythropoiesis. Megakaryocytes are reduced but of normal morphology. Despite the apparent distinctiveness of the morphology, the diagnosis can be difficult, with AML showing maturation (FAB M2) as the principal differential diagnosis. The most useful rapid confirmatory test is by nuclear immunofluorescence showing the diagnostic micro-particulate pattern of nuclear PML protein (Fig. 20.6). Cases with t(11;17) show the normal (wild-type) pattern of discrete nuclear bodies.[108]

Cytochemistry is helpful in confirming difficult cases. The promyelocytes show heavy MPO or SBB positivity, filling the cytoplasm. Multiple Auer rods are well shown by the MPO stain, but are often difficult to see on SBB staining because of the overwhelming intensity of the granule staining. Chloroacetate esterase positivity is usual in the majority of cells, and Auer rods stain positively. A variable proportion of cells show some non-specific esterase positivity in addition to chloroacetate esterase positivity, and rarely this may be the predominant esterase present.[109] The cytoplasm exhibits a deep pink blush on PAS staining.

The hypogranular (microgranular) type (FAB M3v) accounts for 20–30% of cases (Fig. 20.7). In contrast to hypergranular forms, there is frequently a leukocytosis greater than 10×10^9/l. The cells are large, with abundant cytoplasm and variable, sometimes intense cytoplasmic basophilia. The characteristic bilobed nuclei are the main morphologic clue to the diagnosis. The nuclear lobes may be irregular, of different sizes and give an impression of folding rather than the classical figure-of-eight. Fine dust-like granules may be present. Careful scrutiny of the blood and marrow smears usually reveals rare typical hypergranular or 'faggot' cells. The principal differential diagnosis is monocytic leukemia with maturation (FAB M5B) or myelomonocytic leukemia (FAB M4). Cytochemical stains show the same heavy MPO and SBB positivity. CAE is positive, but in fewer cells than the hypergranular form, and non-specific esterase may be strongly positive. Rarely, it is the presence of multiple chloroacetate positive Auer rods that clinches the morphologic diagnosis.[110]

Treatment response and overall survival are poorer in patients presenting with a leukocyte count greater than 10×10^9/l, which includes most patients with hypogranular disease.[111] A positive PCR result on marrow cells after consolidation chemotherapy is predictive for relapse.[111] In patients that achieve PCR-negative marrows, reappearance of PML/RARα transcripts is predictive of relapse, and retreatment at this point improves the prognosis.[112]

AML with inv(16) and t(16;16)

This form of AML, usually myelomonocytic, with specifically abnormal eosinophil precursors and associated with abnormalities of the long arm of chromosome 16 was first recognized in 1983.[113,114] Inv(16)(p13;q22), t(16;16)(p13;q22) and del(16)(q22) all give rise to the same morphologic findings and are associated with a good prognosis.[94,115] The specific cytochemical findings in the abnormal eosinophils were described in 1984,[116] although earlier reports had described such cases but without accompanying cytogenetic data.[117,118] Inv(16) and t(16;16) result in a fusion gene created by fusion of the CBFβ gene at 16q22 with the MYH11 gene at 16p13. This fusion gene is detectable by both RT-PCR and FISH, with both methods detecting the presence of the fusion gene when not detected by metaphase cytogenetics.[119,120]

The pathognomonic cell is an eosinophil precursor that is large, with a low nuclear:cytoplasmic ratio (Fig. 20.8). The nucleus may be 'monocytoid' (i.e. lobular or horseshoe shaped), with chromatin that is less clumped than in normal eosinophils. The cytoplasm contains abnormal eosinophil granules (varied size and coloration) in addition to the very large, sometimes irregular, purple/black granules specific to this entity. These granules, although resembling basophil granules in color on the Romanowsky stain, are not stained by toluidine blue. Their ultrastructural appearances are of eosinophil granules. These cells have been termed 'hybrid' cells or 'eosinobasophils'. The percentage of eosinophils in the marrow ranges from <1% to >50%. The blue/black

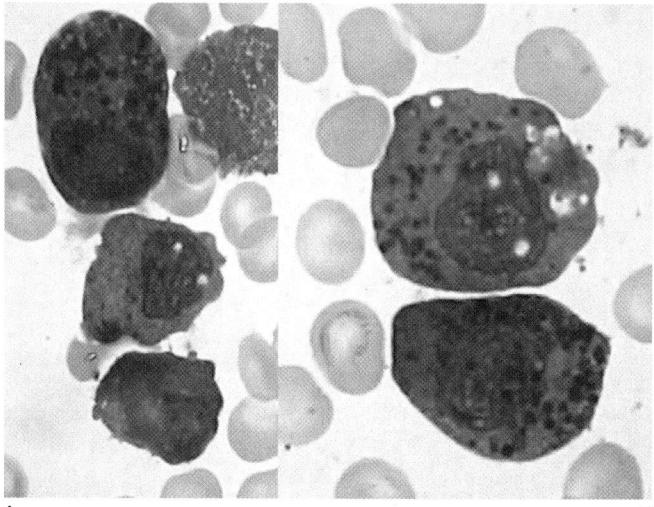

Fig. 20.8 AML with inv(16). (A) May–Grünwald–Giemsa stain. The top cell with a monocytoid nucleus, abundant basophilic cytoplasm and a mixture of small eosinophil granules and large irregular purple/black granules is typical. (B) Two further examples of typical 'eosinobasophils'.

granules are present only in the eosinophil promyelocytes and myelocytes and not in the more mature eosinophils. Auer rods are usually present but may be scarce, and may be seen in maturing granulocytic cells. There is often severe dysplasia of maturing monocytes and granulocytes, and esterase stains often show fewer non-specific esterase-positive cells than expected. The blasts usually show a mixture of heavy (myeloblastic) and scattered granular (monocytic) positivity with MPO or SBB stains. Auer rods are better shown than on the Romanowsky stain. The principal cytochemical abnormalities of the eosinophil granules are PAS positivity (never present in normal eosinophils) and CAE positivity, which is unique to this subtype. Although the vast majority of cases are myelomonocytic, some are classifiable as monocytic (< 20% granulocytes) or myeloblastic (< 20% monocytes). The common link between these cases, irrespective of the overall morphologic classification is the abnormal eosinophil precursors. Although rare, there are occasional cases with a classical inversion, deletion or translocation of 16q22 where no abnormal eosinophils are detectable.

AML with t(v;11)(v;q23)

Translocations and deletions of chromosome 11q23 involve disruption of the MLL gene. Over 40 partner reciprocal chromosomes/genes have been identified. The commonest reciprocal chromosome partners are 9, 17, 19, 6, 10 and 1 in descending order of frequency. There are no specific cytologic correlates of 11q23 abnormalities but there is preponderance of monocytic or myelomonocytic morphology. Although most translocations are identifiable by RT-PCR, the number of partner genes makes this impractical as a screening tool. Disruption of the MLL gene can be shown by interphase FISH.

AML with multilineage dysplasia

The WHO classification subdivides this category according to the presence or absence of a preceding myelodysplastic syndrome. Multilineage dysplasia in AML is defined by severe dysplastic features in two or more cell lines. This effectively means either dyserythropoiesis and/or dysmegakaryopoiesis in addition to dysplasia of the granulocyte/monocyte lineages (Figs 20.9 and 20.10, also see Figs 20.5 and 20.15). Multilineage dysplasia is usual in AML developing as a progression of myelodysplasia. It occurs in *de novo* AML in a minority of cases at all ages, with a progressive increase with age over 60 years. The incidence of trilineage myelodysplasia (TMDS) in *de novo* AML is between 10 and 20%, with the incidence of bilineage or single lineage dysplasia being much

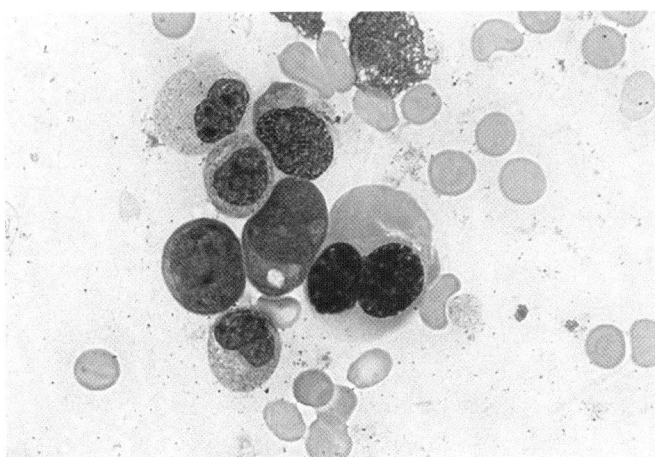

Fig. 20.9 May–Grünwald–Giemsa stain. Bone marrow smear showing two basophilic blast cells, a giant binucleate erythroid precursor and three dysplastic granulocytes. The granulocytes show mature clumped chromatin but no nuclear segmentation. Cytoplasmic granules are variably reduced.

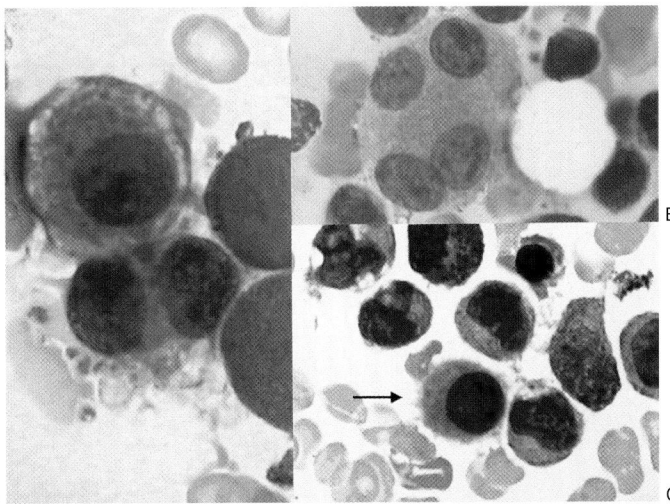

Fig. 20.10 Dysplastic megakaryocytes, May–Grünwald–Giemsa stains. (A) Small mononuclear megakaryocyte and small binucleate form budding platelets. (B) Nuclear lobe separation in a normal-sized granular megakaryocyte. (C) Micromegakaryocyte with dense nuclear chromatin and eccentric cytoplasm with platelet granules.

higher.[121–125] The morphologic and cytogenetic abnormalities in *de novo* AML with TMDS are similar to those encountered in AML secondary to alkylating agents or a preceding myelodysplastic syndrome. Dysgranulopoiesis is defined by the presence of 50% of neutrophils showing hypogranularity or nuclear abnormalities, mainly bilobed or mononuclear (pseudo-Pelger–Huët). Abnormally coarse chromatin clumping and hypersegmentation are less definite features. Erythroid abnormalities are multinuclearity, nuclear fragmentation, nuclear rosetting and karyorrhexis. Megaloblastoid erythropoiesis is relatively common, and includes giant late normoblasts. Iron stains are not routinely carried out at diagnosis in AML, but the

presence of greater than 15% ringed sideroblasts constitutes evidence of significant dyserythropoiesis. Normal erythroid precursors are negative on PAS staining. Detectable erythroid PAS positivity occurs in one-fifth of AML cases, including the majority of M6 cases, and is evidence of dyserythropoiesis.[126] Significant dyserythropoiesis was originally defined as 25% of erythroid precursors showing abnormalities,[121,125] but some studies have used a figure of 50%, in line with the criteria for granulocytes and megakaryocytes.[122–124] Megakaryocyte abnormalities are defined as the presence of at least 3 or greater than 50% micromegakaryocytes or larger megakaryocytes showing multiple separated nuclei or round 'mononuclear' nuclei. Megakaryocytes are frequently too scanty for assessment on aspirate smears. Small studies suggest that assessment of megakaryocyte size on trephine biopsies is useful, with small megakaryocytes denoting a poor prognosis.[127,128] The complete remission rate is generally worse in AML patients with TMDS, but the effect on overall survival is often less clear. Outcome is probably more closely related to adverse cytogenetic findings than the morphologic features.[122,124]

AML therapy related

AML following treatment with cytotoxic agents has been recognized since 1970.[129] Radiation treatment, either alone or combined with chemotherapy, is also a cause of AML. A significant proportion of cases show a preceding period of myelodysplasia of generally short duration before transformation to AML.[130] Two main syndromes are recognized by the WHO classification; namely alkylating-agent-related AML and topoisomerase-II-inhibitor (epipodophyllotoxin) related AML. Alkylating-agent-related disease is characterized by a peak incidence 3–6 years after exposure, frequent preceding myelodysplasia, multilineage morphologic abnormalities (panmyelosis), frequent abnormalities of chromosomes 5 and 7, complex karyotypes and chromosomal evidence of clonal evolution. Morphologic classification is often difficult, and response to treatment is poor.[130–133] The dysplastic features are usually severe. Abnormal basophils are frequent and Auer rods are generally absent from the blasts.[131]

Epipodophyllotoxin-related leukemias differ from the alkylating-agent-related cases in three main respects.[134] The time from treatment to leukemia is shorter, generally less than 3 years.[135] There is seldom a preceding myelodysplastic phase, and trilineage myelodysplasia is rare, with most cases exhibiting monocytic or myelomonocytic morphology. There is a high frequency of 11q23 chromosome abnormalities, which are not generally associated with alkylating-agent-related AML.[135] Children show the same features as adults.[136] Acute promyelocytic leukemia has been identified as occurring after epipodophyllotoxin treatment, particularly in children treated for Langerhans' cell histiocytosis.[137]

AML not otherwise categorized

All cases of AML not defined by the specific categories above fall into this group. This section of the WHO classification is morphology based, with appropriate cytochemistry and immunophenotyping, and is essentially an extension of the FAB system. Since the boundaries between subtypes are defined by morphologic interpretation and percentage criteria which are observer dependent, this group of AML cases is prone to interobserver disagreement. In 1976, after considerable discussion, the FAB group reached a consensus diagnosis in only 85% of the 150 cases (AML and ALL) on which the initial classification was based.[1]

Acute myeloblastic leukemia, minimally differentiated (FAB M0)

By definition this form of AML has no diagnostic morphologic or cytochemical features (Fig. 20.11). Auer rods are absent on Romanowsky, MPO and SBB staining. Less than 3% of blasts are MPO or SBB positive (FAB definition), and there is no esterase evidence of a monocytic origin. The blast cell count is usually high in the marrow. The definition of this subtype is oriented to the blasts only, and occasional cases occur where there is clear evidence of dysplastic granulopoiesis, dyserythropoiesis (e.g. PAS-positive erythroblasts) or dysmegakaryopoiesis, consistent with a myeloid origin. The diagnosis is dependent on demonstrating a myeloid immunophenotype (see below).

Acute myeloblastic leukemia without maturation (FAB M1)

Myeloblasts are the majority population of marrow cells. The blasts are usually medium or large in size with eccentric nuclei, fine open chromatin and multiple nucleoli. Nuclear folding or irregularity can occur, but monocytic lobulation is absent. Small blasts with scanty cytoplasm may predominate. Granules (type II blasts) may be present. Fewer than 10% of marrow cells are promyelocytes and more mature granulocytes. This should be confirmed with CAE staining which provides a useful method of identifying promyelocytes and later granulocytes. There is no significant monocytic component.

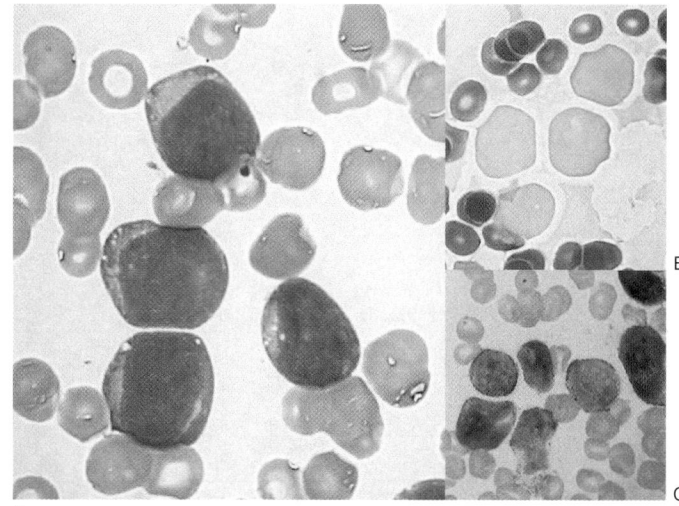

Fig. 20.11 AML minimally differentiated (FAB M0). (A) May–Grünwald–Giemsa stain. Blasts are large and agranular. No Auer rods present. (B) Myeloperoxidase stain. Blasts negative. (C) Immunoreactive cytoplasmic myeloperoxidase (red) in the blasts, alkaline phosphatase-anti-alkaline phosphatase technique.

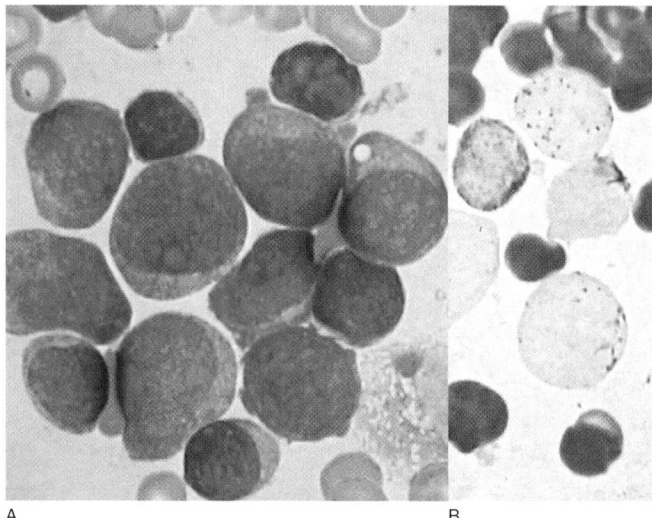

Fig. 20.12 AML without maturation (FAB M1). (A) May–Grünwald–Giemsa stain. Blasts show variable size, eccentric nuclei, no granules or Auer rods and multiple nucleoli. (B) Myeloperoxidase (diaminobenzidine). Blasts show variable positivity, including one Auer rod.

Erythroid precursors are usually scanty. The number of MPO- or SBB-positive blasts varies from the minimum 3% required to virtually 100% (Fig. 20.12). Auer rods are present in about half the cases (Romanowsky, MPO or SBB stains). Multilineage dysplasia is by definition absent.

Acute myeloblastic leukemia with maturation (FAB M2)

The marrow shows more than 20% blasts and more than 10% maturing granulocytes, with a highly variable balance between blasts and maturing cells (Fig. 20.5). The blast morphology and cytochemistry is similar to that in AML without maturation. There may be difficulty in separating granular blasts (type II and type III) from promyelocytes. Promyelocytes are generally larger, with a distinctly eccentric oval nucleus, and concentration of the granules in the Golgi region. Auer rods are present in three-quarters of cases. The maturing granulocytes are frequently dysplastic. Erythropoiesis is variable in amount. Minor dyserythropoietic changes are common (e.g. nuclear irregularity), but more major changes such as multinuclearity, giant normoblasts or PAS positivity should raise the possibility of multilineage dysplasia. Megakaryocytes are usually scanty, but should be carefully assessed for signs of dysplasia. If there is clear evidence of multilineage dysplasia the case should be reclassified as AML with multilineage dysplasia.

Acute myelomonocytic leukemia (FAB M4)

Acute myelomonocytic leukemia shows greater than 20% each of maturing granulocytes and monocytic cells (monoblasts, promonocytes and monocytes). The proportions of each are variable. Maturation may be marked or minimal. The blast cell component may show marked

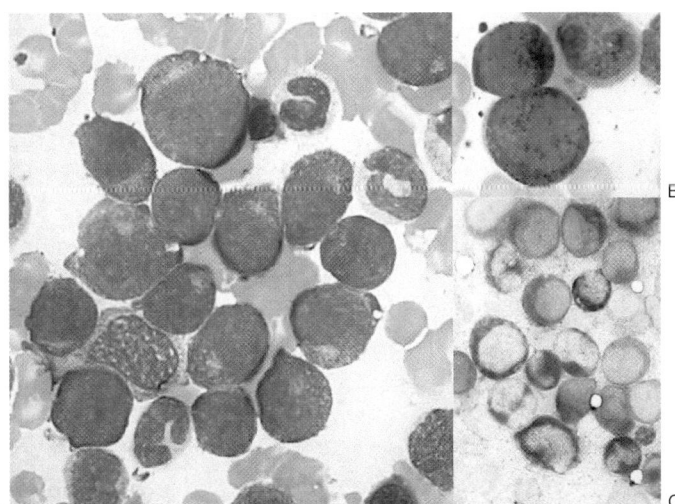

Fig. 20.13 Acute myelomonocytic leukemia (FAB M4).
(A) May–Grünwald–Giemsa stain. Blasts are variable in size and nuclear/cytoplasmic ratio. Dysplastic neutrophils are present. (B) Sudan black B stain showing one blast with localized (myeloblastic) positivity and one with scattered granules (monocytic pattern). The dysplastic neutrophil stains poorly. (C) Combined esterase stain. Almost equal numbers of non-specific esterase positive cells (brown, monocytes) and chloroacetate esterase (blue, granulocytes) positive cells. The chloroacetate positivity indicates more cytoplasmic maturation than is apparent on the May–Grünwald–Giemsa stain.

variation in size and morphology. There is usually a spectrum from smaller myeloblasts with eccentric nuclei touching the cytoplasmic membrane to large monoblasts with abundant cytoplasm and central nuclei. Many blasts cannot be categorized with certainty by morphology alone. The maturing granulocyte component may be dysplastic. Promonocytes may be granular and difficult to distinguish from promyelocytes. Nuclear folding or lobulation is often abnormal in the more mature monocytic cells. Cytochemistry is essential in defining the myelomonocytic nature of the leukemia. Myeloperoxidase and SBB staining tends to be stronger and localized in the myeloblasts and negative or finely granular in the monoblasts/monocytes. Auer rods occur in about half the cases, and are generally confined to the myeloblast population. Combined esterase stains show chloroacetate-positive (granulocyte) and non-specific esterase-positive (monocytic) components, and are confirmatory for the diagnosis (Fig. 20.13). Double-staining of myelocytes and occasionally neutrophils may be present and reflects dysplastic maturation. A search for multilineage dysplasia should be carried out, and the case reclassified if this is present.

Acute monocytic leukemias (FAB M5A and M5B)

In acute monocytic leukemias the marrow is usually almost entirely replaced by the monocytic cells. These may be a homogeneous population of blast cells (FAB M5A, monoblastic, undifferentiated), or there may be considerable maturation to abnormal promonocytes and monocytes (FAB M5B, monocytic, differentiated). In acute monoblastic leukemia (M5A) the blasts are large, up to 50 μm in diameter. Nuclei are round, centrally placed and often show a single prominent nucleolus. Mitoses are generally frequent. Cytoplasmic basophilia is highly variable. Fine or coarse azurophilic granules may be present in large numbers. Small peripheral vacuoles may be present, and occasional large vacuoles (phagosomes) are seen. Cytoplasmic projections or buds may be prominent, and it is not uncommon to find fragments of cytoplasm free on the smear. Myeloperoxidase and SBB stains may be entirely negative, and if positive takes the form of fine widely scattered granules. Auer rods are extemely rare in monoblastic leukemias. The vast majority of cases show diffuse cytoplasmic positivity with non-specific or butyrate esterase (Fig. 20.14). There is cell-to-cell variation in intensity and rarely only a few cells are weakly positive. Care should be taken in diagnosing acute monoblastic leukemia in the absence of esterase positivity. True histiocytic lymphomas, AML minimally

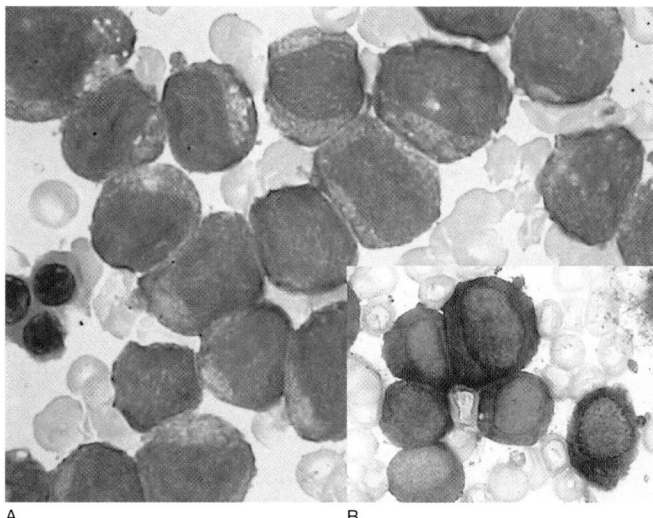

A   B

Fig. 20.14 Acute monoblastic leukemia (FAB M5A).
(A) May–Grünwald–Giemsa stain. The monoblasts are large with basophilic cytoplasm. The nuclei are central with open chromatin and prominent nucleoli. No granules or Auer rods present. (B) Typical strong non-specific esterase (brown) cytoplasmic positivity.

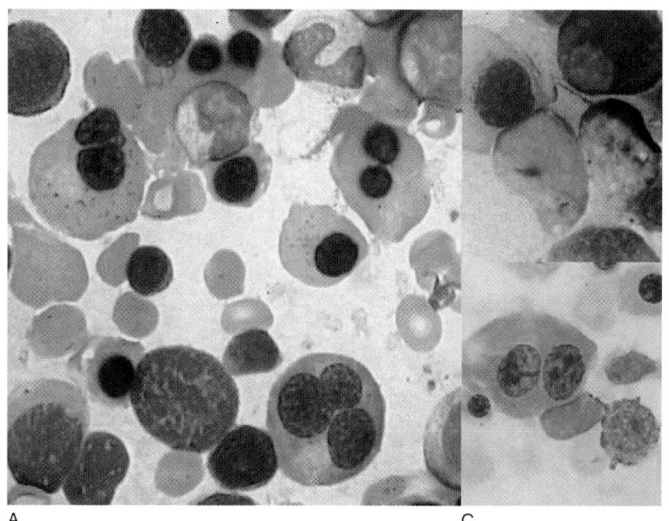

A   C

Fig. 20.15 Acute erythroid leukemia, erythroid/myeloid type (FAB M6). (A) May–Grünwald–Giemsa stain. Mainly large binucleate and multinucleate late normoblasts, with a proerythroblast at top left. Part of two myeloblasts are present at top right. (B) Sudan black B stain. Myeloblast with positive Auer rod. (C) Periodic acid-Schiff stain. Normoblasts are strongly positive.

differentiated (FAB M0), and anaplastic lymphomas are differential diagnoses. Immunophenotyping is essential to resolve these disorders.

Acute monocytic leukemia (FAB M5B) is distinguished by the presence of substantial maturation to promonocytes and monocytes. The cell population is heterogeneous. Blasts are usually not as homogeneous as in M5A, and always comprise less than 80% of the total monocytic population. The maturing monocytes show aberrant folding or lobulation of the nucleus. A small (< 20%) granulocyte component may be present together with some myeloblasts, and Auer rods are more likely to be detected in such cases. Erythrophagocytosis is a rare phenomenon seen in approximately 1% of AML, and may be associated with a t(8;16)(p11;p13).[138]

Acute erythroid leukemia (FAB M6)

Predominantly erythroid *de novo* acute leukemias are rare, comprising less than 5% of AML cases. Myelodysplastic syndromes are the principal differential diagnosis, and other causes of erythroid hyperplasia need to be excluded. The principal diagnostic criteria are: (1) 50% or more of all the marrow cells are erythroid precursors of all stages; and (2) 20% of the non-erythroid cells are myeloblasts (Fig. 20.15). In the WHO system this is termed 'erythroleukemia (erythroid/myeloid)'. Multilineage dysplasia is common.[139] Erythroid presursors of all stages are present. Dyserythropoiesis may be marked, with multinucleate cells at any stage of maturation, nuclear

rosetting, cytoplasmic vacuolation, macronormoblasts, basophilic stippling and Pappenheimer bodies. The peripheral blood usually shows circulating erythroid precursors, but is pancytopenic. Red cell anisopoikilocytosis and macrocytosis are usual. Storage iron is usually increased and ringed sideroblasts may be plentiful. The majority of cases show some PAS positivity in erythroid precursors, varying from only occasional cells to virtually all. Proerythroblasts show coarse peripheral circular PAS-positive granules, with later normoblasts and mature red cells showing diffuse cytoplasmic staining. Myeloblasts may contain Auer rods, and show variable positivity on MPO and SBB stains. Granulocytes are usually dysplastic, and neutrophils may be MPO and SBB negative. Megakaryocyte numbers are variable, and hypolobation or nuclear-lobe separation may be apparent. Cytogenetic abnormalities often seen in myelodysplastic syndromes (MDS) and therapy-related AML are common particularly 5q- and 7q-.[140]

In rare cases the marrow is virtually replaced by erythroid precursors without an identifiable myeloblastic component. The WHO system recognizes these cases as 'pure erythroid leukemia' (Fig. 20.16). These cases show a preponderance of erythroblasts and basophilic intermediate forms.[141] An extremely rare form of blastic erythroid leukemia without recognizable morphology and identifiable only by specialized flow cytometry, exists. It may occur *de novo* or following MDS, but is usually associated with blast crisis of CML or Down's syndrome and often contains a megakaryocytic element.[142,143]

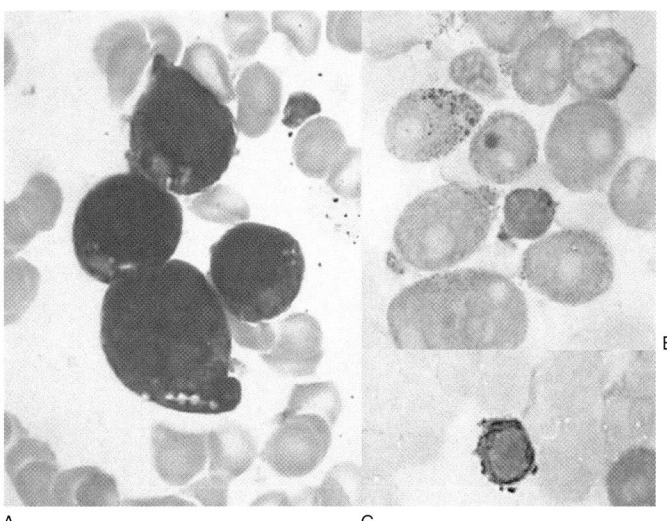

A   C

Fig. 20.16 Pure erythroid leukemia. (A) May–Grünwald–Giemsa stain. Basophilic proerythroblasts showing minor vacuolation and budding. (B and C) Periodic acid-Schiff stain. (B) Proerythroblasts show coarse granular positivity. (C) A late normoblast showing diffuse and granular positivity.

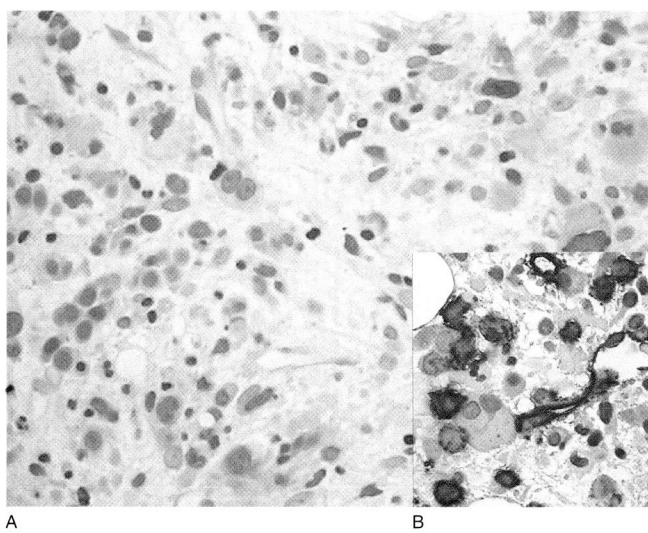

A   B

Fig. 20.17 Acute megakaryocytic leukemia. (A) Hematoxylin and eosin stain. The marrow shows intense fibrosis, atypical megakaryocytes and blast cells. There is no significant erythroid or granulocyte activity. (B) CD34+ blast cells.

Acute megakaryocytic leukemia (FAB M7)

This uncommon form of AML accounts for approximately 3% of cases. It occurs at any age with clustering in infants and young children including some with Down's syndrome. The diagnostic criteria are 20% or more blasts in the blood or marrow, with evidence of megakaryocytic lineage in 50% or more cells in the marrow. The peripheral blood frequently shows leukopenia and anemia, with variable platelet numbers. The marrow is usually fibrotic, particularly if there is much megakaryocyte maturation, and may be inaspirable, precluding cytologic assessment. The diagnosis frequently relies on trephine biopsy analysis. The megakaryocytes and blasts should be the dominant cell lineage present (Fig. 20.17). Megakaryoblasts are frequently small, with scanty cytoplasm showing small spiky projections or blebs.

Micromegakaryocytes, which show dense mature chromatin, cytoplasmic projections and frequently platelet granules, should not be counted as blasts. There are no definitive cytochemical appearances. The blasts are MPO- and SBB-negative, but the presence of small PAS-positive granules, sometimes concentrated in cytoplasmic buds, and focal non-specific esterase is suggestive.[144] The establishment of megakaryocytic lineage requires the demonstration of surface platelet glycoproteins; IIIa (CD61), IIb/IIIa (CD41) or Ib (CD42) by flow cytometry, immunocytochemistry on smears or immunohistochemistry on trephine biopsy sections. Demonstrating

Factor VIII is useful, but blasts and some more mature megakaryocytes may be negative. Ultrastructural demonstration of platelet peroxidase in the blasts is also diagnostic, but has largely been superseded by immmunologic diagnosis. The differential diagnosis includes acute panmyelosis with marrow fibrosis (see below), transforming myelofibrosis (usually associated with substantial splenomegaly), myelodysplastic syndromes with myelofibrosis, metastatic tumors and blast transformation of chronic myeloid leukemia. In young children and infants the disease may present with hepatosplenomegaly and abdominal masses in association with t(1;22)(p13;q13).

Acute basophilic leukemia

AML with some or many basophils, including blasts with scanty basophil granules and basophil myelocytes, is extremely rare. Toluidine blue is a specific stain for basophil and mast-cell granules, not routinely used in the diagnosis of AML. A systematic study of the Romanowsky stains from 750 patients with AML showed 1% or more (maximum 27%) basophils in only 34 cases, an incidence of 0.5%.[145] Toluidine blue staining confirmed the presence of basophils in all cases with available slides. This incidence may be a slight underestimate as some leukemic basophils are agranular and recognizable only on electron microscopy when the characteristic granules showing scrolls and lamellae are visualized.[146] Blast cells may show a few clustered basophil granules (type II equivalent

369

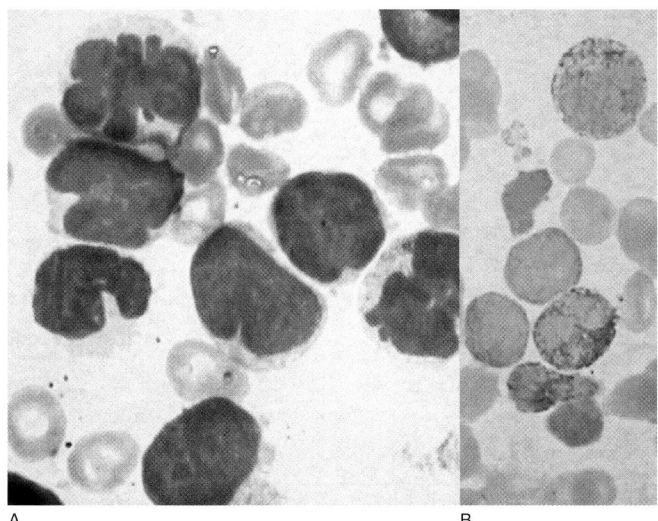

A   B

Fig. 20.18 Acute basophilic leukemia. (A) May–Grünwald–Giemsa stain. The blasts are devoid of granules or Auer rods. The dysplastic mature basophils show nuclei with multiple overlapping segments, pink cytoplasm and scanty ill-defined granules. (B) Toluidine blue stain. Three cells show distinctive metachromatic granule positivity.

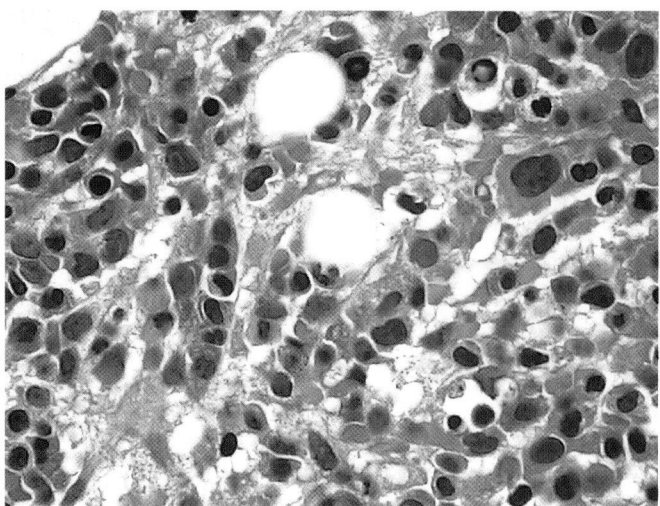

Fig. 20.19 Acute panmyelosis with marrow fibrosis. Hematoxylin and eosin. The marrow shows marked fibrosis with many atypical megakaryocytes. Blasts, erythroid precursors and granulocytes are present.

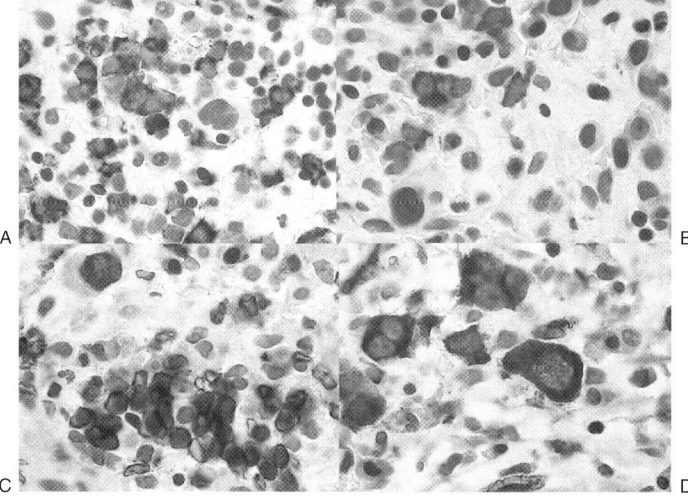

A   B

C   D

Fig. 20.20 Same case as Figure 20.19. Immunoperoxidase stains. (A) Anti-CD34 identifying blast cells. (B) Anti-myeloperoxidase showing granulocyte precursors. (C) Anti-glycophorin C showing left-shifted erythroid precursors. (D) Anti-Factor VIII highlighting the atypical megakaryocytes of various sizes.

of myeloblasts), and promyelocytes and myelocytes show increased numbers of basophil granules, with a basophilic background cytoplasm. Mature basophils may be dysplastic and show scanty or small granules. Their cytoplasm may be reticular and vacuolated. Mature basophils show overlapping 'flower-like' nuclear segments, and this feature in agranular segmented cells should prompt a toluidine blue stain (Fig. 20.18). There is a common but not absolute association of increased basophils with the t(6;9)(p23;q34) and possibly with chromosome 12p abnormalities.[147,148] Basophils of all stages may be scanty. Unless specifically sought, small numbers of basophils in AML may be overlooked. Blast cells are negative for MPO and SBB, but positive blasts are present if there is a significant granulocyte component, and Auer rods may be present. The PAS stain may show large irregular positive blocks or lakes of brightly positive material in mature basophils but not the blasts.[149] Chloroacetate staining is negative, but may be difficult to interpret in the presence of granulocytes. The majority of reported cases with increased basophils have been classified as M2 or M4 in the FAB classification and trilineage dysplasia may be present. Patients may exhibit skin and gut symptoms suggestive of histamine excess.[149] Prognosis is uncertain, with poor outcomes reported, but no significant difference was found in a large randomized trial.[145] The WHO defines acute basophilic leukemia as 'an acute myeloid leukemia in which the primary differentiation is to basophils' but without specifying a minimum percentage of identifiable basophil lineage cells.

Acute panmyelosis with marrow fibrosis

This rare entity is characterized by an acute clinical onset, pancytopenia, minimal organomegaly, and a fibrotic marrow containing more than 20% blasts and significant trilineage hemopoiesis which is usually dysplastic (Figs 20.19 and 20.20). It differs from megakaryocytic leukemia (M7), in which granulopoiesis and erythropoiesis are reduced and abnormal megakaryocytes and blasts predominate. Myelofibrosis is distinguishable by the presence of substantial splenomegaly and absence of the requisite blast component.

The marrow is generally not aspirable, and the blast component is quantified by immunohistochemical staining of the biopsy for CD34[+] cells. The unequivocal demonstration of more than 20% blasts is critical to the diagnosis. Some of the cases described as malignant myelosclerosis,[150,151] acute myelodysplasia with myelofibrosis[152] and acute myelofibrosis[153] correspond to acute panmyelosis with myelofibrosis. The importance of blast cell immunohistochemistry in distinguishing this entity from M7 has been emphasized.[153] The borderline between fibrotic forms of AML and myelodysplastic syndromes with marrow fibrosis also presents difficulties, but the majority of difficult cases can be resolved by appropriate immunohistochemistry identifying blasts, megakaryocytes, granulocytes and erythroid precursors.[154,155]

Hypocellular forms of AML

Up to 10% of patients with AML have a hypocellular marrow at the time of diagnosis. They are predominantly older male patients with severe leukopenia and frequently pancytopenia.[156,157] Overall marrow cellularity is less than 50%. Typically marrow architecture and fat cells are preserved, with the blasts replacing normal hemopoiesis, particularly the granulocytes (Fig. 20.21). Blasts are required to be more than 20% of nucleated cells, and are frequently small and agranular, with scanty or absent myeloperoxidase positivity.[157,158] Multilineage

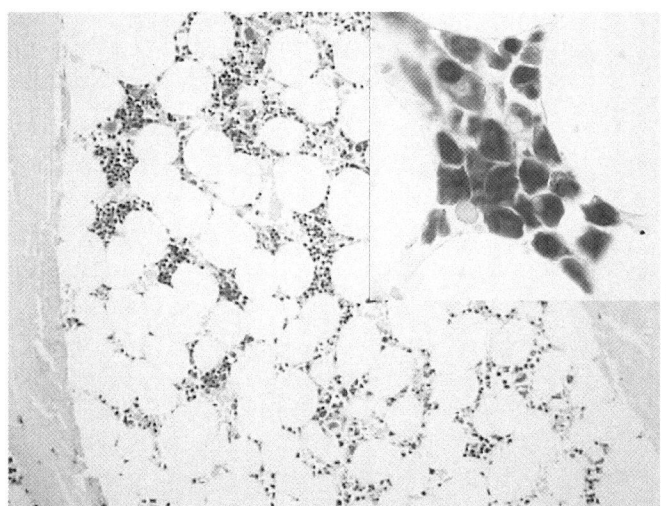

B

A

Fig. 20.21 Hypocellular AML. (A) Hematoxylin and eosin stain. Trephine biopsy from a 76-year-old man with anemia and neutropenia, showing reduced cellularity but preserved fat and architecture. The more cellular areas show preservation of megakaryocytes. (B) A cluster of small blast cells replacing normal hemopoiesis.

dysplasia may be present,[156] but cytogenetic abnormalities are not typical of those seen in MDS.[158]

Extramedullary AML (chloromas, granulocytic sarcomas)

Extramedullary AML may occur prior to any evidence of marrow disease, concurrently with marrow and blood disease or as a manifestation of relapse. Any part of the body may be affected, and detection is biased towards sites that are superficially obvious or cause symptoms, particularly neurological. Children may be more commonly affected, with up to 25% showing evidence of extramedullary disease (including the central nervous system), at diagnosis,[159] but much lower incidence figures have been found in other large studies.[160] Monocytic and myelomonocytic AML, particularly with hyperleukocytosis, tend to cause skin, gum, lymph node and hepatosplenic infiltrates, whereas granulocytic or multilineage disease tends to give rise to solid deposits (chloromas, granulocytic sarcomas). The t(8;21) is the most frequently reported association with solid leukemic deposits, followed by cases with inv(16) and its variants. When extramedullary AML presents prior to marrow disease there is a significant rate of misdiagnosis.[161] Tumors without hemopoietic cell maturation are more easily misdiagnosed, with lymphoma the most frequent inaccurate diagnosis.[162]

Typically, extramedullary AML shows a diffuse infiltrate of mononuclear cells. Maturing granulocytes and eosinophils may be present, but in their absence the leukemic cells may be confused with large cell lymphomas or atypical carcinomas. The diagnosis, once suspected, can be established in virtually all cases by immunohistochemistry with a panel of monoclonal antibodies that recognize CD45, CD43, CD34, CD13, CD33, CD117, myeloperoxidase, lysozyme, CD68, CD14, CD15, Factor VIII or CD61 and glycophorin A.[163] Myeloperoxidase, HLA-DR and CD68 are the most frequently positive antigens.[163] Antibodies to CD3, CD79a and CD20 should be included as negative controls and to identify lymphoid tumors; occasional CD3 positivity in AML tumors has been reported by some authors[164] but not others.[162]

CNS leukemia in AML

Involvement of the central nervous system (CNS) with blast cells in the cerebrospinal fluid (CSF) is rare in AML. The incidence in patients of all ages was found to be 0.5% in one large study, which also showed the ineffectiveness of CNS chemoprophylaxis.[165] The incidence in children is higher, approximately 5%.[159,160] In the presence of a high peripheral blood blast count, any contamination of the CSF with blood precludes accurate diagnosis of CNS disease. The diagnosis is usually obvious on CSF cytology, but when blast cells are scanty cytochemical MPO or immunohistochemical evidence of immunoreactive MPO is usually diagnostic. In monocytic leukemias NSE positivity should be sought. Viral encephalitis can mimic CNS disease, in which case immunohistochemistry for CD3 and CD79 is helpful. Isolated CNS disease may occur as a first indication of relapse, with inevitable subsequent marrow relapse.

Immunophenotypic diagnosis of AML

Multiparameter flow cytometry forms a major component of the diagnostic strategy for the investigation, diagnosis and post-treatment monitoring of AML. The effective use of flow cytometry requires a detailed knowledge of the normal distribution and strength of expression of membrane antigens or clusters of differentiation (CD) on all hematopoietic cells. Immunophenotyping results should always be interpreted in the context of morphologic, cytochemical and clinical findings before a definitive diagnosis is established. In most cases multiparameter flow cytometry can provide precise phenotypic data on the leukemic cells, often on a background of residual normal hematopoietic cells. This is achieved using a variety of gating procedures based on either physical characteristics of blasts cells (forward and sideways light scatter), immunophenotypic characteristics (fluorescence) or a combination of both, usually side scatter versus either CD45 or CD34.[166] As leukemic blast cells show weaker CD45 expression than residual normal hematopoietic cells, the most reliable approach is to use CD45/SSC gating to identify blast cells. The alternative strategy of using CD34/SSC plots is unsuitable for CD34⁻ cases. CD34/SSC gating is extremely effective for characterizing small populations of blast cells typically seen in myelodysplasia, CML and in the detection of minimal residual disease in AML.

Immunophenotyping studies using a comprehensive standardized panel of monoclonal antibodies should be routinely applied to all new presentation cases of AML. The use of extensive panels is less important for establishing initial diagnosis than for uncovering aberrant phenotypes that can be applied to minimal residual disease (MRD) detection following chemotherapy. Although no international standard or guideline exists that specifies which antibodies to use or which combi-

nations are most effective, it is essential that a wide range of well-characterized antigens be studied. These should include lymphoid as well as myeloid antigens. Platelet and erythroid antigens should also be included, along with those antigens also only normally expressed on mature myeloid cells.

In the majority of cases, immunophenotyping can distinguish lymphoid from myeloid blast cells if appropriate panels of monoclonal antibodies are used. The cases that present the most diagnostic difficulty are those of undifferentiated stem cells which show no lineage commitment and those cases of acute lymphoblastic leukemia with coexpression of myeloid antigens. However, as progenitor differentiation pathways become more clearly defined, it is apparent that antigens previously regarded as myeloid or lymphoid specific are expressed on progenitor cells prior to lineage commitment or in the very early stages of precursor cell differentiation.

In the absence of a clinically relevant immunophenotypic classification of AML, immunophenotypic findings are discussed in the context of morphologic subtypes, including correlations between specific cytogenetic abnormalities, morphology and immunophenotype.

Poorly differentiated AML

The FAB types M0 and M1 are probably indistinguishable by membrane immunophenotype, with the majority of cases expressing CD34, CD13 and/or CD33, CD117 and HLA-DR. A proportion of cases also express CD7 and/or TdT. A CD7⁺ TdT⁺ phenotype in AML is associated with a poor prognosis.[167]

AML with evidence of maturation (AML-M2)

This morphologic subtype of AML characteristically shows myeloid maturation and fewer blast cells than in M1. By flow cytometry this can be seen as fewer CD34⁺ blasts and an increase in CD15⁺ mature myeloid cells. Of major importance for this group of patients is identification of the t(8;21) which is a good prognostic marker in adults. It has been reported that CD19 expression in this subtype correlates with the presence of t(8;21).[168,169] However, CD56 expression in AML with t(8;21) is associated with shorter remission duration and survival.[170,171]

Acute promyelocytic leukemia (AML-M3)

Rapid, definitive diagnosis of both hyper- and hypogranular variants of acute promyelocytic leukemia

(APML) is essential. It is usually recognized by its distinct morphologic appearance, though a proportion of cases present where morphologic appearances are not clear-cut as is often seen with the hypogranular variant. In these cases, flow cytometry can be useful in confirming diagnosis. Previous studies demonstrated a CD9+CD15– phenotype for the abnormal promyelocytes though this phenotype is not unique to APML.[172] Similarly, a CD34– HLA-DR-phenotype is commonly seen, but again this is not specific. Orfao and co-workers report that expression of CD13, the existence of a single major blast cell population and a characteristic CD15/CD34 staining pattern can provide a reliable method for the differential diagnosis of APML from other AML types.[173] An alternative approach is to use an immunofluorescent technique using an antibody to identify the specifically abnormal intranuclear pattern of the PML-RARα fusion protein created as a consequence of the t(15;17). Though not applicable to flow cytometry, the slide technique is rapid (results available within 2 h), shows good correlation with PCR- and FISH-based reference methods and appears specific for APML.[174]

Acute myelomonocytic leukemia (AML-M4)

In contrast to the previous categories of AML where only a single population of myeloid cells is present, M4 is characterized by an increase in abnormal monocytes and myeloid blast cells. Flow cytometry studies of M4 highlight two distinct populations (Fig. 20.22), a monocytic component exhibiting some CD14 and strong HLA-DR expression, and a myeloid component that may be undifferentiated as in M0/M1 or show differentiation as in M2.

Acute monocytic leukemia (AML-M5)

There are no satisfactory immunophenotypic markers that discriminate monoblasts from promonocytes or monocytes. The majority of acute monocytic leukemias are strongly CD33+, CD15+ and HLA-DR+ with variable expression of CD14. CD64 (FcRI) is strongly expressed and the majority of cases are CD13– and CD34–.

Acute myeloid leukemia M6 and M7

AML M6 and M7 are rare subtypes and particularly for M6 (erythroid) not well characterized by flow cytometry. Expression of erythroid antigens such as the glycophorin molecules or CD71 on blast cells is evidence of erythroid

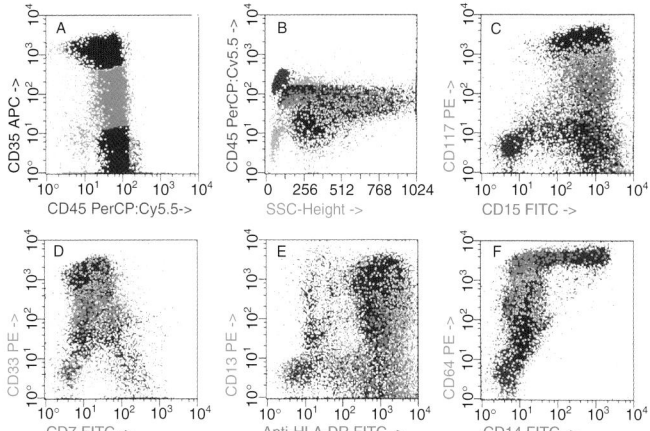

Fig. 20.22 Four color flow cytometry analysis of an acute myelomonocytic leukemia with inv(16). Four combinations of directly conjugated monoclonal antibodies were used to characterize the blast cells: (i) CD15/CD117/CD45/CD34; (ii) CD7/CD33/CD45/CD34; (iii) HLA-DR/CD13/CD45/CD34; (iv) CD14/CD64/CD45/CD34. Analysis of CD34 versus CD45 expression (plot a) and CD45 versus Sideways Light Scatter (plot b) allows clear delineation of (i) undifferentiated blast cells (CD34+++CD45+++); (ii) differentiating blast cells (CD34intermediate+CD45+); (iii) monocytic component (CD34negativeCD45+) and (iv) lymphocytes (CD45+++SSClow). Plot (c) shows the undifferentiated and differentiating myeloid blast cell components to be CD117+CD15+. In contrast, the monocytic component is mainly CD15+CD117–. Plot (d) shows heterogeneous expression of the myeloid antigen CD33 on all leukemic populations. Plot (e) shows the undifferentiated myeloid blast cells to be CD14+HLA-DR+. The differentiating component is losing CD13 expression though retaining HLA-DR expression. The monocytic component is HLA-DR+ with weaker CD13 expression. Plot (f) shows the undifferentiated blast cells to be weakly CD64+, and the differentiating component has intermediate levels of CD64 expression. The monocytic component is heterogeneous with immature forms.

lineage commitment. Acute megakaryoblastic leukemia is well recognized in the context of *de novo* AML or arising from transforming CML. Expression of the platelet antigens CD41, CD42b and/or CD61 by blast cells can be shown by flow cytometry, though it is essential that positive results are confirmed by alkaline phosphatase anti-alkaline phosphatase (APAAP) techniques as platelet adherence to leukemic blasts is a frequent cause of false-positive results.

Detection of residual disease

Standard morphologic criteria for assessing remission attainment are insensitive and subjective. As many as 1×10^{10} residual leukemic blasts may still be present at the end of treatment.[35] The more sensitive molecular methods for monitoring the minority of patients with known cytogenetic abnormalities have gained wide acceptance. Although there are no leukemia-specific antigens that can be studied by flow cytometry, the presence of aberrant phenotypes in many cases of AML provides a marker with which to distinguish these cells from their normal counterparts.[36] Many of the combinations of antibodies used for detecting MRD in AML are customized for individual patients and rely on using an extensive panel of antibodies at presentation.[175] Studies have shown that patients with greater than 5 leukemic cells per 1000 normal cells in first remission show a higher rate of relapse and shorter median relapse-free survival than patients with less than 5 leukemic cells per 1000 normal bone marrow cells.[175]

Cytogenetics in AML

Chromosomal abnormalities are detectable by metaphase cytogenetics in approximately 60% of patients. The two commonest balanced translocations t(8;21) and t(15;17) confer a better prognosis. Abnormalities of 16p13, either inv(16) or t(16;16) probably confer a moderate advantage. In contrast, complex (> 5) abnormalities, monosomy 5, 5q deletions and monosomy 7, whether occurring in *de novo* or therapy-related AML, confer a poor prognosis.[94] Abnormalities of 3q21/q26 are also an adverse finding. The t(9;22)(q34;q11) is an extremely rare occurrence in *de novo* AML and is an adverse feature. Other rare recurring translocations, for example t(6;9)(p23;q34) and t(8;16) (p11;p13), are of indeterminate prognostic significance. Numerical abnormalities are generally of neutral prognostic significance, including trisomy 8 which is present as the sole or additional abnormality in 10% of AML cases. Less than 50% of patients with AML have a prognostically significant cytogenetic abnormality.[94] Table 20.5 summarizes the main abnormalities in AML.

Table 20.5 Principal chromosomal abnormalities in acute myeloid leukemia (AML)

Chromosomal abnormality	Genes involved	Methods of detection	Clinicopathologic correlations
t(8;21)(q22;q22)	AML1-ETO	Metaphase PCR FISH	Younger age Distinctive morphology (M2, M1, MDS) Good prognosis
t(15;17)(q22;q21)	PML-RARα	Metaphase PCR FISH	Younger age Distinctive morphology Good prognosis Response to ATRA
Inv(16)(p13;q22) t(16;16)(p13;q22)	CBFβ-MYH11	Metaphase PCR FISH	Younger age Distinctive morphology Good prognosis
Complex (> 5) abnormalities, –7, 5q–, –5		Metaphase	Secondary and *de novo* AML Multilineage dysplasia Poor prognosis
t(v;11)(v;q23)	MLL	Metaphase FISH Multiple PCR	Mainly monocytic/myelomonocytic AML Secondary to topoisomerase II inhibitors Average prognosis in adults Poor prognosis in infants
Inv(3)(q21;q26) t(3;3)(q21;q26)	EVII (3q26)	Metaphase	Often megakaryoblastic Platelets normal or raised in 30–50% Additional abnormalities frequent
t(6;9)(p23;q34)	DEK-CAN	Metaphase PCR FISH	Associated basophilia, multilineage dysplasia
t(9;22)(q34;q11)	BCR-ABL	Metaphase PCR FISH	Undifferentiated, M1, M2 Poor prognosis Rare < 1%
t(8;16)(p11;p13)	MOZ-CBF	Metaphase FISH	Monocytic/myelomonocytic AML Erythrophagocytosis Prognosis uncertain
t(1;22)(p13;q13)		Metaphase	Megakaryoblastic disease Predominantly infants, some children Additional abnormalities common

ATRA, All-trans-retinoic acid; FISH, fluorescent *in situ* hybridization; MDS, myelodysplastic syndrome; PCR, polymerase chain reaction.

Molecular diagnosis in AML

In the last 15 years the majority of commonly occurring acute leukemia-associated translocations have been cloned. Although Southern hybridization is still considered the gold standard for the molecular detection of gene rearrangements it is now seldom used due to the labor-intensive nature of the procedure and the time constraints within a clinical setting. With the advent and widespread use of PCR techniques the rapid demonstration of significant translocations is possible. Three abnormalities in particular have become diagnostic hallmarks in AML. The t(15;17) is always associated with acute promyelocytic leukemia.[176] Cases of AML with inv(16) or less commonly a t(16;16) show characteristic morphology and CBFβ/MYH11 fusion transcripts.[177] A close morphologic association is also seen in cases of AML with a t(8;21), particularly if stringent morphologic criteria are adhered to.[102] There is clear evidence that metaphase cytogenetics does not always detect these translocations, mainly due to obtaining only normal metaphases, or less commonly failure to obtain any metaphases.[94,96,178] Normal metaphases in AML may be the result of division of residual normal cells, for example erythroid precursors, or the presence of cryptic translocations and insertions.[108]

The t(15;17) results in the disruption of the RARα gene, located at 17q21 and its subsequent fusion to amino terminal sequences derived from the PML gene at 15q22. 'Variant' translocations where RARα is fused to a partner gene other than PML occur extremely rarely, but do not give rise to the typical morphology of APML.[107,179] Analogous to its use in Ph¹-positive ALL, RT-PCR provides information on the configuration of the breakpoints in APML.[180] Demonstration of the reciprocal RARα/PML fusion gene has also been used to provide important confirmatory information.[181]

The inv(16) fuses the core binding factor β (CBFβ) gene at 16q22 to the myosin heavy chain 11 gene (MYH11) at 16p13. The metaphase appearances of the translocation are subtle, and may be difficult to identify, particularly if not suspected morphologically. Breakpoints within CBFβ are generally conserved, although a number of different breakpoints within MYH11 have been reported.[182] A robust RT-PCR has recently been developed capable of detecting the majority of breakpoints associated with this abnormality.[62] Although invariably positive in cases of M4Eo, the translocation has also been described in other AML subtypes.[119,183]

The t(8;21)(q22;q22) fuses the AML1 gene on chromosome 21q22 to the ETO (previously designated MTG-8) gene on 8q22. Breakpoints are conserved in both genes, occurring between exons 5 and 6 in AML1 and exons 1 and 2 in the ETO gene. Design of a simple RT-PCR strategy for this aberration is possible due to the conservation of these breakpoints. The AML1 gene is also involved in a number of other translocations associated with acute leukemia including the t(12;21), t(3;21) and t(16;21).[184,185]

Disruption of the MLL gene is also frequently detectable in cases of AML, and as in ALL, the gene fuses with a large number of partner chromosomes. Disruption of this gene is best demonstrated by FISH-based techniques.[66]

Residual disease monitoring in AML

Leukemia-associated chimeric fusion genes offer a sensitive and specific target for residual disease monitoring in AML. RT-PCR can routinely detect one leukemic cell in 10^5 normal cells, except in the t(15;17) where the sensitivity is of the order of one cell in 10^4. However detection of the PML/RARα fusion gene following the third course of chemotherapy in the current MRC AML clinical trials predicts a poor outcome.[111] Serial quantification of the level of residual disease in these patients gives predictive information and is able to distinguish patients destined to relapse. In contrast, PCR monitoring in AML with the t(8;21) is less informative, as long-term survivors frequently remain PCR positive.[186,187] Competitive PCR has been used to quantify the level of residual disease in AML using a number of molecular targets.[183,188] Preliminary data monitoring the level of AML1/ETO transcripts in remission has identified a threshold of residual disease above which relapse is inevitable.[189] As with quantification of residual disease in ALL, competitive PCR is likely to be superseded by RQ-PCR.

Acute biphenotypic leukemia

In the early and mid-1980s it became apparent that antigens thought to be lineage restricted (myeloid or lymphoid) could be found unexpectedly on leukemic blasts in both ALL and AML. Considerable confusion was caused by the finding of TdT, initially thought to be specific for lymphoblasts, in cases of AML. This gave rise to the concepts of lineage 'infidelity' or 'promiscuity'.[190,191] Increasing numbers of apparently lineage-specific monoclonal antibodies further complicated matters. Some of the confusing data were due to technical variations, some to the cut-off points for designating blast

Table 20.6 Scoring system for defining biphenotypic acute leukemia. Cases scoring 2 points or more from two separate lineages are defined as biphenotypic

Points scored	B lineage	T lineage	Myeloid lineage
2	CD79a cyt IgM cyt CD22	cyt CD3 or surface CD3 anti-TCRα/β anti-TCRγ/δ	Anti-MPO (anti-lysozyme)
1	CD19 CD10 CD20	CD2 CD5 CD8 CD10	CD13 CD33 CDw65
0.5	TdT CD24	TdT CD7 CD1a	CD14 CD15 CD64 CD117

cells as positive or negative (e.g. 10%, 20% etc.), and some due to the limitations of single color flow cytometry or immunocytochemistry. This led to marked variation in the percentage of cases designated as biphenotypic. Recognition of the key roles of surface or cytoplasmic CD3 (T-lineage), CD79 (B-lineage) and myeloperoxidase (cytochemical or anti-MPO positive), led to structured scoring systems where these three features counted more heavily than other surface or internal antigens, which were recognized to be less strictly lineage specific.[192] In 1995 the European Group for the Immunological Characterization of Leukemias (EGIL) proposed a scoring system for defining acute biphenotypic leukemias (Table 20.6).[193] Biphenotypic leukemias appear to show a high frequency of chromosome abnormalities, particularly the t(9;22) and 11q23 abnormalities.[194] The commonest lineage combination was the coexpression of B-lineage and myeloid markers, with less frequent expression of T-lineage and myeloid markers. Cases with mixed T- and B-lineage markers or all three lineages are rare. Approximately 5% of acute leukemias meet the criteria for biphenotypic disease.[195,196] Response to treatment is poor, in keeping with the unfavorable cytogenetic abnormalities that are common in this group of patients.[195,196] Establishing the true incidence of biphenotypic acute leukemia will require large studies utilizing multicolor flow cytometry routinely including all the antibodies required by the scoring system, with systematic inclusion of techniques for detecting cytoplasmic expression of CD3, MPO and CD79, and nuclear TdT.

REFERENCES

1. Bennett JM, Catovsky D, Daniel MT et al 1976 Proposals for the classification of the acute leukaemias. British Journal of Haematology 33: 451–458

2. Bennett JM, Catovsky D, Daniel MT et al 1985 Proposed revised criteria for the classification of acute myeloid leukaemia. Annals of Internal Medicine 103: 626–629

3. Bennett JM, Catovsky D, Daniel MT et al 1985 Criteria for the diagnosis of acute leukemia of megakaryocytic lineage (M7). A report of the French–American–British Cooperative Group. Annals of Internal Medicine 103: 460–462

4. Bennett JM, Catovsky D, Daniel MT et al 1991 proposals for the recognition of minimally differentiated acute myeloid leukaemia (AML-M0). British Journal of Haematology 78: 325–329

5. Harris NL, Jaffe ES, Diebold J et al 1999 World Health Organization classification of neoplastic diseases of the hematopoietic and lymphoid tissues: Report of the Clinical Advisory Committee meeting-Airlie House, Virginia, November 1997. Journal of Clinical Oncology 17: 3835–3849

6. Jaffe E, Harris N, Stein H, Vardiman J (eds) 2001 World Health Organization classification of tumours. Pathology and genetics of tumours of haematopopietic and lymphoid tissues. IARC Press, Lyon

7. Breatnach F, Chessells JM, Greaves MF et al 1981 The aplastic presentation of childhood leukaemia: a feature of common-ALL. British Journal of Haematology 49: 387–393

8. Hasle H, Heim S, Schroeder H et al 1995 Transient pancytopenia preceding acute lymphoblastic leukemia (pre-ALL). Leukemia 9: 605–608

9. Lessard M, Fenneteau O, Sainty D et al 1993 Translocation t(1;19) in acute lymphoblastic leukemia patients with cytological presentation simulating L3-ALL (Burkitt-like). Leukemia and Lymphoma 11: 149–152

10. Harris NL, Jaffe ES, Stein H et al 1994 A revised European–American classification of lymphoid neoplasms: a proposal from the International Lymphoma Study Group. Blood 84: 1361–1392

11. Catovsky D, Bernasconi C, Verdonck PJ et al 1980 The association of eosinophilia with lymphoblastic leukaemia or lymphoma: a study of seven patients. British Journal of Haematology 45: 523–34

12. Bottone E, Macchia P, Consolini R et al 1982 Acute lymphoblastic leukaemia first appearing as hypereosinophilia. European Journal of Pediatrics 138: 85–88

13. Baumgarten E, Wegner RD, Fengler R et al 1989 Calla-positive acute leukaemia with t(5q;14q) translocation and hypereosinophilia – a unique entity? Acta Haematologica 82: 85–90

14. Tricot G, Broeckart-van Orshoven A, van Hoof A, Verwilghen RL 1982 Sudan black B positivity in acute lymphoblastic leukaemia. British Journal of Haematology 51: 615–621

15. Stass SA, Pui C-H, Melvin S et al 1982 Sudan black B positive acute lymphoblastic leukaemia. British Journal of Haematology 57: 413–421

16. Crockard AD 1984 Cytochemistry of lymphoid cells: a review of findings in the normal and leukaemic state. Histochemical Journal 16: 1027–1050

17. Hayhoe FGJ, Quaglino D 1988 Haematological cytochemistry. Churchill Livingstone, Edinburgh

18. McKenna RW, Parkin J, Brunning RD 1979 Morphological and ultrastructural characteristics of T-cell acute lymphoblastic leukemia. Cancer 44: 1290–1297

19. Hann IM, Evans DIK, Marsden HB et al 1978 Bone marrow fibrosis in acute lymphoblastic leukaemia of childhood. Journal of Clinical Pathology 31: 313–315

20. Wallis JP, Reid MM 1989 Bone marrow fibrosis in childhood acute lymphoblastic leukaemia. Journal of Clinical Pathology 42: 1253–1254

21. Habboush HW, Hann IM 1987 Bone marrow necrosis in acute lymphoblastic leukaemia. Scottish Medical Journal 32: 177–180

22. Groeneveld K, te Marvelde JG, van den Beemd MWM et al 1996 Flow cytometric detection of intracellular antigens for immunophenotyping of normal and malignant leukocytes. Leukemia 10: 1383–1389

23. Kappelmayer J, Gratama JW, Karaszi E et al 2000 Flow cytometric detection of intracellular myeloperoxidase, CD3 and CD79a. Interaction between monoclonal antibody clones, fluorochromes and sample preparation protocols. Journal of Immunological Methods 242: 53–65

24. Hann IM, Richards SM, Eden OB, Hill FG 1998 Analysis of the immunophenotype of children treated on the Medical Research Council United Kingdom Acute Lymphoblastic Leukaemia Trial XI (MRC UKALLXI). Medical Research Council Childhood Leukaemia Working Party. Leukemia 8: 1249–1255

25. De Zen L, Orfao A, Cazzaniga G et al 2000 Quantitative multiparametric immunophenotyping in acute lymphoblastic

leukemia: correlation with specific genotype. I. ETV6/AML1 ALLs identification. Leukemia 7: 1225–1231

26. Borowitz MJ, Rubnitz J, Nash M et al 1998 Surface antigen phenotype can predict TEL-AML1 rearrangement in childhood B-precursor ALL: a Pediatric Oncology Group study. Leukemia 11: 1764–1770

27. Pui CH, Raimondi SC, Hancock ML et al 1994 Immunologic, cytogenetic, and clinical characterization of childhood acute lymphoblastic leukemia with the t(1;19) (q23;p13) or its derivative. Journal of Clinical Oncology 12: 2601–2606

28. Borowitz MJ, Hunger SP, Carroll AJ et al 1993 Predictability of the t(1;19)(q23;p13) from surface antigen phenotype: implications for screening cases of childhood acute lymphoblastic leukemia for molecular analysis: a Pediatric Oncology Group study. Blood 82: 1086–1091

29. Behm FG, Smith FO, Raimondi SC et al 1996 Human homologue of the rat chondroitin sulfate proteoglycan, NG2, detected by monoclonal antibody 7.1, identifies childhood acute lymphoblastic leukemias with t(4;11)(q21;q23) or t(11;19)(q23;p13) and MLL gene rearrangements. Blood 87: 1134–1139

30. Tabernero MD, Bortoluci AM, Alaejos I et al 2001 Adult precursor B-ALL with BCR/ABL gene rearrangements displays a unique immunophenotype based on the pattern of CD10, CD34, CD13 and CD38 expression. Leukemia 15: 406–414

31. Klobusicka M, Babusikova O 1998 Immunophenotypic characteristics of T-acute lymphoblastic leukemia cells in relation to DPP IV enzyme expression. Neoplasma 45: 237–242

32. Thiel E, Kranz BR, Raghavachar A et al 1989 Prethymic phenotype and genotype of pre-T (CD7+/ER–)-cell leukemia and its clinical significance within adult acute lymphoblastic leukemia. Blood 73: 1247–1258

33. Schott G, Sperling C, Schrappe M et al 1998 Immunophenotypic and clinical features of T-cell receptor gammadelta+ T-lineage acute lymphoblastic leukaemia. British Journal of Haematology 101: 753–755

34. Vervoordeldonk SF, Merle PA, Behrendt H et al 1996 Triple immunofluorescence staining for prediction of relapse in childhood precursor B acute lymphoblastic leukaemia. British Journal of Haematology 92: 922–928

35. Campana D, Pui CH 1995 Detection of minimal residual disease in acute leukemia: methodological advances and clinical significance. Blood 85: 1416–1434

36. Campana D, Coustan-Smith E 1999 Detection of minimal residual disease in acute leukemia by flow cytometry. Cytometry (Communications in Clinical Cytometry) 38: 139–152

37. Porwit-MacDonald A, Bjorklund E, Lucio P et al 2000 BIOMED-1 concerted action report: flow cytometric characterization of CD7+ cell subsets in normal bone marrow as a basis for the diagnosis and follow-up of T cell acute lymphoblastic leukemia (T-ALL). Leukemia 14: 816–825

38. Ciudad J, San Miguel JF, Lopez-Berges MC et al 1999 Detection of abnormalities in B-cell differentiation pattern is a useful tool to predict relapse in precursor-B-ALL. British Journal of Haematology 104: 695–705

39. Secker-Walker LM, Prentice HG, Durrant J et al 1997 Cytogenetics adds independent prognostic information in adults with acute lymphoblastic leukaemia on MRC trial UKALL XA. British Journal of Haematology 96: 601–610

40. Reider H, Bonwetsch C, Janssen LA et al 1998 High rate of chromosome abnormalities detected by fluorescence in situ hybridization using BCR and ABL probes in adult acute lymphoblastic leukemia. Leukemia 12: 1473–1481

41. Groupe Francais de Cytogenetique Hematologique 1996 Cytogenetic abnormalities in adult acute lymphoblastic leukemia: correlations with hematologic findings and outcome. A collaborative study of the Groupe Francais de Cytogenetique hematologique. Blood 87: 3135–3142

42. Chessels JM, Swansbury GJ, Reeves B et al 1997 Cytogenetics and prognosis in childhood lymphoblastic leukaemia: results of MRC UKALL X. British Journal of Haematology 99: 93–100

43. Pui C-H, Evans WE 1998 Acute lymphoblastic leukaemia. New England Journal of Medicine 339: 605–615

44. Pui CH 2000 Acute lymphoblastic leukaemia in children. Current Opinion in Oncology 12: 3–12

45. Ludwig WD, Reider H, Bartram CR et al 1998 Immunophenotypic and genotypic features, clinical characteristics and treatment outcome of adult pro-B acute lymphoblastic leukaemia: results of the German multicenter trials GMALL 03/87 and 04/89. Blood 92: 1898–1909

46. Heerema NA, Sather HN, Sensel MG et al 2000 Prognostic significance of cytogenetic abnormalities of chromosome arm 12p in childhood acute lymphoblastic leukaemia: a report from the Children's Cancer Group. Cancer 88: 1945–1954

47. Heerema NA, Sather HN, Sensel MG et al 2000 Clinical significance of deletions of chromosome arm 6q in childhood acute lymphoblastic leukaemia: a report from the Children's Cancer Group. Leukemia and Lymphoma 36: 467–478

48. Arico M, Valsecchi MG, Camitta B et al 2000 Outcome of treatment in children with Philadelphia chromosome positive acute lymphoblastic leukemia. New England Journal of Medicine 342: 998–1006

49. Heerema NA, Sather HN, Ge J et al 1999 Cytogenetic studies of infant acute lymphoblastic leukemia: poor prognosis of infants with t(4;11) – a report of the Children's cancer Group. Leukemia 13: 679–696

50. Crist WM, Carroll AJ, Shuster JJ et al 1990 Poor prognosis of children with pre-B acute lymphoblastic leukemia is associated with the t(1;19)(q23;p13): a pediatric oncology group study. Blood 76: 117–122

51. Uckun FM, Sensel MG, Sather HN et al 1998 Clinical significance of translocation t(1;19) in childhood acute lymphoblastic leukemia in the context of contemporary therapies: a report from the Children's Cancer Group. Journal of Clinical Oncology 16: 527–535

52. Heerema NA, Nachman JB, Sather HN et al 1999 Hypodiploidy with less than 45 chromosomes confers adverse risk in childhood acute lymphoblastic leukemia: a report from the children's cancer group. Blood 94: 4036–4045

53. Harbott J, Viehmann S, Borkhardt A et al 1997 Incidence of TEL/AML1 fusion gene analyzed consecutively in children with acute lymphoblastic leukemia in relapse. Blood 90: 4933–4937

54. Heerema NA, Sather HN, Sensel MG et al 1998 Frequency and clinical significance of cytogenetic abnormalities in pediatric T-lineage acute lymphoblastic leukemia: a report from the Children's Cancer Group. Journal of Clinical Oncology 16: 1270–1278

55. Schneider NR, Carroll AJ, Shuster JJ et al 2000 New recurring cytogenetic abnormalities and association of blast cell karyotypes with prognosis in childhood T-cell acute lymphoblastic leukemia: a Pediatric Oncology Group report of 343 cases. Blood 96: 2543–2549

56. Bernards A, Rubin CM, Westbrook CA et al 1987 The first intron in the human c-abl gene is at least 200 kilobases long and is a target for translocations in chronic myelogenous leukemia. Moleleculc Cell Biology 7: 3231–3236

57. Hermans A, Gow J, Selleri L et al 1988 bcr-abl oncogene activation in Philadelphia chromosome-positive acute lymphoblastic leukemia. Leukemia 2: 628–633

58. Heisterkamp N, Stam K, Groffen J et al Structural organization of the bcr gene and its role in the Ph' translocation. Nature 315: 758–761

59. Catovsky D 1979 Ph1-positive acute leukaemia and chronic granulocytic leukaemia: one or two diseases? British Journal of Haematology 42: 493–498

60. Williams DL, Look AT, Melvin SL et al 1984 New chromosomal translocations correlate with specific immunophenotypes of childhood acute lymphoblastic leukemia. Cell 36: 101–109

61. Carroll AJ, Crist WM, Parmley RT et al 1984 Pre-B cell leukemia associated with chromosome translocation 1;19. Blood 63: 721–724

62. van Dongen JJ, Macintyre EA, Gabert JA et al 1999 Standardized RT-PCR analysis of fusion gene transcripts from chromosome aberrations in acute leukemia for detection of minimal residual disease. Report of the BIOMED-1 Concerted Action: investigation of minimal residual disease in acute leukemia. Leukemia 13: 1901–1928

63. Ziemin-van der Poel S, McCabe NR, Gill HJ et al 1991 Identification of a gene, MLL, that spans the breakpoint in 11q23 translocations associated with human leukemias. Proceedings of the National Academy of Science USA 88: 10735–10739

64. Biondi A, Rambaldi A, Rossi V et al 1993 Detection of ALL-1/AF4 fusion transcript by reverse transcription-polymerase chain reaction for diagnosis and monitoring of acute leukemias with the t(4;11) translocation. Blood 82: 2943–2947

65. Pallisgaard N, Hokland P, Riishoj DC et al 1998 Multiplex reverse transcription-polymerase chain reaction for simultaneous screening of 29 translocations and chromosomal aberrations in acute leukemia. Blood 92: 574–588

66. van der Berg M, Beverloo HB, Langerak AW et al 1999 Rapid and sensitive detection of all types of MLL gene translocations with a single FISH probe set. Leukemia 13: 2107–2113

‎

67. Romana SP, Le Coniat M, Berger R 1994 t(12;21): a new recurrent translocation in acute lymphoblastic leukemia. Genes Chromosomes Cancer 9: 186–191

68. Golub TR, Barker GF, Bohlander SK et al 1995 Fusion of the TEL gene on 12p13 to the AML1 gene on 21q22 in acute lymphoblastic leukemia. Proceedings of the National Academy of Science USA 92: 4917–4921

69. Shurtleff SA, Buijs A, Behm FG et al 1995 TEL/AML1 fusion resulting from a cryptic t(12;21) is the most common genetic lesion in pediatric ALL and defines a subgroup of patients with an excellent prognosis. Leukemia 9: 1985–1989

70. Janssen JW, Ludwig WD, Sterry W, Bartram CR 1993 SIL-TAL1 deletion in T-cell acute lymphoblastic leukemia. Leukemia 7: 1204–1210

71. Hoelzer D, Gale RP 1987 Acute lymphoblastic leukemia in adults: recent progress, future directions. Seminars in Hematology 24: 27–39. Review

72. Gale RP, Butturini A 1991 Maintenance chemotherapy and cure of childhood acute lymphoblastic leukaemia. Lancet 338: 1315–1318

73. Cross NC, Hughes TP, Feng L et al 1993 Minimal residual disease after allogeneic bone marrow transplantation for chronic myeloid leukaemia in first chronic phase: correlations with acute graft-versus-host disease and relapse. British Journal of Haematology 84: 67–74

74. Cross NC, Feng L, Chase A et al 1993 Competitive polymerase chain reaction to estimate the number of BCR-ABL transcripts in chronic myeloid leukemia patients after bone marrow transplantation. Blood 82: 1929–1936

75. van Rhee F, Marks DI, Lin F et al 1995 Quantification of residual disease in Philadelphia-positive acute lymphoblastic leukemia: comparison of blood and bone marrow. Leukemia 9: 329–335

76. Miyamura K, Morishima Y, Tanimoto M et al 1990 Prediction of clinical relapse after bone marrow transplantation by PCR for Philadephia-positive acute lymphoblastic leukaemia. Lancet 336: 890

77. Cimino G, Elia L, Rivolta A et al 1996 Clinical relevance of residual disease monitoring by polymerase chain reaction in patients with ALL-1/AF-4 positive-acute lymphoblastic leukaemia. British Journal of Haematology 92: 659–664

78. Hunger SP, Fall MZ, Camitta BM et al 1998 E2A-PBX1 chimeric transcript status at end of consolidation is not predictive of treatment outcome in childhood acute lymphoblastic leukemias with a t(1;19)(q23;p13): a Pediatric Oncology Group study. Blood 91: 1021–1028

79. Nakao M, Yokota S, Horiike S et al 1996 Detection and quantification of TEL/AML1 fusion transcripts by polymerase chain reaction in childhood acute lymphoblastic leukemia. Leukemia 10: 1463–1470

80. d'Auriol L, Macintyre E, Galibert F, Sigaux F 1989 *In vitro* amplification of T cell gamma gene rearrangements: a new tool for the assessment of minimal residual disease in acute lymphoblastic leukemias. Leukemia 3: 155–158

81. Macintyre E, d'Auriol L, Amesland F et al 1989 Analysis of junctional diversity in the preferential V delta 1-J delta 1 rearrangement of fresh T-acute lymphoblastic leukemia cells by *in vitro* gene amplification and direct sequencing. Blood 74: 2053–2061

82. Biondi A, Francia di Celle P, Rossi V, Casorati G et al 1990 High prevalence of T-cell receptor V delta 2-(D)-D delta 3 or D delta 1/2-D delta 3 rearrangements in B-precursor acute lymphoblastic leukemias. Blood 75: 1834–1840

83. Deane M, Norton JD 1991 Immunoglobulin gene 'fingerprinting': an approach to analysis of B lymphoid clonality in lymphoproliferative disorders. British Journal of Haematology 77: 274–281

84. Evans PA, Short MA, Owen RG et al 1998 Residual disease detection using fluorescent polymerase chain reaction at 20 weeks of therapy predicts clinical outcome in childhood acute lymphoblastic leukemia. Journal of Clinical Oncology 16: 3616–3627

85. Goulden NJ, Knechtli CJ, Garland RJ et al 1998 Minimal residual disease analysis for the prediction of relapse in children with standard-risk acute lymphoblastic leukaemia. British Journal of Haematology 100: 235–244

86. van Dongen JJ, Seriu T, Panzer-Grumayer ER et al 1998 Prognostic value of minimal residual disease in acute lymphoblastic leukaemia in childhood. Lancet 352: 1731–1738

87. Brisco MJ, Condon J, Sykes PJ et al 1991 Detection and quantitation of neoplastic cells in acute lymphoblastic leukaemia, by use of the polymerase chain reaction. British Journal of Haematology 79: 211–217

88. Sykes PJ, Neoh SH, Brisco MJ et al 1992 Quantitation of targets for PCR by use of limiting dilution. Biotechniques 13: 444–449

89. Verhagen OJ, Willemse MJ, Breunis WB et al 2000 Application of germline IGH probes in real-time quantitative PCR for the detection of minimal residual disease in acute lymphoblastic leukemia. Leukemia 14: 426–435

90. Bruggemann M, Droese J, Bolz I et al 2000 Improved assessment of minimal residual disease in B cell malignancies using fluorogenic consensus probes for real-time quantitative PCR. Leukemia 14: 1419–1425

91. Hillestad L 1957 Acute promyelocytic leukemia. Acta Medica Scandinavica 157: 189–194

92. Rowley JJ, Golomb H, Dougherty C 1977 15/17 translocation. A consistent chromosomal change in acute promyelocytic leukaemia. Lancet I: 549–550

93. Greenberg P, Cox C, LeBeau MM et al 1997 International scoring system for evaluating prognosis in myelodysplastic syndromes. Blood 89: 2079–2088

94. Grimwade D, Walker H, Oliver F et al 1998 The importance of diagnostic cytogenetics on outcome in AML: analysis of 1,612 patients entered into the MRC AML 10 trial. Blood, 92: 2322–2333

95. Raimondi S, Chang M, Ravindranath Y et al 1999 Chromosomal abnormalities in children with acute myeloid leukemia: clinical characteristics and treatment outcome in a Cooperative Pediatric Oncology Group study – POG 8821. Blood 94: 3707–3716

96. Langabeer S, Walker H, Rogers J et al 1997 Incidence of AML1/ETO fusion transcripts in patients entered into the MRC AML trials. MRC adult leukaemia working party. British Journal of Haematology 99: 925–928

97. Swirsky D, Li Y, Mattews J et al 1984 8;21 translocation in acute granulocytic leukaemia: cytological cytochemical and clinical features. British Journal of Haematology 56: 199–213

98. Ishibashi T, Kimura H, Abe R et al 1986 Involvement of eosinophils in leukemia: cytogenetic study of eosinophilic colonies from acute myelogenous leukemia associated with translocation t(8;21). Cancer Genetics and Cytogenetics 22: 189–194

99. Jacobsen R, Temple M, Sacher R et al 1984 Acute myeloblastic leukaemia and t(8;21) translocation. British Journal of Haematology 57: 539–540

100. Berger R, Bernheim A, Daniel M-T et al 1982 Cytologic characterization and significance of normal karyotypes t(8;21) acute myeloblastic leukemia. Blood 59: 171–178

101. Van Lom K, Hagemeijer A, Vandekerckhove F et al 1997 Clonality analysis of hematopoietic cell lineages in acute myeloid leukemia and translocation (8;21): only myeloid lineages are part of the malignant clone. Leukemia 11: 202–205

102. Nucifora G, Dickstein J, Torbenson V et al 1994 Correlation between cell morphology and expression of the AML1/ETO chimeric transcript in patients with acute myeloid leukemia without the t(8;21). Leukemia 8: 1533–1538

103. Golomb H, Rowley J, Vardiman J et al 1980 'Microgranular' acute promyelocytic leukemia: a distinct clinical, ultrastructural and cytogenetic entity. Blood 55: 253–259

104. Licht J, Chomienne C, Goy A et al 1995 Clinical and molecular characterization of a rare syndrome of acute promyelocytic leukemia associated with translocation (11;17). Blood 85: 1083–1094

105. Redner R, Rush E, Faas S et al 1996 The t(5;17) variant of acute promyelocytic leukemia expresses a nucleophosmin-retinoic acid receptor fusion. Blood 87: 882–886

106. Huang M, Ye Y, Chen S et al 1988 Use of all-trans retinoic acid in the treatment of acute promyelocytic leukemia. Blood 72: 567–572

107. Bennett J, Catovsky D, Daniel M-T et al 2000 Hypergranular promyelocytic leulemia: correlation between morphology and chromosomal translocations including t(15;17) and t(11;17). Leukemia 14: 1197–1200

108. Grimwade D, Gorman P, Duprez E et al 1997 Characterization of cryptic rearrangements and variant translocations in acute promyelocytic leukemia. Blood 90: 4876–4885

109. Tomonaga M, Yoshida Y, Tagawa M et al 1985 Cytochemistry of acute promyelocytic leukemia (M3): leukemic promyelocytes exhibit heterogeneous patterns in cellular differentiation. Blood 66: 350–357

110. Edelman B, Grossman N 1983 Microgranular acute promyelocytic leukemia – a case with multiple Auer rods demonstrable only after staining for chloroacetate esterase. American Journal of Clinical Pathology 79: 621–625

111. Burnett A, Grimwade D, Solomon E et al 1999 Presenting white blood cell count and kinetics of molecular remission predict prognosis in

112. Lo Coco F, Diverio D, Avvisati G et al 1999 Therapy of molecular relapse in acute promyelocytic leukemia. Blood 94: 2225–2229

113. Arthur D, Bloomfield C 1983 Partial deletion of the long arm of chromosome 16 and bone marrow eosinophilia in acute nonlymphocytic leukemia: a new association. Blood 61: 994–998

114. Le Beau M, Larson R, Bitter M et al 1983 Association of an inversion of chromosome 16 with abnormal marrow eosinophils in acute myelomonocytic leukemia. A unique cytogenetic–clinicopathological association. New England Journal of Medicine 309: 630–636

115. Larson R, Williams S, Le Beau M et al 1983 Acute myelomonocytic leukemia with abnormal eosinophils and inv(16) or t(16;16) has a favourable prognosis. Blood 68: 1242–1249

116. Bitter M, Le Beau M, Larson R et al 1984 A morphologic and cytochemical study of acute myelomonocytic leukemia with abnormal marrow eosinophils associated with inv(16)(p13q22). American Journal of Clinical Pathology 81: 733–741

117. Leder L 1970 Akute myelo-monozytare Leukaemia mit atypischen naphthol-AS-D-chloroacetatesterase-positiven Eosinophilen. Acta Haematologica 44: 52–62

118. Liso V, Troccoli G, Specchia G, Magno M 1977 Cytochemical 'normal' and 'abnormal' eosinophils in acute leukemias. American Journal of Hematology 2: 123–131

119. Langabeer S, Walker H, Gale R et al 1997 Frequency of CBF beta/MYH11 fusion transcripts in patients enetered into the U.K. MRC AML trials. The MRC adult leukaemia working party. British Journal of Haematology 96: 736–739

120. Reddy K, Wang S, Montgomery P et al 2000 Fluorescence *in situ* hybridization identifies inversion 16 masked by t(10;16(q24;q22), t(7;16)(q21;q22) and t(2;16)(q37;q22) in three cases of AML-M4Eo. Cancer Genetics and Cytogenetics 116: 148–152

121. Brito-Babapulle F, Catovsky D, Galton D 1987 Clinical and laboratory features of de novo acute myeloid leukaemia with trilineage myelodysplasia. British Journal of Haematology 66: 445–450

122. Goasguen J, Matsuo T, Cox C, Bennett J 1992 Evaluation of the dysmyelopoiesis in 336 patients with *de novo* acute myeloid leukaemia: major importance of dysgranulopoiesis for remission and survival. Leukemia 6: 520–525

123. Kuriyama K, Tomonaga M, Matsuo T et al 1994 Poor response to intensive chemotherapy in *de novo* acute myeloid leukaemia with trilineage myelodysplasia. British Journal of Haematology 86: 767–773

124. Gahn B, Haase D, Unterhalt M *et al* 1996 De novo AML with dysplastic hematopoiesis: cytogenetic and prognostic significance. Leukemia 10: 946–951

125. Tamura S, Takemoto Y, Wada H et al 1998 Significance of trilineage myelodysplasia in de novo acute myeloid leukaemia during remission rather than at diagnosis. British Journal of Haematology 101: 743–748

126. Swirsky D, de Bastos M, Parish S et al 1986 Features affecting outcome during remission induction of acute myeloid leukaemia in 619 adult patients. British Journal of Haematology 64: 435–453

127. Jackson C, Dahl G 1983 Relationship of megakaryocyte size at diagnosis to chemotherapeutic response in children with acute nonlymphocytic leukemia. Blood 61: 867–870

128. Brody P, Krause J 1986 Morphometric study of megakaryocyte size and prognosis in adults with acute non-lymphocytic leukemia. Leukemia Research 10: 475–480

129. Smit C, Meyler L 1970 Acute myeloid leukaemia after treatment with cytostatic agents. Lancet 2: 671–672

130. Michels S, McKenna R, Arthur D, Brunning R 1985 Therapy-related acute myeloid leukemia and myelodysplastic syndrome: a clinical and morphologic study of 65 cases. Blood 65: 1364–1372

131. Foucar K, McKenna R, Bloomfield C et al 1979 Therapy related leukemia. Cancer 23: 1285–1296

132. Le Beau M, Albain K, Larson R et al 1986 Clinical and cytogenetic correlations in 63 patients with therapy-related myelodysplastic syndromes and acute nonlymphocytic leukemia: further evidence for characteristic abnormalities of chromosomes no. 5 and 7. Journal of Clinical Oncology 4: 325–345

133. Hoyle C, de Bastos M, Wheatley K et al 1989 AML associated with previous cytotoxic therapy, MDS or myeloproliferative disorders: results from the MRC's 9th AML trial. British Journal of Haematology 72: 45–53

134. Ellis M, Ravid M, Lishner M 1993 A comparative analysis of alkylating agent and epipodophyllotoxin-related leukemias. Leukemia and Lymphoma 11: 9–13

135. Whitlock J, Greer J, Lukens J 1991 Epipodophyllotoxin-related leukemia. Identification of a new subset of secondary leukemia. Cancer 68: 600–604

136. Pui C-H, Relling M, Rivera G et al 1995 Epipodophyllotoxin-related acute myeloid leukemia: a study of 35 cases. Leukemia 9: 1990–1996

137. Kudo K, Yoshida H, Kiyoi H et al 1998 Etoposide-related acute promyelocytic leukemia. Leukemia 12: 1171–1175

138. Liso V, Specchia S, Capalbo R et al 1995 Cytophagocytosis by the blast cells in acute myeloid leukemia. Leukemia and Lymphoma 18(suppl 1): 65–68

139. Davey F, Abraham N, Brunetto V et al 1995 Morphologic characteristics of erythroleukemia (acute myeloid leukemia; FAB-M6): A CALGB study. American Journal of Hematology 49: 29–38

140. Olopade O, Thangavelu M, Larson R et al 1992 Clinical, morphological, and cytogenetic characteristics of 26 patients with acute erythroblastic leukemia. Blood 80: 2837–2882

141. Mazzella F, Kowal-Vern A, Shrit M et al 1998 Acute erythroleukemia: evaluation of 48 cases with reference to classification, cell proliferation, cytogenetics, and prognosis. American Journal of Clinical Pathology 110: 590–598

142. Villeval J, Cramer P, Lemoine F et al 1986 Phenotype of early erythroblastic leukaemias. Blood 68: 1167–1174

143. Garand R, Duchayne E, Blanchard D et al 1995 Minimally differentiated erythroleukaemia (AML M6 'variant'): a rare subset of AML distinct from AML M6. Groupe Francais d'Hematologie Cellulaire. British Journal of Haematology 90: 868–875

144. Den Ottolander G, te Velde J, Brederoo P et al 1979 Megakaryoblastic leukaemia (acute myelofibrosis): a report of three cases. British Journal of Haematology 42: 9–20

145. Hoyle C, Sherrington P, Fischer P, Hayhoe F 1989 Basophils in acute myeloid leukaemia. Journal of Clinical Pathology 42: 785–792

146. Peterson L, Parkin J, Arthur D, Brunning R 1991 Acute basophilic leukemia. A clinical, morphologic, and cytogenetic study of eight cases. American Journal of Clinical Pathology 96: 160–170

147. Pearson M, Vardiman J, Le Beau M et al 1985 Increased numbers of marrow basophils may be associated with a t(6;9) in ANLL. American Journal of Hematology 18: 393–403

148. Daniel M-T, Bernheim A, Flandrin G, Berger R 1985 Leucemie aigue myeloblastique (M2) avec atteinte de la ligne basophile et anomalies du bras court du chromosome 12 (12p). Comptes Rendu de L'academie des Sciences 301: 299–301

149. Wick M, Li C-Y, Pierre R 1982 Acute non-lymphocytic leukemia with basophilic differentiation. Blood 60: 38–45

150. Lewis S, Szur L 1963 Malignant myelosclerosis. British Medical Journal 2: 472–477

151. Lubin J, Rozen S, Rywlin A 1976 Malignant myelosclerosis. Archives of Internal Medicine 136: 141–145

152. Sultan C, Sigaux F, Imbert M, Reyes F 1981 Acute myelodysplasia with myelofibrosis: a report of eight cases. British Journal of Haematology 49: 11–16

153. Hruban R, Kuhajda F, Mann R, et al 1987 Acute myelofibrosis: immunohistochemical study of four cases and comparison with acute megakaryocytic leukemia. American Journal of Clinical Pathology 88: 578–588

154. Imbert M, Nguyen D, Sultan C 1992 Myelodysplastic syndromes (MDS) and acute myeloid leukemias (AML) with myelofibrosis. Leukemia Research 16: 51–54

155. Rosati S, Anastasi J, Vardiman J 1996 Recurring diagnostic problems in the pathology of the myelodysplastic syndromes. Seminars in Hematology 33: 111–126

156. Howe R, Bloomfield C, McKenna R 1982 Hypocellular acute leukemia. American Journal of Medicine 72: 391–395

157. Gladson C, Naeim F 1986 Hypocellular bone marrow with increased blasts. American Journal of Hematology 21: 15–22

158. Nagai K, Kohno T, Chen Y et al 1996 Diagnostic criteria for hypocellular acute leukemia: a clinical entity distinct from overt acute leukemia and myelodysplastic syndrome. Leukemia Research 20: 563–574

159. Bisschop M, Revesz T, Bierings M et al 2001 Extramedullary infiltrates at diagnosis have no prognostic significance in children with acute myeloid leukaemia. Leukemia 15: 46–49

160. Chang M, Raimondi S, Ravindranath Y et al 2000 Prognostic factors in children with acute myeloid leukemia (excluding children with Down

syndrome and acute promyelocytic leukemia): univariate and recursive partitioning analysis of patients treated on Pediatric Oncology Group (POG) Study 8821. Leukemia 14: 1201–1207

161. Byrd J, Edenfield W, Shields D, Dawson N 1995 Extramedullary myeloid cell tumors in acute nonlymphocytic leukemia: a clinical review. Journal of Clinical Oncology 13: 1800–1816

162. Menasce L, Banerjee S, Harris M 1999 Extra-medullary myeloid tumour (granulocytic sarcoma) is often misdiagnosed: a study of 26 cases. Histopathology 14: 391–398

163. Chang C-C, Eshoa C, Kampalath B et al 2000 Immunophenotypic profile of myeloid cells granulocytic sarcoma by immunohistochemistry. American Journal of Clinical Pathology 114: 807–811

164. Hudock J, Chatten J, Miettinen M 1994 Immunohistochemical evaluation of Myeloid leukemia infiltrates (granulocytic sarcomas) in formalin-fixed paraffin-embedded tissue. American Journal of Clinical Pathology 102: 55–60

165. Rees J, Gray R, Swirsky D, Hayhoe F 1986 Principal results of the Medical Research Council's 8th acute myeloid leukaemia trial. Lancet 2: 1236–1241

166. Borowitz MJ, Guenther KL, Shults KE, Stelzer GT 1993 Immunophenotyping of acute leukemia by flow cytometric analysis. Use of CD45 and right-angle light scatter to gate on leukemic blasts in three-color analysis. American Journal of Clinical Pathology 100: 534–540

167. Vendetti A, Del Poeta G, Buccisano F et al 1998 Prognostic relevance of the expression of Tdt and CD7 in335 cases of acute myeloid leukemia. Leukemia 12: 1056–1063

168. Ferrara F, Di Noto R, Annunziata M et al 1998 Immunophenotypic analysis enables the correct prediction of t(8;21) in acute myeloid leukaemia. British Journal of Haematology 102: 444–448

169. Andrieu V, Radford-Weiss I, Troussard X et al 1996 Molecular detection of t(8;21)/AML1-ETO in AML M1/M2: correlation with cytogenetics, morphology and immunophenotype. British Journal of Haematology 92: 855–865

170. Baer MR, Stewart CC, Lawrence D et al 1997 Expression of the Neural Cell Adhesion Molecule CD56 is associated with short remission duration and survival in acute myeloid leukaemia with t(8;21)(q22;q22). Blood 90: 1643–1648

171. Daniels JT, Davis BJ, Houde-McGrail L, Byrd JC 1999 Clonal selection of CD56+ t(8;21) AML blasts: further suggestion of the adverse clinical significance of this biological marker? British Journal of Haematology 107: 381–383

172. Erber WN, Asbahr H, Rule SA, Scott CS 1994 Unique immunophenotype of acute promyelocytic leukaemia as defined by CD9 and CD68 antibodies. British Journal of Haematology 88: 101–104

173. Orfao A, Chillon MC, Bortoluci AM et al 1999 The flow cytometric pattern of CD34, CD15 and CD13 expression in acute myeloblastic leukaemia is highly characteristic of the presence of PML-RARalpha gene rearrangements. Haematologica 84: 405–412

174. O'Connor SJM, Forsyth PD, Dalal S et al 1997 The rapid diagnosis of acute promyelocytic leukaemia using PML (5E10) monoclonal antibody. British Journal of Haematology 99: 597–604

175. San Miguel JF, Martinez A, Macedo A et al 1997 Immunophenotyping investigation of minimal residual disease is a useful approach for predicting relapse in acute myeloid leukemia patients. Blood 90: 2465–2470

176. Diverio D, Riccioni R, Mandelli F, Lo Coco F 1995 The PML/RAR alpha fusion gene in the diagnosis and monitoring of acute promyelocytic leukemia. Haematologica 80: 155–160

177. Poirel H, Radford-Weiss I, Rack K, Troussard X et al 1995 Detection of the chromosome 16 CBF beta-MYH11 fusion transcript in myelomonocytic leukemias. Blood 85: 1313–1322

178. Lo Coco F, Pelicci PG, Biondi A 1994 Clinical relevance of the PML/RAR-a gene rearrangement in acute promyelocytic leukaemia. Leukemia and Lymphoma 12: 327–332

179. Chen Z, Brand NJ, Chen A et al 1993 Fusion between a novel Kruppel-like zinc finger gene and the retinoic acid receptor-alpha locus due to a variant t(11;17) translocation associated with acute promyelocytic leukaemia. EMBO Journal 12: 1161–1167

180. Pandolfi PP, Alcalay M, Fagioli M et al 1992 Genomic variability and alternative splicing generate multiple PML/RAR alpha transcripts that encode aberrant PML proteins and PML/RAR alpha isoforms in acute promyelocytic leukaemia. EMBO Journal 11: 1397–1407

181. Grimwade D, Howe K, Langabeer S et al 1996 Establishing the presence of the t(15;17) in suspected acute promyelocytic leukaemia: cytogenetic, molecular and PML immunofluorescence assessement of patients entered into the M.R.C. ATRA trial. M.R.C. Adult Leukaemia Working Party. British Journal of Haematology 94: 557–573

182. Liu PP, Hajra A, Wijmenga C, Collins FS 1995 Molecular pathogenesis of the chromosome 16 inversion in the M4Eo subtype of acute myeloid leukemia. (Published Erratum: Blood 1997 Mar 1;89(5): 1842) Blood 85: 2289–2302

183. Evans PA, Short MA, Jack AS et al 1997 Detection and quantitation of the CBFbeta/MYH11 transcripts associated with the inv(16) in presentation and follow-up samples from patients with AML. Leukemia 11: 364–369

184. Okuda T, van Deursen J, Hiebert SW et al 1996 AML1, the target of multiple chromosomal translocations in human leukemia, is essential for normal fetal liver hematopoiesis. Cell 84: 321–330

185. Gamou T, Kitamura E, Hosoda F et al 1998 The partner gene of AML1 in t(16;21) myeloid malignancies is a novel member of the MTG8(ETO) family. Blood 91: 4028–4037

186. Nucifora G, Larson RA, Rowley JD 1993 Persistence of the 8;21 translocation in patients with acute myeloid leukemia type M2 in long-term remission. Blood 82: 712–715

187. Hebert J, Cayuela JM, Daniel MT et al 1994 Detection of minimal residual disease in acute myelomonocytic leukemia with abnormal marrow eosinophils by nested polymerase chain reaction with allele specific amplification. Blood 84: 2291–2296

188. Tobal K, Liu Yin JA 1998 Molecular monitoring of minimal residual disease in acute myeloblastic leukemia with t(8;21) by RT-PCR. Leukemia and Lymphoma 31: 115–120

189. Tobal K, Newton J, Macheta M et al 2000 Molecular quantitation of minimal residual disease in acute myeloid leukemia with t(8;21) can identify patients in durable remission and predict clinical relapse. Blood 95: 815–819

190. Smith LJ, Curtis JE, Messner HA et al 1983 Lineage infidelity in acute leukemia. Blood 61: 1138–1145

191. Greaves MF, Chan LC, Furley AJ et al 1986 Lineage promiscuity in hemopoietic differentiation and leukemia. Blood 67: 1–11

192. Buccheri V, Matutes E, Dyer MJS et al 1993 Lineage commitment in biphenotypic acute leukemia. Leukemia 7: 919–927

193. Bene MC, Castoldi G, Knapp W et al 1995 Proposals for the immunological classification of acute leukemia: European Group for the Immunological Characterization of Leukemias (EGIL). Leukemia 9: 1783–1786

194. Matutes E, Morilla R, Farahat N et al 1997 Definition of acute biphenotypic leukemia. Haematologica 82: 64–66

195. Legrand O, Perrot J-V, Simonin G et al 1998 Adult acute biphenotypic acute leukemia: an entity with poor prognosis which is related to unfavourable cytogenetics an P-glycoprotein over-expression. British Journal of Haematology 100: 147–155

196. Killick S, Matutes E, Powles RL et al 1999 Outcome of biphenotypic leukemia. Haematologica 84: 699–706

The chronic lymphoid and myeloid leukemias and systemic mastocytosis

21

DM Clark   BJ Bain

Chronic lymphocytic leukemia

Clinical features

Pathologic features
Peripheral blood
Bone marrow
Supplementary investigations

Prolymphocytic leukemia

Clinical features

Pathologic features
Peripheral blood
Bone marrow
Other tissues
Supplementary investigations

Prolymphocytic leukemia

Clinical features

Pathologic features
Peripheral blood
Bone marrow
Other tissues
Supplementary investigations

Splenic lymphoma with villous lymphocytes

Clinical features

Pathologic features
Peripheral blood
Bone marrow
Other tissues
Supplementary investigations

T-lineage prolymphocytic leukemia

Clinical features

Pathologic features
Peripheral blood
Bone marrow
Other tissues
Supplementary investigations

Leukemias of large granular lymphocytes

Clinical features

Pathologic features
Peripheral blood
Bone marrow
Other tissues

Sézary syndrome/mycosis fungoides

Clinical features

Pathologic features
Peripheral blood
Bone marrow
Other tissues
Supplementary investigations

Adult T-cell leukemia/lymphoma

Clinical features

Pathologic features
Peripheral blood
Bone marrow
Other tissues
Supplementary investigations

Chronic granulocytic leukemia

Clinical features

Pathologic features
Peripheral blood
Bone marrow
Other tissues
Supplementary investigations

Atypical chronic myeloid leukemia

Clinical features

Pathologic features
Peripheral blood
Bone marrow
Other tissues
Supplementary investigations

Chronic myelomonocytic leukemia

Clinical features

Pathologic features
Peripheral blood
Bone marrow
Other tissues
Supplementary investigations

Juvenile chronic myelomonocytic leukemia

Clinical features

Pathologic features
Peripheral blood
Bone marrow
Other tissues
Supplementary investigations

Eosinophilic leukemia

Clinical features

Pathologic features
Peripheral blood
Bone marrow
Other tissues
Supplementary investigations

Systemic mastocytosis

Clinical features

Pathologic features
Peripheral blood
Bone marrow
Other tissues
Supplementary investigations

The leukemias are neoplastic conditions, resulting from mutation in a myeloid, lymphoid or pluripotent stem cell, in which neoplastic cells derived from the mutant stem cell replace normal hemopoietic cells in the bone marrow. The neoplastic cells often also circulate in the blood stream. The chronic leukemias differ from the acute leukemias in that there is a greater degree of maturation of cells of the leukemic clone. Normal hemopoiesis is less disrupted and the rate of disease progression is slower. If untreated, the chronic leukemias are compatible with survival, in most cases, for a number of years.

In this chapter we deal with the chronic lympho-proliferative disorders that usually present as leukemia. Chronic lymphoid neoplasms more often presenting as lymphoma are dealt with in Chapter 22. We discuss these conditions using the French–American–British (FAB)[1] and World Health Organization (WHO)[2] classifications as a framework. We also deal with all the chronic myeloid leukemias including those that the WHO expert group[2] has assigned to the myeloproliferative/myelodysplastic category. For conditions that are classified by the WHO group as myelodysplastic the reader is referred to Chapter 19.

Chronic lymphocytic leukemia

Chronic lymphocytic leukemia (CLL) is a chronic leukemia resulting from the proliferation of a neoplastic clone of mature B-lymphocytes with a very characteristic immunophenotype. Recent molecular evidence suggests that the mutation that results in this disease may occur either in a naive B-lymphocyte with immunoglobulin V_H genes in germline configuration or from a postgerminal center antigen-experienced B-lymphocyte with somatic mutation of V_H genes.[3]

In the WHO classification, CLL falls into the category designated B-cell CLL/small lymphocytic lymphoma. Cases of small lymphocytic lymphoma differ from CLL only in that there is no peripheral blood lymphocytosis at presentation and often not during the course of the disease. The WHO classification recognizes a variant of CLL in which there is plasmacytoid differentiation or a paraprotein is present.

CLL often pursues a very indolent course with many elderly patients dying from unrelated causes rather than from the leukemia. Patients with advanced-stage disease may die from disease progression or, in a minority, following prolymphocytoid or large cell transformation (Richter's syndrome).

Clinical features

CLL is mainly a disease of the middle-aged and elderly with an incidence of the order of 6/100 000/year and a male:female ratio of approximately 2:1. It is quite uncommon among the Chinese and Japanese.

In the majority of cases the diagnosis of CLL is an incidental one, made when a blood count is performed without there having been any clinical suspicion of leukemia. Most of these patients have no abnormal physical findings nor any symptoms resulting from the leukemia. In other patients with more advanced disease the typical clinical findings are lymphadenopathy, splenomegaly and, less often, hepatomegaly. In some patients the initial presentation is with herpes zoster or with symptoms and signs of anemia resulting from auto-immune hemolytic anemia.

Pathologic features

Peripheral blood

In early-stage disease, the only peripheral blood abnormality is lymphocytosis with an increase of mature small lymphocytes which are relatively uniform in their cytologic features (Fig. 21.1). The lymphocytes typically have a high nucleocytoplasmic ratio, condensed chromatin and an inapparent or barely apparent nucleolus; sometimes the chromatin is condensed into a mosaic pattern. Smear cells are typically seen in blood films, but are not pathognomonic. The presence of some plasmacytoid lymphocytes and small numbers of cells with cleft or irregular nuclei is compatible with a diagnosis of chronic lymphocytic leukemia. There may be up to 10% prolymphocytes

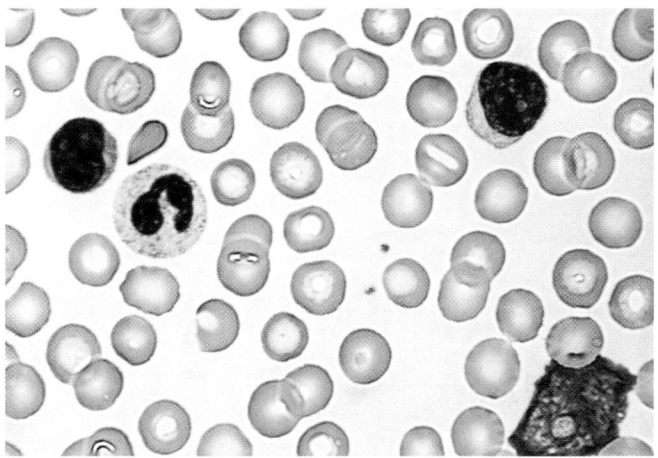

Fig. 21.1 Peripheral blood in chronic lymphocytic leukemia showing two mature small lymphocytes and a smear cell. MGG, × 100 objective.

(atypical cells with larger, more prominent nucleoli) but the presence of more than 10% prolymphocytes or of a spectrum of cells from small to large, with cytoplasmic basophilia, is indicative of a worse prognosis and leads to the case being categorized, according to FAB criteria, as 'chronic lymphocytic leukemia, mixed-cell type'. Mixed-cell type CLL needs to be distinguished from pro-lymphocytoid transformation in which there is a rising percentage of prolymphocytes associated with disease progression.

In patients with more advanced disease, there is anemia and thrombocytopenia. The anemia is usually normocytic and normochromic with no specific morphologic features. In those patients with complicating auto-immune hemolytic anemia there are spherocytes and polychromasia. Neutropenia is uncommon.

Bone marrow

The bone marrow aspirate is hypercellular as the result of an increase in small mature lymphocytes with the same cytologic features as those in the circulating blood. The bone marrow trephine biopsy shows infiltration in all cases. The neoplastic infiltrate is composed predominantly of small lymphocytes with smaller numbers of prolymphocytes and para-immunoblasts (Fig. 21.2). The small lymphocytes have coarsely clumped chromatin and scanty cytoplasm. Prolymphocytes are slightly larger than small lymphocytes with a dispersed chromatin pattern and a small central nucleolus. Para-immunoblasts are medium-sized cells with an open chromatin pattern, prominent central nucleolus and moderate amounts of basophilic cytoplasm. Prolymphocytes and para-immunoblasts may be present in greater numbers in

some areas of the infiltrate (proliferation centers) (Fig. 21.3). Four patterns of infiltration are seen – interstitial, nodular, nodular-interstitial and diffuse.[4] The interstitial pattern is characterized by neoplastic cells infiltrating individually between normal hemopoietic precursors and fat cells. Nodular infiltrates focally replace fat and hemopoietic cells (Fig. 21.4). Nodular–interstitial infiltration is a combination of the nodular and interstitial patterns. In cases with diffuse infiltration there is complete replacement of hemopoietic precursors and fat cells (Fig. 21.5). Cases with a diffuse pattern have a worse prognosis than cases with other patterns of infiltration.[5,6] Unlike many other bone marrow lymphoid infiltrates, there is usually little or no increase in reticulin associated with infiltration by CLL.

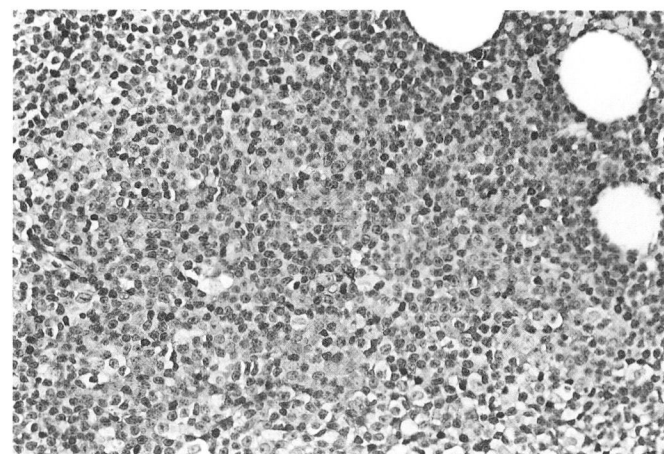

Fig. 21.3 Trephine-biopsy section in chronic lymphocytic leukemia showing a nodular infiltrate containing a proliferation center in which there are increased numbers of prolymphocytes and small numbers of para-immunoblasts. Giemsa, × 40 objective.

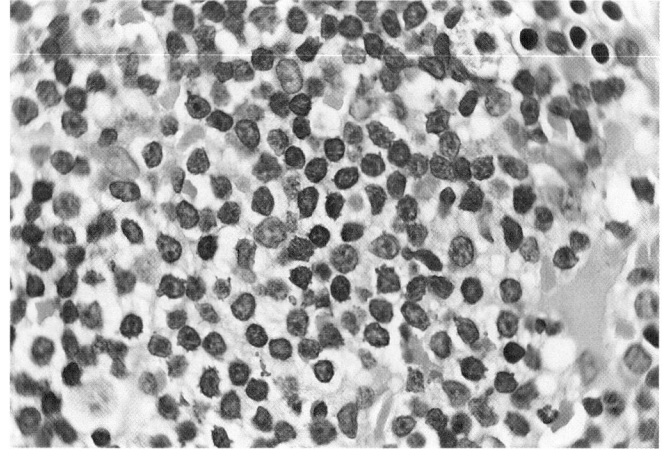

Fig. 21.2 Trephine-biopsy section in chronic lymphocytic leukemia showing infiltration by small lymphocytes with smaller numbers of prolymphocytes. H&E, × 100 objective.

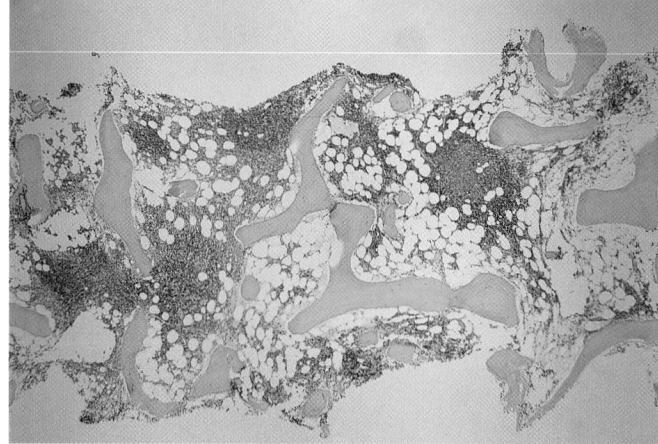

Fig. 21.4 Trephine-biopsy section in chronic lymphocytic leukemia showing focal random nodules of small lymphocytes (nodular pattern). H&E, × 4 objective.

Other tissues

Lymph nodes involvement in CLL is characterized by effacement of nodal architecture by a diffuse infiltrate of small lymphocytes with the formation of proliferation centers in which there are increased numbers of pro-lymphocytes and para-immunoblasts. At low power proliferation centers appear paler than the surrounding areas, and if numerous can give the infiltrate an appearance of nodularity (Fig. 21.6).

In the spleen, infiltration leads to expansion of the white pulp, with some cases also having involvement of the red pulp[7] (Fig. 21.7). Infiltration of the liver involves both portal tracts and sinusoids. Rarely there may be symptomatic infiltration of the skin,[8] lung,[9] CNS[10] or urinary tract;[11] in all these tissues the infiltrate is made up predominantly of small lymphocytes.

Rapid development of an extramedullary tumor is the typical presentation of Richter's transformation of CLL. The neoplastic cells in Richter's syndrome are large B-cells with pleomorphic nuclei, open chromatin and prominent nucleoli.[12] In some patients there is bone marrow infiltration by large pleomorphic B-cells (Fig. 21.8). There is often necrosis of the tumor, a feature not otherwise seen in tissues infiltrated by CLL.

Supplementary investigations

The immunophenotype of CLL is very different from that of all other chronic lymphoproliferative disorders (with the exception of small lymphocytic lymphoma). There is weak surface membrane expression of monotypic (kappa or lambda) immunoglobulin, usually IgM with or without IgD. There is weak expression of certain B-cell

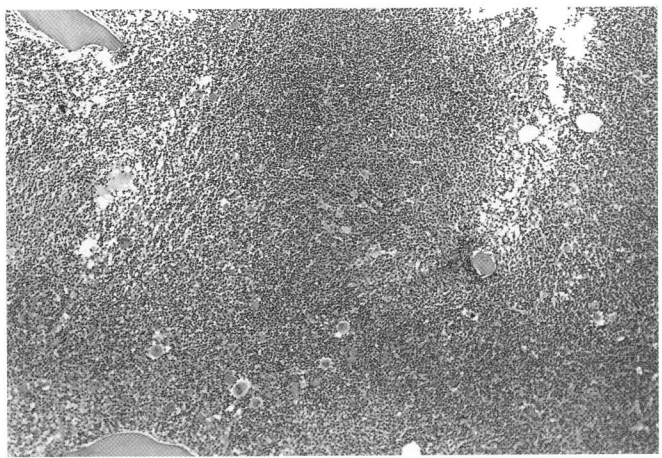

Fig. 21.5 Trephine-biopsy section in chronic lymphocytic leukemia showing complete replacement of fat cells and hemopoietic precursors by an infiltrate of small lymphocytes (diffuse pattern). H&E, × 10 objective.

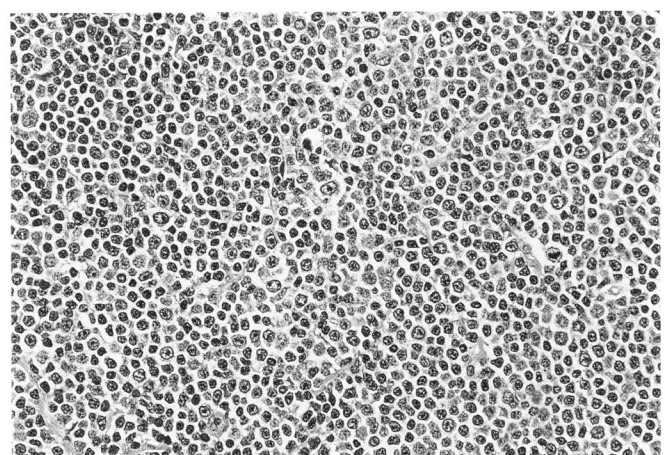

Fig. 21.6 Lymph-node biopsy section in chronic lymphocytic leukemia showing diffuse effacement of nodal architecture with central proliferation center. H&E, × 40 objective.

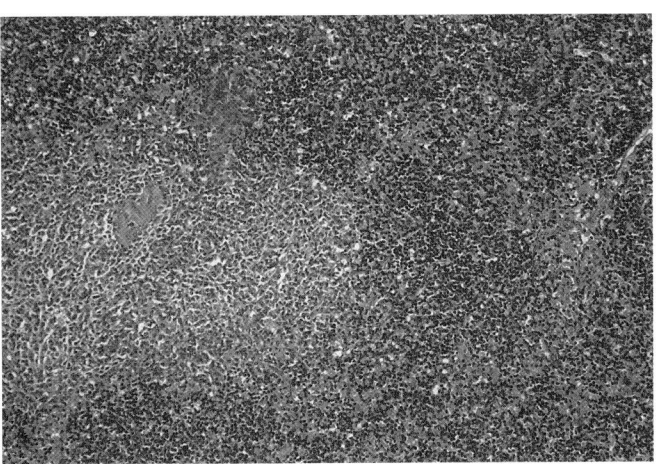

Fig. 21.7 Spleen in chronic lymphocytic leukemia with expansion of the white-pulp areas and infiltration of red-pulp cords by neoplastic cells. H&E, × 10 objective.

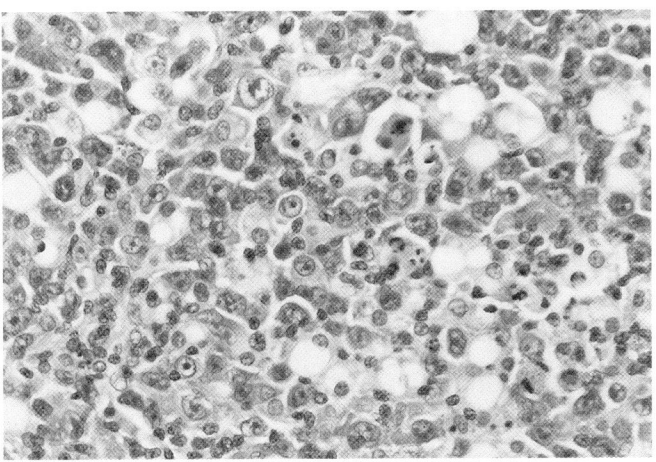

Fig. 21.8 Trephine-biopsy section in Richter's transformation of chronic lymphocytic leukemia showing pleomorphic large lymphocytes. H&E, × 40 objective.

markers, specifically CD20, CD22 and CD79b. Other B-cell markers, such as CD19 and CD79a are more strongly expressed. CLL is unusual among B-cell neoplasms in that there is expression of CD5 (also expressed by cells of mantle cell lymphoma) and CD23. FMC7, which is expressed by most mature B-cell neoplasms, is weak or negative. The immunophenotype is more likely to be atypical in patients with the mixed cell type of CLL.

There is a reduction of normal serum immunoglobulins, particularly in patients with advanced disease. A minority of patients have a paraprotein. A minority of patients, particularly those with more advanced disease, have a positive direct antiglobulin test.

There are no cytogenetic or molecular genetic abnormalities that are pathognomonic of CLL and when abnormalities are found they are often present in only a proportion of cells of the leukemic clone, this indicating that the cytogenetic abnormality does not reflect the initial leukemogenic event. The karyotypic abnormalities most often present are trisomy 12, translocations involving 13q and deletions of 13q-, 6q- and 11q-. Deletions and translocations of 13q usually involve 13q14. Deletions of chromosome 11 are usually large, including 11q23. The most typical molecular genetic abnormalities are deletion of various genes on 13q, including the *RB1* cancer-suppressing gene, and mutations in the *BCL6* gene.

Prolymphocytic leukemia

Prolymphocytic leukemia (PLL) is an uncommon chronic leukemia resulting from the proliferation of a neoplastic clone of mature B-lymphocytes with specific cytologic features and with an immunophenotype that resembles that of non-Hodgkin's lymphoma.

Clinical features

Prolymphocytic leukemia is usually a disease of the middle-aged and elderly. There is a male preponderance. Typically, there is splenomegaly with only minor lymphadenopathy. In most patients the rate of disease progression is much more rapid than that of CLL. Prognosis is considerably worse than that of CLL with the median survival being about 3 years.

Pathologic features

Peripheral blood

The white cell count is usually markedly elevated as the result of the presence of considerable numbers of quite abnormal lymphoid cells. Prolymphocytes are medium-sized to large cells, characterized by a prominent nucleolus which appears vesicular because of perinucleolar chromatin condensation (Fig. 21.9). In some patients the majority of neoplastic cells are typical large prolymphocytes with large prominent nucleoli. In others there is more of a spectrum of cells with the medium-sized and smaller cells having less prominent nucleoli; nevertheless, in these patients also the prolymphocyte is the dominant cell. Smear cells are not a feature. Anemia and thrombocytopenia are common.

Bone marrow

The bone marrow is infiltrated by cells with similar cytologic features to those in the peripheral blood.

The bone marrow trephine biopsy usually shows an interstitial pattern of infiltration, but nodular–interstitial and diffuse patterns are also seen. The neoplastic cells are slightly larger than the small lymphocytes seen in CLL and have coarsely clumped chromatin and a prominent nucleolus (Fig. 21.10). There is usually an increase in reticulin fibers in the areas of infiltration.[13]

Other tissues

The spleen shows expansion of the white-pulp marginal zone by cells similar to those seen in the bone marrow; there is often also infiltration of the red pulp.[14]

Clinically significant involvement of other tissues, including lymph nodes, is uncommon.

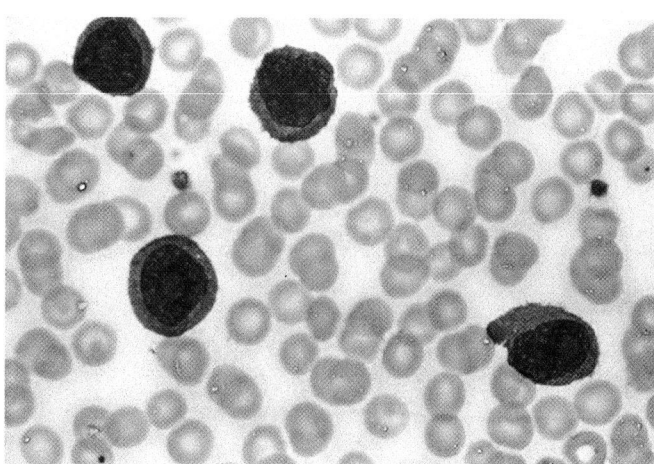

Fig. 21.9 Peripheral-blood film in B-lineage prolymphocytic leukemia showing large lymphoid cells with a regular outline and a round nucleus; each cell has a single large vesicular nucleolus. MGG, × 100 objective.

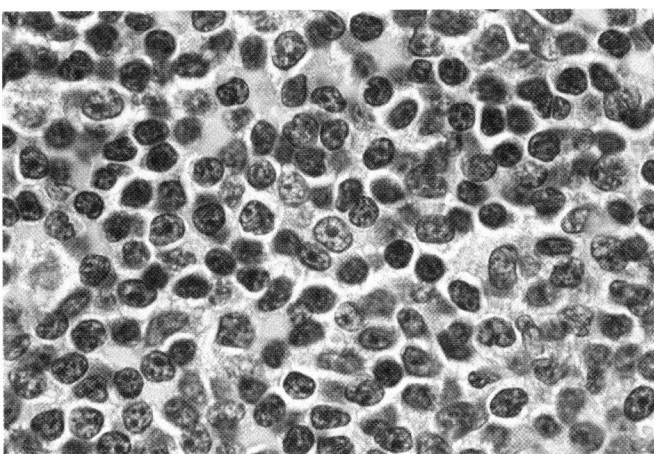

Fig. 21.10 Trephine-biopsy section in B-lineage prolymphocytic leukemia. H&E, × 100 objective.

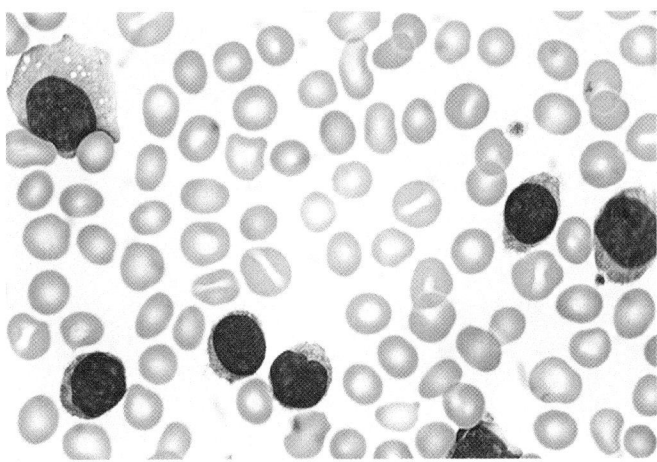

Fig. 21.11 Peripheral-blood film in splenic lymphoma with villous lymphocytes showing mature small lymphocytes; the cytoplasmic margins show fine projections which, in some cells, are at one or both poles of the cell. MGG, × 100 objective.

Supplementary investigations

The neoplastic cells in the majority of patients show strong expression of surface membrane immunoglobulin; this is usually IgM, with or without IgD. CD5 and CD23 are not expressed whereas there is strong expression of CD19, CD20, CD22, CD79a, CD79b and FMC7. In a minority of patients the immunophenotype is closer to that of CLL.

A paraprotein is present in about a third of patients.

There is no specific pathognomonic cytogenetic or molecular genetic abnormality. There are often complex cytogenetic abnormalities which may include trisomy 3, trisomy 12, 6q– and 14q+, the latter sometimes resulting from t(11;14)(q13;q32).

Mutations of the p53 cancer-suppressing gene are common. Patients with t(11;14) have *BCL1* dysregulation.

Splenic lymphoma with villous lymphocytes

Splenic lymphoma with villous lymphocytes is a disease resulting from clonal proliferation of mature small lymphocytes with characterisitic cytologic features and the immunophenotype of non-Hodgkin's lymphoma. Splenic lymphoma with villous lymphocytes is a morphologic variant of splenic marginal zone B-cell lymphoma.

Clinical features

Splenic lymphoma with villous lymphocytes is mainly a disease of the middle-aged and elderly. It may be more common in men than in women. Typically there is spleno-megaly, less often hepatomegaly and lymphadenopathy is not a prominent feature. Disease progression is slow.

Pathologic features

Peripheral blood

The peripheral blood often shows lymphocytosis although this may not be marked. Other patients have cytologically abnormal cells in the absence of lymphocytosis. The neoplastic cells may resemble those of CLL but they are less monomorphic and smear cells are not common. The nucleocytoplasmic ratio is high. Some cells show ragged or villous cytoplasm (Fig. 21.11); the villous projections may be predominantly at one pole of the cell. In some patients there are nucleoli. A minority of cells show plasmacytoid differentiation and there may be increased rouleaux formation resulting from the presence of a paraprotein.

Following splenectomy, recognizable neoplastic cells may disappear from the blood.

Bone marrow

The bone marrow may be normal or there may be minimal or marked infiltration by cells cytologically resembling those in the blood. The trephine biopsy often shows involvement,[15] but infiltration may be subtle and easily overlooked. Interstitial and nodular patterns of infiltration are most common. Some cases have infiltration confined to the sinusoids (intrasinusoidal pattern).[16] The infiltrate consists of small lymphocytes admixed with smaller numbers of plasma cells and plasmacytoid lymphocytes. Immunohistochemical staining for B-cell markers (CD20 and CD79a) is helpful in identifying minor degrees of interstitial and intrasinusoidal infiltration.

Other tissues

The spleen shows expansion of the white-pulp marginal zone by neoplastic cells; these are slightly larger than normal small lymphocytes with dispersed chromatin and moderate amounts of pale cytoplasm. Small aggregates of tumor cells are also present in the red pulp.[7] Involvement of other tissues is infrequent.

Supplementary investigations

The immunophenotype is typical of non-Hodgkin's lymphoma. There is moderate to strong expression of monotypic surface membrane immunoglobulin which is usually IgM with or without IgD. The neoplastic cells express B-cell markers such as CD19, CD20, CD22, CD79a, CD79b and FMC7. They do not express CD5 or CD23. CD38, a marker that is typically expressed by plasma cells, is sometimes expressed. CD11c, a marker that is typical of hairy cell leukemia, is expressed in a significant minority of patients but other markers typical of hairy cells, such as CD25, CD103 and HC2, are not usually expressed.

Imunohistochemical staining for DBA44, a marker expressed in hairy cell leukemia, is often positive.

A serum or urinary paraprotein is often present although the concentration is not usually very high.

The recurrent cytogenetic abnormality most often observed is t(11;14)(q13;q32), an abnormality that is more characteristic of mantle cell lymphoma; it is present in about a fifth of patients. However, the breakpoints differ at a molecular level from those that are characteristic of mantle cell lymphoma. Other recurring cytogenetic abnormalities include i(17q), trisomy 3 and re-arrangements with 2p11, 7q22 and 7q34–36 breakpoints.

Patients with t(11;14) have *BCL1* dysregulation.

T-lineage prolymphocytic leukemia

T-lineage prolymphocytic leukemia (T-PLL) is a rare lymphoproliferative disorder resulting from proliferation of a clone of T-cells with specific cytologic and characteristic immunophenotypic and cytogenetic features. It has no relationship to the B-lineage disease that bears the same name.

Clinical features

The disease occurs in late-middle and old age and is somewhat more common in men than in women. Patients usually present with splenomegaly and in about a half of patients there is also lymphadenopathy and hepatomegaly.[17,18] Skin infiltration occurs in about a third of patients and typically leads to either a papular non-itchy rash on the trunk, face and arms or to a generalized erythroderma. Prognosis is very poor with survival usually being less than a year.

Pathologic features
Peripheral blood

There is moderate to marked lymphocytosis. The pro-lymphocytes of T-PLL are usually readily differentiated from those of B-lineage prolymphocytic leukemia (B-PLL). They are more irregular in shape and may show cytoplasmic basophilia (Fig. 21.12). The nucleolus may be less prominent. Often they are smaller than the cells of B-PLL and in some cases are no larger than the cells of CLL. They can, however, be distinguished from CLL cells by their cytoplasmic basophilia, cytoplasmic blebs and irregular, hyperchromatic nucleus with a nucleolus. The term 'small cell variant' of T-PLL is often used for these cases; they do not differ in any important respect from cases with larger cells.

Bone marrow

The bone marrow is infiltrated by cells with similar cytologic features to those in the blood. Trephine-biopsy histology usually shows a mixed interstitial–diffuse pattern of infiltration.[13,18] The infiltrating cells resemble those of B-PLL although in many cases the cells of T-PLL have more irregular nuclear outlines (Fig. 21.13); immunophenotyping is required to make the distinction on histologic sections. A minority of patients have either very little infiltration or a heavy diffuse infiltrate.

Other tissues

The spleen shows expansion of the white pulp and infiltration of the red pulp.[18] Lymph node architecture is effaced by a diffuse infiltrate that initially replaces the paracortex. An important feature in making a distinction from CLL is the absence of proliferation centers. Skin infiltration is dermal, sometimes with extension into the subcutaneous fat;[18] infiltration is preferentially around skin appendages and blood vessels.[19]

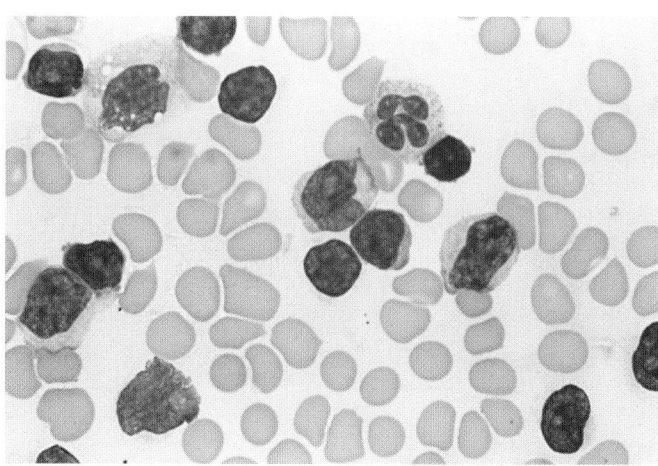

Fig. 21.12 Peripheral-blood film in T-lineage prolymphocytic leukemia showing medium-sized lymphoid cells with irregular outlines and nuclei which are irregular in form; some cells have prominent medium-sized nucleoli. In comparison with B-lineage prolymphocytic leukemia, the cells are smaller and less uniform in appearance and the nucleoli are smaller. MGG, × 100 objective.

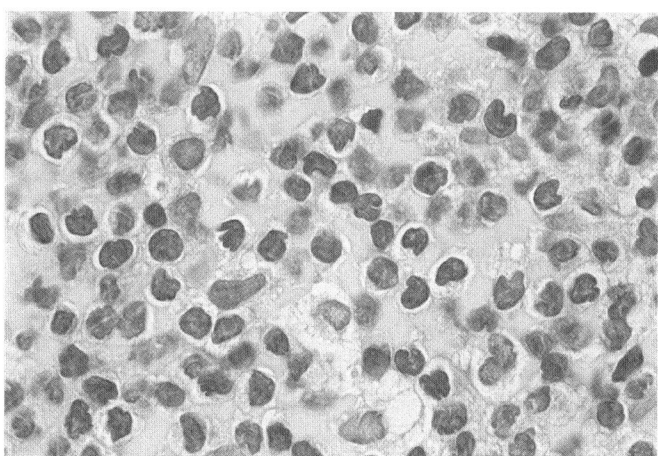

Fig. 21.13 Trephine-biopsy section in T-lineage prolymphocytic leukemia. H&E, × 100 objective.

Supplementary investigations

Leukemic cells are usually CD3 positive although about 20% express cytoplasmic but not surface membrane CD3. They are usually CD4 positive and CD8 negative but in a significant minority of cases cells either express both CD4 and CD8 or are CD4 negative and CD8 positive. Cells usually express CD7, a surface membrane antigen which is much less often expressed in other T-lineage lymphoproliferative disorders. They usually do not express CD25 or express it only weakly, a useful feature in making a distinction from adult T-cell leukemia lymphoma.

The most characteristic cytogenetic abnormalities in T-PLL, observed in about three-quarters of patients, are inv(14)(q11q32) and t(14;14)(q11;q32). Both these re-

arrangements involve the *TCL1* oncogene at 14q32, which is juxtaposed to the T-cell receptor αδ locus at 14q11.

Leukemias of large granular lymphocytes

Leukemias of large granular lymphocytes may be of either T-lineage or natural killer (NK) lineage.[20] The WHO classification recognizes these as separate entities, using the names T-cell granular lymphocytic leukemia and aggressive NK-cell leukemia. Although the leukemic cells may be cytologically similar, these are two distinct conditions. The lack of a readily applicable clonal marker for NK cells means that it is difficult to determine if there are also NK-cell leukemias with less aggressive clinical behavior.

Clinical features

T-cell granular lymphocytic leukemia is a disease of the elderly. It may be an incidental diagnosis or patients may present with recurrent infections, resulting from neutropenia. Hepatomegaly and splenomegaly are common but lymphadenopathy is not. There is an association with rheumatoid arthritis, including Felty's syndrome and it has been estimated that as many as 40% of patients with Felty's syndrome have T-cell granular lymphocyte leukemia.[20] Rare patients have a lymphomatous form of the disease with the peripheral blood and bone marrow being normal.[18] T-cell granular lymphocytic leukemia has a relatively good prognosis with a median survival of approximately 10 years.[20]

Patients with aggressive NK-cell leukemia usually have hepatomegaly and splenomegaly and often have B symptoms. About a third have lymphadenopathy and extranodal involvement may also occur. Patient are, on average, younger than those with T-cell granular lymphocytic leukemia. There is a strong association with Epstein–Barr Virus (EBV) infection with the leukemic cells carrying the virus. This type of leukemia is much commoner in Asia, among Japanese and Chinese, than among Europeans. The prognosis is poor with most patients dying within a few months of diagnosis.[20]

Pathologic features

Peripheral blood

Lymphocytosis is seen in about 50% of patients with T-cell granular lymphocytic leukemia. An increase in large

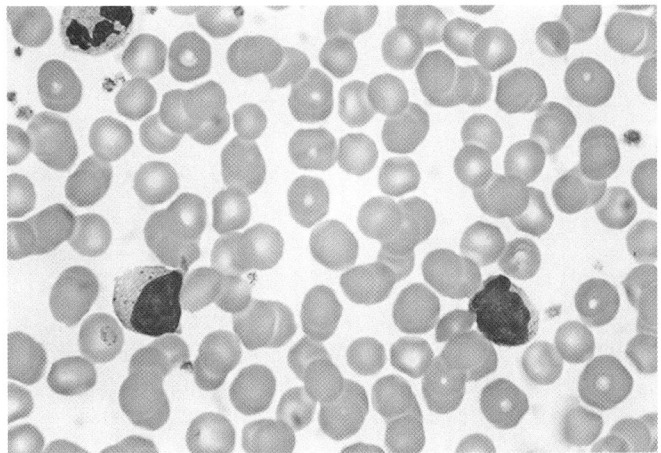

Fig. 21.14 Peripheral-blood film in large granular lymphocyte leukemia showing two leukemia cells, one of which has plentiful cytoplasm containing azurophilic granules. MGG, × 100 objective.

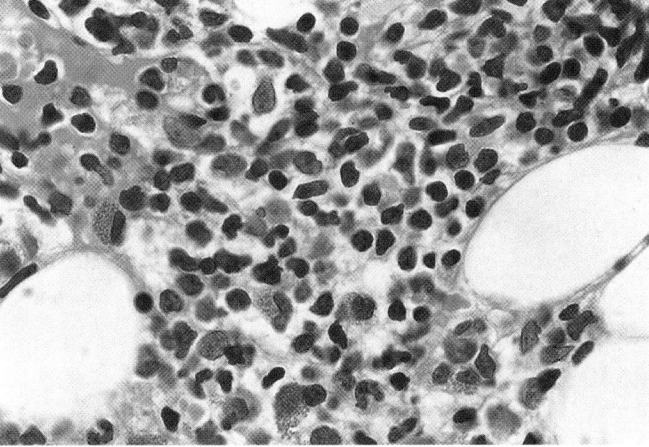

A

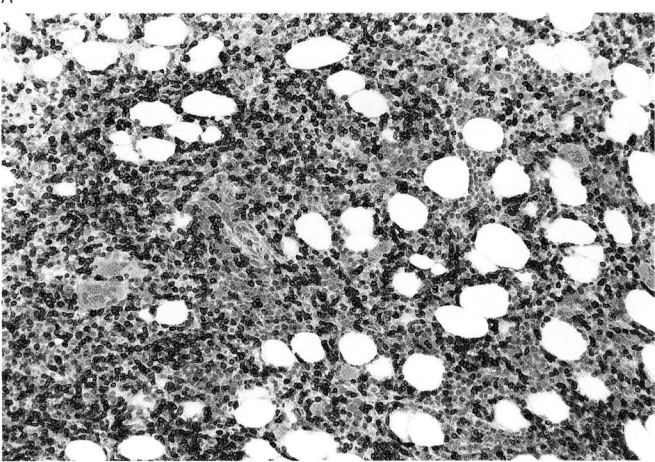

B

Fig. 21.15 Trephine-biopsy section in T-cell granular lymphocytic leukemia showing a nodular–interstitial infiltrate of small/medium sized lymphocytes. (A) H&E, × 40 objective. (B) anti-CD3, immunoperoxidase × 40 objective.

granular lymphocytes is present in virtually all patients (Fig. 21.14). The neoplastic cells are cytologically very similar to normal large granular lymphocytes. They are medium-sized cells with abundant weakly basophilic granular cytoplasm and prominent azurophilic granules. In occasional patients the neoplastic cells lack granules. Around 50% of patients are anemic and about a fifth are thrombocytopenic.[20] There may be associated immunologically-mediated features such as neutropenia and, less often, thrombocytopenia or anemia. The white cell count is not usually greatly elevated but large granular lymphocytes constitute more than 25% of cells.

In aggressive NK-cell leukemia the leukemic cells also resemble normal large granular lymphocytes but they may be cytologically atypical, being larger with a higher nucleocytoplasmic ratio, basophilic cytoplasm of a visible nucleolus. Anemia and thrombocytopenia are common but neutropenia is less common than in T-cell granular lymphocytic leukemia.

Bone marrow

The bone marrow may be infiltrated with cells that are cytologically similar to those in the peripheral blood. Associated abnormalities that may be present in T-cell granular lymphocyte leukemia include pure red cell aplasia and an apparent maturation arrest in the granulocytic series. In aggressive NK-cell leukemia there may be increased hemophagocytic macrophages.

On trephine-biopsy histology the infiltration in T-cell large granular lymphocyte leukemia may be subtle and more readily detected by immunohistochemical staining for the T-cell marker, CD3, than by examination of H&E-stained sections (Fig. 21.15).[18] Infiltration may be inter-

stitial or there may be small focal infiltrates. The neoplastic cells are small to medium sized with irregular nuclear contours and condensed chromatin; cytoplasmic granules are not visible in histologic sections.

Other tissues

Splenic histology in T-cell large granular lymphocyte leukemia shows marked expansion of the red pulp as a result of infiltration predominantly within the sinuses.[7,18] The splenic white pulp is often preserved and some patients have prominent reactive germinal centers. In the liver infiltration is predominantly sinusoidal, but portal tracts may also be infiltrated.[18,21] Lymph nodes are rarely biopsied but have been reported to show paracortical and interfollicular infiltration.[18] In those cases with skin involvement there is dermal infiltration, preferentially around skin appendages.[18]

Supplementary investigations

The typical immunophenotype in T-cell granular lymphocytic leukemia is positivity for CD2, CD3, CD8, CD16 and CD57; CD5 and CD7 are expressed in around 50% of patients.[18,20] Most cases are CD56 negative. In aggressive NK-cell leukemia the typical immunophenotype is positivity for CD2, CD16 and CD56 with variable expression of CD8 and CD57.[20] The essential differences are that in T-cell granular lymphocytic leukemia there is rearrangement of T-cell receptor genes and expression of CD3 whereas in aggressive NK-cell leukemia there is not.

Rheumatoid factor antibodies are present in about 60% of patients with T-cell granular lymphocytic leukemia and antinuclear antibodies in about 40%.[20] A polyclonal hypergammaglobulinemia is usual.

Clonal cytogenetic rearrangements may be detected in both conditions but there are no specific rearrangements that have yet been associated with these diseases. In EBV-associated cases clonality can also be demonstrated by investigation of the length of the episomal form of the virus.

Sézary syndrome/mycosis fungoides

Sézary syndrome and mycosis fungoides are closely related cutaneous lymphomas. Sézary syndrome is characterized by circulating neoplastic cells and an erythrodermic rash whereas mycosis fungoides is initially confined to the skin. Peripheral blood and bone marrow involvement occur late in the course of mycosis fungoides. Large cell transformation may occur in both conditions, including transformation to large cell anaplastic lymphoma.

Clinical features

Sézary syndrome and mycosis fungoides are mainly diseases of the elderly. In Sézary syndrome there is widespread skin infiltration leading to generalized erythroderma with or without plaque-like skin lesions and cutaneous tumors. Mycosis fungoides is characterized initially by pruritic eczematous skin lesions, and later by thickened plaques and tumor formation. In the early stages, lymphadenopathy is usually a result of a type of reactive lymphadenitis that is also seen in association with other non-neoplastic skin conditions (dermatopathic lymphadenopathy). However, later in the disease course there is infiltration of lymph nodes and subsequently hepatomegaly and splenomegaly.

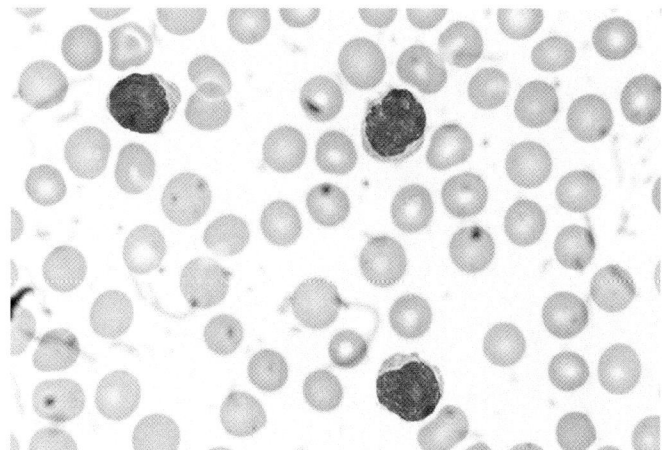

Fig. 20.16 Peripheral-blood film in Sézary syndrome showing small Sézary cells with grooved nuclear surfaces. MGG, × 100 objective.

Pathologic features

Peripheral blood

Circulating neoplastic cells are cytologically very variable between patients. Small Sézary cells have a high nucleocytoplasmic ratio and a 'cerebriform' nucleus with intertwined lobes and hyperchromatic chromatin; the surface of the nucleus often appears grooved (Fig. 21.16). Large Sézary cells have more plentiful cytoplasm and lobulated or cerebriform nuclei. Individual patients may have only small cells, a mixture of large and small cells or mainly large cells. There may be a minority of cells with a flower-shaped nucleus, resembling the cells seen in adult T-cell leukemia/lymphoma. Sometimes Sézary cells have a ring of vacuoles; this appearance, which reflects glycogen in the cytoplasm, has been likened to a string of rosary beads. Reactive eosinophilia is sometimes present.

Bone marrow

Early in the course of the disease bone marrow infiltration is absent or minimal and difficult to detect.[22,23] This may be so even in patients with Sézary syndrome with significant numbers of circulating neoplastic cells. Heavier infiltration is seen late in the disease course. In trephine biopsy sections the neoplastic cells are small with irregular, often convoluted nuclear outlines and condensed chromatin. Some cases also have a population of larger cells with prominent nucleoli.

Other tissues

In the early stages of the disease the histologic changes within the skin are often non-specific, and repeated biopsies may be required to establish the diagnosis. There is a diffuse infiltrate of medium-sized lymphoid cells with irregular convoluted (cerebriform) nuclei in the upper dermis which can obscure the dermo-epidermal junction. Smaller numbers of larger cells with prominent nucleoli are often present. A diagnostically useful feature is infiltration of the epidermis by small groups of neoplastic cells forming Pautrier microabscesses.[24] As the disease progresses with the formation of tumor nodules the number of larger cells within the infiltrate increases.

Dermatopathic lymphadenopathy is characterized by expansion of the lymph node paracortex with numerous Langerhans cells and macrophages containing phagocytosed melanin. In infiltrated lymph nodes, aggregates of small to medium-sized lymphoid cells with cerebriform nuclei are seen in the paracortex.[25] Early involvement is often difficult to recognize, particularly if there are also changes of dermatopathic lymphadenopathy. In the late stages of the disease, other tissues, including liver, spleen and lung, may be infiltrated by neoplastic cells with typical convoluted nuclei.[26]

Supplementary investigations

The typical immunophenotype is positivity for CD2, CD3, CD4, CD5 and CD103. CD7 is expressed in approaching 50% of patients (18). CD8 and CD25 are usually negative; if expressed, CD25 is weak. HLA-DR is sometimes expressed.[18]

Complex cytogenetic abnormalities are common. Tetraploidy or polyploidy may be a feature, particularly in those patients with very large cells.

Adult T-cell leukemia/lymphoma

Adult T-cell leukemia/lymphoma is a disease of adult life. It occurs only in individuals who are carriers of HTLV-I (the human T lymphotropic virus) who have a life-long risk of developing leukemia/lymphoma of at least 1–2%. This disease is necessarily most common in areas where this virus is endemic, particularly Japan and the West Indies, but sporadic cases occur in many other parts of the world where the virus is found, albeit less frequently. The disease may thus occur in the Middle East, Central and West Africa and South America.

Clinical features

About 90% of patients present with leukemia and about 10% with lymphoma. The majority of patients have a sub-acute course with a very poor prognosis but smoldering

and chronic forms of the disease also occur. Common clinical features are skin rash (reflecting cutaneous infiltration), lymphadenopathy, hepatomegaly, splenomegaly and hypercalcemia. The latter manifestation is caused by activation of osteoclasts by cytokines secreted by the neoplastic cells. Opportunistic infections are quite common. They include cryptococcosis, infection with *Pneumocystis carinii* and hyperinfection with *Stronglyloides stercoralis*. Some patients have not only adult T leukemia/lymphoma but also other HTLV-I-related conditions such as tropical spastic paraparesis or uveitis.

Pathologic features
Peripheral blood

In the 90% of patients who present with leukemia rather than lymphoma there are varying numbers of abnormal lymphoid cells in the blood. These cells are very pleomorphic with a moderate amount of cytoplasm and irregularly shaped nuclei that are often nucleolated (Fig. 21.17). A proportion of the cells are lobulated in such a manner that the nuclear shape resembles a flower. A smaller number of cells have a high nucleocytoplasmic ratio and less obvious lobulation so that they resemble Sézary cells. Some cells may have a more diffuse chromatin pattern and some resemble immunoblasts; these are large cells with a prominent nucleolus and plentiful basophilic cytoplasm. There may be reactive eosinophilia and neutrophilia.

Bone marrow

The bone marrow infiltration is often subtle, even in patients who have quite numerous circulating neoplastic

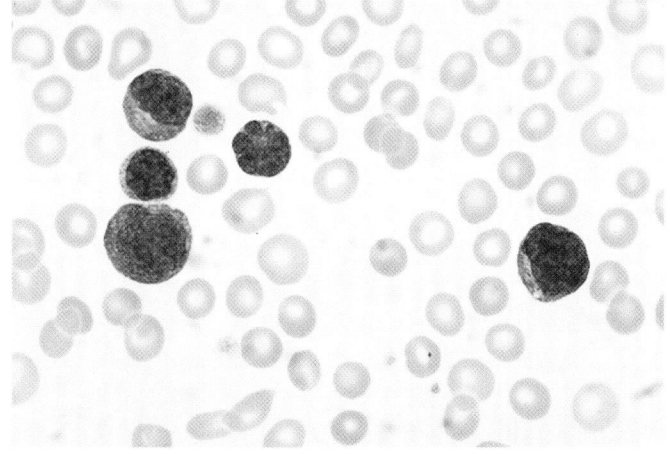

Fig. 20.17 Peripheral-blood film in adult T-cell leukemia/lymphoma showing pleomorphic lymphoid cells, one of which has a flower-shaped nucleolus. MGG, × 100 objective.

cells. In trephine-biopsy sections the pattern of infiltration may be interstitial, focal or diffuse. There is marked variation in the morphology of the neoplastic cells. In most cases the cells have medium-sized or large hyperchromatic nuclei showing marked pleomorphism with irregular, convoluted or lobated outlines and prominent nucleoli (Fig. 21.18).[27,28] Increased numbers of plasma cells and eosinophils are often present within areas of infiltration. Some cases have increased bone resorption with prominent Howship's lacunae containing osteoclasts.

Other tissues

Lymph node infiltration is initially paracortical, but later there is diffuse effacement of the nodal architecture.[27,29] The infiltrate is often polymorphous with a mixture of medium-sized and large cells showing marked nuclear pleomorphism (Fig. 21.19). Some cases have multinucleate tumor cells resembling Reed–Sternberg cells.

Skin infiltration is common.[30] There is a dense lymphoid infiltrate within the dermis often extending into the subcutis. There may be epidermal invasion resembling that seen in mycosis fungoides.[31] The neoplastic cells resemble those seen in the lymph nodes and bone marrow.

Pleural and peritoneal effusions sometimes occur and highly atypical cells are then present in the exudate (Fig. 21.20).

Supplementary investigations

Neoplastic cells usually express CD2, CD3, CD4, CD5 and activation markers such as CD25, CD38 and HLA-DR. Expression of CD3 is weak. Expression of CD25 is the most specific immunophenotypic marker of this disease.

Cytogenetic abnormalities are often complex.

Chronic granulocytic leukemia

Chronic granulocytic leukemia (CGL) (synonyms: chronic myeloid leukemia, chronic myelogenous leukemia) is a chronic myeloproliferative disorder resulting from a specific mutation in a pluripotent (myeloid-lymphoid) stem cell. This type of leukemia was the first neoplastic disease to be defined at a cytogenetic and molecular level when the association with the t(9;22)(q34;q11) translocation and, subsequently, the *BCR-ABL* fusion gene were recognized. In the absence of treatment aimed at eradicating the leukemic clone, chronic granulocytic leukemia shows an almost inevitable progression from a chronic disease to an acute leukemia of myeloid, lymph-

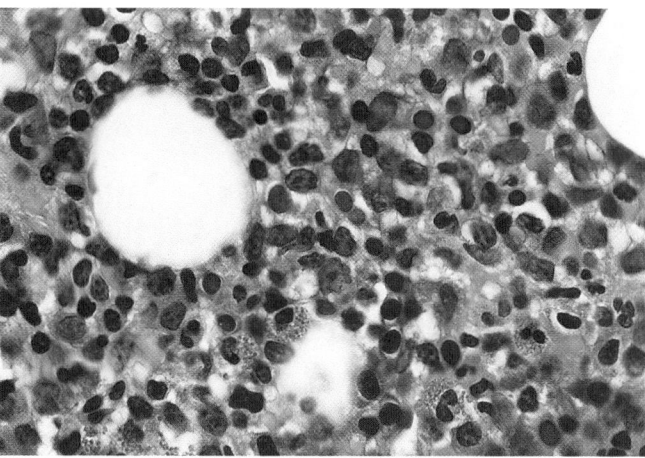

Fig. 20.18 Trephine-biopsy section in adult T-cell leukemia/lymphoma showing infiltration by a pleomorphic population of lymphoid cells with irregular nuclei some containing prominent nucleoli. H&E, × 100 objective.

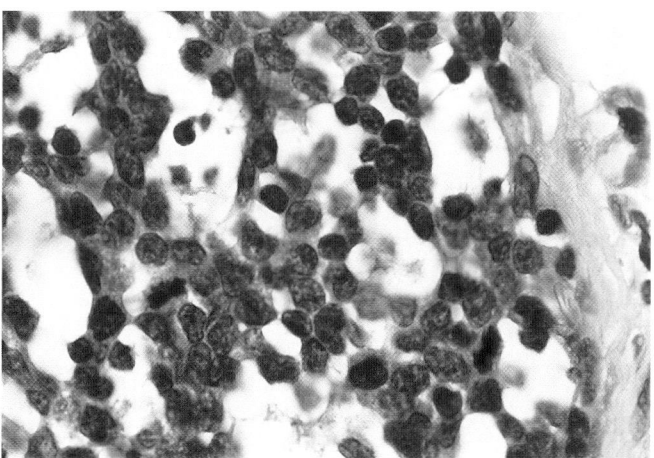

Fig. 20.19 Lymph-node biopsy section adult T-cell leukemia/lymphoma with paracortical infiltration by medium-sized and large lymphoid cells with irregular nuclear outlines. H&E, × 100 objective.

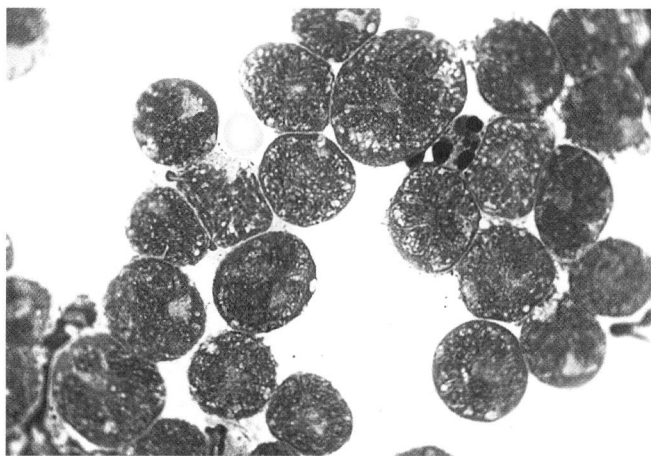

Fig. 20.20 Film of ascitic fluid from a patient with ascites caused by adult T-cell leukemia/lymphoma showing highly pleomorphic medium-sized and large lymphoid cells and one apoptotic cell. MGG, × 100 objective.

oid or biphenotypic lineage, designated blast crisis or blast transformation. There may be an intervening period when the disease enters an accelerated phase.

Clinical features

The usual clinical features of chronic granulocytic leukemia are pallor, hepatomegaly and splenomegaly. Patients who present with more advanced disease have fatigue, weight loss and low-grade fever. However, about a third of patients are diagnosed from an incidental blood count when they are still asymptomatic. With effective treatment, all the clinical features of the disease regress. However, if the disease enters an accelerated phase there may be refractory splenomegaly and the recurrence of signs and symptoms of anemia. In blast transformation there may be a recurrence of hepatomegaly and spleno-megaly and, in addition, lymphadenopathy and tumors at extramedullary sites may develop. Bleeding, bruising and bone pain may also be features of this stage of the disease.

Pathologic features

Peripheral blood

The peripheral blood features are of major importance in the recognition of CGL. Leukocytosis is invariable and is caused by an increase in both mature granulocytes and their precursors (Fig. 21.21). Cells of neutrophil and basophil lineage are almost invariably increased in number and, in the majority of patients, eosinophil numbers are also increased. The two most numerous leukocyte types in the blood are the mature neutrophil and the myelocyte.

Promyelocytes are less numerous than myelocytes and blast cells are, in turn, less numerous than promyelocytes; this reflects the preservation of orderly maturation during the chronic phase of the disease. The platelet count is often elevated, sometimes normal and occasionally reduced. Occasional circulating megakaryocyte nuclei may be seen. Anemia is normocytic and normochromic, without any particular morphologic features. Dysplastic features are absent during the chronic phase of the disease.

When chronic granulocytic leukemia enters an accelerated phase, there may be a recurrence of leukocytosis with the basophil count, in particular, often being elevated. Anemia is also common. Dysplastic features in various lineages may appear.

Blast transformation is generally marked by an increase in peripheral blood blast cells. These are often either megakaryoblasts or agranular myeloblasts but, in a significant minority of patients, they are lymphoblasts. There may also be circulating micromegakaryocytes and dysplastic platelets. The myeloblasts of blast transformation rarely contain Auer rods. Anemia and thrombocytopenia are common at this stage but a minority of patients have thrombocytosis.[32] Absolute basophilia is usual. A minority of patients show the acquired Pelger Huët anomaly or hypogranular neutrophils.[32]

Bone marrow

The bone marrow aspirate is intensely hypercellular as a consequence of granulocytic (neutrophil, eosinophilic, basophilic) hyperplasia (Fig. 21.22). The myeloid:erythroid (M:E) ratio is almost always considerably more than 10:1. In many patients, megakaryocyte numbers are increased. The average size of megakaryocytes is reduced as is

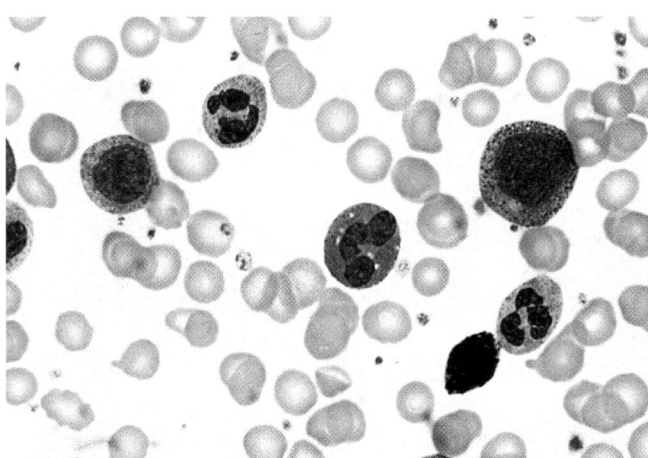

Fig. 20.21 Peripheral blood film in chronic granulocytic leukemia (Ph-positive chronic myeloid leukemia) showing an eosinophil, a basophil, two neutrophils and two neutrophil precursors. MGG, × 100 objective.

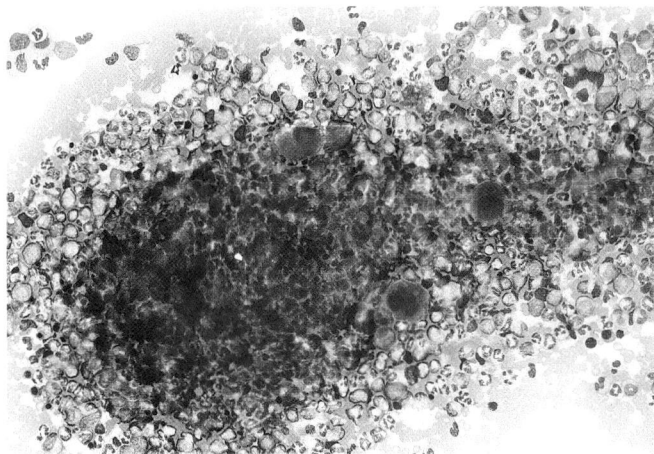

Fig. 20.22 Bone marrow film in chronic granulocytic leukemia showing a fragment which is very hypercellular as the result of both granulocytic and megakaryocytic hyperplasia. MGG, × 20 objective.

the degree of lobulation of the nucleus, but micromega-karyocytes are not features of chronic phase disease.

In the accelerated phase, dysplastic features and a very striking increase in basophils may be seen.

In blast crisis, blast cells with similar cytologic features to those in the blood are increased and soon largely replace all other cells (Fig. 21.23). At this stage of the disease megakaryocyte dysplasia, including numerous micromegakaryocytes, is common and dyserythropoiesis is sometimes marked.

In the chronic phase of CGL the bone marrow trephine biopsy shows marked granulocytic hyperplasia with loss of fat cells[33,34] (Figs 21.24 and 21.25). Eosinophils and eosinophil precursors are often increased. The normal architecture of the marrow is retained with the less mature granulocytic precursors (blasts and promyelocytes) being

found in expanded paratrabecular and peri-arteriolar zones. In the chronic phase, blast cells and promyelocytes are present in small numbers, but as the disease enters an accelerated phase the numbers of blast cells increase (Fig. 21.26); initially this usually occurs focally in the periarteriolar and paratrabecular zones[35] or as random focal aggregates, but later there is a more generalized increase. Immunohistochemical staining for CD34 is useful for highlighting the increased number of blast cells in accelerated phase.[36] There is a variable increase in megakaryocytes, which have smaller more hyperchromatic nuclei with fewer lobes than normal megakaryocytes.[37] In some cases there is striking megakaryocytic hyperplasia. Erythroid precursors are present in normal or reduced numbers. There is usually an increase in reticulin. In a small minority of cases there is also collagen fibrosis

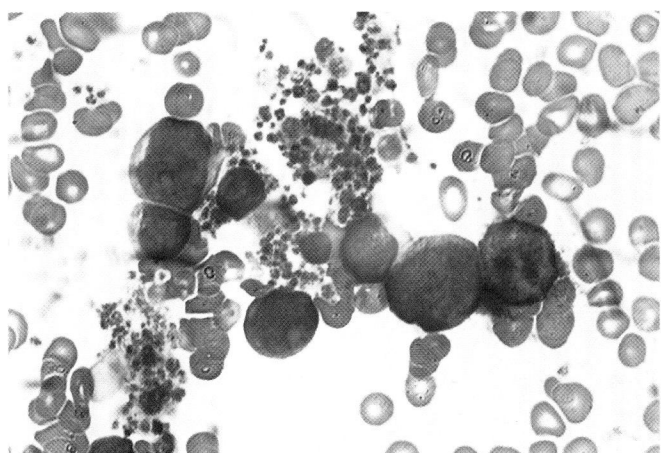

Fig. 20.23 Bone marrow film in megakaryoblastic transformation of chronic granulocytic leukemia showing megakaryoblasts, large platelet clumps and a single Sudan black B-positive neutrophil. Sudan black B stain, × 100 objective.

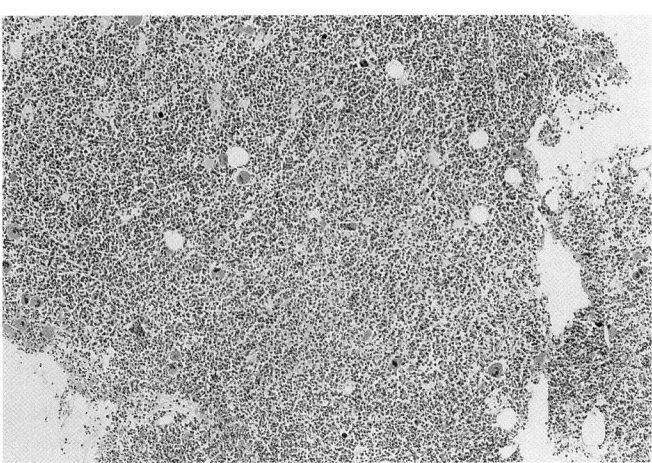

Fig. 20.24 Trephine biopsy section in chronic granulocytic leukemia, chronic phase showing a packed marrow with loss of fat spaces. H&E, × 10 objective.

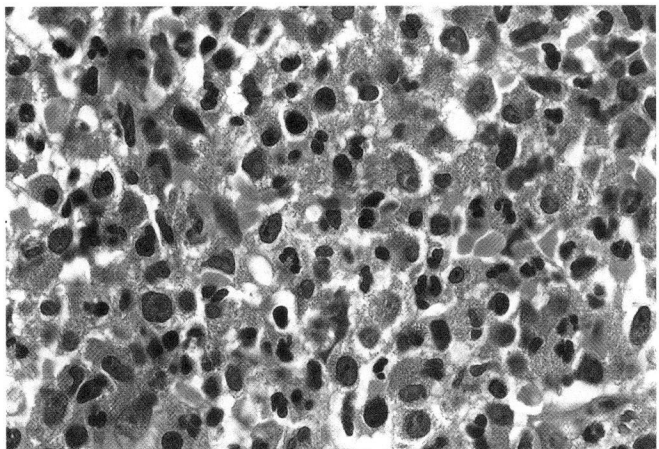

Fig. 20.25 Trephine biopsy section chronic granulocytic leukemia, chronic phase, showing granulocytic hyperplasia. H&E, × 100 objective.

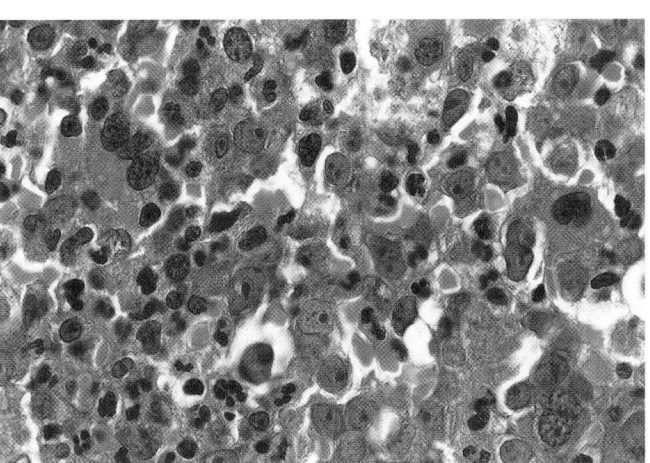

Fig. 20.26 Trephine biopsy section in chronic granulocytic leukemia, accelerated phase showing increased numbers of blast cells. H&E, × 40 objective.

which may be associated with osteosclerosis. The development of marked myelofibrosis may be a feature of the accelerated phase.

Blast crisis is characterized by a diffuse infiltrate of blast cells, replacing more mature hemopoietic cells (Fig. 21.27). It is not possible to distinguish the lineage of the blast cells reliably on routine histologic sections; immuno-histochemical staining, however, will usually allow the blast-cell lineage to be determined.

Other tissues

There is usually marked splenomegaly in CGL as a result of extramedullary hemopoiesis within the splenic red pulp. There is predominance of granulocytic precursors and megakaryocytes. The megakaryocytes in the spleen show similar morphologic abnormalities to those in the bone marrow[7] (Fig. 21.28).

Extramedullary hemopoiesis occurs in many other organs although clinically significant disease is rare; involvement of the liver is common. Blast transformation sometimes occurs at an extramedullary site.

Supplementary investigations

Cytogenetic analysis, most reliably performed on the bone marrow, shows the balanced reciprocal translocation, t(9;22)(q34;q11). The derivative 22q- chromosome, referred to as the Philadelphia (Ph) chromosome, is the hallmark of this disease. As a result of this translocation part of the *ABL* gene from chromosome 9 fuses with part of the *BCR* gene on chromosome 22 to form a hybrid *BCR-ABL* gene. During the accelerated phase and blast transformation there may be clonal evolution with an extra copy of the Ph chromosome and an isochromosome of the long arm of chromosome 17, i(17q), being particularly characteristic.

Neutrophil alkaline phosphatase activity is reduced in more than 90% of patients in the chronic phase of the disease but this investigation is redundant if cytogenetic or molecular genetic analysis is available. Neutrophil alkaline phosphatase activity may increase during the accelerated phase.

Atypical chronic myeloid leukemia

Atypical chronic myeloid leukemia (aCML) is a Ph-negative, *BCR-ABL*-negative condition which has hematologic features that differ from those of CGL. Prognosis is worse. aCML is classified, according to the criteria of the expert group convened by the WHO, as a mixed myeloproliferative/myelodysplastic condition.[2]

Clinical features

Patients often have splenomegaly and signs and symptoms of anemia.

Pathologic features

Peripheral blood

The white cell count is moderately to markedly elevated. As in chronic granulocytic leukemia, there are increased numbers of neutrophils and neutrophil precursors but eosinophilia and basophilia are less often present and

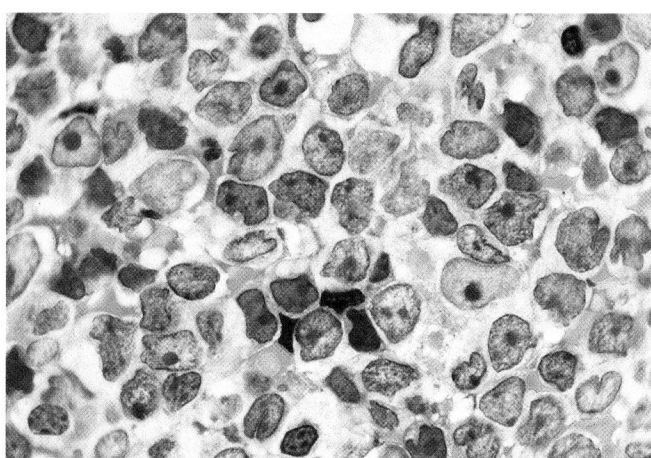

Fig. 20.27 Trephine biopsy section, chronic granulocytic leukemia, blast transformation. There is a diffuse infiltrate of medium-sized blasts with prominent nucleoli. H&E, × 100 objective.

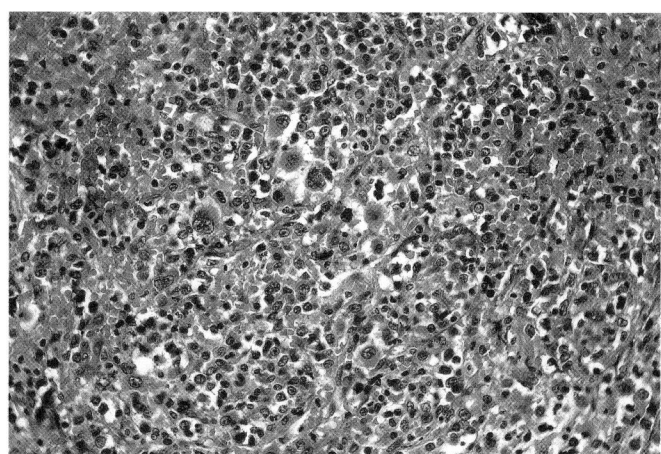

Fig. 20.28 Spleen, chronic granulocytic leukemia. There is extramedullary hemopoiesis within the red pulp. H&E, × 20 objective.

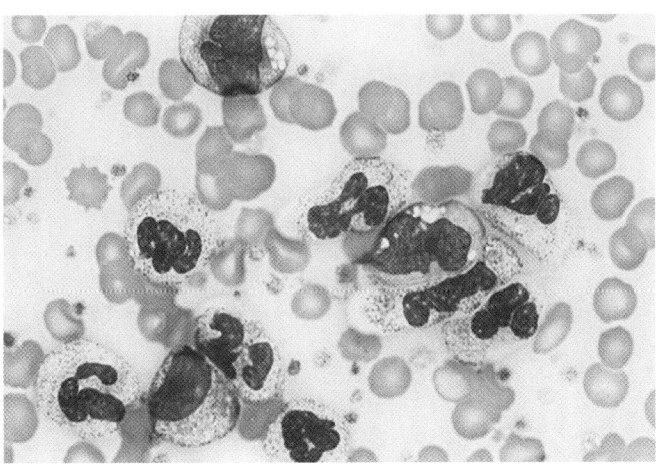

Fig. 20.29 Peripheral blood film in atypical chronic myeloid leukemia showing neutrophils, monocytes and one myelocyte. MGG, × 100 objective.

monocytosis is more marked (Fig. 21.29). There may be dysplastic features in any myeloid lineage. In contrast to CGL, the platelet count is often normal or decreased. Similar diagnostic criteria for distinguishing between aCML and chronic myelomonocytic leukemia (CMML) (see below) have been suggested by the FAB group[38] and by the WHO group.[2] The FAB group suggested that the percentage of granulocyte precursors should be used to make the distinction with these usually being 10–20% in aCML and less than 10% in CMML. In addition, the monocytes were often above 10% in CMML and were usually 3–10% in aCML. Basophils were usually less than 2% in both conditions. The WHO group has also suggested that immature granulocytes should be at least 10%, monocytes should be less than 10% and basophils should be less than 2%.

Bone marrow

The bone marrow aspirate is hypercellular as a result of granulocytic hyperplasia. Granulocytic dysplasia is common. There may also be hyperplasia of cells of monocyte lineage but promonocytes can be difficult to distinguish from promyelocytes unless cytochemistry is employed. Blasts are less than 20%. The M:E ratio is increased but not as markedly as in CGL. Megakaryocytes and erythroblasts may show dysplastic features.

The bone marrow trephine biopsy features are not readily distinguishable from those of typical Ph-positive CGL but dysplasia is generally more marked. The marrow is markedly hypercellular with loss of marrow fat spaces as a result of granulocytic hyperplasia. There is a variable increase in megakaryocytes, which are usually larger and more pleomorphic than those in Ph-positive CGL. Some

cases have increased numbers of monocytes. The monocytes have medium-sized irregular, convoluted nuclei with diffuse chromatin and moderate amounts of pale cytoplasm. Reticulin is often increased.

Other tissues

The spleen shows extramedullary hemopoiesis indistinguishable from that in Ph-positive CGL.

Supplementary investigations

The neutrophil alkaline phosphatase score is variable and this is not a useful test. Clonal cytogenetic abnormalities may be present but the Ph chromosome and *BCR-ABL* fusion gene are not found. The most frequently observed abnormalities are trisomy 8, trisomy 13 and 20q–.

Chronic myelomonocytic leukemia

Chronic myelomonocytic leukemia (CMML) is a Ph-negative, *BCR-ABL* negative condition which has hematologic features that differ both from those of CGL and from those of aCML. In the FAB classification, CMML was classified as one of the myelodysplastic syndromes. In the WHO classification it is assigned to the myeloproliferative/myelodysplastic group of disorders. It is defined by the FAB group as having a monocyte count of greater than $1 \times 10^9/l$ with granulocyte precursors being less than 10% of peripheral blood cells. The second of these criteria distinguishes it from aCML. WHO criteria are similar. CMML is a heterogeneous disorder with some patients having predominantly myelodysplastic features and others predominantly myeloproliferative. The incidence in one study was of the order of 4/100 000/year.[39] Patients are usually elderly and there is a male preponderance.

Clinical features

Patients may have splenomegaly and symptoms of anemia. Hepatomegaly, skin infiltration[40,41] and serous effusions are less common. There may be systemic symptoms including fever, weight loss, night sweats and fatigue. Median survival has differed greatly between various reported series of patients but in most series is several years. Transformation to acute myeloid leukemia (AML) may occur.

Pathologic features

Peripheral blood

The peripheral blood most often shows leukocytosis, monocytosis and neutrophilia (Fig. 21.30) although the total white cell count is sometimes normal and the neutrophil count can be normal or low. Eosinophilia and basophilia are uncommon although there are a subset of patients with t(5;12)(q33;p13) who have CMML with eosinophilia. Blast cells are usually infrequent. If using the FAB classification, blast cells are, by definition, less than 5% of circulating cells; if using the WHO classification, blast cells plus promonocytes are, by definition, less than 20% of circulating cells. Dysplasia in one or more lineages may be present but is not invariable. There may be anemia and thrombocytopenia. The mean cell volume (MCV) is sometimes elevated.

Bone marrow

The bone marrow is hypercellular, usually with both granulocytic and monocytic hyperplasia (Fig. 21.31). The monocytic component may be less apparent in bone marrow aspirate films than in the peripheral blood, partly because monocytes leave the bone marrow soon after production and partly because promonocytes are not always readily distinguished from promyelocytes if cytochemical stains are not used. Blasts may be increased but, by definition, do not exceed 20% of nucleated cells; they are often less than 5%. The WHO group have suggested that cases with fewer than 5% blasts plus promonocytes should be distinguished from cases with 5% or more blasts plus promonocytes since this is of prognostic significance. Bone marrow eosinophils are increased in a subset of patients with CMML. There may be dysplasia in one or more lineages. Erythropoiesis is sometimes sideroblastic.

The trephine biopsy shows granulocytic hyperplasia but, in contrast to CGL, there is often a loss of the normal bone marrow architecture; in some cases immature granulocytic precursors may be seen in a non-paratrabecular position (abnormal localization of immature precursors – ALIP) (Fig. 21.32). Some cases show dysplasia of megakaryocytes with small, hypolobated, hyperchromatic nuclei. The monocytic component is often inconspicuous and difficult to recognize in trephine-biopsy sections. Reticulin is often increased.

Other tissues

Splenomegaly is not usually marked. The spleen shows infiltration of the red pulp by granulocytic precursors

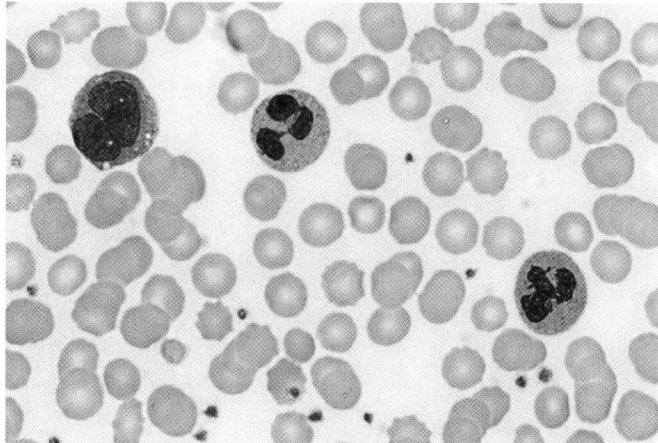

Fig. 20.30 Peripheral blood film in chronic myelomonocytic leukemia showing two neutrophils and a slightly immature monocyte. MGG, × 100 objective.

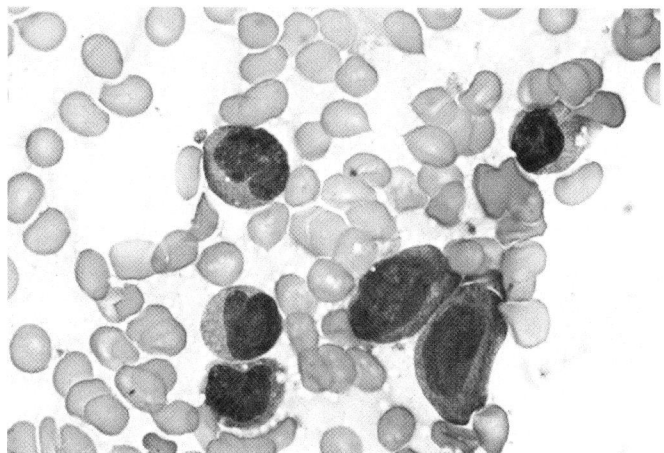

Fig. 21.31 Bone marrow film in chronic myelomonocytic leukemia showing monocyte precursors. MGG, × 100 objective.

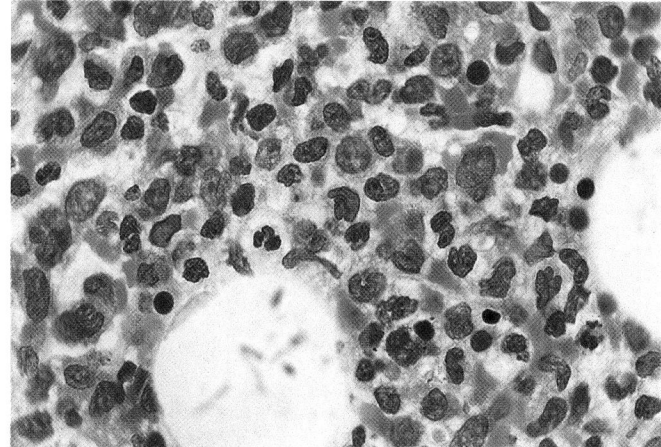

Fig. 21.32 Bone marrow trephine biopsy section, chronic myelomonocytic leukemia showing granulocytic hyperplasia with increased numbers of monocytes and immature monocyte precursors. H&E, × 100 objective.

and megakaryocytes. Cases with skin involvement show dermal infiltration by granulocytic precursors, monocytes and promonocytes. In the late stages of the disease there may be widespread pulmonary infiltrates.[42]

Supplementary investigations

Clonal cytogenetic abnormalities may be present. The most common are +8, –7, 7q– and abnormalities of 12p. *RAS* oncogene mutations are common. In CMML with eosinophilia associated with t(5;12)(q31;p12) a *TEL-PDGFRβ* fusion gene is found.

Juvenile chronic myelomonocytic leukemia

The term juvenile chronic myelomonocytic leukemia (JMML), as defined by the WHO group, is a myelodysplastic/myeloproliferative disorder that encompasses the conditions previously known as juvenile myeloid leukemia and the childhood monosomy 7 syndrome. It results from a mutation in a multipotent myeloid stem cell.

Clinical features

This disorder occurs mainly in infants and is much more common in boys than in girls. The usual clinical features are hepatosplenomegaly, a skin rash and features of anemia. Infection and bleeding are common. There may be lymphadenopathy. The incidence is greatly increased in children with neurofibromatosis type 1 and *café-au-lait*

lesions may be present in children with or without other obvious signs of this disease.

Pathologic features

Peripheral blood

The white cell count is increased with anemia, neutrophilia, monocytosis and thrombocytopenia being usual. There are some circulating granulocyte precursors and small numbers of blast cells (Fig. 21.33). Dysplastic features are common in cells of all lineages. The percentage of hemoglobin F is often increased in relation to what would be expected at the age of the child and there may be other features of fetal hemopoiesis such as reduced carbonic anhydrase and expression of the i antigen.

Bone marrow

The bone marrow is hypercellular as a result of granulocytic and monocytic hyperplasia (Fig. 21.34). There is a variable degree of dysplasia. Blasts cells are, by definition, less than 20% of nucleated cells. Megakaryocytes may be reduced.

Other tissues

Spleen infiltration is in the red pulp with a predilection for trabecular and central arteries.[43] Skin rashes are relatively common, in many cases the histologic features are non-specific resembling a xanthogranuloma or neurofibromatosis, although in some cases abnormal myeloid and monocytic cells are seen in the superficial and deep dermis.[44]

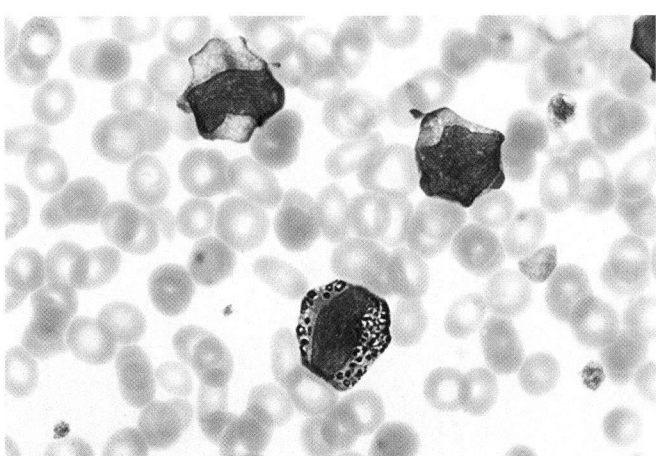

Fig. 21.33 Peripheral blood film in juvenile myelomonocytic leukemia showing a basophil, a blast cell and an abnormal cell which is probably of monocyte lineage. MGG, × 100 objective.

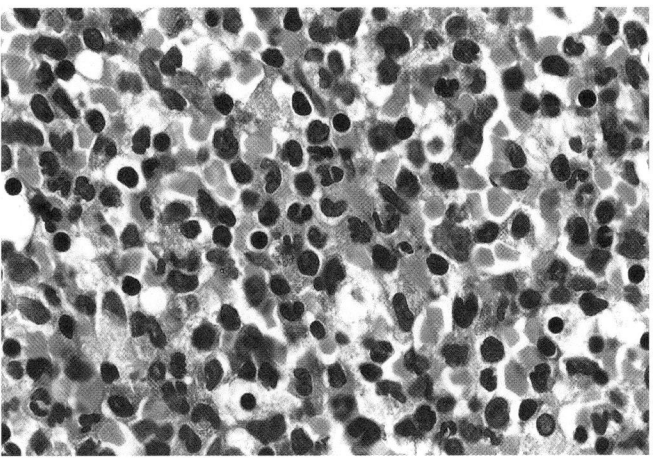

Fig. 21.34 Bone marrow trephine biopsy section, juvenile myelomonocytic leukemia showing granulocytic hyperplasia and increased numbers of monocytes. H&E, × 100 objective.

Supplementary investigations

The Ph chromosome and the *BCR-ABL* fusion gene are absent. Cytogenetic analysis is often normal at onset but clonal abnormalities, including monosomy 7 and trisomy 8, may develop during the course of the disease. Mutations of the *RAS* oncogene are common. Loss of the normal *NF1* gene is common in children with JMML and neurofibromatosis.

Myeloid progenitors show hypersensitivity to granulocyte macrophage colony-stimulating factor (GM-CSF); this has been employed in diagnosis.

Eosinophilic leukemia

Chronic eosinophilic leukemia is a chronic leukemia in which differentiation is predominantly or exclusively eosinophilic. The mutation responsible may, however, be in a multipotent myeloid stem cell or in a pluripotent lymphoid–myeloid stem cell. Eosinophilic leukemia needs to be distinguished from reactive eosinophilia including that due to occult proliferation of neoplastic or other aberrant T-cells. The distinction between eosinophilic leukemia and the idiopathic hypereosinophilic syndrome is also problematical. The latter condition is, by definition, of unknown nature so that cases that can be shown to be clonal or that have an increase of blast cells should be classified as eosinophilic leukemia rather than idiopathic hypereosinophilic syndrome.[45–47] However, some cases initially classified as idiopathic are recognized as leukemic in retrospect when a granulocytic sarcoma develops or transformation to acute leukemia occurs.

Eosinophilic leukemia shows a very striking male preponderance. This is also true of the idiopathic hypereosinophilic syndrome.

Clinical features

There may be hepatomegaly, splenomegaly and symptoms and signs of anemia. Other clinical features result from the release of the contents of eosinophil granules into tissues. Cardiac damage is frequent so that some patients present with cardiac failure or the complications of emboli arising from damaged cardiac valves. Vasculitic rashes and neurological symptoms also occur.

Pathologic features
Peripheral blood

Some patients have eosinophilia as the only significant hematologic abnormality while others have, in addition, other features such as neutrophilia, monocytosis, anemia or thrombocytopenia. There may be small numbers of eosinophil and other granulocyte precursors (Fig. 21.35) including blasts cells. Eosinophils may be cytologically normal but often they are degranulated, vacuolated and hyper- or hypolobulated. Neutrophils may show heavy granulation.

Bone marrow

The bone marrow is hypercellular with a marked increase of eosinophil and precursors and a variable increase of cells of neutrophil and monocyte lineages (Fig. 21.36).

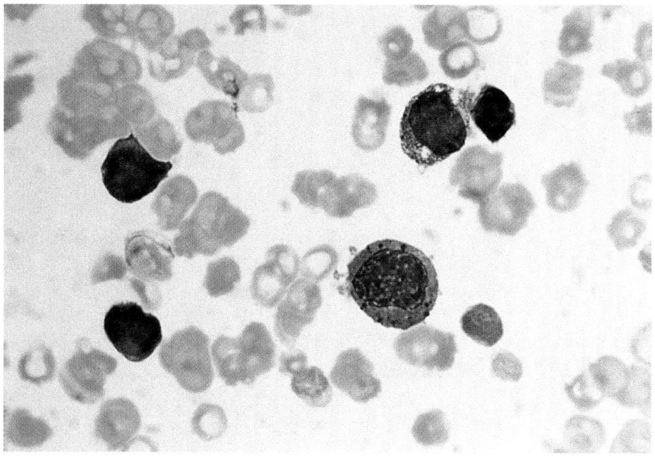

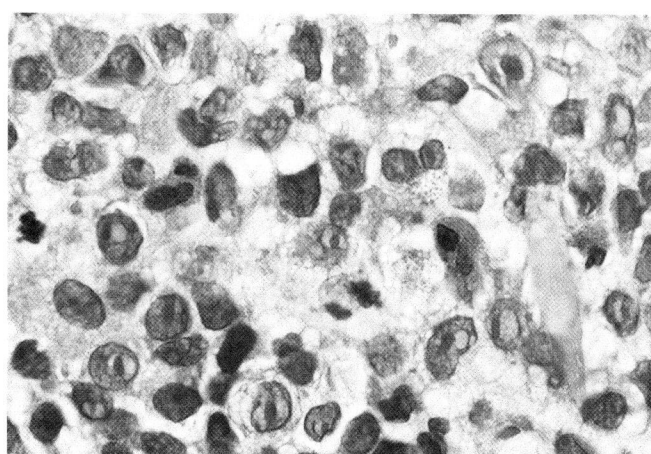

Fig. 21.35 Peripheral blood film in eosinophilic leukemia showing an abnormal non-lobulated eosinophil, an eosinophil myelocyte and three unidentifiable cells. MGG, × 100 objective.

Fig. 21.36 Bone marrow trephine biopsy section in eosinophilic leukemia showing three mature eosinophils and eosinophil precursors (myelocytes and promyelocytes). H&E, × 100 objective.

Blast cells may be normal or increased but, by definition, do not exceed 20%.

Other tissues

In cases with cardiac involvement there is endomyocardial fibrosis with infiltration by eosinophils.[48] The cardiac disease is thought to a direct toxic injury as a result of degranulation of eosinophils.[49]

Supplementary investigations

The Ph chromosome and the *BCR-ABL* fusion gene are absent. Clonal cytogenetic abnormalities that may be present may be either those common in other myeloid neoplasms, such as trisomy 8 and i(17q), or those closely linked with eosinophilic differentiation such as t(8;13)(p11;q12) and the variant translocations with an 8p11 breakpoint, t(8;9)(p11;q32-34) and t(6;8)(q27;p11). The translocation t(5;12)(q33;p13) is more often associated with CMML with eosinophilia but some cases have very marked eosinophilic differentiation.

Not all cases have a clonal cytogenetic abnormality. In those that do not, making the diagnosis of eosinophilic leukemia is more difficult and, unless there is an increase in blast cells, may not be possible.

Systemic mastocytosis

Systemic mastocytosis is a result of neoplastic proliferation of mast cells and is best regarded as a myeloproliferative disorder.[50] The natural history of the disease is variable; some cases have a relatively indolent clinical course while others have an aggressive clinical behavior. Some cases may be associated with myelodysplasia. A minority of cases terminate in AML.

Clinical features

Patients may present with symptoms due to the release of secretory products from mast cell granules. In the most extreme cases this may result in circulatory collapse; more commonly there is abdominal pain, diarrhea, nausea and vomiting, flushing or bronchospasm. Hepatosplenomegaly is common. A minority of patients with systemic mastocytosis have skin rashes due to infiltration by mast cells (urticaria pigmentosa). However, in most patients with urticaria pigmentosa the disease is limited to the skin and there is no evidence of systemic mastocytosis.

Pathologic features

Peripheral blood

The peripheral blood may either be normal or show myeloproliferative or myelodysplastic features. Proliferative features may include monocytosis, eosinophilia, neutrophilia or thrombocytosis. There may be anemia and various cytopenias together with dysplastic feature in cells of any lineage. Small numbers of abnormal circulating mast cells and mast cell precursors may be present (Fig. 21.37).

Bone marrow[50–52]

The bone marrow aspirate shows a variable number of mast cells. Sometimes these remain trapped in the fragments so that they are difficult to recognize. In other patients there are numerous abnormal mast cells also in the trails where their characteristic features are more readily identified. Neoplastic mast cells may be cytologically fairly normal but often they are spindle shaped, have lobulated nuclei or are hypogranular (Fig. 21.38). Mast cell precursors may be recognizable. Other myeloid lineages may show hyperplasia (neutrophilic, eosinophilic or megakaryocytic) or dysplasia (including ring sideroblasts and other features of dyserythropoiesis).

Infiltration is often difficult to recognize in bone marrow trephine biopsy sections in systemic mastocytosis as mast cell granules are not visible on routine H&E stained sections and there is a wide variation in the morphology of neoplastic mast cells. Focal infiltration is most common. The areas of infiltration are ill-defined and often contain eosinophils, lymphocytes, plasma cells and

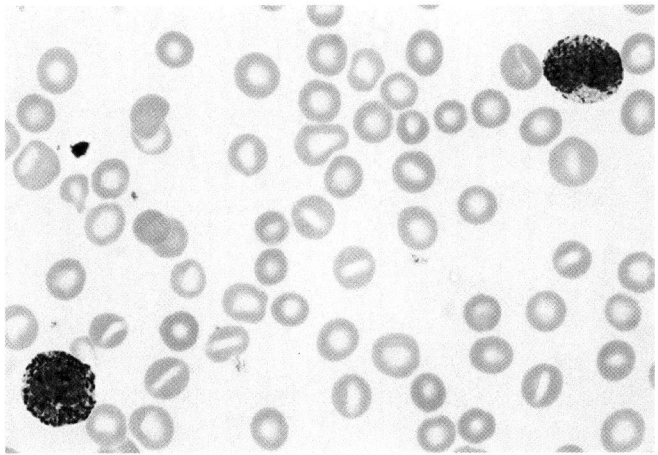

Fig. 21.37 Peripheral blood film in systemic mastocytosis showing two cytologically abnormal circulating mast cells. MGG, × 100 objective.

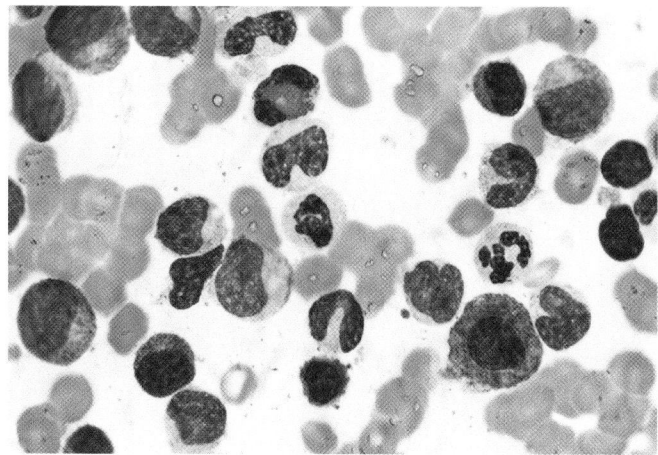

Fig. 21.38 Bone marrow aspirate film in systemic mastocytosis showing a cytologically abnormal mast cells which has fewer and smaller granules than a normal mast cell. MGG, × 100 objective.

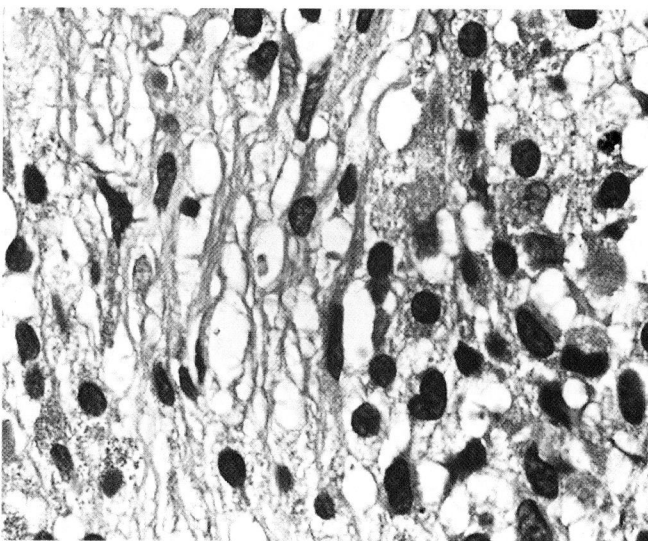

Fig. 21.40 Bone marrow trephine biopsy section in systemic mastocytosis showing spindle shaped and 'histiocyte-like' mast cells. H&E, × 100 objective.

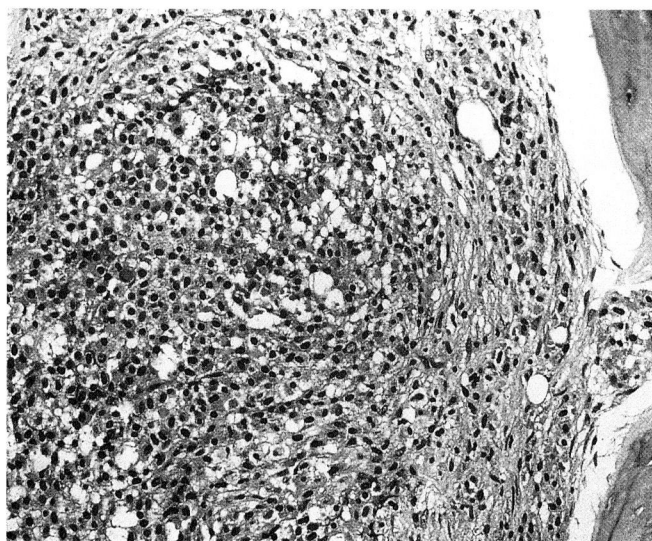

Fig. 21.39 Bone marrow trephine biopsy section in systmic mastocytosis with replacement of the marrow by a diffuse infiltrate of neoplastic mast cells. H&E, × 20 objective.

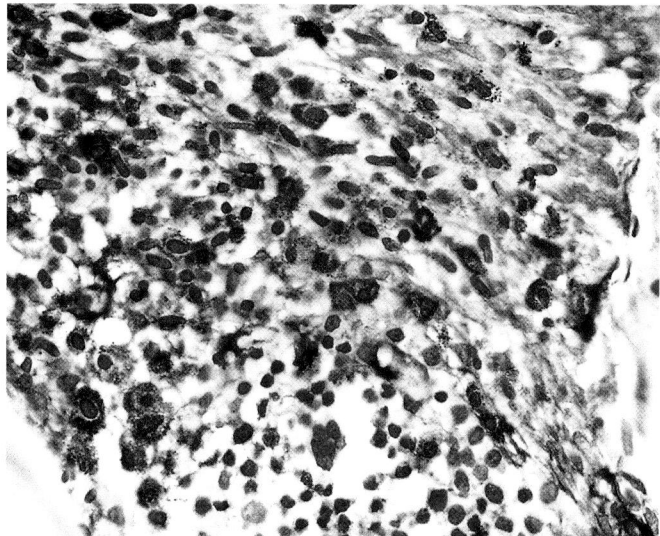

Fig. 21.41 Bone marrow trephine biopsy section in systemic mastocytosis. Anti-mast-cell tryptase, immunoperoxidase, × 40 objective.

macrophages as well as mast cells.[52,53] Infiltration may be random focal or selectively paratrabecular or peri-arteriolar (Fig. 21.39). The neoplastic mast cells show marked variation in morphology and may have plentiful pale cytoplasm and irregular ovoid nuclei, thus closely resembling macrophages, or spindle-shaped nuclei with variable amounts of cytoplasm, causing them to resemble fibroblasts[51] (Fig. 21.40). Reliable identification of the mast cells in histologic sections requires the use of cyto-chemical stains such as Giemsa or toluidine blue, which stain the mast cell granules, or immunohistochemical staining for mast cell tryptase (Fig. 21.41). Immunohisto-chemical staining for mast cell tryptase is more reliable than histochemical stains since neoplastic mast cells may

have few cytoplasmic granules and decalcification of trephine biopsy specimens may reduce the intensity of staining with Giemsa and toluidine blue. The non-infiltrated areas of the biopsy may be relatively normal or show granulocytic hyperplasia and increased numbers of megakaryocytes. The megakaryocytes may show clus-tering and dysplastic nuclear features similar to other myeloproliferative disorders. There is usually a marked increase in reticulin fibers in the areas of infiltration and collagen fibrosis is not uncommon. Osteosclerosis is seen in some cases.

Other tissues

The spleen shows focal infiltration around arterioles and sometimes diffuse infiltration of the red pulp. The areas of infiltration have neoplastic mast cells with associated eosinophils and fibrosis.[54] There may be extramedullary hemopoiesis.

In the liver there is mast cell infiltration and fibrosis within the portal tracts.[55,56] Portal hypertension may occur. Other changes described include nodular regenerative hyperplasia, veno-occlusive disease and cirrhosis.[57,58] Involved lymph nodes show focal infiltration by mast cells associated with fibrosis and the presence of eosinophils.[55] In cases with skin involvement there is a variable infiltrate of mast cells and eosinophils in the dermis.

Supplementary investigations

Clonal cytogenetic abnormalities are sometimes present. The molecular genetic abnormality most often observed is c-*KIT* mutation.

REFERENCES

1. Bennett JM, Catovsky D, Daniel MT et al 1989 Proposals for the classification of chronic (mature) B and T lymphoid leukaemias. French–American–British (FAB) Cooperative Group. Journal of Clinical Pathology 42(6): 567–584
2. Harris NL, Jaffe ES, Diebold J et al 2000 The World Health Organization classification of neoplastic diseases of the haematopoietic and lymphoid tissues: Report of the Clinical Advisory Committee Meeting, Airlie House, Virginia, November 1997. Histopathology 36(1): 69–86
3. Sahota SS, Davis Z, Hamblin TJ et al 2000 Somatic mutation of bcl-6 genes can occur in the absence of V(H) mutations in chronic lymphocytic leukemia. Blood 95(11): 3534–3540
4. Bain BJ, Clark DM, Lampert IA et al 2001 Bone marrow pathology, 3rd edn. Blackwell Science, Oxford
5. Rozman C, Montserrat E, Rodriguez-Fernandez JM et al 1984 Bone marrow histologic pattern – the best single prognostic parameter in chronic lymphocytic leukemia: a multivariate survival analysis of 329 cases. Blood 64(3): 642–648
6. Geisler C, Ralfkiaer E, Hansen MM et al 1986 The bone marrow histological pattern has independent prognostic value in early stage chronic lymphocytic leukaemia. British Journal of Haematology 62(1): 47–54
7. Wilkins BS, Wright DH 2000 Illustrated pathology of the spleen. Cambridge University Press, Cambridge
8. Greenwood R, Barker DJ, Tring FC et al 1985 Clinical and immunohistological characterization of cutaneous lesions in chronic lymphocytic leukaemia. British Journal of Dermatology 113(4): 447–453
9. Berkman N, Polliack A, Breuer R et al 1992 Pulmonary involvement as the major manifestation of chronic lymphocytic leukaemia. Leukaemia and Lymphoma 8(6): 495–499
10. Pohar S, deMetz C, Poppema S et al 1993 Chronic lymphocytic leukemia with CNS involvement. Journal of Neuro-oncology 16(1): 35–37
11. Benekli M, Buyukasik Y, Haznedaroglu IC et al 1996 Chronic lymphocytic leukemia presenting as acute urinary retention due to leukemic infiltration of the prostate. Annals of Haematology 73(3): 143–144
12. Foucar K, Rydell RE 1980 Richter's syndrome in chronic lymphocytic leukemia. Cancer 46(1): 118–134
13. Nieto LH, Lampert IA, Catovsky D 1989 Bone marrow histological patterns in B-cell and T-cell prolymphocytic leukemia. Hematological Pathology 3(2): 79–84
14. Lampert I, Catovsky D, Marsh GW et al 1980 The histopathology of prolymphocytic leukaemia with particular reference to the spleen: a comparison with chronic lymphocytic leukaemia. Histopathology 4(1): 3–19
15. Catovsky D, Matutes E 1999 Splenic lymphoma with circulating villous lymphocytes/splenic marginal-zone lymphoma. Seminars in Hematology 36(2): 148–154
16. Franco V, Florena AM, Campesi G et al 1996 Intrasinusoidal bone marrow infiltration: a possible hallmark of splenic lymphoma. Histopathology 29(6): 571–575
17. Matutes E, Brito-Babapulle V, Swansbury J et al 1991 Clinical and laboratory features of 78 cases of T-prolymphocytic leukemia. Blood 78(12): 3269–3274
18. Matutes E 1999 T-cell lymphoproliferative disorders: classification, clinical and laboratory aspects. In: Polliack A (ed), Advances in blood disorders. Harwood Academic, Australia
19. Mallett RB, Matutes E, Catovsky D et al 1995 Cutaneous infiltration in T-cell prolymphocytic leukaemia. British Journal of Dermatology 132(2): 263–266
20. Lamy T, Loughran TP, Jr 1999 Current concepts: large granular lymphocyte leukemia. Blood Reviews 13(4): 230–240
21. Agnarsson BA, Loughran TP, Jr, Starkebaum G et al 1989 The pathology of large granular lymphocyte leukemia. Human Pathology 20(7): 643–651
22. Salhany KE, Greer JP, Cousar JB et al 1989 Marrow involvement in cutaneous T-cell lumphoma. A clinicopathologic study of 60 cases. American Journal of Clinical Pathology 92(6): 747–754
23. Graham SJ, Sharpe RW, Steinberg SM et al 1993 Prognostic implications of a bone marrow histopathologic classification system in mycosis fungoides and the Sézary syndrome. Cancer 72(3): 726–734
24. Kerl H, Cerroni L, Burg G 1991 The morphologic spectrum of T-cell lymphomas of the skin: a proposal for a new classification. Seminars in Diagnostic Pathology 8(2): 55–61
25. Sausville EA, Worsham GF, Matthews MJ et al 1985 Histologic assessment of lymph nodes in mycosis fungoides/Sézary syndrome (cutaneous T-cell lymphoma): clinical correlations and prognostic import of a new classification system. Human Pathology 16(11): 1098–1109
26. Carney DN, Bunn PA, Jr. Manifestations of cutaneous T-cell lymphoma. Journal of Dermatologic Surgery and Oncology 6(5): 369–377
27. Swerdlow SH, Habeshaw JA, Rohatiner AZ et al 1984 Caribbean T-cell lymphoma/leukemia. Cancer 54(4): 687–696
28. Suchi T, Lennert K, Tu LY et al 1987 Histopathology and immunohistochemistry of peripheral T cell lymphomas: a proposal for their classification. Journal of Clinical Pathology 40(9): 995–1015
29. O'Brien C, Lampert IA, Catovsky D 1983 The histopathology of adult T-cell lymphoma/leukaemia in blacks from the Caribbean. Histopathology 7(3): 349–364
30. Nagatani T, Matsuzaki T, Iemoto G et al 1990 Comparative study of cutaneous T-cell lymphoma and adult T-cell leukemia/lymphoma. Clinical, histopathologic, and immunohistochemical analyses. Cancer 66(11): 2380–2386.
31. Jaffe ES, Blattner WA, Blayney DW et al 1984 The pathologic spectrum of adult T-cell leukemia/lymphoma in the United States. Human T-cell leukemia/lymphoma virus-associated lymphoid malignancies. American Journal of Surgical Pathology 8(4): 263–275.
32. Peterson LC, Bloomfield CD, Brunning RD 1976 Blast crisis as an initial or terminal manifestation of chronic myeloid leukemia. A study of 28 patients. American Journal of Medicine 60(2): 209–220.
33. Schmid C, Frisch B, Beham A et al 1990 Comparison of bone marrow histology in early chronic granulocytic leukemia and in leukemoid reaction. European Journal of Haematology 44(3): 154–158.
34. Knox WF, Bhavnani M, Davson J et al 1984 Histological classification of chronic granulocytic leukemia. Clinical and Laboratory Haematology 6(2): 171–175.
35. Islam A 1988 Prediction of impending blast cell transformation in chronic granulocytic leukaemia. Histopathology 12(6): 633–639.
36. Orazi A, Neiman RS, Cualing H et al 1994 CD34 immunostaining of bone marrow biopsy specimens is a reliable way to clssify the phases of chronic myeloid leukemia. American Journal of Clinical Pathology 101(4): 426–428.
37. Thiele J, Fischer R 1991 Megakaryocytopoiesis in haematological disorders: diagnostic features of bone marrow biopsies. An overview. Virchows Archives A Anatomical Pathology and Histopathology 418(2): 87–97.

38. Bennett JM, Catovsky D, Daniel MT et al 1994 The chronic myeloid leukaemias: guidelines for distinguishing chronic granulocytic, atypical chronic myeloid, and chronic myelomonocytic leukaemia. Proposals by the French–American–British Cooperative Leukaemia Group. British Journal of Haematology 87(4): 746–754.

39. Williamson PJ, Kruger AR, Reynolds PJ et al 1994 Establishing the incidence of myelodysplastic syndrome. British Journal of Haematology 87(4): 743–745.

40. Copplestone JA, Oscier DG, Mufti GJ 1986 Monocytic skin infiltration in chronic myelomonocytic leukaemia. Clinical and Laboratory Haematology 8(2): 115–119.

41. Duguid JK, Mackie MJ, McVerry BA 1983 Skin infiltration associated with chronic myelomonocytic leukaemia. British Journal of Haematology 53(2): 257–264.

42. Yamauchi K, Omata T 1992 Leukemic pneumonitis as a poor prognostic factor in chronic myelomonocytic leukemia. Respiration 59(2): 119–121.

43. Hess JL, Zutter MM, Castleberry RP et al 1996 Juvenile chronic myelogenous leukemia. American Journal of Clinical Pathology 105(2): 238–248.

44. Anzai H, Kikuchi A, Kinoshita A et al 1998 Recurrent annular erythema in juvenile chronic myelogenous leukaemia. British Journal of Dermatology 138(6): 1058–1060.

45. Brito-Babapulle F 1997 Clonal eosinophilic disorders and the hypereosinophilic syndrome. Blood Reviews 11(3): 129–145.

46. Bain BJ 1996 Eosinophilic leukaemias and the idiopathic hypereosinophilic syndrome. British Journal of Haematology 95(1): 2–9.

47. Bain BJ 2000 Hypereosinophilia. Current Opinion Hematology 7(1): 21–25.

48. Kushwaha SS, Fallon JT, Fuster V 1997 Restrictive cardiomyopathy. New England Journal of Medicine 336(4): 267–276.

49. Spry CJ, Take M, Tai PC 1985 Eosinophilic disorders affecting the myocardium and endocardium: a review. Heart Vessels Suppl 1: 240–242.

50. Bain BJ 1999 Systemic mastocytosis and other mast cell neoplasms. British Journal of Haematology 106(1): 9–17.

51. Brunning RD, McKenna RW, Rosai J et al 1983 Systemic mastocytosis. Extracutaneous manifestations. American Journal of Surgery and Pathology 7(5): 425–438.

52. Horny HP, Parwaresch MR, Lennert K 1985 Bone marrow findings in systemic mastocytosis. Human Pathology 16(8): 808–814.

53. Parker RI 1991 Hematologic aspects of mastocytosis: I: Bone marrow pathology in adult and pediatric systemic mast cell disease. Journal of Investigative Dermatology 96(3): 47S–51S.

54. Webb TA, Li CY, Yam LT 1982 Systemic mast cell disease: a clinical and hematopathologic study of 26 cases. Cancer 49(5): 927–938.

55. Metcalfe DD 1991 The liver, spleen, and lymph nodes in mastocytosis. Journal of Investigative Dermatology 96(3): 45S–46S.

56. Yam LT, Chan CH, Li CY 1986 Hepatic involvement in systemic mast cell disease. American Journal of Medicine 80(5): 819–826.

57. Mican JM, Di Bisceglie AM, Fong TL et al 1995 Hepatic involvement in mastocytosis: clinicopathologic correlations in 41 cases. Hepatology 22(4 Pt 1): 1163–1170.

58. Horny HP, Kaiserling E, Campbell M et al 1989 Liver findings in generalized mastocytosis. A clinicopathologic study. Cancer 63(3): 532–538.

Lymphoma

22

BS Wilkins   D Oscier

Introduction

Hematologic consequences of bone marrow involvement by lymphoma

Hematologic consequences of lymphoma unrelated to bone marrow involvement

Indications for bone marrow biopsy in lymphoproliferative diseases
As a diagnostic procedure
As a staging procedure at the time of lymphoma diagnosis
During treatment and follow-up of lymphoma

Blood and bone marrow assessment in diagnosis and follow-up of lymphoma

The laboratory investigation of blood and bone marrow specimens suspected or known to have involvement by lymphoma

Blood

Bone marrow aspirate

Bone marrow trephine

The World Health Organization (WHO) classification of lymphomas

Description of lymphoma entities according to WHO classification

B-cell
Lymphoplasmacytic lymphoma (LPL)

Hairy cell leukemia (HCL) and HCL variant (HCLv)
Extranodal marginal zone lymphoma of mucosa-associated lymphoid tissue (MALT)
Nodal marginal zone lymphoma (+/– monocytoid B-cells)
Follicular lymphoma (FL)
Mantle cell lymphoma (MCL)
Diffuse large B-cell lymphoma (DLC-B)
Burkitt's lymphoma (BL)

T-cell
Extranodal NK/T 'nasal type' lymphoma
Hepatosplenic gamma-delta T-cell lymphoma
Anaplastic large cell lymphoma (ALCL), systemic subtype
Angio-immunoblastic T-cell lymphoma (AILT)
Peripheral T-cell lymphoma, not otherwise characterized (PTCL)

Hodgkin's lymphoma (HL)
Nodular lymphocyte predominant Hodgkin's lymphoma (NLPHL)
Classical Hodgkin's lymphoma

Post-transplant lymphoproliferative diseases (PTLD)

Major issues in the differential diagnosis of blood and bone marrow involvement by lymphoma

Assessment of peripheral blood involvement by lymphoma

Assessment of bone marrow aspirate involvement by lymphoma

Assessment of lymphoid infiltrates in bone marrow trephine biopsy sections
Hematogones
Reactive lymphoid aggregates
Assessing lymphoma grade in bone marrow
Discordance between bone marrow and lymph node (or other site) appearances
Interpreting necrotic deposits of possible lymphoma
Appearances of lymphoma infiltrates following therapy

Bone marrow hyperplastic, dysplastic and stromal reactions to lymphoma
Atypical lymphoid aggregates in chronic myeloproliferative diseases, myelodysplastic syndromes and HIV infection
Classification of lymphoma when bone marrow trephine biopsy provides the sole source of tissue for assessment

Conclusions

Introduction

Blood and bone marrow are relatively frequently involved by lymphomas, particularly those with low-grade clinical behavior.[1] Lymphoproliferative diseases that present with predominantly leukemic behavior have been considered elsewhere (see Chapter 21), as has plasma cell neoplasia (see Chapter 23). In this chapter, blood and bone marrow involvement by lymphomas presenting primarily with lymph node or other solid organ involvement is discussed.

Hematologic consequences of bone marrow involvement by lymphoma

Bone marrow infiltration by lymphoma may be clinically silent or may cause cytopenias due to replacement of hemopoietic tissue. It is uncommon for spread of lymphoma into the bone marrow to be so extensive and severe as to cause marrow failure. Exceptions occur mainly in relation to chronic lymphocytic leukemia (CLL) and mantle cell lymphoma (MCL), whose leukemic behavior may include packing of the marrow with virtually complete replacement of normal hemopoiesis. Knowledge of the extent of marrow involvement is of increasing consequence as novel treatments for lymphoma such as radio-immunotherapy become established; excessive bystander irradiation of hemopoietic tissue and marrow stroma may occur if high doses of radiolabeled antitumor antibodies are taken up by extensive lymphoma deposits. Decisions regarding stem cell transplantation may also be influenced by the extent of residual lymphoma present after chemotherapy. As yet, there are insufficient data to indicate whether or not a 'safe' threshold exists below which residual lymphoma poses no significant risk for contamination of stem cell harvests for autografting. Also unknown are the upper and lower thresholds of bone marrow tumor burden between which purging may be desirable and effective to eliminate mobilized lymphoma cells from such harvests.

Hematologic consequences of lymphoma unrelated to bone marrow involvement

Other hematologic manifestations of low-grade lymphomas include phenomena such as autoimmune blood cell destruction and the presence of a paraprotein in the serum. Features of hypersplenism may be seen accompanying lymphomas that involve the spleen and cause splenomegaly. Cytotoxic effects of lymphoma therapy may lead to prolonged bone marrow hypoplasia in some patients and, in a few, secondary myelodysplasia, acute leukemia or lymphoma may develop months to years after treatment.

Indications for bone marrow biopsy in lymphoproliferative diseases

As a diagnostic procedure

Patients with lymphoma do not always present with lymph node enlargement or obvious tumor formation at other sites. Instead, they may have unexplained cytopenias, a leuko-erythroblastic blood picture, paraprotein, immune paresis or fever requiring examination of bone marrow for diagnostic purposes. Diagnostic lymph node biopsy may not be feasible in frail or elderly patients with disease involvement only at deep sites. Bone marrow examination for diagnostic purposes may also be necessary in patients with peripheral blood lymphocytosis if circulating cells do not show distinctive morphologic or immunophenotypic features. Trephine biopsy in addition to aspiration is always recommended since lymphoma infiltrates may be poorly sampled by the latter technique if they are small or firmly adherent to the marrow stroma.

As a staging procedure at the time of lymphoma diagnosis

Bone marrow aspiration and trephine biopsy are currently performed as part of the staging of most patients with non-Hodgkin's lymphomas and in selected patients with Hodgkin's lymphoma. Criteria for patient selection to undergo these procedures vary between treatment centers and will undoubtedly be revised as imaging techniques such as magnetic resonance imaging and positron emission tomography are refined to permit non-invasive assessment of disease spread. Evidence that bone marrow involvement influences clinical outcome varies for different disease entities within the spectrum of lymphoproliferative disorders. Bone marrow involvement, and its extent, can be important factors in making clinical decisions concerning use of chemotherapy or radiotherapy and selection of radio-immunotherapy dosage. When there is involvement, bone marrow represents a readily accessible source of neoplastic cells for confirmation of diagnosis, assessment of prognosis, development of tumor vaccines and research into disease biology.

During treatment and follow-up of lymphoma

In patients with known lymphoma, bone marrow aspiration and trephine biopsy may be required during or after treatment to investigate cytopenias which may result from complications of treatment, intercurrent illness, relapse or progression of disease. Bone marrow examination may also be performed to assess the extent of any residual disease after treatment, particularly before stem cell harvesting for autograft transplantation.

Blood and bone marrow assessment in diagnosis and follow-up of lymphoma

The full blood count, blood film, bone marrow aspirate and trephine biopsy have complementary roles in the investigation of bone marrow involvement by lymphoma. In different lymphoproliferative diseases, each of these types of specimen may be of greater or lesser value. In lymphomas that do not readily display leukemic behavior, bone marrow trephine biopsy sections are frequently found to contain lymphoma when none is evident in the blood or aspirated marrow.

Where circulating lymphoma cells are available in sufficient number in the peripheral blood, these give the most consistent morphology and immunofluorescent phenotyping. Aspiration of bone marrow without accompanying trephine biopsy may be valuable if representation of disease in the peripheral blood is inadequate for diagnosis, permitting cytologic and immunocytochemical assessment of larger numbers of neoplastic cells. However, aspiration for the evaluation of bone marrow involvement by lymphoma has a high false-negative rate. Deposits of disease frequently occupy sites within the marrow microenvironment that are suboptimally sampled by aspiration (e.g. paratrabecular zones). They may also be adherent to stromal components and less readily aspirated than hemopoietic elements within the marrow. For these reasons trephine biopsy in addition to aspiration is always recommended for the evaluation of bone marrow involvement by lymphoma. Exceptionally, if bone marrow aspiration alone is possible in some patients for whom trephine biopsy cannot be performed,

the aspirate films can still provide valuable information about hemopoietic reserve and iron stores. If aspiration proves technically difficult or a poor sample is obtained, trephine biopsy should definitely be performed and an imprint or roll preparation made for cytologic assessment.

Aspirated bone marrow provides a potential source of cells for morphologic assessment, immunophenotyping, cytogenetic analysis and molecular genetic studies. The latter investigations include clonality analysis, assessment of immunoglobulin variable gene mutation status, reverse transcription-polymerase chain reaction (RT-PCR), fluorescent *in situ* DNA hybridization (FISH) and studies of loss of heterozygosity. Aspirated cells may also be a source of material for DNA vaccine development for the treatment of lymphomas.

Trephine biopsy sections are primarily used for morphologic assessment, including analysis of the spatial distribution and extent of lymphomatous deposits. Spatial and cytologic assessment often provide clues to lymphoma subtype (e.g. the pattern of paratrabecular infiltration typical of follicular lymphoma) and can, as a minimum, be used to assess whether disease involvement represents low-grade or intermediate/high-grade lymphoma. Histologic sections can also be used for immunohistochemistry, FISH and PCR; these ancillary investigations are particularly useful if peripheral blood or aspirated marrow cells do not provide adequate representation of lymphoma. Methods of trephine biopsy processing for histology, including decalcification, are important variables in determining the success with which immunohistochemical and molecular genetic techniques can be applied. For immunophenotyping of lymphoid cell infiltrates in trephine biopsy sections a similar, but somewhat more restricted, range of antibodies is employed to that used for immunofluorescence. Antibodies reactive with antigens such as CD79a and cyclin D1 are also available which have been developed specifically for immunohistochemical use; these are referred to individually in the text below, where relevant.

The laboratory investigation of blood and bone marrow specimens suspected or known to have involvement by lymphoma

Morphology, immunophenotype and genetic features of individual subtypes of lymphoma involving the bone marrow are described below. However, it is appropriate here to outline the general principles of investigations that should be performed using blood and bone marrow specimens in all cases of suspected involvement by lymphoma.

Blood

A full blood count and differential white-cell count should always be performed. The blood film should be stained using May–Grünwald–Giemsa (MGG) or Wright's method to assess cytologic features. When circulating abnormal cells are known or suspected to be present, immunofluorescent phenotyping by flow-activated cell sorting (FACS) should be performed; a useful basic antibody panel is shown in Table 22.1. Peripheral blood cells should also be analysed by classical cytogenetic and/or molecular genetic methods when the differential

diagnosis includes lymphomas known to be associated consistently with abnormal genetic features. Table 22.2 summarizes currently known common genetic associations of lymphomas.

Bone marrow aspirate

A minimum of three films should be prepared and air-dried, using MGG stain for cytologic assessment and differential cell count. A Perls' stain is also desirable as a routine, for assessment of iron stores. Aspirated bone marrow cells should also be sent in suspension for FACS immunophenotyping and genetic analysis.

Bone marrow trephine

Cores of tissue should be collected that will contain at least 1 cm of interpretable, uncrushed bone marrow after

Table 22.1 Typical antigen expression patterns found in subtypes of peripheral B-cell non-Hodgkin's lymphoma

Disease	Antibodies						
	SmIg	*CD79B*	CD5	CD10	CD23	*FMC7*	Other
CLL	w	–/w	+	–	+	–/+	*CD38⁺⁄⁻*
PLL	st	+	–/+	–	–/+	+	
LPL	st	+	–	–	–	+	
HCL	st	+	–	–	–	+	CD103⁺ *CD25⁺*
HCLv	st	+	–	–	–	+	CD103⁺⁄⁻ *CD25⁻*
Extranodal MZL of MALT type	st	+	–	–	–	+	CD21⁺ CD35⁺
Nodal MZL	st	+	–	–	–	+	CD21⁺ CD35⁺
SMZL	st	+	–	–	–/+	+	
FL	st	+	–	+	–/+	+	
MCL	st	+	+	–	–	+	Cyclin D1⁺
DLC-B	st	+	–/+	+/–	–	+	
BL	st	+	–	+	–	–	> 90% of cells Ki67⁺

Abbreviations: diagnostic categories abbreviated as in main text. *SmIg*, surface membrane immunoglobulin; W, weak positive staining; St, strong positive staining. Antibodies denoted in italics currently available for FACS but not fixed tissue immunohistochemistry.

Table 22.2 Commonly observed genetic associations of peripheral B-cell non-Hodgkin's lymphoma

Disease	Cytogenetic abnormalities	Genes involved	V gene status	Clonal heterogeneity
CLL	del 13q, del 11q, +12	?	G/M	No
LPL	t(9;14)	Ig/*PAX5*	M	No
HCL	?	?	M	No
HCLv	?	?	M	No
Extranodal MZL of MALT type	t(11;18)	AP12/*MLT*		
	t(1;14)	Ig/*BCL10*	M	Yes
Nodal MZL	?	?	M	Yes
SMZL	del7q, +3	?	M	No
FL	t(14:18)	Ig/*BCL2*	M	Yes
MCL	t(11;14)	Ig/*BCL1*	G	No
DLC-B	t(14:18)	Ig/*BCL2*	M	Variable
	t(8;14)	Ig/*MYC*	M	Variable
	t(3q27)	*BCL6*	M	Variable
BL	t(8;14)	Ig/*MYC*	M	Yes

Abbreviations: diagnostic categories abbreviated as in main text. G, germline; M, mutated; V gene, immunoglobulin variable region gene.

histologic processing. In practice, because of likely inclusion of cortex at the outer end and crushed tissue at the inner end, plus shrinkage that occurs during processing, unfixed cores at the time of collection should be at least 1.5 cm long.[2] If aspiration has been unsuccessful, touch preparations should be made using the trephine biopsy core by rolling it gently between two slides and then staining both air-dried slides with MGG. After processing the core for histology, thin sections (1–2 μm for plastic-embedded specimens; 3–4 μm for decalcified, wax-embedded ones) should be cut and stained with hematoxylin and eosin (H&E) from a minimum of three levels through the core. Levels are usually cut 25–50 μm apart, depending on local practice and the diameter of the specimen. On the middle level, reticulin, periodic acid-Schiff (PAS) and Giemsa stains should be performed routinely. H&E provides a basic and familiar stain with which to assess cell morphology. Lymphoid infiltrates are often associated with increased reticulin deposition and a disturbance of the normal pattern of reticulin fiber distribution. PAS stain highlights carbohydrate-rich molecules and consequently stains immunoglobulin if it is of the IgM class and sufficiently abundant. IgM is richly glycosylated; consequently, intracytoplasmic and, occasionally, extracellular accumulation of this immunoglobulin can be detected in some cases of lymphoplasmacytic lymphoma. The key importance of high-quality Giemsa staining in trephine biopsy sections cannot be over-emphasized. The broad color spectrum of this metachromatic stain highlights the presence of lymphoid infiltrates by virtue of the cells having less cytoplasm than the background hemopoietic cells. The latter have abundant cytoplasm that varies from deeply basophilic (erythroid precursors) to lilac/pink (neutrophil granulocyte precursors; megakaryocytes) and bright orange/red (eosinophil granulocyte precursors). Most nuclei stain turquoise/blue with Giemsa in fixed tissue sections and, consequently, any collection of lymphoid cells will stand out as being turquoise/blue in color, against a generally mauve/pink background (Fig. 22.1). Immunohistochemistry can be useful in confirming the precise diagnosis of lymphoma involving bone marrow and in assessing its grade at this site but is of little value in differentiating reactive lymphoid aggregates from small deposits of low-grade lymphoma. For the latter task, molecular genetic analysis is gaining importance[3,4] but technical factors relating to decalcification methods and plastic-embedding processes currently limit the quality of nucleic acid preservation; false-negative results are common.

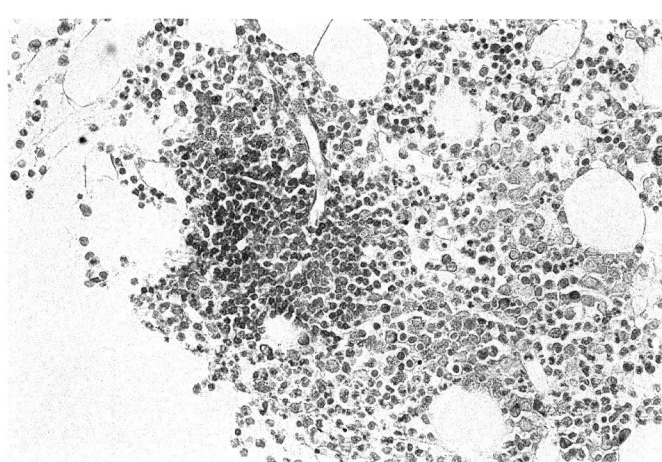

Fig. 22.1 Lymphoid nodule in a bone marrow trephine biopsy section demonstrated with a Giemsa stain. Closely packed lymphoid cell nuclei result in intense blue staining of the nodule relative to the background hemopoietic tissue, which has a mauve/pink tone overall. Note also the reactive eosinophils around the margin of the nodule, which stain orange/red with Giemsa. Eosinophil aggregation at the periphery of lymphoid nodules is more commonly seen accompanying reactive nodules than neoplastic lymphoid infiltrates but may also occur with the latter, especially following chemotherapy. Decalcified, wax-embedded bone marrow trephine biopsy; Giemsa stain, original magnification × 200.

A detailed discussion of technical matters is beyond the scope of this chapter and only brief comments are made here. In general, high-quality, thin sections from either paraffin-embedded or plastic-embedded trephine biopsy specimens are suitable for morphologic assessment of lymphoma involvement. Plastic-embedded specimens (usually in methyl or glycol methacrylate resin) require modifications to be made to standard tinctorial and immunohistochemical methods that may be difficult to incorporate into automated staining schedules but a wide range of immunostains can none the less be performed in laboratories specialized to handle these specimens. With paraffin-embedded specimens, decalcification with ethylene diamine tetra-acetic acid (EDTA) may theoretically be preferable to formic acid decalcification for antigen preservation in tissues but, in practice, few antigens of relevance to current immunohistochemistry are affected detrimentally by the latter. Formic acid decalcification is preferred by many laboratories as it can be achieved more rapidly than decalcification by chelation with EDTA. However, the increasing desirability of applying molecular genetic techniques, including FISH and PCR, to trephine biopsy specimens may increase use of EDTA in future since it undoubtedly preserves nucleic acids better than exposure to formic acid.[5,6]

The World Health Organization (WHO) classification of lymphomas

At the end of 1999, an outline version of a new lymphoma classification was published as a result of the WHO lymphoma classification project.[7] This embodied the principles of the revised European–American lymphoma (REAL) classification,[8] which was published in 1994 and has since become widely accepted in lymphoma diagnostic practice. A fundamental principle of the REAL classification was the definition of lymphomas as according to their distinctive clinical, as well as pathologic, features. Most of the REAL classification remains unchanged by the WHO, except for minor alterations in terminology. Some lymphomas considered as provisional entities in the REAL system are now accepted as definite entities within the WHO classification. Table 22.3 summarizes the lymphoma categories recognized by the WHO scheme. Areas of uncertainty in lymphoma classification remain, however, and an important feature of the WHO classification is that it has flexibility to allow for further evolution in the understanding of lymphoma (and leukemia) so that it should be able serve us for many years to come. Emerging information about the mutational status of immunoglobulin variable region genes in B-cell lymphomas[9,10] will almost certainly necessitate refinement of the classification, as the biological significance of such data becomes clearer. However, while immunophenotypic, cytogenetic and molecular genetic features are addressed by the REAL

Table 22.3 Summary of the proposed World Health Organization classification of lymphomas

B-cell neoplasms
Precursor B-cell origin:
Precursor B-lymphoblastic leukemia/lymphoma

Peripheral (mature) B-cell origin:
B-cell chronic lymphocytic leukemia/small lymphocytic lymphoma
B-cell prolymphocytic leukemia
Lymphoplasmacytic lymphoma
Splenic marginal zone B-cell lymphoma, with or without villous lymphocytes
Hairy cell leukemia (and hairy cell leukemia variant)
Plasmacytoma and plasma cell myeloma
Extranodal marginal zone B-cell lymphoma of MALT type
Nodal marginal zone lymphoma, with or without monocytoid B-cells
Follicular lymphoma (grades 1–3; with or without diffuse areas)
Mantle cell lymphoma
Diffuse large B-cell lymphoma
    (with specified subtypes mediastinal large B-cell lymphoma and primary effusion lymphoma)
    (morphologic variants – centroblastic, immunoblastic, anaplastic, etc.)
Burkitt's lymphoma/Burkitt cell leukemia
    (with specified subtypes endemic, sporadic and HIV-associated)
    (morphologic variant – Burkitt-like lymphoma)

T- and NK-cell neoplasms
Precursor T-cell origin:
Precursor T-lymphoblastic lymphoma/leukemia

Peripheral (mature) T-cell origin:
T-cell prolymphocytic leukemia
T-cell granular lymphocytic leukemia
Aggressive NK-cell leukemia
Adult T-cell lymphoma/leukemia
    (associated with HTLV-1 infection)
Extranodal NK/T-cell lymphoma of nasal type
Enteropathy-type T-cell lymphoma
Hepatosplenic gamma-delta T-cell lymphoma

Subcutaneous panniculitis-like T-cell lymphoma
Mycosis fungoides and Sezary syndrome
Anaplastic large cell lymphoma
    (with specified primary systemic and primary cutaneous subtypes, in each case further classified as T-cell or null phenotype)
Angio-immunoblastic T-cell lymphoma
Peripheral T-cell lymphoma, not otherwise characterised

Hodgkin's lymphoma
Nodular lymphocyte predominance Hodgkin's lymphoma
Classical Hodgkin's lymphoma, subtyped as:
    Nodular sclerosis Hodgkin's lymphoma
    Lymphocyte-rich Hodgkin's lymphoma
    Mixed cellularity Hodgkin's lymphoma
    Lymphocyte depletion Hodgkin's lymphoma

Post-transplant lymphoproliferative disorders
Early lesions:
Reactive plasma cell hyperplasia
Infectious mononucleosis-like lymphoproliferation

Polymorphic types:
Polyclonal
Monoclonal

Monomorphic types:
B-cell lymphomas (classified as for B-cell lymphomas, above)
    Diffuse large B-cell lymphoma
    Burkitt's lymphoma
    Plasma cell myeloma
T-cell lymphomas (classified as for T-cell lymphomas, above)
    Peripheral T-cell lymphoma, not otherwise characterized
    Other classifiable subtypes

Other types:
Hodgkin's lymphoma-like lymphoproliferations (methotrexate therapy-associated)
Plasmacytoma-like lesions

HTLV-1, human T-lymphocytotrophic virus-1; MALT, mucosa-associated lymphoid tissue.

and WHO classifications, neither specifically encompasses features of bone marrow involvement in the definition of lymphoma entities. An advance, in the WHO system, is the recognition of subtypes of lymphoma that tend to exhibit leukemic behavior. Other valuable information, particularly that relating to patterns of lymphoma distribution within the bone marrow, does not yet have a recognized place in lymphoma classification.

Description of lymphoma entities according to WHO classification

B-cell

Lymphoplasmacytic lymphoma (LPL)

(REAL; lymphoplasmacytoid lymphoma)

Clinical features, pathology, blood and bone marrow aspiration

Lymphoplasmacytic lymphoma is an indolent lymphoid neoplasm comprising 1–2% of all non-Hodgkin's lymphomas.[11] Bone marrow involvement is common at presentation and 30% of patients have splenomegaly and/or lymphadenopathy. The clinical presentation usually reflects the presence of a circulating paraprotein (IgM in almost all cases) with or without hyperviscosity symptoms, an associated peripheral neuropathy that is believed to be a paraneoplastic phenomenon[12] or con-

sequences of tumor burden such as bone marrow failure. Blood involvement is rare, except in advanced disease; it is characterized by the presence in the circulation of plasmacytoid cells with an eccentric nucleus and basophilic cytoplasm. Bone marrow aspirate films show a mixture of small lymphocytes, lymphoplasmacytoid cells and mature plasma cells (Fig. 22.2). There is frequently an accompanying increase in mast cells. Typical immunofluorescence findings are summarized in Table 22.1.

A t(9;14)(p13;q32) translocation has been reported in association with LPL.[13,14] This translocation juxtaposes the paired-box transcription factor gene *PAX5* with the immunoglobulin heavy chain gene but it is not yet clear how this influences the plasmacytic differentiation that is characteristic of LPL.

Bone marrow trephine biopsy

Bone marrow is frequently the predominant site of disease involvement in LPL and trephine biopsy histology is positive in over 50% of patients, often with more extensive involvement than suggested by aspirate films.[1] The cells are predominantly small lymphocytes with varying numbers of plasma cells and cells having intermediate (plasmacytoid) features. The plasma cells may contain Dutcher bodies, which are inclusions of immunoglobulin that invaginate the nuclear membrane and appear intranuclear in histologic sections (Fig. 22.3). Less commonly, intracytoplasmic immunoglobulin inclusions (Russell bodies) are found. Scattered blast cells may be seen but no true para-immunoblasts are present and no proliferation centers are formed; finding the latter would indi-

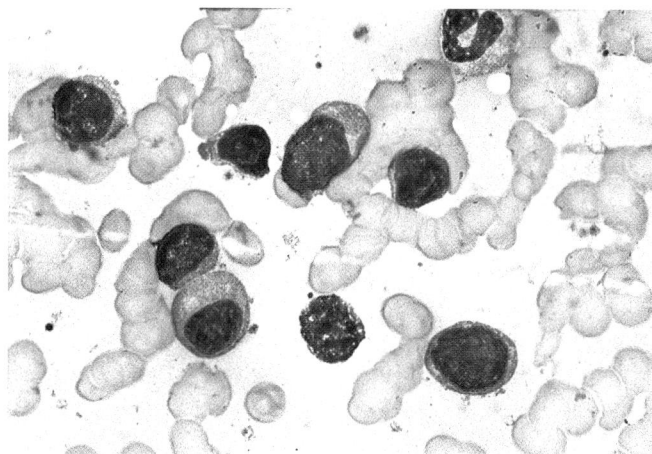

Fig. 22.2 Aspirated bone marrow showing cell mixture typical of LPL, with small lymphocytes, lymphoplasmacytoid cells and mature plasma cells represented. Bone marrow aspirate film; MGG stain, original magnification × 1000.

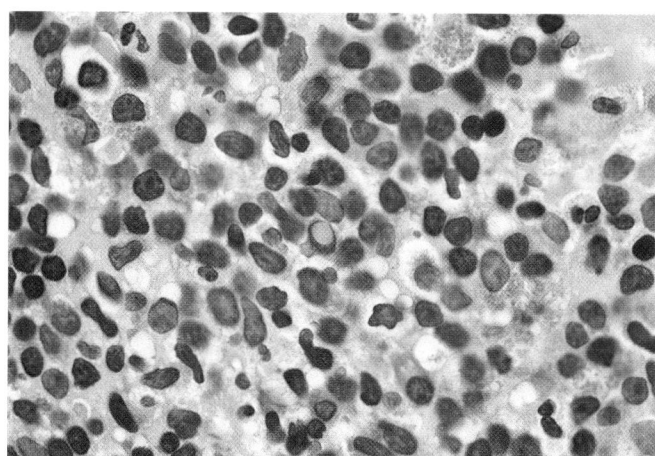

Fig. 22.3 Bone marrow infiltrate of LPL showing a prominent Dutcher body within a nucleus in the center of the field. Section of decalcified, wax-embedded bone marrow trephine biopsy; H&E stain, original magnification × 1000.

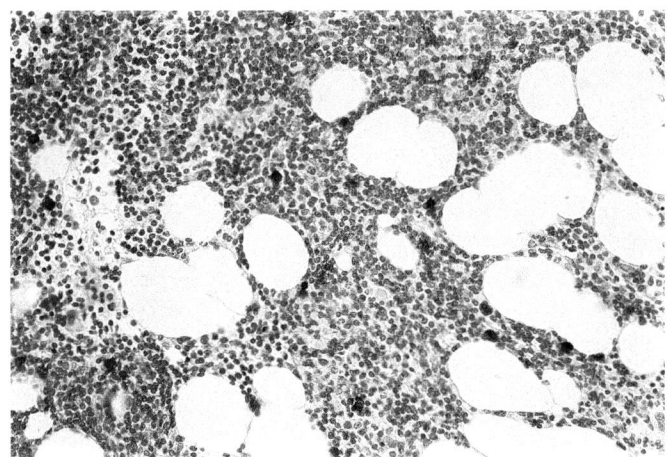

Fig. 22.4 Infiltrate of LPL in bone marrow accompanied by numerous mast cells, which have purple granular cytoplasm in this section stained with buffered thionin (a metachromatic stain similar to toluidine blue). Section of decalcified, wax-embedded bone marrow trephine biopsy; original magnification × 200.

cate a diagnosis of B-cell chronic lymphocytic leukemia (B-CLL) with plasmacytic differentiation, rather than LPL. The presence of increased numbers of reactive mast cells in the marrow interstitium, sometimes located preferentially in the periphery of lymphoid infiltrates, may be helpful in supporting a diagnosis of LPL (Fig. 22.4). This phenomenon, however, is also seen in a minority of cases of CLL and is possibly related to IgM expression rather than to other properties of either disease.[15] The pattern of infiltration is usually irregular, paratrabecular or diffuse throughout the interstitium; mixtures of these patterns are common in individual cases. Well-defined nodular infiltrates are unusual and should prompt consideration of CLL, marginal zone lymphoma (usually of splenic type, with or without circulating villous lymphocytes) or MCL as alternative diagnoses. The paratrabecular infiltrates of LPL are not usually as extensive or regular as those found in follicular lymphoma. In some patients who have an IgM paraprotein, sinusoids contain PAS-positive proteinaceous material that represents plasma rich in IgM and there may also be interstitial deposits of PAS-positive IgM crystals.

In trephine biopsy sections, immunohistochemistry shows that the small B-lymphocytes of LPL express CD20, CD79a and CD45RA but lack expression of CD5 and CD10. In occasional cases, a proportion of the neoplastic cells expresses CD23. Plasma cell differentiation is often highlighted by staining for CD79a and can be demonstrated even more clearly using the antibody VS38c, reactive with rough endoplasmic reticulum-associated p63 protein.[16] Expression of monotypic immunoglobulin in the cytoplasm of cells showing plasmacytic differentiation is usually easily demonstrated,

most commonly IgM kappa,[15] and light chain mRNA production can also be shown by *in situ* hybridization.

Hairy cell leukemia (HCL) and HCL variant (HCLv)

(REAL: hairy cell leukemia; the variant was not classified as a distinct entity)

Clinical features and pathology in the spleen

Hairy cell leukemia is predominantly a disease of middle-aged men. The clinical presentation is with anemia, bleeding or infection (often with opportunistic organisms), reflecting peripheral blood cytopenias caused by hypersplenism and/or bone marrow failure. Sixty per cent of patients at presentation have splenomegaly and 40% have hepatomegaly.[11] In the spleen, HCL is recognized by the presence of a diffuse infiltrate of typical hairy cells (see below), causing effacement of normal red and white pulp architecture. As in the bone marrow, splenic infiltration is accompanied by reticulin deposition, interstitial hemorrhage and vascular ectasia. Cases of HCL variant (HCLv) more closely resemble B-cell prolymphocytic leukemia (B-PLL) in their pattern of splenic involvement.

Blood and bone marrow aspiration

Most patients with HCL have circulating hairy cells. These are large lymphoid cells which have abundant, pale blue cytoplasm and hair-like projections from the cell surface.[17] The nucleus is frequently indented and has a smooth chromatin pattern with indistinct nucleoli. Typical immunofluorescent phenotyping results are summarized in Table 22.1. Peripheral cytopenias are common in HCL, particularly monocytopenia. Bone marrow aspiration is often unsuccessful due to increased marrow reticulin associated with HCL infiltration.

The variant form of hairy cell leukemia is characterized by a higher white blood cell count, different morphology, with prominent nucleoli in the hairy cells, and different immunophenotype (see Table 22.1).

Current knowledge of genetic abnormalities associated with HCL and HCLv is extremely limited.

Bone marrow trephine biopsy

The degree of bone marrow involvement is usually extensive at presentation, with large areas of marrow showing almost complete replacement of normal

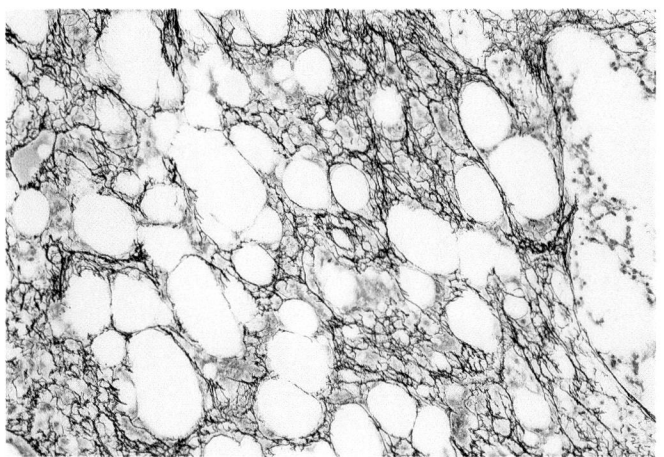

Fig. 22.5 Markedly increased stromal reticulin (grade III/IV) in bone marrow accompanying relatively subtle interstitial infiltration by HCL. Section of decalcified, wax-embedded bone marrow trephine biopsy; Gordon & Sweet's stain for reticulin, original magnification × 200.

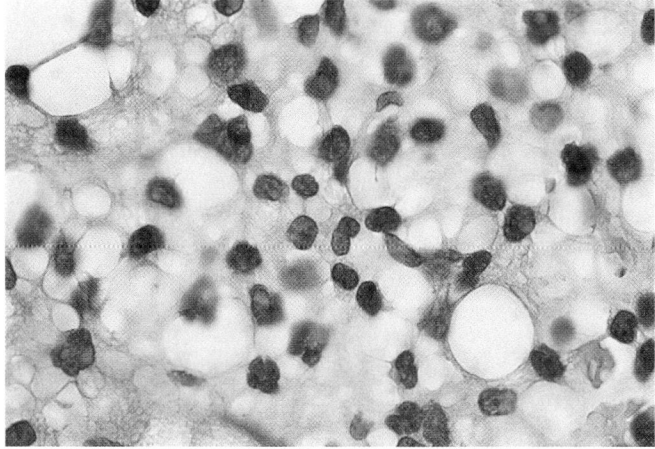

Fig. 22.6 High-power view of cells in HCL. They are widely spaced with abundant, pale cytoplasm and irregular nuclei. One cell with a bi-lobed nucleus is present in the center of the field. Section of decalcified, wax-embedded bone marrow trephine biopsy; H&E stain, original magnification × 1000.

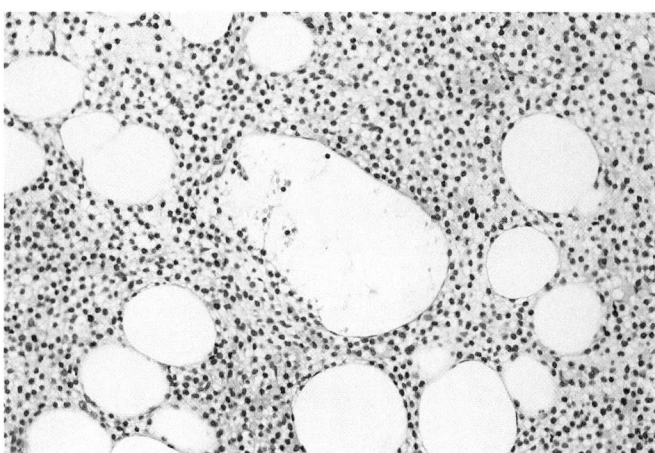

Fig. 22.7 Infiltrate of HCL causing a sinusoid to gape because of increased stromal reticulin deposition. The sinusoid can be distinguished from fat spaces elsewhere in the section by virtue of its larger size and its more irregular outline. Higher-power examination would also allow its lining of flattened endothelium to be seen and blood cells within its lumen to be identified. Section of decalcified, wax-embedded bone marrow trephine biopsy; H&E stain, original magnification × 200.

hemopoiesis by infiltrating hairy cells. Occasionally, the marrow appears hypoplastic, with a subtle pattern of diffuse interstitial infiltration and partial preservation of hemopoiesis; granulopoiesis is often disproportionately reduced and this picture should not be confused with hypoplastic/aplastic anemia or a hypoplastic myelodysplastic syndrome. In subtle as well as extensively involved examples of HCL, interstitial reticulin is greatly increased (Fig. 22.5), which is rarely the case in other hypoplastic states. The infiltrating cells are of medium size with round, oval or bi-lobed nuclei and abundant, empty-looking cytoplasm (Fig. 22.6). Occasionally, they appear spindle-shaped. The abundant cytoplasm gives an appearance of the cells being widely spaced from one another. Extravasation of red cells into the interstitium is common and sinusoids appear prominent, with gaping lumens, as a result of the background of increased reticulin fibers (Fig. 22.7). Collagen fibrosis is rare and only isolated reports exist of osteosclerosis in association with HCL.[18,19] Transformation of HCL to a more aggressive, large B-cell lymphoma occurs infrequently. Assessment of residual disease during and after therapy can be difficult in HCL, in which small interstitial clusters of scattered neoplastic cells may be all that remain, with or without persistent increased reticulin; immunohistochemistry usually reveals more disease than is readily apparent from standard tinctorial stains. The histologic features of HCLv are quite different from those described above for HCL. They resemble those seen in B-CLL or B-PLL, with focal nodular and interstitial infiltration by small lymphoid cells, some having nucleoli. Cells in HCLv lack the distinctive nuclear and cytoplasmic characteristics of classical hairy cells and any increase in stromal reticulin is less marked than in the usual form of HCL.

In trephine biopsy sections, hairy cells can be shown by immunohistochemistry to express CD20, CD79a and CD45RA but not CD5, CD10 or CD23. Dot-like cytoplasmic expression of CD68 may also be demonstrable. Hairy cells also react well with the monoclonal antibody DBA44, which recognizes an as yet uncharacterized HCL-associated antigen[20] but is not entirely specific.[21] In addition, monoclonal antibodies reactive with tartrate-resistant acid phosphatase in fixed tissue sections are now available and appear promising for diagnostic confirmation and follow-up of HCL.[22,23] Cells in HCLv are generally tartrate-resistant acid phosphatase (TRAP)-negative.

After treatment, HCL infiltration usually appears dramatically reduced and the increased reticulin resolves rapidly in most patients. However, immunohistochemistry is important in the evaluation of post-treatment trephine biopsies in HCL because, at least with conventional treatments such as interferon, it generally reveals considerably more residual disease than can be appreciated from standard tinctorial stains.

Extranodal marginal zone lymphoma of mucosa-associated lymphoid tissue (MALT)-type

(REAL: marginal zone lymphoma, extranodal, MALT-type)

Clinical features and pathology at presenting sites

Extranodal marginal zone lymphomas of MALT-type are indolent lymphoproliferative disorders with a 10-year survival of more than 80%. The most common primary sites of MALT-type extranodal marginal zone lymphoma are within the gastrointestinal tract. Salivary glands, skin, orbit, lung and urogenital organs are the sites of origin in smaller numbers of patients. At presentation, 30% of patients have involvement of more than one mucosal site.[11] As defined in the WHO classification, these lymphomas are low grade and arise in the context of normal or induced (e.g. by *Helicobacter pylori* infection in the stomach) lymphoid tissue in the organs involved. The neoplastic cell is typically a centrocyte-like cell with a tendency to infiltrate epithelial structures, forming lympho-epithelial lesions. Trisomy 3 has been detected in more than 60% of cases using FISH and comparative genomic hybridization;[24,25] less common are trisomies of chromosomes 7 and 12.[24] The translocation t(11;18) (q21;q21) has been found in some cases, associated with the formation of an *AP12-MLT* fusion gene.[26] This fusion gene is of uncertain functional significance at present but is absent from node-based and splenic forms of marginal zone lymphoma. Genetic features of MALT-type extranodal marginal zone lymphoma are summarized in Table 22.3.

In some cases, progression to large B-cell lymphoma can be seen in MALT-type lymphoma, indicating requirement for more aggressive management. In order to avoid confusion for patient management, the large cell component is classified separately (as diffuse large B-cell lymphoma), so that the need for consideration of more intensive treatment is made clear.

Blood and bone marrow aspiration

Bone marrow involvement has been reported in 15–40% of cases.[11] Fifteen per cent of patients are anemic at presentation but circulating lymphoma cells are not seen. Bone marrow aspiration rarely reveals the presence of lymphoma cells, even when trephine biopsy shows histologic evidence of involvement. In those few patients with a positive aspirate, immunofluorescence findings are as summarized in Table 22.1.

Bone marrow trephine biopsy

When present, infiltrates of extranodal marginal zone lymphomas of MALT-type are usually nodular but paratrabecular and interstitial involvement has been described.[27,28] A differential diagnosis of follicular lymphoma (FL) should be considered carefully if paratrabecular infiltration is the predominant finding but such infiltrates are rarely as extensive or well developed in MALT-type lymphoma as in FL. If nodular infiltrates are present, B-CLL and MCL should be considered. These differential diagnoses can usually be excluded if the clinical features and immunophenotype of the lymphoma at its primary site are known.

The infiltrating cells are small but their centrocyte-like morphology can be difficult to appreciate due to admixture of reactive lymphocytes. For the same reason, immunohistochemistry is often difficult to interpret but the neoplastic cells express CD20 and CD79a while lacking expression of CD5, CD10, CD23 and cyclin D1.

Nodal marginal zone lymphoma (+/– monocytoid B-cells)

(REAL: provisional entity – nodal marginal zone lymphoma +/– monocytoid B-cells)

Clinical features and lymph node pathology

Nodal marginal zone lymphoma is rare, comprising less than 2% of all non-Hodgkin's lymphomas. Presentation is usually with advanced disease characterized by peripheral and para-aortic lymphadenopathy. Five-year survival is 50–60%.[11]

The histologic appearances in lymph nodes can be similar to those of nodal involvement secondary to extranodal lymphoma of MALT-type and may also require distinction from reactive monocytoid B-cell hyperplasia. Monocytoid B-cells are medium-sized cells that are quite similar to hairy cells in histologic sections, having oval or bi-lobed nuclei and abundant, clear cytoplasm; however, infiltrates in nodal marginal zone lymphoma (MZL) are usually heterogeneous, including centrocyte-like cells and others showing marginal zone cell or plasmacytoid differentiation.

Blood and bone marrow aspiration

The blood is involved in 10% of patients but up to 30% have bone marrow involvement. The appearance of circulating cells varies between patients; they may resemble small lymphocytes or be larger, with monocytoid appearances. The immunophenotype is indistinguishable from extranodal, MALT-type marginal zone lymphoma (see Table 22.1). Little is known about underlying genetic abnormalities; trisomy 3 has been found in up to 50% of cases[11] but, like most numerical chromosomal abnormalities found in lymphomas, is probably a secondary phenomenon.

Bone marrow trephine biopsy

Few descriptions have been published recording histologic features of bone marrow involvement in nodal marginal zone lymphoma. Nodular and paratrabecular patterns of infiltration have been described.[29] The infiltrating cells are a mixture of lymphocytes, centrocyte-like cells, monocytoid cells and plasma cells. A differential diagnosis of follicular lymphoma requires consideration if paratrabecular infiltration is predominant. If infiltration is nodular, alternative diagnoses of B-CLL, MCL and splenic marginal zone lymphoma (SMZL) should be excluded. Clinical features, knowledge of the lymph node or splenic histology and immunophenotype usually exclude these other diagnoses. In histologic sections, the neoplastic cells can be shown to express CD20, CD79a but not CD5, CD10, CD23 or cyclin D1. A dot-like pattern cytoplasmic expression of CD68 may be found in cases with monocytoid differentiation.

Follicular lymphoma (FL)

(REAL: follicle center cell lymphoma, grades I–III)

Clinical features and lymph node pathology

Follicular lymphoma comprises approximately 35% of non-Hodgkin's lymphoma. Disease is frequently wide-spread at diagnosis; lymph nodes, spleen, bone marrow and peripheral blood are involved in 10% of cases. The median survival is around 7–9 years and up to 60% of cases transform to diffuse large B-cell lymphoma.[11]

In lymph nodes, FL typically replaces normal structures with well-defined, uniformly sized neoplastic germinal centers containing neoplastic centrocytes and centroblasts. Preservation of mantle zones and interfollicular components is variable and a minority of patients have significant additional diffuse infiltration by lymphoma cells. Completely diffuse lymph node involvement by FL is rare and controversy remains as to the true nature of diffuse lymphomas composed predominantly of centrocytes. The REAL and WHO classifications divide FL into three grades, depending on the relative proportions of centrocytes and centroblasts present; precise details of how this grading is achieved are available elsewhere.[30,31] Assessment of grade in FL is of prognostic value; grades I and II behave as low-grade lymphomas with a chronic course but long survival, while grade III disease is more aggressive and has an outcome equivalent to diffuse large B-cell lymphoma.

Most cases of FL have a t(14;18)(q32;q21) translocation which dysregulates the *BCL2* oncogene by placing it under the influence of the immunoglobulin heavy chain gene promoter. Variant translocations involving kappa and lambda light chain genes occur in a few patients; t(2;18)(p12;q21) and t(18;22)(q21;q11), respectively (see Table 22.3).

Blood and bone marrow aspiration

Follicular lymphoma cells, when present in the circulation, are usually centrocytes which appear smaller than those seen in bone marrow or lymph nodes and which have little or no cytoplasm. Nuclear chromatin is condensed and uniformly distributed; in typical cases a deep nuclear cleft can be seen (Fig. 22.8). Circulating centroblasts, which are larger cells with prominent nucleoli, are usually only seen in advanced disease. Aspirated bone marrow contains detectable centrocytes and/or centroblasts only infrequently, even when trephine biopsy shows clear evidence of histological involvement. Typical immunofluorescence findings in FL are summarized in Table 22.1.

Bone marrow trephine biopsy

Trephine biopsy sections from patients with FL show involvement in the majority of cases but deposits of disease may be small and focal. If no lymphomatous infiltration is detected in initial sections, examination of

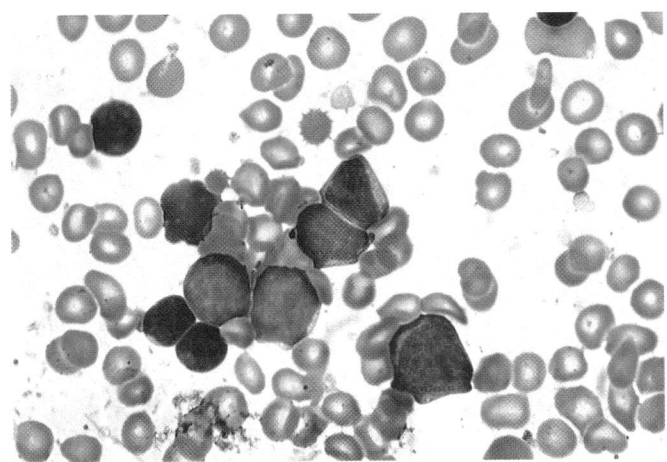

Fig. 22.8 Cytology of FL in a bone marrow aspirate film. A mixed population of atypical lymphoid cells is present, including large and small cells with irregular nuclear indentations. MGG stain, original magnification × 1000.

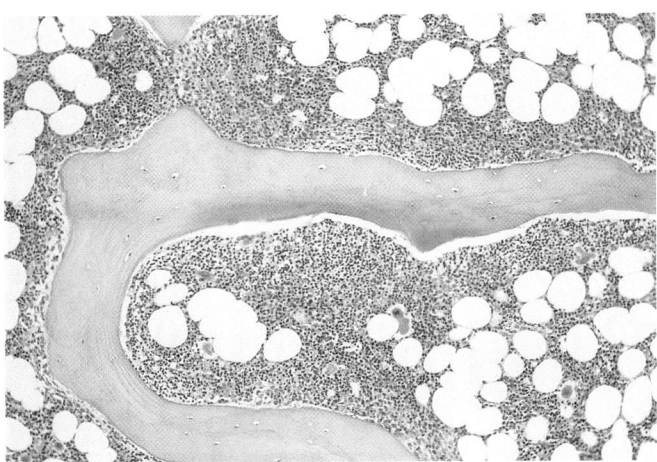

A

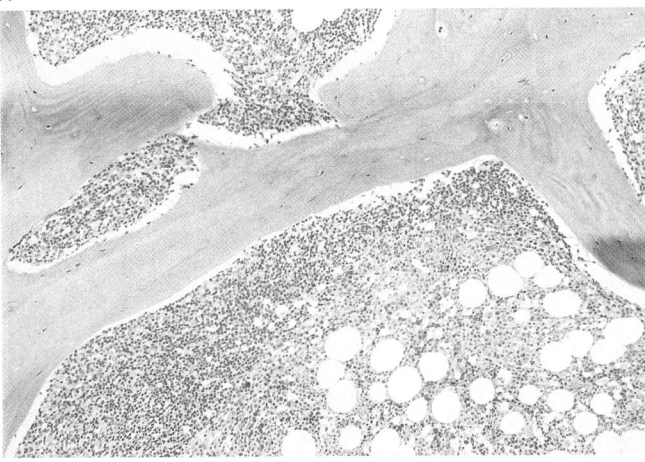

B

Fig. 22.9 Classical band-like paratrabecular infiltration of bone marrow by FL. (A) H&E stain; (B) Giemsa stain. At low magnification, loss of fat spaces and condensation of cellular tissue around the trabecular margin is a clue to the presence of lymphoma at this site and Giemsa staining highlights the presence of closely packed small lymphoid cells forming the paratrabecular infiltrates. Section of decalcified, wax-embedded bone marrow trephine biopsy, original magnification × 100.

further sections representing deeper parts of the tissue core is mandatory to avoid missing focal deposits.

The classical pattern of bone marrow infiltration by FL is paratrabecular. Well-developed paratrabecular infiltrates form bands or 'crescent moon' shapes with the longest axis abutting and lying parallel to the trabecular surface (Figs 22.9 and 22.10). Nodular infiltrates are found less often and diffuse interstitial involvement is distinctly uncommon; in either case, typical areas of paratrabecular infiltration are usually also seen, providing the biopsy core is of adequate size. In contrast with the lymph node features, neoplastic germinal centers are rarely formed in bone marrow deposits of FL. If they are present (Fig. 22.11), care must be taken not to mistake them for focal transformation to large cell lymphoma, since they may contain prominent centroblasts. In paratrabecular infiltrates, the cells present are predominantly non-neoplastic small T-lymphocytes, with only small numbers of centrocytes and even fewer centroblasts usually being present. Consequently, immunohistochemistry may be misleading in trephine biopsy sections and greater reliance should be placed on recognition of the distinctive paratrabecular distribution of FL infiltrates. The differential diagnosis of FL in trephine biopsy sections includes B-CLL, LPL, SMZL and MCL; paratrabecular infiltration is almost never found in B-CLL and is usually less well developed in the others than in FL. However, clinical features, immunophenotype and cytologic details usually permit the correct diagnosis to be established without difficulty. It is much more

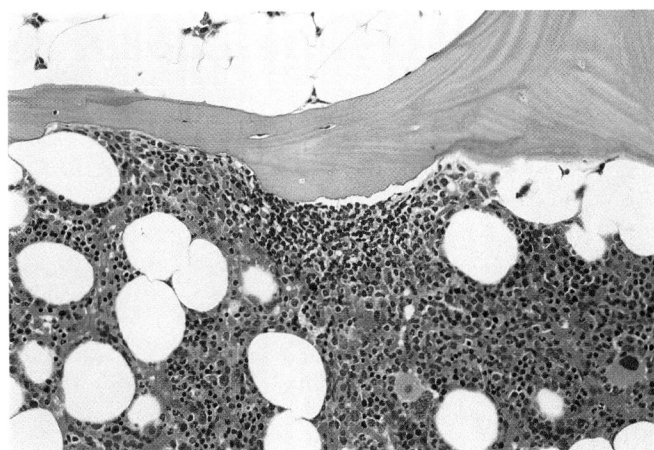

Fig. 22.10 Subtle involvement of bone marrow by FL. In contrast to the extensive linear paratrabecular infiltrates shown in Fig. 22.9, lymphoma in this example is represented by a small 'crescent moon' deposit of lymphoma. Although tiny, this deposit can still be seen clearly to be associated with the surface of the adjacent bony trabecula, having its longest axis along the trabecular margin. Section of decalcified, wax-embedded bone marrow trephine biopsy; H&E stain, original magnification × 200.

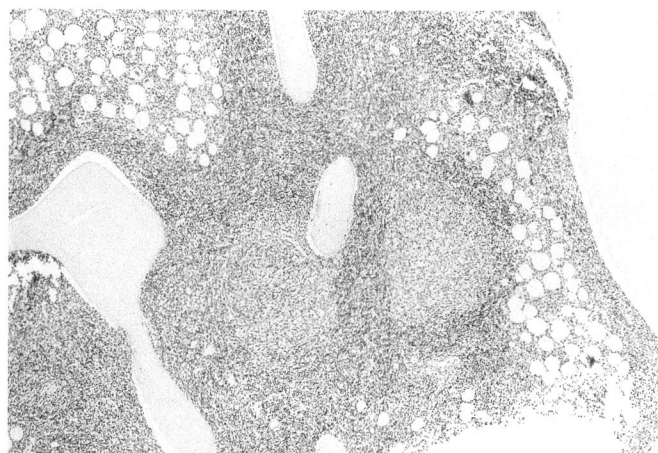

Fig. 22.11 Formation of neoplastic germinal centers within an infiltrate of FL in bone marrow. Note the additional component of paratrabecular infiltration in the background. Paler staining of the germinal centers relative to paratrabecular infiltrates in this example reflects the lesser admixture of small, non-neoplastic lymphocytes in the former. Paratrabecular infiltrates are almost always accompanied by numerous reactive T-lymphocytes. Section of decalcified, wax-embedded bone marrow trephine biopsy; H&E stain, original magnification × 50.

difficult, and is currently impossible in some cases, to distinguish minimal non-paratrabecular infiltrates of FL from non-neoplastic lymphoid nodules.

By immunohistochemistry, neoplastic cells in FL are seen to express CD20, CD79a and CD10 but not CD5 or cyclin D1. They also usually lack CD23 expression. Use of immunostaining to demonstrate BCL2 protein is not recommended in trephine biopsy sections, since this antigen is expressed strongly by reactive T-cells; the latter, as described above, often outnumber and obscure the neoplastic cells.

Following treatment, deposits of FL in bone marrow trephine biopsy sections may appear hypocellular and fibrotic or may be difficult to distinguish from reactive lymphoid aggregates. It can be very difficult to determine the significance of such residual disease. Application of immunohistochemistry and molecular genetic techniques has, to date, been too limited to determine their value in this context.

Mantle cell lymphoma (MCL)

Clinical features and lymph node pathology

MCL comprises approximately 6% of non-Hodgkin's lymphoma. The median age at diagnosis is 60 years and most patients present with widespread disease involving lymph nodes, spleen and, sometimes, the gastro-intestinal (GI) tract ('lymphomatous polyposis'). Median survival is only 3 years.[11]

MCL in lymph nodes grows in a diffuse or vaguely nodular fashion, sometimes showing a tendency to expand mantle zones around residual, non-neoplastic germinal centers. The cytology of MCL varies from lymphocytic to centrocytic but is usually uniform in any individual patient; occasional patients have a so-called 'blastoid' variant of MCL, in which cells resemble lymphoblasts. Growth in the spleen or at MALT sites within the GI tract has essentially similar characteristics.

The translocation t(11;14)(q13;q32) is strongly associated with MCL (see Table 22.3) and places the *BCL1* oncogene, which encodes cyclin D1, under regulation of the immunoglobulin heavy chain gene promoter. This leads to inappropriate expression of cyclin D1, a cell cycle regulatory protein that is not usually detectable in cells of lymphoid origin. A variant translocation, t(11;22)(q11;q13), juxtaposes *BCL1* with the lambda light chain gene in a minority of patients with MCL. Cells of MCL rarely show evidence of immunoglobulin variable region gene hypermutation.

Blood and bone marrow aspiration

Sixty per cent of patients have bone marrow involvement at diagnosis and circulating lymphoma cells are present in the blood in 30%, particularly those with advanced disease.[11] However, there is a subgroup of patients who present with lymphocytosis ± splenomegaly but with no lymphadenopathy and in whom the disease pursues a more indolent course.

Circulating cells, when present, are pleomorphic; the predominant cell type is medium-sized with moderately abundant chromatin, an irregular nuclear outline and dispersed chromatin. Similar features identify the cells in bone marrow aspirate films (Fig. 22.12) and they have a distinctive immunophenotype when analysed by FACS (see Table 22.1). In the blastoid form of MCL, nucleoli are seen within tumor cell nuclei.

Bone marrow trephine biopsy

Histologic evidence of bone marrow involvement is found in more than 70% of patients with MCL.[32] The pattern of infiltration varies widely between patients; nodular, interstitial, diffuse and paratrabecular patterns have been described. Nodular infiltration (Fig. 22.13), with or without an additional interstitial component is probably the most commonly seen pattern. Paratrabecular infiltration occurs fairly frequently but, in contrast with FL, is less extensive and is almost always overshadowed by other patterns of involvement.[29] The cells are small and, as in lymph nodes, may be lymphocyte-like, may

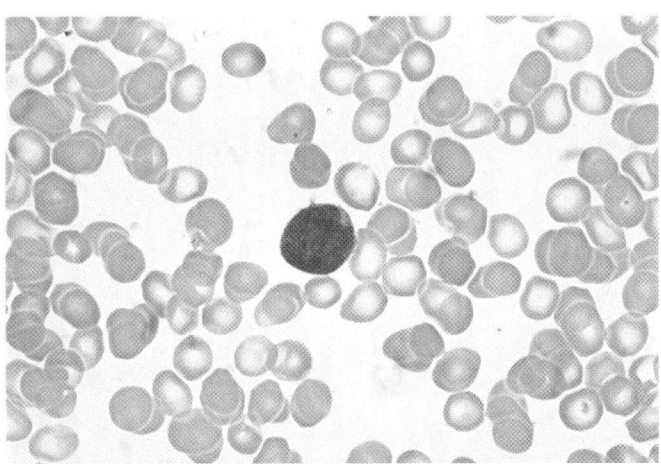

Fig. 22.12 Cytology of MCL in aspirated bone marrow. A typical neoplastic mantle cell; medium-sized with scanty cytoplasm and an irregular nuclear outline. Bone marrow aspirate film; MGG stain, original magnification × 1000.

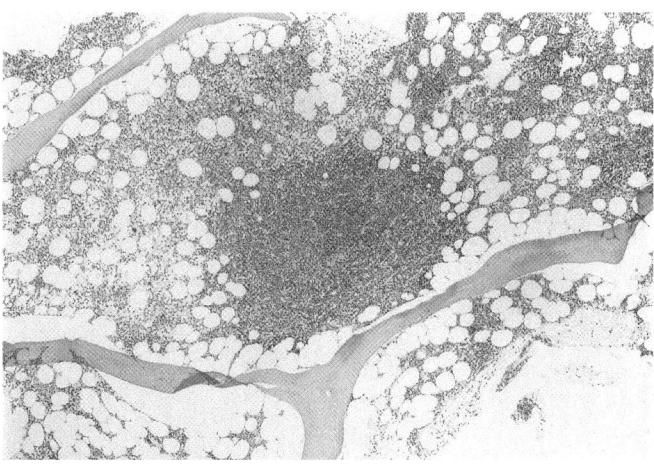

Fig. 22.13 Nodular infiltration of bone marrow by MCL. AT this magnification, a minor degree of interstitial infiltration cannot be confirmed or excluded but predominance of the nodular pattern is clear. Section of decalcified, wax-embedded bone marrow trephine biopsy; H&E stain, original magnification × 50.

resemble centrocytes or, in a minority of cases, have lymphoblast-like features.

The main differential diagnoses are B-CLL, B-PLL, SMZL and, when paratrabecular infiltration is present, LPL and FL. The blastoid variant requires distinction from Burkitt's lymphoma and acute lymphoblastic leukemia. Immunohistochemistry is valuable for demonstration of cyclin D1 expression in the nuclei of neoplastic cells in MCL but is technically demanding. The cells of B-CLL, SMZL and FL do not express this molecule and only rare cases of B-PLL are positive. The cells of MCL also express CD20, CD79a and CD5 but not CD10, CD23 or terminal deoxynucleotidyl transferase (TdT).

Diffuse large B-cell lymphoma (DLC-B)

Clinical features and pathology at presenting sites

Diffuse large B cell lymphoma (DLC-B) comprises 30% of non-Hodgkin's lymphomas. Presentation may be with node-based or extranodal disease. Thirty per cent of patients have B symptoms (fever, weight loss, night sweats) at the time of diagnosis. Assessment of prognostic factors is important for therapy; such factors include age, stage of disease, performance status and serum lactate dehydrogenase (LDH) concentration. Patients with good prognosis disease have an 83% 5-year survival while in those with poor prognosis disease this drops to 32%.[11]

DLC-B usually causes total or near-total loss of normal lymph node architecture and replacement by large blast cells. Most commonly these are centroblasts but a variable proportion of immunoblasts and plasmablasts

may be present. The infiltrating cells may be monotonous or exhibit marked pleomorphism; in occasional cases, cells resembling Reed–Sternberg cells may be found. Other morphologic variants include those rich in non-neoplastic T-cells and macrophages (sometimes referred to as 'T-cell-rich B-cell lymphoma'). Cases of DLC-B also arise *de novo* at extranodal sites, particularly the central nervous system, mediastinum, GI system and testis. Intravascular large B-cell lymphoma is another variant of DLC-B, which usually presents as a result of CNS or subcutaneous vascular infiltration; however, patients with primary presentation of this lymphoma in bone marrow have also been described.[33,34] At present, it is unclear whether variants of DLC-B with primary extranodal presentation are related pathogenetically to low-grade node-based or extranodal lymphomas.

Genetic findings in DLC-B are complex; aneuploidy is common and complex aberrant clones are often found. Cells may show t(14;18)(q32;q21), with *BCL2* dysregulation, as in FL. The translocation t(3;14)(q27;q32), and others involving 3q27 breakpoints, are also relatively common in DLC-B of all morphologic varieties; these genetic alterations lead to inappropriate expression of the *BCL6* oncogene.[35] Immunoglobulin variable region genes show evidence of hypermutation with ongoing changes, implying continued exposure to somatic mutator mechanisms.[36]

Blood and bone marrow aspiration

Blood involvement in DLC-B is rare and, when present, circulating lymphoma cells are usually large, with a large

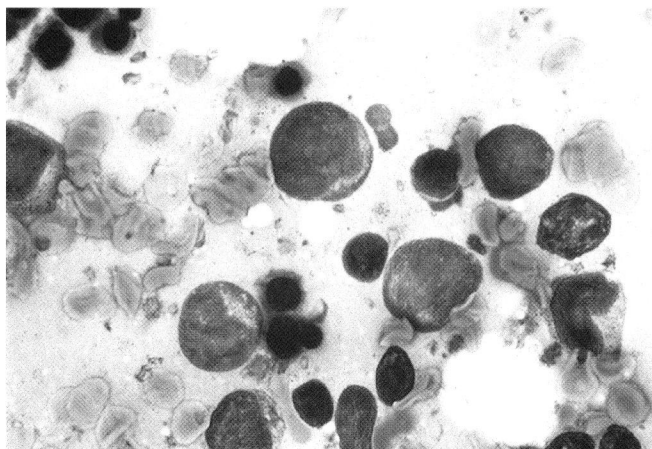

Fig. 22.14 Cytology of DLC-B in aspirated bone marrow. Cells are large with varying amounts of cytoplasm, irregular nucear outlines and prominent nucleoli. Bone marrow aspirate film; MGG stain, original magnification × 1000.

nucleus, prominent multiple nucleoli and abundant cytoplasm. Bone marrow aspirate involvement can be recognized by the presence of cells with these features (Fig. 22.14); immunophenotypic findings do not permit their distinction from some other subtypes of non-Hodgkin's lymphoma (NHL).

Bone marrow trephine biopsy

Involvement of the bone marrow by DLC-B is uncommon. There are no characteristic patterns of distribution of DLC-B within intertrabecular spaces; infiltrates usually form random, solid patches or are dispersed in the interstitium. The intravascular variant is unusual, with bone marrow infiltration being predominantly intrasinusoidal (Fig. 22.15); the marrow interstitium and lumens of larger vessels are involved less conspicuously. The cellular morphology of large blast cells in bone marrow infiltrates of DLC-B generally matches that seen at the primary site(s). In some cases, bone marrow infiltration may be discordant and show low-grade histologic features, even when no accompanying low-grade lymphoma has been found in sections from a lymph node or other diagnostic specimen. This is occasionally helpful in providing evidence to support origin of an apparently *de novo* DLC-B from FL, if typical paratrabecular infiltrates of FL are found in the bone marrow trephine biopsy sections. The presence of discordant low-grade lymphoma in the bone marrow of patients with DLC-B does not appear to influence prognosis significantly, whereas the concordant presence of DLC-B in the bone marrow is an adverse factor. Examples of discordance involving low-grade lymphoma elsewhere and DLC-B in the bone marrow are very rare.

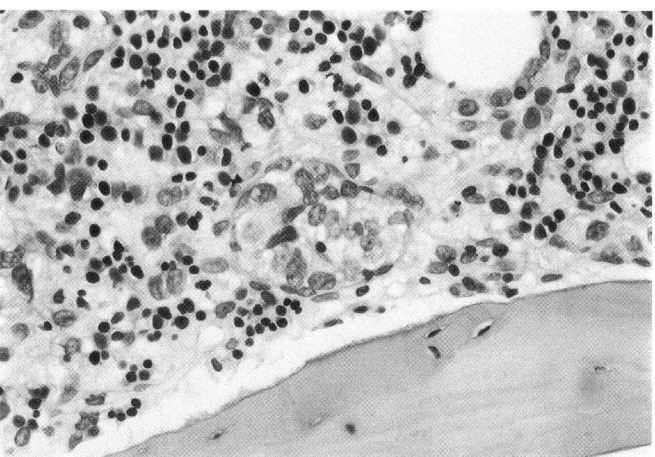

A

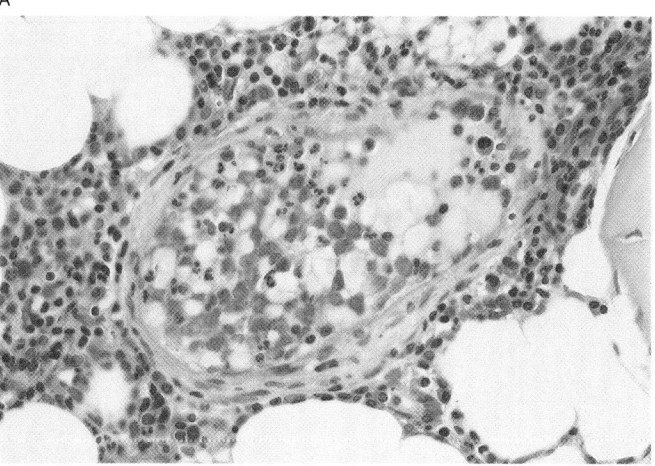

B

Fig. 22.15 Intravascular DLC-B in bone marrow. (A) Large malignant lymphoid cells apparently forming a cluster because of their confinement within a sinusoidal lumen. (B) Larger blood vessels within bone marrow, in this case probably a venule, can also contain malignant lymphoid cells in this variant of DLC-B. Sections of decalcified, wax-embedded bone marrow trephine biopsy; H&E stain, original magnification × 400.

The differential diagnosis of DLC-B in bone marrow includes Burkitt's lymphoma, myeloma, acute lymphoblastic leukemia and acute myeloid leukemia. Occasionally, a rich admixture of non-neoplastic T-cells and macrophages in bone marrow infiltrates of DLC-B, as in T-cell-rich large B-cell lymphoma at other sites, suggests an alternative diagnosis of Hodgkin's lymphoma. Attention to clinical features, cytologic detail in the infiltrating cells and the appearances of hemopoietic tissue in the background usually permit discrimination between these alternatives. Immunohistochemistry can be used to confirm the B-cell phenotype of neoplastic cells, which express CD20 and CD79a. Less consistently, there may be expression of CD10, BCL2 or BLC6 but staining for myeloid markers and TdT will be negative. Occasionally, cells will be found to express CD30; in the context of a B-cell immunophenotype, this is of no clinicopathologic significance.

Burkitt's lymphoma (BL)

(REAL: Burkitt's lymphoma and Burkitt-like lymphoma)

Clinical features and pathology at presenting sites

Burkitt's lymphoma is rare, accounting for fewer than 1% of all case of NHL. Cure is possible with highly intensive chemotherapy regimes and hemopoietic stem cell transplantation.

The WHO classification recognizes three clinical subtypes of Burkitt's lymphoma (endemic, sporadic and immunodeficiency-related) and incorporates Burkitt-like lymphomas as morphologic variants. Endemic BL is a disease of childhood in sub-Saharan Africa and is frequently extranodal at presentation, with a high incidence of jaw tumors. Sporadic BL occurs in all parts of the world and has a wide age distribution; ileocaecal tumor formation in young males is a common presentation. Burkitt's lymphoma in the context of immuno-deficiency is most commonly seen in association with human immunodeficiency virus (HIV) infection but may also occur as a form of post-transplant lymphoprolifer-ative disease; its histologic features resemble those of the sporadic disease. The endemic and immunodeficiency-associated subtypes of BL are very strongly associated with latent Epstein–Barr virus (EBV) infection of neo-plastic cells, believed to be important in pathogenesis, while sporadic cases of BL are less consistently associated with EBV latency. All subtypes of BL are characterized histologically by diffuse proliferation of medium-sized cells that have a round nucleus, small or inconspicuous nucleoli and a rim of basophilic cytoplasm that may contain lipid vacuoles. The designation 'Burkitt-like' implies the presence of cells that are somewhat more heterogeneous than usual, including some that bear resemblance to centroblasts or have more irregular nuclear outlines than typical BL. Cells in BL associated with immunosuppression may show more evidence of plasmablastic differentiation than those in the other subtypes. High cell turnover in all subtypes is reflected by the presence of abundant tingible body macrophages, responding to the high rate of apoptotic cell death and providing the well-known 'starry sky' appearance. It should be noted that this feature is not specific to BL but may also be found in other aggressive lymphomas with high rates of apoptotic cell death.

At a genetic level, BL cells characteristically have trans-locations involving the *cMYC* oncogene and the immuno-globulin heavy or light chain genes; t(8;14)(q24;q32), t(2;8)(p12;q24), t(8;22)(q24;q11). The precise breakpoints vary between endemic, sporadic and immunodeficiency-associated subtypes. The subtypes also vary in their association with clonal latent infection by EBV; endemic BL is highly associated with EBV latency in tumor cells, sporadic BL less so and, of the immunodeficiency-asso-ciated cases, EBV latency is most frequently encountered in those arising in HIV-positive patients. Immunoglobulin variable region genes are hypermutated in BL.

Blood and bone marrow aspiration

Circulating tumor cells are present in a minority of patients with BL; in effect, these patients have mature B-cell acute lymphoblastic leukemia (B-ALL) of ALL-L3 subtype as defined by the French–American–British group.[37] The cells are large, with cytoplasmic basophilia and vacuolation. Nuclear chromatin is dispersed and nucleoli are indistinct. The same morphology is re-presented in bone marrow aspirate films, when involved, and the immunophenotype is distinguished from other B-ALL by absence of nuclear terminal deoxynucleotidyl transferase (TdT) expression.

Bone marrow trephine biopsy

The bone marrow is not commonly involved by BL, ex-cept those patients who present with acute lymphoblastic leukemia (ALL) of ALL-L3 subtype; the latter is essentially a leukemic presentation of BL. When present, BL cells in trephine biopsy sections resemble those seen at other sites of disease involvement, being medium-sized with round nuclei, inconspicuous nucleoli and basophilic cytoplasm. Vacuolation of the cytoplasm is difficult to appreciate in histologic sections, even when prominent in cytology preparations. Mitotic figures are usually numerous. Infiltration may be interstitial, nodular or diffuse[1] and may be accompanied by tingible body macrophages, giving a similar 'starry sky' appearance to that seen at other sites of involvement. The differential diagnosis includes ALL, blastoid variants of MCL and aggressive morphologic variants of DLC-B. The clinical context and immunophenotype are usually discrimi-natory. The cells of BL express CD20 (sometimes only weakly) CD79a and CD10 but not CD5, cyclin D1 or TdT. In the absence of cytogenetic or molecular genetic con-firmation of a rearrangement involving *cMYC*, immuno-histochemical demonstration of Ki67 antigen expression provides indirect evidence that cell cycle control has been dysregulated to leave all BL cells active in the cell cycle. Essentially 100% of tumor cells in BL express Ki67 antigen, a picture that is very uncommon in all other lymphomas. The presence of EBV in tumor cells can be demonstrated in trephine biopsy sections by immunohistochemistry for latent membrane protein-1 (LMP-1) or EBV nuclear antigen-2 (EBNA-2), or by *in situ* hybridization to demonstrate EBV early RNA species (EBER). As mentioned above, however, EBV is less commonly associated with sporadic BL than with endemic and HIV-associated cases.

T-cell

Extranodal NK/T 'nasal type' lymphoma

(REAL: angiocentric T-cell lymphoma)

Enteropathy-type T-cell lymphoma
Subcutaneous panniculitis-like T-cell lymphoma

Clinical features and pathology at presenting sites

These are rare subtypes of natural killer (NK) and T-cell lymphomas presenting in adults with distinctive clinical features but rarely involving bone marrow; for this reason they are considered only briefly here. Lymphomas of NK/T 'nasal type' are much more common in the Far East than anywhere else and are associated with latent EBV infection in most cases. It is important to note that, although the classical presentation is with a necrotizing mid-facial neoplasm, these lymphomas also occur at other body sites. Inflammatory features frequently mask the presence of neoplastic cells and the diagnosis may be difficult to establish. Enteropathy-type T-cell lymphoma usually presents in adults with small bowel obstruction due to constricting tumor or with perforation due to tumor ulceration; multiple sites of small bowel tumor formation may be found at laparotomy. Most cases show histologic features of gluten-sensitive enteropathy in non-neoplastic small bowel tissue and a proportion of patients have clinically overt celiac disease, usually of adult onset. As its name implies, subcutaneous panniculitis-like T-cell lymphoma presents with clinical features of panniculitis and also has striking inflammatory histologic features accompanying dispersed malignant cells in subcutaneous tissue. The neoplastic T/NK-cells in these lymphoma subtypes are large and frequently pleomorphic. The clinical course is usually aggressive.

Blood and bone marrow aspirate findings

Rare patients with disseminated NK/T-cell nasal type lymphomas may have pancytopenia; circulating or aspirated neoplastic cells have some resemblance to those of T-cell large granular lymphocyte leukemia but have a higher nucleocytoplasmic ratio and are more pleomorphic. Blood and bone marrow aspirate samples virtually never contain neoplastic cells in enteropathy-type or subcutaneous panniculitis-like T-cell lymphomas but peripheral blood cytopenias, accompanied by prominent bone marrow aspirate features of hemophagocytosis, may be seen in the latter disease.

Bone marrow trephine biopsy

Bone marrow trephine histology rarely shows evidence of direct involvement by these subtypes of T-cell lymphoma. In those few cases with involvement, appearances are indistinguishable from peripheral T-cell lymphomas of no specific subtype. Random or diffuse patterns of infiltration may be present, with cells of medium to large size, often with high nucleocytoplasmic ratios and irregular nuclear outlines. Immunohistochemistry is needed to demonstrate expression of T-cell-associated antigens such as CD3, CD45RO and CD5. There may be admixed inflammatory cells, including macrophages, and increased stromal reticulin may accompany the infiltrates. Subcutaneous panniculitis-like T-cell lymphoma may be accompanied by a severe hemophagocytic syndrome. The latter is represented in trephine biopsy sections by prominence of large, round stromal macrophages containing abundant phagocytosed hemopoietic cells and other debris.

Hepatosplenic gamma-delta T-cell lymphoma

Clinical features, pathology, blood and bone marrow aspirate findings

This is a rare lymphoma with a median age at presentation of approximately 30 years. Most patients present with hepatosplenomegaly and have systemic symptoms. Most are pancytopenic at presentation and approximately half have circulating lymphoma cells. The presence of the latter heralds aggressive, end-stage disease in some patients, although prognosis in all cases is poor;[38–40] currently, there is no effective treatment for this lymphoma.

Liver and spleen are diffusely enlarged by intra-sinusoidal lymphoid cell infiltration with little tendency for solid accumulation of neoplastic cells. The cells vary somewhat in morphology from patient to patient; they may be small, medium-sized or large with regular or folded nuclei, a condensed chromatin pattern and inconspicuous nucleoli. They have moderately abundant, pale cytoplasm. In the terminal stages of disease, transformation to blast cells with prominent nucleoli may occur. Identical cells are present in the bone marrow and, when involved, in peripheral blood. Molecular genetic studies have shown monoclonal rearrangements of either gamma or beta or both sets of T-cell receptor genes in individual patients. It appears that neoplastic cells in this disease can express the alpha-beta T-cell receptor in some cases[38,41,42] and this does not alter clinical behavior compared with cases showing gamma-delta T-cell receptor expression.

Bone marrow trephine biopsy

Histologic sections show erythroid and megakaryocytic hyperplasia, with interstitial and intrasinusoidal infiltration by neoplastic cells. The latter are of variable size, as described above, and are often pleomorphic; immunohistochemical stains reveal that they express CD3 and CD56 but usually neither CD4 nor CD8. If involvement is slight, immunohistochemical staining of sinusoidal endothelium for von Willebrand factor, CD31 or CD34 may be useful to highlight the location of infiltrating cells. The presence of prominent intrasinusoidal infiltration permits distinction of this disease from other T-cell lymphomas. The marrow reaction, T-cell phenotype of the neoplastic cells and their mixed cytology distinguish it from intravascular large B-cell lymphoma. A T-cell phenotype, cellular pleomorphism and absence of nodular infiltrates also distinguish hepatosplenic gamma-delta T-cell lymphoma from SMZL, which may also show predominantly intrasinusoidal infiltration.

Anaplastic large cell lymphoma (ALCL), systemic subtype

Clinical and pathologic features

Anaplastic large cell lymphoma (ALCL) accounts for 2% of adult and 13% of pediatric non-Hodgkin's lymphoma.[11] Approximately 50% express the anaplastic lymphoma-associated kinase (ALK; see below). Those patients with ALK-positive disease have different clinical features from those whose lymphoma cells are ALK-negative. Positive ALK expression is associated with younger age, male sex, combinations of nodal and extranodal involvement and

the occurrence of 'B' symptoms. Patients with ALK-positive disease have significantly better survival following intensive chemotherapy than do patients with ALK-negative disease.[43–45]

In ALCL, involved lymph nodes are infiltrated, sometimes only to a minor extent, by clusters and sheets of pleomorphic large cells. Reactive changes may be prominent, dominating the histologic picture. Skin infiltrates are frequently present and are indistinguishable histologically from those found in localized cutaneous ALCL. The neoplastic cells usually resemble Reed–Sternberg cells of Hodgkin's lymphoma but variants of ALCL occur that are characterized by smaller, mononuclear neoplastic cells (small cell variant) or by admixture of abundant non-neoplastic lymphocytes and macrophages (lymphohistiocytic variant). Such morphologic variation does not appear to influence prognosis. The neoplastic cells of ALCL typically express CD30 in association with epithelial membrane antigen (EMA) and a range of antigens associated with either T- or NK-cell differentiation. Cells in a minority of cases appear null, lacking expression of T- and NK-cell markers. These immunophenotypic variations are not associated with significant differences in clinical behavior. By contrast with Hodgkin's lymphoma, immunohistochemical staining for CD45 is usually positive and for CD15 is usually negative.

Variation in the precise nature of the underlying chromosomal translocation pairs the *ALK* gene with one of several alternative partner genes. The nature of the fusion partner influences subcellular localization of the ALK enzyme but this is not known to influence clinical behavior of the disease.[46] Immunohistochemistry can reveal the distribution of ALK within neoplastic cells, correlating in most patients with the cytogenetic and molecular genetic findings.[47]

Blood and bone marrow aspiration

Peripheral blood cytopenias occur and correlate with the presence of bone marrow involvement but circulating tumor cells are not seen. Neoplastic cells are occasionally represented in aspirated bone marrow; they can be recognized by their large size, abundant moderately basophilic cytoplasm and large irregular, sometimes multiple, nuclei with prominent nucleoli. Reactive hemophagocytosis may be found.[48]

Bone marrow trephine biopsy

Trephine biopsy sections reveal evidence of bone marrow infiltration in only a minority of patients. Involvement is possibly more common in the elderly. Infiltration is usually interstitial or focal and may be subtle, with only small clusters or single cells present.[49] Cell morphology resembles that at the primary site, with Reed–Sternberg cell-like features in most cases but small cell variants and admixed inflammatory cells may confuse the picture. Immunohistochemical staining for CD30 and ALK is helpful, although ALK expression is found less frequently in older patients than in younger ones. The major differential diagnosis is with Hodgkin's lymphoma but metastatic melanoma, carcinoma and Langerhans cell histiocytosis require consideration in some cases and a panel of several immunohistochemical stains, including cytokeratins, S100 protein, HMB45, CD1a, CD15, CD45, EMA and ALK may be needed to establish the correct diagnosis.

Angio-immunoblastic T-cell lymphoma (AILT)

(REAL: angio-immunoblastic lymphadenopathy-like T-cell lymphoma)

Clinical features and lymph node pathology

Patients are usually adults and present with lymphadenopathy, often disseminated although not bulky. Additional features of fever, auto-immune phenomena, drug hypersensitivities and hypergammaglobulinemia (usually polyclonal) are common.

Lymph nodes involved by angio-immunoblastic T-cell lymphoma (AILT) usually show T-zone expansion with inactive B-cell follicles. The expanded paracortex may contain vaguely nodular, expansile areas of infiltration. High endothelial venules and other arborizing small blood vessels are usually prominent and are seen well with PAS staining. The latter may also show deposits of extravascular PAS-positive material, of uncertain origin. Cells within infiltrated areas are mixed, with scattered blast cells, macrophages, plasma cells and single or clustered medium-sized cells that have abundant clear cytoplasm. The clear cells may appear to be clustered around small blood vessels; immunostaining reveals these cells to be of T-cell phenotype, usually of CD4 subtype, while the scattered blasts are a mixture of T- and B-cells. In most cases an irregular meshwork of dendritic cells expressing CD21 and CD23 is present underlying expanded areas of paracortex. Evidence of latent EBV infection can be demonstrated in most cases.

Blood and bone marrow aspiration

Direct involvement of peripheral blood is very rare in AILT but there may be cytopenias involving erythroid cells, platelets, granulocytes and lymphocytes in various combinations. Reactive increases in plasma cells, plasmacytoid cells and atypical lymphocytes may be seen. The presence of a leuko-erythroblastic blood picture may reflect marrow infiltration. Bone marrow aspirate films usually show similar non-specific findings but neoplastic T-cells can occasionally be found; FACS and/or molecular genetic analysis are required for confirmation if suspicious cells are seen.

Bone marrow trephine biopsy

Trephine biopsy sections show evidence of infiltration relatively frequently in AILT, although the reported incidence varies widely between different studies (e.g. Schnaidt *et al* 1980, Ghani and Krause 1985). Involvement is usually focal, with infiltrates distributed randomly within marrow spaces (Fig. 22.16).[50,51] Infiltrates have a similar mixed composition to those found in affected lymph nodes and the underlying stroma usually has increased reticulin present, sometimes with a locally increased number of capillaries. Extracellular PAS-positive material is rarely seen. The background hemopoietic tissue frequently shows dysplastic features, with abnormalities of cell distribution within marrow spaces. Megakaryocytes and erythroid cells may show cytological atypia and granulopoiesis may be left-shifted, with relatively increased numbers of immature cells (promyelocytes and myelocytes).

Immunohistochemistry may be helpful to confirm the presence of atypical T-cells and to exclude alternative

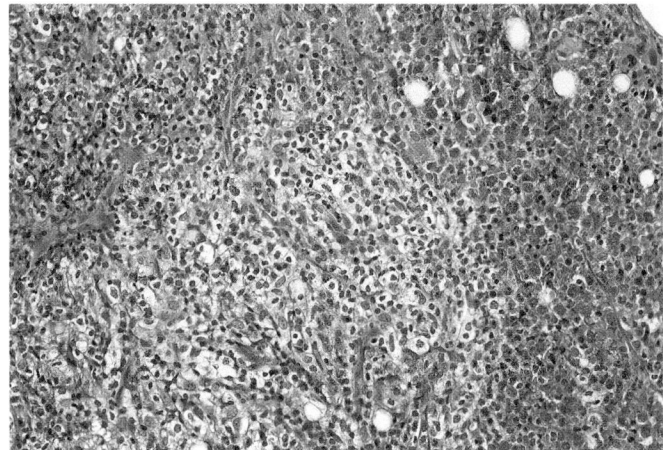

Fig. 22.16 Bone marrow infiltrated by AILT. The marrow is hypercellular and disorderly with an irregular area of infiltration by a mixture of medium-sized and large pale cells. A hint of cell 'streaming' is present due to accompanying increased stromal reticulin and vascularity (reticulin staining would be needed for confirmation of these secondary features). Section of decalcified, wax-embedded bone marrow trephine biopsy; H&E stain, original magnification × 200.

diagnoses such as Hodgkin's lymphoma and T-cell-rich forms of diffuse large B-cell lymphoma. The histologic and immunohistochemical features of AILT in bone marrow show considerable overlap with those found in other peripheral T-cell lymphomas, particularly those of no specified subtype, and a conclusive diagnosis can only be made by lymph node biopsy.

Peripheral T-cell lymphoma, not otherwise characterized (PTCL)

Clinical features and lymph node pathology

These lymphomas account for approximately 6% of NHL and occur in a wide age range of patients (median 61 years; range 17–90 years). There is usually extensive nodal involvement at presentation, with 65% of patients having stage IV disease.[11] Extranodal involvement occurs more frequently than in B-cell NHL and systemic features, such as fever, are also common. Peripheral T-cell lymphomas in this category are probably a mixture of different entities that cannot currently be distinguished into defined prognostic groups; overall, they are aggressive neoplasms with worse prognoses than DLC-B.

Lymph node histology in peripheral T-cell lymphomas, not otherwise characterized (PTCL) varies considerably between cases. Underlying lymph node architecture is usually preserved and a mixed infiltrate replaces normal components to a variable extent. Frequently, but not always, the paracortex is preferentially involved. Reactive cells, including macrophages, eosinophils, lymphocytes and plasma cells are usually present and may be sufficiently numerous to obscure neoplastic T-cells. The latter may be small, medium or large in size, in differing proportions, and may have aberrant T-cell phenotypes such as absent expression of both CD4 and CD8. Immunohistochemistry and molecular genetic demonstration of a monoclonal T-cell receptor gene rearrangement are usually needed to confirm the diagnosis.

Blood and bone marrow aspiration

Peripheral blood involvement by PTCL occurs only rarely and, in keeping with lymph node cytologic features, the cells may vary in size from small to large or be highly pleomorphic. Bone marrow involvement is also recognized only infrequently in aspirate films or by FACS analysis of aspirated cells, despite the fact that trephine biopsy is positive relatively frequently.

Bone marrow trephine biopsy

While PTCL accounts for only a minority of non-Hodgkin's lymphomas, bone marrow involvement in this category of lymphoma is frequent, with the majority of reported cases in several series having positive bone marrow staging biopsies (e.g. Caulet *et al* 1990, Gaulard *et al* 1991).[52,53] Some cases of PTCL present with bone marrow as the sole or predominant site of disease. Infiltration is usually focal and patchy or diffuse throughout the interstitium. Reactive cells are frequently admixed with the infiltrates, as in AILT, but the neoplastic cells in PTCL are usually larger and more obviously atypical, with marked pleomorphism. There is usually a patchy or diffuse increase in reticulin, sometimes with increased capillaries in areas of focal infiltration. Dysplastic hemopoietic features may be seen in non-infiltrated areas of marrow,[54] as in AILT. Lymph node histology is required to distinguish PTCL from AILT. Immunohistochemistry may be necessary to exclude possible alternative diagnoses of bone marrow involvement by Hodgkin's lymphoma, large B-cell lymphoma or ALCL. The bone marrow histology may also mimic a post-transplant lymphoproliferative disorder or the polymorphous lymphoid aggregates found in some patients with HIV infection; clinical context usually suggests the likelihood of one or other of these latter types of infiltration.

Hodgkin's lymphoma (HL)

Nodular lymphocyte predominant Hodgkin's lymphoma (NLPHL)

Clinical features and lymph node pathology

Nodular lymphocyte predominant Hodgkin's lymphoma (NLPHL) comprises approximately 5% of all Hodgkin's lymphoma. The median age at presentation is mid-30s and males are affected significantly more often than females. The disease usually involves peripheral lymph nodes (neck, axillary or inguinal groups) and approximately 80% of patients have stage I or II disease at diagnosis. The prognosis is good; 90% of patients remain alive at 10 years from diagnosis, mostly having had removal of involved lymph nodes with or without adjunctive local radiotherapy as their sole treatment.[11] There is, however, a higher risk of late disease relapse than in classical Hodgkin's lymphoma and relapse may involve disease transformation into DLC-B.

In lymph nodes, NLPHL is characterized histologically by replacement of normal structures with expanded, B-cell-rich nodules enclosing scattered CD30-negative large blast cells. These large cells have distinctive 'popcorn cell' appearances, express CD45 and are positive for B-cell markers such as CD20 and CD79a; they are typically accompanied by scattered or loosely clustered macrophages and rosettes of T-lymphocytes. True Reed–Sternberg cells are not present and the features of NLPHL may be accompanied by progressive transformation of germinal centers, a histologically distinctive reactive process. Immunoglobulin variable region genes have been shown to be mutated, with intraclonal heterogeneity, and functional immunoglobulin is produced.

Blood and bone marrow aspiration

Peripheral blood involvement by NLPHL essentially does not occur. Bone marrow examination for staging is not usually performed in NLPHL and, consequently, involvement has rarely been reported in marrow aspirate films.

Bone marrow trephine biopsy

Involvement of the bone marrow is distinctly uncommon in NLPHL and, like aspiration, marrow trephine biopsy for staging is performed infrequently. The finding of lymphoid or lymphohistiocytic infiltrates in bone marrow trephine biopsy sections from a patient diagnosed as having NLPHL should prompt review of the original diagnosis, since stage IV disease occurs rarely. Most such cases, upon review, are found to represent lymphocyte-rich classical Hodgkin's lymphoma.[55] In true NLPHL, the bone marrow is usually entirely normal.

Classical Hodgkin's lymphoma:

Nodular sclerosing subtype (NSHL)
Mixed-cellularity subtype (MCHL)
Lymphocyte-depleted (LDHL)
Lymphocyte-rich classical subtype (LRCHL)

Clinical features and lymph node pathology

Classical Hodgkin's lymphoma occurs with approximately one-third of the frequency of non-Hodgkin's lymphomas. Typical presentation is with supradiaphragmatic lymphadenopathy and approximately 30% of patients have 'B' symptoms. The disease has a bi-modal age incidence, with peaks in childhood and after the age of 55 years. Disease spread occurs: (1) locally with extranodal infiltration; (2) contiguously between adjacent lymph node groups; and (3) hematogenously to bone marrow, liver and spleen.

All variants of classical Hodgkin's lymphoma are characterized histologically by the presence of Reed–Sternberg (RS) cells. These cells frequently have distinctive lacunar morphology in nodular sclerosing Hodgkin's lymphoma (NSHL) but, in the other subtypes, classical binucleate and multinucleate RS cells are found. They express CD30 and, in a majority of cases, CD15; they generally lack expression of CD45 and EMA. Markers of B-cells, such as CD20 and CD79a, may be positive but there is usually no demonstrable production of immunoglobulin or J-chain. Mononuclear Hodgkin's cells sharing these immunophenotypic properties are present in most cases and predominate in some. In all subtypes of classical Hodgkin's lymphoma, RS cells are accompanied by reactive lymphoid cells, macrophages and eosinophils. Bands of fibrosis separating nodular areas of mixed, cellular infiltration are present in NSHL. Lymphocyte-depleted Hodgkin's lymphoma (LDHL) is much less frequently diagnosed now than in pre-immunohistochemistry days, since many cases previously categorized as LDHL can now be shown to be variants of anaplastic large cell lymphoma. Lymphocyte-rich classical Hodgkin's lymphoma (LRCHL) is a newly described subtype, first identified as a provisional entity in the REAL classification. It is characterized by appearances superficially resembling NLPLH, as described above, but with true RS cells and clinical behavior more in keeping with mixed-cellularity Hodgkin's lymphoma (MCHL).

Cases of classical Hodgkin's lymphoma have been shown to have immunoglobulin variable region gene mutations without intraclonal heterogeneity. Immunoglobulins are not transcribed, due either to crippling mutations or defective regulatory elements.

Blood and bone marrow aspiration

A full blood count frequently shows normocytic, normochromic anemia and the erythrocyte sedimentation rate is often raised. In 10% of patients there is peripheral blood eosinophilia and there may be leukopenia due to a reduction in circulating CD4$^+$ T-lymphocytes. Bone marrow is involved in 10–14% of patients; usually those with advanced disease. Reed–Sternberg cells are exceptionally uncommon in aspirate films, since infiltrates of disease contain few neoplastic cells and are typically densely fibrotic (see below); representative cells are only rarely yielded upon aspiration. Non-involved bone marrow usually has reactive appearances with granulocytic and megakaryocytic hyperplasia, with or without increased cells of the eosinophil lineage.

Bone marrow trephine biopsy

Trephine biopsy is much more sensitive than aspiration for detection of bone marrow involvement by HL, at least in part because the infiltrates cause stromal fibrosis and are difficult to aspirate. Depending on patient selection criteria, different studies have reported up to 15% of bone marrow trephine biopsies performed for staging in HL to be positive.[56–58] This figure is undoubtedly an overestimate, since many patients with clinical stage IA or IIA disease do not undergo bone marrow examination. Bilateral biopsies or single long-core biopsy increase the positive detection rate in HL and in non-Hodgkin's lymphomas.[56] However, the clinical value of bone marrow staging in HL has been questioned,[57,58] since patient management is rarely influenced directly by the outcome. Occasionally, bone marrow is the primary or sole site of involvement by HL; this is particularly the case in patients with HIV-associated HL.

Involvement of bone marrow by HL is rarely subtle; the infiltrates usually form sizeable, irregular patches with dense underlying fibrosis. Occasionally, all or most of the biopsy core is replaced; extensively involved bone marrow may contain areas of necrosis, even in previously untreated patients. Classical RS cells may or may not be found and mononuclear Hodgkin's cells are usually few, scattered widely within irregular areas of macrophage and lymphocyte infiltration (Fig. 22.17). Plasma cells and eosinophils are usually also present in these infiltrates but the number of these cells varies considerably between patients. Sometimes, the infiltrates appear densely fibrotic, with few cells of any type other than fibroblasts

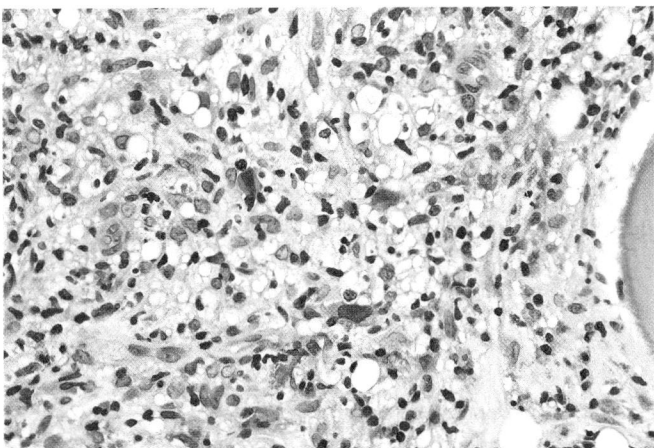

Fig. 22.17 Extensive infiltration by a mixed population of cells in bone marrow involved by HL. Occasional large cells representing mononuclear Hodgkin's cells are present although classical Reed–Sternberg cells are uncommon. Section of decalcified, wax-embedded bone marrow trephine biopsy; H&E stain, original magnification × 400.

evident, and remodeling of trabecular bone may be seen; this pattern is relatively common in specimens taken for re-staging after treatment.

Criteria for interpretation of these features differ depending upon whether or not trephine biopsy has been performed in a patient with a known diagnosis of HL, confirmed histologically at another site. If the diagnosis has already been established, it is generally regarded as adequate to see atypical large cells in an appropriate lymphohistiocytic background in order to confirm bone marrow involvement. If the diagnosis has not been made by histologic study of tissue from a lymph node or other site, a diagnosis of HL in the bone marrow can only be made with certainty if true RS cells are identified. This may require examination of multiple sections, cut at different levels from the tissue core. Identification of RS cells and mononuclear Hodgkin's cells is also assisted by immunohistochemistry for CD30, CD15, B- and T-cell-associated antigens and markers of anaplastic large cell lymphoma.

Appearances of NSHL, MCHL and LDHL in bone marrow trephine biopsy sections are similar and it is not possible to subtype classical HL variants on the basis of bone marrow histology. The differential diagnosis includes ALCL, other T-cell lymphomas, T-cell-rich variants of diffuse large B-cell lymphoma and the polymorphous reactive lymphohistiocytic infiltrates which occur in some HIV-positive patients. If fibrosis is severe, idiopathic myelofibrosis and metastatic carcinoma also require consideration. Infiltrates of LRCHD are usually composed predominantly of reactive small lymphocytes, with few macrophages or other inflammatory cells and very infrequent RS or mononuclear Hodgkin's cells. They may be mistaken for deposits of low-grade non-Hodgkin's lymphoma unless sections from multiple levels and immunohistochemical stains are examined.

It is important to realize that, in focally involved and uninvolved bone marrow from patients with HL there is frequently marked granulocytic and megakaryocytic hyperplasia, often with increased eosinophil production. Erythropoiesis is usually normal or somewhat reduced. Prominent megakaryocytes should not be mistaken for RS cells. These reactive changes, presumably cytokine-mediated, are most marked in younger patients but should not be overlooked in older individuals, in whom overall hemopoietic cellularity may not appear to be greatly increased. Common findings in association with these hyperplastic appearances are scattered sarcoid-like granulomas and aggregates of apoptotic neutrophil nuclei within the cytoplasm of stromal macrophages. Rarely, generalized marrow hypoplasia is found, without evidence of infiltration by disease.

Post-transplant lymphoproliferative disease (PTLD)

Clinical and pathologic features

The clinical presentation of post-transplant lympho-proliferative disease (PTLD) is very variable. Patients presenting in the early post-transplant period often have an infectious mononucleosis-like disease characterized by constitutional symptoms and rapid enlargement of tonsils and cervical lymph nodes. Patients with PTLD of late onset, usually a year or more after transplantation, have less severe constitutional symptoms and frequently have extranodal disease similar to the HIV-related lymphomas. The cumulative incidence of PTLD at 10 years is in the order of 5% following heart transplantation and 1% following renal or bone marrow transplantation.[59,60] The incidence of PTLD is higher in patients who are sero-negative for EBV at the time of transplantation, compared with those who are seropositive.

Lymphoproliferative disorders arising after solid organ or bone marrow transplantation also vary greatly in histologic appearance and immunophenotype between individuals.[61] Although they may appear to arise from either T- or B-cells, EBV infection is associated with the majority of cases, through reactivation of latent infection in the graft recipient or as a result of primary infection acquired from graft tissue. Similar EBV-associated lymphoid proliferations occur in other acquired and inherited immune deficiency states. Morphologically, examples of PTLD have been reported that are equivalent to most subtypes of large B-cell, Burkitt's, peripheral T-cell and Hodgkin's lymphomas, plus plasmacytic pro-liferations. Also well described in the spectrum of PTLD are polymorphous lymphoid infiltrates composed of complex mixtures of inflammatory cells and atypical lymphoid cells, including B-cells at all stages of maturation.

Cases of PTLD may be polyclonal or monoclonal, and their clonal status does not necessarily indicate their likely aggressiveness. Factors predicting responsiveness to modulation of immunosuppressive therapy versus requirement for cytotoxic chemotherapy are under active investigation.[62]

Blood and bone marrow aspiration

Peripheral blood rarely contains detectable disease and bone marrow aspiration is also usually negative. In examples equivalent to subtypes of transplant-unrelated NHL, there may occasionally be involvement with the same cytologic features as those described in individual

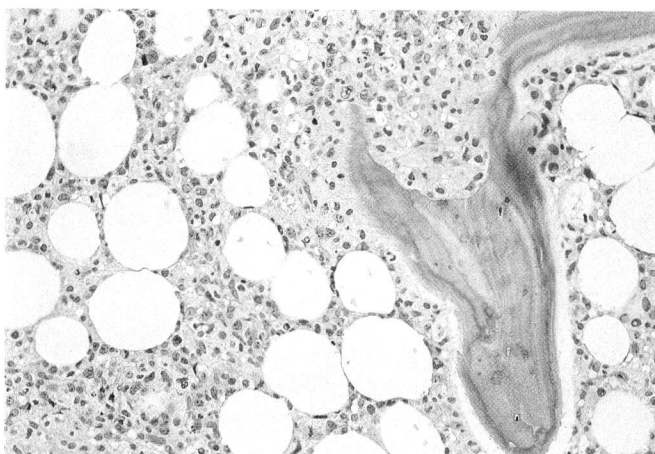

Fig. 22.18 Poorly-defined interstitial and nodular replacement of bone marrow by a polymorphous infiltrate of PTLD, in this example showing erosion of trabecular bone. Section of decalcified, wax-embedded bone marrow trephine biopsy; H&E stain, original magnification × 200.

sections above. Blood or bone marrow plasmacytosis (polyclonal or monoclonal) may be encountered in cases with plasma cell-predominant lymphoid proliferations.

Bone marrow trephine biopsy

Approximately 50% of patients with polymorphous PTLD have involvement of the bone marrow, seen in trephine biopsy sections as poorly-defined irregular or nodular infiltrates of mixed cells (Fig. 22.18).[63] Bone marrow involvement by PTLD in patients who have variants equivalent to B-cell, T-cell or Hodgkin's lymphomas shares the morphology of the primary tumor and has features as described above for the equivalent lymphomas seen in immunocompetent individuals.

Major issues in the differential diagnosis of blood and bone marrow involvement by lymphoma

Assessment of peripheral blood involvement by lymphoma

It can be difficult to determine whether peripheral blood lymphocytosis is reactive or neoplastic in some patients, particularly when the lymphocyte count is only modestly raised. Abnormal cytology is usually evident if circu-lating cells are larger than normal or have very irregular nuclear morphology but can be hard to appreciate in small cells. Hairy or villous cytoplasm in small lymphoid cells is exaggerated in slightly thicker areas of the blood film, where cells are less well spread, and looking in such areas can be helpful in cases with few cells present. Obviously, FACS immunophenotyping and molecular genetic clonality studies can usually confirm the diagnosis.

Reactive B lymphocytosis may occur in smokers, characterized by the presence of circulating B-lymphocytes with abundant cytoplasm and, in a proportion of cases, distinctive bi-lobed nuclei.[64] The lymphocytes appear polyclonal by FACS immunophenotyping and are typically accompanied by a polyclonal increase in serum IgM. However, a clonal origin for this phenomenon is suggested by the finding of a hundred-fold increase in rearrangements between immunoglobulin heavy or light chain genes and *BCL2*, relative to control subjects, and the occurrence of an isochromosome 3q in both kappa- and lambda- expressing cells.[65–67]

Assessment of bone marrow aspirate involvement by lymphoma

As described in the individual sections above, aspiration is relatively insensitive for detection of bone marrow involvement by many lymphomas. False-negative results are particularly likely in the presence of stromal fibrosis or focal, minor degrees of infiltration. Trephine biopsy is therefore always recommended as a component of any bone marrow staging examination but information from aspirated bone marrow is maximized by performance of FACS immunophenotyping in all cases, with additional cytogenetic and molecular genetic analyses where practical.

Normal bone marrow during infancy contains many more lymphoid cells than are present in later life,[68] predominantly due to developing B-lymphoid cells, known as hematogones, that resemble dispersed or clustered lymphoblasts. These cells may comprise as many as 40% of bone marrow cells and, when abundant, may be mistaken for blast cells of ALL. Their phenotype is similar to ALL blast cells but expression of cell-surface antigens such as CD19 and CD10 is generally weak, unlike leukemic cells in most cases of ALL. When bone marrow is aspirated during follow-up investigations after chemotherapy for ALL in young children, it is important not to confuse regenerating hematogones with residual or relapsed acute leukemia. In adults, hematogones are seen rarely, even during hemopoietic regeneration after myelo-ablative therapy, but their presence has been reported in occasional patients.[69]

In the bone marrow of adults there are usually few B-lymphocytes and rather more T-cells. The latter are predominantly CD8+ and are dispersed throughout the interstitium. NK-cells are not normally present. Aggregates of B-cells occur in many adults, particularly in association with systemic infections and other inflammatory processes. These may cause confusion in interpretation of bone marrow aspirate films if the needle fortuitously enters one. Examination of trails behind a number of particles on different slides usually makes it clear that a focal lymphocyte-rich lesion has been sampled. Immunocytochemistry may be informative but the same cells are often not represented in the marrow suspension sent for FACS. Trephine biopsy histology is needed to confirm the presence of architectural features indicating a reactive rather than lymphomatous infiltrate but the sections may not include the precise site sampled by aspiration and an inference has to be drawn from the appearances of other lymphoid aggregates, if present.

Assessment of lymphoid infiltrates in bone marrow trephine biopsy sections

Hematogones

Hematogones in infancy are less readily identifiable in histologic sections than in aspirate films; consequently, they rarely cause diagnostic difficulty in these preparations. However, they may be seen in hypocellular, regenerating bone marrow following chemotherapy in children and, in this context, they should not be mistaken for residual leukemic cells of ALL. Hematogones are usually dispersed among other hemopoietic cells, whereas leukemic blast cells are more likely to be present in clusters or confluent sheets. The phenotype of hematogones as demonstrated by immunohistochemistry in fixed tissue sections (CD10+ve and TdT+ve, with variable expression of CD20 and CD79a) cannot distinguish them reliably from ALL blast cells.

Reactive lymphoid aggregates

Nodular aggregates of small lymphoid cells may be found in trephine biopsy sections as a reactive phenomenon, unrelated to any neoplastic lymphoid proliferation. Criteria for distinguishing such aggregates from neoplastic lymphoid infiltrates remain imperfect and controversial.[3,70,71] Immunostaining is helpful in only occasional examples and morphologic features currently remain the best guide. Improved application of molecular genetic techniques, such as PCR amplification and IgH/TcR gene rearrangement studies, may offer clearer answers in future. However, initial reports suggest that new areas of uncertainty are raised in relation to the sensitivity and specificity of the methods employed.[3,4]

The position of a lymphoid aggregate within the bone marrow is important in assessing whether it is reactive or neoplastic. It is never normal for lymphoid cells to aggregate at trabecular margins or the edges of sinusoids. As discussed earlier, paratrabecular lymphoid infiltrates are most likely to represent FL, with the differential diagnosis being LPL, SMZL and MCL. Perisinusoidal infiltrates may be subtle but declare themselves on low-power histologic examination because they distort and pull open the lumen of the adjacent sinusoid, as a result of an accompanying increase in stromal reticulin (Fig. 22.19).

To be accepted as reactive, lymphoid nodules should be few in number, centrally placed within intertrabecular spaces, small and round in profile with well-demarcated margins. A small capillary may be present, running from the periphery into the center of the nodule (see Fig. 22.1) and there may be reactive changes such as aggregation of eosinophils in the adjacent hemopoietic tissue. An underlying meshwork of reticulin or CD23+ follicular dendritic cells may be present or absent, probably more dependent on the size of a particular nodule than on its reactive or neoplastic nature. The subjective nature of these criteria will be obvious to the reader but, to date, an objective gold-standard for assessment of bone marrow lymphoid nodules remains elusive.

The cytologic composition of lymphoid infiltrates is also critical to their interpretation. Most non-neoplastic aggregates consist of small lymphocytes with only occasional large blast cells; they show little evidence of plasma cell differentiation. Reactive germinal center formation is distinctly uncommon but, when it occurs, the composition of the lymphoid follicle recapitulates that found in lymph nodes and other organized lymphoid tissues (Fig. 22.20). Centroblasts, centrocytes and occasional tingible body macrophages occupy the germinal center and a mantle of small lymphocytes is present around the periphery. Formation of reactive germinal centers within bone marrow lymphoid aggregates is said to be increased in patients with rheumatoid arthritis and other systemic chronic inflammatory disorders.[72] It should be remembered that neoplastic germinal centers are very rarely found in bone marrow infiltrates of follicular lymphoma and, in almost all such cases, the neoplastic follicles are accompanied by areas of

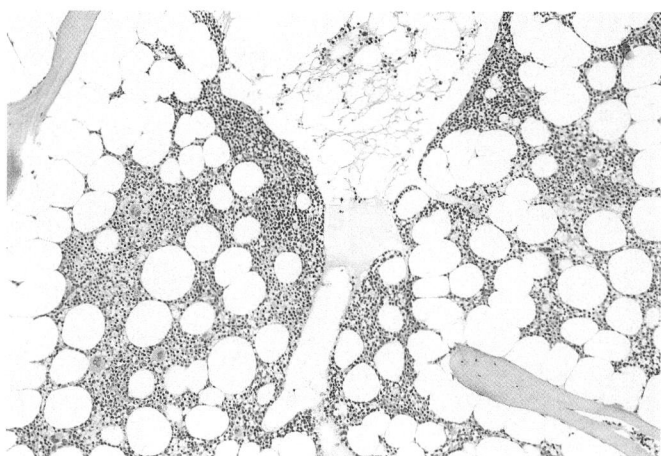

Fig. 22.19 Perisinusoidal lymphoid aggregates causing the adjacent sinusoid to gape open. Section of decalcified, wax-embedded bone marrow trephine biopsy; H&E stain, original magnification × 100.

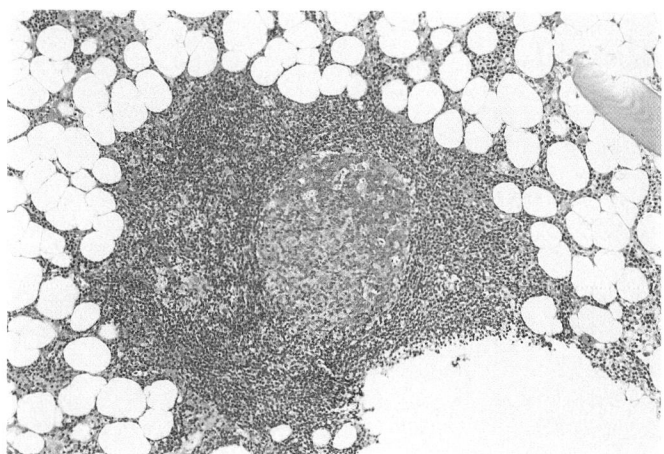

Fig. 22.20 Reactive germinal center in a bone marrow lymphoid nodule. This particular example was an incidental finding in a patient with no history of rheumatoid arthritis or other chronic inflammatory disease. Note the well-formed germinal center and mantle zone with clear demarcation between these two components of the nodule. Section of decalcified, wax-embedded bone marrow trephine biopsy; H&E stain, original magnification × 100.

classical paratrabecular infiltration. Reactive lymphoid aggregates also require distinguishing from nodular infiltrates of B-CLL, a pattern found particularly frequently, in the absence of significant interstitial infiltration, in so-called 'nodular partial remission' in patients receiving chemotherapy.

Assessing lymphoma grade in bone marrow

Bone marrow involvement in low-grade lymphomas is much more common than in intermediate and high-grade lymphomas, with the exception MCL (intermediate grade), in which marrow involvement is frequently present. In DLC-B and BL, morphologic features are usually distinctive and predictive of clinical behavior (intermediate- and high-grade, respectively). Involvement by low-grade lymphoma or MCL is manifest in trephine biopsy sections by infiltrates composed exclusively or predominantly of small cells; immunophenotyping assists in establishing the diagnosis in cases of MCL, as described earlier. However, the presence of increased numbers of large cells occasionally causes difficulty in the assessment of grade in bone marrow infiltrates of FL and B-CLL. In these contexts, confluent sheets of large blast cells may be seen in rare instances, representing Richter's transformation in B-CLL and, in FL, transformation to DLC-B. In other examples, with higher than usual blast cell numbers present in infiltrates that are otherwise typical of low-grade lymphoma, the significance of the blast cell component is not known. For example, a high content of para-immunoblasts may be found in nodular areas of B-CLL infiltration but this does not necessarily indicate progression to prolymphocytic leukemia and is entirely compatible with a typical picture of B-CLL.

Discordance between bone marrow and lymph node (or other site) appearances

Sometimes bone marrow trephine biopsy for lymphoma staging reveals marrow involvement by lymphoma of higher or lower grade than that present in the diagnostic lymph node or extranodal tissue biopsy specimen. Usually, the picture is one of paratrabecular or nodular infiltration by low-grade lymphoma in the bone marrow of a patient known to have intermediate-grade lymphoma elsewhere. This pattern is important to recognize as it has little influence on patient survival; it does not have the adverse prognostic significance that bone marrow involvement by intermediate-grade lymphoma would have.[73] In addition, in patients with evidence only of diffuse large B-cell lymphoma elsewhere, the finding of characteristic paratrabecular low-grade lymphoma infiltrates in bone marrow can be helpful in establishing origin from FL. Patients with DLC-B arising by transformation from low grade FL may have a worse prognosis than those in whom it arises *de novo*, although use of modern intensive treatment regimes can eliminate such differences.[74]

The finding of intermediate- or high-grade lymphoma in bone marrow trephine biopsy sections from a patient with low-grade lymphoma elsewhere is evidence of disease progression or transformation in the bone marrow.

Interpreting necrotic deposits of possible lymphoma

Occasionally, the situation is encountered, usually in patients with large cell or high-grade lymphomas, in which extensive marrow infiltration is present but represented only by necrotic tissue. That the marrow is infiltrated and the picture is not one of infarction of normal hemopoietic tissue can be suspected in most cases from the loss of fat spaces in areas of necrosis. Reticulin staining generally confirms an underlying disturbance of stromal architecture. Stains such as H&E, Giemsa and PAS offer little further insight into the nature of necrotic tissue in the bone marrow but immunostaining, applied with care, can be very helpful. In particular, CD20 is well preserved in necrotic lymphoid cells and can demonstrate the B-cell nature of a lymphomatous infiltrate, often highlighting the size and outline of individual cells so that at least a partial impression of cell morphology can be gained. Since most cases of necrotic lymphoma in the bone marrow are examples of DLC-B, this is of considerable practical value.

Demonstration of most T-cell-associated antigens in this context is unreliable, since they are not well preserved on lymphoid cells and the antibodies used for their detection will cross-react with myelomonocytic cells, including macrophages attracted to the site in response to the presence of necrosis. Alone of the T-cell markers, CD3 may be adequately preserved and false-positive results are not generally found. For the differential diagnosis of HL, use of CD30 and CD15 immunostaining is unreliable. In rare cases of metastatic carcinoma mimicking necrotic lymphoma, high- and low-molecular weight cytokeratins may be stained successfully without non-specific positive results. Immunostaining for melanoma markers is unreliable in necrotic tissue due to poor antigen preservation and, in the case of S100 protein, cross-reactivity with macrophages.

Appearances of lymphoma infiltrates following therapy

Apart from quantitative changes in the degree of bone marrow infiltration by lymphoma following chemotherapy, there may also be changes in the morphology of cell infiltrates. At present, it remains controversial whether nodular lymphoid infiltrates, not occupying paratrabecular or perisinusoidal locations, are reactive phenomena or residual deposits of low-grade lymphoma. A prominent, hypercellular rim of granulocytes, particularly eosinophils, often surrounds such nodules and they are usually composed predominantly of small T-lymphocytes, with few B-cells, regardless of the original lymphoma diagnosis. It is relatively common to see such nodules following anti-CD20 immunotherapy of low-grade lymphoma and, while some authors claim they are not neoplastic,[75] confirmatory evidence to date is incomplete.

Bone marrow hyperplastic, dysplastic and stromal reactions to lymphoma

Hemopoiesis in the bone marrow often appears remarkably unaffected by significant levels of infiltration by lymphoma. However, certain types of lymphoma are regularly associated with spatial and cytologic abnormalities of hemopoiesis, often with increased stromal reticulin, presumably secondary to cytokine production by the neoplastic cells themselves or inflammatory cells stimulated by their presence. Infiltration of the bone marrow by T-cell lymphomas of angio-immunoblastic or unspecified subtypes has particularly been reported in association with such phenomena.[51-54,76] However, occasional cases of B-cell lymphoma, of various subtypes, are also accompanied by marked hemopoietic cell hyperplasia and/or by stromal edema and fibrosis. In these cases, the presence of lymphomatous infiltrates is usually obvious; attention to megakaryocyte morphology usually excludes a true myeloproliferative disorder but it can be difficult to determine whether or not a myelodysplastic syndrome is represented. Hematological follow-up, with bone marrow aspiration and cytogenetic studies ± trephine biopsy may be helpful.

Atypical lymphoid aggregates in chronic myeloproliferative diseases, myelodysplastic syndromes and HIV infection

Lymphoid infiltrates that are atypical by virtue of their size, distribution or number are occasionally found in bone marrow trephine biopsy sections from patients with chronic myeloproliferative disease (CMPD) or myelodysplastic syndrome (MDS). The prognosis for individual patients does not seem to be altered by the presence of such aggregates and reflects the progress of their underlying hemopoietic disorder. In most cases, these infiltrates contain a mixture of small T- and B-lymphocytes and

appear reactive; in some cases, T- and or B-cell populations have been demonstrated which share clonal cytogenetic abnormalities with myeloid cells.[77-79] Rare examples of coincidental B-CLL and CMPD/MDS have been recorded (e.g. Lai et al 1999),[80] which is not surprising considering the relatively advanced age of most patients with these types of diseases.

Lymphoid aggregates, which may be nodular or irregular, are found commonly in HIV-positive individuals undergoing bone marrow examination for assessment of cytopenias or symptoms suggestive of opportunistic infection. Provided that they are few in number, composed predominantly of small cells and do not have an obviously lymphomatous pattern of infiltration (e.g. paratrabecular infiltration) these can generally be considered reactive and monitored by follow-up with repeat biopsies. Poorly-formed granulomas and loose polymorphous lymphohistiocytic infiltrates may mimic higher-grade lymphomas; immunohistochemistry may be needed to demonstrate the mixed, macrophage-rich nature of these infiltrates. Most lymphomas associated with immunocompromise due to HIV infection are of Burkitt's type, and have obviously malignant cytologic features, rather than resembling polymorphous PTLD.

Classification of lymphoma when bone marrow trephine biopsy provides the sole source of tissue for assessment

Occasionally, lymphoma presents with bone marrow as the sole site of disease or as the most accessible site for diagnostic biopsy. As an additional problem, bone marrow aspiration frequently yields no lymphoma cells in patients in whom trephine biopsy sections show definite evidence of lymphoma infiltration, so that immunofluorescence data cannot be obtained to support the diagnosis. In each of these circumstances, bone marrow histology is crucial to diagnosis. The spatial distribution and cellular composition of lymphoma infiltrates, supplemented by judicious use of immunohistochemistry, permits accurate WHO categorization in most cases. The various spatial patterns of lymphoma in different diagnostic categories have been described in earlier sections of this chapter. No single pattern is unique to any lymphoma entity but it is possible to make some helpful generalizations. Paratrabecular infiltration is highly suggestive of FL although it may also be seen in LPL, MCL and SMZL; in the latter conditions, paratrabecular infiltrates are rarely as extensive or linear as in FL. Paratrabecular infiltration occurs with exceptional rarity, if ever, in B-CLL. The latter usually exhibits nodular infiltration with greater or lesser degrees of interstitial spread. The presence of scattered or clustered para-immunoblasts in nodular areas of small lymphoid cell infiltration strongly suggests B-CLL. The presence of occasional blast cells in LPL or the rare formation of neoplastic follicles in FL can mimic para-immunoblasts but FL will generally show at least some areas of para-trabecular infiltration while infiltrates of LPL are usually more irregular in shape and less well defined than those of B-CLL. The presence of numerous plasma cells and formation of Dutcher bodies supports a diagnosis of LPL, both features being rare in B-CLL. Nodular infiltration is also a frequent pattern in MCL but the nodules in this disease appear monotonous cytologically, without blast cells or plasma cells. Immunohistochemistry for CD5, CD10, CD23 and cyclin D1 (plus CD20 or CD79a and CD3 to assess overall T- and B-cell numbers) usually distinguishes between these various small B-cell lymphomas (see Table 22.1). The 'spaced out' infiltrates of HCL are histologically distinctive and are rarely confused with other small cell subtypes of lymphoma; reticulin staining and immunohistochemistry for TRAP provide confirmation, if needed.

Infiltrates of large lymphoid cells require distinction from increased numbers of immature myelomonocytic cells, poorly differentiated plasma cell neoplasms and, rarely, metastatic cancer. Immunohistochemistry is highly valuable in this context, as described above in relation to DLC-B. As at other sites, recognition and classification of peripheral T-cell lymphomas in the bone marrow is more difficult. A high index of suspicion and careful assessment of any clinical or laboratory findings suggesting T-cell lymphoma are important. Unexplained or disproportionate histologic features of myelodysplasia in this context should prompt a detailed search for lymphoma infiltrates. The latter are generally randomly distributed and contain abundant reactive cells (macrophages, endothelium, fibroblasts, plasma cells, etc.) as well as neoplastic T-cells. Differential diagnosis from HL, T-cell-rich variants of DLC-B and polymorphous forms of PTLD necessitates immunohistochemistry, as described in the relevant sections above.

Conclusions

Examination of blood, aspirated bone marrow and bone marrow trephine biopsy specimens provides complementary information in the assessment of patients with known or suspected lymphoma. Bone marrow sampling is important, predominantly in contributing to the

planning of treatment and monitoring of disease response to treatment. It may be essential for diagnosis if disease at other sites is inaccessible, the patient is too frail to undergo lymph node biopsy or bone marrow is the only site of disease. Trephine biopsy has a particularly important role in this context; since histologic patterns of bone marrow involvement in trephine biopsy sections permit most lymphomas to be assigned to their WHO categories, especially if supplemented by FACS or immunohistochemical immunophenotyping. However, morphologic discrimination between reactive lymphoid nodules and minimal involvement by lymphoma in bone marrow remains an important unsolved problem. It is to be hoped that wider application of molecular genetic techniques such as FISH and PCR will improve the accuracy of this distinction and aid the assessment of minimal residual disease following treatment.

REFERENCES

1. Bain BJ, Clark DM, Lampert IA, Wilkins BS 2001 Bone marrow pathology, 3rd edn. Blackwell Science, Oxford, 231–331
2. Bishop PW, McNally K, Harris M 1992 Audit of bone marrow trephines. Journal of Clinical Pathology 45: 1105–1108
3. Kröber SM, Horny H-P, Greschniok A, Kaiserling E 1999 Reactive and neoplastic lymphocytes in human bone marrow: morphological immunohistological and molecular biological investigations on biopsy specimens. Journal of Clinical Pathology 52: 521–526
4. Brinckmann R, Kafmann O, Reinartz B, Dietel M 2000 Specificity of PCR-based clonality analysis of immunoglobulin heavy chain gene rearrangements for the detection of bone marrow involvement by low-grade B-cell lymphomas. Journal of Pathology 190: 55–60
5. Wickham CL, Boyce M, Joyner M et al 2000 Amplification of PCR products in excess of 600 base pairs using DNA extracted from decalcified, paraffin-embedded bone marrow trephine biopsies. Journal of Clinical Pathology Molecular Pathology 53: 19–23
6. Wickham CL, Sarsfield P, Joyner MV et al 2000 Formic acid decalcification of bone marrow trephines degrades DNA: alternative use of EDTA allows amplification and sequencing of relatively long PCR products. Journal of Clinical Pathology Molecular Pathology 53: 336
7. Harris NL, Jaffe ES, Diebold J et al 1999 Commentary: The World Health Organization classification of neoplastic diseases of the hematopoietic and lymphoid tissues. Report of the Clinical Advisory Committee Meeting, Airlie House, Virginia, November 1997. Histopathology 36: 69–86
8. Harris NL, Jaffe ES, Stein H et al 1994 A revised European–American classification of lymphoid neoplasms: a proposal from the International Lymphoma Study Group. Blood 84: 1361–1392
9. Klein U, Goossens T, Fischer M et al 1998 Somatic mutation in normal and transformed human B cells. Immunological Reviews 162: 261–280
10. Dunn-Walters D, Thiede C, Alpen B, Spencer J 2001 Somatic hypermutation and B cell lymphoma. Philosophical Transactions of the Royal Society of London B 356: 73–82
11. Armitage JO, Weisenberger DD 1998 New approach to classifying non-Hodgkin's lymphomas: clinical features of the major histologic subtypes. Journal of Clinical Oncology 16: 2780–2795
12. Dimopoulos MA, Alexanian R 1994 Waldenström's macroglobulinaemia. Blood 83: 1452–1459
13. Iida S, Rao PH, Nallasivam P et al 1996 The t(9;14)(p13;q32) chromosomal translocation associated with lymphoplasmacytoid lymphoma involves the PAX-5 gene. Blood 88: 4110–4117
14. Ohno H, Ueda C, Akasaka T 2000 The t(9;14)(p13;q32) translocation in B-cell non-Hodgkin's lymphoma. Leukemia and Lymphoma 36: 435–445
15. Wilkins BS, Buchan SL, Webster J, Jones DB 2001 Tryptase-positive mast cells accompany lymphocytic as well as lymphoplasmacytic

lymphoma infiltrates in bone marrow trephine biopsies. Histopathology 39: 150–155

16. Banham AH, Turley H, Pulford K et al 1997 The plasma cell associated antigen detectable by antibody VS38 is the p63 rough endoplasmic reticulum protein. Journal of Clinical Pathology 50: 485–489

17. Bain BJ 1995 Blood cells. A practical guide, 2nd edn. Blackwell Science, Oxford, 298–300

18. VanderMolen LA, Urba WJ, Longo DL et al 1989 Diffuse osteosclerosis in hairy cell leukemia. Blood 74: 2066–2069

19. Verhoef GE, de Wolf-Peeters C, Zachee P, Boogaerts MA 1990 Regression of diffuse osteosclerosis in hairy cell leukaemia after treatment with interferon. British Journal of Haematology 76: 150–151.

20. Hounieu H, Chittal SM, al Saati T et al 1992 Hairy cell leukemia. Diagnosis of bone marrow involvement in paraffin-embedded sections with monoclonal antibody DBA.44. American Journal of Clinical Pathology 98: 26–33

21. Salomen Nguyen N, Valensi F, Troussard X, Flandrin G 1996 The value of monoclonal antibody DBA44 in the diagnosis of B-lymphoid disorders. Leukemia Research 20: 909–913

22. Janckila AJ, Cardwell EM, Yam LT, Li CY 1995 Hairy cell identification by immunohistochemistry of tartrate-resistant acid phosphatase. Blood 85: 2839–2844

23. Hoyer JD, Li CY, Yam LT et al 1997 Immunohistochemical demonstration of acid phosphatase isoenzyme 5 (tartrate-resistant) in paraffin sections of hairy cell leukemia and other hematologic disorders. American Journal of Clinical Pathology 108: 308–315

24. Brynes RK, Almaguer PD, Leathery KE et al 1996 Numerical cytogenetic abnormalities of chromosomes 3, 7 and 12 in marginal zone B-cell lymphomas. Modern Pathology 9: 995–1000

25. Dierlamm J, Rosenberg C, Stul M et al 1997 Characteristic pattern of chromosomal gains and losses in marginal zone B cell lymphoma detected by comparative genomic hybridization. Leukemia 11: 747–758

26. Rosenwald A, Ott G, Stilgenbauer S et al 1999 Exclusive detection of the t(11;18)(q21;q21) in extranodal marginal zone B cell lymphomas (MZBL) of MALT type in contrast to other MZBL and extranodal large B cell lymphomas. American Journal of Pathology 155: 1817–1821

27. Griesser H, Kaiser U, Augener W et al 1990 B-cell lymphoma of the mucosa-associated lymphatic tissue (MALT) presenting with bone marrow and peripheral blood involvement. Leukemia Research 14: 617–622

28. Schmid C, Isaacson PG 1992 Bone marrow trephine biopsy in lymphoproliferative disease. Journal of Clinical Pathology 45: 745–750

29. Henrique R, Achten R, Maes B et al 1999 Guidelines for subtyping small B-cell lymphomas in bone marrow biopsies. Virchows Archiv 435: 549–558

30. Mann R, Berard C 1982 Criteria for the subclassification of follicular lymphomas: a proposed alternative method. Hematological Oncology 1: 187–192

31. Nathwani BN, Metter GE, Miller TP et al 1986 What should be the morphologic criteria for the subdivision of follicular lymphomas? Blood 68: 837–845

32. Perry DA, Bast MA, Armitage JO, Weisenburger DD 1990 Diffuse intermediate lymphocytic lymphoma. A clinicopathologic study and comparison with small lymphocytic lymphoma and diffuse small cleaved cell lymphoma. Cancer 66: 1995–2000

33. Dufau JP, le Tourneau A, Molina T et al 2000 Intravascular large B cell lymphoma with bone marrow involvement at presentation and haemophagocytic syndrome: two Western cases in favour of a specific variant. Histopathology 37: 509–512

34. Parrens M, Dubus P, Agape P et al 2000 Intrasinusoidal bone marrow infiltration revealing intravascular lymphomatosis. Leukemia and Lymphoma 37: 219–223

35. Schlegelberger B, Zwingers T, Harder L et al 1999 Clinicopathogenetic significance of chromosomal abnormalities in patients with blastic peripheral B-cell lymphoma. Kiel-Wien-Lymphoma Study Group. Blood 94: 3114–3120

36. Ottensmeier CH, Thompsett AR, Zhu D et al 1998 Analysis of VH genes in follicular and diffuse lymphoma reveals ongoing somatic mutation and multiple isotype transcripts in early disease, with changes during progression. Blood 91: 4292–4299

37. Bennett JM, Catovsky D, Daniel MT et al 1976 Proposals for the classification of the acute leukaemias. French–American–British (FAB) co-operative group. British Journal of Haematology 33: 451–458

38. Cooke CB, Krenacs L, Stetler-Stevenson M et al 1996 Hepatosplenic T-cell lymphoma: a distinct clinicopathologic entity of cytotoxic gamma delta T-cell origin. Blood 88: 4265–4274

39. Sallah S, Smith SV, Lony LC et al 1997 Gamma/delta T-cell hepatosplenic lymphoma: review of the literature, diagnosis by flow cytometry and concomitant autoimmune hemolytic anemia. Annals of Hematology 74: 139–142

40. Weidmann E 2000 Hepatosplenic T cell lymphoma. A review on 45 cases since the first report describing the disease as a distinct lymphoma entity in 1990. Leukemia 14: 991–997

41. Lai R, Larratt LM, Etches W et al 2000 Hepatosplenic T-cell lymphoma of alphabeta lineage in a 16-year-old boy presenting with hemolytic anemia and thrombocytopenia. American Journal of Surgical Pathology 24: 459–463

42. Macon WR, Levy NB, Kurtin PJ et al 2001 Hepatosplenic alphabeta T-cell lymphomas: a report of 14 cases and comparison with hepatosplenic gammadelta T-cell lymphoma. American Journal of Surgical Pathology 25: 285–296

43. Benharroch D, Meguerian-Bedoyan Z, Lamant L et al 1998 ALK-positive lymphoma: a single disease with a broad spectrum of morphology. Blood 91: 2076–2084

44. Falini B, Pileri S, Zinzani PL et al 1999 ALK+ lymphoma: clinico-pathological findings and outcome. Blood 93: 2697–2706

45. Stein H, Foss HD, Durkop H et al 2000 CD30(+) anaplastic large cell lymphoma: a review of its histopathologic, genetic and clinical features. Blood 96: 3681–3695

46. Falini B, Pulford K, Pucciarini A et al 1999 Lymphomas expressing ALK fusion protein(s) other than NPM-ALK. Blood 94: 3509–3515

47. Pulford K, Lamant L, Morris SW et al 1997 Detection of anaplastic lymphoma kinase (ALK) and nucleolar protein nucleophosmin (NPM)-ALK proteins in normal and neoplastic cells with the monoclonal antibody ALK1. Blood 89: 1394–1404

48. Wong KF, Chan JK, Ng CS et al 1991 Anaplastic large cell Ki-1 lymphoma involving bone marrow: marrow findings and association with reactive hemophagocytosis. American Journal of Hematology 37: 112–119.

49. Fraga M, Brousset P, Schlaifer D et al 1995 Bone marrow involvement in anaplastic large cell lymphoma. Immunohistochemical detection of minimal disease and its prognostic significance. American Journal of Clinical Pathology 103: 82–89

50. Schnaidt U, Vykoupil KF, Thiele J, Georgii A 1980 Angioimmunoblastic lymphadenopathy. Histopathology of bone marrow involvement. Virchows Archiv [Pathology: Anatomy] 389: 369–380

51. Ghani AM, Krause JR 1985 Bone marrow biopsy findings in angioimmunoblastic lymphadenopathy. British Journal of Haematology 61: 203–213

52. Caulet S, Delmer A, Audouin J et al 1990 Histopathological study of bone marrow biopsies in 30 cases of T-cell lymphoma with clinical, biological and survival correlations. Hematological Oncology 8: 155–168

53. Gaulard P, Kanavaros P, Farcet JP et al 1991 Bone marrow histologic and immunohistochemical findings in peripheral. T-cell lymphoma: A study of 38 cases. Human Pathology 22: 331–338

54. Hanson CA, Brunning RD, Gajl-Peczalska KJ et al 1986 Bone marrow manifestations of peripheral T-cell lymphoma. A study of 30 cases. American Journal of Clinical Pathology 86: 449–460

55. Sextro M, Diehl V, Franklin J et al 1996 Lymphocyte predominant Hodgkin's disease – a workshop report. Annals of Oncology 4 (suppl 6): S61–S65

56. Bartl R, Frisch B, Burkhardt R et al 1982 Assessment of bone marrow histology in Hodgkin's disease: correlation with clinical factors. British Journal of Haematology 51: 345–360

57. Macintyre EA, Vaughan Hudson B, Linch DC et al 1987 The value of staging bone marrow trephine biopsy in Hodgkin's disease. European Journal of Haematology 39: 66–70

58. Ellis ME, Diehl LF, Granger E, Elson E 1989 Trephine needle bone marrow biopsy in the initial staging of Hodgkin disease: sensitivity and specificity of the Ann Arbor staging procedure criteria. American Journal of Hematology 30: 115–120

59. Thomas JA, Crawford DH, Burke M 1995 Clinicopathologic implications of Epstein–Barr virus related B cell lymphoma in immunocompromised patients. Journal of Clinical Pathology 48: 287–290

60. Swinnen LJ 2000 Diagnosis and treatment of transplant-related lymphoma. Annals of Oncology 11 (suppl 1): 45–48

61. Harris NL, Ferry JA, Swerdlow SH 1997 Posttransplant lymphoproliferative disorder: summary of Society for

Hematopathology Workshop. Seminars in Diagnostic Pathology 14: 8–14

62. Swinnen LJ 2000 Transplantation-related lymphoproliferative disorder: a model for human immunodeficiency virus-related lymphomas. Seminars in Oncology 27: 402–408

63. Koeppen H, Newell K, Baunoch DA, Vardiman JW 1998 Morphologic bone marrow changes in patients with posttransplantation lymphoproliferative disorders. American Journal of Surgical Pathology 22: 208–214

64. Troussard X, Flandrin G 1996 Chronic B-cell lymphocytosis with binucleated lymphocytes (LWBL): a review of 38 cases. Leukemkia and Lymphoma 20: 275–279

65. Mossafa H, Troussard X, Valensi F et al 1996 Isochromosome i(3q) and premature chromosome condensation are recurrent findings in chronic B-cell lymphocytosis with binucleated lymphocytes. Leukemia and Lymphoma 20: 267–273

66. Delage R, Roy J, Jacques L et al 1997 Multiple bcl-2/Ig gene rearrangements in persistent polyclonal B-cell lymphocytosis. British Journal of Haematology 97: 589–595

67. Delage R, Roy J, Jacques L, Darveau A 1998 All patients with persistent polyclonal B cell lymphocytosis present bcl-2/Ig gene rearrangements. Leukemia and Lymphoma 31: 567–574

68. Rego EM, Viana SR, Falcao RP 1998 Age-related changes of lymphocyte subsets in normal bone marrow biopsies. Communications in Clinical Cytometry 201: 22–29

69. Davis RE, Longacre TA, Cornbleet PJ 1994 Hematogones in the bone marrow of adults. Immunophenotypic features, clinical settings and differential diagnosis. American Journal of Clinical Pathology 102: 202–211

70. Faulkner Jones BE, Howie AJ, Boughton BJ, Franklin IM 1988 Lymphoid aggregates in bone marrow: study of eventual outcome. Journal of Clinical Pathology 41: 768–775

71. Thiele J, Zirbes TK, Kvasnicka HM, Fischer R 1999 Focal lymphoid aggregates (nodules) in bone marrow biopsies: differentiation between benign hyperplasia and malignant lymphoma – a practical guideline. Journal of Clinical Pathology 52: 294–300

72. Farhi DC 1989 Germinal centres in the bone marrow. Hematological Pathology 3: 133–136

73. Conlan MG, Bast M, Armitage JO, Weisenburger DD 1990 Bone marrow involvement by non-Hodgkin's lymphoma: the clinical significance of morphologic discordance between the lymph node and bone marrow. Nebraska Lymphoma Study Group. Journal of Clinical Oncology 8: 1163–1172

74. Williams CD, Harrison CN, Lister TA et al 2001 High-dose chemotherapy and autologous stem cell support for chemosensitive transformed low-grade follicular non-Hodgkin's lymphoma: a case-matched study from the European Bone Marrow Transplant Registry. Journal of Clinical Oncology 19: 727–735

75. Douglas VK, Gordon LI, Goolsby CL et al 1999 Lymphoid aggregates in bone marrow mimic residual lymphoma after rituximab therapy for non-Hodgkin lymphoma. American Journal of Clinical Pathology 112: 844–853

76. Auger MJ, Nash JR, Mackie MJ 1986 Marrow involvement with T cell lymphoma initially presenting as abnormal myelopoiesis. Journal of Clinical Pathology 39: 134–137

77. White NJ, Nacheva E, Asimakopoulos FA et al 1994 Deletion of chromsome 20q in myelodysplasia can occur in a multipotent precursor of both myeloid cells and B cells. Blood 83: 2809–2816

78. Kroef MJ, Fibbe WE, Mout R et al 1993 Myeloid but not lymphoid cells carry the 5q deletion: polymerase chain reaction analysis of loss of heterozygosity using mini-repeat sequences on highly purified cell fractions. Blood 81: 1849–1854

79. Mongkonsritragoon W, Letendre L, Li CY 1998 Multiple lymphoid nodules in bone marrow have the same clonality as underlying myelodysplastic syndrome recognized with fluorescent *in situ* hybridization technique. American Journal of Hematology 59: 252–257

80. Lai R, Arber DA, Brynes RK et al 1999 Untreated chronic lymphocytic leukemia concurrent with or followed by acute myelogenous leukemia or myelodysplastic syndrome. A report of five cases and review of the literature. American Journal of Clinical Pathology 111: 373–378

Abnormalities in immunoglobulin synthesizing cells

F Davies   K Anderson

Multiple myeloma

Epidemiology and etiology

Biology
The cell of origin
IL-6 is a major growth and survival
factor for myeloma cells
Other cytokines involved in
myeloma growth and survival
Adhesion molecule expression and
disease progression
Cytogenetic and molecular abnormalities
Pathogenesis of bone disease

Diagnostic criteria

Clinical features
Bone disease
Hyperviscosity
Recurrent infections
Renal failure
Neurological features

Staging and prognostic factors

Pathology

Treatment
Conventional treatment
Radiation therapy
Bisphosphonate therapy
Interferon therapy
High-dose therapy – autologous
transplantation
High-dose therapy – allogeneic
bone marrow transplantation

Novel therapies – thalidomide
Novel therapies – antibody-
mediated therapies
Novel therapies – immune-
based therapies

**Monoclonal gammopathy of
undetermined significance**

Clinical features

Biology

Pathology

**Treatment/management/
disease progression**

Plasma cell leukemia

Clinical features

Biology

Pathology

**Treatment/management/
disease progression**

Solitary bone plasmacytoma

Clinical features

Pathology

**Treatment/management/
disease progression**

Extramedullary plasmacytoma

Clinical features

Pathology

Treatment/management/disease progression

POEMS syndrome

Lymphoproliferative disorders associated with IgM paraprotein

Biology

Clinical features

Pathology

Treatment/management

Disease progression

Light-chain-associated amyloidosis

Biology

Clinical features

Pathology

Treatment/management

Disease progression

Heavy-chain disorders

α-heavy-chain disease
Clinical features
Pathology
Treatment/management/disease progression

γ-heavy-chain disease
Clinical features
Pathology
Treatment/management/disease progression

μ-heavy-chain disease
Clinical features
Pathology
Treatment/management/disease progression

Cryoglobulinemia

Clinical features

Pathology

Treatment, management/disease progression

Multiple myeloma

Multiple myeloma is a clonal B-cell neoplasm that affects terminally differentiated B-cells (i.e. plasma cells). The clinical picture of multiple myeloma involves a combination of bone destruction, immune deficiency, bone marrow failure and renal failure. The diagnosis requires the presence of at least two of three characteristic features: (1) a paraprotein or monoclonal immunoglobulin in the blood and/or the urine; (2) bone marrow infiltration by malignant plasma cells; and (3) the presence of osteolytic bone lesions. The outlook for patients is poor with a median survival of approximately 3.5 years, which has not changed in the last 30 years despite the introduction of new therapies.

Epidemiology and etiology

Multiple myeloma represents 10–15% of all hematologic malignancies and 1% of all cancers, with an incidence of 2/100 000 population in the UK. The incidence increases with age, with approximately 40% of patients presenting under the age of 60 years and only 2% of cases occurring before the age of 40 years. There is a moderate excess in males. Geographic and racial differences play an important role, as the disease is more common in blacks than Caucasians and has a low incidence in Chinese. The high rates of myeloma among black populations and the low rates in Chinese appear to be retained after migration to new countries, suggesting an inherited rather than environmental explanation for the differences.[1] Epidemiological studies have been carried out to identify environmental risks factors. An association with radiation exposure is seen in survivors of the World War II atomic bombs, as well as in occupationally and therapeutically exposed groups. There is also a suggestion of an association with farming, paper production, wood work and the exposure to a variety of chemicals including petroleum, benzene and materials associated with plastic and rubber manufacture.[2,3] The effect of inherited polymorphic variations within cytokine genes has also been investigated with regard to the predisposition to myeloma. Genetic polymorphisms associated with a high production of tumor necrosis factor α or lymphotoxin α confer a significant risk of developing monoclonal gammopathy of uncertain significance (MGUS) and myeloma, whereas there is no influence of the polymorphism associated with a high production of IL-6.[4,5]

Biology

The cell of origin

The main phenotypic features of myeloma plasma cells include abnormal localization within the bone marrow, replacement of normal bone marrow elements, and dysregulation of immunoglobulin secretion. There is much debate and controversy, however, regarding the exact site of origin and nature of the proliferating cell. Normal bone marrow plasma cells are derived from cells that have passed through a germinal center in a lymph node or other organ. Within the germinal center cells undergo somatic hypermutation, class switching of the immunoglobulin gene, and selection by antigen-binding affinity; only cells with high binding affinity survive to become plasma cells. In myeloma the immunoglobulin genes from individual plasma cells show the same pattern of somatic hypermutation,[6] consistent with the clonal expansion of a single postgerminal center B-cell. The high incidence of translocations involving the switch region on chromosome 14 would also indicate that the final molecular oncogenic event occurs late in B-cell development. A number of studies have detected clonal variable, diversity, joining (VDJ) sequences linked to the μ heavy chain, suggesting the presence of a preswitched cell or a marginal zone memory B-cell as part of the myeloma clone.[7] This contrasts with MGUS where there is intraclonal variation in the pattern of mutation,[8] suggesting transformation of a virgin or memory B-cell with progeny which continue to pass through the normal process of germinal center selection before becoming plasma cells (Fig. 23.1).

IL-6 is a major growth and survival factor for myeloma cells

IL-6 is a multifunctional cytokine originally identified as a B-cell differentiation factor inducing the final differentiation of B-cells into antibody-producing cells. In contrast, in myeloma evidence suggests that IL-6 is the major growth factor promoting cell proliferation and cell survival. Multiple reports support an autocrine IL-6-mediated growth mechanism, since some myeloma cells and derived cell lines both produce and respond to IL-6 *in vitro*.[9] Moreover, autocrine IL-6 mediated myeloma cell growth can be induced by triggering tumor cells via their cell surface CD40.[10] An IL-6-mediated paracrine growth mechanism has also been postulated based upon observations that bone marrow stromal cells (BMSCs) are the

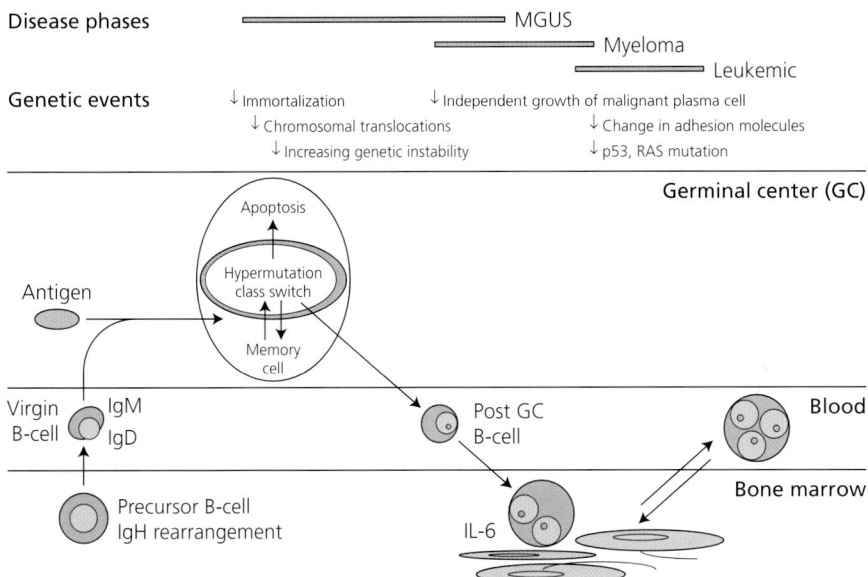

Fig. 23.1 A model of myeloma pathogenesis. After encountering cognate antigen, a virgin B-cell transforms to form a germinal center (GC). The initial event in the development of MGUS is immortalization of such a cell, which is then at an increased risk of developing chromosomal translocations into the IgH switch region and of increased genetic instability. In MGUS there is a continual passage of clonally related cells through the GC, where the cells continue to acquire mutations within their clonally related IgH regions. These cells subsequently migrate to the bone marrow where they differentiate into plasma cells. The development of myeloma is associated with the independent growth of one such clone that proliferates within the bone marrow. During the early phases of myeloma, plasma cells pass into the blood and subsequently home back to the marrow. In the later stages of the disease, changes in adhesion molecules result in a leukemic phase that is associated with the acquisition of p53 and *RAS* mutations.

major source of IL-6 in myeloma, freshly isolated myeloma cells cultured without exogenous IL-6 rapidly stop proliferating, and adhesion of myeloma cells to BMSCs upregulates IL-6 secretion by BMSCs[11,12] (Fig. 23.2).

The action of IL-6 is dependent on an 80 kD membrane-bound specific receptor, IL6-R and a transmembrane signal transducer, gp130. A soluble receptor molecule (sIL6-R) can mediate the binding of IL-6 to gp130 and hence signal transduction in cells that lack membrane-bound IL-6R. Soluble IL6-R and membrane-bound IL6-R have a similar affinity for circulating IL-6. The gp130 receptor also exists in a soluble non-membrane bound form in the plasma, and at high levels may competitively bind and inhibit the growth-promoting effects of IL-6/sIL6-R complexes.[13] The downstream effects of the binding of IL-6 to the IL-6 receptor results in tyrosine phosphorylation and association with gp130, the signal transducing subunit of the IL6-R, leading to the subsequent formation of gp130 homodimers. The homodimerization of gp130 results in activation of the Janus kinase (JAK) family of tyrosine kinases JAK1, JAK2 and/or Tyk2, and the phosphorylation of gp130. Following the activation of these tyrosine kinases, three down-

stream pathways are activated. First, phosphorylated gp130 binds to STAT3, which is phosphorylated by JAK family kinases; homodimers of phosphorylated STAT3 rapidly migrate to the nucleus and bind to IL-6 response elements on the promoter of IL-6-induced genes. Second, IL-6 phosphorylates STAT1, and the heterodimer of tyrosine-phosphorylated STAT1 and STAT3 binds the nuclear DNA sequence termed interferon α activated sequence (GAS) or *sis*-inducible element (SIE). Finally, the Ras-dependent mitogen-activated protein kinase (MAPK) cascade is also activated with sequential activation of Shc (Src homology 2/α-collagen related), Grb, Son of sevenless 1 (Sos 1), Ras, Raf, MEK and MAPK. Activation of this cascade ultimately leads to activation of the transcription factors NF-IL-6 and AP-1 complex (Jun/Fos)[13–16] (Fig. 23.3).

IL-6 is not only a growth factor but also a survival factor for myeloma cells. Apoptosis induced by Fas and γ-irradiation is associated with activation of various serine/threonine kinases, in particular stress activated protein kinase (SAPK) and p38 kinase. In contrast, dexamethasone-induced apoptosis is associated with a significant decrease in the activities of MAPK and p70[RSK],

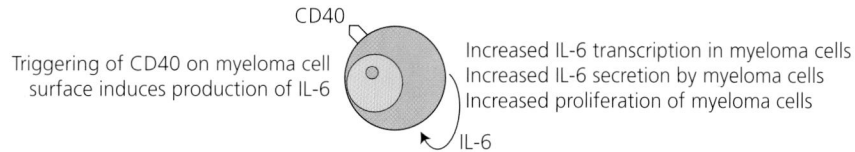

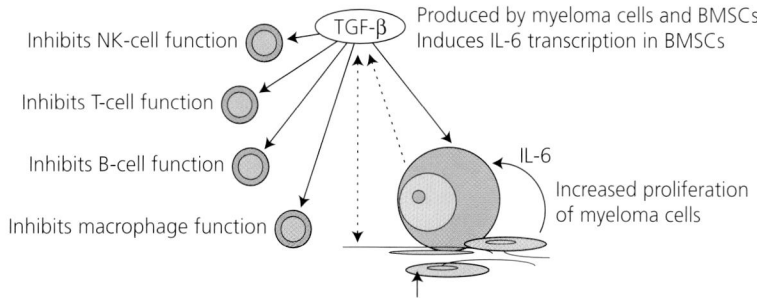

Fig. 23.2 IL-6 mediated myeloma cell growth. Autocrine IL-6 myeloma cell growth can be triggered by CD40 on the myeloma cell surface. IL-6 paracrine myeloma cell growth results from the adhesion of myeloma cells to bone marrow stroma, leading to an upregulation of IL-6 transcription and secretion by the stromal cells due to both cell to cell contact the secretion of TGF-β by myeloma cells.

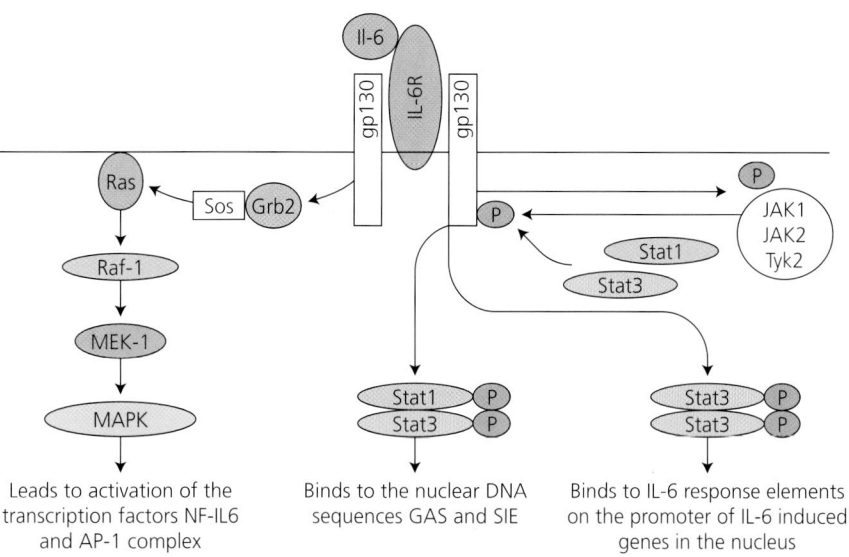

Fig. 23.3 IL-6 signaling cascades in myeloma. The binding of IL-6 to its receptor results in the activation of the Janus kinase family of tyrosine kinases and the further activation of three downstream pathways involving STAT1, STAT3 and the Ras-dependent mitogen-activated protein kinase (MAPK) cascade.

without activation of SAPK and p38 stress kinases.[17,18] IL-6 inhibits dexamethasone-induced apoptosis and the associated downregulation of MAPK, whereas it does not inhibit either apoptosis or activation of SAPK induced by irradiation. In addition irradiation-induced apoptosis is associated with release of the mitochondrial apoptogenic protease cytochrome C into the cytosol, whereas apoptosis induced by dexamethasone or anti-FAS has no detectable effect on cytochrome C release.[19] Recently, the cascades mediating dexamethasone-induced multiple myeloma cell death, as well as resistance to apoptosis conferred by IL-6, have been further characterized.

Dexamethasone-induced apoptosis in myeloma cells is associated with tyrosine phosphorylation and kinase activity of related adhesion focal tyrosine kinase (RAFTK), also known as proline-rich tyrosine kinase 2 (PYK2).[20] IL-6 blocks both the dexamethasone-induced RAFTK tyrosine phosphorylation and apoptosis and activates Src homology protein tyrosine phosphatase 2 (SHP2), which modulates RAFTK activity. Taken together, these data demonstrate that apoptotic stimuli utilize two distinct signaling pathways. One pathway is induced by dexamethasone, RAFTK dependent, cytochrome C independent, and inhibited by IL-6. The other is induced by irradiation and anti-Fas, RAFTK independent, associated with cytochrome C release, and unaffected by IL-6 (Fig. 23.4).

Abnormalities in cell cycle regulatory proteins also contribute to myeloma cell growth. Mutations in the retinoblastoma (Rb) gene or abnormalities on the Rb protein (pRb) have been noted in up to 70% of myeloma patients and 80% of myeloma-derived cell lines. Studies suggest that both dephosphorylated and phosphorylated pRb are present in myeloma cells and that the latter predominates. IL-6 further shifts pRb from its dephosphorylated form in responsive myeloma cells, thereby promoting tumor-cell growth via two mechanisms: (1) by decreasing binding of dephosphorylated pRb to E2F and releasing G1 growth arrest; and (2) by upregulating IL-6 secretion by myeloma cells and IL-6-mediated autocrine tumor cell growth.[21] Abnormalities in other cell cycle associated proteins also underlie abnormalities in myeloma cell growth regulation. For example, with progression to plasma cell leukemia (PCL), loss of p16 protein is observed due to transcriptional inactivation of p16 gene by methylation.[22] In addition p21 protein is constitutively

expressed in the majority of myeloma cells independent of the status of p53, and its expression is upregulated by dexamethasone and downregulated by IL-6; moreover, IL-6 inhibits the increase in p21 triggered by dexamethasone.[23]

Dexamethasone also induces G1 growth arrest in myeloma cells, whereas IL-6 facilitates G1 to S phase transition; moreover, the effect of dexamethasone may also be blocked by IL-6. The correlation of changes in p21 expression and in cell cycle implicate p21 in the coupling of dexamethasone and IL-6-related signals to cell cycle regulation in myeloma. Finally, murine double minute 2 (MDM2) is constitutively expressed in myeloma cells and may enhance cell cycle progression in tumor cells both by activating E2F-1 and by downregulating wild type p53 and p21.[24]

There is also extensive evidence supporting a role for IL-6 in the growth and survival of myeloma cells *in vivo*. Serum IL-6 and sIL-6 receptor levels correlate with disease activity and survival.[25–27] Patients with MGUS have serum IL-6 levels similar to normal individuals, in contrast to the high serum IL-6 levels observed in some patients with myeloma or PCL. Retrospective investigations into the mechanism of action of a number of effective conventional drugs show that they exert their effects, at least in part, via disruption of IL-6-dependent myeloma cell growth, further supporting a major role for this cytokine in myeloma pathogenesis. γ interferon leads to the inhibition of growth via downregulation of the IL6-R;[28,29] all-*trans* retinoic acid (ATRA) inhibits growth, decreases IL-6 production by myeloma cells and stromal cells, and downregulates IL6-R and gp 130 expression on myeloma cells;[30] and α interferon inhibits growth by the downregulation of IL6-R and gp 130.[31]

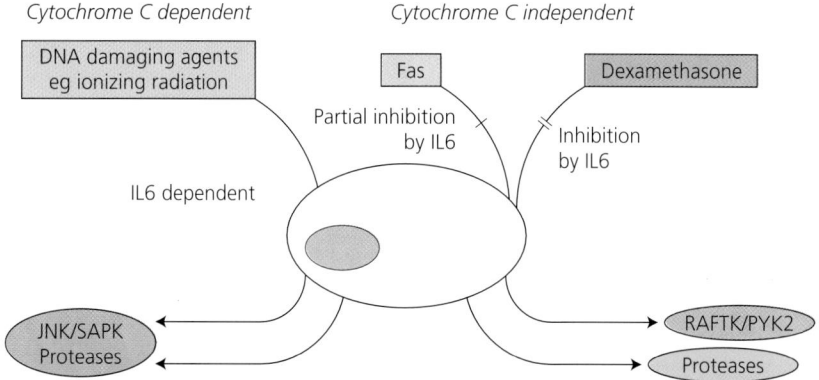

Fig. 23.4 Apoptosis signaling in myeloma. There are at least two distinct signaling cascades for apoptosis in myeloma. One pathway is induced by dexamethasone, RAFTK dependent, cytochrome C independent, and inhibited by IL-6. The other is induced by irradiation and anti-Fas, RAFTK independent, associated with cytochrome C release, and unaffected by IL-6.

Other cytokines involved in myeloma growth and survival

A number of other cytokines have been implicated in myeloma cell growth and survival either directly or indirectly via upregulation of IL-6 secretion. Transforming growth factor β (TGFβ) is produced by patient myeloma cells and induces IL-6 transcription and secretion in bone marrow stromal cells.[32] TGFβ-mediated upregulation of IL-6 secretion in bone marrow stromal cells results in tumor-cell proliferation, in contrast to the inhibitory effect of TGFβ on normal B-, T- and NK cells. Interleukin-1β induces paracrine IL-6 production and myeloma cell growth, mediates bone resorbing activity in myeloma via osteoclast-activating factors, and increases the expression of the adhesion molecules VCAM-1 and ICAM-1 on the myeloma cell surface.[33,34] Interleukin-1α stimulates myeloma cells to produce IL-6, which consequently augments proliferation of myeloma cells in an autocrine manner.[35] Peripheral blood mononuclear cells isolated from patients with myeloma and cultured with IL-3 and IL-6 for 6 days *in vitro* give rise to a population of proliferating B-cell blasts that differentiate into idiotypic cytoplasmic immunoglobulin positive plasma cells.[36] Interleukin-4 inhibits the growth of myeloma cells *in vitro* perhaps by blocking endogenous IL-6 synthesis.[37] Granulocyte macrophage colony-stimulating factor (GM-CSF) has been reported to enhance the IL-6 responsiveness of myeloma cells *in vitro* and has been utilized to facilitate the development of IL-6-dependent human myeloma lines.[38] Recently, vascular endothelial growth factor (VEGF) and basic fibroblastic growth factor (bFGF) have also been implicated as growth and survival factors for myeloma cells following the unexpected finding of increased angiogenesis in human myeloma bone marrow. Bone marrow neovasculaturization parallels the progression of myeloma, with low levels in stable disease and higher levels in active disease;[39] and low microvessel density has been identified as a favorable prognostic feature.[40–42] Initial studies suggest a paracrine mechanism of action where VEGF and bFGF secreted by plasma cells induces an upregulation of IL-6 secretion by stromal cells that express the VEGF receptor, resulting in tumor cell growth.[43,44] Patients with active myeloma have elevated levels of these angiogenic cytokines, and a positive correlation has been demonstrated between the degree of bone marrow plasmacytosis and VEGF expression[39,42]

Adhesion molecule expression and disease progression

Adhesion molecules mediate both homotypic adhesion of tumor cells as well as heterotypic adhesion of tumor cells to either extracellular matrix (ECM) proteins or BMSC (Table 23.1). Membrane phenotypic studies reveal a number of differences in the adhesion molecule profile between myeloma plasma cells and their normal counterparts. Both normal and myeloma plasma cells have a high expression of CD44, CD29, CD49d (VLA-4), and CD54 in contrast, CD56 (NCAM) and CD58 (LFA-3) are expressed at higher levels on myeloma cells.[45,46] These differences reflect the way that malignant cells interact

Table 23.1 Adhesion molecule profile in multiple myeloma

Adhesion molecule on myeloma cell	Adhesion molecule on BMSC or ECM	Receptor on myeloma cell	Receptor on BMSC or ECM
ICAM 1 (CD54)	ICAM 1	LFA 1	–
–	ICAM 2 (CD102)	LFA 1	–
ICAM 3 (CD50)	–	LFA 1	–
–	VCAM 1 (CD106)	VLA 4/NCAM	–
NCAM (CD56)	–	VCAM 1	Heparan sulfate proteoglycan
VLA 1 (CD29/49a)	–	–	Laminin, collagen
VLA 4 (CD29/49d)	–	–	VCAM 1, fibronectin
VLA 5 (CD29/49e)	–	–	Fibronectin
LFA 1 (CD11a/18)	–	ICAM 1,2,3	ICAM 1
LFA 3 (CD58)	–	ICAM 1	ICAM 1, fibronectin
CD44	–	–	Hyaluronate
Syndecan 1 (CD138)	–	–	Type 1 collagen fibronectin

BMSC, bone marrow stromal cell; ECM, extracellular matrix; CD cluster designation; ICAM, intracellular adhesion molecule; LFA, lymphocyte function associated; NCAM, neural cell adhesion molecule; VCAM, vascular cell adhesion molecule; VLA, very late activation.

with the bone marrow microenvironment and both the growth and migration of malignant plasma cells are altered by the pattern of expression of adhesion markers[47,48] (Fig. 23.5). After class switching in the lymph node, adhesion molecules (e.g. CD44, VLA-4, VLA-5, LFA-1, CD56, CD138 and MPC-1) mediate homing of myeloma cells to the bone marrow. Subsequently, binding of myeloma cells to BMSC occurs mediated by VLA-4 to VCAM-1 and ECM, CD138 to type I collagen and VLA-4 to fibronectin interactions. Such binding not only localizes tumor cells to the bone marrow microenvironment but also stimulates IL-6 transcription and secretion from BMSCs with related paracrine growth of myeloma cells.[12] Triggering via CD40 found on tumor cells induces increased expression of known cell surface

adhesion molecules including CD11a, CD11b, CD11c and CD18, and both augments their adhesion to BMSC, and induces IL-6 transcription, secretion and related autocrine myeloma growth.[10] Adhesion can also induce the production of matrix metalloproteinase-1, which favors bone resorption and tumor invasion. As disease progresses, the development of plasma cell leukemia is characterized by decreased expression of certain adhesion molecules (e.g. CD56, VLA-5, MPC-1 and CD138), which facilitates tumor cell mobilization within the peripheral blood.[45,46,49,50] The acquisition of other adhesion molecules on myeloma cells (CD11b, CD44 and receptor for hyaluronan-mediated motility (RHAMM) assists transit through the endothelium during egress from the bone marrow. Extramedullary spreading of myeloma cells is facilitated by the reappearance of CD56, VLA-5, MPC-1, and CD138. Several groups have assessed the mechanisms and relevance of adhesion and related triggering of IL-6 for the *in vivo* growth of multiple myeloma cells using murine models. In severe combined immunodeficient mice implanted with human fetal bone grafts, human multiple myeloma cells specifically home to human, and not murine, bone marrow, where they proliferate and trigger human IL-6 secretion, just as observed *in vitro*.[51]

Cytogenetic and molecular abnormalities

Cytogenetic and molecular genetic techniques have allowed the identification of genes which play a central part in the pathogenesis of many types of lymphoproliferative disorders. In myeloma this has been difficult because of the low proliferation rate of the tumor cells and hence the yield of analyzable metaphases. Newer techniques utilizing metaphase and interphase cells have overcome some of these problems. An abnormal karyotype is present in 30–50% of patients;[52,53] however, using fluorescent *in situ* hybridization (FISH), abnormalities can be detected in up to 90% of patients.[54,55] Numerous studies have demonstrated an increased incidence of cytogenetic abnormalities later in the disease process, suggesting that chromosomal abnormalities are fundamental in the disease pathogenesis and may be useful as prognostic factors.[56,57] Numerical chromosomal abnormalities are common: 61–68% of patients show hyperdiploidy, 9–20% pseudodiploidy and 10–30% hypodiploidy.[56] The most common abnormalities are trisomy 3, 7, 9 and 11; monosomy 13; and in females, monosomy X.[54–56,58] Data using traditional cytogenetic methods and flow cytometry for DNA ploidy demonstrate that patients with hyperdiploidy have a survival

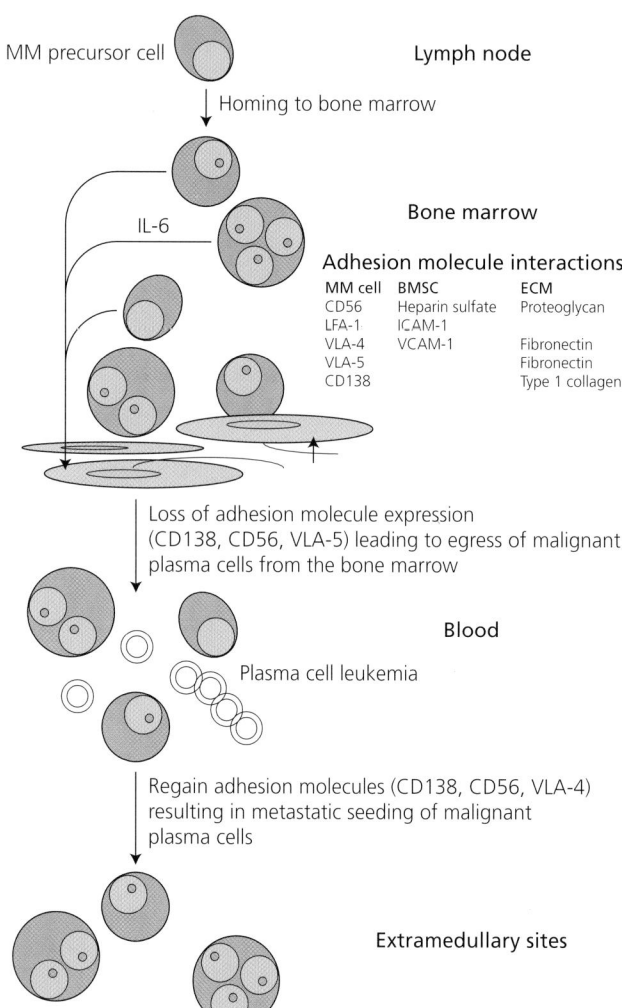

Fig. 23.5 Adhesion molecules and disease progression. Myeloma cells (mm) home to the bone marrow where they adhere to bone-marrow stromal cells and extracellular matrix proteins, resulting in an increase in IL-6 secretion and myeloma cell growth and survival. In the terminal phase of disease and plasma-cell leukemia changes in adhesion molecule profile lead to the egression of myeloma cells into the peripheral blood and extravascular sites.

advantage.[59] FISH has also been used to determine the effect of aneuploidy of individual chromosomes on prognosis and demonstrates that trisomies of chromosome 6, 9 and 17 are associated with prolonged survival, whereas monosomy 13 is associated with poor overall survival.[60] Complex structural abnormalities including translocations and deletions are also well described, with chromosome 1, 6, 14, 16 and 19 being most commonly affected.[61] Patients with partial or complete deletions of chromosome 13 and 11q have an unfavorable prognosis with a median survival of 11 and 12 months, respectively.[62]

The hallmark genetic lesion for many B-lineage tumors involves dysregulation of an oncogene as a consequence of a translocation involving either the immunoglobulin heavy chain (IgH) locus (14q32), or less frequently, variant translocations involving one of the immunoglobulin light chain loci (2p12 kappa or 22q11 lambda). In myeloma abnormalities involving chromosome 14 are common, with a reported frequency of 10–40% using karyotype analysis.[53,56,61] The incidence is higher in end-stage and extramedullary disease.[52] Extensive Southern blot analysis of myeloma cell lines has shown that the translocations involve the switch region of the IgH gene, rather than the VDJ region as in other B-cell malignancies. A number of genes have been reported to be involved including translocations into bcl-1 and bcl-2, events rarely seen in clinical myeloma.[63] Novel genes have also been identified including MUM1/IRF4 involved in t(6;14)[64] and FGFR3 involved in t(4;14).[65] A noteworthy feature is the number of potential chromosomal sites at which genes have been found, rather than a single consistent abnormality. FISH techniques identify translocations involving this area as a universal event in primary patient material, suggesting a central role for illegitimate switch recombination in the pathogenesis of myeloma (Table 23.2).[66,67]

The central role of IL-6 as a growth factor in myeloma and the importance of RAS in the IL-6 signaling pathway suggests that mutations in this oncogene may be important in myeloma pathogenesis. Early in the disease process myeloma plasma cells are dependent on external IL-6 for both growth and survival. It would therefore be predicted that mutations resulting in IL-6 independence would occur late in the disease process. Indeed this appears to be the case, with mutations of the N and K RAS gene seen in up to 47% of cases of myeloma, with the incidence rising to 67% in end-stage disease.[68,69] The retinoblastoma gene (Rb) is a key regulator of the cell cycle as well as IL-6 transcription: IL-6 promotes the dephosphorylation of Rb and thereby enhances IL-6 transcription. Mutations of the Rb gene or abnormalities in pRb have been described in up to 70% of myeloma patients and 80% of myeloma cell lines. The Rb gene is located on chromosome 13q, a region that is frequently deleted in myeloma and associated with a poor prognosis;[62] however, the deletions detected by karyotyping on chromosome 13q are large and likely involve other relevant genes. P53 functions at the GIS cell cycle checkpoint, mediating cell cycle arrest in the presence of DNA damage. It has been implicated in both tumor progression and chemotherapy resistance in a number of other malignancies. Studies of p53 in myeloma show a mutation rate of 2–4%,[70,71] although the frequency in end-stage disease and in myeloma cell lines increases to 40%. This is reflected in studies of serial samples from myeloma patients: p53 mutations were identified in the terminal stages of disease which were not present in plateau phase disease,[72] suggesting a multistep process with p53 mutation as a late event in tumor progression.

Pathogenesis of bone disease

Bone destruction in multiple myeloma is a prominent feature and causes considerable morbidity. Bone remodeling is a continuous process of resorption by osteoclasts and the subsequent formation of new bone by osteoblasts. Osteoclasts are dependent on stromal osteoblasts for cytokines such as IL-6 and IL-11 which are required for their development.[73] In myeloma there is an increase in the number of osteoclasts and bone resorption in areas of the marrow adjacent to abnormal plasma cells,

Table 23.2 Incidence of switch region translocations of chromosome 14 in myeloma[63–67]

Translocation	Oncogene	Function	Incidence
t(4;14)(p16;q32)	FGFR3/MMSET	Growth factor receptor	5/21 cell lines 15–25% patient samples
t(6;14)(p25;q32)	MUM1/IRF4	Transcription factor	2/11 cell lines rare in patients
t(8;14)(q24;q21)	c-myc	Growth/apoptosis	1/11 cell lines 2% patient samples
t(11;14)(13;q32)	Cyclin D1	Growth	6/12 cell lines 16% patient samples
t(14;16)(32;q23)	Cmaf	Transcription factor	5/12 cell lines 1% patient samples

FGFR3, fibroblastic growth factor 3; MMSET, multiple myeloma SET domain; MUM1, multiple myeloma oncogene 1; IRF4, insulin response factor 4.

but not in those areas adjacent to normal marrow cells.[74] New bone formation is also reduced when the tumor burden in the marrow is high,[75] and the combination of increased resorption and decreased formation leads to an uncoupling of normal bone remodeling. This imbalance of bone remodeling is reflected in serum osteocalcin levels, which are low in patients with advanced myeloma, frequent osteolytic lesions and poor prognosis.[76] Lymphotoxin, tumor necrosis factor α(TNFα), and IL-1β can also stimulate osteoclastic bone resorption *in vitro,* and IL-6 appears to have a major role in mediating bone resorption by acting as an osteoclast activator and inducer of TNFα and IL-1β production in marrow cells.[77,78] These cytokines stimulate the bone marrow stromal cells and osteoblasts to produce TNF-related activation-induced cytokine (TRANCE), a TNF family member, resulting in the differentiation and maturation of osteoclast progenitors. The increased osteoclast activity results in the secretion of TGFβ, IL-6, bFGF and insulin-like growth factor (ILG-F) from the bone marrow matrix in turn leading to further myeloma cell growth. Osteoprotegerin, a TNF-receptor superfamily member, is produced by a number of cell types and acts as an alternative receptor for TRANCE, leading to direct regulation of osteoclast activity. In myeloma this balance is disturbed due to an increase in TRANCE and the inactivation of osteoprotegerin by syndecan-1 (CD138), which is present in large amounts and actively shed from myeloma cells.[79] Matrix metalloproteinases (MMP), a family of proteolyic enzymes, are also involved in the development of bone disease. *In vitro* coculture experiments suggest that MMP-7 and MMP-9 secreted by myeloma cells result in the activation of MMP-1 and MMP-2 in BMSC, leading to further bone destruction.[80] These *in vitro* data are further supported by clinical studies that show that MMP-2 levels correlate with disease activity.[39] Macrophage inflammatory protein 1 α (MIP-1α), a recently described osteoclast stimulatory factor, has also been shown to be elevated in myeloma bone marrow compared to normal marrow, suggesting an important role for this chemokine in myeloma bone disease.[81]

Diagnostic criteria

Both major and minor criteria for the diagnosis of myeloma have been identified. These include the presence of excess monotypic marrow plasma cells, monoclonal immunoglobulin in either the serum or urine, decreased normal immunoglobulin levels, and lytic bone lesions (Table 23.3). Myeloma must be distinguished from other disorders characterized by monoclonal gammopathies,

Table 23.3 Criteria for the diagnosis of multiple myeloma

Major criteria
1. Plasmacytoma on tissue biopsy
2. Bone marrow plasmacytosis (> 30% plasma cells)
3. Monoclonal immunoglobulin spike on serum electrophoresis: IgG> 3.5 g/dl or IgA > 2.0 g/dl; kappa or lambda light chain excretion > 1.0 g/day on 24 h urine electrophoresis

Minor criteria
a. Bone marrow plasmacytosis (10–30% plasma cells)
b. Monoclonal immunoglobulin spike present but of lesser magnitude than above
c. Lytic bone lesions
d. Normal IgM < 50 mg/dl, IgA < 100 mg/dl or IgG < 600 mg/dl

Any of the following criteria will confirm the diagnosis:
- Any two major criteria.
- Major criteria 1 plus minor criteria b, c or d.
- Major criteria 3 plus minor criteria a or c.
- Minor criteria a, b and c or a, b and d.

both malignant and otherwise. These include MGUS, Waldenström's macroglobulinemia, non-Hodgkin's lymphoma, light-chain amyloid, idiopathic cold agglutinin disease, essential cryoglobulinemia, and heavy-chain disease. These disorders are discussed later in this chapter.

Clinical features

The clinical picture of myeloma both at presentation and during its clinical course is a complex of bone destruction leading to pain or fracture with hypercalcemia; infection due to immune deficiency; marrow failure leading to anemia and less commonly thrombocytopenia; and renal failure due to hypercalcemia, direct damage from paraprotein or precipitation of light chain in renal tubules. These features, at times associated with plasmacytoma, hyperviscosity and biochemical disturbances, dominate the clinical course of most myeloma patients.

Bone disease

The accumulation of myeloma cells within the cavity of bones in the axial skeleton produces bone pain and destruction. The pain arises in the axial skeleton, and loss of height due to collapse of vertebrae and kyphosis are common. Although bone pain may be gradual in onset, pathologic fractures are frequent and usually indicated by the sudden onset of local tenderness and pain. In almost all cases bone lesions are osteolytic, but a minority (2%) of patients have osteosclerotic lesions (Fig. 23.6). The majority of patients also have diffuse osteopenia.

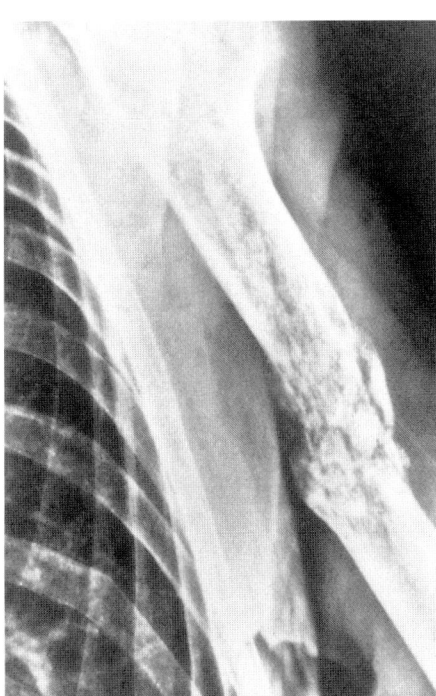

Fig. 23.6 Radiograph showing a typical osteolytic lesion and pathologic fracture of the left humerus.

Bone resorption leads to an increased calcium in 20–40% of patients.

Hyperviscosity

Hyperviscosity syndrome occurs in 5–10% of patients and is usually associated with an IgA paraproteinemia, due of the tendency of the IgA paraprotein to polymerize. Clinical features include a predisposition to bleeding from mucosal surfaces, dilatation and segmentation of retinal and conjunctival veins, and central nervous system disturbances including headache, drowsiness, weakness and confusion which may progress to epileptic fits, paralysis and coma. Symptoms improve with vigorous plasmapheresis to reduce both the paraprotein concentration and serum viscosity. Specific therapy to control the underlying disease should follow immediately.

Recurrent infections

Susceptibility to infection is a prominent feature of myeloma and the mechanisms responsible for the failure of the immune response are complex. Streptococcal pneumoniae and *Hemophilus* infections usually occur early during response to chemotherapy. Gram-negative infections occur in refractory and advancing disease or in the setting of previous antibiotic therapy, medical intervention and hospitalization. The role of prophylactic antibiotics is controversial.

Renal failure

Fifty per cent of myeloma patients will develop some form of renal impairment during their illness. The specific renal lesions are due to the formation of intratubular casts of paraprotein or the diffuse precipitation of paraprotein in renal tissue. Many other factors also contribute to the development of renal failure including infection, hypercalcemia, hyperuricemia, direct plasma cell infiltration of the kidneys, dehydration, antibiotic therapy and amyloidosis. Free light chains (Bence Jones proteins) are inherently nephrotoxic, with lambda light chains more nephrotoxic than kappa. The most important aspect of the management of renal failure in myeloma is preventative by the maintenance of a high fluid throughput. Acute episodes of renal failure may be reversible, and even the clinical syndrome of chronic renal failure can be improved by vigorous hydration and reduction of the myeloma cell mass by intensive chemotherapy.

Neurological features

Disorders of the central and peripheral nervous system may also play a prominent part in the clinical presentation and disease course. Non-specific higher cerebral dysfunction can result from hypercalcemia, hyperviscosity, anemia or uremia and requires urgent treatment. Spinal cord or nerve root compression occurs in 10% of patients and may be due to compression by a plasmacytoma. A symmetrical distal sensory or sensorimotor neuropathy may also occur, associated with axonal degeneration with or without amyloid deposition; there is no specific therapy. In some cases this is associated with monoclonal antibodies directed against peripheral nerve myelin. Myelomatous meningitis is rare and is usually associated with rapidly progressive, widespread disease.

Staging and prognostic factors

Two traditional staging systems reliably separate patients into prognostic groups using simple laboratory measurements. Performance status, renal function and hemoglobin level all emerged as important prognostic factors in the UK Medical Research Council's studies and form the basis of the MRC staging system.[82] The extent of bone lesions and the presence of hypercalcemia are also thought to reflect the aggressiveness of the disease and these elements are incorporated in the Durie and Salmon staging system (Table 23.4).[83] These systems remain widely used in the clinic to determine which patients should receive therapy, although few physicians would use them to direct specific therapy decisions.

Table 23.4 Durie and Salmon staging system[83]

	Low (stage I)	Intermediate (stage II)	High (stage III)
Requirements	All of A,B,C and D		At least one of A,B,C,D
A. Hemoglobin	> 10 g/dl		< 8.5 g/dl
B. Serum calcium	Normal		> 3 mmol/l
C. Isotype		Not stage I or stage III	
IgG	< 5 g/dl		> 7g/dl
IgA	< 3 g/dl		> 5 g/dl
BJ	< 4 g/day		> 12 g/day
D. Skeletal survey	None/Solitary lesion		Advanced lytic disease

At present beta 2 microglobulin (β2m) is the single most important prognostic variable in multiple myeloma.[84] It is a polypeptide that forms that extracellular portion of the light chain of the class I histocompatibility complex, which is present on all nucleated cells. It is released into the blood as cells turnover and is excreted by the kidney. In myeloma patients with normal renal function, rising serum β2m levels predict progression of disease. Serum levels also correlate with tumor stage and with response to therapy. The extent and type of bone marrow infiltration also has prognostic significance: patients with a plasmablastic morphology have a median survival of 16 months, compared to a median survival of 35 months for patients with other morphologic subtypes.[85] Measures of tumor-cell proliferation such as the plasma cell labeling index (PCLI), are also useful.[86] PCLI is usually low (< 1%) at diagnosis, higher at relapse, and lower in patients with MGUS. A high PCLI correlates with a shorter survival time independent of tumor-cell mass. The absolute number of circulating peripheral blood cells with the phenotype of myeloma plasma cells varies with disease status in individual patients: a decrease occurs with response to treatment, levels remain stable in plateau phase, and a marked increase occurs at relapse.[49] The percentage of circulating plasma cells at diagnosis has also been shown to be an independent prognostic variable.[87] The presence of certain cytogenetic abnormalities also has prognostic significance, for example patients with partial or complete deletions of chromosome 13 or abnormalities of 11q have an adverse outcome.[62] The identification of more accurate prognostic factors is necessary both to select patients for whom aggressive therapy is indicated, and to provide accurate assessment of the outcome of treatment approaches.

Pathology

A normochromic normocytic anemia is often present, with rouleaux formation and a high non-specific background staining on the blood smear due to the presence of circulating paraprotein. In patients with more advanced disease, thrombocytopenia and neutropenia may also be present. Occasional circulating plasma cells with a phenotype similar to those within the marrow can be demonstrated, and the absolute number of these cells is of prognostic importance.[49,87] In the majority of cases plasma cells will exceed 10% of the nucleated cells within the bone marrow. Plasma cells usually appear moderately to severely dysplastic with large eccentrically placed nuclei, which may be either multiple or cleaved[88] (Fig. 23.7A,B). Nucleoli are prominent and nuclear inclusions may be present, including Dutcher bodies and Russell bodies (Fig. 23.7C). Cytoplasm may be sparse or foamy or vacuolated. Plasma cells from IgA myeloma often have a characteristic flame-cell appearance (Fig. 23.7D). Approximately 8% of myeloma cases demonstrate plasmablastic features, with more than 2% of cells having a plasmablastic morphology (Fig. 23.7E). Plasmablasts have a fine reticular chromatin pattern, large nucleoli and less abundant cytoplasm (less than half of the nuclear

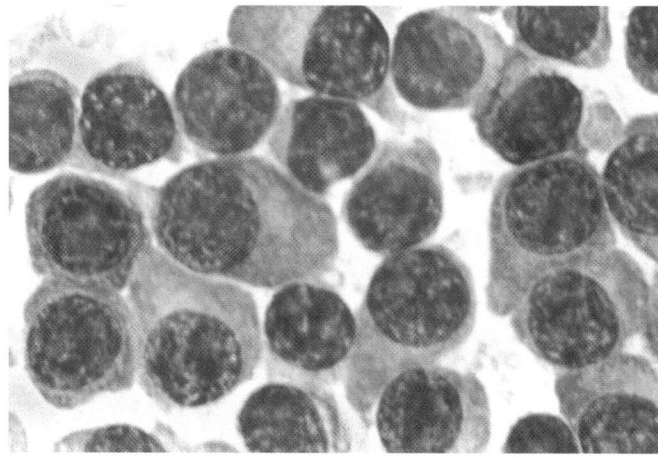

A

Fig. 23.7 Bone-marrow plasma cell morphology in myeloma. (A) Atypical plasma cells with varying degree of nuclear size and cytoplasmic volume.

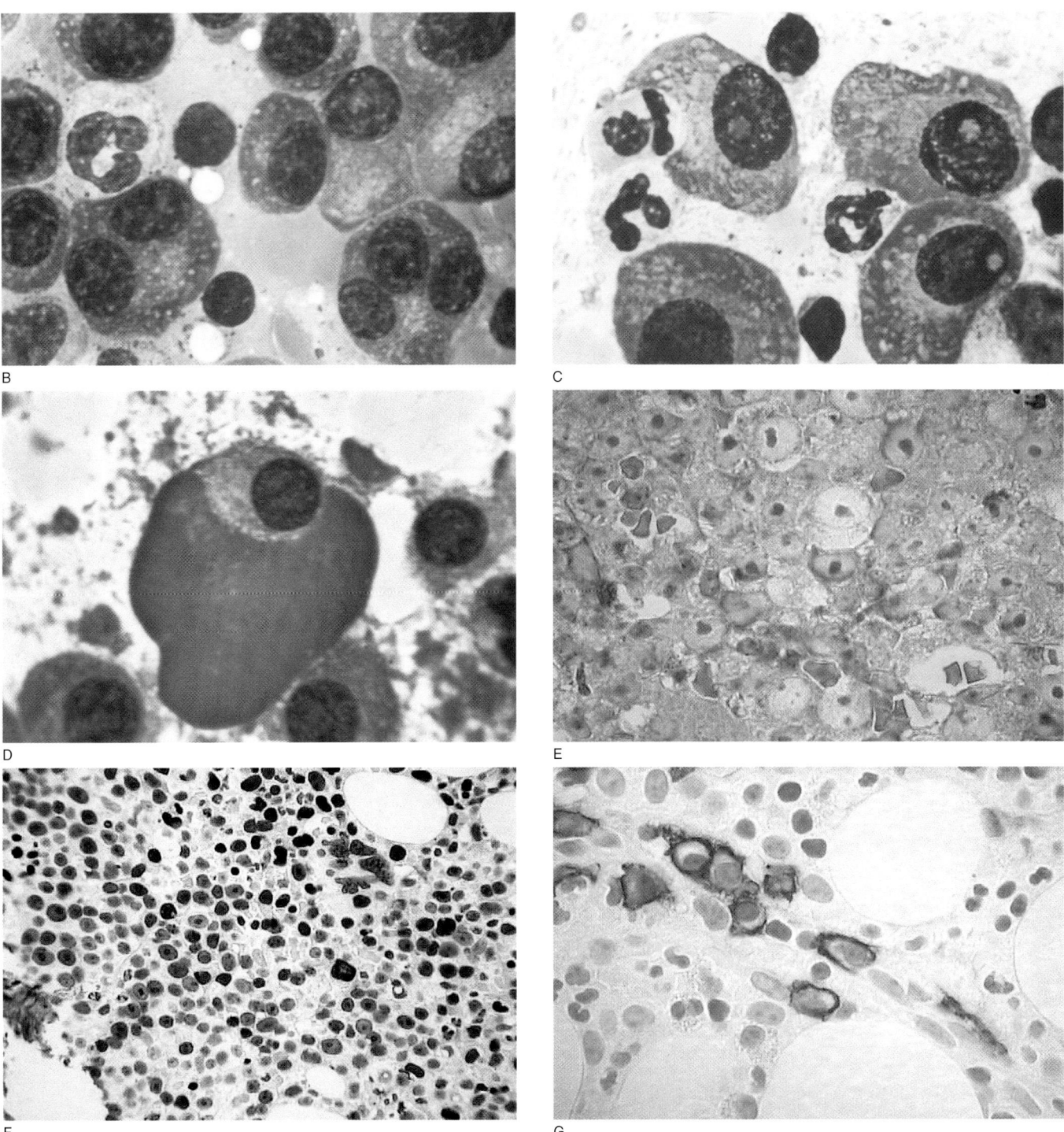

Fig. 23.7 *(Cont'd)* (B) Large multinucleated plasma cells. (C) Plasma cells with inclusion bodies. (D) Flame cell from a patient with IgA myeloma. (E) Plasmablastic cells. (F) Plasmablastic cells with high Ki67 expression. (G) Normal perivascular plasma cells.

area). This morphologic subset is associated with a high PCLI, more advanced and aggressive disease, and a worse prognosis (Fig. 23.7F).[85] A reactive plasmacytosis due to chronic inflammation or infection may also present with an increase in plasma cells in the bone marrow. This can be readily distinguished from multiple myeloma by the normal morphology as well as phenotype of the

plasma cells and an increase in eosinophils, mast cells and megakaryocytes (Fig. 23.7G).

Plasma cells are terminally differentiated B-cells and hence express a number of B-cell antigens as well as myeloma-associated antigens. Both normal and malignant plasma cells express CD38 and CD138, but lack CD10, CD20, CD23, CD34 and CD45RO. The most reliable antibodies used to detect plasma cells by flow cytometry are therefore CD38, CD138 and CD45RO. It is possible to distinguish myeloma plasma cells from their normal counterparts, since the former express significantly higher levels of the important adhesion molecules CD56 and CD138 and significantly lower levels of CD19, CD38 and CD45 than the latter. Plasma cells from normal individuals are consistently CD19+ CD56 low; whereas 65% of myeloma cases have a plasma cell phenotype of CD19− CD56+, 30% CD19− CD56 low, and 5% CD19+ CD56.+[49] Immunocytochemical studies confirm the monclonality of the plasma cells, and the type of immunoglobulin secreted should correlate with the serum paraprotein and urinary light chain.

On bone marrow biopsy plasma cells normally accumulate around blood vessels. However, in multiple myeloma this pattern is lost and the myeloma cells are found as single cells or small clusters between adipocytes. As the disease progresses, diffuse marrow replacement occurs, resulting in a packed marrow with complete loss of normal marrow architecture (Fig. 23 8A–C). Occasionally, there is a paratrabecular distribution similar to follicular center lymphoma, and in some patients with aggressive disease tumor nodules containing abnormal plasma cells may be seen. Assessing the degree of marrow infiltration is often difficult due both to the patchy nature of the disease and the presence of either hypoplastic or hyperplastic areas. There may be a discrepancy between the percentage of plasma cells in the aspirate compared to the biopsy, due either to the presence of fibrosis or nodular infiltration resulting in a low number of plasma cells on the smear.

Bone changes evident on the biopsy include diffuse osteoporosis and increased reticulin deposition. Recent reports demonstrate an increase in neoangiogenesis in the bone marrow from myeloma patients,[39,40] confirmed using immunochemical staining for von Willebrand's factor (factor VIII-related antigen), CD31 or CD34.

Treatment

Current therapy for multiple myeloma includes the use of conventional low-dose chemotherapy or high-dose chemotherapy with autologous or allogeneic stem cell transplantation. The mechanisms of action of the commonly used drugs are summarized in Table 23.5. Although these regimens are able to reduce tumor burden, complete molecular remission of disease is rare and all patients eventually relapse. Novel pharmacologically and immunologically based treatment approaches are currently being evaluated which will be used either alone or in combination with conventional and high-dose

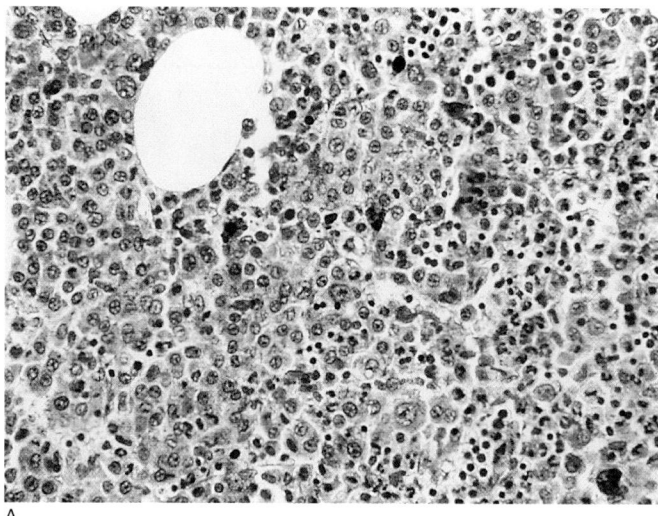

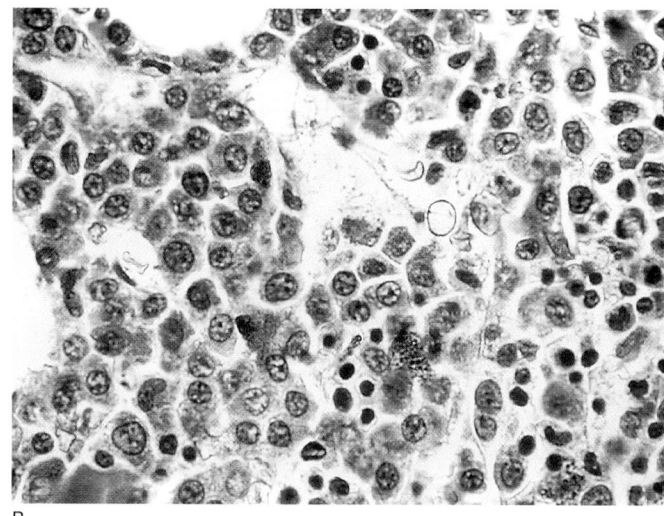

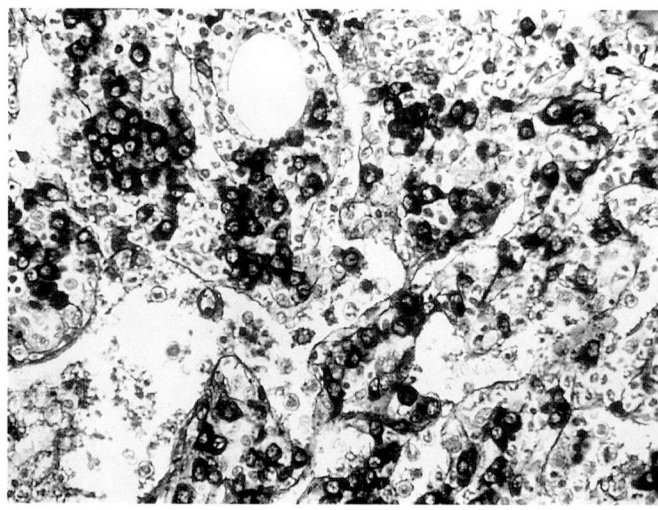

Fig. 23.8 Bone marrow biopsy in myeloma. (A–B). Heavily infiltrated marrow. (C). Immunohistochemistry demonstrating monoclonal kappa positive plasma cells.

chemotherapy to improve response and outcome (Fig. 23.9). Importantly, *in vitro* and *in vivo* studies of the mechanisms of action of these novel approaches are also providing new insights into the biology of myeloma.

Conventional treatment

The development of chemotherapy for multiple myeloma began in the 1950s with the use of single alkylating agents, principally oral melphalan. Prior to this there was no specific therapy available, and the prognosis of patients was extremely poor with median survival times ranging from 3.5 to 11.5 months.[89] Treatment with melphalan improved the median survival of patients to

between 24 and 36 months, with approximately 50% of patients responding to therapy. However, only a minority (5%) of patients attained a true complete response (CR), with the disappearance of paraprotein and a normal marrow.[90] A series of prospective randomized trials has been carried out in which combination chemotherapy regimens including cyclophosphamide, melphalan, BCNU, CCNU, adriamycin, vincristine and prednisolone in various combinations have been compared to treatment with melphalan and prednisolone alone. In a recent Myeloma Trialists Collaborative Group overview of worldwide randomized trials (a total of 27 trials), there was no significant difference in mortality in patients treated with melphalan/prednisolone therapy versus

Table 23.5 Mechanisms of action of commonly used antimyeloma drugs

Drug	Mechanism of action
Alkylating agents (melphalan, cyclophosphamide, BCNU)	x-linking DNA strands in resting and dividing cells
Glucocorticoids (dexamethasone)	Increased apoptosis of myeloma plasma cells with associated phosphorylation of RAFTK
Vinca alkaloids (vincristine)	Inhibition of microtubule formation resulting in the arrest of dividing cells in metaphase
Anthracyclines (adriamycin)	Binds to nucleic acids by intercalation with base pairs of the DNA double helix interfering with DNA synthesis
Interferon α	Direct cytotoxicity Inhibition of IL-6 secretion and downregulation of IL-6 receptor Increase in tumor cell surface antigens and expansion of specific T-cells
Bisphosphonates (pamidronate, zoledronate)	Reduced osteoclastic activity and decreased bone absorption Myeloma plasma cell and bone-marrow apoptosis Decreased production of IL-6 and metalloproteinases
Thalidomide	Growth arrest or increased apoptosis of myeloma plasma cells Alteration in adhesion molecule profile Alteration in cytokine secretion and/or bioavailability (IL-6 and VEGF) Decreased angiogenesis Altered immune response

RAFTK, related adhesion focal tyrosine kinase; VEGF, vascular endothelial growth factor.

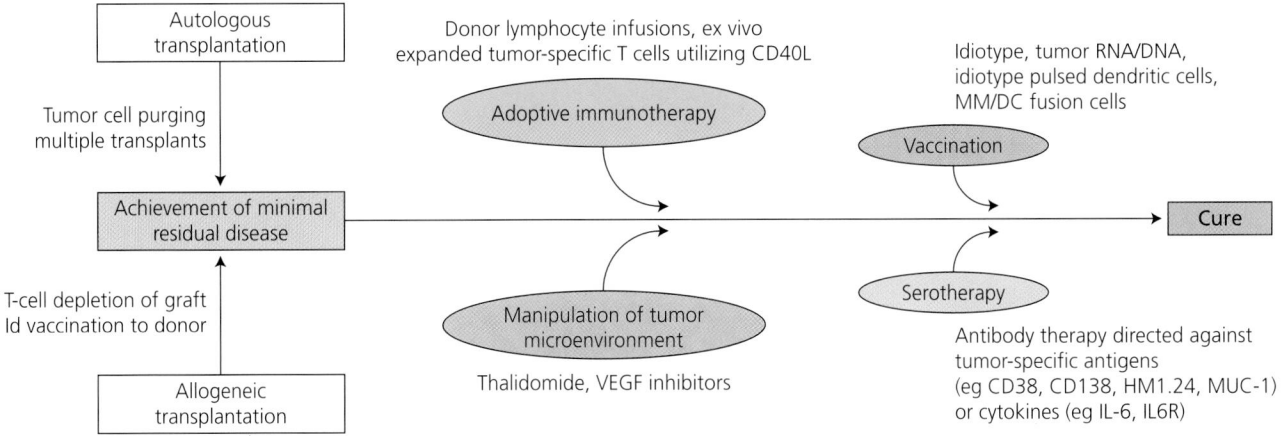

Fig. 23.9 Novel treatment model. In the future novel, pharmacologically and immunologically based treatment approaches may be used alone or in combination with high-dose chemotherapy to achieve a minimal disease state, improve survival, and eventually achieve cure.

combination chemotherapy, although an improved response rate was observed in the combination chemotherapy group.[91] In the early 1980s, it was noted that high doses of glucocorticoid steroids were capable of producing remission in patients with refractory or relapsed disease.[92] The addition of adriamycin and vincristine given as a continuous infusion over 4 days to dexamethasone (VAD) or methylprednisolone (VAMP), achieved responses in these patients.[93,94] Both of these regimens (VAD and VAMP) have now been used as primary therapy in myeloma patients and achieved high overall (70–80%) and complete response rates (8–28%).[95,96]

Radiation therapy

Radiation therapy is an effective treatment modality in myeloma. Its role in established disease is to palliate disease-related skeletal complications, including impending cord compression due to a spinal plasmacytoma, pathologic fracture from long bone plasmacytomas, and pain related to bone lesions.

Bisphosphonate therapy

Skeletal complications are a major source of morbidity in myeloma, since bone healing occurs uncommonly and is delayed in patients responding to chemotherapy. Bisphosphonates such as pamidronate inhibit osteoclastic activity and reduce bone resorption. They have been evaluated in a number of randomized clinical trials, and their efficacy in reducing bone complications is well documented.[97,98] *In vitro* reports suggest that these drugs have a direct antimyeloma effect, inducing apoptosis in both myeloma plasma cells and bone marrow stromal cells, as well as inhibiting secretion of IL-6 and MMP-1.[99,100] A recent report also suggests an immunomodulatory action by the stimulation $\gamma\delta$T-cells and the induction of myeloma-specific cytotoxicity.[101]

Interferon therapy

Interferon α has been therapeutically tested in several clinical trials, and a recent meta-analysis of individual patient data reveals a small but significant survival advantage for patients treated with interferon α as maintenance treatment or in combination with conventional chemotherapy for remission induction.[102]

High-dose therapy – autologous transplantation

A number of groups have shown an improvement in response rates and survival using high-dose melphalan with transplantation of either bone marrow (ABMT) or peripheral blood stem cell (PBSCT) in both relapsed/refractory and newly diagnosed patients when compared to historic controls[103–105] (Table 23.6). There are currently a number of ongoing prospective randomized trials comparing high-dose therapy with either PBSCT or ABMT support to conventional combination therapy, notably South Western Oncology Group (SWOG), Intergroupe

Table 23.6a Representative studies of autologous transplantation for newly diagnosed myeloma

	Patients *(n)*	TRM (%)	Complete response (CR) (%)	OS (median)	EFS (median)
Attal et al[103]	100	2	22	52% at 5 years	27 months
Barlogie et al[104]	231	3	41	68 months	43 months
Powles et al[107]	195	4.9	53	54 months	25 months
Lenhoff et al[105]	274	4	34	61% at 4 years	27 months
Algere et al[106]	259	4	51	35 months	23 months

Table 23.6b Representative studies of allogeneic transplantation for newly diagnosed myeloma

	Patients *(n)*	TRM (%)	Complete response (CR) (%)	OS (actuarial)	EFS (actuarial)
Gahrton et al[112]	162	41	44	28% at 84 months	45% at 60 months
Bensinger et al[113]	80	44	36	20% at 54 months	24% at 54 months
Anderson[114]	61[a]	5	28	40% at 36 months	20% at 38 months

[a] T-cell depleted.
EFS, event-free survival; OS, overall survival; TRM, transplant-related mortality.

Français du Myeloma (IFM) and Medical Research Council (MRC) VII trial. To date the only published trial (IFM) shows an improved response rate (81% vs 57%), progression free survival (27 months vs 18 months) and overall survival (probability at 5 years of 52% vs 12%) in patients undergoing high-dose treatment compared to conventional treatment.[103] The relative merits of high-dose therapy either early or as salvage therapy for relapse after conventional therapy have also been examined in a randomized trial; overall survival was 64 months for patients receiving either early or late (relapse) high-dose therapy; however, the Time Without Symptoms and Toxicity (TwisTT) favored the early transplant cohort.[108] Although the results from these studies of autografting in myeloma are encouraging, the survival curves show no obvious plateau and suggest that high-dose therapy with stem cell support is not a curative procedure. Several additional strategies are therefore currently being evaluated to improve the outcome, including methods to either deplete tumor cells or select normal hematopoietic progenitor cells by virtue of CD34 expression from autologous bone marrow or peripheral blood stem cells prior to transplantation.[109,110] Although these methods may achieve up to a 5 log depletion of tumor cells without affecting engraftment, their clinical benefit is unproven since residual tumor cells are detectable within both the graft and the patient post-transplantation. Other groups are adopting an approach of multiple high-dose therapies with stem cell transplantation. Barlogie and colleagues[104] report increased response rates compared to historic controls, although the impact on disease-free survival requires further follow-up. Early results from the French randomized trial of single versus double autologous transplantation suggest no difference in response rates or overall survival.[111]

High-dose therapy – allogeneic bone marrow transplantation

Allogeneic bone marrow transplantation has not been widely used in the treatment of multiple myeloma because of the high associated morbidity and mortality of up to 40%, especially in older patients (Table 23.6).[112–114] Experience drawn from the European Group for Bone Marrow Transplantation (EBMT – 1983–1993) on data from 162 patients showed 44% complete responses, with some of the responses durable.[112] The stage at diagnosis, preconditioning remission status, extent of previous treatment, and serum β2 microglobulin level were important prognostic factors; males and patients with IgG myeloma faired less well. The overall actuarial survival was 32% at 4 years and 25% at 7 years. Residual clonal myeloma cells are, however, still detectable by polymerase chain reaction (PCR) post-transplantation, consistent with the lack of a plateau in the survival curves and the continued late relapses.[115] The assumption that this mode of treatment is most likely to eradicate myeloma cells and the possibility of a significant graft versus myeloma effect has encouraged its further consideration. Data from multiple centers have shown that patients with relapsed hematologic malignancies after allogeneic BMT can achieve marked clinical responses after infusions of lymphocytes collected from the marrow donor (DLI) due to a graft versus leukemia effect. A recent study has reported the results of donor lymphocyte infusion for the treatment of relapsed myeloma after allogeneic BMT.[116] In this study there was evidence of response to DLI in 62% of cases, providing further support for a graft versus myeloma effect; however, graft-versus-host disease (GVHD) occurred in 66% of patients and contributed to a procedure-related mortality of 15%. By utilizing CD8 depleted DLI, we have recently demonstrated that the graft-versus-myeloma (GVM) effect can be preserved and GVHD abrogated.[117] Patients who receive DLI have a markedly abnormal T-cell repertoire detected by molecular analysis of T-cell receptor (TCR) Vβ gene rearrangements in peripheral T-cells. Following infusion of CD4+ DLI, analysis of TCR utilization identified the expansion of clonal and oligoclonal T-cell populations that coincide with the elimination of myeloma cells from the marrow and decreases in levels of circulating monoclonal paraprotein.[118] Further analysis of these T-cell responses will allow the identification of T-cell clones and myeloma-specific antigens important in tumor immune surveillance. Attempts are also underway to immunize the allogeneic marrow donor to the patient's specific idiotypic myeloma protein and thereby transfer specific immunity against myeloma at the time of allografting.[119] Finally, low-dose radiotherapy in combination with chemotherapy is undergoing evaluation in the setting of non-myeloablative transplantation.[120] This approach can be used in older individuals or patients who otherwise would not be eligible for conventional high-dose transplantation due to underlying morbidity. The goal of this strategy is to reduce the conditioning regimen-related toxicity whilst attempting to take advantage of the graft versus myeloma effect of allogeneic transplantation.

Novel therapies – thalidomide

The recent reports of increased bone marrow angiogenesis, coupled with the known anti-angiogenic properties of thalidomide, provided the rationale for the use of this drug for the treatment of relapsed or refractory myeloma, and an impressive response rate of over 30% has been reported.[121] In our own experience, the dramatic and rapid responses seen in patients suggest that mechanisms besides the anti-angiogenic effects may be important in the drug's antimyeloma activity. From experiments performed within our laboratory and knowledge drawn from the use of thalidomide in other diseases, a number of mechanisms of antimyeloma activity can be postulated (Fig. 23.10). We have documented a direct effect of thalidomide on the myeloma plasma cell and the bone marrow stromal cell, leading to an inhibition of tumor-cell growth and survival.[122] Thalidomide may also modulate the adhesion of myeloma cells to the bone marrow stroma, leading to a reduction in the secretion of cytokines that augment myeloma cell growth and survival and confer drug resistance.[123] It may alter the secretion and bioactivity of cytokines that are secreted into the bone marrow microenvironment by myeloma and/or stromal cells, such as IL-6, IL-1β, IL-10 and TNFα, and thereby inhibit myeloma cell growth and survival. Finally, thalidomide may also act against myeloma via immunomodulatory effects, such as the induction of a CD8 Th1 T-cell response with the secretion of interferon γ and IL-2 or by increasing natural killer (NK) cell cytolytic activity.[124,125]

Novel therapies – antibody-mediated therapy

The introduction of therapeutic monoclonal antibodies has permitted the development of effective tumor-targeted therapies with minimal host toxicity. In myeloma, however, there are relatively few antigens present on tumor cells that make suitable targets. The majority of known antigens are either not selectively expressed, shed, or secreted. A number of antibody-based therapies are being investigated both *in vitro* and *in vivo* either to target antigens on the myeloma cell surface, for example CD38,[126,127] CD138, MUC1,[128] HM1.24,[129] or to inhibit cytokine mediating growth and survival signaling, for example antibodies directed against IL-6[130] and the IL-6 receptor complex.[131,132]

Novel therapies – immune-based strategies

One of the major obstacles to curing myeloma is the persistence of minimal residual disease post high-dose therapy and stem cell transplantation, and a number of approaches are being developed for the generation and enhancement of allogeneic and autologous antimyeloma immunity post-transplantation. T-cell recognition of myeloma is suggested by the restricted usage of Vα and

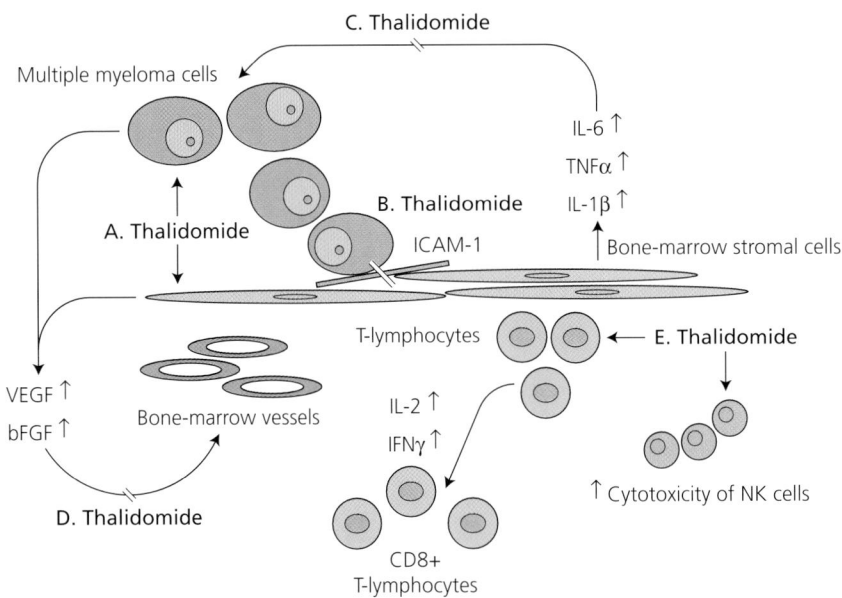

Fig. 23.10 Although the exact mechanism of action of thalidomide in myeloma is unclear, it can be postulated that its pharmacological effects may be mediated via a number of pathways involving both the tumor cell and the bone marrow microenvironment: (A) a direct effect on tumor or bone marrow stromal cells, (B) an alteration in the adhesion profile between myeloma and bone marrow stromal cells, (C) an inhibition of cytokine release from bone marrow stromal cells, (D) an anti-angiogeneic effect, or (E) an immunomodulatory effect.

Vβ segments in the peripheral blood, the presence of activated idiotype reactive CD8+ cells, the growth of T-cell clones by stimulation with IL-2 and F(ab')2 fragments derived from autologous idiotypic protein, and the production of cytokines such as IFNγ, IL-2 and IL-4 after stimulation with autologous idiotypic protein.[133–135] A variety of vaccination strategies are therefore currently under investigation utilizing patient specific idiotype, RNA, and DNA; or autologous myeloma cells treated *ex vivo* with CD40 ligand to enhance antigen presentation.[136] Immunization with dendritic cells pulsed with patient-specific idiotypic protein or immunization with fusions of myeloma cells with autologous dendritic cells represents an alternative strategy.[137,138] Other immuno-therapeutic approaches being evaluated in the post-transplant setting include the use of donor lymphocyte infusions or the infusion of autologous T-cells expanded *ex vivo* against patient tumor cells.[139]

Monoclonal gammopathy of undetermined significance

MGUS describes a condition characterized by the presence of a low level of paraprotein in the absence of other clinical features of multiple myeloma, Waldenström's macroglobulinemia, or other B-cell lymphoproliferative disorders. The previous term 'benign monoclonal gammopathy' is a misleading description of the disease, since a proportion of patients will develop a more aggressive plasma cell disorder.

Clinical features

The incidence of MGUS increases with age, with 1% of the population under the age of 60 years and between 4–5% of the population over the age of 80 years being affected.[140,141] The demonstration of a paraprotein in the serum or urine is often an incidental finding and patients are typically asymptomatic. The serum paraprotein is usually less than 3 g/dl, with little or no urinary component, and may be present despite normal total protein or globulin levels. Bone lesions, hypercalcemia, renal impairment, lymphadenopathy or organomegaly should suggest a diagnosis of myeloma or Waldenström's macro-globulinemia. There is an association of MGUS with a number of disorders including chronic lymphocytic leukemia, peripheral neuropathy and myopathy, derma-tologic disorders (pyoderma granulosum), and immuno-supression (AIDS and transiently post bone marrow or renal transplantation).

Biology

The main features of the biology of the disease have been discussed in detail above. Immunoglobulin heavy chain sequence analysis demonstrates an intraclonal variation in the pattern of mutation,[8] suggesting transformation of a virgin or memory B-cell with progeny continuing to pass through the normal process of germinal center selection before becoming plasma cells. Cytogenetic analysis reveals findings similar to myeloma, including a complex karyotype with trisomies and monosomies, structural abnormalities, and translocations involving chromosome 14.[142]

Pathology

The peripheral blood picture is normal, with no evidence of increased circulating plasma cells or anemia. Clonal plasma cells are present within the bone marrow in an interstitial distribution and represent less than 5–10% of the total nucleated cells. Using flow cytometry it is possible to identify plasma cells with both a normal and 'myeloma' phenotype (CD38++, CD19+ and CD56− vs CD38+, CD19− and CD56+).[49]

Treatment/management/disease progression

There is no specific treatment for patients with MGUS. Long-term surveillance is recommended since approxi-mately 25% of cases will develop an overt plasma cell disorder. Data regarding disease progression have been derived from a cohort of 241 patients with MGUS at the Mayo clinic who have been followed for 24–38 years.[143] The majority of patients who progress develop myeloma, although some show symptoms or signs of amyloid or Waldenström's macroglobulinemia. There are currently no predictive factors to determine which patients will progress although recent data demonstrate that IL-1β expression may distinguish patients with myeloma from patients with MGUS: > 95% of myeloma patients have elevated IL-1β levels compared to < 25% of MGUS patients. Continued follow-up of MGUS patients will determine whether aberrant expression of IL-1β is a critical genetic event in the progression of MGUS to myeloma and whether it may be used prognostically.[33] Overall, 50% of patients with MGUS will die from an unrelated cause; the remaining 25% of patients will continue with stable paraprotein levels, but may develop disease over a longer follow-up period.

Plasma cell leukemia

Plasma cell leukemia (PCL) is a rare plasma cell disorder characterized by the presence of more than $2 \times 10^9/1$ circulating plasma cells which constitute 20% of all peripheral blood cells. The majority (60%) of cases are *de novo* or primary, in which a leukemic picture develops in the absence of a documented preceding plasma cell disorder. Forty per cent of cases are secondary and occur in a minority of myeloma patients (1%) with terminal disease.[144–146]

Clinical features

The median age at diagnosis of primary PCL is 55 years, approximately 10 years younger than for myeloma. Although patients with primary PCL present with symptoms similar to those of myeloma, the disease course is often more aggressive with symptoms relating to extramedullary disease including plasmacytomas and hepatosplenomegaly. Anemia, hypercalcemia and renal failure are also more common.[144–146]

Patients with secondary disease usually have advanced myeloma that is refractory to treatment and may present with worsening symptoms related to bone marrow failure including anemia, infections, bleeding or plasmacytomas.

Biology

The adverse biological prognostic factors usually associated with end-stage myeloma are invariably present at diagnosis in cases of primary PCL. These include a high PCLI; complex cytogenetic abnormalities including deletions of chromosome 13; amplification of c-myc; as well as mutations of RAS and p53.[59,62,68] Other features, including changes in adhesion-molecule profile and the importance of IL-6 as a growth factor, are discussed above.

Pathology

The peripheral blood is characterized by the presence of a large number of circulating plasma cells, which may be morphologically normal or have blastic features (Fig. 23.11). Anemia is invariably present, and both neutropenia and thrombocytopenia are common. Rouleaux formation is usually also present with a high non-specific background staining, especially in secondary PCL cases where the level of paraprotein is often high. The bone marrow is heavily infiltrated with plasma cells morpho-

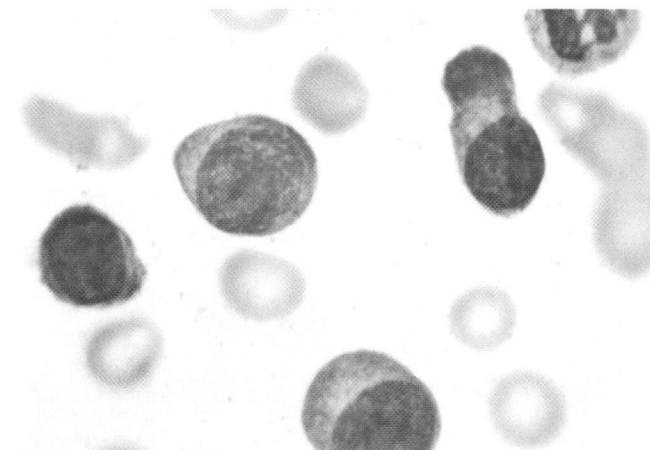

Fig. 23.11 Peripheral blood film of plasma cell leukemia.

logically similar to those within the peripheral blood. Other normal hematopoietic elements are reduced. Occasionally cells can be of lymphocyte size without obvious evidence of plasma cell morphology. In these cases other phenotypic features of plasma cell differentiation must be sought, such as loss of B-cell markers and gain of CD38 and CD138.

Treatment/management/disease progression

There are no clinical trials addressing the best treatment approaches for patients with PCL. Combination chemotherapy followed by either allogeneic or autologous transplantation seems the most appropriate strategy, due to the aggressive nature of the disease with an overall survival of less than 1 year. A number of groups also use more traditional acute leukemia regimens. Patients with underlying myeloma who have developed PCL tend to have end-stage disease resistant to conventional therapy; therefore more experimental treatment approaches are appropriate. The median survival for these patients is extremely poor.[144–146]

Solitary bone plasmacytoma

Some patients present with a single solitary painful bone lesion due to a plasma cell infiltrate, and further studies reveal no evidence of systemic disease.

Clinical features

The bone lesions are commonly in the axial skeleton, particularly in the vertebrae. The median age at presentation is 55 years and a monoclonal protein may be present, although at a level lower than is usual in myeloma. Full clinical staging is required in order to differentiate solitary plasmacytoma from myeloma and reveals a negative skeletal survey, absence of clonal plasma cells on bone marrow examination, and lack of anemia, hypercalcemia or renal involvement.[147–150]

Pathology

Biopsy of the lesion demonstrates a clonal infiltration of typical myeloma plasma cells (Fig. 23.12A). Histologic examination of the peripheral blood or bone marrow should reveal no evidence of plasmacytosis, although more sensitive techniques such as flow cytometry and PCR may detect abnormal clonal cells.

Treatment/management/disease progression

The treatment of choice is radiotherapy. Local control is achieved in 90% of patients, with an accompanying fall in paraprotein level. The majority (two-thirds) of patients will go on to develop overt myeloma at a median time to progression of 2–3 years, although some patients remain stable for more than 10 years.[148–151] The recent introduction of magnetic resonance imaging (MRI) has

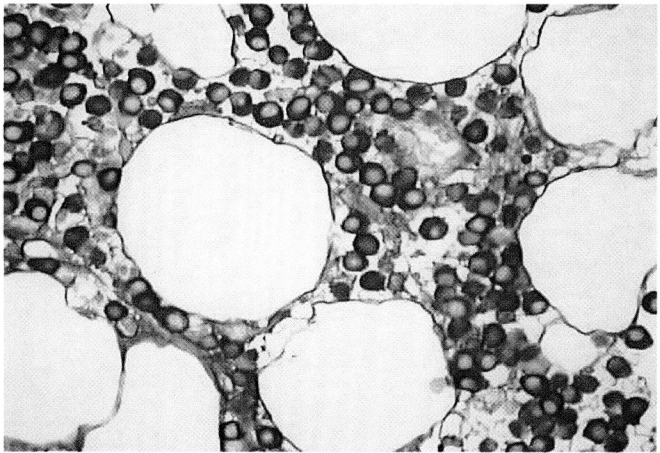

A

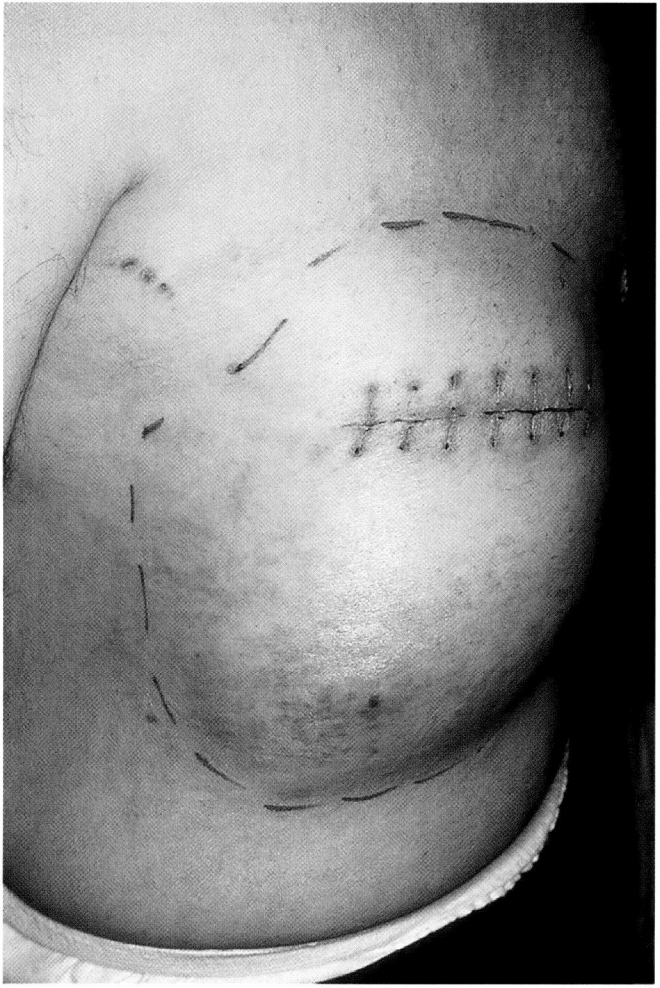

B

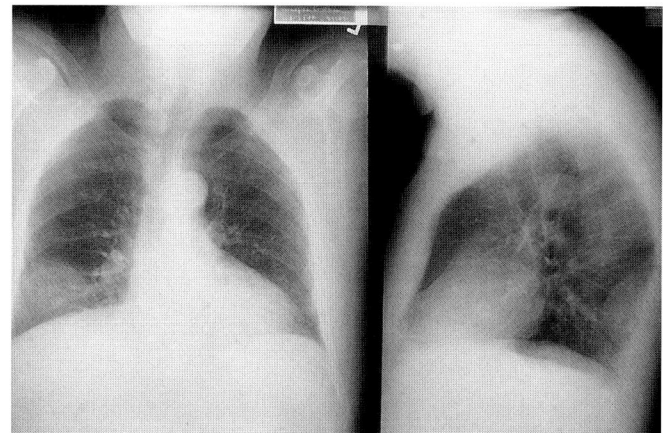

C

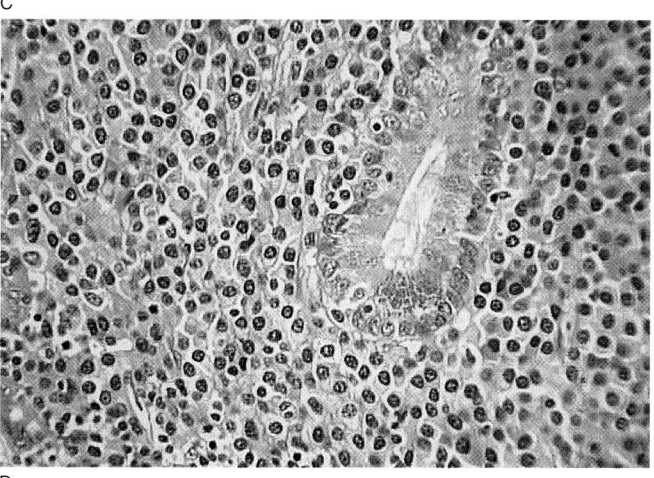

D

Fig. 23.12 (A) Isolated bone plasmacytoma (λ light chain). (B–C.) Soft tissue plasmacytoma in a patient with end-stage disease with corresponding PA and lateral chest radiograph. (D) Isolated plasmacytoma of small intestine.

revealed unsuspected bone lesions in approximately 30% of patients, and there is a suggestion that this technique may be able to distinguish patients who will progress to multiple myeloma from those patients with a more benign clinical course.[152] There is no definitive evidence that systemic treatment delays the onset of myeloma, and it may increase the likelihood of developing secondary leukemia.

Extramedullary plasmacytoma

Clinical features

Isolated extramedullary plasmacytoma may also occur. Ninety per cent lesions are in the upper respiratory tract and present with epistaxis, nasal discharge, hoarseness or sore throat, although lesions may also occur in the thyroid, skin and thymus. Twenty-five per cent of patients will have a monoclonal protein present in the serum or urine. It is important to distinguish patients with solitary extramedullary plasmacytoma from patients with soft tissue spread of advanced myeloma due to differences in clinical disease course[147,148] (Fig. 23.12B–D).

Pathology

Lesions are characteristically submucosal and contain a clonal plasma cell infiltrate. Some lesions reflect marginal cell lymphoma which have undergone extensive plasma cell differentiation.

Treatment/management/disease progression

For solitary extramedullary plasmacytoma, radiotherapy is the treatment of choice and is associated with a less than 5% risk of local recurrence. This risk is further decreased if adjacent lymph nodes are included in the radiation field.[151] Disease progression may occur occasionally either to myeloma with typical bone lesions, plasmacytosis and monoclonal protein, or to a disease characterized by multiple extramedullary lesions with no bone marrow plasmacytosis.

POEMS syndrome

The acronym polyneuropathy (P), organomegaly (O), endocrinopathy (E), M-protein (M) and skin changes (S)

describes a syndrome associated with plasma cell disorders, particularly but not exclusively osteosclerotic myeloma.[153,154] It is most frequently reported in Japanese males aged 40–50 years. A monoclonal protein is demonstrable in the plasma or urine in 75% of patients, usually of IgAλ isotype. Clinical features include a demyelinating polyneuropathy (more motor than sensory); hepatomegaly, splenomegaly and lymphadenopathy; diabetes mellitus, primary gondal failure, hypothyroidism and Addison's disease; and skin hyperpigmentation, thickening and hypertrichosis. Sixty per cent of patients will have pathologic changes consistent with multiple myeloma, although the extent of bone marrow infiltration by plasma cells may be low. The increase in plasma cells is usually associated with osteosclerosis. Lymph node involvement is common, and pathologic features resemble the hyaline-vascular variant of Castleman's disease with follicular hyperplasia, vascular proliferation, and an interfollicular infiltration of lymphocytes, plasma cells and immunoblasts. The median survival is approximately 2 years, and treatment is of the underlying plasma cell disorder.

Lymphoproliferative disorders associated with an IgM paraprotein

Waldenström's macroglobulinemia (WM) is a chronic B-cell lymphoproliferative disorder in which most of the clinical manifestations are due to the presence of an IgM paraprotein. The disorder is characterized by bone marrow infiltration with small lymphocytes, lymphoplasmacytoid cells and plasma cells, and a high level of IgM paraprotein. Both the Revised European American Lymphoma (REAL) and the World Health Organization (WHO) classifications consider WM as a clinical syndrome associated with the diagnosis of lymphoplasmacytoid lymphoma/immunocytoma. However, the presence of an IgM paraprotein is not specific for WM. The differential diagnosis includes other indolent lymphoproliferative disorders, for example chronic lymphocytic leukemia with IgM paraprotein, splenic lymphoma with villous lymphocytes (SLVL), and splenic marginal zone lymphoma (SMZL). Differences in the level of paraprotein, lymphocytic morphology, and degree of marrow involvement in relation to spleen size may help to distinguish WM from SLVL and SMZL, since the malignant cells within these disorders share the same phenotype. Other conditions associated with an IgM paraprotein include MGUS and, rarely, true IgM myeloma.[155]

Biology

Sequence analysis of the immunoglobulin heavy-chain gene demonstrates the presence of somatic mutations within the variable region without intraclonal diversity, suggesting that the malignant cell of origin has traversed the germinal center.[156] Immunophenotypic analysis also supports this hypothesis since the cells express monoclonal surface and cytoplasmic IgM; pan B-cell markers CD19, 20 and 22; and late B-cell differentiation markers such as CD38 and FMC7; but lack CD5, 10 and 23.[157] Complex abnormal karyotypes have been described, including trisomy and monosomy of a number of chromosomes and structural aberrations of 6q and 11q.[158,159] Although there is no characteristic translocation, a t(9;14)(p13;q32) has been described in which the PAX-5 gene, which encodes for a B-cell-specific transcription factor, is juxtaposed to the immunoglobulin heavy-chain locus.[160]

Clinical features

WM is 10–20% less common than multiple myeloma. It is predominantly a disease of the elderly, with a median age at presentation of 65 years. It is more common in Whites than Blacks, with a slight male predominance. Symptoms may occur due to tumor cell infiltration of bone marrow (cytopenia, increased infections and bleeding), splenomegaly, hepatomegaly and lymphadenopathy. Other clinical features include hyperviscosity in 20% of patients and type 1 cryoglobulinemia, although clinically relevant cryoglobulinemia causing Raynaud's phenomenon, purpura and glomerulonephritis occurs in less than 5% of patients. Cold agglutinin anemia may occur in 10% of patients when the monoclonal IgM behaves as a cold reactive antibody that interacts with erythrocyte antigens at low temperatures and results in the development of acrocyanosis, Raynaud's phenomenon, and episodic or chromic hemolysis. Neurological manifestations are present in 10% of patients related to infiltration of peripheral nerves with paraprotein, antibodies against various glycoproteins and glycolipids of the peripheral nerves, and amyloid deposition. In contrast to other plasma cell disorders, there is an absence of bony changes and lytic lesions. Occasionally, renal involvement may be present, due either to glomerular abnormalities or to amyloid deposition resulting in a non-selective proteinuria. Diagnosis requires the presence of an IgM paraprotein in the serum and the infiltration of characteristic cells within the bone marrow. As in myeloma, the presence of an IgM paraprotein may be an incidental finding, and the distinction between MGUS and WM is often controversial. MGUS is defined as IgM paraprotein <3g/dl associated with no constitutional symptoms, organomegaly or anemia and approximately 10% of patients with MGUS will develop WM at a median follow-up of 8 years.[161] Prognostic features for WM are not well characterized, although the response to treatment appears to be the most important variable in a number of studies. Age >60 years, the presence of cytopenias, as well as initial tumor burden and IgM level, have been identified as adverse prognostic features.[162,163]

Pathology

Most patients have disseminated disease with peripheral blood, bone marrow, lymph node, liver and spleen infiltration. Examination of the peripheral blood usually demonstrates a normochromic normocytic anemia with increased rouleaux formation, increased background staining consistent with a raised ESR/PV, and a serum IgM paraprotein (often with reduced IgG and IgA). When the paraprotein has the characteristic of a cold agglutinin or a cryoglobulin, either red cell aggregates or a cryoglobulin precipitate may be demonstrated. The lymphocyte count is usually normal, although monoclonal circulating cells can be demonstrated using flow cytometry. Some patients may present with pancytopenia. Bone marrow aspirate demonstrates an increased cellularity with an infiltration of small lymphocytes, lymphoplasmacytoid cells (cells with abundant basophillic cytoplasm but with lymphocyte-like nuclei), or plasma cells (Fig. 23.13). Other common features include hyperplasia of mast cells and the presence of Dutcher bodies, lymphocytes containing periodic acid-Schiff (PAS) positive intranuclear and intracytoplasmic inclusions consisting of IgM. Bone biopsy reveals an extensive

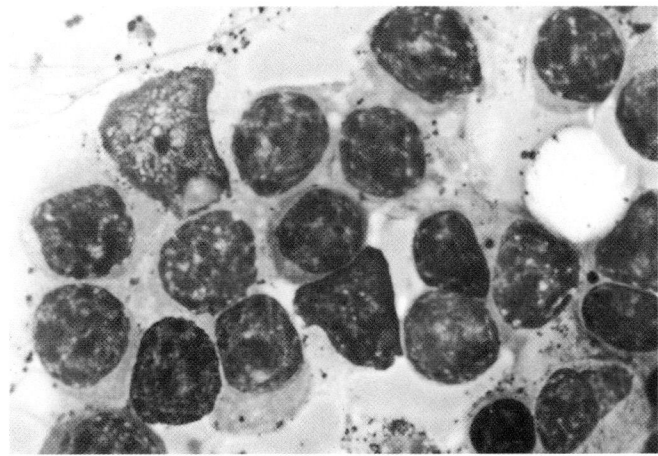

Fig. 23.13 Bone marrow aspirate of Waldenström's macroglobulinemia.

diffuse infiltrate of cells separated by hypoplastic marrow (Fig. 23.14A–C). Lymph node biopsy demonstrates an interfollicular infiltration with sparing of the sinuses. Occasionally lung, renal, gastrointestinal and leptomeningeal involvement may be seen.

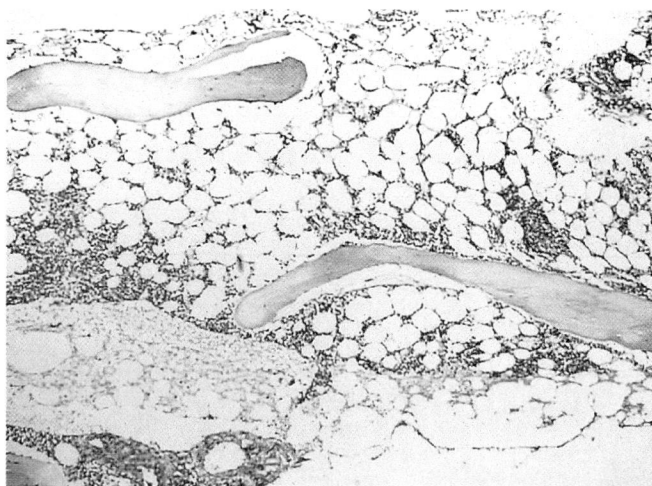

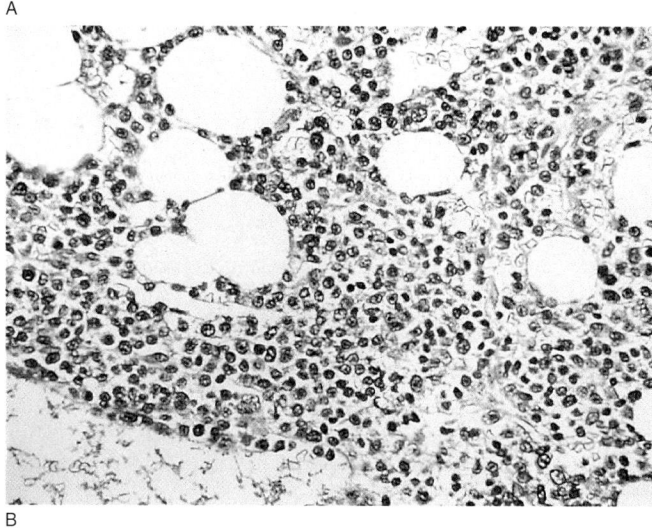

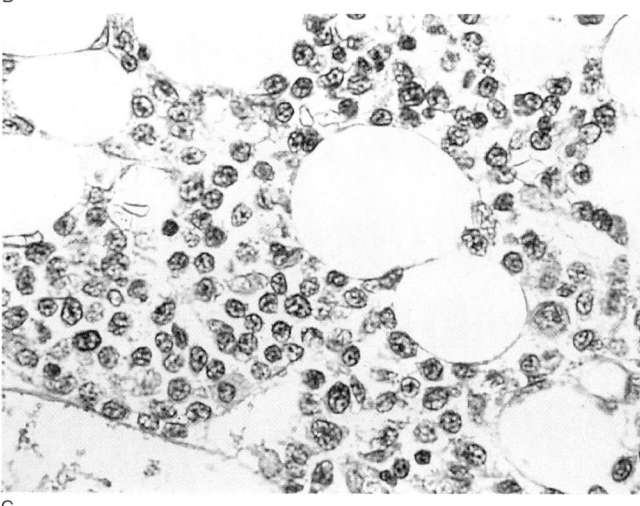

Fig. 23.14 Bone biopsy of Waldenström's macroglobulinemia (A–C).

Treatment/management

Initial management includes the correction of the raised plasma viscosity using plasmapheresis. A single plasmapheresis can result in a reduction of IgM of 35% and a decrease in plasma viscosity of 50–60%. Since 80% of the IgM paraprotein is intravascular, this effect can last for up to 6 weeks. This treatment is offered as a short-term measure whilst concomitant chemotherapy to reduce the tumor burden becomes effective. Traditionally, first-line chemotherapy has been with alkylating agents, particularly chlorambucil. The addition of steroids may be of particular value in patients with immune hemolytic anemia, cold agglutinin disease and cryoglobulinemia. Response rates of up to 60% are observed, although the rate of response is often slow.[162,164] Combination chemotherapy has also been used (CHOP, CAP); although response rates and survival appear to be superior, there is no direct comparison with chlorambucil. Recently purine analogs (fludarabine/2 chlorodeoxyadenosine (2 CDA)) as primary therapy have resulted in response rates of 40–85%.[165–167] Responses are usually more rapid than with alkylating agents, and these drugs are therefore the treatment of choice in patients with serious complications due to the disease. There are no data to suggest that patients with MGUS or stable disease benefit from treatment, and hence therapy should be reserved for symptomatic patients or for patients where there is evidence of disease progression. In the relapse setting patients are likely to respond again to the initial induction regimen, and studies of purine analogs suggest that they are able to induce responses in approximately one-third of patients resistant to alkylating agent.[165] Patients in resistant relapse are candidates for treatment with novel therapeutic agents. There have been promising reports of high (20–50%) response rates in heavily pretreated cases to either α interferon or tumor-directed antibody therapy using anti-CD20.[168,169] There are also a number of reports using high-dose therapy with either autologous or allogeneic transplantation.[170,171] These anecdotal reports suggest that most patients do seem to respond to treatment, although results need to be interpreted with caution due to small numbers and short follow-up.

Disease progression

WM remains incurable with a median survival of 5 years. The majority of patients die from infection, bone marrow failure or progressive disease that has become resistant to treatment. Approximately 20% of patients will die from an incidental cause. In a minority of patients, WM may transform into a high-grade B-cell lymphoma (Ritcher's syndrome), characterized by unexplained fever, weight loss, rapidly enlarging lymph nodes, extranodal involvement, and a reduction in IgM consistent with tumor dedifferentiation. The outcome for these patients is extremely poor.[155,161–163]

Light-chain-associated amyloidosis

Amyloidosis is a spectrum of diseases associated with the deposition of extracellular protein in major organs to form characteristic fibrillar sheets that disrupt organ structure and function. Light-chain amyloid, previously called primary amyloid, is characterized by the extracellular deposition of fibrillar protein derived from monoclonal light chains. The light chains are cleaved into fragments that consist of whole or part of the variable domain of the molecule, although occasionally intact light chains may also be deposited. The fragments form beta-pleated sheets which become insoluble and resistant to degradation following the deposition of glycosaminoglycans and the normal protein serum amyloid P component (SAP). A number of other types of proteins may also be deposited, leading to the formation of beta pleated sheets; however, these types of amyloid are not associated with plasma cell abnormalities. The proteins deposited include the circulating acute phase reactant protein serum amyloid A, an apolipoprotein of high-density lipoprotein. The deposition of this protein is usually a long-term complication of chronic inflammation or infective states, and the condition was previously known as reactive or secondary amyloid. Other proteins are deposited in association with Alzheimer's, type II diabetes and dialysis arthropathy (Table 23.7).[172,173]

Biology

The exact reason for the deposition of protein is unknown, although it is thought that the aberrant structure of the light chain confers the amyloidogenic potential. Mouse studies demonstrate that repeated injections of immunoglobulin from amyloid patients lead to the development of amyloid deposits within the mouse, whereas injections of immunoglobulins from myeloma patients result in no deposits.[174] The hypothesis that it is a unique amino-acid sequence which renders the protein amyloidogenic is also supported by the fact that γVI subclass of light chains seems to be uniquely associated with amyloidosis.[175]

Clinical features

This is a rare disorder with an annual incidence of 3000 cases in the US. The clinical features depend on the spectrum of organ involvement, with the most commonly affected organs being the heart, kidneys and peripheral nerves.[172,173,176,177] Cardiac features are present in one-third of patients at diagnosis and include cardiomegaly, restrictive cardiomyopathy, cardiac failure and arrythmias. Renal features include nephrotic syndrome and renal failure. Forty percent of patients have carpal tunnel syndrome, and peripheral neuropathy is present in 20%. Other features include macroglossia (infrequent but pathognomonic), gastrointestinal malabsorption, hepatosplenomegaly, and skin involvement including papular and nodular lesions and characteristic purpura around the eyes. Rarely, deficiency in factor IX and X may be present, resulting in bleeding disorders due to the binding of calcium-dependent clotting factors to the amyloid deposits. A monoclonal component is present in the serum or urine in 65% and 86% of cases respectively, although immunofixation is often required to demonstrate its presence as the peak may be small. The

Table 23.7 Classification of amyloidosis

Fibril protein	Syndrome
Immunoglobulin light chain	Systemic disease. Associated with myeloma or Waldenström's. Previously known as primary amyloid
Serum amyloid A protein	Systemic disease usually reactive and associated with chronic inflammation
Transthyretin	Familial and senile systemic disease
β2 microglobulin	Hemodialysis-associated disease, carpal tunnel syndrome and localized senile prostate disease
β protein derived from β-amyloid protein precursor	Alzheimer's disease
Islet amyloid polypeptide, amylin	Type II diabetes

monoclonal component may be either κ or λ light chains, but the majority are λ (4:1). Amyloid may occur as a long-term complication of most clonal B-cell disorders, especially myeloma (15%) and less commonly Waldenström's macroglobulinemia.

Pathology

The peripheral blood picture is usually normal, although Howell–Jolly bodies are present in 25% of cases suggesting hyposplenism due to amyloid infiltration of spleen. A low-level plasmacytosis is present on the bone marrow aspirate, and in some cases plasma cells may account for more than 20% of the total nucleated cells. Even if the plasma cell number is normal there is often an imbalance in κ:λ ratio suggesting the presence of abnormal cells, and immunoglobulin heavy chain PCR will confirm a clonal picture. When amyloid occurs in association with Waldenström's macroglobulinemia, lymphoplasmacytoid cells will be present. The bone biopsy reveals similar findings to those in the aspirate, but in addition demonstrates amyloid deposits within the small blood vessel walls or extravascularly. On electron microscopy these fibrils are linear, non-branching, and 10–15 nm in length. Examination with bipolarized light following staining with Congo red demonstrates apple green birefringence. This is pathognomonic for light-chain amyloid and is the standard for diagnosis. Amyloid also stains metachromically with crystal violet, fluoresces after staining with thioflavine-T, and is pink and homo-

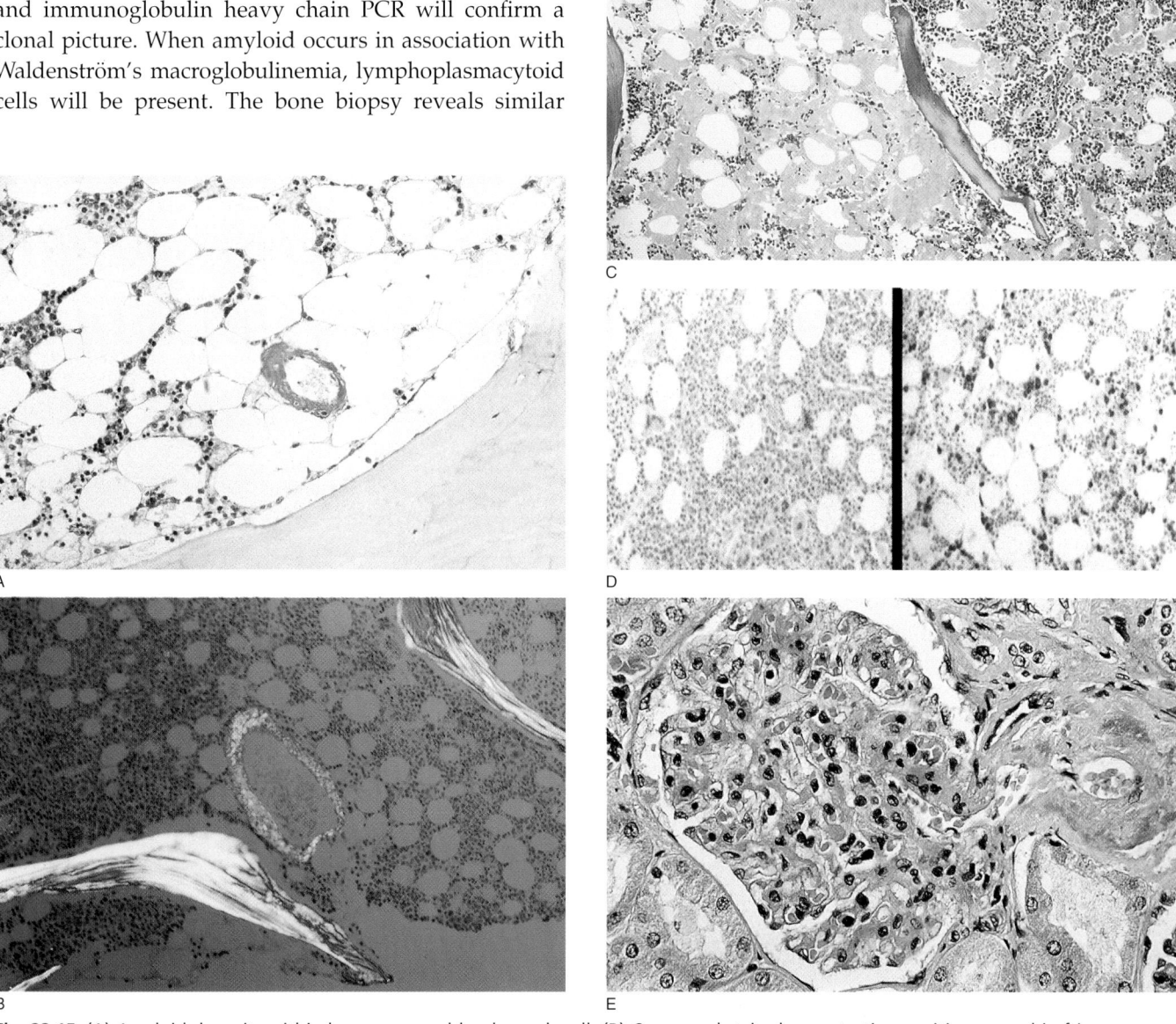

Fig. 23.15 (A) Amyloid deposits within bone marrow blood vessel wall. (B) Congo red stain demonstrating positive green birefringence within the blood vessel wall. (C) Interstitial amyloid. (D) Immunohistochemistry demonstrating monoclonal lambda positive plasma cells. (E) Renal amyloid.

genous on H&E staining (Fig. 23.15A–D). Light-chain amyloid may be distinguished from other types of amyloid immunochemically using type specific anti-light-chain sera, although this may be negative since a number of antibodies react with parts of the molecule that have been degraded during formation of the protein deposit. Light-chain amyloid may also be distinguished from other types of amyloid, as there is no abolition of Congo red staining by prior treatment with potassium permanganate. The characteristic amyloid deposition can be demonstrated in all affected organs on biopsy (Fig. 23.15E). If biopsy of the primary organ is dangerous, then a fine-needle aspirate of abdominal fat or a rectal biopsy are less invasive ways to demonstrate the presence of disease and are commonly positive (80% of cases). Scintigraphy using radio-labeled SAP is useful to determine the extent of disease and organ involvement.[178]

Treatment/management

Supportive therapy is directed toward alleviating symptoms and improving the function of affected organs (i.e. controlling heart failure, renal failure). Specific treatment is also required to reduce or eliminate the plasma cell clone, as there is a suggestion that amyloid may regress when the primary source of protein is removed. The combination of melphalan and prednisolone is associated with a moderate survival benefit, although response to therapy can take up to 6 months and complete elimination of the plasma clone with improvement in amyloid-related organ dysfunction is rarely observed.[177,179,180] Recent reports suggest that high-dose melphalan with autologous peripheral blood stem cell support is able to induce complete remissions that are associated with an improvement in organ dysfunction and increased survival.[181,182] Owing to an increased risk of peri-transplant related mortality, current guidelines suggest that this therapy should be offered only to patients with less than three organs involved and reasonable cardiac function. Patients with predominantly cardiac or renal involvement should be considered for organ transplantation.

Disease progression

Because amyloid is deposited in key viscera, such as the heart and liver, the disease may progress rapidly. The median survival of untreated patients is 12–15 months, with 50% of deaths occurring from a cardiac cause.[172,173] Prognosis is dependent on the pattern of organ involvement: if the heart is the main affected organ at presentation, then the median survival is 6 months; whereas survival is 21 months when there is primary involvement of the kidney.[177] Other poor prognostic variables include renal failure, jaundice, and large total body amyloid deposition demonstrated by SAP scintigraphy.

Heavy-chain disorders

This group of rare plasma cell disorders is characterized by the production of a monoclonal immunoglobulin that is formed from truncated heavy chains with no associated light chains. The diagnosis depends on the detection of structurally abnormal immunoglobulin in patient serum or urine which consists mainly of the Fc region of the molecule. The actual length of the chain varies between patients but is usually one-half to three-quarters of the normal counterpart, with the majority of cases having complete deletion of the C_H1 domain. The mechanisms leading to the production of the abnormal protein are not clearly understood. The analysis of rearranged gene sequences demonstrates a high level of somatic mutation with deletions and insertions of sequences of unknown origin. This suggests that cells producing the abnormal heavy chains arise during somatic hypermutation in the germinal center, and that further genetic alterations are required at a later stage in the developmental process for malignant transformation to occur.[183–185] The abnormal immunoglobulin is not evident by serum electrophoresis in a high proportion of cases, and identification may therefore require more sensitive techniques such as serum immunoelectrophoresis or immunofixation. The presenting clinical features depend on the type of heavy chain involved.

α-heavy-chain disease

α-heavy-chain disease predominantly affects the bowel and is associated with the production of the heavy chain of IgA, usually α1 subtype that forms polymers which are secreted into the serum and bowel lumen.

Clinical features

Of the 400 cases reported to date, the majority are from the Mediterranean or the Middle East. Presentation is usually in the third decade of life with a slight male predominance. Environmental factors in early infancy are important in the etiology of the disease, especially low socio-economic status and poor hygiene leading to the development of recurrent infectious diarrhea and chronic parasitic infections.[186] The main clinical features include diarrhea, weight loss, abdominal pain, vomiting and evidence of malabsorption. Abdominal masses may also be present. Occasionally, the disease may present with respiratory symptoms due to infiltrations in the respiratory tract.[187]

Pathology

Intestinal lesions characteristically affect segments of the duodenum and the jejunum with no intervening normal mucosa. Initially a plasmacytic or lymphoplasmacytic infiltrate involving the mucosal lamina propria is present (stage A). With disease progression atypical cells extend to the submucosa, and villous atrophy may occur (stage B). Some cases evolve into large cell lymphoma of immunoblastic type (stage C) which may present as discrete ulcerating tumors or extensive infiltrates of long segments of bowel wall. The mesenteric lymph nodes are usually involved. Infiltration of the bone marrow, liver and spleen is rare, but may occur with stage-C disease. A mild to moderate anemia may be present due to the malabsorption of iron, folate and vitamin B12.

Treatment/management/disease progression

In the absence of therapy, the disease is generally progressive with the initial benign lesions evolving into immunoblastic lymphoma. In early stage disease treatment with antibiotics (metronidazole and ampicillin) results in complete clinical, histologic and immunologic remission in about 40% of patients, supporting the hypothesis of an underlying infectious etiology. CHOP-based chemotherapy regimens are recommended for more advanced disease, although the median overall survival is poor.[188]

γ-heavy-chain disease

This heterogeneous group of disorders presents with a variety of clinical and pathologic features that are characterized by the secretion of abnormal IgG heavy chains. It is an extremely rare disorder, and only 100 cases have been reported in the literature.[189]

Clinical features

γHCD predominantly occurs in blacks and Asians with a median age at presentation of 60 years, although a number of cases have been reported in children. The clinical features include lymphadenopathy, hepatomegaly and splenomegaly with associated constitutional symptoms such as weight loss and fever. Autoimmune disorders occur frequently and include rheumatoid arthritis, systemic lupus erythematosus, vasculitis and myasthenia gravis.

Pathology

There is no consistent morphologic pattern corresponding to the serologic diagnosis of γHCD.[190] The bone marrow is usually infiltrated with lymphocytes, lymphoplasmacytoid cells or plasma cells. Lymph node biopsy may show evidence of a lymphoplasmacytoid proliferation, a plasma cell infiltrate, or non-Hodgkin's lymphoma. Unusual pathologic features include eosinophila or multinucleated giant cells, suggesting the presence of an atypical granulomatous lesion. The peripheral blood may show evidence of a moderate normochromic normocytic anemia, lymphocytosis with atypical lymphoplasmacytoid cells or plasma cells, and eosinophilia.

Treatment/management/disease progression

The clinical disease course varies. If the abnormal heavy chain is an incidental finding, then no therapy is required. For symptomatic patients therapy with agents that are active in other plasma cell disorders should be utilized.

μ-heavy-chain disease

This type of heavy-chain disease is extremely rare, with only 29 cases reported worldwide. It is characterized by the secretion of abnormal heavy chains of IgM and is usually associated with the presence of other lymphoproliferative disorders, particularly chronic lymphocytic leukemia (CLL) and less commonly Waldenström's macroglobulinemia and myeloma.[189]

Clinical features

Presenting features included hepatomegaly, splenomegaly and abdominal lymphadenopathy. Unlike other types of heavy-chain disorders, light-chain secretion may also occur and give rise to an amyloid-like picture.[191]

Pathology

The majority of patients have morphologic and phenotypic features indistinguishable from CLL on peripheral blood smear. A lymphocytosis or plasmacytosis is present within the bone marrow.

Treatment/management/disease progression

The mainstay of treatment is therapy directed at the underlying lymphoproliferative disorder.

Cryoglobulinemia

The presence of an underlying plasma cell disorder may lead to the development of cryoglobulinemia. In type I cryoglobulinemia the paraprotein secreted, usually IgG or IgM, has the characteristics of a cryoglobulin. In type II and type III cryoglobulinemia the paraprotein, usually IgM, has antibody activity against another immunoglobulin, often polyclonal IgG, and results in immune complex formation. In 75% of patients, no pathologic manifestations other than those due to the characteristic of the immunoglobulin are present at the time of diagnosis and the term 'essential cryoglobulinemia' is appropriate.[192,193] Over a 10-year period of follow-up, approximately 25% of patients will go on to develop symptoms and signs associated with a lymphoproliferative disorder. In the remaining 25% of cases, the cryoglobulinemia is a manifestation of an overt lymphoproliferative disorder including myeloma, Waldenström's macroglobulinemia, immunocytoma, mucosal-associated lymphoid tissue lymphoma (MALToma) and follicular lymphoma. In this subset of patients 25% will have type I, 70% type II and 5% type III cryoglobulinemia.[194]

Clinical features

The clinical features depend on the type of cryoglobulin formed and result from either the precipitation of the immunoglobulin at reduced body temperatures or to the deposition of immune complexes in major organs or the periphery. The most common presenting features include vasculitis of the skin, arthralgia, peripheral neuropathy, proliferative glomerulonephritis and hepatitis.

Pathology

The peripheral blood film is usually normal. In a minority of cases a cryoglobulin precipitate is present, usually demonstrable as a weakly basophilic globular mass, less often as crystals or a fibrillar deposit. Occasionally, cryoglobulin precipitates are ingested by neutrophils or monocytes and are seen as globular, variably basophillic intracytoplasmic inclusions. Within the bone marrow a lymphocytosis is common in essential cryoglobulinemia, and in up to 40% of cases clonality can be demonstrated using either immunohistochemistry or flow cytometry. In cases associated with an underlying lymphoproliferative disorder, the histologic features of that disorder will dominate. On biopsy of the kidney, membranoproliferative glomerulonephritis (60%) and mesangial proliferative glomerulonephritis (20%) can be demonstrated. Chronic active hepatitis with periportal lymphoid infiltrates is often present on liver biopsy.

Treatment/management/disease progression

Cytotoxic therapy including cyclophosphamide and steroids, along with plasmapheresis is the mainstay of treatment for symptomatic essential cryoglobulinemia. If an underlying lymphoproliferative disorder is present, then therapy must be directed at reducing tumor-cell burden.

Acknowledgments

We are extremely grateful to Dr Arthur Skarin (Dana Farber Cancer Institute, Boston, USA), Dr Carl O'Hara, (Boston, Boston Medical Center, USA), Dr Andrew Jack and Professor Gareth Morgan (Haematolgolgical Malignancy Diagnostic Service, Leeds General Infirmary, Leeds, UK) for the illustrations.

REFERENCES

1. Bergsagel D 1995 The incidence and epidemiology of plasma cell neoplasms. Stem Cells 13(supp 12): 1–9
2. Cuzick J, De Stavola B 1988 Multiple myeloma – a case control study. British Journal of Cancer 57: 516–520
3. Herrington LJ, Weiss NS, Olsham AF 1998 Epidemiology of myeloma. In: Malpass JS, Bergsagel DE, Kyle R, Anderson K (eds), Myeloma: biology and management. Oxford Medical Publications, Oxford, 150–186
4. Davies FE, Rollinson SJ, Rawstron AC et al 2000 High producer haplotypes of tumour necrosis factor α and lymphotoxin α are associated with an increased risk of myeloma and have an improved progression free survival after treatment. Journal of Clinical Oncology 18: 2843–2851
5. Zheng C, Huang DR, Bergenbrant S et al 2000 Interleukin-6, tumour necrosis factor α, interleukin-1β and interleukin-1 receptor antagonist promoter or coding gene polymorphisms in multiple myeloma. British Journal of Haematology 109: 39–45
6. Bakkus, MHC, Heirman C, Van Riet I et al 1992 Evidence that multiple myeloma Ig heavy chain VDJ genes contain somatic mutations but show no intraclonal variation. Blood 80: 2326–2335
7. Billadeau D, Ahmann G, Greipp P et al 1993 The bone marrow of multiple myeloma patients contains B cell populations at different stages of differentiation that are clonally related to the malignant plasma cell. Journal of Experimental Medicine 178: 1023–1031
8. Sahota SS, Leo R, Hamblin TJ et al 1996 Ig VH gene mutational patterns indicate different tumour cell status in human myeloma and

monoclonal gammopathy of undetermined significance. Blood 87: 746–755

9. Kawano M, Hirano T, Matsuda T et al 1988 Autocrine generation and requirement of BSF-2/IL-6 for human multiple myelomas. Nature 332: 83–85

10. Urashima M, Chauhan D, Uchiyama H et al 1995 CD40 ligand triggered interleukin-6 secretion in multiple myeloma. Blood 85: 1903–1912

11. Klein B, Zhang XG, Jourdan M et al 1989 Paracrine rather than autocrine regulation of myeloma cell growth and differentiation by interleukin 6. Blood 73: 517–526

12. Uchiyama H, Barut BA, Mohrbacher AF et al 1993 Adhesion of human myeloma derived cell lines to bone marrow stromal cells stimulates IL-6 secretion. Blood 82: 3712–3720

13. Kishimoto T, Akira S, Narazaki M et al 1995 Interleukin 6 family of cytokines and gp 130. Blood 86: 1243–1254

14. Kishimoto T, Taga T, Akira S 1994 Cytokine signal transduction. Cell 76: 253–262

15. Ogata A, Chauhan D, Teoh G et al 1997 Interleukin 6 triggers cell growth via the ras dependent mitogen-activated protein kinase cascade. Journal of Immunology 159: 2212–2221

16. Ogata A, Chauhan D, Urashima M et al 1997 Blockade of mitogen activated protein kinase cascade signaling in interleukin 6 independent multiple myeloma cells. Clinical Cancer Research 3: 1017–1022

17. Chauhan D, Kharbanda S, Ogata A et al 1997 Interleukin 6 inhibits Fas induced apoptosis and stress activated protein kinase activation in multiple myeloma cells. Blood 89: 227–234

18. Chauhan D, Pandey P, Ogata A et al 1997 Dexamethasone induced apoptosis of multiple myeloma cells in a JNK/SAP kinase independent mechanism. Oncogene 15: 837–843

19. Chauhan D, Pandey P, Ogata A et al 1997 Cytochrome c dependent and independent induction of apoptosis in multiple myeloma cells. Journal of Biological Chemistry 272: 29995–29997

20. Chauhan D, Pandey P, Hideshima T et al 2000 SHP2 mediates the protective effects of interleukin-6 against dexamethasone induced apoptosis in multiple myeloma cells. Journal of Biological Chemistry 275: 27845–27850

21. Urashima M, Ogata A, Chauhan D et al 1996 Interleukin-6 promotes multiple myeloma cell growth via phosphorylation of retinoblastoma protein. Blood 88: 2219–2227

22. Ng MHL, Chung YF, Lo KW et al 1997 Frequent hypermethylation of p16 and p15 genes in multiple myeloma. Blood 87: 2500–2506

23. Urashima M, Teoh G, Chauhan D et al 1997 Interleukin-6 overcomes p21WAF1 upregulation and G1 growth arrest induced by dexamethasone and interferon in multiple myeloma cels. Blood 90: 279–289

24. Teoh G, Urashima M, Ogata A et al 1997 MDM2 protein overexpression promotes proliferation and survival of plasma cell leukemia cells. Blood 90: 1982–1992

25. Bataille R, Jourdan M, Zhang XG et al 1989 Serum levels of interleukin 6, a potent myeloma cell growth factor, as a reflect of disease severity in plasma cell dyscrasias. Journal of Clinical Investigation 84: 2008–2011

26. Kyrtsonis MC, Dedoussis G, Zervas C et al 1996 Soluble interleukin-6 receptor (sIL-6R), a new prognostic factor in multiple myeloma. British Journal of Haematology 93: 398–400

27. Pulkki K, Pelliniemi TT, Rajamaki A et al 1996 Soluble interleukin-6 receptor as a prognostic factor in multiple myeloma. British Journal of Haematology 92: 370–374

28. Jernberg-Wiklund H, Pettersson M, Nilsson K 1991 Recombinant interferon-gamma inhibits the growth of IL-6 dependent human multiple myeloma cell lines *in vitro*. European Journal of Haematology 46: 231–239

29. Portier M, Zhang XG, Caron E et al 1993 Gamma-interferon in multiple myeloma: inhibition of interleukin-6 dependent myeloma cells growth and downregulation of IL-6 receptor expression in vitro. Blood 81: 3076–3082

30. Ogata A, Nishimoto N, Shima Y et al 1994 Inhibitory effect of all-trans retinoic acid on the growth of freshly isolated myeloma cells via interference with interleukin-6 signal transduction. Blood 84: 3040–3046

31. Schwabe M, Brini AT, Bosco MC et al 1994 Disruption by interferon α of autocrine IL6 growth loop in IL6 dependent U266 myeloma cells by homologous and heterologous downregulation of the IL-6 receptor alpha and beta chains. Journal of Clinical Investigation 94: 2317–2325

32. Urashima M, Ogata A, Chauhan D et al 1996 Transforming growth factor beta: differential effects on multiple myeloma versus normal B cells. Blood 87: 1929–1938

33. Lust JA, Donovan KA 1999 The role of IL-1β in the pathogenesis of multiple myeloma. Hematology and Oncology Clinics of North America 13: 1117–1125

34. Kawano M, Yamamoto I, Iwato K et al 1989 Interleukin-1 beta rather than lymphotoxin as the major bone resorbing activity in human multiple myeloma. Blood 72: 1646–1649

35. Kawano M, Tanaka H, Ishikawa H et al 1989 Interleukin-1 accelerates autocrine growth of myeloma cells thorough interleukin-6 in human myeloma. Blood 73: 2145–2148

36. Bergui L, Schena M, Gaidano G et al 1989 Interleukin 3 and interleukin 6 synergistically promote the proliferation and differentiation of malignant plasma cell precursors in multiple myeloma. Journal of Experimental Medicine 170: 613–618

37. Hermann F, Andreeff M, Gruss HJ et al 1991 Interleukin-4 inhibits growth of multiple myelomas by suppressing interleukin-6 expression. Blood 78: 2070–2074

38. Zhang XG, Bataille R, Jourdan M et al 1990 Granulocyte macrophage colony stimulating factor synergizes with interleukin-6 in supporting the proliferation of human myeloma cells. Blood 76: 2599–2605

39. Vacca A, Ribatti D, Presta M et al 1999 Bone marrow neovascularisation, plasma cell angiogenic potential and matrix metalloproteinase-2 secretion parallel progression of human multiple myeloma. Blood 93: 3064–3073

40. Munshi N, Wilson CS, Penn J et al 1998 Angiogenesis in newly diagnosed multiple myeloma: poor prognosis with increased microvessel density in bone marrow biopsies. Blood 92 (suppl 1): 400

41. Rajkumar SV, Fonseca R, Witzig TE et al 1999 Bone marrow angiogenesis in patients achieving complete response after stem cell transplantation for multiple myeloma. Leukemia 13: 469–472

42. Sjak-Shie N, Sulur G, Said J et al 2000 Angiogenesis and vascular endothelial growth factor expression correlate with the degree of bone marrow involvement in multiple myeloma patients. Blood 94 (suppl 2): 4590

43. Bellamy WT, Richter L, Frutiger Y et al 1999 Expression of vascular endothelial growth factor and its receptors in hematopoietic malignancies. Cancer Research 59: 728–733

44. Dankbar B, Padro T, Leo R et al 2000 Vascular endothelial growth factor and interleukin 6 in paracrine tumour-stromal cell interaction in multiple myeloma. Blood 95: 2630–2636

45. Van Camp B, Durie BGM, Spier C et al 1990 Plasma cells in multiple myeloma express a natural killer cell associated antigen: CD56. Blood 76: 377–382

46. Pellat-Deceunynck C, Barille S, Puthier D et al 1995 Adhesion molecules on human myeloma cells: Significant changes in expression related to malignancy, tumour spread and immortilisation. Cancer Research 55: 3647–3653

47. Uchiyama H, Barut BA, Chauhan D et al 1992 Characterisation of adhesion molecules in human myeloma cell lines. Blood 80: 2306–2314

48. Teoh G, Anderson KC 1997 Interaction of tumour and host cells with adhesion and extracellular matrix molecules in the development of multiple myeloma. Hematology and Oncology Clinics of North America 11: 27–42

49. Rawstron AC, Owen RG, Davies FE et al 1997 Circulating plasma cells in multiple myeloma: characterisation and correlation with disease status. British Journal of Haematology 97: 46–55

50. Rawstron AC, Barrans SI, Blythe D et al 1999 Distribution of myeloma plasma cells in peripheral blood and bone marrow correlates with CD56 expression. British Journal of Haematology 104: 138–143

51. Urashima M, Chen BP, Chen S et al 1997 The development of a model for the homing of multiple myeloma cells to human bone marrow. Blood 90: 754–765

52. Liang W, Hopper JE, Rowley JD 1979 Karyotypic abnormalities and clinical aspects of patients with multiple myeloma and related paraproteinemic disorders. Cancer 44: 630–644

53. Weh HJ, Gutensohn K, Selbaach J et al 1993 Karyotype in multiple myeloma and plasma cell leukaemia. European Journal of Cancer 29A: 1269–1273

54. Drach J, Schuster J, Nowotny H et al 1995 Multiple myeloma: high incidence of chromosomal aneuploidy as detected by interphase fluorescent *in situ* hybridisation. Cancer Research 55: 3854–3859

55. Flactif M, Zandecki M, Lai JL et al 1995 Interphase fluorescent insitu

hybridisation (FISH) as a powerful tool in the detection of aneuploidy in multiple myeloma. Leukaemia 9: 2109–2114

56. Lai JL, Zandecki M, Mary JY et al 1995 Improved cytogenetics in multiple myeloma: a study of 151 patients including 117 patients at diagnosis. Blood 85: 2490–2497

57. Smadja V, Louvet C, Isnard F et al 1995 Cytogenetic study in multiple myeloma at diagnosis: comparison of two techniques. British Journal of Haematology 90: 619–624

58. Tabernero D, San Miguel JF, Garcia-Sanz R et al 1996 Incidence of chromosome numerical changes in multiple myeloma. American Journal of Pathology 149: 153–161

59. Garcia-Sanz R, Orfao A, Gonzaalez M et al 1995 Prognostic implications of DNA aneuploidy in 156 untreated multiple myeloma patients. British Journal of Haematology 90: 106–112

60. Perez-Simon JA, Garcia-Sanz R, Tabernero MD et al 1998 Prognostic value of numerical chromosome aberrations in multiple myeloma: A FISH analysis of 15 different chromosomes. Blood 91: 3366–3371

61. Sawyer JR, Waldron JA, Jaganath S et al 1995 Cytogenetics findings in 200 patients with multiple myeloma. Cancer, Genetics and Cytogenetics 82: 41–49

62. Tricot G, Barlogie B, Jaganath S et al 1995 Poor prognosis in multiple myeloma is associated only with partial or complete deletions of chromosome 13 or abnormalities involving 11q and not with other karyotype abnormalities. Blood 86: 4250–4256

63. Chesi M, Bergsagel PL, Brents LA et al 1996 Dysregulation of Cyclin D1 by translocation into the IgH gamma switch region in two multiple myeloma cell lines. Blood 88: 674–681

64. Iida S, Rao PH, Butler M et al 1997 Deregulation of MUM1/IRF4 by chromosomal translocation in multiple myeloma. Nature Genetics 17: 226–230

65. Chesi M, Nardini E, Brents LA et al 1997 Frequent translocation t(4;14)(p16.3;q32.3) in multiple myeloma: association with increased expression and activating mutations of fibroblast growth factor receptor 3. Nature Genetics 16: 260–264

66. Avet-Loiseau H, Li JY, Facon T et al 1998 High incidence of translocations t(11;14)(q13;q32) and t(4;14)(p16;q32) in patients with plasma cell malignancies. Cancer Research 58: 5640–5645

67. Avet-Loiseau H, Brigaudeau C, Morineau N et al 1999 High incidence of cryptic translocations involving the Ig heavy chain gene in multiple myeloma as shown by fluorescence *in situ* hybridization. Genes Chromosomes Cancer 24: 9–15

68. Portier M, Moles JP, Makars GR et al 1992 P53 and RAS gene mutations in multiple myeloma. Oncogene 7: 2539–2543

69. Corradini P, Ladetto M, Voena C et al 1993 Mutational activation of N- and K-ras oncogenes in plasma cell dyscrasias. Blood 81: 2708–2713

70. Owen RG, Davis SAA, Randerson J et al 1997 P53 gene mutations in multiple myeloma. Molecular Pathology 50: 18–20

71. Preudhomme C, Facon T, Zanddecki M et al 1992 Rare occurrence of p53 gene mutations in multiple myeloma. British Journal of Haematology 81: 440–443

72. Neri A, Baldini L, Trecca D et al 1993 P53 gene mutations in multiple myeloma are associated with advanced forms of malignancy. Blood 81: 128–135

73. Manolagas SC, Jilka RL 1995 Bone marrow, cytokines and bone remodelling. New England Journal of Medicine 332: 305–311

74. Bataille R, Chappard D, Klein B 1992 Mechanisms of bone lesions in multiple myeloma. Haematology and Oncology Clinics of North America 6: 285–295

75. Taube T, Beneton MN, McCloskey EV et al 1992 Abnormal bone remodelling in patients with myelomatosis and normal biochemical indices of bone resorption. European Journal of Haematology 49: 192–198

76. Bataille R, Delmas PD, Chappard D et al 1990 Abnormal serum bone gla protein levels in multiple myeloma: crucial role of bone formation and prognostic implications. Cancer 66: 167–172

77. Cozzolino F, Torcia M, Aldinucci D et al 1989 Production of interleukin- 1 by bone marrow myeloma cells: its role in the pathogenesis of lytic bone lesions. Blood 74: 380–387

78. Garrett IR, Durie BGM, Nedwin GE et al 1987 Production of lymphotoxin, a bone resorbing cytokine by cultured human myeloma cells. New England Journal of Medicine 317: 526–532

79. Tricot G 2000 New insights into the role of microenvironment in multiple myeloma. Lancet 335: 248–249

80. Barille S, Akhoundi C, Colette M et al 1997 Metalloproteinases in multiple myeloma: production of matrix metalloproteinase-9,

activation of proMMMP-2 and induction of MMP-1 by myeloma cells. Blood 90: 1649–1655

81. Choi SJ, Cruz JC, Craig F et al 2000 Macrophage inflammatory protein 1-alpha is a potential osteoclast stimulatory factor in multiple myeloma. Blood 96: 671–675

82. Medical Research Council's Working Party on Leukaemia in Adults 1980 Prognostic features in the third MRC myelomatosis trial. British Journal of Cancer 42: 831–840

83. Durie BGM, Salmon SE 1975 A clinical staging system for multiple myeloma. Correlation of measured cell mass with presenting clinical features, response to treatment and survival. Cancer 36: 842–854

84. Norfolk DN, Child JA, Cooper EH et al 1980 Serum β2 microglobulin in myelomatosis: potential value in stratification and monitoring. British Journal of Cancer 42: 510–515

85. Greipp PR, Leong T, Bennett JM et al 1998 Plasmablastic morphology – an independent prognostic factor with clinical and laboratory correlates. Blood 91: 2501–2507

86. Greipp PR, Katzman JA, O'Fallon WM et al 1988 Value of β2 microglobulin level and plasma cell labeling indices as prognostic factors in patients with newly diagnosed myeloma. Blood 72: 219–223

87. Witzig TE, Gertz MA, Lust JA et al 1996 Peripheral blood monoclonal plasma cells as a predictor of survival in patients with multiple myeloma. Blood 88: 1780–1787

88. Bartl R, Frisch B, Fateh-Moghadam A et al 1987 Histological classification and staging of multiple myeloma. A retrospective and prospective study of 674 cases. American Journal of Clinical Hematology 87: 342–355

89. Love EM 1986 The chemotherapy of multiple myeloma. In: Delamore IW (eds), Multiple myeloma and other proteinaemias. Churchill Livingstone, Edinburgh, 353–375

90. MacLennan IC, Chapman C, Dunn J et al 1992 Combined chemotherapy with ABCM versus melphalan for treatment of myelomatosis. The Medical Research Council Working Party for Leukaemia in Adults. Lancet 25: 200–205

91. Myeloma Trialists Collaborative Group 1998 Combination chemotherapy versus melphalan plus prednisolone as treatment for multiple myeloma: an overview of 6633 patients from 27 randomised trials. Journal of Clinical Oncology 16: 3832–3842

92. Alexanian R, Barlogie B, Dixon D 1986 High dose glucocorticoid treatment of resistant myeloma. Annals of Internal Medicine 105: 8–11

93. Alexanian R, Barlogie B, Tucker S 1990 VAD based regimens as primary treatments for multiple myeloma. American Journal of Hematology 33: 86–89

94. Forgeson GV, Selby P, Lakhani S et al 1988 Infused vincristine and adriamycin with high dose methylprednisolone (VAMP) in advanced previously treated multiple myeloma patients. British Journal of Cancer 58: 469–473

95. Samson D, Gaminara E, Newland A et al 1989 Infusion of vincristine and doxorubicin with oral dexamethasone as first line therapy for multiple myeloma. Lancet 2: 882–885

96. N Raje, R Powles, S Kullarni et al 1997 A comparison of vincristine and doxorubicin infusional chemotherapy with methylprednisolone (VAMP) with the addition of weekly cyclophosphamide (C-VAMP) as induction treatment followed by autografting in previously untreated myeloma. British Journal of Haematology 97: 153–160

97. Berenson J, Lichtenstein A, Porter L et al 1996 Efficacy of pamidronate in reducing skeletal events in patients with advanced multiple myeloma. New England Journal of Medicine 334: 488–493

98. McCloskey EV, Maclennan ICM, Drayson MT et al 1998 A randomized trial of the effect of clodronate on skeletal morbidity in multiple myeloma. British Journal of Haematology 100: 317–325

99. Derenne S, Amiot M, Barille S et al 1999 Zoledronate is a potent inhibitor of myeloma cell growth and sectretion of IL-6 and MMP-1 by the tumoral environment. Journal of Bone Mineralisation Research 14: 2048–2056

100. Shipman CM, Rogers MJ, Apperley JF et al 1998 Anti tumour activity of bisphosphonates in human myeloma cells. Leukemia and Lymphoma 32: 129–138

101. Kunzmann V, Bauer E, Fouria J et al 2000 Stimulation of γδT cells by aminobisphosphonates and induction of anti-plasma cell activity in multiple myeloma. Blood 96: 384–392

102. Peest D 1999 The role of alpha interferon in multiple myeloma. Pathol Biol (Paris) 47: 172–177

103. Attal M, Harousseau JL, Stoppa AM et al 1996 Autologous bone marrow transplantation versus conventional chemotherapy in

multiple myeloma: a prospective randomised trial. New England Journal of Medicine 335: 91–97

104. Barlogie B, Jagannath S, Vesole DH et al 1997 Superiority of tandem autologous transplantation over standard therapy for previously untreated multiple myeloma. Blood 89: 789–793

105. Lenhoff S, Hjorth M, Holmberg E et al 2000 Impact on survival of high dose therapy with autologous stem cell support in patients younger than 60 years with newly diagnosed multiple myeloma: a population based study. Blood 95: 7–11

106. Algere A, Diaz Mediavilla J, San Miguel J et al 1998 Autologous peripheral blood stem cell transplantation for multiple myeloma: a report of 259 cases from the Spanish Registry. Bone Marrow Transplant 21: 133–140

107. Powles R, Raje N, Milan S et al 1997 Outcome assessment of a population based group of 195 unselected myeloma patients under 70 years of age offered intensive treatment. Bone Marrow Transplant 20: 435–443

108. Fermand JP, Ravaud P, Chevret S et al 1998 High dose therapy and autologous peripheral blood stem cell transplantation in multiple myeloma: upfront or rescue treatment. Results of a multi-centre sequential randomised clinical trial. Blood 92: 3131–3136

109. Johnson RJ, Owen RG, Smith GM et al 1996 Peripheral blood stem cell transplantation in myeloma using CD34 selected cells. Bone Marrow Transplant 17: 723–727

110. Vescio R, Schiller G, Stewart AK et al 1999 Multicentre phase III trial to evaluate CD34+ selected versus unselected autologous peripheral blood progenitor cell transplantation in multiple myeloma. Blood 93: 1858–1868

111. Attal M, Harousseau JL, Facon T et al 1999 Single vs double transplantation in myeloma – a randomised trial of the intergroupe francais du myeloma (IFM). Blood 84 (suppl 1): 3152

112. Gahrton G, Tura S, Ljungman P et al 1995 Prognostic factors in allogeneic bone marrow transplantation for multiple myeloma. Journal of Clinical Oncology 13: 1312–1322

113. Bensinger WI, Buckner CD, Anasetti C et al 1996 Allogeneic marrow transplantation for multiple myeloma: an analysis of risk factors on outcome. Blood 88: 2787–2793

114. Anderson KC 2000 Plasma cell tumors. In: Bast, Kufe, Pollock et al (eds), Cancer medicine, 5th edn BC Decker, Hamilton, 2066–2085

115. Corradini P, Voena C, Tarella C et al 1999 Molecular and clinical remissions in multiple myeloma: Role of autologous and allogeneic transplantation of hematopoietic cells. Journal of Clinical Oncology 17: 208–215

116. HM Lokhurst, A Schattenberg, JJ Cornelissen et al 1997 Donor leucocyte infusions are effective in relapsed multiple myeloma after allogeneic bone marrow transplantation. Blood 90: 4206–4211

117. Alyea EP, Soiffer RJ, Canning C et al 1998 Toxicity and efficacy of defined doses of CD4+ donor lymph for treatment of relapse after allogeneic bone marrow transplantation. Blood 91: 3671–3680

118. Orsini E, Ayea EP, Schlossman R et al 2000 Changes in T cell receptor repertoire associated with graft versus tumour effect and graft versus host disease in patients with relapsed multiple myeloma after donor lymphocyte infusion. Bone Marrow Transplant 25: 623–632

119. Kwak LW, Taub DD, Duffey PL et al 1995 Transfer of myeloma idiotype-specific immunity from an active immunised marrow donor. Lancet 345: 1016–1020

120. Carella AM, Champlin R, Slavin S et al 2000 Mini allografts; ongoing trials in humans. Bone Marrow Transplant 25: 345–350

121. Singhal S, Mehta J, Desikan R et al 1999 Antitumor activity of thalidomide in refractory multiple myeloma. New England Journal of Medicine 18: 1565–1571

122. Hideshima T, Chauhan D, Shima Y et al 2000 Thalidomide and its analogues overcome drug resistance of human multiple myeloma cells to conventional therapy. Blood 96: 2943–2950

123. Geitz H, Handt S, Zwingenberger K 1996 Thalidomide selectively modulates the density of cell surface molecules involved in the adhesion cascade. Immunopharmacology 31: 213–221

124. Haslett PAJ, Corral LG, Albert M et al 1998 Thalidomide costimulates primary human T lymphocytes, preferentially inducing proliferation, cytokine production, and cytokine responses in the CD8+ subset. Journal of Experimental Medicine 187: 1885–1892

125. Corral LG, Haslett PAJ, Muller GW et al 1999 Differential cytokine modulation and T cell activation by two distinct classes of thalidomide analogues that are potent inhibitors of TNFα. Journal of Immunology 163: 380–386

126. Vooijs WC, Schuurman HJ, Bast EJ et al 1995 Evaluation of CD38 as target for immunotherapy in multiple myeloma. Blood 85: 2282–2284

127. Stevenson FK, Bell AJ, Cusack R et al 1991 Preliminary studies for an immunotherapeutic approach to the treatment of human myeloma using chimeric anti-CD38 antibody. Blood 77: 1071–1079

128. Treon SP, Mollick JA, Urashima M et al 1999 Muc-1 core protein is expressed on multiple myeloma cells and is induced by dexamethasone. Blood 93: 1287–1298

129. Ozaki S, Kosaka M, Wakatsuki S et al 1997 Immunotherapy of multiple myeloma with a monoclonal antibody directed against a plasma cell-specific antigen, HM1.24. Blood 90: 3179–3186

130. Klein B, Widjenes J, Zhang XG et al 1991 Murine anti interleukin 6 monoclonal antibody therapy for a patient with plasma cell leukaemia. Blood 78: 1198–1204

131. Tsunernari T, Koishihara Y, Nakamura A et al 1997 New xenograft model of multiple myeloma and efficacy of a humanised antibody against human interleukin 6 receptor. Blood 90: 2437–2444

132. Suzuki H, Yasukawa K, Saito T et al 1992 Anti human interleukin 6 receptor antibody inhibits human myeloma growth *in vivo*. European Journal of Immunology 22: 1989–1993

133. Moss P, Gillespie G, Frodsham P et al 1996 Clonal populations of CD4+ and CD8+ T cells in multiple myeloma and paraprotinemia. Blood 87: 3297–3306

134. Dianzani U, Pileri A, Boccadoro M et al 1988 Activated idiotype-reactive cells in suppressor/cytotoxic subpopulations of monoclonal gammopathies: correlation with diagnosis and disease status. Blood 72: 1064–1068

135. Lefvert AK, Yi Q, Osterborg A et al 1995 Idiotypic reactive T cell subsets and tumour load in monoclonal gammopathies. Blood 86: 3043–3049

136. Stevenson FK, Link CJ, Traynor A et al 1999 DNA vaccination against multiple myeloma. Seminars in Hematology 36 (suppl 1): 38–42

137. Reichardt VL, Okada CY, Liso A et al 1999 Idiotype vaccination using dendritic cells after autologous peripheral blood stem cell transplantation for multiple myeloma – a feasibility study. Blood 93: 2411–2419

138. Raje N, Hideshima T, Teoh G et al 1999 Multiple myeloma/dendritic cell fusions as a vaccination strategy for multiple myeloma. Blood 94 (suppl 1): 538

139. Schultze JL, Anderson KC, Gilleece MH et al 1998 Autologous adoptive T cell transfer for a patient with plasma cell leukemia: results of a pilot phase 1 trial. Blood 92 (suppl 1): 446

140. Axelsson U, Bachmann R, Hallen J 1966 Frequency of pathological proteins in 6995 sera from an adult population. Acta Medica Scandinavica 179: 235–247

141. Kyle RA, Finkelstein S, Elveback LR et al 1972 Incidence of monoclonal proteins in a Minnesota community with a cluster of multiple myeloma. Blood 40: 719–724

142. Drach J, Angerler J, Schuster J et al 1995 Interphase fluorescence *in situ* hybridisation identifies chromosomal abnormalities in plasma cells from patients with monoclonal gammopathy if undetermined significance. Blood 86: 3915–3921

143. Kyle RA 1993 Benign monoclonal gammopathy – after 20–35 years of follow up. Mayo Clinic Proceedings 68: 26–36

144. Garcia-Sanz R, Orfao A, Gonzalez M et al 1999 Primary plasma cell leukemia: clinical, immunophenotypic, DNA ploidy and cytogenetic characteristics. Blood 93: 1032–1037

145. Noel P, Kyle RA 1987 Plasma cell leukaemia: an evaluation of response to therapy. American Journal of Medicine 83: 1062–1068

146. Dimopoulos MA, Palumbo A, Delasalle KB et al 1994 Primary plasma cell leukemia. British Journal of Haematology 88: 754–759

147. Dimopoulos MA, Kiamouris C, Moulopoulos LA 1999 Solitary plasmacytoma of bone and extramedullary plasmacytoma. Hematology and Oncology Clinics of North America 13: 1249–1257

148. Knowling MA, Harwood AR, Bergsagel DE 1983 Comparison of extramedullary plasmacytomas with solitary and multiple plasma cell tumors of bone. Journal of Clinical Oncology 1: 255–262

149. Liebross RH, Ha CS, Cox JD et al 1998 Solitary bone plasmacytoma: outcome and prognostic factors following radiotherapy. International Journal of Radiation Oncology Biology and Physics 441: 1063–1067

150. Frassica DA, Frassica FJ, Schray MF et al 1989 Solitary plasmacytoma of bone: Mayo clinic experience. International Journal of Radiation Oncology Biology and Physics 16: 43–48

151. Holland J, Trenker DA, Wasserman TH et al 1992 Plasmacytoma. Treatment results and conversion to myeloma. Cancer 69: 1513–1517

152. Moulopouos LA, Dimopoulos MA, Weber D et al 1993 Magnetic resonance imaging in the staging of solitary plasmacytoma of bone. Journal of Clinical Oncology 11: 1311–1315

153. Bardwick PA, Zvaifler NJ, Gill GN et al 1980 Plasma cell dyscrasia with polyneuropathy, organomegaly, endocrinopathy, M protein and skin changes: the POEMS syndrome. Medicine 59: 311–322

154. Iwashita H, Ohnishi A, Asada M et al 1977 Polyneuropathy, skin hyperpigmentation, edema and hypertrichosis in localised osteosclerotic myeloma. Neurology 27: 675–681

155. Dimopoulos MA, Panayiotidis P, Moulopoulos LA et al 2000 Waldenstroms macroglobulinemia: clinical features, complications and management. Journal of Clinical Oncology 18: 214–226

156. Wagner SD, Martinelli B, Luzzato L et al 1994 Similar patterns of Vk gene usage but different degrees of somatic mutation in hairy cell lymphoma, prolymphocytic leukemia, Waldenstroms macroglobulinema and myeloma. Blood 83: 3647–3653

157. Owen RG, Parapia LA, Richards SJ et al 1999 Waldenstroms macroglobulinaemia: bone marrow marginal zone lymphoma. British Journal of Haematology 105 (suppl 1): 89

158. Carbone P, Caradonna F, Granata F et al 1990 Chromosomal abnormalities in Waldenstroms macroglobulinaemia. Cancer, Genetics and Cytogenetics 61: 147–151

159. Louviaux I, Michaux L, Hagenmeijer A et al 1998 Cytogenetic abnormalities in Waldenstroms disease: a single centre study on 45 cases. Blood 92 (suppl 1): 184b

160. Iida S, Rao PH, Nallasivarn P et al 1996 The t(9;14)(p13;q32) chromosome translocation associated with lymphoplasmacytoid lymphoma involves the PAX-5 gene. Blood 88: 4110–4117

161. Kyle RA, Garton JP 1987 The spectrum of IgM monoclonal gammopathy in 430 cases. Mayo Clinic Proceedings 62: 719–731

162. Facon T, Brouillard M, Duhamer A et al 1993 Prognostic factors in Waldenstroms macroglobulinemia: a report of 167 cases. Journal of Clinical Oncology 11: 1553–1558

163. Gobbi P, Bettini R, Montecucco C et al 1994 Study of prognosis in Waldenstroms macroglobulinemia: a proposal for a simple binary classification with clinical and investigational utility. Blood 83: 2939–2945

164. Kyle RA, Greipp PR, Gertz MA et al 2000 Waldenstroms macroglobulinemia: a prospective study comparing daily with intermittent oral chlorambucil. British Journal of Haematology 108: 737–742

165. Leblond V, Ben-Othmann T, Deconinck E et al 1998 Activity of fludarabine in previously treated Waldenstroms macroglobulineamia: a report of 71 cases. Journal of Clinical Oncology 16: 2060–2064

166. Dimopoulos MA, Kantarjian H, Weber D et al 1994 Primary therapy for Waldenstroms macroglobulinaemia with 2-chlorodeoxyadenosine. Journal of Clinical Oncology 12: 2694–2698

167. Foran JM, Rohatiner AZ, Coiffer B et al 1999 Multicentre phase II study of fludarabine phosphate for patients with newly diagnosed lymphoplasmacytoid lymphoma, Waldenstroms macroglobulinemia and mantle cell lymphoma. Journal of Clinical Oncology 17: 546–553

168. Rotoli B, DeRenzo A, Frigeri F et al 1994 A phase II trial on alpha interferon effect in patients with monocloncal IgM gammopathy. Leukemia and Lymphoma 13: 463–469

169. Treon SP, Agus DB, Link B et al 2000 Rituximab is an active agent in Waldenstroms macroglobulinemia. Journal of Clinical Oncology 19: abstr 13

170. Desikan R, Dhodapkar M, Siegel D et al 1999 High dose therapy with autologous peripheral blood stem cell support for Waldenstroms macroblobulinemia: a pilot study. British Journal of Haematology 105: 993–996

171. Martino R, Shah A, Romero P et al 1999 Allogeneic bone marrow transplantation for advanced Waldenstroms macroglobulinemia. Bone Marrow Transplant 23: 747–749

172. Gilmore JD, Hawkins PN, Pepys MB 1997 Amyloidosis: a review of recent diagnostic and therapeutic developments. British Journal of Haematology 99: 245–256

173. Falk RH, Comenzo RL, Skinner M 1997 The systemic amyloidoses. New England Journal of Medicine 337(13): 898–909

174. Solomon A, Weiss DT, Pepys MB 1992 Induction in mice of human light chain associated amyloidosis. American Journal of Pathology 140: 629–637

175. Solomon A, Frangione B, Franklin EC 1982 Bence Jones proteins and light chains of immunoglobulins. Preferential association of the V lambda subgroup of human light chains with amyloidosis AL. Journal of Clinical Investigation 70: 453–460

176. Kyle RA, Gertz MA 1995 Primary systemic amyloidosis: clinical and laboratory features. Seminars in Hematology 32: 45–59

177. Skinner M, Anderson J, Simms R et al 1996 Treatment of 100 patients with primary amyloidosis: a randomised trail of melphalan, prednisolone and colchicine versus colchicine alone. American Journal of Medicine 100: 290–298

178. Hawkins PN, Myers MJ, Epenetos AA et al 1988 Specific localisation and imaging of amyloid deposits *in vivo* using 131 I-labeled serum amyloid P component. Journal of Experimental Medicine 167: 903–913

179. Kyle R, Gertz M, Greipp et al 1997 A trial of three regimens for primary amyloidosis: colchicine alone, melphalan and prednisolone and melphalan, prednisolone and colchicine. New England Journal of Medicine 336: 1202–1207

180. Gertz MA, Lacy MQ, Lust JA et al 1999 Prospective randomised trail of melphalan and prednisolone versus vincristine, carmustine, melphalan, cyclophosphamide and prednisolone in the treatment of primary systemic amyloidosis. Journal of Clinical Oncology 17: 262–267

181. Comenzo RL, Sanchorawala V, Fisher C et al 1998 Dose intensive melphalan with blood stem cell support for the treatment of AL amyloidosis; survival and responses in 25 patients. Blood 91: 3662–3670

182. Moreau P, Leblond V, Bourquelot P et al 1998 Prognostic factors for survival and response after high dose therapy and autologous stem cell transplantation in systemic AL amyloidosis: A report on 21 patients. British Journal of Haematology 101: 766–769

183. Cogne M, Silvain C, Khamlichi AA et al 1992 Structurally abnormal immunoglobulins in human immunoproliferative disorders. Blood 79: 2181–2195

184. Fermand JP, Brouet JC 1999 Heavy chain diseases. Hematology and Oncology Clinics of North America 13(6): 1281–1294

185. Seligmann M, Mihaesco E, Preud'homme JL et al 1979 Heavy chain diseases: current findings and concepts. Immunology Reviews 48: 145–167

186. Rambaud JC, Brouet JC Seligmann M et al 1994 Alpha chain disease and related lymphoproliferative disorders. In: Ogra P, Mestecky J, Lamm ME et al (eds), Handbook of mucosal immunology. Academic Press, San Diego, 425

187. Florin-Christensen A, Doniach D Newcomb PB 1974 Alpha chain disease with pulmonary manifestations. British Medical Journal 2: 413–415

188. Ben-Ayed F, Halphen M Najjar T 1989 Treatment of alpha chain disease. Results of a prospective study of 21 Tunisian patients by the Tunisian–French Intestinal Lymphoma Study group. Cancer 63: 1251–1256

189. Fermand JP, Brouet JC 1999 Heavy chain diseases. Hematology and Oncology Clinics of North America 13: 1281–1294

190. Wester SM, Banks PM, Li CY 1982 The histopathology of γ heavy chain disease. American Journal of Clinical Pathology 78: 427–436

191. Pred'homme JL, Bauwens M, Dumont G et al 1997 Cast nephropathy in μ heavy chain disease. Clinical Nephrology 48: 118–121

192. Brouet JC, Clauvel JP, Danon et al 1974 Biological and clinical significance of cryoglobulins. A report of 86 cases. American Journal of Medicine 57: 775–788

193. Monti G, Galli M, Invernizzi F et al 1995 Cryoblobulinaemias: a multicentre study of the early clinical and laboratory manifestations of primary and secondary disease. Q J M 88: 115–126

194. Invernizzi F, Pioltelli P, Cattaneo R et al 1979 A long term follow up study in essential cryoglobulinemia. Acta Haematological 61: 93–99

Abnormalities of hemostasis

Hemostatis: principles of investigation 473

Disorders affecting megakaryocytes and platelets: inherited conditions 493

Acquired disorders affecting megakaryocytes and platelets 525

Inherited disorders of coagulation 557

Acquired bleeding disorders 577

Natural anticoagulants and thrombophilia 599

Hemostasis: principles of investigation

24

DH Bevan

Introduction

Physiology of hemostasis applied to diagnosis

Primary hemostatis – formation of the platelet plug
Platelet adhesion
Platelet aggregation

Secondary hemostasis – generation of fibrin clot by the coagulation pathway
Clot initiation: the tissue factor/factor VIIa complex
Clot amplification: the 'tenase' complex
Clot propagation: the prothrombinase complex

Clot regulation and removal: the protein C and fibrinolytic pathways
Clot regulation: the protein C system and antithrombin
Fibrinolysis: the plasmin system

The clinical approach to the patient with a possible hemostatic disorder

History

Key questions
Surgical challenges
Epistaxis
Gastrointestinal or urogenital bleeding

Menstruation
Bruising
'Third space' bleeds
Summation and duration of bleeding episodes
Pattern of bleeding
Drug history
Family history

Clinical examination
Skin
Mucosae
Musculoskeletal system
Nervous system
Active bleeding

On defining the pretest probability of a bleeding disorder

Screening tests of hemostasis – two warnings
On venepuncture
On screening tests

Laboratory investigation of hemostasis

Tests of primary hemostasis
Screening tests
Diagnostic tests

Coagulation tests
Coagulation screening tests
Diagnostic coagulation tests

Introduction

The hemostatic system, a complex defense against bleeding, is critical to survival. Its integrity is compromised by inherited or acquired failure of its individual components, or by deregulation of the entire system provoked by organ failure, the inflammatory response, or exposure to cancer cell surfaces. Hemostasis also acts (in the wrong place, at the wrong time) as thrombosis. Bleeding is always a threat, while thrombosis increases due to age-related changes in coagulation factors and blood vessels to become the dominant hemostatic risk in later life.

The extreme complexity of hemostasis revealed by scientific scrutiny induces a degree of alienation in many clinicians practicing at the bedside and in the operating theatre. The hematologist must be their translator of basic knowledge into clinically useful advice, and guide to the increasing menu of potent drugs and biological agents available for the therapy of bleeding and thrombosis.

To do this work a reliable toolkit of investigational methods is essential. These include a focused approach to the patient's personal and familial medical history, a set of rapid laboratory tests to indicate the presence and general nature of any hemostatic malfunction, and the ability to extend this inquiry to measurement of specific proteins and analysis of DNA if required. The principle underlying these 'nested' methods of investigation is common to all disciplines in clinical pathology: provide data that increases (or decreases) the likelihood that a particular pathologic state – a diagnosis – is present and needs specific therapy or other intervention.

Hemostatic tests retain unique features and problems in interpretation. Even coagulation screening tests (the only commonly requested tests that require explicit co-reporting of control experiments) are complex bioassays in miniature. An abnormal value can have diametrically opposed meanings for patient care depending on the clinical context. Expressing clinical pretest probability in an intelligible way and using test results to modify this probability is the best way of avoiding potential confusion and error.[1]

The application of meta-analysis of randomized studies ('evidence-based medicine') to diagnostic laboratory testing has been limited,[2] and hemostatic testing is no exception. It is therefore not possible yet to claim evidence-based validation, in its strict sense, for many of the principles discussed below. However, the writings of many expert clinician–scientists over the years are the best guide we have to these principles, and should certainly form a starting-point for further analyses.

Physiology of hemostasis applied to diagnosis

The clinical approach to the patient who may have a hemostatic disorder is informed by knowledge of the physiology of hemostasis. Hemostatic reactions operate in a clock-like sequence, the first two phases being termed 'primary' and 'secondary' hemostasis.

A careful clinical history and examination (see below) can tentatively locate the potential defect in one of these phases, guiding the selection of initial investigations. The pretest probability of a defect involving primary hemostasis rises if abnormal bleeding follows a 'mucosal' pattern (see below), while a history of muscle or joint bleeding increases the likelihood of a coagulation deficiency. Disorders of the regulatory protein C pathway tend to manifest as venous thromboembolism. Abnormalities of the final phase of hemostasis, fibrinolysis, tend to contribute to bleeding in specific clinical settings, for example disseminated intravascular coagulation (DIC) and hepatic failure.

To assist this diagnostic thinking, it helps to keep in mind a simplified map of the hemostatic system, whatever knowledge of its complexity one possesses (or not, as the case may be). These simple maps are caricatures: readers are referred to fuller versions[3,4] and to other chapters in this volume.

Primary hemostasis – formation of the platelet plug[5] (Fig. 24.1)

Platelets, highly structured and excitable anucleate cellular bodies, circulate in the blood at a concentration of $150–400 \times 10^9/l$.

Platelet adhesion

Vessel wall damage provokes a variety of signals from damaged or activated vascular endothelial cells and/or exposure of the underlying subendothelial matrix. Platelets first adhere to the signaling site via adhesive ligands. The dominant interaction is between platelet membrane receptor glycoprotein Ib-IX and the giant polymer von Willebrand factor (vWF), particularly its most adhesive high molecular weight forms.

Platelet aggregation

Adherent platelets flatten and activate membrane fibrinogen receptors (glycoprotein IIb-IIIa) that bind

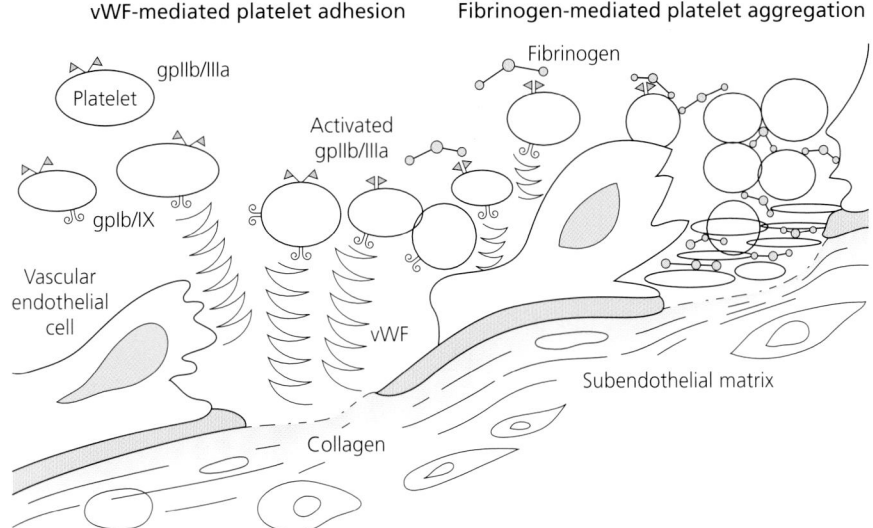

vWF-mediated platelet adhesion   Fibrinogen-mediated platelet aggregation

Fig. 24.1 Platelet adhesion and aggregation at sites of vascular damage (schematic).

plasma fibrinogen (Fb). The resulting syncytical platelet aggregate provides a reactive surface composed of platelet membranes. This activated membrane flips inside out, exposing the negatively charged phospholipid, phosphatidylserine (PS). By binding the tenase and prothrombinase complexes, PS allows coagulation reactions to proceed. This altered ('activated') platelet membrane is sometimes termed platelet factor 3.

Secondary hemostasis – generation of fibrin clot by the coagulation pathway (Fig. 24.2)

Unless underpinned by a fibrin net, primary platelet plugs disintegrate under the shear stress of flowing blood. The complex coagulation pathway that generates fibrin can be divided into three substages:

Clot initiation: the tissue factor/factor VIIa complex

The receptor tissue factor (TF), exposed on adventitial cells, activated endothelial cells and leukocytes in the damage zone, then binds and activates factor VII. TF/VIIa complexes bind and activate factor X. Resulting FXa moves to the platelet surface.

This is a regulatory 'decision point'. If this burst of FXa cleaves sufficient thrombin from its precursor (prothrombin), thrombin-mediated activation of the cofactors factor VIII and factor V, and the enzyme factor IX – together with recruitment of more thrombin-

activated platelets – assemble a 'critical mass' that allows coagulation to proceed. If thrombin generation falls short, tissue factor pathway inhibitor (TFPI) suppresses the TF/VIIa/Xa complex and coagulation is stalled.

Clot amplification: the 'tenase' complex

If the 'decision' is positive, sufficient FVIIIa and FIXa are formed to make the intrinsic tenase complex, in which FVIIIa acts as a rate-enhancing cofactor in the cleavage of FX to FXa by FIXa, providing a sustained source of FXa. The location of this FXa on the platelet surface enables it to move to the nascent prothrombinase complex.

Clot propagation: the prothrombinase complex

The surge of FXa forms prothrombinase complexes with FVa on platelet surfaces, speeding thrombin generation from prothrombin. Thrombin cleaves fibrinogen to form a durable fibrin clot, and binds to it, promoting further clot growth. This is a secure barrier against bleeding.

Clot regulation and removal: the protein C and fibrinolytic pathways

Two further systems regulate and eventually remove the clot (in the context of tissue repair and neoangiogenesis) (also see Chapter 28):

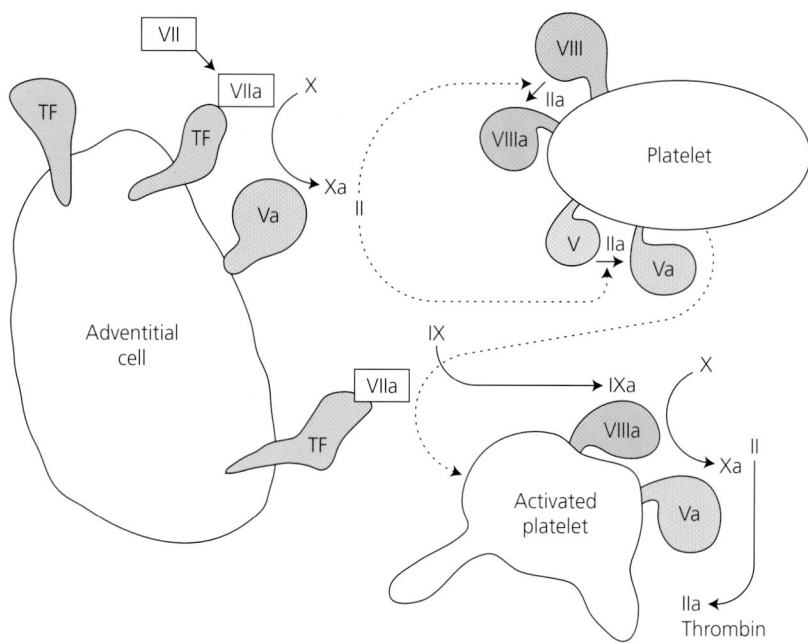

Fig. 24.2 Thrombin generation in-vivo: coagulation factor interactions mediated by cell surfaces (schematic).

Clot regulation: the protein C system[6] and antithrombin

Thrombin formed around healthy vascular endothelial cells puts a brake on coagulation by binding to a receptor, thrombomodulin, which retargets it to protein C. Thrombin/thrombomodulin activates aPC, which inactivates FVa and FVIIIa, slowing thrombin formation. To target FVa and FVIIIa in their membrane complexes, aPC needs a cofactor, protein S.

Thrombin activity is restricted to the platelet surface and the fibrin matrix of the clot by a conformation-dependent inhibitor, antithrombin (AT)[7] that inactivates fluid-phase thrombin. To work efficiently, AT must bind to heparin-like proteoglycans on healthy endothelial cells.

Fibrinolysis: the plasmin system[8]

Clots contain the seeds of their own destruction in the form of a clot-bound protein, plasminogen. This is cleaved by tissue plasminogen activator (tPA) secreted by healthy vascular endothelial cells, or urokinase on the surface of macrophages, to the fibrinolytic enzyme plasmin. Plasmin cleaves fibrin into fibrin degradation products, notably the D-dimer fragment specific to cleavage of cross-linked fibrin.[9] This removes the clot, and activates matrix metalloproteinases that initiate remodeling of vessels (angiogenesis).

One problem in the investigation of coagulation is the artificial nature of available laboratory tests, which commence by separating plasma from the very cell surfaces crucial to *in vivo* hemostasis – particularly platelets. These absent membranes are then simulated by adding back tissue extracts or recombinant proteins with properties similar (but rarely identical) to the physiologic substrates. In addition, as is seen below, the coagulation 'screen' – the crucial bridge between the clinical perception that something is wrong and its laboratory definition – invokes an obsolete model of hemostasis. A clear mental distinction must be made between the current model of *in vivo* hemostasis and the older model applied *in vitro*.

The clinical approach to the patient with a possible hemostatic disorder

If you prick us, do we not bleed?

Shakespeare, 'The Merchant of Venice'

The question of a possible hemostatic disorder occurs in two main settings. An individual is referred because they have presented with, or self-reported, clinical phenomena suggesting excess bleeding. Investigation can proceed in a structured elective style. In the second case, excess bleeding occurs acutely in a patient undergoing treatment in the hospital, emergency department or surgical theater. The tempo, urgency and completeness of the diagnostic work-up (before recourse to therapeutic action) are then different, but the principles are shared.

Experts writing about the investigation of possible bleeding disorders unanimously stress the importance of a carefully taken history.[10–12] They also recommend specific questions, answers to which alter the pretest probability of a bleeding disorder. The discussion below draws on this consensus. Similarly, key findings on clinical examination may aid the diagnostic process, although they are less frequent than narrative clues.

It must be conceded that these narrative and clinical signs have not been formally tested, either singly or in clusters, for their relative value in predicting the presence of hemostatic disorders. Such testing has refined and simplified the use of clinical clues in other contexts,[13] and may be of future benefit in hemostasis. Until such clarification becomes available, the shared insight of experienced clinicians is our best guide.

History

The role of the history-taker is to determine if the patient's account is consistent with excessive bleeding. After initial open questioning related to the presenting complaint, a systematic inquiry is made with the help of key questions intended to elicit quantitative information about the bleeding in question. People (including doctors) tend to over-estimate, by eye, volumes of blood lost from the body, so it is more informative to focus questioning on the duration of a bleeding episode and what had to be done about it.

Key questions
Surgical challenges
Dental surgery

Surgical trauma to the incompressible tooth socket sitting in the fibrinolytic milieu of the oral cavity is a stiff challenge to the hemostatic system. Useful questions about the effect of extractions focus on the duration of bleeding and the actions compelled by it. Compare the two accounts in Table 24.1. The second account gives a much clearer indication of excessive blood loss. Most people (in the UK, at least) are disinclined to make an early return to the dentist without a pressing reason.

Other types of surgery

Questions about blood loss after circumcision and tonsillectomy are traditional, but the timing and selectivity of the former, and decreasing popularity of the

Table 24.1 Two accounts of bleeding after dental extraction

1.
Q: How much did you bleed?
A: Loads. A cupful ... the pillow was red...
Q: The whole pillow?
A: Well, where my mouth was, you know...

2.
Q: When was the tooth pulled?
A: About 3 p.m.
Q: How long did the bleeding last?
A: Still going lunchtime the next day.
Q: What did you do?
A: I had to go back to the dentist. She put stitches in, but she wasn't happy, so she sent me to hospital...

latter, mean that only a small minority of individuals (or their parents) will give a useful response. As in the case of dental extraction, questions should focus on duration of bleeding and subsequent medical actions.

Many individuals are referred for investigation of a possible bleeding disorder as a result of excess blood loss after major surgery, although the commonest cause of this is purely 'surgical' – a transected blood vessel evading the hemostat. Large and/or late wound hematomata or generalized 'oozing' from a tissue surface or organ bed are more likely to indicate a hemostatic disorder. The patient's own recall of these events is likely to be hazy, and documentation of the amount, duration and clinical reaction to peri- and postoperative bleeding should be sought in the patient's medical records.

Epistaxis

Nosebleeds are a universal experience in childhood, so the usefulness of enquiring about them (nearly everyone will recall some) depends on the questions asked. In bleeding disorders, epistaxes tend to run 'like a tap' rather than to drip; require a bowl to catch the blood rather than a tissue; and resist arrest (or reroute via the mouth) on pinching the nares. Frequently recurring epistaxes that provoke multiple nasal cauterizations also increase the possibility of a bleeding disorder.

Gastrointestinal or urogenital bleeding

Rectal bleeding compels a search for colorectal disease even if a systemic bleeding disorder is present. Coumarin-induced rectal bleeding has led to the early detection and cure of cancers. Similar action must follow hematemesis, hematuria or vaginal bleeding. Occasional prolonged episodes of spontaneous hematuria occur in hemophilia, sometimes in mildly affected individuals.

Menstruation

As with other perceptions of bleeding symptoms by both sexes, women accustomed only to their own menstrual loss may not regard it as abnormally heavy. Bleeding for >7 days per month, bleeding that regularly 'breaks through' sanitary protection, the need to wear both tampons and pads (or double pads), and the need to protect the bed with a towel, or to cancel social engagements due to bleeding, are reliable indications of menorrhagia. Questioning should be sensitive and preceded by an explanation of its relevance.

Bruising

A sizeable minority of the population will answer 'yes' to 'do you bruise easily?' and many older people bruise the sun-thinned skin of their hands and forearms, so this question is not helpful. A semi-quantitative approach is useful: the bruises can be compared to some common object (in the UK the 50 pence coin, about 2 cm in diameter). Having frequent bruises larger than this is significant. Most normal ('simple') bruises occur on the outer surfaces of the upper arms and thighs, 'bumpers' in contact with the environment: bruises on the trunk, neck or face, or on the inner aspects of limbs are more significant, as are palpable bruises (hematomata). Solar or simple bruises are rarely pathologic.

A patient complaining of easy bruising who cannot show a single bruise at the time of the consultation, or one who agrees that there are fewer days with bruises than days without,[11] is less likely to have a bleeding disorder. Thrombocytopenic purpura crop around the ankles, where venous pressure is highest, and are more likely to be perceived as 'a rash' than as bruises.

'Third space' bleeds

In the hemophilias (inherited and acquired), over-anticoagulation with heparins or coumarins, and other systemic bleeding disorders, the presenting complaint may be hemorrhage into joints, muscles, or other deep tissue compartments. These events may not be perceived as bleeds by the patient or even by the attending clinical team, since they present with pain, swelling, nerve entrapment or other space-occupying features rather than with evident blood loss. By mimicking tumors, or presenting as acute monoarthritis, they may provoke biopsy or drainage attempts with potentially catastrophic results. In the context of anticoagulant therapy, failure to recognize such bleeds, and consequent 'pushing on' with heparin or warfarin, is equally dangerous.

The first-line clinicians called upon to deal with these events are rarely experienced in their recognition, so the best protection lies in local in-service education and guidelines, together with constant availability of hematologic advice and the freedom to access it.

Summation and duration of bleeding episodes

All types of blood loss should be summated. A patient with a credible history of significant bruising *and* epistaxis is more likely to have a bleeding disorder than one with bruising alone. Bleeding symptoms that go back to childhood or adolescence are likely to be inherited, and prompt a family history, while if recently developed they point to an acquired cause and a general enquiry for systemic disease.

Pattern of bleeding

A 'mucosal' pattern of bleeding episodes (epistaxis, menorrhagia, bleeding after dental surgery) may guide the initial investigation towards platelet and vWF analysis since it suggests a problem with primary hemostasis. Presentation with hemarthrosis or other third-space bleeds is classical in hemophilia. However, this is hardly a clear distinction, since hemophilia also causes mucosal hemorrhage and dental disasters: stating that menorrhagia is more likely in primary bleeding disorders than in hemophilia is tautologic. In general, it is necessary to perform at least screening tests (q.v.) of both primary hemostasis and coagulation in people who bleed too much.

Drug history

A full list of all prescribed or across-the-counter medication (including herbal and other complementary medicines) taken by the individual should be compiled. Aspirin remains the most prevalent agent causing bleeding symptoms and abnormal platelet function test results: in addition to being prescribed widely for its anti-thrombotic effect, it is a component of many preparations on sale to the public. Some of these preparations have names that advertize the presence of aspirin (e.g. Aspro®) while others (e.g. Nurse Sykes' Powders®) do not: a full list of such products is given in the British National Formulary.[14] Other non-steroidal anti-inflammatory agents share the aspirin effect. Antibiotics, major tranquillizers and antidepressive agents may all be associated with bleeding via antiplatelet function effects. Platelet function testing should be performed first with the patient taking the drug, then 2 weeks after stopping, in order to demonstrate its effect.

Family history

A reliable family history entails documenting a pedigree chart including all known family members with their names and dates. The key questions illustrated above are asked about each member in turn, seeking confirmation of any said to have a bleeding tendency. Any described as having hemophilia should, if possible, be traced to the Hemophilia Center carrying out their care: a relative famous for 'hemophilia' often turns out to have no evidence of the disorder at all.

Taking a family history of this quality is time-consuming, may take more than one session, and suits the elective better than the emergency setting. It often extends the individual's historical knowledge of their family beyond its limit. Furthermore, a negative family history excludes nothing, since many bleeding disorders, including severe hemophilia, occur sporadically.

Clinical examination

Skin

The whole skin surface should be inspected for purpura and bruising, documenting the distribution, size and age of lesions and correlating them with the clinical history. Palpation of bruises will detect hematomata, while palpable purpura suggests vasculitis. Close attention should be paid to the ankles, where venous and capillary pressure is highest: petechiae first appear here in thrombocytopenia, and signs of venous or arterial insufficiency may be evident. Large bruises (ecchymoses) typical of hemophilia or anticoagulant overdose may be found tracking into dependant parts of the body such as the scrotum.

The surface of lesions should be inspected. Edema may indicate the urticarial component of anaphylactoid purpura. Lesions of hereditary hemorrhagic telangiectasia may be seen in finger pulps and ear lobes, spreading over the face in later life. Bruises with abrasions or thermal trauma, that follow the outline of a blunt object, or are associated with other signs of abuse or self-harm may indicate non-accidental injury or factitious bruising.

Scars should be examined. Keloid formation might rule out a skin bleeding time. In Ehlers–Danlos syndrome they pucker like tissue paper on sideways compression, and may show central breakdown with fresh exudation. Poor scar quality may also be seen in hypo- or a-fibrinogenemia.

Non-hemorrhagic lesions mistaken for signs of bleeding include cherry-red Campbell de Morgan spots, stretch marks, livedo reticularis, and Majocchi's purpura or other 'dermatological' purpuras.

Mucosae

The oral cavity should be inspected for the petechiae or 'blood blisters' of 'wet' thrombocytopenia. Gingival bleeding is usually associated with gingivitis. Oral hemorrhage in the hemophilias occurs at sites of minor trauma or dental surgery, and may consist of a small but persistent bleeding point, a friable oozing clot, or a tumor-like sublingual swelling.

Musculoskeletal system

Joints should be examined for warmth, effusion, synovitis, reduced range of movement and misalignment. Muscle groups should be examined for wasting and contractures. These signs of cumulative damage due to hemarthrosis and intramuscular hematomas are characteristic of the hemophilias, but are also seen in rare disorders such as type 3 von Willebrand disease, deficiency or severe recessive disorders such as homozygous factor XIII, factor VII or factor X deficiency. Intramedullary hemorrhage of the long bones is a feature of afibrinogenemia and α2-antiplasmin deficiency, both very rare: it mimics lytic bone disease.[15]

Nervous system

Evidence of nerve compression injuries may be evident combined with damage to the musculoskeletal system identified above. Retinoscopy should be performed in all patients with purpura, particularly involving the oral mucosa: retinal hemorrhages indicate active CNS bleeding and the need for urgent therapy.

Active bleeding

The postoperative or traumatized patient with excessive bleeding should be examined for the signs itemized above, but sites of blood loss should be directly observed if possible. External losses, including those via surgical drains, should be assessed: dilution with tissue exudate can exaggerate blood losses. Similar over-estimation can occur in hematuria. If in doubt in either of these situations, a hemoglobin estimate on the drain fluid or urine can be helpful. Tracking hematomata should be sought. All intravascular access points, together with other skin incisions pre- or postdating the main episode of blood loss, should be inspected for evidence of bleeding or rebleeding after earlier closure. Fresh bleeding from such sites is a sign of DIC in its consumptive phase.

On defining the pretest probability of a bleeding disorder

Using information from the history and examination the clinician can work out a broad pretest probability (e.g. low, moderate or high) that the patient has a clinical bleeding disorder. The accuracy and precision of the history and examination described above in defining this pretest probability have not been tested by methods that have provided such information in other contexts.[13] Such studies are feasible and desirable in bleeding disorders, but even in their absence, a rational estimate of pretest probability is a crucial step towards interpreting the results of laboratory testing. Without it, tests of hemostasis can be frankly misleading.

Screening tests of hemostasis – two warnings

Armed with an estimate of pretest probability, the next step is to perform screening tests of hemostasis to generate further data capable of increasing or decreasing it.

On venepuncture

This requires a blood sample, which should be taken by an expert venepuncturist – especially in the case of a child – from a peripheral vein with minimal venous stasis. On no account should the jugular, subclavian or femoral veins be approached if there is any possibility of a bleeding disorder. Many inexperienced clinicians seem drawn to perform a 'femoral stab' on patients covered in bruises: this can result in a massive compartment bleed in the femoral triangle. Multiple attempts to obtain samples from the antecubital fossa can likewise result in severe bleeds. An expert hand is vital.

On screening tests

These tests 'screen' hemostasis, not people – a source of considerable misunderstanding and futile testing. They do not meet the epidemiological standard of true screening tests because they are not sensitive or specific enough to screen a population for bleeding disorder. They *only* work in concert with the history and examination as described above.

The 250 'clotting screen' requests typically made every day in a large teaching hospital represent educational failure. This futile attempt to screen the population entering hospital for surgery (or other intervention) for bleeding risk depends partly on misinterpretation of the ambiguous term 'screen'. Even more misleading – and potentially wasteful – is the lazy application of the term 'thrombophilia screen' to detailed testing for inherited and acquired thrombophilia (q.v.). When the term 'screen' is unavoidable, it is used below strictly to refer to tests performed as the result of a clinical history of bleeding or thrombosis.

Initial screening tests, usually applied whatever the pattern of abnormal bleeding, consist of a multiparameter blood count including the platelet count, and coagulation tests: a prothrombin time (PT), activated partial thromboplastin time (APTT), and sometimes a thrombin clotting time (TT).

If the pretest probability of a bleeding disorder is possible or probable, normal results in these initial tests should be followed by a skin bleeding time estimation or whole blood platelet function analysis. The need for further platelet function tests, specific assays of hemostatic proteins or genes, or further clinical tests for systemic disorders depend in part on the results of 'global' tests of hemostasis, but should also proceed if the full history is convincing, even if initial tests are normal. Below, tests of primary hemostasis and coagulation are grouped together for coherency, but they are also ranked into 'screening' and 'diagnostic' categories.

Laboratory investigation of hemostasis

Tests of primary hemostasis

Screening tests

The platelet count

Methods In the current laboratory, platelet counting is performed on an anticoagulated venous blood sample as part of the multiparameter 'full blood count' generated by automated cytometers. Current systems count particles of platelet-like size (2–$37\,\mu M^3$) by electrical aperture impedence or laser light scattering. To censor 'noise' at the low end and red cells at the high end of this range, devices fit a lognormal distribution curve to this raw count or otherwise manipulate it to calculate the reported platelet count.

The validity of the platelet count accordingly depends on instrument standardization, calibration and quality control: details of these procedures can be found elsewhere.[15] Because instruments count particles by size, blast cell fragments (in acute leukemia) or schistocytic red cells (in thrombotic thrombocytopenic purpura) may lead to over-estimation, and large platelets (in immune thrombocytopenia or myelofibrosis) to underestimation, of the true platelet count.

A commoner source of error in platelet counting is ethylenediamine tetracetic acid (EDTA)-induced platelet clumping, an *in vitro* artifact confirmed by microscopy of a blood film of EDTA-anticoagulated blood and a recount in citrate-anticoagulated blood. A low platelet count should also be checked by examining the specimen tube for clot formation.

Normal and abnormal platelet counts The normal ('Gaussian') reference range for the concentration of platelets in venous blood ('the platelet count') is 150–400 $\times 10^9$/l. By definition, 5% of normal individuals have platelet counts outside this range. To regard and investigate asymptomatic individuals with isolated, stable, mild thrombocytopenia (100–150 $\times 10^9$/l) as if they had a disease may be to confound 'Gaussian' and 'diagnostic' concepts of normality.[1] However, evidence to justify abandoning this seemingly unproductive practice is lacking.

By contrast, in a sick patient, *falling* platelet counts in the range 150–400 $\times 10^9$/l, or even from $> 400 \times 10^9$/l into the normal range, may indicate the early, reversible stages of dangerous hemostatic disorders (e.g. DIC or heparin-induced thrombocytopenia). A falling platelet count in the normal range may also be a clue to the presence of sepsis, falciparum malaria or other systemic diseases. Any fall of $> 50 \times 10^9$/l in a 24-h period should alert the hematologist and be communicated to the clinical team.

Correlating the platelet count with the clinical situation The action taken in response to the finding of a low platelet count depends on the presence or risk of bleeding, since the two are not always correlated. In many patients with immune thrombocytopenia (ITP), clinical bleeding may be minor or absent even at very low counts ($< 10 \times 10^9$/l), and precipitant therapy may not be necessary. However, the presence of mucosal bleeding in ITP indicates early therapy.

Lesser degrees of thrombocytopenia (20–50 $\times 10^9$/l) are dangerous when combined with reduced platelet function (e.g. antiplatelet agents, myelodysplasia, myelofibrosis); abnormal coagulation (e.g. DIC); leukemia (e.g. acute promyelocytic leukemia); cerebral vasculopathy in sickle cell anemia, or with severe anemia of any cause. In these situations, aggressive therapy including intensive platelet transfusion support is often needed.

When confronting a reduced platelet count, an apparently simple variable, potential laboratory error or artifact must be sought, and the platelet count must be placed firmly in the clinical context. These are core principles in all hemostatic testing.

Platelet function testing

If a history of excess bleeding suggests a defect in primary hemostasis but the platelet count is normal, or insufficiently reduced to account for it ($> 100 \times 10^9$/l), tests of platelet function are indicated. Recent technological developments have changed the range and sequence of tests applied for this purpose. It is logical first to perform 'global' tests of platelet function: skin bleeding time and whole blood platelet function analysis. If either or both give results consistent with abnormal platelet function, further definition of the defect by platelet aggregometry and other tests should be attempted. The limited sensitivity of these methods, and the myriad defects that can occur in the platelet's parallel activation, transduction and secretion systems,[16] often mean that no definitive diagnosis can be made outside a research laboratory. A degree of diagnostic uncertainty is tolerable, however, because therapeutic modalities for disorders of primary hemostasis tend to be broadly applicable across them all.

Whole blood platelet function analysis Many workers have attempted to develop devices that mimic (and therefore test) the linked phases of platelet adhesion and aggregation in uncentrifuged whole blood.[17] Recent automated devices appear to accomplish this in a valid and reproducible way. By eliminating the need to prepare platelet-rich plasma, they reduce both sample volume and the time needed to do the test. These methods appear to be more sensitive to subtle platelet function defects, possibly because they eliminate *ex-vivo* platelet activation during centrifugation.

The most widely used device is the PFA-100® (Dade-Behring)[18] which draws a citrated blood sample through paired filters impregnated with platelet agonists and measures the time taken by resulting platelet aggregates to occlude them, providing two numerical end-points. One filter contains collagen and adenosine diphosphate (ADP): occlusion of this (at the high shear rate achieved by the device) is dependant on vWF – platelet gpIb/IX interaction and therefore the vWF content of the blood sample. The second filter combines collagen with epinephrine, and the rate of occlusion tests platelet granule function and signal transduction. Occlusion of the collagen/epinephrine filter is also very sensitive to the effect of aspirin and other antiplatelet agents. Use of this device is now widespread in laboratories testing for von Willebrand disease and platelet function disorders. PFA-100 analysis, where available, is also tending to replace the skin bleeding time for evaluating the response of primary bleeding disorders to therapy with desmopressin, sources of vWF, or platelet concentrates.[18]

The skin bleeding time (SBT)

Previously a major criterion for the diagnosis of defects in primary hemostasis, prolongation of the skin bleeding time (even in its most reliable form, the Ivy template method) lost some of this status after being shown to lack sensitivity, reproducibility and operator-independence[19] in general use. In expert hands it can still produce useful evidence in equivocal cases,[11] and it remains part of the constellation of tests helpful in the diagnosis of von Willebrand's disease (vWD), although PFA-100 analysis is probably more sensitive.[18]

The Ivy method is recommended. A sphygmomanometer cuff is applied above the elbow and kept inflated to 40 mmHg to increase distal capillary pressure uniformly. Using a disposable device (e.g. Simplate®), a 5-mm long × 1-mm deep incision is made on the volar surface of the forearm, and a stopwatch started. Emerging blood is traditionally lifted off with the edge of a Whatman® filter paper, without applying pressure to the incision. The watch is stopped when the cut stops bleeding, and the time recorded as the SBT. Using this technique, an SBT > 10 min is abnormal, indicating a primary bleeding disorder.

Measuring the size of the blots, or further observation of the cut for rebleeding, are no longer thought to add useful data. The procedure is uncomfortable for many patients, especially children, and leaves a small scar even if properly dressed with skin closures. Patients should be warned about this before giving valid consent to the procedure. After one instance of reflex withdrawal of the forearm that extended the cut from 5 mm to 3 cm, the author always keeps one hand gently but firmly on the patient's wrist when doing this test.

Diagnostic tests

Classical platelet aggregometry

This elegant but demanding technique was introduced by Born.[20] Platelet-rich plasma (PRP) prepared by cen-

trifugation of citrated blood is subsampled into warmed plastic cuvettes, stirred, and exposed to platelet agonists in doses that provoke aggregation of normal platelets. Consequent aggregation (or the lack of it) is detected by increasing light transmission through the cuvette, the time-course and extent of which are recorded on paper in the form of a curve. Interpretation combines inspection of the shape of this curve with a value for % aggregation, 100% being taken as the difference in light transmission between stirred PRP and buffer solution ('blank').

Platelet agonists (collagen, thrombin, epinephrine, arachidonate) cause aggregation by binding to receptors on the platelet surface and provoking the platelet release reaction, or by serendipitous interaction with the gpIb/IX receptor and vWF in the patient plasma (ristocetin). The combined response of an individual's platelets to a panel of these reagents may form a pattern characteristic of a specific disorder (e.g. Glanzmann's thrombasthenia), a narrow differential diagnosis (e.g. Bernard–Soulier disease versus vWD), or a broad class of disorders (e.g. δ- and α-storage-pool disorders). Aggregometry is therefore indispensable in the diagnosis of severe platelet function disorders, but requires expert performance and interpretation.

In practice, the investigation of individuals with convincing histories of excess bleeding is often frustrated by normal findings using classical aggregometry. This suggests that the technique is relatively insensitive to mild platelet function disorders. In about half such cases, PFA-100® analysis (see above) detects a prolonged closure time, usually of the collagen–epinephrine filter.

Investigations of platelet granule structure and function

Measurement of the release of effector molecules from δ-granules (e.g. ADP by the luciferase method, or ^{14}C-serotonin release) or α-granules (e.g. β-thromboglobulin by ELISA) after platelet stimulation by agonists may further define disorders with findings on aggregometry or whole blood analysis consistent with storage pool disorders.

Transmission electron microscopy of platelets may demonstrate abnormal granule number or ultrastructure.

Fluorescence-activated cell sorting (FACS) analysis of platelets labeled with monoclonal antibodies specific for cell membrane epitopes (e.g. glycoproteins Ib/IX and IIb/IIIa) are useful in the diagnosis of Bernard–Soulier disease and Glanzmann's thrombasthenia respectively.

These techniques straddle the boundary between diagnostic and research laboratory methods. They are appropriate only for reference laboratories that have sufficient expertise, technical resources and experience to correctly interpret their results.

Coagulation tests

Coagulation screening tests

This venerable set of simplified bioassays is performed on platelet-poor plasma centrifuged from a citrated sample of blood. In the modern laboratory, coagulometers detect the assay end-point of fibrin clot formation by mechanical or optical means.

Prothrombin time (PT) and the international normalized ratio

As invented by Quick,[21] a source of tissue factor ('thromboplastin': an aqueous extract of mammalian brain or, increasingly, a recombinant version)[22] is added to citrated test plasma at 37°C and the mixture recalcified. Maximal stimulation of the clot initiation ('extrinsic') pathway results in clot formation in 12–15 s.

The PT depends on: (1) concentrations and activity of coagulation factors VII, X, V, II and fibrinogen in the test plasma; and (2) the sensitivity of the chosen thromboplastin to these activities and their inhibition. The PT is more sensitive to early-acting factors, particularly FVII, than to FII and fibrinogen (Fig. 24.3).

The end-point (clot formation) is timed and compared to the mean result obtained testing normal plasmas. If the PT (performed for diagnosis) is prolonged, a 50:50 mixing test (see below for the APTT) can be performed to indicate whether factor deficiency or inhibition is more likely to be responsible, although inhibitors affecting the PT alone are rare.

The PT is reported as a time (the control time coreported) or, increasingly, as a ratio (PT test plasma: PT normal plasma). Ratios obtained with different thromboplastins are transformed ('normalized') by the international sensitivity index (ISI) assigned to the test thromboplastin to correct for its sensitivity to factors VII, X and II by comparing its performance to that of an international reference thromboplastin.[23] The transformed ratio is reported as the international normalized ratio (INR):

$$INR = (PTpatient/MNPT)^{ISI}$$

where MNPT = the geometric mean PT of the population (in practice, 20 normal plasma samples).

The INR was introduced to harmonize coumarin anticoagulation, but it also functions as the prothrombin time for diagnosis ratio (PTDr) if a suitably sensitive thromboplastin is used. The closer the ISI of a thromboplastin to 1.0, the more likely it is to be reliable in both settings.

Interactions between thromboplastins and automated coagulometers performing the PT introduce more complexity. A large laboratory should not only determine its own reference range for the INR/PTDr, but also the 'system ISI' of its coagulometer/thromboplastin combination(s).[24]

INR > 1.2 indicates a defect in the TF/VII clot initiation pathway to thrombin. This could be due to deficiency or inhibition (anticoagulant or antibody) of any or all of factors VII, X, V, II, or fibrinogen (if < 1 g/l) (Table 24.2). Coumarin therapy rapidly reduces FVII levels and the INR is sensitive to FVII. The INR is therefore used to monitor coumarin therapy (therapeutic range 2–4).

Activated partial thromboplastin time (APTT)

This mini-assay of the clot amplification ('intrinsic') pathway was introduced by Langdell *et al.*[25] A phospholipid reagent that mimics the activated platelet surface (i.e. rich in PS,[26] although to supraphysiologic levels)[27] is incubated with test plasma at 37°C. Erratic contact activation is over-ridden by adding a strong activator such as kaolin, and the mixture recalcified. Sequential reactions provoked by contact activation in the presence of PS result in clot formation in 30–40 s.

Table 24.2 Causes of ↑ INR/PTDr (> 1.2)

Hepatocellular disease
Vitamin K malabsorption (cholestasis, steatorrhea)
Vitamin K deficiency (neonates, anorexia, hospitalization, intensive care)
Vitamin K antagonist (coumarins e.g. Warfarin)
Inherited deficiency of FII, FVII, or FX
Disseminated intravascular coagulation
Inhibitors to FII, FVII, or FX (autoantibodies or anticoagulants [e.g. hirudin, heparin])

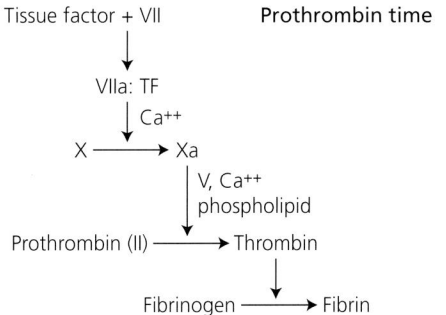

Fig. 24.3 Sequence of reactions in the Prothrombin TIme (PT) test.

The clotting end-point is measured by a coagulometer and expressed as the APTT in seconds, compared to the locally derived reference range. The APTT is also expressed as a ratio (APTTr) when used as a monitoring test for therapy with unfractionated heparin (UFH), and the use of this ratio in diagnostic work is acceptable.

This end-point depends on: (1) the concentrations and activities of contact factors prekallikrein, high-molecular-weight kininogen (HMWK) and factor XII; (2) the concentrations and activities of coagulation factors XI, IX, VIII, X, V, II and fibrinogen; and (3) the sensitivity of the whole test system to these activities and their inhibition. The APTT is more sensitive to contact and early-acting coagulation factors than to prothrombin and fibrinogen (Fig. 24.4). Elevated acute-phase proteins (factor VIII and fibrinogen) shorten the APTT and may obscure the effect of mild deficiencies and inhibitors in pregnancy and sepsis.

The APTT is an important test in three clinico-pathologic situations. First, it detects inherited and acquired hemophilia A and B because of its sensitivity to factors VIII and IX, and their inhibition, in plasma. Second, it detects the presence of 'lupus-like' (phospholipid-dependant) inhibitors because of its sensitivity to PS in the test reagent. Third, it detects the presence and concentration of heparin in plasma, and is therefore used to monitor unfractionated (but not low-molecular-weight) heparin therapy.

A reagent/coagulometer system sensitive to all three of these variables should be employed if possible, but the key function of the APTT – its role in the coagulation screen – is to detect hemophilia. Sensitivity to factor VIII and IX (i.e. the ability to detect levels of either factor below 45 iu/dl) is paramount, the practical convenience of a multifunctional APTT notwithstanding. A reference laboratory might opt for different APTT systems for different roles, rather than compromise any of them.

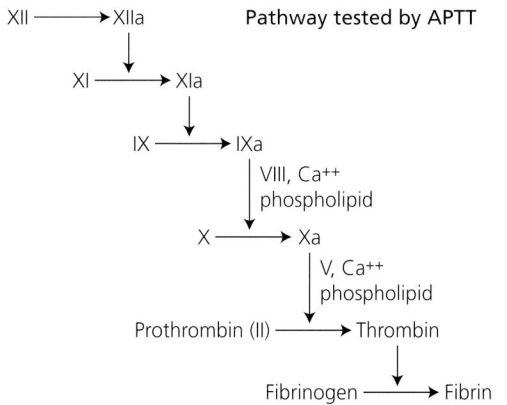

Fig. 24.4 Sequence of reactions in the Activated Partial Thromboplastin Time (APTT) test.

APTT correction tests

The sensitivity of the APTT to inhibitors of coagulation dictates that further information is gained by repeating the APTT on a 50:50 mixture of test plasma and normal pooled plasma. This correction test should be performed in most instances of prolonged APTT or APTTr not due to heparin therapy or contamination (see below).

A prolonged APTT due to contact or coagulation factor deficiency corrects on addition of an equal volume of pooled normal plasma to the test sample. For example, the factor IX content of a normal pool suffices to bring the mixture up to a level giving a near-normal APTT, even if the test plasma has < 1% normal factor IX. In contrast, an inhibitor in the test plasma will inactivate coagulation factors in the added normal plasma, preventing correction.

'Correction' has been defined as the APTT of the mixture 'being near to that of normal'[28] but using current reagents, most authors imply that correction of the APTT in a 50:50 mix means 'to normal'[12,29,30] (i.e. APTTr < 1.2). As with all coagulation tests, local criteria based on the performance of reagents and coagulometers and the experience of expert laboratory staff should be determined and applied. Since full, partial or absent correction (i.e. all possible results of the test) will all lead to more sensitive assays of coagulation factors and inhibitors, correction tests only indicate where to start.

If the clinical situation and/or screening tests suggest a possible factor VIII inhibitor, a modified method reflects inhibitor kinetics and identifies mild but clinically significant inhibitors. Unlike phospholipid-dependent antibodies, allo- and autoimmune anti-FVIII antibodies may need incubation with the target proteins for up to 2 h at 37°C to inhibit them. Extended incubation of the mixture therefore avoids illusory correction of a slow-acting inhibitor. An extra control (test and normal plasmas incubated separately and mixed just before testing) corrects for loss of factor VIII activity due to incubation alone.[31]

Classic mixing experiments

Correction studies employing absorbed plasma reagents, aged serum, or plasmas from patients with severe deficiencies, are popular thought-experiments in practical examinations in hematology. Laboratories that have the time, staff and expertise to prepare, store, and maintain stringent quality control of, a library of such reagents still find their differential correction of patient APTT a rapid route to specific diagnosis.[11] However, these requirements, and incompatibility with the automated coagulometers used to confirm the specific diagnosis of coagulation factor deficiencies, mean that they are no longer part of current routine practice. In any event, findings in classic mixing experiments must always be confirmed by specific factor assays.

Diagnostically misleading APTT prolongation

APTT sensitivity extends to components of the test plasma that are clinically irrelevant (prekallikrein, HMWK and factor XII) and the frequent contamination of coagulation samples with heparin from intravenous lines. The APTT is therefore prone to diagnostic false positives when used as an indiscriminate screening test in hospital practice, potentially causing delay and cost while the cause of a long APTT is tracked down. For these reasons, and its sensitivity both to states causing severe bleeding (hemophilia) and dangerous thrombosis (lupus anti-coagulant), the APTT can only be interpreted in the light of the clinical history (Table 24.3).

APTT detects UFH but not low-molecular-weight heparins (LMWH). APTTr monitors UFH therapy (therapeutic range APTTr 1.5–2.5). Samples taken via heparin-flushed lines are useless: heparin cannot be flushed out.

Thrombin time (TT)

This simple test (Fig. 24.5) adds thrombin to test plasma and times the resulting clot end-point. TT is expressed in seconds and compared to a normal control range (e.g. TT 15 s, control = 11 s). An abnormal TT (> 15 s) is due to: (1) deficiency of fibrinogen; (2) an inhibitor capable of

Table 24.3 Causes of ↑ APTT ratio (> 1.2)

Hemophilia (inherited FVIII or FIX deficiency)
von Willebrand disease (↓ FVIII due to reduced vWF carrier function)
Factor XI deficiency
Acquired deficiency of FII, FV, FVIII, FIX (e.g. consumption in DIC)
Acquired hemophilia (autoantibody to FVIII or FIX)
Contact factor deficiencies
Phospholipid-dependent ('lupus') inhibitors
Unfractionated heparin (UFH)

Table 24.4 Causes of ↑ TT (> 3 s > control)

Afibrinogenemia
Hypofibrinogenemia
Dysfibrinogenemia
Inhibitors of fibrin polymerization: paraproteins, fibrin–fibrinogen degradation products (FDPs)
Heparin (unfractionated)

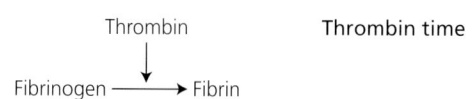

Fig. 24.5 The Thrombin Time (TT) test reaction.

inhibiting exogenous thrombin (e.g. heparin, hirudin); or (3) inhibition of fibrinogen polymerization due to an abnormal fibrinogen molecule (dysfibrinogenemia) or interfering substances (fibrin/fibrinogen degradation products, paraproteins). Some laboratories add calcium to the thrombin solution used in the TT to narrow the normal range and improve reproducibility, but this entails a loss of sensitivity to dysfibrinogens and is not recommended.

Heparin interference with coagulation screening tests: the reptilase time

Heparin contamination is common in samples from wards, theaters and intensive care units – anywhere that intravenous access devices are used for blood sampling. It is therefore reasonable to exclude it before pursuing a diagnosis of DIC (see below), which it mimics. Reptilase (the venom of *Bothrops atrox*) clots fibrinogen in a heparin-insensitive way while retaining sensitivity to other abnormalities that prolong the TT. A reptilase time (normal 10–12 s) is therefore a helpful and necessary adjunct to the coagulation screen.

Fibrinogen assay

Measuring the concentration of fibrinogen in plasma can be regarded as an extension of the initial coagulation screen: the PT and APTT are relatively insensitive to moderate hypofibrinogenemia and a prolonged TT requires explanation if heparin contamination has been excluded by a reptilase time. The most reliable method for the automated routine laboratory is the Clauss method,[32] a parallel-line bioassay based on the TT performed on serial dilutions of patient plasma and control. Fibrinogen estimates 'derived' from automated PT or APTT analysis can be misleading in the very states (e.g. DIC) in which fibrinogen assay is most useful, and are not recommended.

Fibrin–fibrinogen degradation products (FDPs) and D-dimer assay

In several clinical situations it is helpful to detect the presence of plasmin-digested cleavage products of cross-linked fibrin and fibrinogen termed fibrin–fibrinogen degradation products (FDP). An elevated FDP concentration (> 100 mg/ml) suggests DIC (see below) or rarer primary fibrinolytic states.

A variety of commercial immunoassays use polyclonal antibodies to detect and quantify molecules expressing fibrinogen epitopes, for example by coated latex bead agglutination. These include native fibrinogen and its direct plasmin cleavage products, as well as fragments that signify plasmin digestion of intravascular fibrin. This lack of specificity necessitates testing serum produced by *ex vivo* clotting in the presence of an inhibitor of fibrinolysis (e.g. aprotinin) to prevent *ex vivo* generation of FDP, requiring a separate and specific FDP sample tube.

Recently developed assays employ monoclonal antibodies that recognize the D-dimer fragment produced by plasmin digestion of cross-linked fibrin (i.e. thrombus).[11] The increased sensitivity and specificity of this assay allows detection of the relatively low levels of D-dimer circulating in the presence of deep vein thrombosis and pulmonary embolism (venous thromboembolic disease, VTED). D-dimer assay combined with the pretest probability estimate derived from a clinical scoring system is useful in the diagnosis of VTED.[33] Since the D-dimer assay retains sensitivity to DIC and uses the citrated coagulation screen sample it has largely replaced older polyspecific assays for serum FDP.

Logical use of the coagulation screen

Combining the results of the PT, APTT and TT tests, and using them as a logical 'circuit tester' (see Fig. 24.6) maximizes the information provided by the coagulation screen, particularly when considered with the platelet count. The logic of the coagulation screen combined with platelet testing has been expressed in algorithmic form[34] and as a web-based interactive computer program,[35] but is probably straightforward enough to keep in one's head.

For example, if the APTT ratio is increased and corrects to normal with 50:50 normal plasma, but the INR, TT and platelet count are normal, the probable deficiency is restricted to one of the factors tested only by the APTT: FXII, FXI, FIX or FVIII. The exact deficiency is determined by specific assays of single factors, starting with a factor VIII assay because this is the commonest cause of severe hemophilia (see Table 24.5).

A single gene lesion *typically* reduces the function of a single coagulation factor, and therefore *usually* prolongs a single coagulation screen test. Exceptions to this rule of thumb are, in the first case, genetic disorders causing

Table 24.5 Logical use of the clotting screen and pretest probability

A 66-year-old male bled for 48 h after surgery. Excess bleeding was noted from surgical drains *and* as a wound hematoma. Pretest probability of a bleeding disorder (from history and examination) ∴ = high

Platelet count = 245 × 10⁹/l

APTTr ↑ (1.9) corrects with 50:50 normal plasma. INR and TT normal.

∴ There is a deficiency (it corrects) of one or more factors tested only by the APTT: a contact factor, or clotting factors VIII, IX or XI.

Pretest probability suggests FVIII, FIX or FXI deficiency: all can cause excess bleeding after surgery. Contact factor deficiencies do not cause excess bleeding.

Specific activity assays of these factors are performed, starting with FVIII-C (the commoner of the two potentially severe deficiencies).

Result: FVIII:C = 190 iu/dl (normal 50–150 iu/dl)
FIX:C = 13 iu/dl (normal 50–150 iu/dl)

∴ The patient has mild hemophilia B (Christmas disease). This may not become manifest as bleeding until a major surgical challenge occurs, perhaps for the first time in later life. In the context of surgery no hemophilia is 'mild'.

∴ therapy is needed to raise the FIX level.

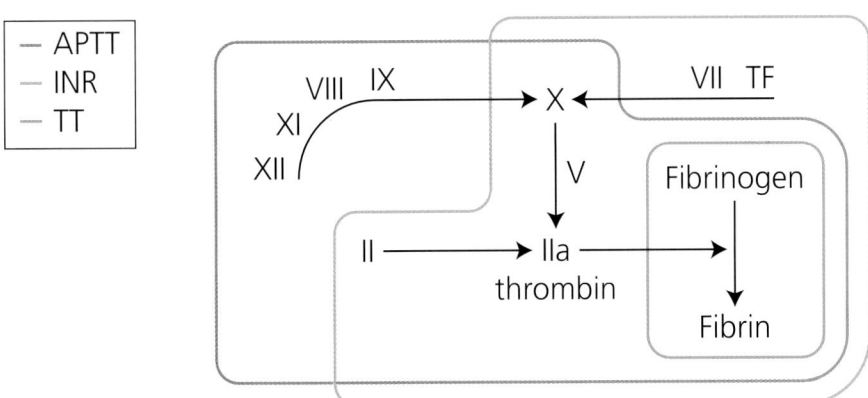

Fig. 24.6 The coagulation screen as a "circuit tester".

combined factor deficiencies (e.g. FV + FVIII deficiency);[36] in the second case severe FX, FV, prothrombin or fibrinogen deficiencies; these are all rarities.

In contrast, systemic diseases or drugs alter the synthesis, postsynthetic processing or function of several clotting factors and may reduce the platelet count. They are therefore reflected by abnormalities of several screening tests. For example, hepatocellular failure: (1) reduces the plasma concentration of all coagulation factors; (2) induces a hyperfibrinolytic state further consuming them; and (3) is often associated with portal hypertension causing splenic pooling of platelets.

The dangerous clinical disorder of hemostasis designated DIC also causes abnormalities in several screening tests because coagulation factors and platelets are consumed by chaotic activation of the whole hemostatic system. The APTTr may be misleadingly low in DIC, either because DIC is occurring on the background of an acute phase response (in sepsis or pregnancy) or due to circulating activated coagulation factors. Whenever the clinical situation and/or the pattern of abnormalities seen in the coagulation screen are consistent with DIC, an FDP or D-dimer assay (q.v.) should be added to the screen to detect the high levels of fibrin/fibrinogen degradation products characteristic of DIC. A fibrinogen assay should also be done to guide supportive transfusion therapy.

Heparin, by blocking the function of several clotting factors, mimics the effect of these serious global disorders of hemostasis by prolonging all three coagulation screening tests. It mainly confounds when samples for coagulation screening are drawn from vascular access devices flushed with heparin to keep them patent. Although such contamination can be partly excluded by performing a reptilase time test (q.v.), this causes delay in critical situations. It is better to establish a general rule that all coagulation samples must be taken by direct venepuncture.

Disorders of hemostasis that may not affect screening tests

von Willebrand disease (vWD) This common disorder may prolong the APTT, but this depends on a secondary effect on FVIII/vWF binding. Clinically significant type I vWD is often associated with a normal APTT. If the pretest probability of a bleeding disorder is moderate or high, whole blood platelet function (see above) should be measured. This procedure will also ensure that platelet function disorders, also 'silent' in the coagulation screen, are not missed. vWF assays should be done if whole blood platelet function analysis is not available.

Mild but clinically significant deficiencies of coagulation factors Depending on reagent/coagulometer system sensitivities, mild deficiencies (i.e. factor levels 10–40 iu/dl) may not be detected by the APTT. When normal coagulation screening tests and platelet function are found in the context of a high pretest likelihood of a clinical bleeding disorder, exclusion of factor VIII, factor IX and factor XI deficiencies finally depends on specific assays (see Table 24.6).

Factor XIII deficiency This transglutaminase stabilizes fibrin polymer by catalyzing fibrin cross-linking. Factor XIII deficiency, a rare autosomal recessive disorder, presents classically as bleeding from the umbilical cord stump or delayed bleeding after surgical challenge.

Clots formed from the plasma of individuals with severe factor XIII deficiency (< 0.03 units/ml) differ from normal by dissolving in 5M urea, monochloroacetic acid or 2% acetic acid. This simple screening test should be applied to individuals with a high pretest probability of a bleeding disorder who give negative results with all other tests, supplemented by more sensitive immunoassays for factor XIII.

Diagnostic coagulation tests

Specific assays of individual clotting factors

The final diagnostic step in the investigation of an individual with a potential bleeding disorder is assay of the biological activity and/or molecular concentration of individual coagulation factors in their plasma. Knowledgeable interpretation of the results of screening tests will narrow the range of likely defects and the first assays performed should follow this logic. This is preferable to 'shotgun' analyses because coagulation assays are expensive tests that consume the scarce resource of expert technical attention. Clearly, the labeling of an individual as having an inherited severe coagulation disorder has

Table 24.6 Final words on screening tests of hemostasis

If the clotting screen or full blood count is abnormal, refocus the history and examination (e.g. to look for malignancy or hepatic disease).

Clinical findings always take precedence over negative laboratory screening.

If there is moderate or high pretest probability of a bleeding disorder, ignore negative screening tests and proceed to assays of specific coagulation factors and platelet function.

If these in turn find nothing, refer the problem to an expert in the field of hemostasis.

such profound implications for them, their family and the healthcare system that the investigation must attain the highest possible degree of certainty at this stage.

Functional bioassays

The most clinically relevant assay of a coagulation factor tests its ability to promote clot formation in human plasma – its 'activity'. Testing function in a biological system (e.g. human plasma) is termed bioassay. In exchange for clinical relevance, the complexity of bioreagents imposes limits on accuracy and reproducibility. To keep these limits within tolerable bounds the use of a hierarchy of plasma standards to calibrate and control assays is essential, as is constant participation in quality control exercises. These are discussed in the next section.

The activity of a coagulation factor is determined by bioassay, in which the potency of the patient's plasma – its ability to correct the prolonged clotting time of plasma missing the factor in question – is compared to that of a plasma standard. Since the plasma standard has a known content of the factor, the unknown content of the patient's plasma can be calculated by comparison. The resulting activity is indicated by the suffix [:C], for example factor VIII:C.

If the calibration trail of the assay standard leads eventually to the current International Standard, the result can be expressed in international units (iu). Strictly, the activity of a coagulation factor in plasma should be expressed as iu/ml (normal 0.5–1.5 iu/ml), but is often expressed as iu/dl (normal 50–150 iu/dl) in order to match the intuitive convention of 'per cent normal'.

One-stage assays The simplest assay design is the one-stage method which depends on correction of the clotting time (e.g. using the APTT as the 'marker system' in a FVIII:C assay) of a plasma from which the factor in question is absent. This reagent is termed the substrate plasma. Individuals with severe inherited deficiencies remain a major source of substrate plasma (which accordingly is a potential infection risk), although the availability of commercial reagents reliably depleted of single coagulation factors by immunoadsorption has broadened the applicability of one-stage assays. As a result, because of their conceptual simplicity, adaptability to automation, and use of everyday (i.e. APTT, PT) reagents, one-stage assays are commoner in practice than more complex designs, except in special situations.

All one-stage assays share the same design apart from their marker system, which may be the PT (for prothrombin, FV:C, FVII:C and FX:C assays) the APTT (for FVIII:C, FIX:C, FXI:C or contact factor assays) or snake venom clotting times (Taipan for prothrombin [not in the context of coumarin therapy], Russell's Viper for FX:C).

Serial dilutions (at least three) of patient plasma are added to substrate plasma. The same is done with the assay standard. Clot end-points are measured for each dilution.

The manual method plots clotting times on the vertical axis against dilution on the horizontal axis, using logarithmic graph paper. This results in two 'curves' (which should form parallel straight lines) – a standard curve and an unknown (patient) curve. From the standard curve, a horizontal line ('of equal potency') is drawn to where it intercepts the unknown curve: a vertical line dropped to the horizontal axis from this point marks the potency of the patient plasma relative to the standard. Full descriptions of this method, including the requirements for parallelism on which its validity rests, can be found elsewhere.[37–39]

Even when controlled and standardized, it remains a bioassay with irreducible limits on precision and reproducibility. A single assay can only be relied upon to give an answer within 20% of the 'true' value (the idealized mean value of an infinite number of tests). This is one basis (the other being the variation of plasma FVIII levels in individuals) of the common rule that at least three assays (reducing the error to ± 10%) are required to define the severity of hemophilia. To reduce the error to ± 2.5% would theoretically require 64 assays.[37] These sources of within-laboratory error are compounded by inter-laboratory variance, which in external quality control exercises can give a CV (coefficient of variation) of 30–50%.[40]

In modern routine laboratories the potency is calculated mathematically by computer modules linked to automated coagulometers.

Two-stage assays This form of assay differs by eliminating the substrate plasma and phospholipid reagent of the APTT-based assay: instead, a reaction mixture is prepared (containing excess FIX and FX) in which the formation of factor Xa is proportionate to the concentration of FVIII:C or FIX:C in dilutions of unknown and assay standard plasmas as above. FXa thus generated is measured by its action in a second reaction mixture (using a clot end-point) or directly by its action on a chromogenic substrate (see below). Potency calculations are then carried out as for one-stage assays.

Chromogenic assays Rather than using a clotting end-point in a two-stage assay as above, the availability of synthetic amidolytic substrates sensitive to factor Xa enable the use of a color reaction detectable and quantifiable by spectrophotometry. This chromogenic method has been adapted to measure several hemostatic enzymes and their inhibitors, and is highly compatible with automation.[41] One theoretical advantage of the chromogenic method is that it directly measures the first product (FXa) of the FVIII/FIX interaction, rather than requiring the participation of several other factors in the production of a clotting end-point. This increases the precision and reproducibility of the assay. In addition, lack of dependence on phospholipid reagents makes the chromogenic method more reliable in the assay of therapeutic concentrates, both in the vial and in the patient.[27]

Immunoassays

Immunoassays use poly- or monoclonal antibodies to detect and quantify coagulation proteins. Except in the special case of 'functional' epitopes (i.e. immunologic determinants linked so closely to the functional site of a molecule that they are assumed to act as a reliable marker of its activity), immunoassays detect the presence of a protein rather than its function. Immunoassays may therefore give normal results in disorders due to loss-of-function mutations that result in normal or slightly reduced amounts of protein (e.g. type 2A vWD). However, immunoassay remains a cornerstone of diagnosis in vWD because of the continued lack of a reliable non-surrogate functional assay of vWF.

The ability to stick purified monoclonal antibodies to plastic or latex surfaces, together with ubiquitous chromogenic reactions derived from the alkaline phosphatase/anti-alkaline phosphatase (APAAP) method, have transformed immunoassay technology. Enzyme-linked immunosorption assay (ELISA) and recent latex agglutination assays are rapidly supplanting the older radiometric and immunoelectrophoretic methods (e.g. Laurell electroimmunoassay).[42] Such immunoassays are most often used in the diagnosis of vWD and thrombophilia (q.v.).

Molecular diagnosis in disorders of hemostasis

The diagnostic chain may now be continued to DNA sequencing and the direct detection of gene mutations or deletions affecting genes encoding coagulation proteins, particularly carrier detection and antenatal diagnosis in the hemophilias (q.v.). However, gene analysis has not yet become part of the standard clinical diagnostic criteria for coagulation and platelet disorders as it has for some types of thrombophilia.

The problem of testing the fibrinolytic system

The fibrinolytic system is of vital importance to the organism, and scientific investigation and exploitation of its components has led to important therapeutic agents with major impact in common life-threatening thrombotic disorders. None the less, it remains the 'Cinderella' of hemostatic testing.[43] Partly, this is due to the evanescent nature of most clinical disturbances of fibrinolysis. Compared to chronic disorders of coagulation, the fibrinolytic system rarely 'sits still' for long enough to study it. In addition, a fibrinolytic equivalent to the coagulation screen does not really exist: the euglobulin clot lysis time (ECLT) is insensitive and poorly reproducible. Immunoassays of key fibrinolytic enzymes and inhibitors are available, but interpreting their results in thrombotic syndromes is difficult and currently unproductive.[43] In acute clinical situations fibrinogen and D-dimer assays will give clues to the presence of hyperfibrinolysis. α2-Antiplasmin deficiency, the only well-documented inherited bleeding disorder attributed to chronic excess plasmin activity, does not declare itself in any screening test: clinical suspicion should lead to measurement of α2-antiplasmin by ELISA.[44]

Minimizing error in hemostatic testing, interpretation and process

The hematologist must identify potential sources of imprecision, error or misinterpretation in laboratory testing that could impede correct diagnosis and patient safety. Tests of hemostasis are fertile ground for such errors: no hematologist can afford to be a passive consumer of their results. Areas that require constant vigilance are:

The pre-analytical phase Traumatic venepuncture, stop-flow blood drawing, and suboptimal mixing or filling of sodium citrate-containing coagulation sample tubes are all potential sources of error. Polycythemia (by decreasing the plasma:citrate ratio) and anemia (the reverse effect) can alter results. Coagulation samples should be tested as soon as possible: any sample waiting more than 3 h (>2 h for FVIII:C assays) for analysis will give misleading results. Coagulation bioassays should preferably be done on fresh rather than frozen-thawed plasma, although pressures on the modern laboratory often prevent observance of this rule.

Test methodology Written standard operating procedures (SOPs) for every test in its repertoire must be held in the laboratory – and used. SOPs must be regularly updated and externally peer-reviewed as part of an inspection by an accrediting agency. Training must ensure observation of SOPs by all workers performing or validating tests during the laboratory 24 h cycle, and by operators of any point-of-care devices under supervision by the laboratory.

Test reagents and calibration: the hierarchy of standards Bioassays impose a requirement for reference materials, including thromboplastin reagents, assay standards,[40] and drugs. Plasma or concentrate standards are freeze-dried aliquots of plasma or concentrate with a certified content of the factor in question. These secondary standards are in turn assayed (calibrated) against primary International Standard materials held by national biological standards agencies such as the National Institute for Biological Standards and Controls in the UK, and ultimately the World Health Organization and other international bodies.[45] Tracing a calibration trail through this hierarchy of standards ensures that results obtained in different laboratories and in different countries are comparable.

Internal quality control and external quality assurance Laboratories must perform regular internal quality control procedures, particularly after introducing new tests, methods or machines or when established versions give cause for concern. They must also participate in external quality assurance schemes commensurate with their function: a Hemophilia Center laboratory would be expected to participate in an extended scheme that focused on assays of single coagulation factors, the detection and quantification of coagulation inhibitors, etc. Regular participation in the exercises provided by such a scheme registers a 'running score' of the performance of a laboratory that indicates the reliability of its results. This cumulative performance indicator must be available for inspection by the users of these results. The collated results of such exercises, published among users as surveys, provide useful information on the performance of current tests.

Potential confounding effects The influence of age on hemostatic variables must always be considered, and age-specific reference ranges consulted, particularly interpreting results obtained in infants and children, whose levels of vitamin K-dependant factors and natural anticoagulants differ from those in adults. Pregnancy, particularly during the third trimester and in the peripartum, is associated with marked changes in the levels of both procoagulant and anticoagulant proteins, with potential under- or over-diagnosis of hemostatic abnormalities. The ABO blood group status of an individual must be considered when interpreting vWF levels, which can also be affected by age, exercise, the acute-phase response, or needle-phobia. vWF levels may also change throughout the menstrual cycle, although this is not a universal finding.

Maximizing the clinical utility of hemostatic testing

New responsibilities: multidisciplinary audit and clinical governance It is no longer enough for the laboratory simply to issue a reliable test result. An additional responsibility is to provide the result to the end-user as rapidly as required and with all the interpretation required to maximize its utility.

A frequent practical problem, particularly in the investigation of mild bleeding disorders, is failure to provide a diagnostic decision even after a lengthy series of tests and repeat measurements. This situation arises most often when vWD or platelet function disorders are in question, and results in frustration for the patient and referring clinician. A patient left in diagnostic limbo may be subjected to delays in surgical or other treatment, or even unnecessarily exposed to blood products.

To minimize this problem, the diagnostic process (including confirmatory testing) should be planned and carried out as a single sequence, preferably under the supervision of a single clinician (nurse or doctor), rather than as a piecemeal affair subject to the vagaries of clinic appointments and changing staff. An experienced clinician should evaluate the resulting evidence, including personal and family histories, make a clear probabilistic judgement on the presence or absence of a hemostatic disorder, explain it to the patient and document it. In addition, a clear plan of action in the event of surgery should be formulated, even if this is merely to observe blood loss carefully, and communicated to the surgical team. By these means even patients in whom no objective cause can be found despite credible histories of excess bleeding can be helped.

The performance of the diagnostic pathway for disorders of hemostasis should be continually evaluated and improved by the multidisciplinary team, using the methods of clinical audit. In this way it is possible to avoid leaving patients and their physicians uncertain of the outcome of the diagnostic process.

Combining test results with clinical scoring systems Clinical scoring systems can be used to refine the crude pretest probability estimate described above. The most striking example of this in current practice is the combination of a simple but validated clinical risk assessment with laboratory measurement of the D-dimer concentration in a blood sample. The predictive power of this combination allows secure diagnosis and treatment of venous thromboembolic disease.[33] It is likely that similar combinations of clinical and laboratory methods would be valuable in other contexts. Validated clinical decision rules have great potential value in medicine,[1] and hemostatic testing stands to gain considerable value by inclusion in similar models.

REFERENCES

1. Sackett DL, Straus SE, Richardson WS et al 2000 Diagnosis and screening. In: Sackett DL, Straus SE, Richardson WS et al (eds), Evidence-based medicine, 2nd edn. Churchill Livingstone, Edinburgh, 67–93
2. Deeks JJ 2001 Systematic reviews of evaluations of diagnostic and screening tests. British Medical Journal 323: 157–162
3. Mann KG 1999 Biochemistry and physiology of blood coagulation. Thrombosis and Haemostasis 82(2): 165–174
4. Hoffman M, Monroe DM 2001 A cell-based model of haemostasis. Thrombosis and Haemostasis 85: 958–965
5. Ruggeri ZM 1997 Mechanisms initiating platelet thrombus formation. Thrombosis and Haemostasis 78(1): 611–616
6. Esmon CT 2001 Protein C, protein S, and thrombomodulin. In: Colman RW, Hirsh J, Marder VJ et al (eds), Hemostasis and thrombosis: basic principles and clinical practice, 4th edn. Lippincott Williams & Wilkins, Philadelphia, 335–353
7. Carrell RW, Huntington, JA, Mushunje A, Zhou A 2001 The conformational basis of thrombosis. Thrombosis and Haemostasis 86: 14–22
8. Bachmann F 2001 Plasminogen–plasmin enzyme system. In: Colman RW, Hirsh J, Marder VJ et al (eds), Hemostasis and thrombosis; basic principles and clinical practice, 4th edn, Lippincott Williams & Wilkins, Philadelphia, 275–320
9. Bounameaux H, de Moerloose P, Perrier A, Reber G 1994 Plasma measurement of D-dimer as a diagnostic aid in suspected venous thromboembolism: an overview. Thrombosis and Haemostasis 71: 1–6
10. Nilsson I-M 1987 Assessment of blood coagulation and general haemostasis. In: Bloom AL, Thomas DP (eds), Haemostasis and thrombosis, 2nd edn. Churchill Livingstone, Edinburgh, 922–932
11. Bowie EJW, Owen CA 1996 Clinical and laboratory diagnosis of hemorrhagic disorders. In: Ratnoff OD, Forbes CD (eds), Disorders of hemostasis, 3rd edn. W.B. Saunders, Philadelphia, 53–78
12. Greaves M, Preston FE 2001 Approach to the bleeding patient. In: Colman RW, Hirsh J, Marder VJ et al (eds), Hemostasis and thrombosis: basic principles and clinical practice, 4th edn. Lippincott Williams & Wilkins, Philadelphia, 783–793
13. Richardson WS, Wilson MC, Guyatt GH et al 1999 Users' guides to the medical literature: XV. How to use an article about disease probability for differential diagnosis. Journal of the American Medical Association 281: 1214–1219
14. British National Formulary 42. 2001 London: British Medical Association and Royal Pharmaceutical Society of Great Britain, 210
15. Groner W, Simson E 1995 Standardization. In: Groner W, Simson E (eds), Practical guide to modern hematology analyzers. John Wiley, Chichester, 95–117
16. Rao AK 2001 Congenital disorders of platelet secretion and signal transduction. In: Colman RW, Hirsh J, Marder VJ et al (eds), Hemostasis and thrombosis: basic principles and clinical practice, 4th edn. Lippincott Williams & Wilkins, Philadelphia, 893–904
17. Salzman EW 1963 Measurement of platelet adhesiveness: a simple *in vitro* technique demonstrating an abnormality in von Willebrand's disease. Journal of Laboratory and Clinical Medicine 62: 724–735
18. Jilma B 2001 Platelet function analyser (PFA-100): a tool to quantify congenital or acquired platelet dysfunction. Journal of Laboratory and Clinical Medicine 138: 152–163
19. Rodgers RPC, Leven J 1990 A critical reappraisal of the bleeding time. Seminars in Thrombosis and Hemostasis 16: 1–20
20. Born GVR, Cross MJ 1963 The aggregation of blood platelets. Journal of Physiology (London) 168: 178–195
21. Quick AJ 1940 The thromboplastin reagent for the determination of prothrombin. Science 92: 113–114
22. Tripodi A, Arbini A, Chantarangkul V, Mannucci PM 1992 Recombinant tissue factor as a substitute for conventional thromboplastin in the prothrombin time test. Thrombosis and Haemostasis 67: 42–45
23. WHO Expert Committee on Biological Standardization (1999) Guidelines for thromboplastins and plasma used to control oral anticoagulant therapy. Technical Report Series 889, forty-eight report, Geneva, Switzerland
24. Chantarangkul V, Tripodi A, Mannucci PM 1992 The effect of instrumentation on thromboplastin calibration. Thrombosis and Haemostasis 67: 588–589
25. Langdell RD, Wagner RH, Brinkhous KM 1953 Effect of antihemophilic factor in one-stage clotting tests. A presumptive test for hemophilia and simple one-stage hemophilic factor assay procedure. Journal of Laboratory and Clinical Medicine 41(4): 637–647
26. Kelsey PR, Stevenson KG, Poller L 1984 The diagnosis of lupus anticoagulants by the activated partial thromboplastin time – the central role of phosphatidyl serine. Thrombosis and Haemostasis 52: 172–175
27. Mikaelson M, Oswaldson U, Jankowski MA 2001 Measurement of Factor VIII activity of B-domain deleted recombinant Factor VIII. Seminars in Haematology 38(2) (suppl 4): 13–23
28. Austen DEG, Rhymes IL 1984 Laboratory diagnosis of blood coagulation disorders. In: Biggs R, Rizza CR (eds), Human blood coagulation, haemostasis and thrombosis, 3rd edn. Blackwell Scientific, Oxford, 175
29. Giddings JC 1980 The investigation of hereditary coagulation disorders. In: Thompson JM (ed), Blood coagulation and haemostasis: a practical guide, 2nd edn. Churchill Livingstone, Edinburgh, 48–116
30. Greaves M, Cohen H, Machin SJ, Mackie I 2000 Guidelines on the investigation and management of the antiphospholipid syndrome. British Journal of Haematology 109: 704–715
31. Kaspar CK, Ewing NP 1982 Measurement of inhibitor to factor VIIIC (and IXC). In: Bloom AL (ed), The hemophilias. Churchill Livingstone, Edinburgh, 39–50
32. Clauss A 1957 Gerrinnungsphysiologische schnellmethode zur bestimmung des fibrinogens. Acta Haematologica 17: 237–246
33. Wells PS, Anderson DR, Rodger M et al 2001 Excluding pulmonary embolism at the bedside without diagnostic imaging: management of patients with suspected pulmonary embolism presenting to the emergency department by using a simple clinical model and D-dimer. Annals of Internal Medicine 135: 98–107
34. Favoloro EJ 1994 Assessment of haemostatic function: follow up evaluation of abnormal screening coagulation tests and possible outcomes. Australian Journal of Medical Science 15: 39–45
35. Nguyen AND, Uthman MO, Johnson KA 2000 A web-based teaching program for laboratory diagnosis of coagulation disorders. Archives of Pathology and Laboratory Medicine 124: 588–593
36. Seligsohn U, Zivelin A, Zwang E 1982 Combined factor V and factor VIII deficiency among non-Ashkenazi Jews. New England Journal of Medicine 307: 1191–1195
37. Rizza CR, Rhymes IL 1982 Coagulation assay of VIIIC and IXC. In: Bloom AL, (ed), The hemophilias. Churchill Livingstone, Edinburgh, 18–38
38. Barrowcliffe TW, Curtis AD 1987 Principles of bioassay. In: Bloom AL, Thomas DP (eds), Haemostasis and thrombosis, 2nd edn. Churchill Livingstone, Edinburgh, 996–1004
39. Mannucci PM, Tripodi A 1999 Factor VIII clotting activity. In: Jespersen J, Bertina RN, Haverkate F (eds), E.C.A.T. assay procedures, 2nd edn. Kluwer Academic, London, 107–119
40. Barrowcliffe TW 1990 Standardization of assays of factor VIII and factor IX. Ricerca in Clinica e in Laboratorio 20(2): 155–165
41. Hutton L 1987 Chromogenic substrates in haemostasis. Blood Reviews 1: 201–206
42. Giddings JC 1987 Immunoanalysis of haemostatic components. In: Bloom AL, Thomas DP (eds), Haemostasis and thrombosis, 2nd edn. Churchill Livingstone, Edinburgh, 982–995
43. Bauer KA 2001 Conventional fibrinolytic assays for the evaluation of patients with venous thrombosis: don't bother. Thrombosis and Haemostasis 85: 377–378

44. Favier R, Aoki N, de Moerloose P 2001 Congenital α2-antiplasmin deficiencies: a review. British Journal of Haematology 114: 4–10

45. Hubbard AR, Rigsby P, Barrowcliffe TW 2001 Standardization of factor VIII and von Willebrand factor in plasma: callibration of the 4th International Standard (97/586). Thrombosis and Haemostasis 85(4): 634–638

Disorders affecting megakaryocytes and platelets: inherited conditions

25

JG White

Introduction

Structure

Disorders of megakaryocytes

Congenital megakaryocyte hypoplasia

Thrombocytopenia and absent radii (TAR) syndrome

Fanconi anemia

Disorders of platelets

Platelet organelle defects
Dense bodies – general aspects

Hermansky–Pudlak syndrome (HPS)

Storage pool deficiency (SPD)

Chediak–Higashi syndrome (CHS)

Alpha granules

Gray platelet syndrome

Alpha-granule, dense-body deficiency

Heterogeneous storage organelle deficiency

Enlarged alpha granules
Jacobsen–Paris–Trousseau syndrome

Lysosomes

Chediak–Higashi syndrome

Giant dense body disorder

Disorders of platelet membranes and membrane organization

Small platelets
Wiskott–Aldrich syndrome

Giant platelet disorders
Mediterranean macrothrombocytopenia
May–Hegglin anomaly (MHA)
Epstein's syndrome (ES)
Hereditary nephritis associated with May–Hegglin syndrome
Gray platelet syndrome (GPS)
Montreal platelet syndrome (MPS)
Bernard-Soulier syndrome (BSS)

Membrane inclusion disorders

Enyeart anomaly (EA)

Medich giant inclusion disorder

Summary

Introduction

The blood platelet is a deceptively simple cell. Though the smallest of the circulating blood elements, it derives from the largest cell in bone marrow, the megakaryocyte. Its diminutive appearance, lack of a nucleus and clear hyaloplasm (cytoplasm) made it difficult for early microscopists to recognize the platelet as a distinct entity.[1–4] As a result it was the last of the circulating cellular elements to be identified.[5] Anonymity, however, suited the platelet well. The cell prefers to remain nondescript, and seeks its refuge as far from the center of the column of flowing blood as possible.[6] Other blood cells carry oxygen, remove carbon dioxide, supply nutrients, transport waste, and leave the circulation to participate in immune and inflammatory reactions as required, but not the platelet. It remains as quiet as possible for its 10–12 day life span. If the cell can retire in the spleen without becoming involved in any of the useful activities served by other blood elements, the platelet's life can be considered a complete success.

Thus the platelet has no function in the circulation, except one: to keep blood flowing. It is the sentinel on guard at all times to react immediately with sites of vascular injury as soon as subendothelium is exposed. Within seconds platelets fill an injured site with a hemostatic plug that prevents further loss of blood and ultimately, with other cell systems, restores the integrity of the vascular system for normal blood flow.[7–10]

The platelet serves its function as the silent sentinel of the circulation very well, but, unfortunately, it does have a blind side. It does not distinguish its role in hemostasis from involvement in thrombosis. As a result participation of platelets in vaso-occlusive events leading to heart attacks, strokes or other ischemic phenomena often overshadows its value as the basic cellular unit of hemostasis.[11]

While normal platelets contribute significantly to hemostasis and thrombosis, abnormal platelets cause bleeding disorders that may express mild symptoms or life-threatening hemorrhage. The study of individuals with platelet-related bleeding disorders has been very important. Not only has it helped to provide appropriate treatment for the bleeding patient, but it has also greatly improved our knowledge of normal hemostasis and the mechanisms of thrombosis. The present chapter focuses on the inherited disorders of platelets and their parent megakaryocytes.

Structure

Before discussing pathology, aspects of normal megakaryocyte and platelet morphology will be considered. The megakaryocyte develops in human bone marrow from the same stem cell as do other cellular elements.[12] However, its transformation from a megakaryoblast into a multinucleated giant cell is unique. The nucleus undergoes a process of endoreduplication without cell division. As a result the cell enlarges dramatically and contains many unseparated nuclear lobes (Fig. 25.1). The final number of lobes is variable, but is usually 16–32. During this process of maturation the megakaryocyte begins to form organelles including alpha granules, dense bodies and lysosomes. The surface of the giant cell invaginates into the cytoplasm forming demarcation membranes, and converts the matrix into incomplete, platelet-sized subunits. Megakaryocytes may rest at stages during maturation, but ultimately complete their development and move to endothelial cells of the bone marrow sinuses. There they extend pseudopods between endothelial cells and deliver platelets to the circulation.

The product of this beautiful developmental sequence is rather unimpressive. It is the smallest of the cellular elements in blood and on peripheral smears resembles a speck of dirt rather than a cell. Yet, closer examination in

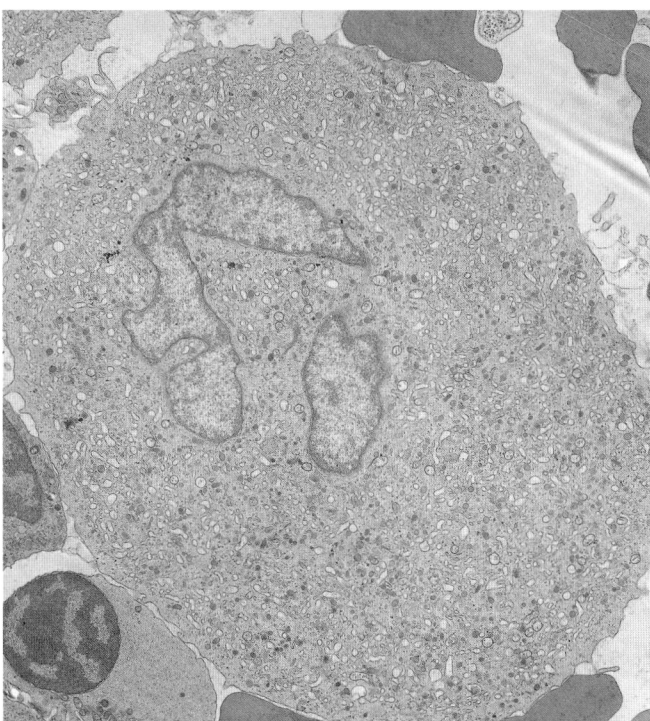

Fig. 25.1 Megakaryocyte. Human megakaryocyte from a trephine sample fixed immediately after removal from the needle. The large cell in thin section has a relatively spherical shape and smooth surface contours. Internal membranes and organelles are randomly distributed throughout the cytoplasm, but are separated from the surface by a thin margin. The appearance suggests a mature cell in the resting state, and not in the process of proplatelet formation or platelet shedding. × 4350.

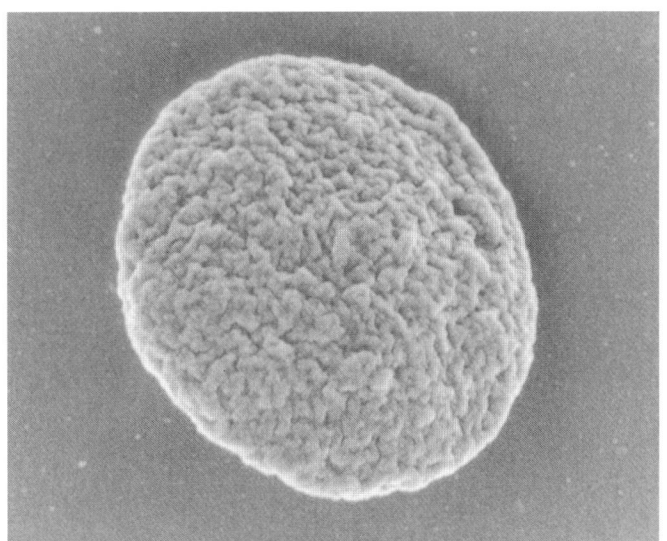

Fig. 25.2 Washed platelet from a suspension incubated at 37°C mounted on a 4 × 8 mm glass slide fragment, fixed with glutaraldehyde and dried by the critical point method for study in the low-voltage, high-resolution scanning electron microscope (LVHR-SEM). The cell has retained its characteristic discoid form. Convolution of the rugose surface membrane resembles the gyri and sulci on the brain. × 25 000.

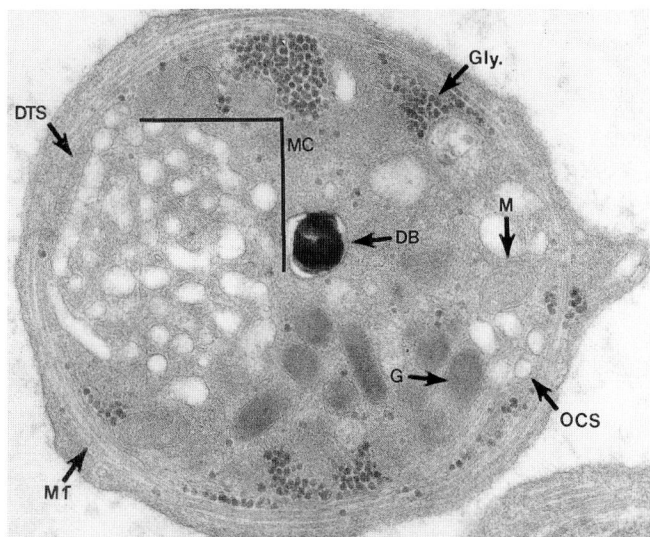

Fig. 25.3 Thin section of a discoid human platelet. A circumferential microtubule (MT) lying just under the cell wall supports the lentiform shape. Elements of the open canalicular system (OCS) and channels of the dense tubular system (DTS) are randomly dispersed in the cytoplasm and also closely associated in some areas to form membrane complexes (MC). Organelles, including alpha granules (G), dense bodies (DB) and mitochondria (M) are evenly spread throughout the cell. Gly, glycogen. × 37 000.

the electron microscope reveals that the platelet is a disc similar in appearance to the discus hurled by athletes. At high magnification in the low-voltage high-resolution scanning microscope the plasma membrane is furrowed, resembling the surface of the brain[13] (Fig. 25.2). Dimples appearing on the exposed surface and in replicas of freeze-fractured platelets are openings of the surface-connected open canalicular system (OCS). Thin sections in the equatorial plane reveal a circumferential coil of microtubules supporting platelet discoid form lying just below the surface membrane[14] (Fig. 25.3). A large number of alpha granules, a few dense bodies and occasional lysosomes are randomly dispersed in the cytoplasm, along with mitochondria and masses of glycogen particles. Elements of the dense tubular system (DTS) of channels are also scattered randomly with two exceptions. One channel is closely associated with the circumferential coil of microtubules (Fig. 25.4). Other DTS channels are interwoven with elements of the OCS to form membrane complexes (MC). The similarity of this organization to the sarcoplasmic reticulum of embryonic muscle cells has been noted.[15] Cytoplasm surrounding the organelles and other formed structures is a featureless protein matrix in thin section, but even in the resting state contains some actin filaments. Alpha granules are the most numerous of the formed organelles. They vary somewhat in size and shape, but are generally round. A nucleoid, more dense than the matrix of the alpha granule, is often seen in thin

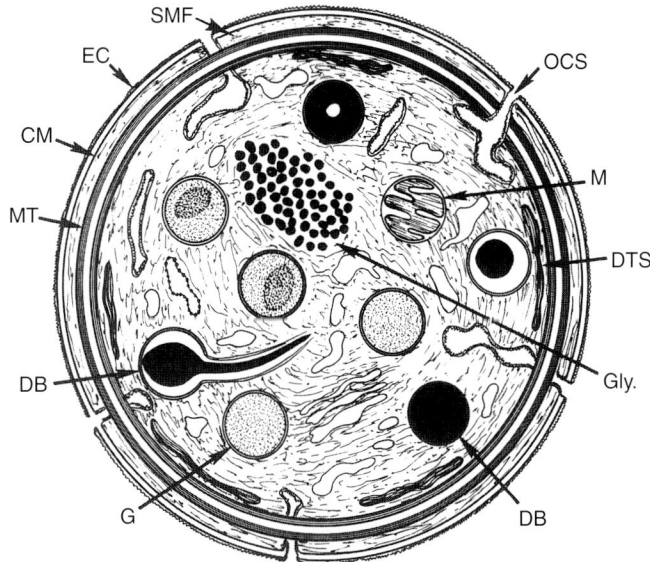

Fig. 25.4 The diagram summarizes ultrastructural features observed in thin sections of discoid platelets cut in the equatorial plane. Components of the peripheral zone include the exterior coat (EC), trilaminar unit membrane (CM) and submembrane area containing specialized filaments (SMF) which form the wall of the platelet and line channels of the surface-connected canalicular system (CS). The matrix of the platelet interior is the sol-gel zone containing actin microfilaments, structural filaments, the circumferential band of microtubules (MT) and glycogen (Gly). Formed elements embedded in the sol-gel zone include mitochondria (M), granules (G) and dense bodies (DB). Collectively, they constitute the organelle zone. The membrane systems include the surface-connected canalicular system (OCS) and the dense tubular system (DTS), which serve as the platelet sarcoplasmic reticulum.

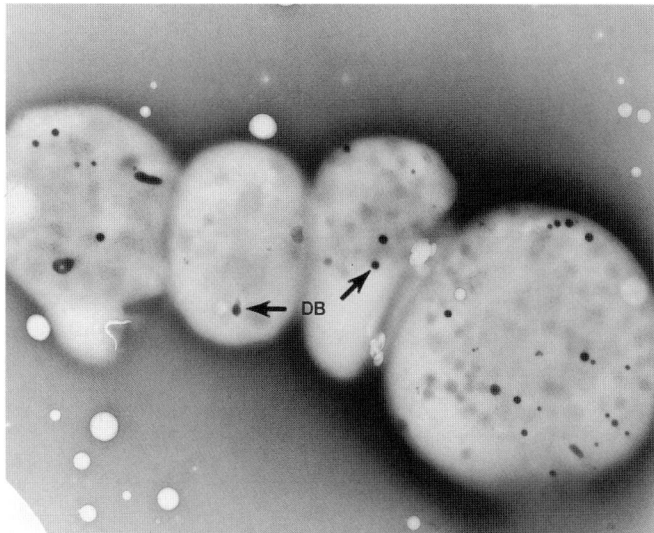

Fig. 25.5 Human platelets examined unfixed and unstained in the transmission electron microscope. Dense bodies (DB) inside the cytoplasm are inherently electron opaque, permitting visualization and enumeration by this technique. × 10 000.

sections. Cross-sections of a few tubular elements in the matrix are von Willebrand factor concentrated in alpha granules. Dense bodies often have a typical bull's eye appearance with the inherently opaque central core separated from the enclosing membrane by a clear space. The morphology of dense bodies, however, is extremely variable (Fig. 25.5). Some dense bodies have long, tail-like extensions or appear to be localized in alpha granules. The basis for the structural variation in dense bodies is unknown.

Disorders of megakaryocytes

In a very real sense, all of the conditions affecting the parents are visited on the progeny. Thus, except for immune thrombocytopenias, all platelet abnormalities are found in megakaryocytes. It has been easier in the past, however, to characterize the problems in platelets from circulating blood than on megakaryocytes from bone marrow. Defects in such conditions as the TAR (thrombocytopenia and absent radii) syndrome,[16] therefore, remain ill defined.

Congenital megakaryocyte hypoplasia

Amegakaryocytic thrombocytopenia and congenital megakaryocyte hypoplasia are rare conditions in newborn infants.[17] The cause for inability to promote conversion of stem cells into megakaryocytes is unknown, since some cases have had normal levels of thrombopoietin. Hemorrhagic complications may be mild or life-threatening. Steroids appear to be of little value, but supportive care and platelet transfusion may be successful in some cases until megakaryocyte production begins.

Thrombocytopenia and absent radii (TAR) syndrome[16-18]

Megakaryocyte hypoplasia is a characteristic feature of the TAR syndrome. The basis for the hypoplasia is unknown. Occasional patients will have a leukemoid blood picture, but this eventually disappears and megakaryocyte production increases. Chromosomal abnormalities have not been reported, but are undoubtedly present in this disorder. Circulating platelets in patients with the TAR syndrome appear normal.

Fanconi anemia

Most interest has focused on the anemia in this disorder, but it should be realized that Fanconi anemia is a major cause of heritable thrombocytopenia due to megakaryocytic hypoplasia.[19] It is characterized by the association of bone marrow failure and pancytopenia with other congenital anomalies affecting the musculoskeletal and genitourinary systems (see Chapter 13). While the congenital anomalies are evident at birth, the pancytopenia may be delayed for several years. Thrombocytopenia and megakaryocytic hypoplasia may be the first signs of impending bone marrow failure in Fanconi anemia.

Disorders of platelets

Inherited platelet disorders are, in reality, megakaryocyte disorders, as indicated above. The platelets have been studied intensively in these conditions while the megakaryocytes remain a mystery. Therefore our efforts in this chapter are focused on platelets and megakaryocytes are introduced where possible.

Platelet organelle defects

Dense bodies – general aspects

In 1951, Rand and Ried[20] found that 5-hydroxytryptamine (5-HT, serotonin) was a normal constituent of platelets, and Baker *et al*[21] were able to demonstrate that subcellular particles separated from platelets were rich in this amine, as well as in adenosine triphosphate (ATP). Many workers subsequently confirmed the observation of Baker *et al*[21] and added the findings that serotonin, ATP, and ADP were located either in vacuoles or the granule fraction.[22] The subcellular localization of 5-HT at the ultrastructural level, utilizing methods which had been successful in differentiating catecholamine-containing organelles in the adrenal gland, was reported by Wood.[23] Employing an initial fixation in glutaraldehyde followed by exposure to potassium dichromate at low or high pH, he was able to identify organelles rich in different amines, including 5-HT. One of the cells in his report which demonstrated localization of serotonin in very dense organelles was the blood platelet. The association of serotonin with dense bodies was confirmed by ultrastructural autoradiography[24] and by chemical determinations on isolated platelet subcellular organelles prepared by density gradient centrifugation.

An examination of thin sections of glutaraldehyde-osmic acid-fixed platelets in our laboratory revealed a different frequency of serotonin storage organelles.[25] An average of 1–1.4 dense bodies per thin sectioned platelet was found in counts on 100 cells from five normal human donors (see Fig. 25.3). Some sectioned platelets had no dense bodies in their cytoplasm. This deficiency, however, was compensated for by a significant number of cells containing 4–8 opaque organelles.

Evaluation of platelets by the whole-mount technique supported the findings made in thin-sectioned material.[26] Inherently electron-opaque dense bodies were easily counted in the unstained whole mounts (see Fig. 25.5). An average of 6.15 dense bodies per platelet was found with a range of 0–24 per cell in platelets from 10 donors.

The origin of platelet dense bodies has not been specifically defined. Early work had suggested that formation of the organelles was directly related to the uptake of serotonin.[23,27] Dense bodies were found only in circulating platelets, never in megakaryocytes. Later, however, it was shown that dense bodies are present in megakaryocytes from normal human bone marrows. If dense bodies are present in megakaryocytes, then some mechanism must exist for their development in the parent cell. Ultrastructural studies have suggested that such a mechanism does exist. Employing the uranaffin reaction introduced by Richards and Da Prada,[28] Daimon and Gotoh[29] confirmed the presence of dense bodies in megakaryocytes.

Hermansky–Pudlak syndrome (HPS)

The Hermansky–Pudlak syndrome (HPS) is a recessively inherited autosomal disease in which the triad of

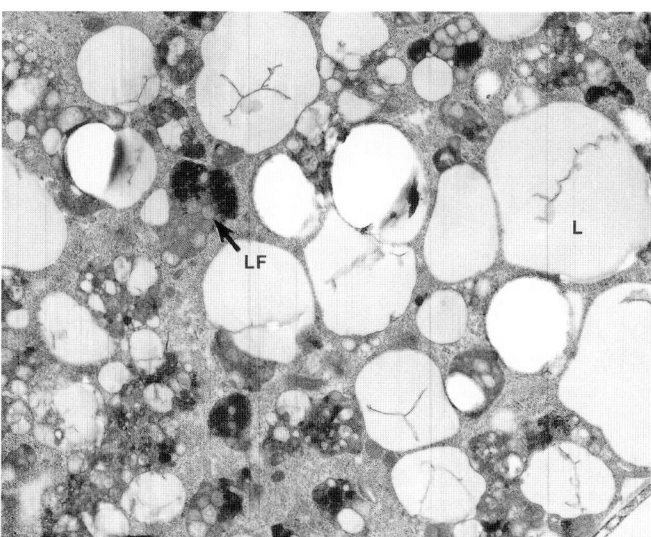

Fig. 25.6 Hermansky–Pudlak syndrome (HPS). Bone marrow macrophage from a patient with HPS. Erythrocytes and other cells are in various stages of digestion. Products resulting from their destruction include lipid droplets (L) and inclusions resembling ceroid-lipofuscin (LF). The appearance is similar to that of the 'sea blue histiocyte' observed in various storage diseases. × 11 000.

tyrosinase-positive oculocutaneous albinism, accumulation of ceroidlike material in reticuloendothelial cells of bone marrow (Fig. 25.6) and other tissues, and a hemorrhagic diathesis due to defective platelets are constantly associated.[30] HPS occurs in patients of diverse ethnic extraction. It has been observed in American Caucasian and black populations, Argentinians, Belgians, Canadians, Czechs, Dutch, English, Finns, Germans, East Indians, Irish, Italians, Japanese, Hasidic and Ashkenazi Jews, Mexicans, Poles, Puerto Ricans, Swiss and Ukrainians.[31] HPS occurs in isolates in Holland, Switzerland and Madras, India. It is estimated that HPS occurs in approximately 1 in 2000 Puerto Ricans in the northwestern quarter of the island. The pigmentary phenotype of Puerto Rican and non-Puerto Rican HPS patients is extremely variable. Some resemble tyrosinase-negative albinos with no clinically detectable pigment in skin, hair and eyes. Most have some pigment in skin, hair and eyes and resemble tyrosinase-positive, oculocutaneous albinos. A few have deeply pigmented skin and hair, but depigmented ocular fundi and resemble ocular albinos. However, all phenotypes include nystagmus, hypoplasia of the fovea, albinotic fundi, and decreased visual acuity.

Ceroid storage has been associated with restrictive lung disease, kidney failure and cardiomyopathy. However, not all HPS patients develop these problems. The youngest patient we have seen with storage disease was a six-year-old boy with restrictive lung disease and granulomatous colitis, while the oldest patient without clinical evidence of storage disease was 54 years of age.

The major cause of death in patients with HPS is fibrotic restrictive lung disease, which occurred in 43% of deceased subjects.[32] All deaths from this cause occurred between 35 and 46 years of age. The second leading cause of death is hemorrhage in the perinatal period or in mothers at delivery. Sixteen per cent died from this cause. While morbidity data show that 21.6% of HPS patients have evidence of granulomatous colitis, sequelae of this condition resulted in death in only 8.1% of the deceased subjects. Thus, 67.6% died from causes directly associated with the syndrome, while 32.4% died from causes unrelated to HPS.

A granular, yellow, autofluorescent material which resembles ceroid-lipofuchsin histochemically and ultrastructurally accumulates in tissues of HPS patients. The amount of accumulation is age dependent, and the tissues in which it accumulates vary in different patients. The organs most frequently affected and in which the largest amounts of material accumulate are initially the epithelium of proximal renal tubules and later the distal tubules with little in glomeruli or the collecting tubules, bone marrow macrophages (Fig. 25.6), spleen and liver, predominantly in the portal area and in Kupfer cells. Ceroid was stored in lysosome-like structures as a granular amorphous material or occasionally with a tendency to form curvilinear or fingerprint patterns. The amount of ceroid in tissues did not always correlate with the amount of tissue damage. Tissue damage was primarily limited to gut and lung, tissues normally associated with active macrophages.

As a result of their platelet defects, HPS patients usually have a mild bleeding diathesis with ease of bruising, epistaxis and prolonged bleeding following injury, delivery or tooth extraction.[30–32] Fatal hemorrhagic episodes have occurred and are often associated with the use of cyclooxygenase inhibitors such as acetylsalicylic acid. In previous reviews of ultrastructural defects in congenital disorders of platelet function it was suggested that HPS was the first disorder in which an abnormality detectable in the electron microscope could be correlated directly with a specific biochemical deficiency, impaired platelet function *in vitro*, and clinical bleeding problems in patients.[33] The population of electron-dense bodies in HPS platelets was greatly reduced and in some cases virtually absent (Fig. 25.7). Biochemical analysis revealed that HPS platelets had very low levels of serotonin and a marked reduction in the non-metabolic pool of adenine nucleotides. However, earlier studies had shown that neither serotonin nor adenine nucleotides were responsible for the inherent opacity of platelet dense bodies, but that a concentration of heavy metal, such as calcium, impaired passage of the electron beam.[26] Subsequent

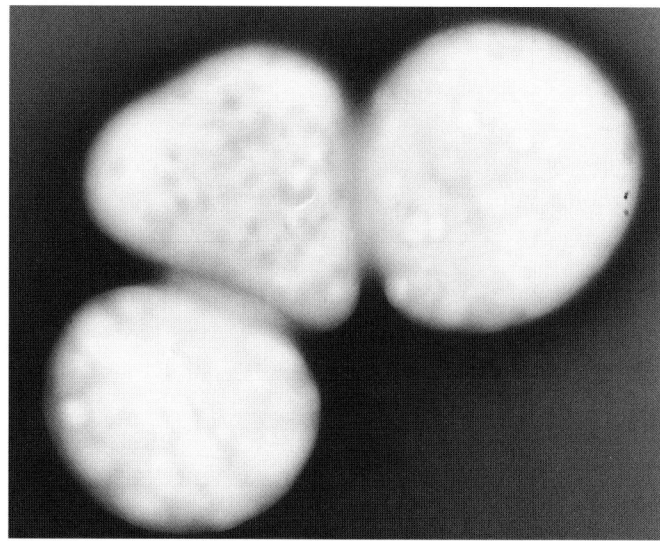

Fig. 25.7 Hermansky–Pudlak syndrome (HPS). Unstained, unfixed, whole-mount preparation of platelet from an HPS patient reveal complete absence of dense bodies. × 13 500.

studies have shown that normal platelet dense bodies are rich in calcium, and that HPS platelets contain significantly less calcium than do normal cells.

HPS platelets develop the same sequential changes as normal platelets when stimulated by aggregating agents, including shape change, internal transformation, and molding of cell surfaces together in tightly packed, small aggregates. Owing to the marked deficiency in ADP, the amount of nucleotide secreted by activated HPS cells is insufficient to bring uninvolved platelets into large aggregates and sustain the platelet–platelet association long enough to establish irreversible aggregation. As a result, HPS platelets do not develop second waves of aggregation when exposed to concentrations of ADP, epinephrine and thrombin, which cause biphasic, irreversible aggregation of normal cells on the aggregometer. However, they will form irreversible aggregates if exposed to a high concentration of exogenous ADP. In addition, they can form irreversible aggregates, in some instances, even when stirred with epinephrine alone.

Other defects reported in HPS platelets may be partly responsible for the elevated threshold of activation. Abnormalities in prostaglandin synthesis and formation of thromboxane A_2 have been noted. These have been related to defective malondialdehyde formation or decreased liberation of arachidonic acid from membrane phospholipids. The abnormalities may influence the aggregation response to arachidonate, although some patients have a normal response to this agent. Some have noted that secretion of acid hydrolases is delayed in HPS platelets, and the defect can be corrected by adding back ADP, a product normally stored in dense bodies. Thus, the defective function of HPS platelets may not be due to storage pool deficiency alone, but to other facets of platelet regulatory physiology that may be directly or indirectly involved.

Storage pool deficiency (SPD)

Patients with mild bleeding problems seemingly related to abnormal platelet secretion were recognized before the HPS was reported.[34] Weiss *et al*[35] described six members of a family in whom secretable ADP was decreased. They postulated that their aggregation defects might be due to a specific deficiency in the non-metabolic pool of ADP. Subsequent studies of this family and other patients with a similar history and laboratory findings confirmed that defective platelet function was due to platelet storage pool deficiency (SPD). The platelet abnormality in SPD is very similar, if not identical, to that observed in HPS, even though SPD patients have normal pigmentation and no evidence of ceroid-lipofuchsin storage. As a result, it is difficult to relate the absence of dense bodies in HPS platelets to defects in melanosome formation or storage of aging pigment.

Platelets from patients with SPD are normal in size and number. Structural features of their platelets are normal, other than the marked deficiency (Fig. 25.8) or absence of dense bodies. Weiss *et al*[36] pointed out that the deficiency of adenine nucleotides and serotonin is less profound in SPD than in HPS platelets, and often quite variable. The bleeding in SPD patients has been found

to correlate inversely with the dense body content of ATP and ADP, but appears more closely tied to the ADP level. Incubation of normal platelets with ^{14}C-serotonin results in rapid uptake of the amine and concentration in dense bodies. In patients with SPD, the initial rate of uptake is normal, but saturation levels are decreased.[36] Normal platelets retain ^{14}C-serotonin in dense bodies for many hours, while SPD platelets lacking dense bodies rapidly lose the radioactive amine. The lost serotonin is quickly converted to 5-hydroxyindolacetic acid and 5-hydroxytryptophal by monoamine oxidases.

Failure of SPD platelets to retain serotonin has been attributed to a failure to form metal–nucleotide complexes necessary to bind 5-HT. The reason they are unable to develop metal–nucleotide complexes, however, is unknown. The origin of dense bodies in the parent megakaryocyte was discussed above. It is possible that HPS and SPD megakaryocytes fail to generate vesicles from the Golgi apparatus destined to become dense bodies. If they do make them, the vesicles may be defective and unable to transport calcium, nucleotides, or both to their interior. Since a variable number of dense bodies are present in platelets from many patients with SPD, it is probable that they make the membrane precursor, but it does not function properly. The nature of the defect remains unknown.

Platelet storage disease (SPD) has been reported to be less frequent than HPS.[36] However, it may be more common. Since bleeding symptoms are mild and the pseudoalbinism and ceroidlipofuchsin accumulation characteristic of HPS are absent, individuals with SPD may not come to the attention of physicians. Also, the degree of adenine nucleotide and serotonin deficiency in SPD platelets is variable and usually not as severe as in the HPS, resulting in further moderation of the disease. As a result, many patients with SPD may go undetected during their lifetimes.

Weiss *et al*[36] have provided an excellent analysis of this condition. Of 18 patients with various granule disorders, four were found to have dense body deficiency without other clinical features of HPS. In at least one family the disorder appeared to be inherited as an autosomal dominant. The hemorrhagic symptoms in SPD patients were generally mild, and they lacked the severe gastrointestinal bleeding seen in some patients with HPS. Depletion of dense body contents and electron-opaque organelles was less in SPD platelets compared to individuals with HPS. Weiss *et al.*[36] noted that serotonin levels in SPD platelets were reduced in proportion to the reduction in platelet ADP. SPD platelets may also be deficient in their ability to synthesize intermediates of prostaglandin biosynthesis. After stimulation by collagen,

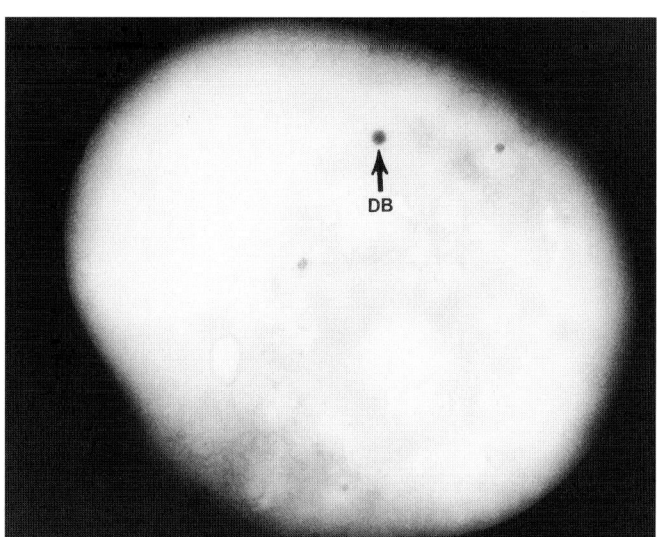

Fig. 25.8 Storage pool deficiency (SPD). Unstained, unfixed, wholemount preparation reveal a single dense body (DB) in one platelet. The frequency in this patient was one dense body for every 20 platelets. × 16 000.

SPD platelets produced less than 20% of the PGE_2 and PGF_2 synthesized by normal cells.

The decrease in dense bodies in SPD correlates with the deficiency in serotonin and adenine nucleotides, the impaired response of the cells to aggregating agents, and the clinical symptoms of the patient. Thus, SPD is the second disorder in which impaired platelet function can be directly associated with an ultrastructural defect in the cells. However, the normal pigmentation of individuals with this disorder and the absence of an unusual accumulation of ceroid or lipofuchsin in macrophages suggest that the cause is basically different than that responsible for platelet storage pool deficiency in HPS. The genetic basis for the SPD found in other inherited disorders, such as Wiskott–Aldrich syndrome[37] and TAR syndrome[38] remains to be determined.

Chediak–Higashi syndrome (CHS)

The Chediak–Higashi syndrome (CHS)[39,40] is a rare, autosomally inherited disorder characterized clinically by photophobia, nystagmus, pseudoalbinism, marked susceptibility to infection, hepatosplenomegaly, lymphadenopathy and malignancy.[41] Laboratory diagnosis is based on the presence of giant organelles in nearly all leukocytes on Wright-stained peripheral blood smears[42] (Fig. 25.9; also see Chapter 17). The massive granules have been found in neutrophils, eosinophils, lymphocytes and monocytes from blood and in their bone marrow precursors.[43]

Despite the presence of thrombocytopenia, which develops during the accelerated phase of CHS, and an early report describing two patients with markedly decreased platelet serotonin,[44] blood platelets have not been considered a major problem in this disease. However, several studies have shown that platelets express the genetic falut of the disorder.[45–47] Platelets from patients with CHS are biochemically, physiologically and functionally abnormal.[45] The defect has been related to a marked reduction in platelet-dense bodies.[48,49] Elevated levels of cyclic 3',5'-adenosine monophosphate (cAMP) were noted in platelets from one infant with CHS.[45] However, the level of cAMP was corrected to normal by treatment with ascorbate with out apparent improvement in platelet function.[50] Thus, the platelet appears to be involved in the expression of the CHS along with other blood cells containing cytoplasmic granules.

As attractive as these findings were when first reported, there is little enthusiasm for them at present. Elevations in levels of cAMP or decreased concentrations of cGMP were not found in blood cells of other patients with CHS.[51] Reversal of clinical symptoms by treatment

with large amounts of vitamin C has not been found in most patients with the disease. Observations of a decrease in microtubule numbers in CHS cells[52] that led to the studies of cyclic nucleotides and the suggestion to use ascorbate[50] to treat the disease were not confirmed.[51]

Involvement of platelets in CHS appears variable. A patient with characteristic clinical and laboratory features of the disease has been followed in this laboratory for 20 years.[53] His platelets are functionally, biochemically and morphologically very close to normal (Fig. 25.10). We

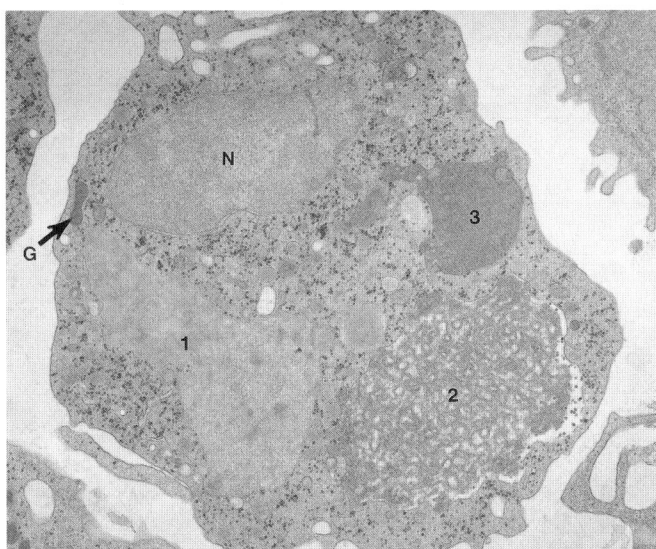

Fig. 25.9 Chediak–Higashi syndrome (CHS). Neutrophil from a patient with CHS. A nuclear lobe (N) and normal-sized granule (G) are dwarfed by greatly enlarged lysosomes (1,2,3). ×16 000.

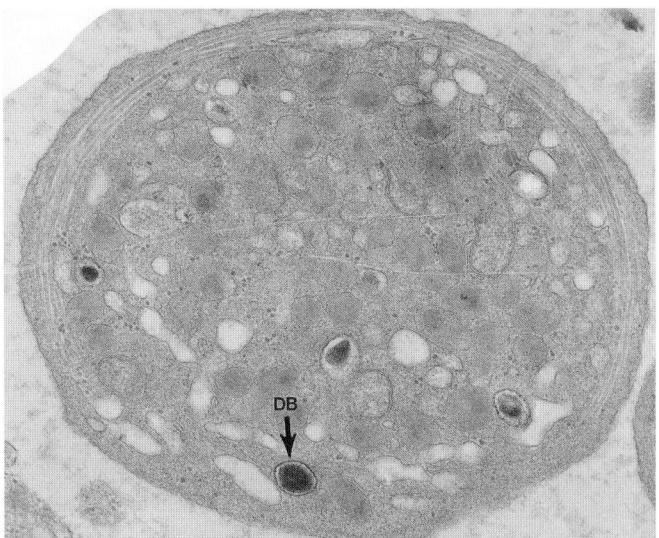

Fig. 25.10 Chediak–Higashi syndrome (CHS). Platelets from most patients with CHS are storage-pool deficient. However, some patients are only mildly abnormal. The cell in this illustration is from a patient with all of the features of CHS. However, his platelets contain about half the normal number of dense bodies (DB). × 30 000.

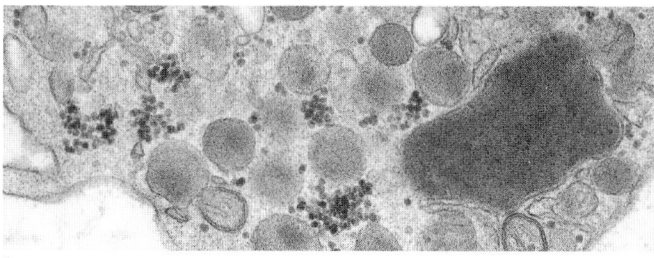

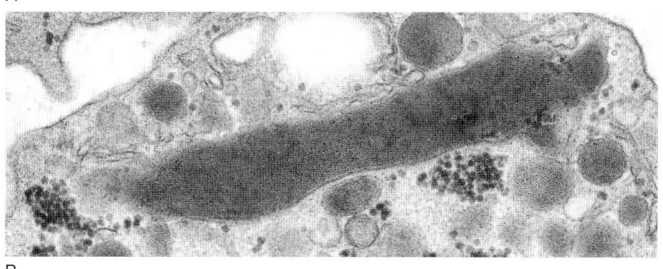

Fig. 25.11 (A,B) Chediak–Higashi syndrome (CHS). About 5% of platelets from patients with CHS contain giant granules. Incubation for acid phosphatase activity has shown that the giant granules in CHS platelets are lysosomes. A,B × 44 000.

have studied several other patients with CHS who have storage pool deficiency, and their platelets are almost, but not completely, devoid of dense bodies.

In addition to storage pool deficiency, platelets from patients with CHS have been found to contain the giant granule anomaly.[46] Giant granules of a type not seen in normal platelets or in other platelet disorders were found in platelets from our patient with CHS in a ratio of about 1:100 cells in thin sections (Fig. 25.11a,b). Parmley *et al*[47] have confirmed this observation in another patient and have shown that the giant granules in CHS platelets are acid phosphatase positive. The relationship of the giant granule anomaly to the storage pool deficiency of CHS platelets has not been defined.

Alpha granules

Alpha granules are the most numerous of the three types of platelet storage organelles destined for secretion[14,54] (see Fig. 25.3) They vary in size from 0.2 to 0.3 μm in diameter, but an occasional large granule is not uncommon in normal platelets. Alpha granules are round to oval in shape when viewed in thin sections. However, rod- and spindle-shaped alpha granules are not rare. Two zones of differing opacity are evident in the matrix of the organelle. The nucleoid is the more electron dense, and frequently has the opacity of a platelet dense body.

The lighter zone of the alpha-granule matrix usually appears unorganized. However, an occasional spindle- or rod-shaped granule can have a periodic substructure,

suggesting an orderly arrangement of constituent proteins.[55] Since fibrinogen is present in alpha granules, the periodicity has been related to this protein.[56] Direct evidence for this, however, is lacking. Periodicity is far more apparent in whole-mount preparations than in thin sections of human and animal platelet alpha granules. For example, whole mounts of bovine platelets reveal periodicity in the substructure of every alpha granule. Tubular elements resembling microtubules in cross section are present in alpha granules.[57] Ultrastructural immunocytochemistry has shown that the tubular structures are von Willebrand factor (vWF) or that vWF is very closely associated with them.[58]

Biochemical studies together with evaluation of platelets from patients who lack alpha granules have provided a long list of proteins concentrated within them.[59] Fibrinogen and vWF have been mentioned. Beta-thromboglobulin (β-TG), platelet factor 4 (PF-4), thrombospondin, platelet-derived growth factor (PDGF), Factor V, and high-molecular-weight kininogen are also present. The list grows longer each year. Some of the alpha-granule proteins are synthesized by megakaryocytes, while others may be taken up from blood into either megakaryocytes or platelets. The ability of platelets to take up foreign particulates from plasma and transfer them to apparently intact alpha granules was reported several years ago.[60] Recently, megakaryocytes have been shown to take up transfused horseradish peroxidase into alpha granules and the organelles can be detected subsequently in circulating platelets by cytochemical techniques. Recognition of this pathway is important because it appears to resolve a long-standing argument concerning the origin of platelet fibrinogen. Defibrination of animal models, followed by histochemical and cytochemical studies of bone marrow and platelets, has shown that platelet fibrinogen originates from blood.[61,62]

Secretion of alpha-granule contents is a characteristic feature of the platelet response to potent aggregating agents. The process of secretion has been characterized as a transfer of chemical substances confined in storage organelles of resting platelets to the exterior plasma without simultaneous loss of cytoplasmic constituents.[63] Platelet release is highly selective, involving some organelles and not others, and physiologic, since it does not result from non-specific injury.[64,65]

Several mechanisms have been proposed to explain how substances confined to the storage organelles in resting platelets are discharged to the exterior during the platelet release reaction. One theory suggests that organelles move to the periphery of activated platelets, fuse with the cell membrane at any point, and extrude their contents to the outside. A similar sequence of events has been observed during the process of secretion in many endocrine systems.[66] However, the evidence advanced to support this mechanism in platelets is quite meager.

Ginsberg *et al*[67] have suggested a different mechanism for secretion of products from platelet organelles. Based on immunocytochemical and ultrastructural studies of PF$_4$ secretion, they suggested that platelet alpha granules fuse together in the activated platelet, resulting in the formation of a large compound granule or sealed vacuole. Their evidence indicated that the sealed vacuole formed by granule fusion moves to the periphery of activated cells and fuses with the plasma membrane, resulting in release.

Small vacuoles do develop in thrombin-activated platelets.[68] Yet the actual fusion of granules to form a compound vacuole and its movement to the cell surface as proposed by Ginsberg *et al.* have not been observed in activated samples. There is a swelling of the OCS and dilatation of granule membranes after communication and discharge of contents into the OCS. Granule fusion is rarely seen under these conditions, but can occur under others.[69] It has been noted in platelets from patients with certain leukemias[70] (Fig. 25.12), and regularly develops in platelets during long-term storage under mildly alkaline conditions[71] (Fig. 25.13). Granule fusion in leukemic platelets or during storage, however, does not appear related to the release reaction.

In recent studies we have examined the release reaction in bovine platelets[72] and re-evaluated the secretory pathway in human cells.[73] Tannic acid, often used as an electron-dense stain, was employed to delineate the

process of secretion. The chemical dye was found in a preliminary investigation to precipitate fibrinogen and selectively deposit osmic acid on fibrinogen and fibrin. Samples of citrate platelet-rich plasma (C-PRP) and washed human platelets stimulated by thrombin in the presence of ethylenediamine tetracetic acid (EDTA) develop dramatic changes in their morphology. The cells lose their lentiform appearance, become irregular in form, and extend numerous pseudopods. Platelet organelles become concentrated in cell centers and enclosed within rings of constricted microtubules (Fig. 25.14). Higher concentrations of thrombin cause rapid discharge of granule contents and reduction in their number. As a result, dense spots of actomyosin, in which centrally concentrated organelles are enclosed in less activated platelets, appear more prominent in strongly stimulated cells.[74]

Tannic-acid-stained platelet aggregates from C-PRP were identical in appearance to unstained control aggregates, except for the presence of osmium black precipitate. Amorphous black material surrounded the aggregates and was deposited between the cells. Electron-dense material was also present in normal-sized and swollen granules in many platelets. Connections between channels and granules and direct communication between canaliculi and the surrounding plasma were evident.

Amorphous precipitate was not present outside the thrombin-activated cells from samples of washed platelets resuspended in the presence of EDTA, and aggregates were absent. The platelets, however, revealed the same physical changes observed in thrombin-aggregated cells from platelet-rich plasma (PRP). Many granules were

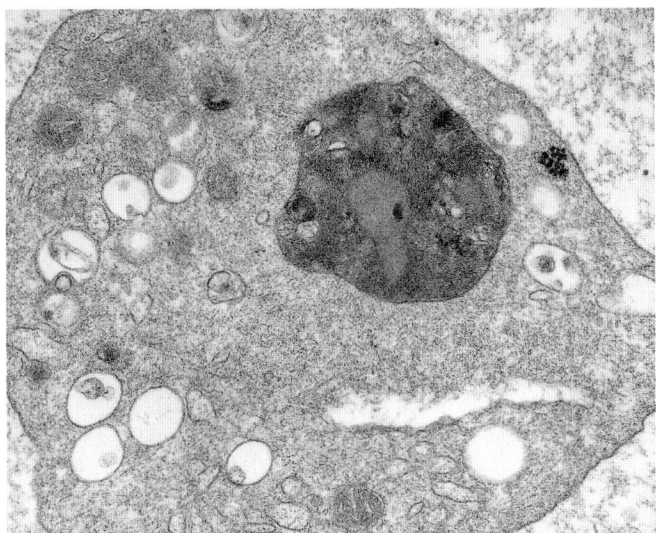

Fig. 25.12 Giant alpha granules. Alpha-granule fusion resulting in the formation of giant organelles is common in patients with myeloproliferative syndromes or myelomonocytic leukemia. × 29 000.

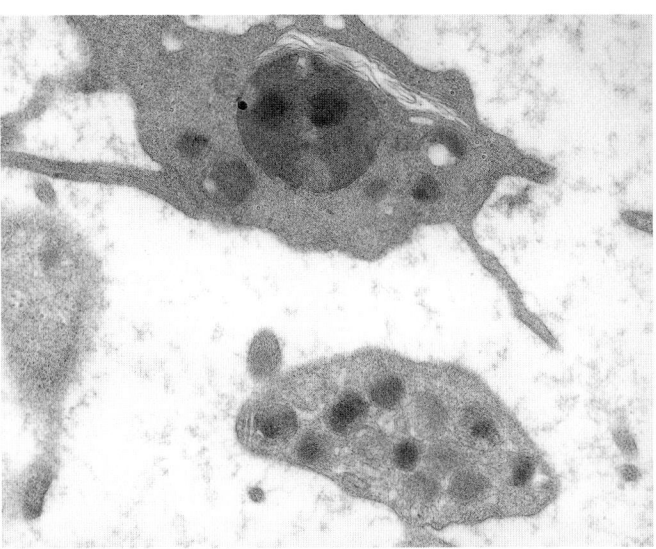

Fig. 25.13 Giant alpha granules. Platelets from a sample of platelet-rich plasma (PRP) stored under mildly alkaline conditions for 2 weeks. Fusion of alpha granules to form giant organelles is common during long-term storage. × 23 000.

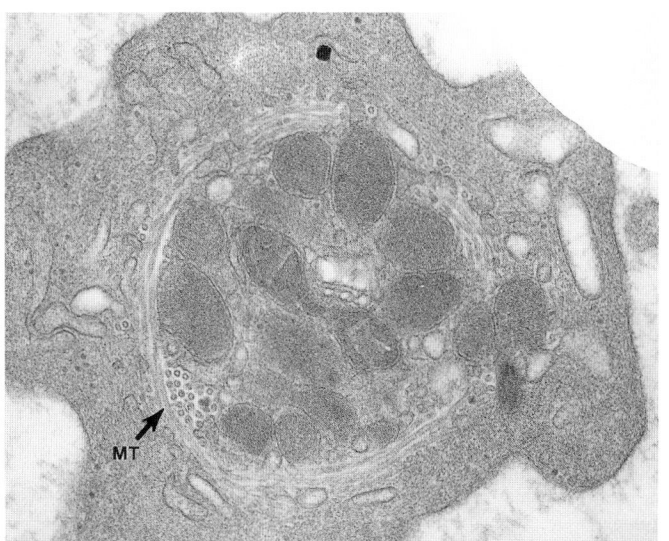

Fig. 25.14 Internal transformation. Shape change and pseudopod formation following exposure to agonists are accompanied by internal changes. Organelles move from random positions and concentrate in platelet centers. The closely associated granules are encircled by constricted rings of the circumferential microtubule (MT) and microfilaments not visible in this thin section. × 45 000.

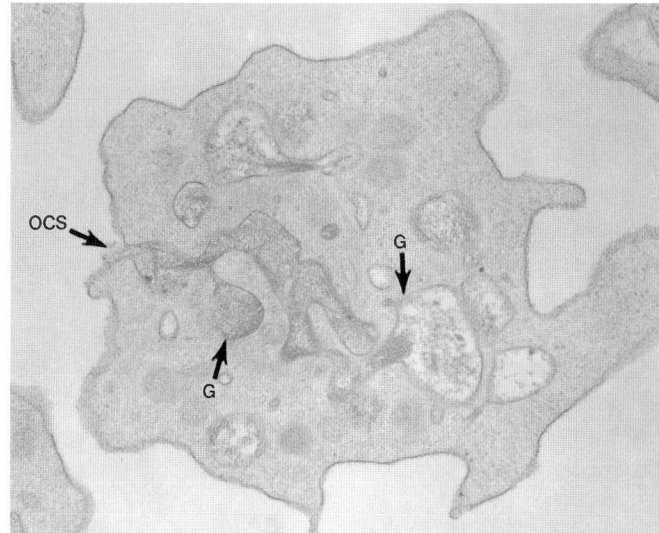

Fig. 25.15 Platelet secretion. Platelet from a sample of washed cells suspended in a buffer containing EDTA and stimulated by 3 U/ml of thrombin. The sample was fixed in glutaraldehyde containing tannic acid 3 min after exposure to the agonist without stirring. Tannic acid acts as a selective mordant, binding osmic acid to fibrin and fibrinogen under these conditions, permitting ultrastructural identification of the secretory process. In this example at least two granules (G) have fused with one channel of the open canalicular system (OCS) and their content of fibrinogen–fibrin is in the process of extrusion from the platelet. × 33 000.

stained intensely by tannic acid-osmium. Other granules were swollen and their content of amorphous stained material appeared diluted. Channels of the OCS were also delineated by electron-dense stain. Some channels were tortuous and narrow and contained little tannic acid. Others were filled by electron-dense material and widely dilated. Communications between granules and OCS channels were evident in many platelets (Fig.25.15). The connection appeared to foster swelling of the granules and dilation of the channels, so that recognition of the site of fusion was often obscured. More than one granule was frequently in communication with the same OCS channel. This relationship often resulted in extensive dilation of the OCS and granules fused to it. Occasionally, channel openings on to the surface were dilated, but usually remained constricted as in resting platelets. In some examples a single channel opened in more than one place on to the surface membrane of an activated platelet. The electron-dense material present in channels frequently appeared in the process of extrusion into the surrounding medium.

The difference in the mechanism of secretion in bovine compared to human cells may seem confusing. Bovine platelets do not have a well-defined OCS. As a result, they use the surface membrane as the primary route for discharge of products from secretory granules. Human platelets have an extensive system of internalized surface membrane formed into channels of the OCS. It is used as the primary route of secretion in human cells. Bovine platelets can develop primitive canaliculi following

activation and granule products can leave the cell through these conduits. Yet it employs the cell surface as a preferential route for exocytosis. The basis for the species variations in platelet structure resulting in different preferred routes for secretion of granule products remains unknown. However, it is clear that there are significant differences in bovine and human platelet shape change, pseudopod formation, spreading on surfaces, and internal transformation. Differences, therefore, in the mode of platelet secretion are not surprising.

Gray platelet syndrome

The gray platelet syndrome (GPS) is a rare disorder.[75] Since description of the first case, two other patients have been reported in the United States.[59,76] In France, two siblings, a brother and sister, have been characterized with GPS.[77] Recently, a patient from New Zealand, two in Australia, another living in England, and a family in Japan have been found to have GPS.

The original patient[75] was evaluated for thrombocytopenia as a child and found to have large, nearly agranular platelets which appeared gray or blue–gray on Wright-stained blood smears. Splenectomy improved, but did not correct the platelet count to normal. It remained between 100 000 and 125 000/mm³. Most of his platelets retained the large agranular appearance noted before splenectomy, but a small percentage were of normal size and contained some granules. Since his mean platelet volume was increased (11.1 μm³), the thrombocytopenia was probably relative, as it is in other giant platelet syndromes, and the circulating platelet biomass (platelet number × mean platelet volume) was normal.[78]

Aggregation studies revealed an essentially normal response to most aggregating agents. However, the reaction of gray platelets to collagen and thrombin was less than normal.[59] Increasing concentrations of these reagents restored the full response. Levels of serotonin and adenine nucleotides were normal. PF4, β-TG, fibrinogen, thrombomodulin and PDGF were markedly reduced. Lysosomal enzymes and catalase were within normal limits. Ultrastructural studies revealed wide variations in platelet size and morphology. Most platelets were relatively large, vacuolated, and nearly devoid of organelles (Fig. 25.16). Dense bodies, occasional mitochondria, and a few granules were present in the cells.[76] Cytochemical studies with the uranaffin reaction confirmed the presence of dense bodies. A few small granules were positive for catalase and larger granules revealed reaction products for acid phosphatase and β-glucuronidase. The percentage of alpha granules was less than 15% of control platelets. Many cells were filled with elements of the dense tubular system (Fig. 25.17), while others principally contained channels of the OCS. Dilated vacuoles communicating with the OCS were common, and appeared to be sites usually occupied by alpha granules. This observation was important because megakaryocytes in patients with GPS can synthesize the proteins missing in alpha granules, but the products are lost before the large platelets reach circulating blood.

The problem in this disorder appears to be related to packaging.[79] Proteins destined for concentration in alpha granules either do not reach the developing organelles or are lost after inclusion within their membranes. The latter seems to be more likely. Breton-Gorius et al[80] have shown that loss of granule contents and release of PDGF from megakaryocytes may be a major, but not the only, factor involved in development of marrow fibrosis in the GPS, in patients with megakaryocytic leukemia and in myeloproliferative disorders.

In addition to proliferation of reticulin or fibrosis, the marrow of patients with GPS reveals one other abnormal feature. Emperiopolesis, the uptake of other blood cells into the demarcation membrane systems of megakaryocytes, is not a rare finding.[79] Originally, it was considered to be an indication of malignant disease, but it does occur in normal individuals. In GPS it is a striking feature.[79] Some

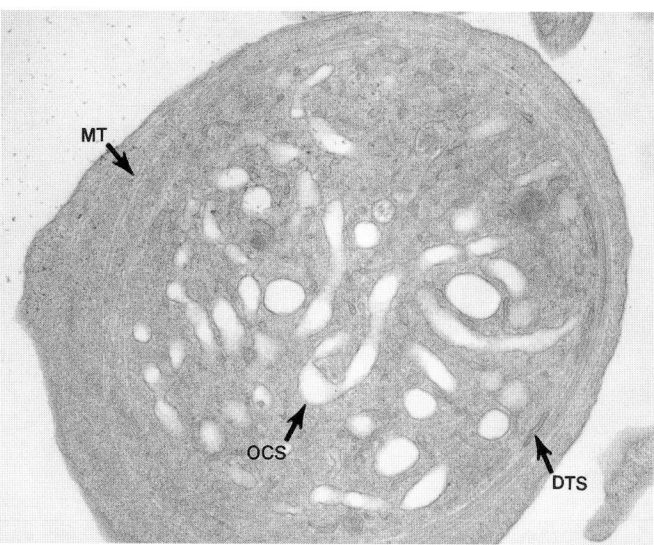

Fig. 25.16 Gray platelet syndrome (GPS). Alpha granules are absent in this platelet from a patient with GPS. Channels of the open canalicular system (OCS) are the dominant feature. DTS, dense tubular system; MT, microtubule. × 15 000.

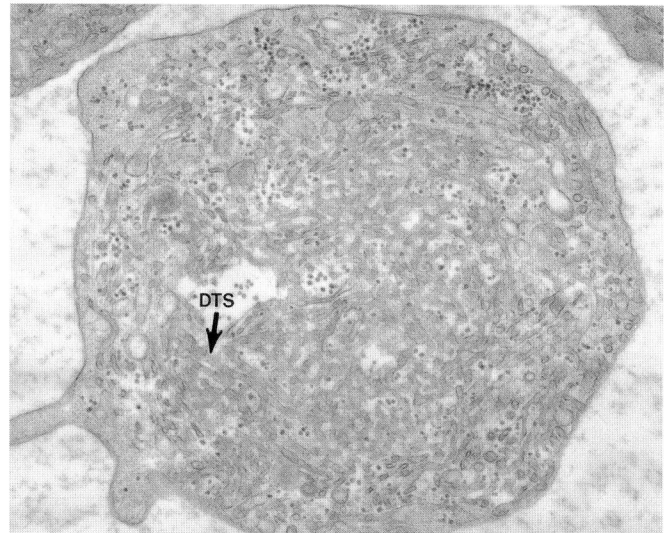

Fig. 25.17 Gray platelet syndrome (GPS). The GPS platelet in this illustration is filled with channels from the dense tubular system (DTS). × 24 000.

megakaryocytes contain 10–12 neutrophils and occasional monocytes. The loss of chemotactic proteins from defective granules through the OCS of developing platelets and demarcation membranes of the parent cell may attract leukocytes to the evolving channel system.

Our second patient with GPS also has Goldenhar's syndrome.[81] Examination of the literature and two other patients with Goldenhar's syndrome failed to reveal gray platelets. Since other patients with GPS do not have the second syndrome, there does not appear to be any direct link between them.

A Japanese family with GPS[82] appears to have a more severe problem with bleeding than the American patients. Also, the response of their platelets to ADP and collagen was abnormal, whereas platelets from both of our patients with GPS aggregated in a normal manner when stirred with these agents. The alpha-granule deficiency and reduction in levels of granule-associated products were significantly less in Japanese kindred compared to the patients studied here. In view of the less-severe platelet alpha-granule deficiency, a plethora of other morphologic defects, reduced production of thromboxane A_2, severe deficiency of platelet factor 3 activity, and low levels of factor VIII subunits, it is possible that the disorder presented by the Japanese family may be a variant of the GPS reported by Raccuglia.[75] The Japanese workers have suggested that the condition found in their kindred may more likely represent a release-type defect[83] than an organelle deficiency disorder. Since other patients with GPS are profoundly deficient in alpha granules compared to the Japanese kindred, the suggestion may be appropriate for their family.

Alpha-granule, dense-body deficiency

Although intermediate forms appear to exist, only one case of combined alpha-granule, dense-body deficiency has been defined.[36] The patient with combined deficiency has hemorrhagic symptoms. No other stigmata are evident in this patient. As a result, there is nothing else to suggest the presence of platelet alpha-granule dense-body deficiency. Since there is only a single case of combined defect, the pattern of inheritance is uncertain. The morphology of platelets with deficiency in both alpha granules and dense bodies is very different from that of gray platelets. Though variable in size, the cells missing both secretory organelles are not significantly increased in mean platelet volume. The large vacuoles commonly observed filling the cytoplasm of gray platelets are virtually absent from cells with the combined defect.[84] This observation suggests that the abnormality responsible for failure to form granules in the combined deficiency disorder differs from that in the GPS. No basis for the decrease in dense bodies was detected in thin sections of platelets from the patient with combined deficiency.

Heterogeneous storage organelle deficiency

Weiss *et al*[36] have described two families with diminution of dense bodies and partial deficiency of alpha granules.

One of the families also had platelets with an increased lecithin to phosphatidyl ethanolamine ratio, increased glycoprotein IV, and decreased adhesion to subendothelium. The inheritance of the combined partial deficiencies of alpha granules and dense bodies in the two families appears to be autosomal dominant.

Enlarged alpha granules

Jacobsen–Paris–Trousseau syndrome

A novel genetic thrombocytopenia with platelet inclusion bodies, dysmegakaryopoiesis, mild congenital anomalies and mental retardation associated with chromosome 11 deletion at 11q23 was recently reported.[85-87] platelet inclusion bodies were found to be giant alpha granules present in 15% of the cells in peripheral blood (Fig. 25.18). This condition had not been described previously, and as a result the authors termed it the Paris–Trousseau syndrome. However, the Jacobsen syndrome is also associated with deletion of chromosome 11 at q23.3.[88-90] Typical anomalies include trigonocephaly, facial dysmorphism, cardiac defects, syndactyly and psychomotor retardation, although none of these features is invariably present.[88] Approximately 47% of the patients with Jacobsen syndrome were found to be thrombocytopenic,[85] but investigation of their platelets by electron microscopy was not reported. Recently, we have evaluated platelets from two patients with Jacobsen syndrome.[91] Both individuals have the same giant alpha granules in their platelets observed in cells from patients with the Paris–

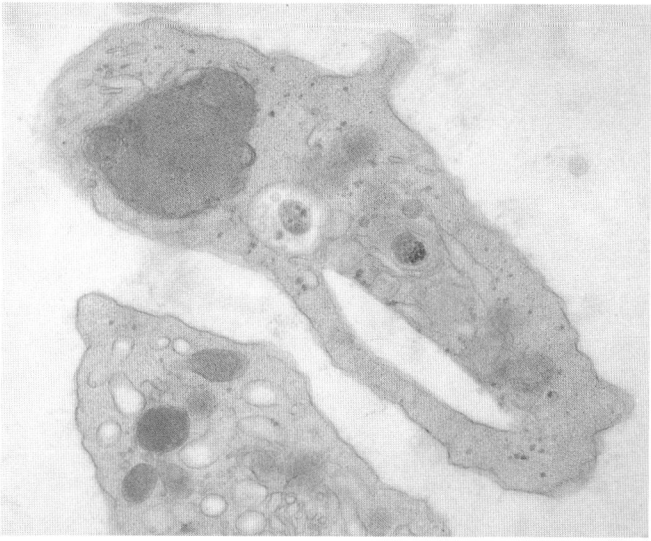

Fig. 25.18 Jacobsen, Paris–Trousseau syndrome. Platelet is from a patient with Jacobsen syndrome whose platelets contain the giant alpha granules identical to those in patients with the Paris–Trousseau syndrome. × 45 000.

Trousseau syndrome (Fig. 25.19). Since patients with the Paris–Trousseau syndrome and Jacobsen syndrome share the same chromosomal defect, we have suggested that the two disorders are the same. The only difference may be that dense bodies were virtually absent in platelets from the two patients with Jacobsen syndrome. Reports on the Paris–Trousseau syndrome have not mentioned the state of platelet dense bodies.[85–87]

Lysosomes

Platelets are known to contain and secrete a variety of hydrolytic enzymes, including acid phosphatase, aryl sulfatase, β-N-acetylgalactoseaminidase, α-arabinosidase, and others.[92] For many years it was believed that hydrolases were confined to alpha granules, but subcellular fractionation suggested they were localized at a different site in the cell.[22] Platelet lysosomes have been difficult to characterize cytochemically, although an early study suggested that acid phosphatase was localized to an organelle similar in size to the alpha granules.[93] Bentfield and Bainton[94] studied the localization of acid phosphatase and aryl sulfatase in rat megakaryocytes and platelets. Their investigations suggested that lysosomes arose as variably-sized vesicles from the Golgi cisternae. The lysosomal vesicles ranged from 175 to 250 nm in diameter and were much smaller than alpha granules.[95]

Recently we have used cerium as the capture ion for phosphate liberated by acid phosphatase, rather than lead phosphate (Fig. 25.20). Results of our experiments support the concept that hydrolytic enzymes are localized to a form of granule in platelets rather than to vesicles. The concept that platelet lysosomes are granules rather than vesicles is supported by other observations. Platelets contain very few, if any, vesicles. Those present are usually covered by barbs typical of clathrin-coated endocytic vesicles.[96] The rest are in reality part of the tortuous open canalicular system, as demonstrated by electron-dense tracers. Thus, the multiple proteins making up the acid hydrolase complement of platelet lysosomes appear to be packaged in organelles similar to those found in phagocytic cells.

Chediak–Higashi syndrome

Characteristic features of the Chediak–Higashi syndrome (CHS) were discussed earlier in this chapter. Most of the circulating leukocytes, including neutrophils, eosinophils, basophils, monocytes and lymphocytes, contain various forms of giant lysosomes (see Fig. 25.9). It was this feature that suggested that CHS is a form of lysosomal disease.[97]

Most of the interest in platelets from patients with CHS has focused on the storage pool deficiency and virtual absence of dense bodies discussed above. Yet, dense bodies are not lysosomes. Why they are absent rather than enlarged like abnormal organelles in other cells in this disorder[98] is unknown. The fact that CHS platelets do contain giant lysosomes has received less attention.[46] Enlarged organelles are present in 1–5% of their platelets (see Figs 25.11a,b). A cytochemical study has

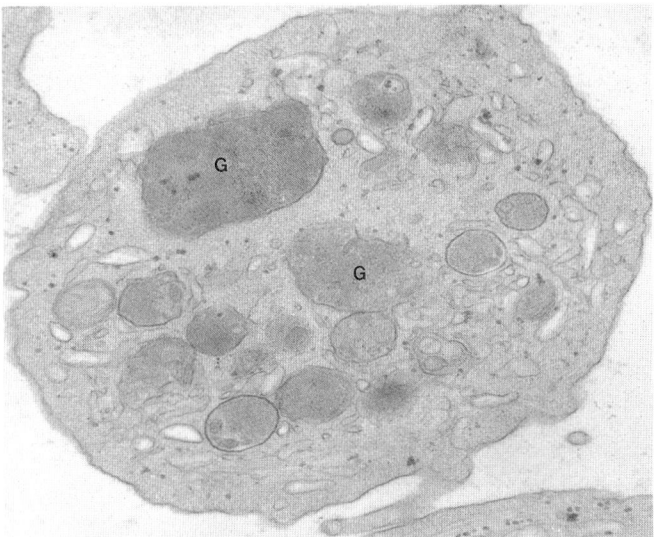

Fig. 25.19 Platelet from another patient with the Jacobsen syndrome containing several giant alpha granules (G) identical to those found in platelets from Paris–Trousseau syndrome patients. × 38 000.

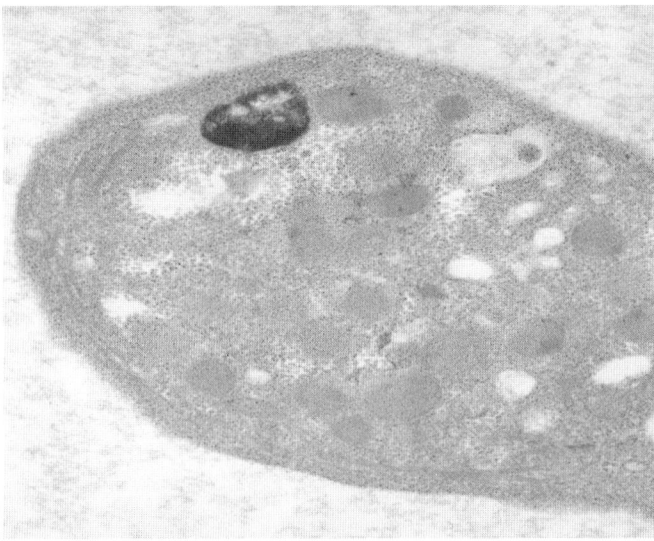

Fig. 25.20 Platelet lysosomes. Cell from a sample of washed platelets incubated for acid phosphatase activity in medium containing cerium as the capture agent. Reaction product is confined to a single organelle. × 35 000.

shown that the giant granules contain acid phosphatase, demonstrating that they are lysosomes[47] (Fig. 25.21). The relationship of the giant lysosomes in CHS platelets to the absence of dense bodies has not been defined. However, the platelet in CHS is the only cell in this disorder shown to have abnormalities in two distinctly different types of organelles.[46,98]

Giant dense body disorder

Recently, we have evaluated an impressive giant-platelet dense body disorder.[84] The child was found to have thrombocytopenia shortly after birth. During the course of evaluating him we found that his mother had a normal platelet count, but the same platelet defects as her child. Platelets from both contain excessive numbers of giant electron-opaque organelles (Fig. 25.22). Despite their increased number and size, the platelets from mother and child contained normal levels of serotonin and adenine nucleotides. Concentrated platelet samples from the child and C-PRP from his mother responded normally to aggregating agents. Siblings and relatives of the propositi had normal platelets. Immunocytochemistry revealed that the giant dense bodies contained peroxidase and were, therefore, lysosomes. The reason why these giant lysosomes are inherently electron opaque is unclear.

Disorders of platelet membranes and membrane organization

Platelet membranes and membrane systems are unique.[99] Surface membranes enclosing all other circulating blood cells develop through a process of maturation and cell division. Platelet membranes are formed within the confines of a single cell which does not undergo division into daughter cells[100] (Fig. 52). The mechanism involved in the formation of platelets within the parent megakaryocyte has been of great interest for many years, but has not been resolved. Behnke[101,102] used electron-dense tracers to demonstrate that the surface of maturing rat megakaryocytes undergoes invagination, resulting in sequestration of the cytoplasm into subunits about the size of platelets (Fig. 25.23). As beautiful as that work was, it did not reveal how tube-like channels from the parent cell surface could develop into flat sheets that form the outer membranes of discoid platelets.[103] Also, it could not be determined in thin sections whether or not

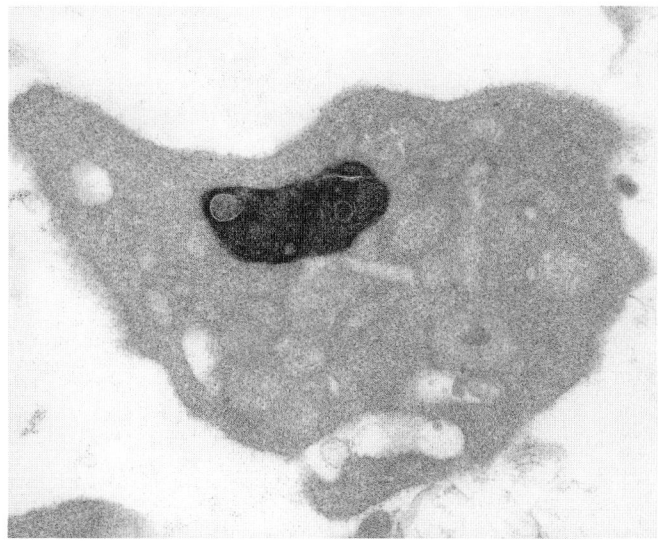

Fig. 25.21 Chediak–Higashi syndrome (CHS). Platelet from patient with CHS reacted for acid phosphatase with cerium as the capture agent. A giant lysosome in the cell cytoplasm is positive for the hydrolytic enzyme activity. × 35 000.

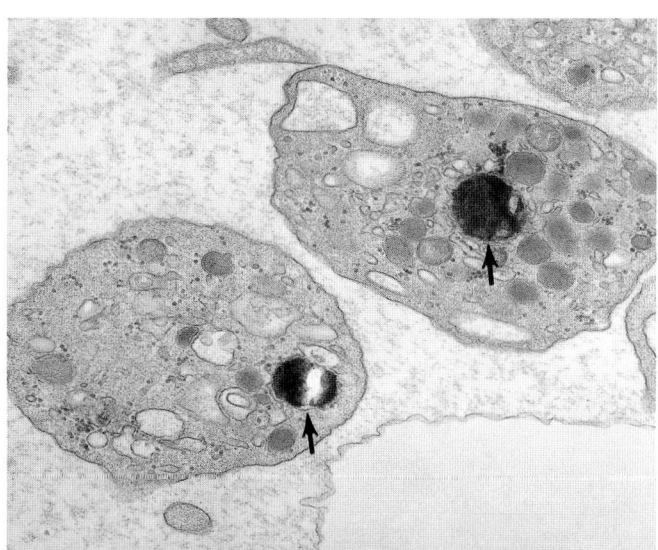

Fig. 25.22 Giant dense body disorder (GDBD). Dense bodies (↑) in two platelets from one of our patients with the GDBD are huge compared to adjacent alpha granules and mitochondria. × 26 000.

individual platelets were completely formed or were parts of membrane-demarcated chains[104] (Fig. 25.23).

Wright[100] was the first to suggest that megakaryocytes in bone marrow produce cytoplasmic processes resembling chains that penetrate into the intravascular compartment and fragment to produce platelets. The *in vitro* study of Thiery and Bessis[105] gave substance to this concept. They demonstrated that future platelets in the cytoplasm of megakaryocytes became arranged in long, ribbon-like structures. The projections elongated progressively, giving the megakaryocyte an octopus-like appearance in the phase contrast microscope. In time, the long processes

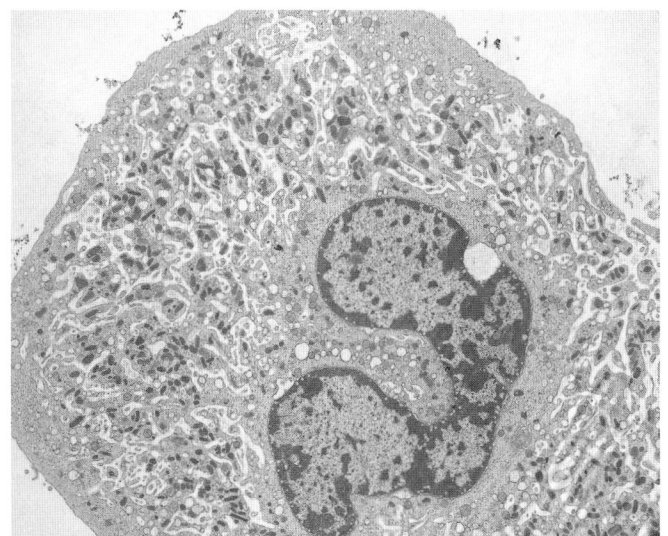

Fig. 25.23 Megakaryocyte. Platelet-forming cell from human marrow. Areas on the left and right sides of the cell appear to be breaking up into platelets or proplatelets. × 4300.

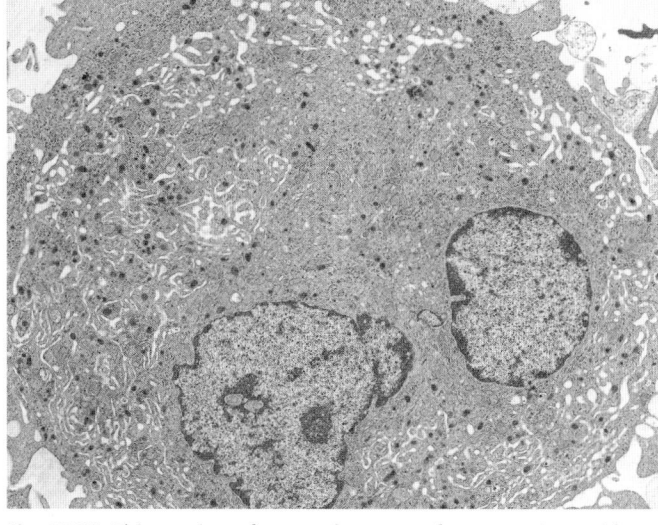

Fig. 25.24 Thin section of a megakaryocyte from a patient with Wiskott–Aldrich syndrome (WAS). The cell is of normal size and all structures, including the demarcation membrane system, resemble similar structures in normal megakaryocytes. × 4500.

developed alternating swellings and constrictions. If the cell at this stage was disturbed, platelets would break loose from their attachment threads to the chain, adhere to glass, and spread in a normal manner.

Support for the observations of Thiery and Bessis was provided by Becker and deBruyn[106] and subsequently by Scurfield and Radley,[107] on fixed samples of bone marrow examined in scanning and transmission electron microscopes. Platelets were derived from long intrasinusoidal extensions originating from extravascularly located megakaryocytes. Release into the circulation was probably initiated by local constrictions in the long processes, yielding either single cells or long segments of proplatelet cytoplasm. Incompletely segmented platelets resembling extended pieces of proplatelet cytoplasm have been recovered from human blood. Thus, the literature provides considerable support for the concept that platelets are delivered from bone marrow matrix to the sinusoids via long processes which constrict segmentally to provide single cells or chains of incompletely separated platelets to circulating blood.[108]

It is hoped that a clear understanding of platelet formation will develop soon. We need the clarification in order to understand why circulating platelets have a nearly identical size, with a mean platelet volume (MPV) of 7–10 fl. It almost seems that platelets are stamped out in a mold and then delivered to blood. Yet the megakaryocyte is no mold. It is a dynamic membrane-forming system and understanding how it works is the key to understanding normal and abnormal platelet membranes and membrane organization.[109]

Small platelets

Wiskott–Aldrich syndrome

The Wiskott-Alrich syndrome (WAS) is an X-linked, recessively inherited disorder characterized by thrombocytopenia, eczema and recurrent infections.[110,111] Immunologic defects include reduced levels of IgM, reduced or absent isoagglutinins to blood groups A and B, reduced lymphocyte counts, impaired lymphocyte responses to certain mitogens, and markedly elevated IgE.[37,112] Platelets, in additions to being present in reduced numbers, are one-half to two-thirds normal size and have been reported to be deficient in granules, dense bodies, mitochondria, adenine nucleotides and serotonin.[37] However, our findings suggest that organelles are normal, even though the cell is small (Fig. 25.24).

After splenectomy, platelet counts may return to normal in many patients, and increase in the number of cells is associated with restoration of normal size and ultrastructural apperance.[113] The results suggest that the platelet defect in WAS may be due to extrinsic factors influencing maturation of megakaryocytes in the bone marrow.[114] Wiskott–Aldrich syndrome is not ordinarily considered to result from an intrinsic membrane defect, although a surface-membrane glycoprotein deficiency was reported.[115] Most workers consider a metabolic abnormality[116] in oxidative phosphorylation to underlie the small size and defective function.[117] However, it is possible that WAS is caused by a membrane maturation defect in the megakaryocyte.

Development of specific zones in cytoplasm destined to become individual platelets follows a definite sequence of events. Deoxyribonucleic acid synthesis and endore-duplication of the nucleus take place first.[118] This is followed by a laying down of a huge system of rough endoplasmic reticulum (RER) for synthesis of proteins.[119] Transfer of synthesized proteins to the Golgi zone is followed by delivery to three different types of storage organelles that fill the cytoplasm of the huge cell. The final event involves invagination of the surface to form demarcation membranes, which delineate a general outline of individual cells.[101] If, for some reason, the process of maturation were interrupted, what might be expected to occur? For example, in idiopathic thrombocytopenic purpura or severe hemorrhage the demand for platelets in circulating blood causes early release of large, young platelets, some of which contain residual elements of RER. The result suggests that the demarcation membranes are incompletely developed before platelets are released, resulting in larger size.

If, on the other hand, maturation is delayed in the marrow by 1 or 2 days, demarcation membranes would have time to overdevelop. As a result, the platelet zones may be one-half normal size. Because the platelets would be 2 or 3 days older than normal cells before leaving the parent cell in the marrow, energy reserves would be decreased and life span shortened.[117] The short life span of platelets and delayed development of megakaryocytes would cause thrombocytopenia. All of these features are characteristics of WAS. Thus, although the hypothesis is speculative, WAS may represent a postmature disorder owing to protracted membrane formation in the megakaryocyte. The observation that splenectomy often restores numbers, size, biochemistry and function to normal[113] supports the possibility that WAS platelets are not intrinsically abnormal, but become so if maturation is delayed.

Giant platelet disorders

Mediterranean macrotherombocytopenia

Large platelets, moderate thrombocytopenia, and splenomegaly have been described in a significant percentage of persons originating from the Italian and Balkan peninsulas and is therefore referred to as Mediterranean macrothrombocytopenia.[78] Erythrocyte stomatocytosis is also observed in high frequency in the population. Individuals with this problem do not have a bleeding tendency. There is an inverse correlation between platelet counts and mean platelet volume, so that individuals

with Mediterranean macrothrombocytopenia have the same platelet biomass in circulating blood as individuals with normal platelet counts. Thus, thrombocytopenia is not due to bone marrow failure. Platelet ultrastructure appears to be normal. The mode of inheritance has not been clearly established. Therefore, Mediterranean macrothrombocytopenia is a benign morphologic variant, reflecting a tendency within every species for the ciruculating platelet biomass to vary within defined limits.[78]

May–Hegglin anomaly (MHA)

May-Hegglin anomaly (MHA) has an autosomal dominant pattern of inheritance.[120,121] Platelet counts are reduced to about $50\,000/mm^3$ in these patients, but the MPV is 5–7 times that of normal cells (Fig. 25.25). If one multiplies the platelet number by MPV to obtain the platelet mass in circulating blood, there is little difference between the values obtained in MHA and normal individuals.[78] Thus, patients with MHA are not really thrombocytopenic. The number of megakaryocytes present in bone marrow of MHA patients is not increased, and their mean volume is similar to that of normal megakaryocytes.

A characteristic feature of MHA, in addition to giant platelets, is the presence of spindle-shaped bodies in all types of granulocytes and in monocytes[122] (Figs 25. 25–27). The inclusions are referred to as Dohle bodies, but are not to be confused with the enlarged azurophilic granules in neutrophils of patients with severe infections[123] (Fig. 25.28), even though they are referred to by the same

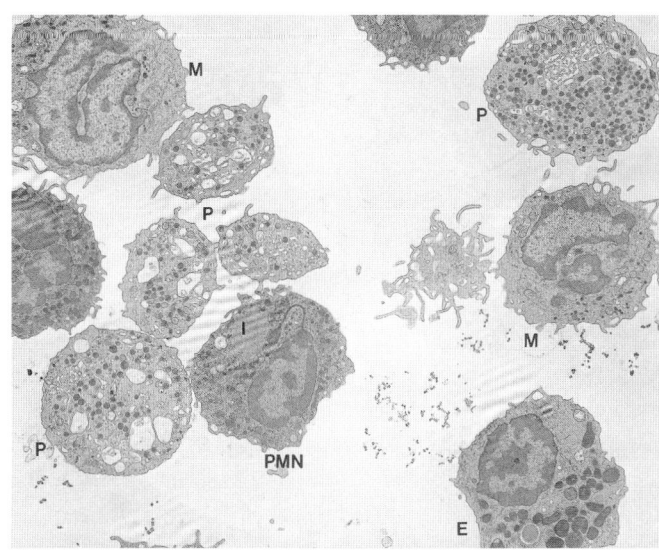

Fig. 25.25 Buffy coat from a patient with May–Hegglin anomaly. Platelets (P) in this thin section are as large as monocytes (M), eosinophils (E), and polymorphonuclear leukocytes (PMN). One PMN contains a May–Hegglin inclusion (I). × 4000.

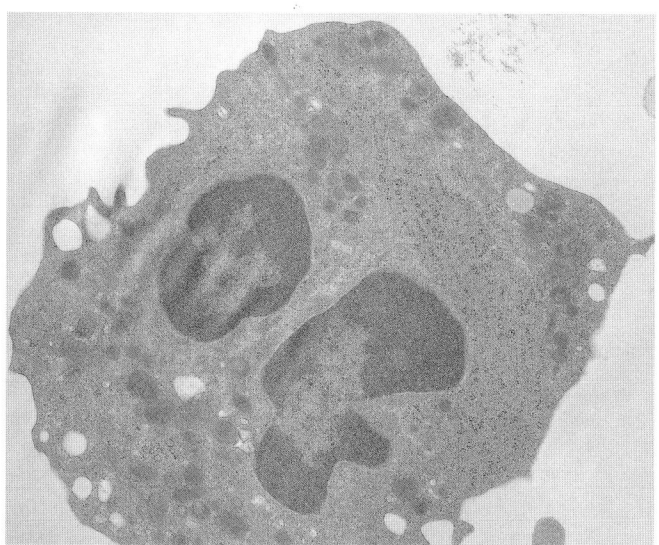

Fig. 25.26 Neutrophil from an individual with May–Hegglin anomaly (MHA) containing a spindle-shaped inclusion typical of the MHA. × 13 000.

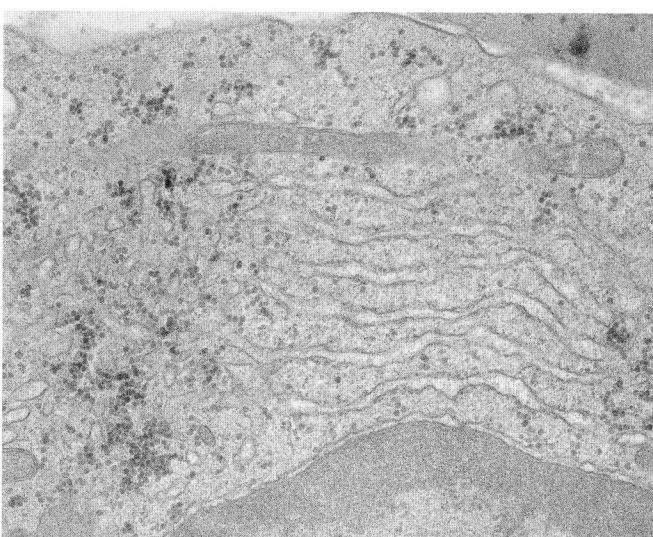

Fig. 25.28 Dohle body. A neutrophil from a patient with septicemia. Parallel stacks of rough endoplasmic reticulum present in this cell give the impression of being a distinct inclusion (Dohle body) when viewed in the light microscope on Wright-stained blood smears. × 33 000.

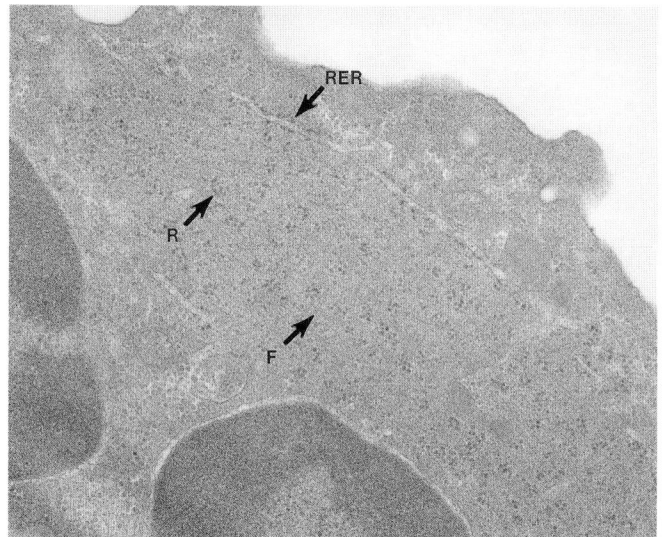

Fig. 25.27 May–Hegglin inclusion. Fragments of rough endoplasmic reticulum (RER) are associated with May–Hegglin anomaly (MHA) inclusions, but the predominant structures are rows of ribosomes (R) dispersed between intermediate filaments (F). The inclusion is not enclosed within a membrane. × 20 000.

name. Dohle bodies in MHA leukocytes are basophilic on Wright-stained blood smears and react positively when stained with methylgreen pyronine.[124] The immature nature of the inclusions suggested by these staining reactions is borne out in ultrastructural studies.[125] Short segments of RER, clusters of ribosomes, and a framework of parallel filaments are the principal constituents of May–Hegglin inclusions viewed in thin section[126] (Fig. 25.27). The filaments are 8–9 nm in diameter and resemble intermediate filaments found in many cell types.[127] Light and electron microscopic studies suggest that MHA

inclusions result from a failure to completely disassemble and resorb the RER and ribosome clusters characteristic of early states in the development of mature circulating cells.

MHA inclusions may also be related in some way to giant platelet formation in the megakaryocyte[128] (Fig. 25.29). Although channels of the demarcation membrane system (DMS) derived from the surface membrane may appear in primitive megakaryocytes, the tortuous mass of membrane does not reach its full stage of development in the form of platelet-sized fields until protein synthesis is virtually complete.[118] At this stage the channels of RER have ordinarily been converted to smooth endoplasmic reticulum (SER), and are distributed evenly throughout the cytoplasm. Only by removal or drastic modification of the massive membrane barrier imposed by the RER is it possible for the surface-derived DMS to penetrate into and subdivide the deepest recesses of megakaryocyte cytoplasm.

Yet the mere disappearance of one membrane system and development of another does not explain the fine balance of interaction between the DMS and SER. In every platelet, close associations between the surface-derived channels and residual elements of SER can be identified. We have called these specialized associations membrane complexes (MC).[53] Since MCs are intrinsic features of normal platelet anatomy, it is clear that their development in the parent megakaryocyte requires a balanced distribution of elements from the two channel systems throughout the cytoplasm.

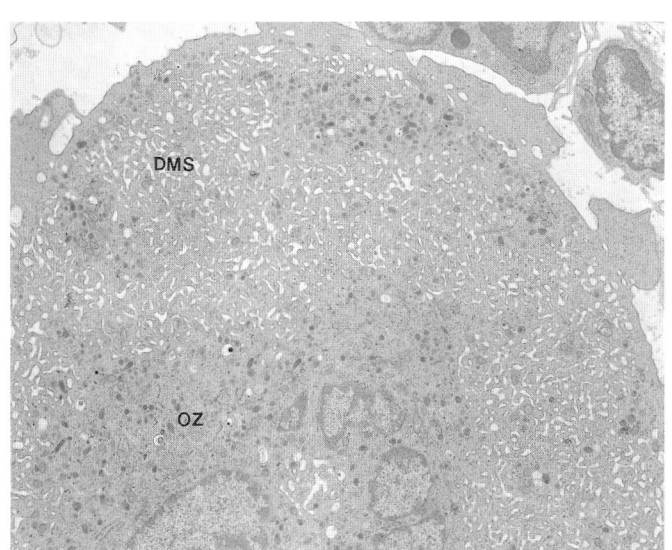

Fig. 25.29 Megakaryocyte from bone marrow of a patient with May–Hegglin anomaly (MHA). The large cells are similar in size to those from normal individuals. However, their internal organization is different. Areas of intense demarcation membrane system (DMS) formation in MHA megakaryocytes are separated from organelle zones (OZ), whereas they are intermixed in normal platelet-forming cells. × 3800.

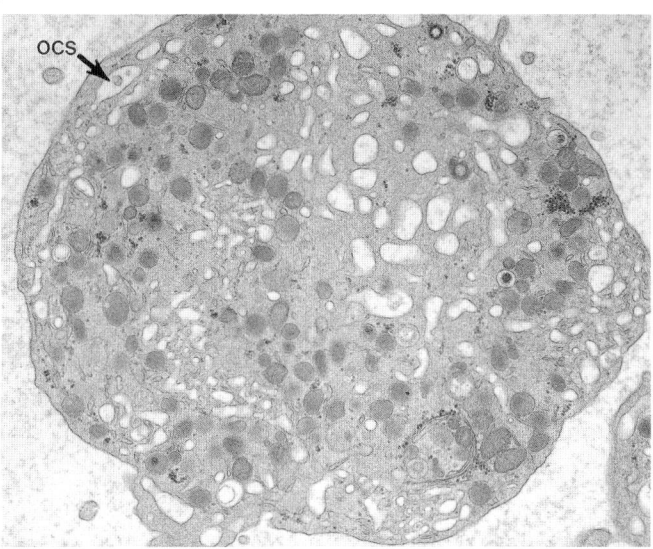

Fig. 25.30 May–Hegglin anomaly (MHA) platelet. Aside from their large size, the morphology of MHA platelets is very similar to that of normal cells. However, they are relatively spherical, rather than discoid in shape, and the open canalicular system (OCS) is more prominent. × 18 000.

What would happen if the timing of these events leading to sequestration of megakaryocyte cytoplasm was thrown off? If demand for platelets was greatly increased so they had to be delivered from immature megakaryocytes to circulating blood before completion of protein synthesis, what would they look like? One would expect their cytoplasm to be less mature and to contain at least some RER. Indeed, the platelets in the peripheral blood of patients with idiopathic thrombocytopenic purpura (ITP) often have this appearance. Also, on the basis of the rationale given above, one would expect ITP platelets to be large. Indeed they are, and the name 'megathrombocyte' was coined to describe them.[129] Thus, shortening of the time interval for development and interaction of the DMS and SER can result in large platelets with immature features.

MHA platelets, despite their large size, do not resemble the megathrombocytes of ITP (Fig. 25.30). The giant MHA thrombocytes are almost uniformly huge, while ITP platelets are irregular in size, with only a few large cells present in peripheral blood.[130] Characteristics of immaturity are lacking in the MHA platelets. Organelles, including alpha granules, lysosomes, dense bodies, mitochondria and peroxisomes, are present in normal numbers and distribution. The basophilia and occasional segments of RER found in left-shifted ITP[129] platelets are absent in MHA cells.

In fact, the only apparent difference between huge MHA platelets and normal-sized cells is the increased

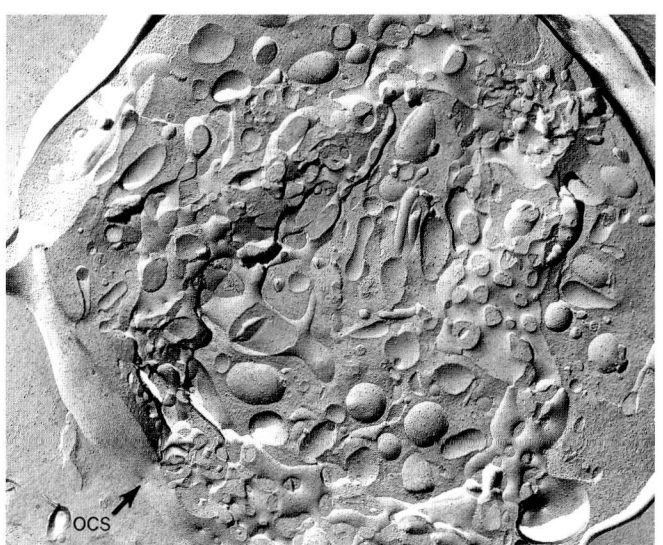

Fig. 25.31 Replica of a freeze-fractured platelet from a patient with May–Hegglin anomaly. The open canalicular system (OCS) is prominent. Channels communicating with the cell surface join each other and pursue tortuous courses throughout the cytoplasm. In some areas they form close associations with elements of the dense tubular system in membrane complexes. × 27 000.

amount of internalized membrane and the size of the membrane complexes (Figs 25.30 and 25.31). Clearly, there is no defect in the ability of MHA megakaryocytes to invaginate the surface membranes and form the DMS; nor does there appear to be a problem of interaction between DMS and SER to form membrane complexes. These intricate mazes formed by the two channel systems in MHA megakaryocytes are very prominent in circulating platelets. Thus, the membrane systems and their interactions appear to be involved in some way in the pathogenesis of the giant platelets of the MHA.[131]

The precise mechanism is still uncertain. Since both the DMS and SER are fully developed in MHA megakaryocytes, an imbalance of some form in their interaction would seem to be a likely possibility.[132] The inclusions in MHA leukocytes may provide a clue to the defective process in the megakaryocytes. MHA inclusions appear to represent collections of RER, ribosomes, and filaments which have failed to disappear during the maturation sequence. Their tendency to remain in aggregates into mature stages may be reflected in developing MHA megakaryocytes. If channels of RER remain associated for prolonged periods during conversion to SER, the interaction with the wave of advancing DMS could be perturbed. As a result, excessive interaction may occur between the two types of channels to form large membrane complexes with a consequent reduction in the interactions of DMS to form sequestration zones. The imbalance could result in giant platelets and increased membrane complex formation, precisely the characteristic features of circulating MHA platelets.

There is a second way in which persistence of channels of RER or clusters of SER could result in giant platelet formation. As mentioned above, the RER during the stage of protein formation presents a formidable barrier to penetration by DMS pushing in from the cell surface. If it fails to disassemble, even though conversion to SER takes place, barriers may remain, and result in a decreased number of very large sequestration zones.[132]

There may be other possible ways in which an imbalance of membrane interaction could result in evolution of the giant MHA platelets. However, the two suggested have the advantage of bringing together the pathogenesis of the MHA inclusions in leukocytes and the development of giant platelets in megakaryocytes. Some of the individuals with MHA have prolonged bleeding times and hemorrhagic symptoms which cannot be explained on the basis of reduced platelet numbers alone. However, tests of platelet function and aggregation have, in general, been normal and the platelet defect responsible for excessive bleeding in MHA has not been defined.[127]

Epstein's syndrome (ES)

Interstitial or mixed nephritis and nerve deafness[133] (Alport's syndrome) represent a well-known and not very rare hereditary disease. Epstein *et al*[134] were first to note that some families with this autosomal dominant disorder were also thrombocytopenic and had giant, abnormal platelets. Affected members had prolonged

bleeding times, defective platelet adhesion, and abnormal aggregation in response to collagen and epinephrine. Another family with hereditary deafness, renal disease and thrombocytopenia reported by Eckstein *et al*[135] had large platelets with normal ultrastructural morphology and *in vitro* function. Eckstein's family was considered a variant of the syndrome reported by Epstein,[134] but the basis for the differences in platelet function and clinical bleeding problems in the separate families has not been explained. More recently Hansen *et al*[136] reported that giant platelets from a family with Epstein syndrome lack microtubules and dense bodies. Neither defect was recorded in previous studies of platelet ultrastructure in patients with ES,[134,137] and we have not encountered these additional defects in our patients.

Platelets from these patients with ES are usually not quite as large as those from individuals with MHA, but are nearly indistinguishable from them in all other respects[138] (see Fig. 25.30). The enlarged platelets are frequently the size of lymphocytes, monocytes and neutrophils, and, like nucleated blood cells, are spherical in shape, rather than discoid (Figs 25.32 and 25.33). Immunofluorescence studies with specific antibodies against tubulin, the subunit protein of microtubules, have shown that the large cells have markedly increased numbers of microtubule coils which are highly disorganized compared to normal platelets.[139] Instead of forming a marginal band consisting of 8–12 closely associated coils lying just inside the surface membrane along its greatest circumference, the ES platelet has 50–100 coils organized like a ball of yarn, rather than a marginal bundle. It is not certain whether the disorganized micro-

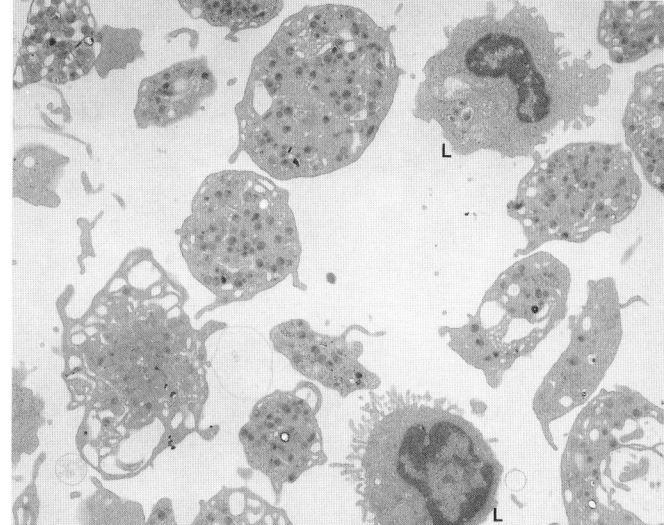

Fig. 25.32 Platelets from a patient with Epstein's syndrome (ES). Most of the platelets in this thin section are as large as the two lymphocytes (L). × 6000.

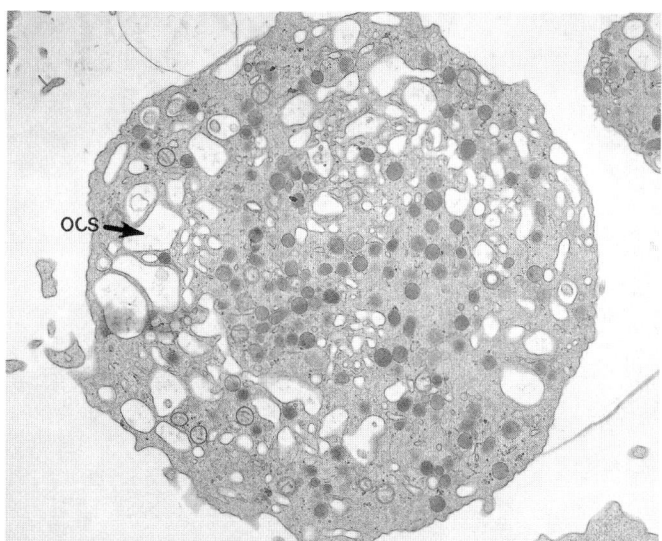

Fig. 25.33 Platelet from patient with Epstein's syndrome (ES). The cell is large, but basic morphologic features are similar to those of normal platelets. Channels of the open canalicular system (OCS) are as prominent in ES cells as they are in May–Hegglin anomaly (MHA) platelets. × 13 000.

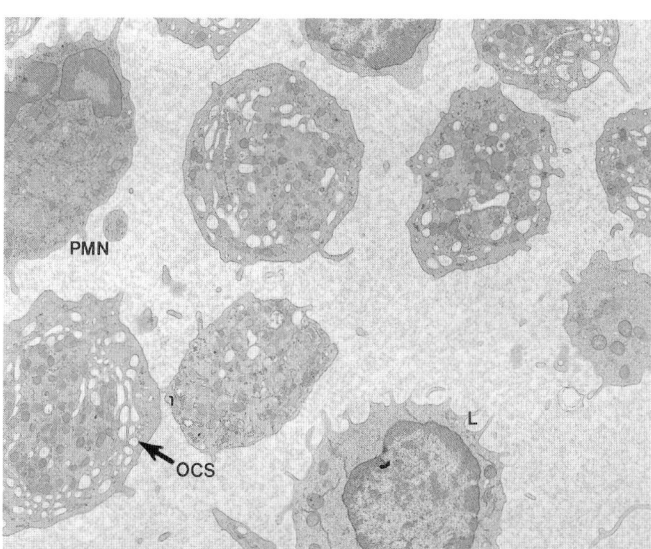

Fig. 25.34 Platelets from a patient with Fechtner syndrome. The cells are nearly as large as the lymphocyte (L) and polymorphonuclear leukocyte (PMN) in the same section. OCS, open canalicular system. × 2000.

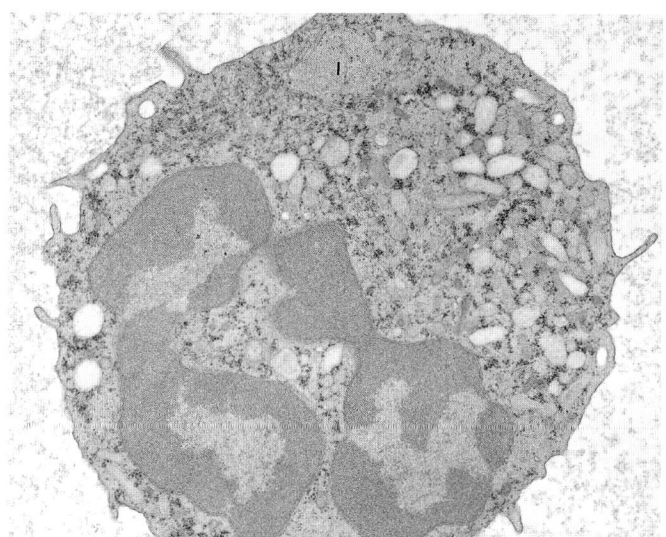

Fig. 25.35 Inclusion (I) body in a neutrophil from a patient with the Fechtner syndrome. Absence of glycogen and organelles are almost the only distinguishing features at this magnification. × 12 000.

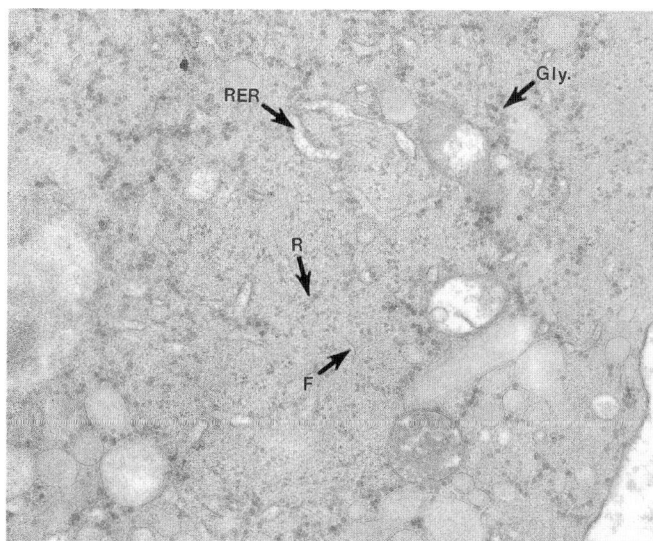

Fig. 25.36 Fechtner neutrophil inclusion body. Bits of rough endoplasmic reticulum (RER) are present with clusters of ribosomes (R). Occasional filaments (F) are also present. The ribosomes are easily distinguished from glycogen (Gly) particles because they are half the size and not as electron dense. × 27 000.

tubule coils cause the spherical shape of ES platelets or are the result of it.

The OCS is prominent in ES platelets, as it is in MHA cells.[138] The association of OCS channels with elements of the dense tubular system results in the formation of large membrane complexes in ES and MHA platelets. Membrane complexes are part of normal anatomy, and therefore are not inherently abnormal in giant platelets.

However, the large size of membrane complexes in ES and MHA platelets has suggested that the huge complexes may be the cause of macrothrombocytopenia.[131,134] Since the precise mechanisms of normal platelet membrane formation and organization in megakaryocytes have not been clearly defined, it is uncertain what the formation of giant membrane complexes has to do with the genesis of giant platelets.

Hereditary nephritis associated with May–Hegglin syndrome

The giant platelets observed in patient with MHA and ES are virtually identical. What separates the syndromes are other features of the hereditary disorders. ES patients are characterized by all of the features of Alport's syndrome[133] in addition to giant platelets, but lack the leukocyte inclusions characteristic of MHA.[140] MHA patients have spindle-shaped inclusions in circulating granulocytes and monocytes, but do not have high-frequency hearing loss. congenital cataracts or interstitial nephritis.

Brivet *et al*[141] have described a family in whom features of MHA and ES appeared together. Basophilic inclusion bodies, referred to as Dohle bodies in their report, were found in granulocytes of three affected family members studied. Clinical deafness and congenital cataracts were not found. Proteinuria, intermittent hematuria and mild elevation in blood pressure were presenting features of the nephritis in an 11-year-old female member of the family. A paternal grand aunt had died while on periodic hemodialysis and the father had proteinuria.

In contrast to the family reported from France, our kindred has characteristic features of Alport's syndrome.[133] High-frequency deafness and congenital cataracts were found in affected members in four generations. Renal biopsies revealed interstitial nephritis typical of ES and Alport's syndrome. One family member has undergone renal transplantation.

Platelets were large, but their light microscopic and ultrastructural appearance was not significantly different from that of normal platelets (Fig. 25.37). Platelet aggregation in response to epinephrine, arachidonate, thrombin, adenosine diphosphate, collagen and restocetin was normal. Levels of nucleotides and serotonin were normal in proportion to cell volume. The concentration of adenosine triphosphate secreted and the percentage of arachidonic acid converted to thromboxane B_2 were also proportional to cell number. Thus, this family represents a variant of Alport's syndrome with cataracts and leukocyte inclusions that, because of the associated macro-thrombocytopenia, may be confused with MHA or ES.

Gray platelet syndrome (GPS)

General features and specific details of GPS were discussed above. Platelets from patients with GPS are very large and often bizarre.[75] Therefore, the syndrome is classified as a giant platelet disorder, as well as a disorder of platelet organelles. The choice of GPS as the appellation for this disorder was based on the appearance of the cells

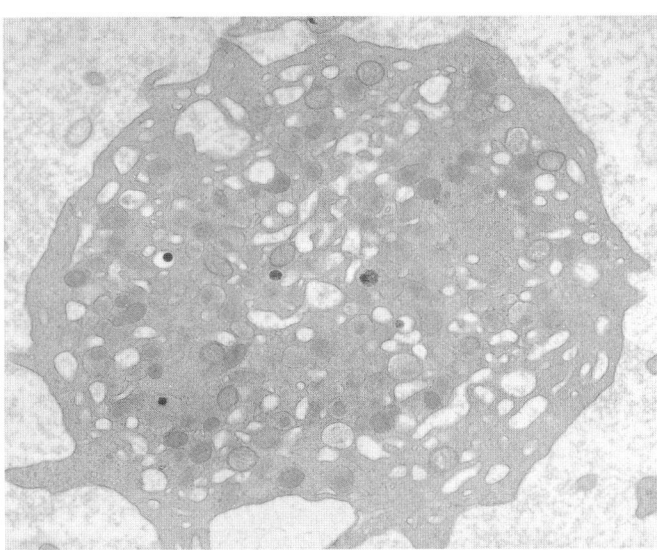

Fig. 25.37 Platelet from a patient with Fechtner syndrome. Channels of the open canalicular system are a prominent feature, but otherwise the morphology is identical to that found in normal platelets. × 16 000.

on Wright-stained blood smears. Absence of alpha granules and relative immaturity provided a grayish cast to the cells when observed in the light microscope. The other main feature was their large size. As a result, Raccuglia felt it necessary to distinguish gray platelets from the large cells found in other giant platelet disorders. Although GPS platelets are big, they are not as large as the cells from patients with MHA or ES.[132,138] As a result, platelet counts are usually higher in GPS patients than in patients with other giant platelet disorders. The morphology of gray platelets is also strikingly different from that of ES and MHA cells.[76] The virtual absence of alpha granules in most platelets is a characteristic feature. Gray platelets are found in other disorders, such as the transient leukemia of infancy in Down's syndrome (Fig. 25.38), in myeloproliferative syndromes, and in certain leukemic states in adults, but usually involve only a small percentage of the cells.

Absence of alpha granules permits the gray platelet to manifest a wide range of morphologic appearances.[76] Sometimes the cytoplasm is a monotonous matrix with a few mitochondria and dense bodies. In other GPS platelets the cytoplasm may be dominated by elements of the DTS, channels of the OCS, or a combination of the two, and the membrane complexes that result from their interaction. Vacuoles similar in size or larger than alpha granules were a common feature of the large gray platelets. The presence in megakaryocytes[109] as well as in platelets and the absence of alpha granules suggested that these structures might have been destined to enclose alpha granules.[76] Studies with electron-dense tracers

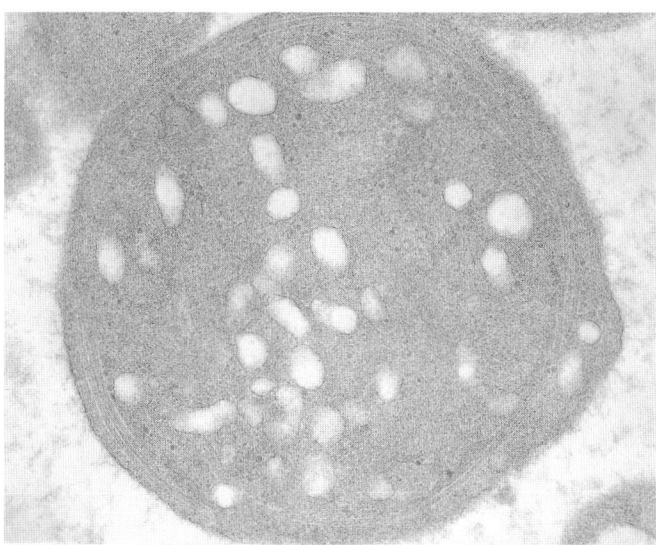

Fig. 25.38 Pseudo-gray platelets. This cell is from a patient with transient leukemia of childhood and Down's syndrome. The cells are of normal size, but devoid of alpha granules. As a result, they strongly resemble platelets from patients with gray platelet syndrome. × 36 000.

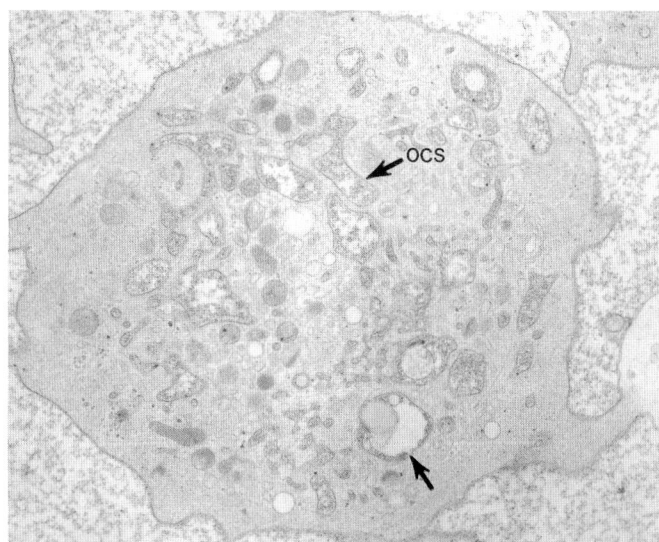

Fig. 25.39 Gray platelets fixed in the presence of an electron-dense tracer, tannic acid. Channels of the open canalicular system (OCS) and putative alpha granules (↑) connected to the OCS are filled with the stain. × 20 000.

demonstrated that the empty, sac-like structures were in direct continuity with surrounding plasma through channels of the OCS (Fig. 25.39).

Recent immunocytochemical studies have confirmed the suggestion that the vacuoles are putative alpha-granule membranes.[144] An antibody, GMP-140, specific for alpha-granule membranes was localized in resting gray platelets to the vacuole membranes by immunogold techniques. Activation of gray platelets by thrombin resulted in redistribution of GMP-140 to the plasma

membrane, just as in normal platelets. Endogenously synthesized PF4 was undetectable in gray platelets, but plasma-derived proteins, albumin and IgG were present in normal amounts and secreted in a normal manner after exposure to thrombin. Therefore, the fundamental defect in GPS appears to be transfer of the endogenously synthesized alpha-granule proteins to their appropriate target, or loss of these proteins to the outside due to premature connection of the organelles to demarcation membranes or channels of the OCS.[109] Our studies favor the latter hypothesis.

Cramer *et al*[145] used an immunogold method to localize fibrinogen and vWF in platelets from three patients with GPS. Both vWF and fibrinogen were distributed homogeneously in the rare normal alpha granules and also in small, abnormal alpha granules. The small structures were similar in size to immature granules present in normal megakaryocytes. Stimulation of GPS platelets by thrombin resulted in the release of fibrinogen from the small organelles to channels of the OCS. These findings add further support to the concept that GPS megakaryocytes make the proteins destined for alpha granules and do target them appropriately. However, the putative alpha granules, for the most part, are unable to retain the proteins and lose them to the surrounding plasma.

Montreal platelet syndrome (MPS)

A giant platelet disorder affecting three generations of a Canadian family has been studied extensively by Frojmovic and his colleagues[146] since it was first reported by Lacombe and d'Angelo.[147] The syndrome is characterized by autosomal dominant inheritance, the presence of giant platelets on peripheral blood smears with absence of leukocyte inclusions, a prolonged bleeding time, greatly reduced platelet counts (< 10 000–15 000/mm³), spontaneous platelet aggregation and normal clot retraction. At first the family members were thought to have the Bernard–Soulier syndrome, but ristocetin-induced platelet aggregation was normal and studies of surface membrane glycoproteins revealed no abnormality. The basis for the spontaneous aggregation of patient platelets was studied in detail without resolving the problem.[148] There may be an undescribed abnormality in MPS cell membranes resulting in the binding of fibrinogen and a calcium-independent form of spontaneous platelet aggregation.

Electron microscopy of MPS platelets revealed increased volume, but nowhere near the size of MHA or ES platelets (Figs 25.40 and 25.41). There was an increased frequency of large alpha granules in these cells, but the

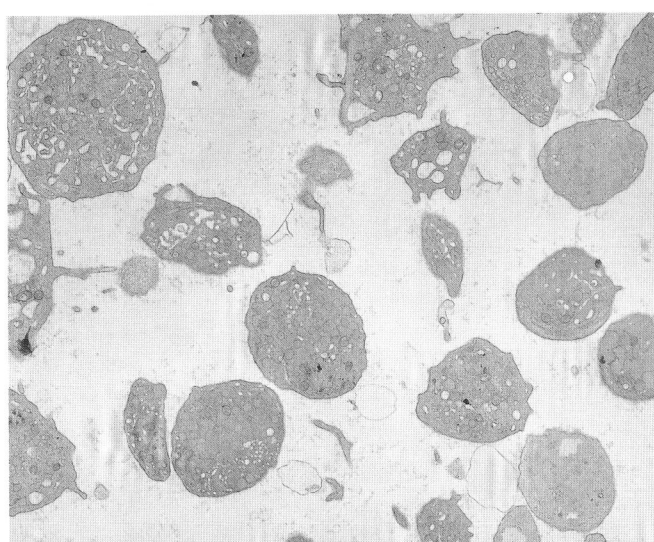

Fig. 25.40 Platelets from a patient with Montreal platelet syndrome (MPS). Except for their large size, MPS platelets resemble normal platelets. × 6000.

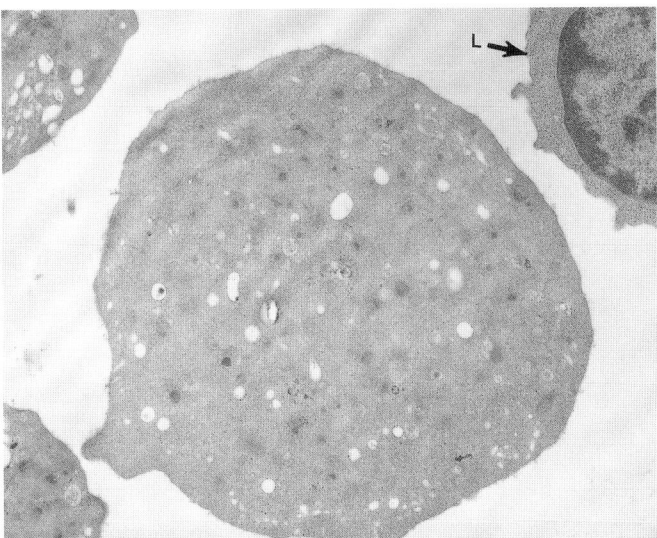

Fig. 25.42 Bernard–Soulier syndrome. Most patients with this disorder have very large platelets. This cell is larger than the adjacent lymphocyte (L). × 15 000.

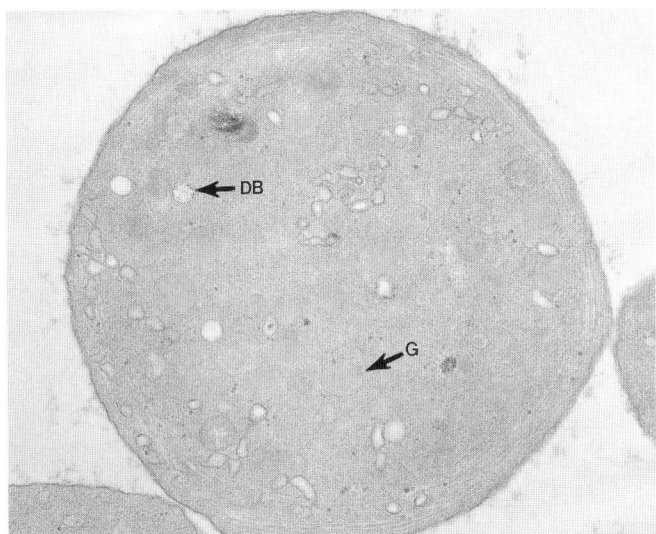

Fig. 25.41 Platelet from a patient with Montreal syndrome. The cell contains a normal component of alpha granules (G) and dense bodies (DB). × 19 000.

difference from normal platelets was not significant. MPS platelets contained elements of the OCS and DTS, as well as membrane complexes, but they were not unusual in size or frequency in comparison to MHA or ES cells. This is of interest because Frojmovic has shown that shape-changing agents produce unusually large platelets when stirred with cells from the family with MPS.[146] The rationale offered to explain hypervolumetric shape change is based on the assumption that MPS platelets contain an excessively well-developed OCS. Stimulation by potent agonists was speculated to cause evagination of the overdeveloped OCS on to the surface, greatly expanding its total surface area. The microscopic studies showing a normal frequency of OCS channels in MPS platelets suggest that the hypothesis may be incorrect. It is possible that the hypervolumetric shape change may be due to other factors influencing MPS platelet membrane resistance to deformation.[149]

Bernard–Soulier syndrome (BSS)

BSS[150] is an autosomal recessively inherited hemorrhagic disorder resulting from platelet inability to adhere to vascular subendothelium as a consequence of a surface membrane defect.[151]

At least three of the major glycoproteins, GPIb, GPIX, and GPV, are modified or absent from the surface membranes of BSS platelets.[152] Patients with BSS are thrombocytopenic and most reports suggest that a significant proportion of their platelets are markedly enlarged (Fig. 25.42). However, Frojmovic has suggested that BSS platelets are not increased in size.[153] Rather, they appear large compared to normal platelets on peripheral blood smears because of a proposed tendency to spread into thin films on contact with glass. The volume of BSS platelets in suspension was found to be normal. Abnormal spreading was related to an increased content of intracellular membrane extruded on to the cell surface during the spreading process (Fig. 25.43).

Characteristic ultrastructural defects have not been observed in thin sections of BSS platelets, but a report based on evaluation of replicas from freeze-fractured BSS platelets has indicated a distinct difference in the size and distribution of intramembranous particles (IMP)

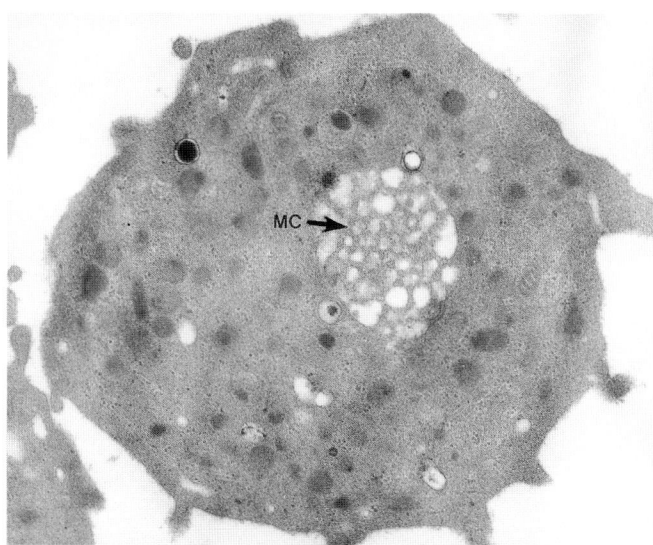

Fig. 25.43 Bernard–Soulier syndrome. The platelet in this example has a membrane complex (MC), but channels of the open canalicular system are not especially prominent in cells from these patients. × 22 000.

compared to normal platelets.[154] IMP are exposed on both the P-face (PF) and the E-face (EF) of freeze-fractured normal platelets and vary in size from about 5 to 13 nm. Approximately 1000 IMP/μm^2 are present on the EF compared to 500 IMP/μm^2 on the PF of human cells, yielding a PF/EF ratio of 0.5. Chevalier *et al*[154] reported an increase in larger IMP in both fracture faces of BSS platelets and a greater concentration of particles on the PF than on the EF, resulting in reversal of the normal PF/EF ratio. Other recent reports have suggested that BSS platelets contain increased numbers of dense bodies, the storage pool of adenine nucleotides.[155] The increase in dense bodies is associated with a five-fold increase in the capacity of BSS platelets to store serotonin.

GPIb, one of the glycoproteins missing from the surface membranes of BSS platelets,[152] is the receptor for vWF. As a result, BSS platelets do not aggregate with ristocetin or bovine factor VIII, which must interact with vWF and platelet GPIb to cause aggregation. BSS platelets also respond less well than normal cells to thrombin, possibly due to their deficiency in another surface-membrane glycoprotein, GPV or GPIX. Thus, the surface-membrane glycoprotein defects in BSS platelets have been closely linked to functional impairment in *vitro* and *in vivo*.

Other studies have raised questions about some of these findings. Examination of platelets from numerous patients with BSS by electronic sizing, ultrastructural and morphometric techniques has revealed that all are enlarged, though there is considerable variation. Some BSS patients have platelets about twice normal size,

while others reveal cells as large as those from families with MHA or ES. Thus, BSS is a giant platelet disorder as originally described, despite the suggestion that BSS platelets were of normal size in suspension.[153]

Frojmovic *et al* proposed that the hypervolumetric shape change and tendency to spread into thin films on glass slides were due to an excessive amount of internalized surface membrane in the form of channels of the open canalicular system.[153] However, careful study of platelets from several BSS patients in the electron microscope after incubation of their cells with electron-dense tracers has failed to reveal an increase in the OCS (Figs 25.42 and 25.43). If anything, the extent of the OCS in BSS platelets is less than in normal cells. Thus, the suggestion that evagination of an overdeveloped OCS is the basis for excess spreading or hypervolumetric shape change observed in BSS platelets appears unwarranted.

Investigations employing the technique of micropipette elastimetry[156] may offer a better explanation for observations described by Frojmovic *et al*. Micropipette elastimetry has been used extensively to evaluate mechanical properties of erythrocyte membranes, but platelets seemed too small to study by this procedure. However, the problems have been overcome, and the technique extended to the investigation of normal and abnormal platelets.[156] Under the same conditions of negative pressure, membrane segments aspirated from BSS platelets are two to three times longer than those drawn from normal cells or other inherited disorders. Deformability of thrombasthenic platelets was normal, indicating that deficiency in a different glycoprotein than that missing on BSS platelets is not sufficient to affect deformability. Other giant platelet disorders, including MHA, ES and GPS, were also as resistant to aspiration as normal platelets, showing that large size is not a significant factor influencing resistance to micropipette aspiration.

A biochemical basis for the marked softness of BSS platelet membranes has been found to be a transmembrane protein.[157] It is connected on the inside surface to a cytoskeletal protein, actin-binding protein. Evaluation of the effects of chilling, cytochalasin B and vincristine on platelet-membrane deformability in micropipettes had shown that the cytoskeleton is very much involved in resistance to deformation.[156] Therefore, the absence of GPIb and its transmembrane link to actin-binding protein of the internal cytoskeleton is the likely explanation for the increased spreading on glass and hypervolumetric shape change of BSS platelets.

The freeze-fracture study that suggested intramembranous particles are larger and distributed differently in a split lipid bilayer of BSS platelets compared to normal cells involved only a single patient with the disorder.[154] In an attempt to confirm this observation, platelets from nine patients with BSS have been evaluated by freeze-fracture. This experience suggests that IMP on both the E-face and P-face of BSS platelets are of normal size and that their distribution yields the same E-face to P-face ratio as on replicas of normal platelet membranes.

Membrane inclusion disorders

Enyeart anomaly (EA)

The literature contains many refrences to single patients or families with giant platelets, thrombocytopenia and mild to severe bleeding problems. We have tried to characterize as many giant platelet disorders as possible in order to define the mechanism of their formation in megakaryocytes. The Enyeart anomaly (EA) is one of these. A mother and her teenaged daughter were referred to us several years ago with lifelong histories of mild bleeding symptoms and congenital thrombocytopenia. Both have giant platelets (Fig. 25.44). The large cells are relatively unresponsive to stimulation by most aggregating agents, but evaluation of membrane glycoproteins failed to reveal deficiencies in GPIb, GPIIb-IIIa, or other surface receptors. A small inclusion was found in a small but significant number of their platelets which had not been reported previously (Figs 25.44 and 25.45).

We held our results on two patients, hoping others would appear, and they have. Dr John O' Brien of Portsmouth, England sent us samples from a patient with giant platelets and both clinical and laboratory findings similar to those for the two women desribed above. Her platelets were found to contain the same inclusion as in those of the other two. A fourth patient from California with giant platelets also has a small, but significant, number of the inclusions in her cells. Thus, EA appears to represent a distinct giant platelet disorder characterized by the presence of a small inculsion body. The nature of the defect leading to giant platelets, defective function, and formation of the inclusion body remians obscure.

Medich giant inclusion disorder

The young woman with this problem has a lifelong history of mild to severe bleeding.[132] She bruises easily and has had severe menorrhagia, requiring transfusion therapy on two occasions. The patient had macrothrombocytopenia. Her platelet count varies from 30 000 to 60 000/mm₃, and her mean platelet volume is 28–35 fl. The platelets are big, but not as large as those from

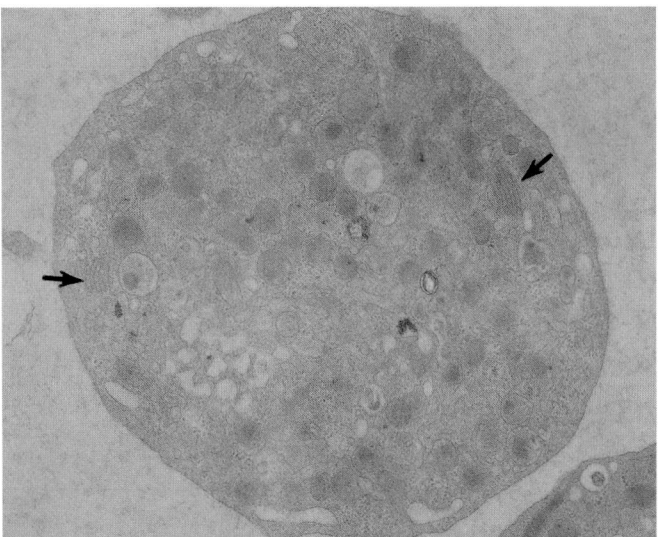

Fig. 25.44 Enyeart anomaly (EA). A platelet from one of our first two patients with this disorder. General features of platelet morphology are normal. However, there are two inclusions (↑) in the cytoplasm that are not found in normal platelets. × 16 000.

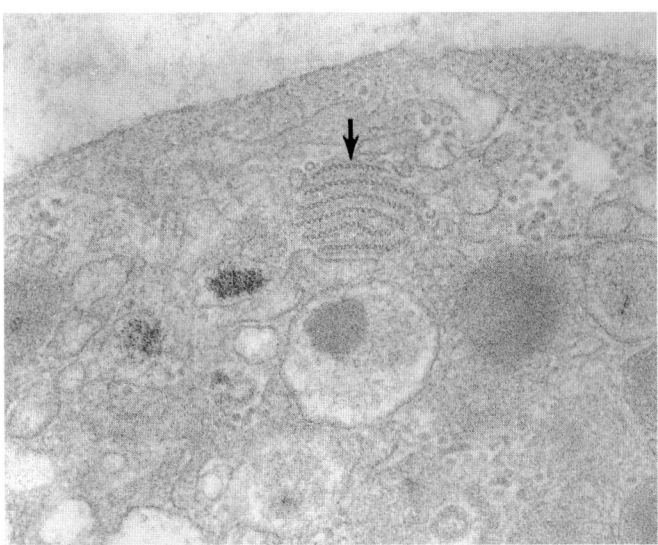

Fig. 25.45 Enyeart anomaly (EA). The EA inclusion (↑) is not membrane enclosed. However, it may resemble stacked membranes separated by amorphous, dense material on some occasions. A peculiar variation is shown here. It resembles a helix formed by a light and a dark string twisted tightly together. The linear helices appear stacked, but the precise nature of their organization and derivation remain obscure. × 60 000.

patients with MHA and ES. They are, however, very abnormal. The principal defects are found in the membrane systems and their organization (Fig. 25.46). Channels of the DTS are arranged in stacks in some cells and in linear arrangements in others. Membrane complexes formed by interaction of channels from the OCS and DTS are often condensed and sometimes enclosed within membranes resembling antophagic vacuoles. The most unusual

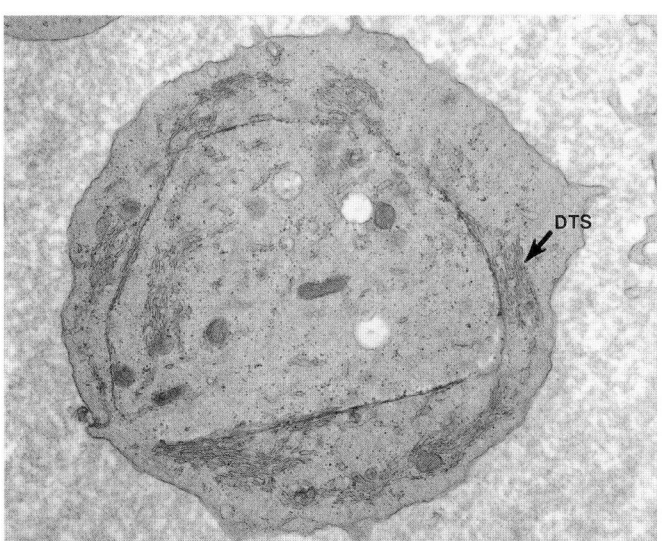

Fig. 25.46 Medich giant platelet inclusion disorder (MGPID). Platelets from this patient are large and reveal considerable variation in morphology. The example shown in this illustration contains primarily elements of the dense tubular system (DTS). One channel appears to encircle the cytoplasm, and has linear and curvilinear segments. × 24 000.

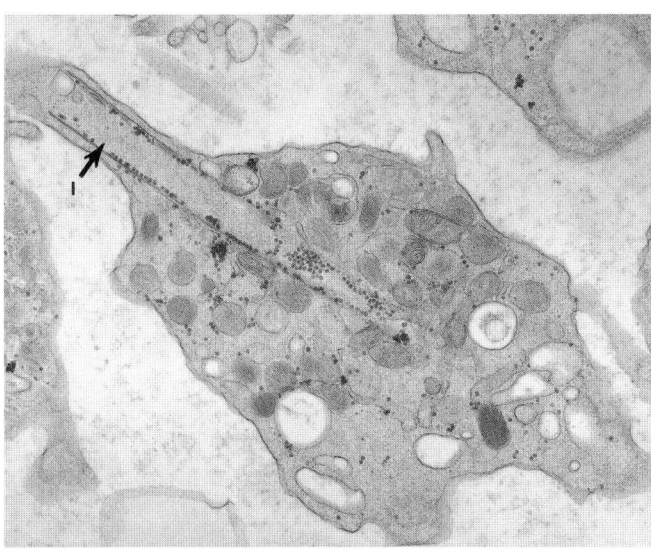

Fig. 25.47 Medich giant platelet inclusion disorder. A membrane inclusion (I) is present in the cytoplasm of this platelet. Glycogen particles are prominent inside the inclusion and along its membranous surfaces. Both ends of the inclusion are open to the cytoplasm. × 20 000.

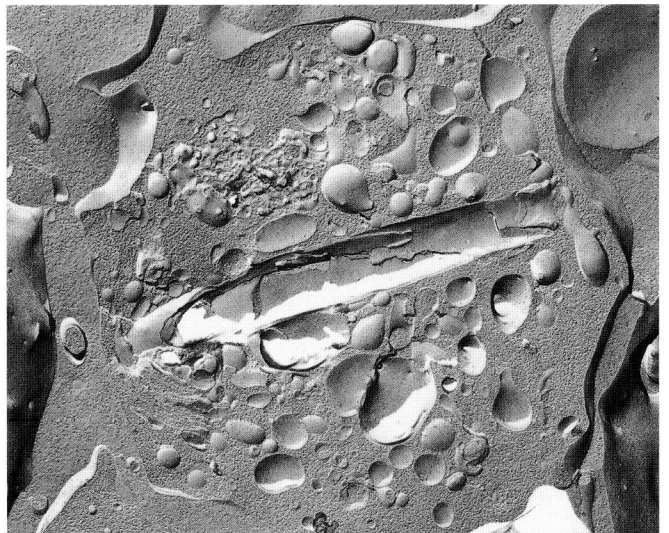

Fig. 25.48 Replica of freeze-fractured Medich giant platelet inclusion disorder cell. The inclusion revealed in the cytoplasm resembles a cigar with several membrane layers. × 17 000.

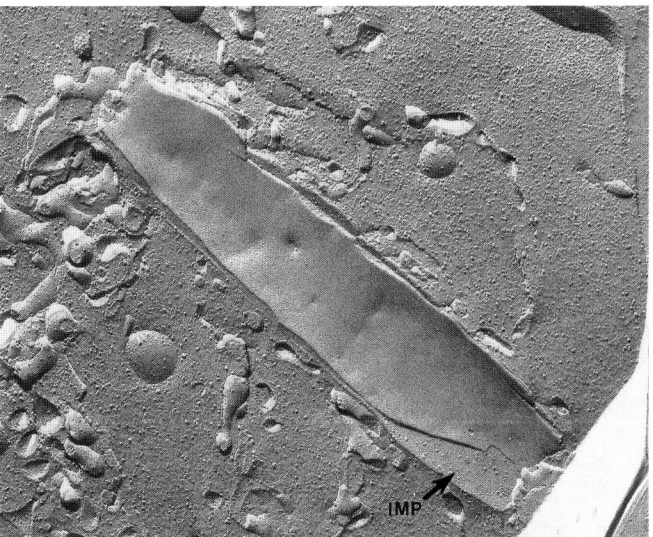

Fig. 25.49 Freeze-fractured platelet from a patient with Medich giant inclusion disorder. Intramembranous particles (IMP) can be seen on one of the exposed membrane faces, but the major membrane lacks IMP. × 32 000.

feature of her platelets, however, is the presence of membranous inclusions not observed previously in human cells (Fig. 25.47). The inclusions are tube-like or cigar shaped, and are composed of membranes wrapped like onion-skin layers around cores of cytoplasm. The inclusion is best seen in freeze-fractured platelets (Fig. 25.48) which reveals another facet of their unusual structure. They are the only membranes in human blood cells and other cell systems which lack intramembranous particles (Fig. 25.49). Our studies suggest that the tubular inclusions result from defective formation of membrane compexes.

At the time we first observed these structures, we considered them unique to the patient and human platelets. However, similar structures are present in platelets from all species of rats we have thus far observed, including the Wistar, Sprague–Dawley and Long–Evans hooded rat and in the giant platelets of the Wistar–Furth rat.[158] Precisely why the inclusions should be a normal constituent of rat platelets and only found in the giant abnormal cells of a single human patient is unknown.

In addition to the morphologic abnormalities, the patient's platelets are relatively unresponsive to aggregating agents, have low baseline calcium levels, and flux calcium poorly when stimulated by thrombin. The defects in calcium metabolism may be directly related to the abnormal organization of the DTS and OCS in her giant platelets.

Summary

As diverse as the group of inherited structural defects and giant platelet disorders presented in this chapter may seem, there is a common thread that ties them together. All appear to represent some form of membrane aberration. Sometimes only a small inclusion identifies the membrane defect, sometimes a massive increase in size. In others, whole populations of organelles are missing or surface membranes lack specific glycoproteins essential for their function. All of them are born in the deep recesses of the bone marrow megakaryocyte. Getting the megakaryocyte out into the light of day, or at least into a culture medium, should certainly lead to the solution of many, if not all, of the disorders of platelet membranes.

REFERENCES

1. Clay RS, Court TH 1932 The history of the microscope. Charles Griffin, London, 20–436
2. Leeuwenhoek A van 1674 Microscopical observations. Philosophical Transactions of the Royal Society of London 121–128
3. Hewson W 1774 Experimental inquiries: Part 1. Containing an inquiry into the properties of the blood, 2nd edn. J Johnson, London
4. Donné A 1842 De l'origine des globules du sang, de leur mode de formation et de leur fin. Comptes Render Seances de L'Academia des Sciences 14: 366–368
5. Bizzozero J 1882 Ueber einen neuen formbestandheil des bleetes und dessen rolle bei der thrombose und der blutgerinnung. Archives in Pathological Anatomy and Physiology 90: 261–332
6. Tocantins LM 1938 The mammalian blood platelet in health and disease. Medicine 17 155–260
7. Roth GJ 1991 Developing relationships: arterial platelet adhesion, glycoprotein Ib, and leucine-rich glycoproteins. Blood 77: 5–19
8. Saelman EUM, Nieuwenhuis HK, Hese KM et al 1994 Platelet adhesion to collagen types I through VIII under conditions of stasis and flow is mediated by GPIa/IIa ($\alpha_2\beta_1$-integrin). Blood 83: 1244–1250
9. Sixma JJ, Wester J 1977 The haemostatic plug. Seminars in Hematology 14: 265–299
10. Sixma JJ, van Zanten GH, Banga JD et al 1995 Platelet adhesion. Seminar in Hematology 32: 1–6
11. White JG 1987 Platelet structural physiology: the ultrastructure of adhesion, secretion and aggregation in arterial thrombosis. In: Mehta JL, Conti CR Brest AN (eds) Thrombosis and platelets in myocardial ischemia. Cardiovascular Clinics 18: 13–33 Breton-Gorius J, Levin J, Nurden AT (eds) 1990
12. Molecular biology and differentiation of megakaryocytes Prog in Clin and Biol Res 356. Wiley-Liss, New York, 1–372
13. White JG, Escolar G 1993 Current concepts of platelet membrane response to surface activation. Platelets 4: 176–189
14. White JG, Gerrard JM 1980 The cell biology of platelets. In: Weissman G (ed), Handbook of inflammation (The cell biology of inflammation). Elsevier/North Holland, New York, 83–143
15. White JG 1975 Is the canalicular system the equivalent of the muscle sarcoplasmic reticulum? Hemostasis 4: 185
16. Dignan PSJ, Maular AM, Frantz C 1967 Phocomelia with congenital hypoplastic thrombocytopenia and myeloid leukemoid reactions. Journal of Pediatrics 70: 561–573
17. O'Gorman-Hughes DW 1967 Neonatal thrombocytopenia: assessment of aetiology and prognosis. Australian paediatric Journal 3: 276
18. Hall JG, Levin J, Kuhn JP et al 1969 Thrombocytopenia with absent radius. Medicine 48: 411
19. Fanconi G 1927 Familiare infantile perniziosa: artige Anamie (Pernizioses Blutbild und Konstitution). Jahrbuch Kinderheilkund 117: 257
20. Rand M, Ried G 1951 Source of serotonin in serum. Nature 168: 385–386
21. Baker RV, Blaschko H, Born GVR 1959 The isolation from blood platelets of particles containing 5-hydroxytryptamine and adenosine triphosphate. Journal of Physiology (London) 149: 55–61
22. Siegel A, Luscher EF 1967 Non-identity of the granules of human blood platelets with typical lysosomes. Nature 215: 745–746
23. Wood JG 1965 Electron microscopic localization of 5-hydroxytryptamine (5-HT). Texas Reports of Biology and Medicine 23: 828–837
24. Davis RB, White JG 1968 Localization of 5-hydroxytryptamine in blood platelets: an autoradiographic and ultrastructural study. British Journal of Haematology 15: 93–99
25. White JG 1968 The origin of dense bodies in the surface coat of negatively stained platelets. Scandinavian Journal of Haematology 5: 371–382
26. White JG 1969 The dense bodies of human platelets: inherent electron opacity of serotonin storage particles. Blood 33: 598–606
27. Tranzer JP, Da Prada M, Pletscher A 1966 Letter to the editor. Ultrastructural localization of 5-hydroxytryptamine in blood platelets. Nature 211: 1547–1575
28. Richards JG, Da Prada M 1977 Uranaffin reaction: a new cytochemical technique for the localization of adenine nucleotides in organelles storing biogenic amines. Journal of Histochemistry and Cytochemistry 25: 1322–1336
29. Daimon T, Gotoh Y 1982 Cytochemical evidence of the origin of the dense tubular system in the mouse platelet. Histochemistry 76: 189–196
30. Witkop CJ Jr, Hill CW, Desnick SJ et al 1973 Ophthalmologic, biochemical, platelet and ultrastructural defects in various types of oculocutaneous albinism. Journal of investigative Dermatology 60: 443–456
31. Witkop CJ Jr 1985 Inherited disorders of pigmentation. Clinical Dermatology 3: 70–134
32. Witkop CJ, White JG, Townsend D et al 1988 Ceroid storage disease in Hermansky–Pudlak syndrome: induction in animal models. In: Nagy ZS (ed) Lipofuchsin-1987: state of art. Elsevier, Amsterdam, 413–436
33. White JG 1972 Ultrastructural defects in congenital disorders of platelet function. Annals of the New York Academy of Science 201: 205–233
34. Weiss HJ 1967 Platelet aggregation, adhesion and ADP release in thrombopathia (platelet factor 3 deficiency) – a comparison with Glanzmann's thrombasthenia and von Willebrand's disease. American Journal of Medicine 43: 570–578
35. Weiss HJ, Chervenick PA, Zalusky R 1969 A familial defect in platelet function associated with impaired release of adenisone diphosphate. New England Journal of Medicine 281: 1264–1268
36. Weiss HJ, Witte LD, Kaplan KL et al 1979 Heterogeneity in storage pool deficiency: studies on granule-bound substances in 18 patients including variants deficient in alpha granules, platelet factor-4, beta-thromboglobulin and platelet-derived growth factor. Blood 54: 1296–1308
37. Grottum KA, Hovig T, Holmsen H et al 1969 Wiskott–Aldrich syndrome: qualitative platelet defects and short platelet survival. British Journal of Haematology 17: 373–388
38. Day HJ, Holmsen H 1972 Platelet adenine nucleotide 'storage pool deficiency' in thrombocytopenia absent radii syndrome. Journal of the American Medical Association 221: 1053
39. Chediak M 1952 Nouvelle anomalie leukocytaire de caractere constitutionnel et familial. Reviews Hematologic Paris 7: 362–372
40. Higashi O 1954 Congenital gigantism of peroxidase granules: the first case ever reported of qualitative abnormality of peroxidase. Tohoku Journal of Experimental Medicine 59: 315–321

41. Wolff SM, Dale DC, Clark RA et al 1972 The Chediak–Higashi syndrome: studies of host defenses. Annals of Internal Medicine 76: 293–306

42. Bequez-Cesar A 1943 Neutropenia cronica maligna familiar con granulaciones atipicas de los leucocitos. Boletin Society Cubana Pediatrica 15: 900–902

43. White JG, Clawson CC 1980 Development of giant granules in platelets during prolonged storage. American Journal of Pathology 101: 635–646

44. Page AR, Berendes H, Warner J, Good RA 1962 The Chediak–Higashi syndrome. Blood 20: 330–338

45. Boxer GJ, Holmsen H, Robkin L et al 1977 Abnormal platelet function in Chediak–Higashi syndrome. British Journal of Haematology 35: 521–533

46. White JG 1978 Platelet microtubules and giant granules in the Chediak–Higashi syndrome. American Journal of Medical Technology 44: 273–278

47. Parmley RT, Poon MC, Crist WM, Molluk A 1979 Giant platelet granules in a child with the Chediak–Higashi syndrome. American Journal of Hematology 6: 51–60

48. Bell TG, Myers KM, Prieur DJ et al 1976 Decreased nucleotide and serotonin storage associated with defective function in Chediak–Higashi syndrome platelets. Blood 48: 175–184

49. Buchanan GR, Handin RI 1976 Platelet function in the Chediak–Higashi syndrome. Blood 47: 941–947

50. Boxer LA, Watanabe AM, Rister M et al 1976 Correction of leukocyte function in Chediak–Higashi syndrome by ascorbate. New England Journal of Medicine 295: 1041–1045

51. Gallin JI, Elin RJ, Hubert RT et al 1979 Efficacy of ascorbic acid in Chediak–Higashi syndrome (CHS): Studies in humans and mice. Blood 53: 226–234

52. Oliver JM 1976 Impaired microtubule function correctable by cyclic GMP and cholinergic agonists in the Chediak–Higashi syndrome. American Journal of Pathology 85: 395–418

53. White JG 1972 Ultrastructural defects in congenital disorders of platelet function. Annals of the New York Academy of Science 201: 205–233

54. White JG 1971 Platelet morphology. In: Johnson SA (ed) The circulating platelet. Academic Press, New York, 45–121

55. White JG, Krivit W 1966 The ultrastructural localization and release of platelet lipids. Blood 27: 167–186

56. Rodman NF, Mason RG, McDevitt NB, Brinkhous KM 1961 Morphological alterations of human blood platelets during early phases of clotting. American Journal of Pathology 40: 271–283

57. White JG 1968 Tubular elements in platelet granules. Blood 32: 148–156

58. Cramer EM, Meyer D, LeMenn R, Breton-Gorius J 1985 Eccentric localization of von Willebrand factor within tubular structure of platelet alpha granules resembling that of Weibel Palade bodies. Blood 66: 710–715

59. Gerrard JM, Phillips DR, Rao GHR et al 1980 Biochemical studies of two patients with the gray platelet syndrome–selective deficiency of platelet alpha granules. Journal of Clinical Investigation 66: 102–109

60. White JG 1968 Transfer of thorium particles from plasma to platelets and platelet granules. American Journal of Pathology 53: 567–575

61. Handagama PJ, George JN, Schuman MA et al 1987 Incorporation of a circulating protein into megakaryocyte and platelet granules. Proceedings of the National Academy of Sciences USA 84: 861–865

62. Handagama PJ, Schuman R, Schuman MA, Bainton DF 1988 *In Vivo* defibrination results in markedly decreased levels of fibrinogen in megakaryocytes and platelets in rats. Abstract, American Society of Hematology Annual Meeting, San Antonio, Texas

63. Grette K 1962 Studies on the mechanism of thrombin-catalyzed hemostatic reaction in blood platelets. Acta Physiological Scandinavian (suppl) 56(195): 1–93

64. Holmsen H (1987) Platelet secretion. In: Colman RW, Hirsh J, Marder VJ (eds), Hemostasis and thrombosis. Lippincott, Philadelphia, 390–403

65. Kaplan K, Brockman MJ, Chernoff A et al 1979 Platelet alpha granule proteins: studies on release and subcellular organization. Blood 53: 604–618

66. Stormorken H 1969 The release reaction of secretion. Scandinavian Journal of Haematology (suppl) 9: 3–24

67. Ginsberg MH, Taylor L, Painter RG 1980 The mechanisms of thrombin-induced platelet factor 4 secretion. Blood 55: 661–669

68. White JG 1983 The morphology of platelet function. In: Harker LA, Zimmerman TS (eds), Methods in hematology, series 8L:

Measurements of platelet function. Churchill-Livingstone, New York, 1–25

69. David-Ferreira JF 1964 The blood platelet: electron-microscopic studies. International Reviews of Cytology 17: 99–148

70. Maldonado JE 1975 Giant platelet granules in refractory anemia (preleukemia) and myelomonocytic leukemia: a cell marker? Blood Cells 1: 129–135

71. White JG, Clawson CC. 1980 Development of giant granules in platelets during prolonged storage. American Journal of Pathology 101: 635–646

72. White JG 1987 The secretory pathway of bovine platelets. Blood 69: 878–885

73. White JG, Krumwiede M 1987 Further studies of the secretory pathway in thrombin stimulated human platelets. Blood 69: 1196–1203

74. White JG, Krivit W, Vernier R 1965 The platelet-fibrin relationship in human blood clots: an ultrastructural study utilizing ferritin conjugated anti-human fibrinogen antibody. Blood 25: 241–249

75. Raccuglia G 1971 Gray platelet syndrome: a variety of qualitative platelet disorder. American Journal of Medicine 51: 818–828

76. White JG 1979 Ultrastructural studies of the gray platelet syndrome. American Journal of Pathology 95: 455–462

77. Levy-Toledano S, Caen JP, Breton-Gorius J et al 1981 Gray platelet syndrome: alpha-granule deficiency, its influence on platelet function. Journal of Laboratory and Clinical Medicine 98: 831–849

78. Von Behrens WE 1972 Evidence of phylogenelic canalization of the circulating platelet mass in man. Thrombosis Diathesis Haemorrhagica 27: 159–163

79. Breton-Gorius J 1981 On the alleged phagocytosis by megakaryocytes. British Journal of Haematology 47: 635–636

80. Breton-Gorius J, Bizet M, Reyes F 1982 Myelofibrosis and acute megakaryoblastic leukemia in a child: topographic relationship between fibroblasts and megakaryocytes with an alpha-granule defect. Leukemia Research 6: 97–110

81. Goldenhar M 1952 Association malformatives de l'oeil et de l'oreille, en perticulier le syndrome dermoide epibulbaire-appendices appendices auriculaires-fistula auris congenita et ses relations avec la dysostose mandibulofaciale. Journal de Genetique Humaine 1: 243–282

82. Mori K, Suzuki S, Sugai K 1984 Electron microscopic and functional studies on platelets in gray platelet syndrome, Tohoku Journal of Experimental Medicine 143: 261–287

83. Rao AK, Holmsen H 1986 Congenital disorders of platelet function. Seminars in Hematology 23: 102–118

84. White JG 1986 Platelet granule disorders. Critical Reviews of Oncology/Hematology 4: 337–377

85. Breton-Gorius J, Favier R, Guichard J et al 1995 A new congenital dysmegakaryopoietic thrombocytopenia (Paris–Trousseau) associated with giant platelet alpha-granules and chromosome 11 deletion at 11q23. Blood 85: 1805–1814

86. Favier R, Douay L, Esteva B et al 1993 A novel genetic thrombocytopenia (Paris–Trousseau) associated with platelet inclusions, dysmegakaryopoiesis and chromosome deletion at 11q23. Comptes Rendus de I'Academic des Sciences (Patis) 316: 698–701

87. Favier R 1997 Paris–Trousseau thrombocytopenia: a new entity and a model for understanding megakaryocytopoiesis (editorial). Pathologie et Biologie (Paris) 45: 693–696

88. Jacobsen P, Hauge M, Henningsen K et al 1973 An (11;21) translocation in four generations with chromosome 11 abnormalities in the offspring. A clinical, cytogenetical, and gene marker study. Human Heredity 23: 568–585

89. Michaelis RC, Velagaleti GV, Jones C et al 1998 Most Jacobsen syndrome deletion breakpoints occur distal to FRA11B. American Journal of Medical Genetics 76: 222–228

90. Penny LA, Dell' Aquila M, Jones MC et al 1995 Clinical and molecular characterization of patients with distal 11q deletions. American Journal of Human Genetics 56: 676–683

91. Krishnamurti L, Neglia JP, Nagarajan R et al (2002) Paris–Trousseau syndrome platelets in a child with Jacobsen's syndrome. American Journal of Hematology (in press)

92. Holmsen H, Day HJ, Stormorken H 1969 The blood platelet release reaction. Scandinavian Journal of Haematology (suppl 8): 326

93. White JG 1971 The ultrastructural cytochemistry and physiology of blood platelets. In: Mostafi FK, Brinkhous KM (eds) William and Wilkins, Baltimore, 873–915

94. Bentfield ME, Bainton DF 1975 Cytochemical localization of

lysosomal enzymes in rat megakaryocytes and platelets. Journal of Clinical Investigation 56: 1635–1649

95. Stenberg PE, Bainton DF 1986 Storage organelles in platelets and megakaryocytes In: Phillips DR, Shuman M (eds), Biochemistry of platelets. Academic Press, New York, 257–294

96. Morgenstern E 1982 Coated membranes in blood platelets. European Journal of Cell Biology 26: 315–318

97. White JG 1966 The Chediak–Higashi syndrome: a possible lysosomal disease. Blood 28: 143–156

98. White JG, Clawson CC 1979 The Chediak–Higashi syndrome: spectrum of giant organelles in peripheral blood cells. Henry Ford Hospital Medical Journal 27: 286–298

99. White JG 1988 Platelet membrane ultrastructural and its changes during platelet activation. In: Harris H, Hirschorn K (eds), Platelet membrane receptors: molecular biology, immunology, biochemistry, and pathology. Alan R Liss, New York, 1032

100. Wright JH 1906 The origin and nature of the blood platelets, Boston Medical Surgical Journal 154: 643–645

101. Behnke O 1968 An electron microscope study of the megakaryocyte of the rat bone marrow. I. The development of the demarcation membrane system and the platelet surface coat. Journal Ultrastructure Research 24: 412–433

102. Behnke O 1969 An electron microscope study of the rat megakaryocyte. II. Some aspects of platelet release and microtubules. Journal of Ultrastructure Research 26: 111–129

103. Tavassoli M 1980 Megakaryocyte–platelet axis and the process of platelet formation and release. Blood 55: 537–545

104. Radley JM, Haller CJ 1982 The demarcation membrane system of the megakaryocyte: a misnomer? Blood 60: 213–219

105. Thiery JP, Bessis M 1956 Mecanisme de la plaquettogenese. Etude *in vitro* par la microinematographie. Reviews Hematologie 11: 162–174

106. Becker RP, deBruyn PPH 1976 The transmural passage of blood cells into myeloid sinusoids and the entry of platelets into the sinusoidal circulation; a scanning electron microscopic investigation. American Journal of Anatomy 145: 183–206

107. Scurfield G, Radley JM 1981 Aspects of platelet formation and release. American Journal of Hematology 10: 285–296

108. Radley JM, Scurfield GT 1980 The mechanism of platelet release. Blood 56: 996–999

109. Breton-Gorius J, Vainchenker W, Nurden A et al 1981 Defective alpha-granule production in megakaryocytes from gray platelet syndrome: ultrastructural studies of bone marrow cells and megakaryocytes growing in culture from blood presursors. American Journal of Pathology 102: 10–19

110. Wiskott A 1937 Familiarer angeborener morbus werlhofii? Monatsschrif Kinderheilkunde 68: 212–215

111. Aldrich RA, Steinberg AG, Campbell DC 1954 Pedigree demonstrating a sex-linked recessive condition characterized by draining ears, eczematoid dermatitis and bloody diarrhea. Pediatrics 13: 133–141

112. Prchal JT, Carroll AJ, Prchal JF et al 1980 Wiskott–Aldrich syndrome: cellular impairments and their implication for carrier detection. Blood 56: 1048–1053

113. Lum LG, Tubergen DG, Carash L, Blaese RM 1980 Splenectomy in the management of thrombocytopenia of the Wiskott–Aldrich syndrome. New England Journal of Medicine 302: 892–896

114. Ochs HD, Slichter SJ, Harker LA et al 1980 The Wiskott–Aldrich syndrome: studies of lymphocytes, granulocytes and platelets. Blood 55: 243–252

115. Parkman R, Kenney D, Remold-O'Donnell E et al 1981 Surface protein abnormalities in lymphocytes and platelets from patients with Wiskott–Aldrich syndrome. Lancet II: 1387–1389

116. Baldinni MG 1972 Nature of the platelet defect in Wiskott–Aldrich syndrome. Annals of the New York Academy of Science 201: 437–444

117. Krivit W, Yunis E, White JG 1966 Platelet survival studies in Wiskott–Aldrich syndrome. Pediatrics 37: 339–341

118. Levine RF 1986 Old and new aspects of megakaryocyte development and function. In: Levine RF, Williams N, Levin J et al (eds), Megakaryocyte development and function. Alan R Liss, New York, 1–20

119. Breton-Gorius J, Vainchenker W 1986 Expression of platelet proteins during the *in vitro* and *in vivo* differentiation of megakaryocytes and morphological aspects of their maturation. Seminars in Hematology 23: 43–67

120. May R 1909 Leukocyteneinschlusse. Deutsch Archiv fur Klincal Medingin 96: 1–6

121. Hegglin R 1945 Gleichzertge Konstitutionelle Veranderungen on Neutrophilen und Thrombocyten. Helvetica Medica Acta 12: 439–440

122. Volpe E, Cuccurullo L, Valente A et al 1974 The May–Hegglin: further studies on leukocytes inclusions and platelet ultrastructure. Acta Haematologica 52: 238–247

123. Dohle V 1912 Leukocyteneinschlussee bei scharlach. Zentralblatt fur Bakteriologie 61: 63–68

124. Jenis EH, Takeuchi A, Dillon DE et al 1971 The May–Hegglin anomaly: ultrastructure of the granulocytic inclusion. American Journal of Clinical Pathology 55: 187–196

125. White JG, Gerrard JM 1976 Ultrastructural features of abnormal blood platelets. American Journal of Pathology 83: 590–632

126. Jordon SW, Larsen WE 1965 Ultrastructural studies of the May–Hegglin anomaly. Blood 25: 921–932

127. Luscher JM, Schneider J, Mizukami I, Evans RK 1968 The May–Hegglin anomaly: platelet function, ultrastructure and chromosome studies. Blood 32: 950–961

128. Godwin HA, Ginsburg AD 1974 May–Hegglin anomaly: a defect in megakaryocyte fragmentation? British Journal of Haematology 26: 117–128

129. Karpatkin S 1985 Autoimmune thrombocytopenic purpura. Seminars in Hematology 22: 260–288

130. Firkin BG, Wright R, Miller S 1969 Splenic macrophages in thrombocytopenia. Blood 33: 240–248

131. Breton-Gorius J 1975 Development of two membrane systems associated in giant complexes in pathological megakaryocytes. Series Hematologica 8: 49–67

132. White JG 1987 Inherited abnormalities of the platelet membrane and secretory granules. Human Pathology 18: 123–139

133. Alport AC 1927 Hereditary familial congenital hemorrhagic nephritis. British Medical Journal i: 504–506

134. Epstein CJ, Sahud MA, Piel CA et al 1972 Hereditary macrothrombocytopathia, nephritis and deafness. American Journal of Medicine 52: 299–310

135. Eckstein JD, Filip DJ, Watts JC 1975 Hereditary thrombocytopenia, deafness and renal disease. Annals of Internal Medicine 82: 639–645

136. Hansen MS, Behnke O, pedersen NT, Videbaek A. 1978 Megathrombocytopenia associated with glomerulonephritis, deafness and aortic cystic medianecrosis. Scandinavian Journal of Haematology 21: 197–205

137. Bernheim J, Dechavanne M, Bryon PA et al 1976 Thrombocytopenia, macrothrombocytopathia, nephritis and deafness. American Journal of Medicine 61: 145–150

138. White JG 1982 Membrane abnormalities in congenital disorders of human blood platelets. In: Sheppard JR, Andetson VE, Eaton JW (eds), Membranes and genetic disease. Alan R Liss, New York, 351–370

139. White JG, Sauk JJ 1984 The organization of microtubules and microtubule coils in giant platelet disorders. American Journal of Pathology 116: 514–522

140. Cawley JC, Hayhoe FGJ 1972 The inclusions of the May–Hegglin anomaly and Dohle bodies of infection: an ultrastructural comparison. British Journal of Haematology 22: 491–496

141. Brivet F, Girot R, Barbanel C et al 1981 Hereditary nephritis associated with May–Hegglin anomaly, Nephron 29: 59–62

142. Peterson LC, Rao KV, Crosson JT, White JG 1985 Fechtner syndrome – a variant of Alport's syndrome with leukocyte inclusions and macrothrombocytopenia. Blood 65: 397–406

143. Rao AK, Holmsen H 1986 Congenital disorders of platelet function. Seminars in Hematology 23: 102–118

144. Rosa JP, George JN, Bainton DF et al 1987 Gray platelet syndrome: demonstration of alpha granule membrane that can fuse with the cell surface. Journal of Clinical Investigation 80: 1138–1146

145. Cramer EM, Meyer D, LeMenn R, Breton-Gorius J 1985 Eccentric localization of von Willebrand factor within a tubular structure of platelet alpha granules resembling that of Weibel Palade bodies. Blood 66: 710–715

146. Milton JG, Frojmovic MM 1979 Shape-changing agents produce abnormally large platelets in a hereditary 'giant platelets syndrome (MPS)'. Journal of Laboratory and Clinical Medicine 93: 154–161

147. Lacombe M, d'Angelo G 1963 Etudes sur une thrombopathie familiare. Neuvo Revue Franc Hematologie 3: 611–614

148. Milton JG, Frojmovic MM, Tang SS, White JG 1984 Spontaneous platelet aggregation in a hereditary giant platelet syndrome (MPS). American Journal of Pathology 114: 336–345

149. White JG, Burris SM, Tukey D et al 1984 Micropipette aspiration of

human platelets: influence of microtubules and actin filaments on deformability. Blood 64: 210–214

150. Bernard J, Soulier JP 1948 Sur une nouvelle variété de dystrophie thrombocytaire hemorragipare congenitale. Semaine des Hopitoux de Paris 24: 317–321

151. Bernard J 1983 History of congenital hemorrhagic thrombocytopathic dystrophy. Blood Cells 9: 179–193

152. Nurden AT 1985 Glycoprotein defects responsible for abnormal platelet function in inherited disorders. In: George JN, Nurden AT, Phillips DR (Eds). Platelet membrane glycoproteins. Plenum Press, New York, 357–387

153. Frojmovic MM, Milton JG, Caen JP 1978 Platelets from 'giant platelet syndrome (BSS)' are discocytes and normal sized. Journal of Laboratory and Clinical Medicine 91: 109–113

154. Chevalier J, Nurden AT, Thiere JM 1979 Freeze-fracture studies on the plasma membranes of normal human, thrombasthenia and Bernard–Soulier platelets. Journal of Laboratory and Clinical Medicine 94: 232–245

155. Rendu F, Nurden AT, Lebret M, Caen JP 1981 Further investigations on Bernard–Soulier platelet abnormalities. A study of 5-hydroxytryptamine uptake and mepacrine fluorescence. Journal of Laboratory and Clinical Medicine 97: 689–697

156. White JG, Burris SM, Hasegawa D, Johnson M 1984 Micropipette aspiration of human blood platelets: a defect in the Bernard–Soulier's syndrome. Blood 63: 1249–1252

157. Fox JEB 1985 Identification of actin-binding protein as the protein linking the membrane skeleton to glycoproteins on platelet plasma membranes. Journal of Biological Chemistry 260: 11970–11977

158. Davis RB 1973 Glycogen distribution in rat platelets. American Journal of Pathology 72: 241–252

Acquired disorders affecting megakaryocytes and platelets

26

D Provan   AC Newland

Introduction

Structure and function of megakaryocytes and platelets

Human platelets

Platelet structure and function
Platelet membrane constituents
The integrin family of proteins
Platelet integrins and related proteins

Platelet alloantigens

Cytoplasmic platelet constituents

Biological function of platelets
Platelet activation
Platelet adhesion
Platelet shape change
Platelet aggregation

Quantitative platelet abnormalities: thrombocytopenia

Pseudothrombocytopenia

Pooling of platelets in the spleen
Mechanism involved

Thrombocytopenia due to failure of platelet production

Acquired amegakaryocytic thrombocytopenia
Causative agents
Drug-induced megakaryocyte hypoplasia

Bone marrow failure syndromes
Aplastic anemia

Pathogenesis
Experimental evidence to date
Which stem cell antigens are involved?
Implicated agents in aplastic anemia
Clinical features
Laboratory findings
Bone marrow examination
Management

Thrombocytopenia due to increased platelet destruction

Non-immunologic causes of thrombocytopenia
Disseminated intravascular coagulation (DIC)
Thrombotic thrombocytopenic purpura and hemolytic uremic syndrome
Pre-eclampsia and HELLP syndrome
Thrombocytopenia caused by massive blood transfusion
Liver disease
Thrombocytopenia caused by infection
Thrombocytopenia due to hematinic deficiencies

Immunologic causes of thrombocytopenia

Alloantibody-mediated thrombocytopenia
Neonatal alloimmune thrombocytopenia
Post-transfusion purpura (PTP)

Autoantibody-mediated thrombocytopenia
Idiopathic thrombocytopenic purpura (ITP)
Acute ITP

Chronic ITP
Secondary immune thrombocytopenia

Drug-induced thrombocytopenia
Heparin-induced thrombocytopenia (HIT)
Other drugs causing immune-mediated
platelet destruction

**Acquired functional abnormalities
of platelets**

Uremia in renal failure
Pathogenesis
Management

Myeloproliferative disorders
Pathophysiology
Platelet abnormalities in the
myeloproliferative disorders
Clinical features
Management

**Platelet abnormalities in leukemia and
myelodysplastic syndromes**

**Platelet dysfunction in patients
with paraproteinemias**

Drugs that interfere with platelet function

Introduction

Platelets play a pivotal role in primary hemostasis, and bleeding may arise through a large number of different pathologies including those that reduce platelet numbers (thrombocytopenia) or render the platelets functionally defective. Therefore, for simplicity we have divided our discussion into those disorders causing quantitative abnormalities of platelets before later discussing qualitative defects that affect the function of platelets. Before examining the pathologic basis of platelet diseases it is useful to review the mechanics of platelet production, as well as the structure and normal function of platelets.

Structure and function of megakaryocytes and platelets

Human platelets

Thrombopoiesis, the generation of platelets from megakaryocytes in the bone marrow, is complex and incompletely understood. Megakaryocytes are large end-stage cells from which platelets bud. The earliest recognized committed progenitor is the burst-forming unit (BFU)-Meg.[1] Figure 26.1 shows megakaryocyte development from stem cell stage through to platelet

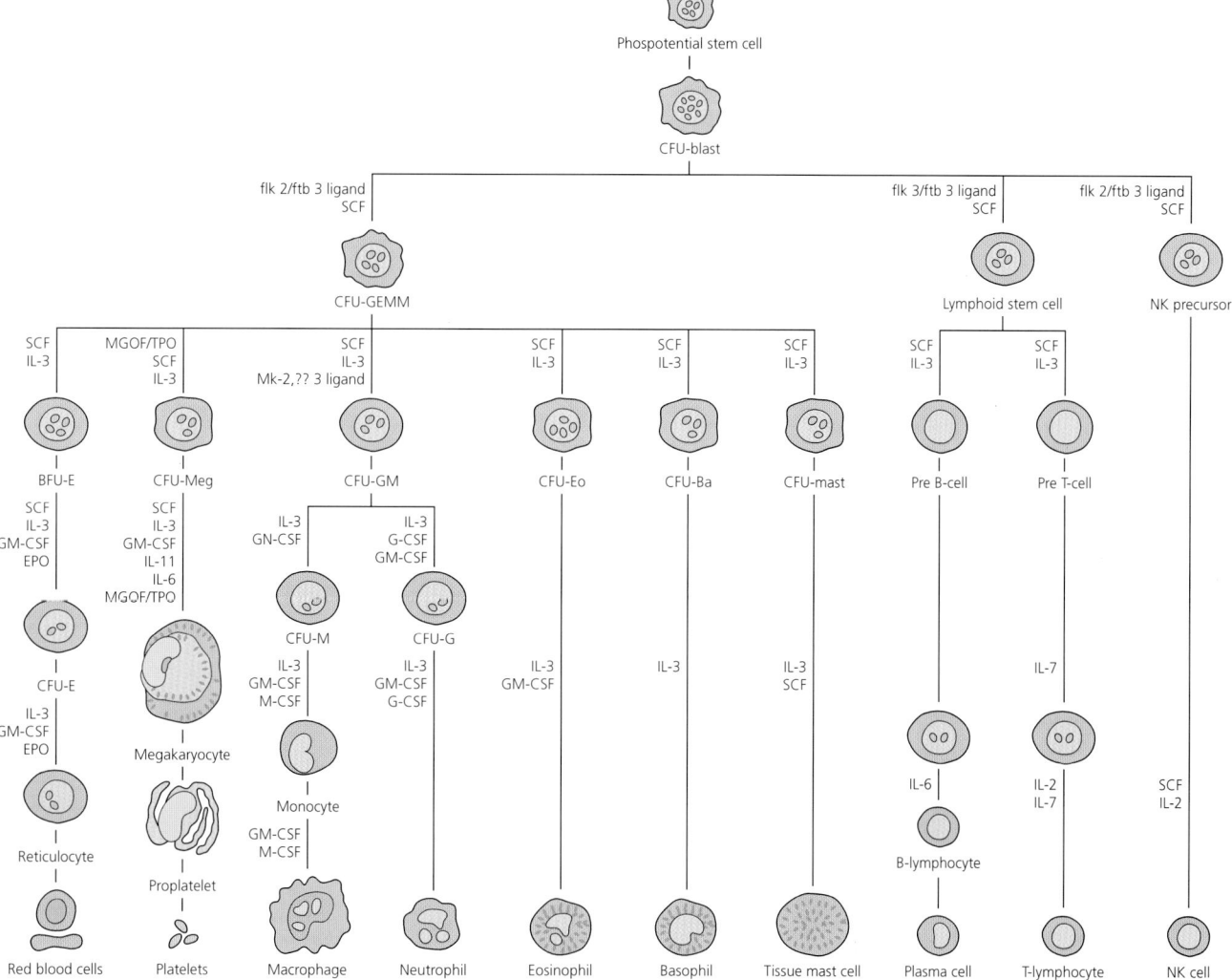

Fig. 26.1 Hematopoietic lineages, showing megakaryocyte development and platelet production. From Provan D, Gribben JG 2000 (eds), *Molecular haematology.* Blackwell Science, Oxford, with permission.

production. BFU-Megs develop into colony-forming unit (CFU)-Megs in the presence of growth factors thrombopoietin (TPO), interleukin-3 (IL-3) and IL-11. Megakaryocyte nuclei are large polyploid structures with chromosome contents between diploid (2N) to 64N. Such polyploid status is achieved through a process termed nuclear endoduplication; that is, successive doubling of chromosome content in the absence of cell division. Platelets are produced from megakaryocytes that are 8N or greater.[2]

A single megakaryocyte can generate around 3000 platelets of which 20–30% are pooled in the spleen. In health the peripheral blood platelet count is 150–400 × 10^9/l but this fluctuates, for example following heavy exercise, 'stress', and around the menstrual cycle. This transient rise in platelet count may be caused by mobilization of platelets pooled in the spleen. There are also racial differences in the 'normal' platelet count and some Mediterranean races have platelet counts as low as 80 × 10^9/l in health. Platelets are produced at a rate of 35 000–44 000 per microlitre per day[3] and have a lifespan of 9–10 days. As platelets age they gradually lose their functional capacity, hence younger platelets are biologically the most active.

Platelet structure and function

Normal platelet function requires the presence of key membrane proteins and two major types of cytoplasmic granule. Because of their limited metabolic activity, and the presence of polymorphic glycoproteins on their exterior surface, platelets are vulnerable to attack by many agents including drugs, toxins, viruses and the immune system. In addition, drugs or diseases that interfere with platelet function do so for the lifetime of the platelet, and for this reason, it may take several days for the effects of any interfering drugs to diminish once the offending agent is stopped, by which point new platelets have entered the peripheral circulation.

Platelet membrane constituents

The platelet plasma membrane contains a variety of polymorphic glycoprotein molecules which interact with ligands such as coagulation factors, vessel wall components and other molecules in order to generate the primary hemostatic plug.

The integrin family of proteins

Integrins are key platelet membrane proteins and have been characterized on a large number of leukocytes and

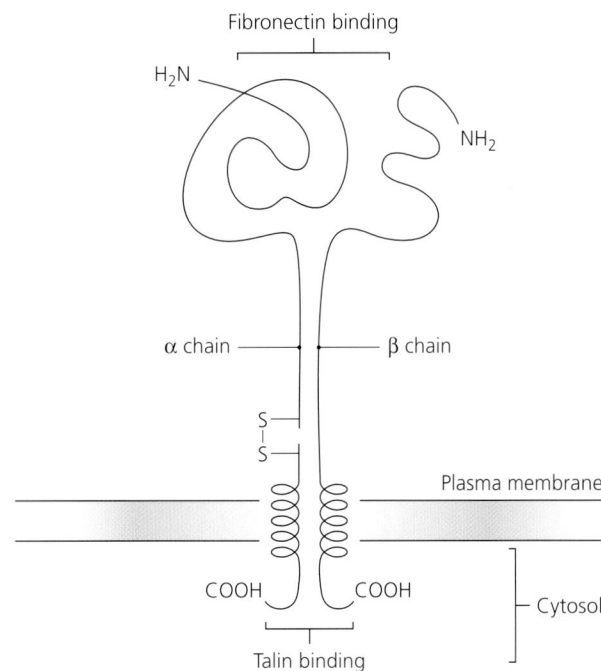

Fig. 26.2 Fibronectin receptor on mammalian fibroblasts: the platelet integrins share homology with the fibronectin receptor.

many other cells. For example, the fibronectin receptor on mammalian fibroblasts is one of the best characterized matrix receptor proteins[4] (Fig. 26.2). This receptor, in common with all other integrins, is a heterodimer consisting of a non-covalently associated complex of two distinct high-molecular-weight polypeptides, α and β. The receptor functions as a transmembrane linker which mediates the interaction between the intracellular actin cytoskeleton and fibronectin in the extracellular matrix. Like all integrins, the fibronectin receptor recognizes so-called RGD (Arg-Gly-Asp) sequences in matrix components. In platelets, integrins recognize and bind a variety of proteins in order to form a hemostatic plug through a complex mechanism of platelet adhesion, shape change, and activation of the clotting pathway.

Platelet integrins and related proteins

Platelets contain five major integrins, which include the collagen receptor (GPIa/IIa), fibronectin receptor (GPIc/IIa), laminin receptor (GPIc'/IIA), vitronectin receptor ($\alpha_v\beta_3$), and the most important glycoprotein IIb/IIIa.[5–7] These are shown in Figure 26.3. Further detail is provided by Table 26.1. These proteins are essential for normal platelet function, and are often the target of immunological attack in disorders such as idiopathic thrombocytopenic purpura (ITP).

Table 26.1 Platelet integrins and related proteins

Glycoprotein		Ligand	Function
Integrins			
Ia/IIa	$\alpha_2\beta_1$, VLA-5, CD49e/CD29	Collagen	Platelet–collagen adhesion
Ic/IIa	$\alpha_5\beta_1$, CD49b/CD29, VLA-2	Fibronectin	
IIb/IIIa	$\alpha_{IIb}\beta_3$, CD41/CD61	Fibrinogen, vWF, vitronectin	Platelet–platelet aggregation
Non-integrin proteins			
Ib/IX	CD42	vWF	Platelet–endothelial microfibril adhesion
IV		Thrombospondin	Platelet aggregation
V			

vWF, von Willebrand factor.

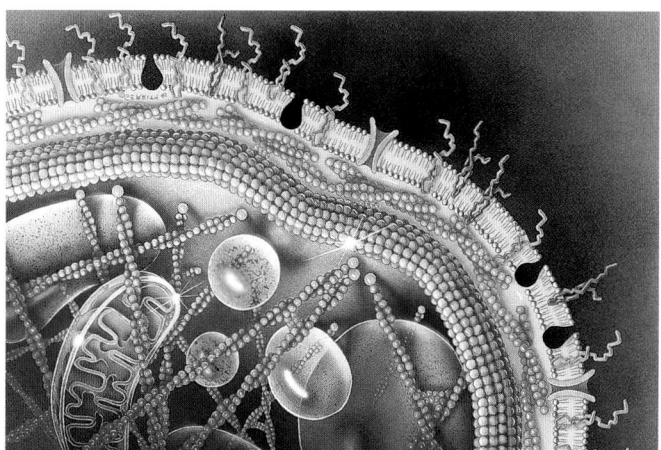

Fig. 26.3 Cartoon of platelet membrane, showing platelet glycoproteins. Peg Berrity, Science Photo Library.

Table 26.2 Human platelet alloantigen system. Modified from Waters[8]

System	Antigen	Antigen frequency (%)	Glycoprotein (GP)
HPA-1	HPA-1a	97.46	IIIa
	HPA-1b	30.80	
HPA-2	HPA-2a	99.79	Ib(α)
	HPA-2b	11.81	
HPA-3	HPA-3a	86.14	IIb
	HPA-3b	62.92	
HPA-4	HPA-4a	> 99.9	IIIa
	HPA-4b	< 0.1	
HPA-5	HPA-5a	989.79	Ia (α)
	HPA-5b	20.65	

Platelet alloantigens

These can be platelet-specific or shared with other cells. Important shared antigens include HLA class I and ABH (blood group A and B) antigens. Platelet-specific antigens fall into five well-defined human platelet antigen (HPA) groups (shown in Table 26.2): HPA-1, HPA-2, HPA-3, HPA-4 and HPA-5, each of which has an a and b allele. Each platelet allotype represents a single amino acid substitution in the platelet glycoprotein molecule. Because some platelet glycoproteins carry epitopes that play a major role in platelet function, platelet alloantibodies may not only cause thrombocytopenia but also affect primary haemostasis.

Cytoplasmic platelet constituents

Platelets contain two principal types of granule: dense bodies and α granules (Fig. 26.4). Dense bodies contain ADP, ATP, 5-HT, calcium and pyrophosphate. The α granules contain PF4, β thrombospondin, PDGF, vWF, fibrinogen, factor V and fibronectin. The contents of these granules are integral components of the platelet's biological activities.

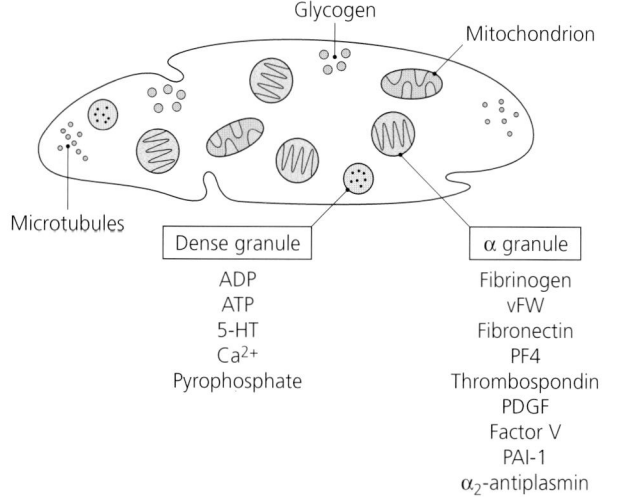

Fig. 26.4 Schematic representation of the platelet showing dense granules and α granules, with details of the contents of each.

Biological function of platelets

The primary role of the platelet is the prevention of blood loss from damaged tissues and vessels. Their main function, therefore, is one of primary hemostasis, which is achieved through platelet activation, adhesion, shape change and aggregation.

Platelet activation

If there is damage to the endothelial lining of blood vessels, platelets become exposed to subendothelial structures. Platelets release a variety of attractants and other chemicals and recruit other platelets which are attracted to the site of injury. The activated platelets provide a strong procoagulant surface which triggers the main clotting cascade, with the final product being the generation of thrombin and the production of a fibrin clot, composed of platelets enmeshed within a fibrin network.

Platelet adhesion (Fig. 26.5a)

This process involves interaction between the platelet integrins, listed above, and the subendothelium. The main integrin involved in platelet adhesion is GPIIb/IIIa which can be activated via a number of signals including exposure to extracellular matrix components such as collagen, in addition to other key activators such as adenosine diphosphate (ADP). Known ligands for platelet integrins include molecules such as fibrinogen, fibronectin and von Willebrand factor.

Platelet shape change

After adhesion to the subendothelium, platelets undergo a major shape change, from a discoid shape to one which is irregular, with projections (Fig. 26.6). This process is initially reversible but ultimately becomes irreversible.

Platelet aggregation (Fig. 26.5b)

There are a number of compounds that can induce platelet aggregation, including ADP, collagen, thrombin, adrenaline, vasopressin and others.

Quantitative platelet abnormalities: thrombocytopenia

Thrombocytopenia, a reduction in platelet count, may be caused by:

- impaired production
- increased destruction
- altered distribution
- combination of these.

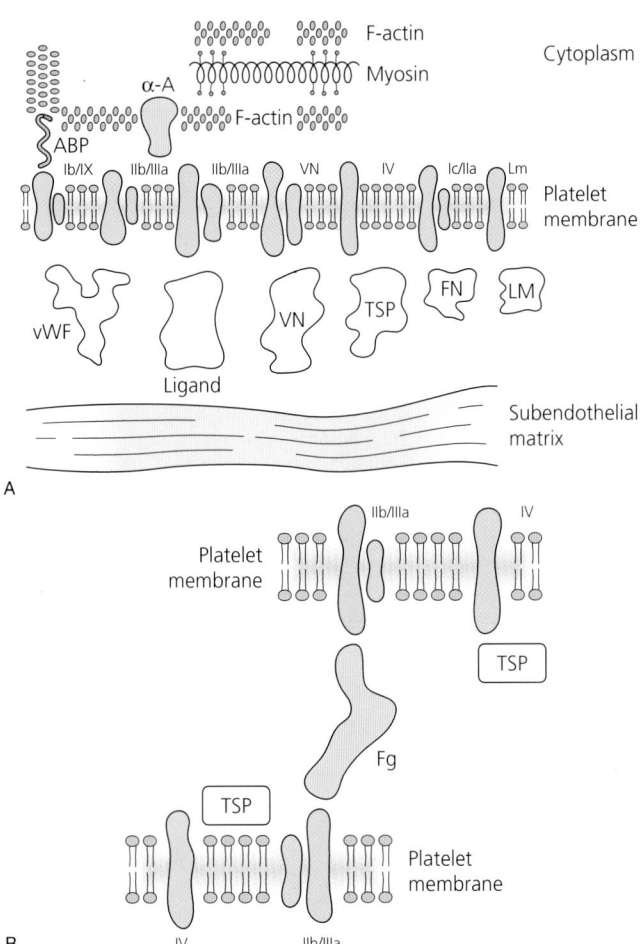

Fig. 26.5 (A) Platelet adhesion to subendothelium: the platelet membrane contains a variety of glycoprotein receptors to adhesive proteins. VN, vitronectin; Lm laminin receptor; ABP, actin-binding protein; α-A, α-actin; vWF, von Willebrand factor; TSP, thrombospondin; FN, fibronectin. From Mackie,[218] with permission. (B) Platelet aggregation: the terminal event in platelet aggregation is thought to be the binding of fibrinogen to GPIIb/IIIa receptors on adjacent platelets. The fibrinogen bridge may be stabilized by thrombospondin bound to its receptor (GPIV). From Mackie,[218] with permission.

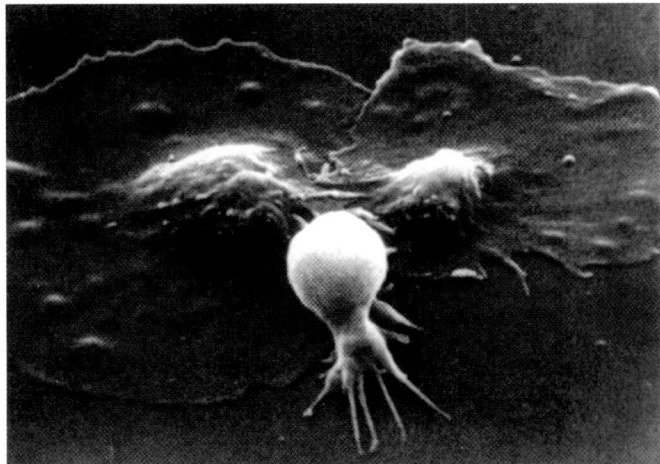

Fig. 26.6 Platelet shape change. Scanning electron micrograph of platelet shape transformation during adhesion to the arterial wall. Assemblies of actin filaments create spike-like attachment points and arrange themselves in an expansive webwork that mantles the neighboring space. From Roth,[220] with permission.

Pseudothrombocytopenia

This term describes patients in whom the peripheral blood platelet count is found to be spuriously low, and is caused by a variety of mechanisms. Platelet clumping caused by the anticoagulant ethylenediamine tetracetic acid (EDTA) is the commonest cause, with an incidence of around 0.1%. EDTA-induced pseudothrombocytopenia is easily excluded by examination of a blood film which will confirm the presence of numerous large platelet clumps.[9,10] Other causes of pseudothrombocytopenia include the presence of giant platelets, which are not counted as platelets by modern automated counters, and platelet satellitism (platelets attach themselves to monocytes or granulocytes) (Fig. 26.7). These anomalies are not clinically important in themselves, but if not recognized at the outset, may result in a patient undergoing unnecessary tests in order to determine the cause for the apparent thrombocytopenia.

Pooling of platelets in the spleen

This mechanism accounts for the thrombocytopenias seen in patients with hepatic cirrhosis and portal hypertension. The term hypersplenism is used for patients in whom there is thrombocytopenia through excessive splenic pooling of platelets.

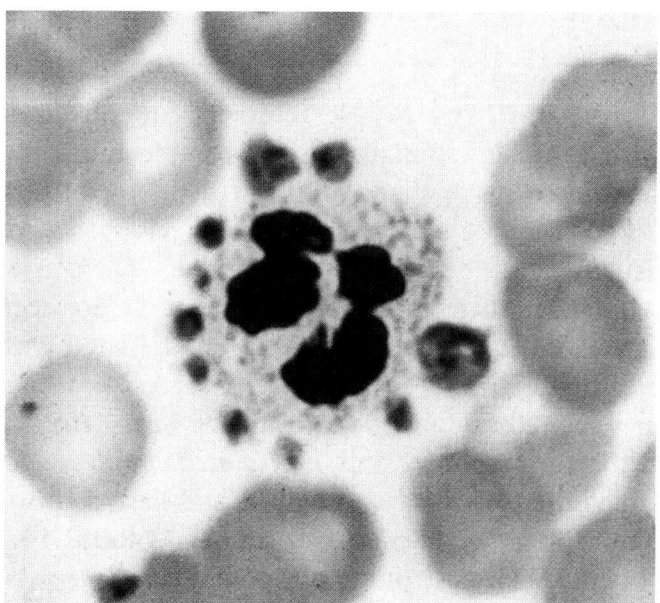

Fig. 26.7 Platelet satellitism. The figure shows a neutrophil surrounded by adherent platelets. From Lewis SM, Bain B, Bates I & Dacie J 2000 (eds), Practical haematology, 9th edn. Churchill Livingstone, Edinburgh, with permission.

Mechanism involved

In health, the spleen may pool up to one-third of the total platelet mass, and in disease states this may rise to 90%.[11] Although the peripheral blood platelet count may only be a fraction of the normal range, the patient generally has an overall normal platelet mass since production is entirely normal but the low peripheral counts simply reflect a larger than normal mass of platelets pooled in the spleen. Evidence for these figures comes from the large rise in the platelet count seen in patients immediately following splenectomy. In addition, the administration of adrenaline causes constriction of the splenic artery which has the effect of reducing blood flow to the spleen five-fold and emptying of the spleen with concomitant rise in peripheral blood platelet count.

Thrombocytopenia due to failure of platelet production

Acquired amegakaryocytic thrombocytopenia

This describes severe thrombocytopenia caused by a selective reduction in megakaryocytes in an otherwise normal bone marrow, and is the result of damage to the megakaryocyte progenitor cell. The disorder is analogous to acquired pure red-cell aplasia (PRCA).

Causative agents

Like PRCA, acquired amegakaryocytic thrombocytopenia may be caused by drugs, toxins and connective tissue disorders.[12–14]

Drug-induced megakaryocyte hypoplasia

All drugs that are myelosuppressive will inhibit megakaryocyte stem cells. Cytosine arabinoside is particularly toxic. In general, agents that are cell cycle phase-specific have the most profound effects on megakaryocytes (e.g. methotrexate and cytosine arabinoside). Other drugs may selectively 'poison' megakaryocytes, and induce profound hypoplasia, for example thiazide diuretics, ethanol and estrogens. The novel antiproliferative drug, anagrelide, used in essential thrombocythemia, inhibits the postmitotic phase of megakaryocyte differentiation, thereby effectively reducing platelet numbers.[15]

Bone marrow failure syndromes

The bone marrow failure (BMF) disorders are those in which there is a failure of production of bone marrow precursor cells in contrast to those disorders such as myelodysplastic syndromes in which normal or increased numbers of abnormal cells are produced, or those in which the survival of the cells is reduced. The BMF syndromes are a diverse groups of disorders with a common endpoint in which there is loss of hematopoietic stem cells. BMF can be acquired or inherited (see Table 26.3).

Aplastic anemia

Aplastic anemia is an uncommon disorder with an incidence of 2–5 per million population per year.[16] Patients present with variable degrees of pancytopenia. Idiopathic aplastic anemia (IAA) is commonest making up at least two-thirds of cases. The disorder is typified by a hypocellular bone marrow and peripheral blood cytopenia. Importantly, there are no abnormal cells in either marrow or peripheral blood and there are no specific diagnostic features. A detailed account of aplastic anemia is provided in Chapter 13.

Pathogenesis

The actual mechanisms whereby toxins or other environmental agents cause aplasia are unknown but, at least for idiopathic aplastic anemia, there is believed to be a strong autoimmune component. This is supported by observations that there is reversal of the pancytopenia using immunosuppressive therapies such as antilymphocyte globulin. In addition, patients with idiopathic aplastic anemia have elevated numbers of activated CD8+ T-cells.

Table 26.3 Acquired bone marrow failure syndromes

Idiopathic (majority)			
Secondary	Drugs	Predictable	Cytotoxics Benzene
		Idiosyncratic	Chloramphenicol Gold
	Viruses	EBV Hepatitis HIV Parvovirus	
	Immune disease Thymoma Pregnancy PNH Radiation		

EBV, Epstein–Barr virus; HIV, human immunodeficiency virus; PNH, paroxysmal nocturnal hemoglobinuria.

Finally, a variety of studies have shown that colony growth of normal bone marrow cultured in the presence of aplastic anemia marrow lymphocytes or mononuclear cells from marrow or blood from patients with IAA, is suppressed.[17–20] It is believed that in IAA self-reactive T-cells attack stem cells causing their destruction which leads to peripheral blood cytopenia. However, as with other autoimmune diseases, the primary initiating event is unknown. This may be viral but the evidence to support this is, at best, circumstantial.

Experimental evidence to date

There are a great deal of observational data which may shed light on the pathogenesis of bone marrow failure due to aplasia. There is believed to be a strong genetic component, with a significantly increased incidence of HLA class II antigens DR2 and DPw3. The actual mechanism of aplasia may be multistep and involve a combination of abnormalities of the stem cell, stroma, growth factor production or immune suppression.[21,22] *In vitro* experimental work has shown that both CFU-GM and BFU-E are reduced in aplastic anemia.[17,18,23,24]

Which stem cell antigens are involved?

These are unknown at present; however, there is evidence to suggest that autoreactive T-cells are driven by IFN-γ and TNF-β, resulting in upregulation of Fas receptors on the stem cells, and ultimately the Fas-dependent apoptotic pathway.[25,26]

Implicated agents in aplastic anemia

Drugs A variety of drugs have been shown to induce aplastic anemia. Benzene was the first drug ever described that was capable of inducing bone marrow aplasia.[27] Other agents include organic compounds related to benzene, which include DDT. In the antibiotic arena, chloramphenicol was the first ever to produce an idiosyncratic aplastic anemia, with an estimated risk of developing aplastic anemia with chloramphenicol of around 1 in 20 000.[16] Chloramphenicol induces two major effects: bone marrow suppression and vacuole formation in red-cell precursor cells.

Radiation Early evidence for the role of radiation in the development of aplasia was provided from patients with ankylosing spondylitis who underwent chronic low-dose radiotherapy as part of their treatment. Such therapy was shown conclusively to induce not only aplastic anemia but also acute leukemia.[28] Larger doses of radiotherapy are also associated with bone marrow aplasia.

Viral infections There are strong associations between viral hepatitis and the development of aplastic anemia,[29,30] which may occur during the recovery period or as long as 1 year following the infection. In earlier reports, patients developing aplastic anemia were predominantly young males with an overall survival of around 10 weeks. Both hepatitis A and B are implicated although most cases are non-A non-B, but not hepatitis C.[31] Other viruses such as Epstein–Barr virus (EBV) and parvovirus may induce aplastic anemia and human immunodeficiency virus (HIV) causes a huge variety of hematologic abnormalities, including aplastic anemia.

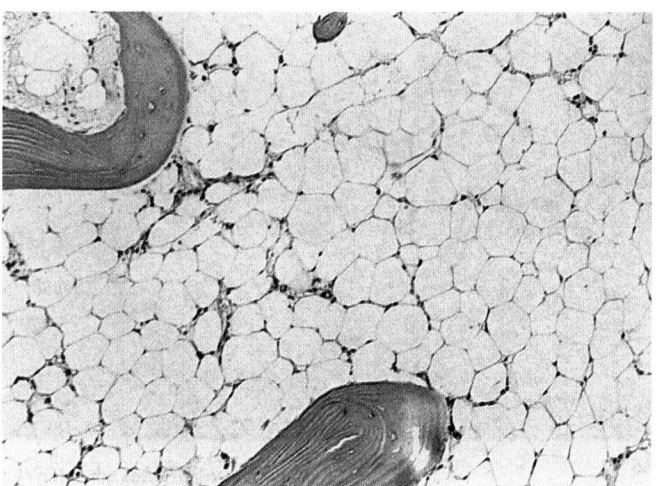

Fig. 26.8 Trephine biopsy in aplastic anemia. The specimen shows a marrow largely replaced by fat cells.

Clinical features

Aplastic anemia has an insidious onset with general symptoms of anemia. Where the thrombocytopenia is marked there may be petechial hemorrhages, bruising or bleeding. The risk of infection is increased if there is profound neutropenia. Apart from pallor and other signs attributable to anemia, physical examination findings are generally unremarkable.

Laboratory findings

Pancytopenia is present and variable. The reticulocytes are low and usually less than 1%.[32] Macrocytosis is a feature and is believed to be due to increased levels of erythropoietin (Epo) stimulating the residual bone marrow erythroblasts.[33] The total white blood count (WBC) is reduced and, of these, the neutrophils are most important in the overall prognosis. Infections are more common as the neutrophil counts drop. The peripheral blood lymphocytes are usually normal or slightly reduced in number, and the platelet count is reduced.

Bone marrow examination

The aspirate usually contains much fat and empty marrow particles. Residual hematopoietic tissue comprises lymphocytes, plasma cells, macrophages and mast cells. For accurate determination of cellularity, a trephine is required and helps define the grade of aplasia (Fig. 26.8). A scoring system has been devised by the International Aplastic Anemia Study Group[34] whereby severe aplastic anemia is defined by: bone marrow of $<25\%$ cellularity, or $<50\%$ cellularity with $<30\%$ hematopoietic cells, plus at least two of: neutrophils $<0.5 \times 10^9/l$, platelets $<20 \times 10^9/l$, and anemia with reticulocyte index $<1\%$.

The overall prognosis for patients with neutrophils $<0.2 \times 10^9/l$ is particularly poor; this group has, by definition, very severe aplastic anemia.[35]

Management

The median survival for patients with aplastic anemia with neutrophils $<0.5 \times 10^9/l$ is 3–6 months.[36] Management comprises supportive care with definitive therapies comprising bone marrow transplantation and immunosuppression. For a full discussion, readers are referred to Chapter 13 and an excellent review by Young and Barrett.[37]

Thrombocytopenia due to increased platelet destruction

These may be immunologic or non-immunologic.

Non-immunologic causes of thrombocytopenia

Disseminated intravascular coagulation (DIC)

DIC is characterized by excessive activation of the coagulation cascade (also see Chapter 28). In most cases DIC is an acute event, but chronic DIC is well described, although clinically less important. The main problem faced in patients with DIC is of bleeding, which may be mild, but is often severe with generalized oozing from venepuncture sites, central lines and other indwelling cannulae, gastrointestinal and genitourinary tracts. Microthrombi are found in 5–10% of cases, often affecting digits, with resulting peripheral gangrene.

Pathogenesis

DIC is triggered by the release of tissue thromboplastins which contain a high concentration of phospholipids following trauma, surgery, mismatched blood transfusion and a variety of other triggers (Table 26.4).

Laboratory diagnosis

The blood count will usually show thrombocytopenia. Coagulation tests are the most important assays for the detection of DIC, and will show prolongation of prothrombin time, activated partial thromboplastin time (APTT), thrombin time with reduced fibrinogen and elevated D-dimers.

Management

Supportive care can be given with fresh-frozen plasma (FFP), cryoprecipitate and platelet transfusions but the most effective treatment is removal of the cause.[38]

Thrombotic thrombocytopenic purpura and hemolytic uremic syndrome

Thrombotic thrombocytopenic purpura (TTP) is a disseminated microangiopathy, and was first described by Moschowitz in 1924.[39] TTP has an incidence of around 1 in 50 000 hospital admissions. TTP and hemolytic uremic syndrome (HUS) were originally believed to be distinct disorders but are now regarded as different expressions of the same disease process; they share many characteristics but HUS is more common in children and

the renal abnormalities are more marked than in TTP (Table 26.5, also see Chapter 10).

Clinical features of TTP

TTP is a rare disorder that previously carried a high mortality and is characterized by the pentad:

- thrombocytopenia
- microangiopathic hemolysis
- neurologic symptoms and signs
- renal function abnormalities
- fever.

TTP can affect any organ system but it is the involvement of the hematopoietic, renal and central nervous systems that leads to the typical clinical features.

The mortality rate has been reduced through effective treatment and good supportive care. The disorder is sporadic, affecting males and females equally. It may develop in pregnancy and in this setting must be differentiated from pre-eclampsia, eclampsia and the HELLP (haemolysis, elevated liver enzymes and low platelets) syndrome.

TTP typically has a sudden onset, with fever and neurologic symptoms including paralysis, coma, fits and

Table 26.4 Triggers for disseminated intravascular coagulation (DIC)

Trauma	Including surgical
Dissemination of cancer cells	Malignancy, following administration of chemotherapy
Massive hemolysis	Post mismatched blood transfusion
Venoms	e.g. snake venoms
Endothelial injury	Gram-negative sepsis
Infections	
Burns	
Septicemia	

Table 26.5 Classification of thrombocytopenic purpura (TTP) and hemolytic uremic syndrome (HUS). Modified from George and El-Harake[46]

Idiopathic TTP/HUS	Classic adult TTP and childhood non-verotoxin-associated HUS-TTP	
Secondary TTP-HUS	Pregnancy-related	TTP, postpartum HUS
	Verotoxin-induced	*Escherichia coli* and *Shigella dysenteriae* I Childhood HUS[40 41] Epidemic adult TTP-HUS
	Malignant disease	Especially metastatic carcinomas
	Drug-induced	Chemotherapy agents e.g. mitomycin C,[42] cisplatin, and other drugs Immunosuppressive agents e.g. cyclosporin[43] quinine,[44] ticlopidine[45]
	Post-marrow/stem cell transplantation	Especially in conjunction with total body irradiation or high-dose (intensive) chemotherapy

psychiatric disturbance. There is usually purpura and the clinical picture is one of a fluctuating course.

Laboratory investigations

A full blood count and blood film will show anemia (hemoglobin ~ 8–9g/dl) with polychromasia and other evidence of hemolysis. The film will usually show red-cell fragments and will confirm the thrombocytopenia (platelet count 20–50 × 10⁹/l) (Fig. 26.9). There is usually evidence of hemoglobinemia reflecting the presence of intravascular hemolysis. Lactate dehydrogenase will be elevated. Clotting tests are generally normal although occasionally there may be features of DIC.

Pathogenesis

Systemic endothelial damage appears to be the key triggering factor for both TTP and HUS.[47] It is believed that oxidant stress results in endothelial damage with resultant decrease in prostacyclin production by endothelial tissues, which leads to a diminution in the fibrinolytic capacity of vessel walls and the production of antiendothelial cell antibodies. There is also an ability of TTP plasma to induce apoptosis of microvascular endothelial cells.[48] Post-mortem examination generally shows characteristic changes in small blood vessels and end-organs. However, these are seldom demonstrated in life. The principal lesions are microthrombi, composed of platelet aggregates throughout the capillary network and small blood vessels of organs affected by the process. The thrombi are composed of platelet plugs, hyaline degeneration and fibrin. The triggering factor is not known but may involve some form of pathologic

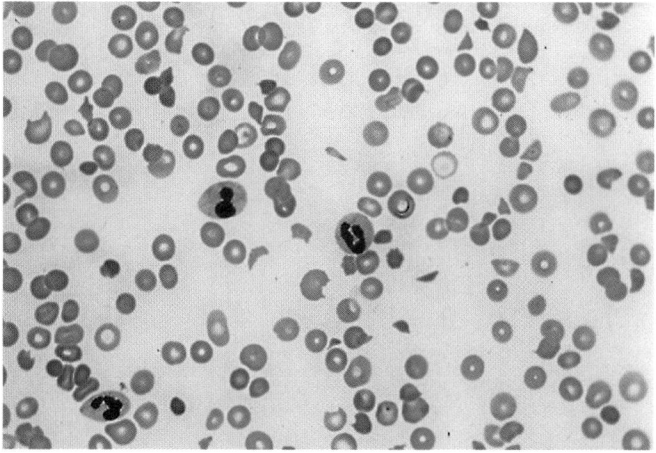

Fig. 26.9 Peripheral blood film from a patient with thrombotic thrombocytopenic purpura (TTP). Note the many fragmented red cells, characteristic of this disorder. Figure kindly provided by Dr John Amess, Barts & The London NHS Trust.

interaction between platelets and vascular endothelium. In addition, endothelial damage may lead to the release of very large von Willebrand factor multimers which may contribute to the disease[49] (this is discussed below).

The role of von Willebrand factor in TTP

In normal plasma von Willebrand Factor (vWF) vWF multimers are present as a series of proteins ranging in size from 500 kDa to 20 000 kDa. The multimers themselves are composed of 250 kDa subunits linked together by disulfide bonds. In health there is proteolytic cleavage of vWF[50] but in some TTP patients there has been shown to be an absence of the vWF cleaving protease.[51] It is possible, therefore, that an absence of vWF cleavage protein, either acquired or constitutional, may predispose to TTP. By contrast, when plasma samples from patients with HUS are assayed, there appears to be normal levels of vWF cleaving protein which may help explain the major pathophysiologic differences between TTP and HUS. Very large vWF multimers are found in the plasma of some patients with TTP, especially those with a relapsing form of the disease. It is believed that these ultra-large vWF multimers may induce platelet aggregation in the microcirculation.[52] Ultra-large vWF multimers, produced by the vascular endothelium, are released into the patient's plasma and may be found in the plasma at the beginning of the acute episode. The vWF multimers are strongly aggregating for platelets and are able to bind GP Ib/IX and IIb/IIIa.

Diagnosis

There is no specific diagnostic test for TTP or HUS, and the diagnosis is clinical, based on the constellation of clinical features and laboratory confirmation of thrombocytopenia and microangiopathic hemolytic anemia.

Management

Prior to 1970 patients often died from TTP, but with the availability of plasma treatment in the form of FFP, with or without plasma exchange, the survival has improved dramatically.[53,54] The disease is highly variable in its course and it is difficult to predict the clinical outcome at the outset. Patients require intensive-care nursing and are generally ventilated. Hemodialysis is often required along with plasma exchange with FFP replacement. Cryosupernatant is also useful. Corticosteroids have also been used.

If TTP is suspected clinically and on laboratory parameters large-volume plasma exchange should be instituted immediately and continued daily until significant clinical improvement and all hematologic parameters have normalized. This form of treatment has markedly reduced the previously high mortality rate from 90% to 10–20%. Aspirin can be started once the platelet count exceeds $50 \times 10^9/l$.

Hemolytic uremic syndrome of childhood

The disorder was first described in 1955 by Gasser,[55] who reported on five patients (all infants) with acute renal failure, who died of renal cortical necrosis. These cases were extreme and would be considered as atypical HUS today. Verotoxin-induced HUS is the classical HUS of childhood, and generally follows an episode of acute gastroenteritis involving verotoxin-producing *Escherichia coli* or *Shigella dysenteriae* I (which produces Shiga toxin.[56] Childhood HUS is seen typically in young children but can also affect adults.[57–59] The disorder has an incidence of around 1 per 100 000 per annum for children below the age of 15 years, but the incidence may be higher in children below this age. There is a seasonal incidence, with the highest number of new cases reported in the summer months.[60,61]

Etiology Verotoxin is produced by the *E. coli* 0157:H7 subtype. This toxin is structurally related to the Shiga toxin produced by *S. dysenteriae*.[62]

Pathogenesis The toxin is cytopathic and there is stimulation of a variety of cytokines including interleukin-8 (IL-8), which activates and attracts neutrophils.[63]

Clinical features Children typically present with diarrhea (often bloody), vomiting and abdominal pain. Because of the large volume of fluid loss, patients are often oliguric or anuric at presentation. Fever, hypertension and fits are also features.

Laboratory findings There is evidence of acute renal failure and features of microangiopathic hemolysis.[64] The blood count will generally show an elevated WBC, most usually neutrophilia; the prognosis is worst for patients with total neutrophil counts exceeding $20 \times 10^9/l$.[60]

Management Around half of the children affected will require hemodialysis for between 1 and 2 weeks. Unlike adult TTP, plasma exchange using FFP replacement is not often required in children. Clinical trials have shown no benefit from the use of plasma infusions.[65]

Outlook Unlike adult TTP, childhood HUS is rarely fatal and the mortality is around 3–5%. In fatal cases deaths are usually in the first week of the illness and are mostly attributable to central nervous system involvement in the HUS process.

Pre-eclampsia and HELLP syndrome

Pre-eclampsia occurs in the third trimester of pregnancy and is associated with hypertension, edema, sodium retention, proteinuria and DIC. Pre-eclampsia may progress to eclampsia which is characterized by convulsions.[66] Previously, pre-eclampsia/eclampsia and HELLP have been considered distinct disorders but it seems more likely that they represent a spectrum of a pathologic process. The underlying mechanism is not clear but there appears to be activation of procoagulant proteins and platelets through endothelial damage.

HELLP syndrome

This disorder, characterized by hemolysis, elevated liver enzymes and low platelet count, occurs in 0.5–0.9% of all pregnancies,[67,68] and is associated with a mortality rate of 1–4%.[69] Perinatal mortality is high and may reach 40%.[70]

Clinical features

HELLP is associated with generalized weakness, nausea and vomiting, right upper quadrant pain, headache and visual upset.[70] In some cases HELLP may occur following delivery.[68]

Pathophysiology

There may be abnormalities of the placental vessels with resulting placental ischemia. This is associated with the systemic release of a thromboxanes, angiotensin, tumor necrosis factor-α (TNF-α) and other procoagulant proteins.[68,71] DIC results leading to thrombi which threaten major end-organs including placenta, renal, hepatic and central nervous system. The thrombi lead to endothelial damage and there is microangiopathic hemolytic anemia (MAHA) and failure of the organs affected by the thrombotic process. Liver failure and occasionally liver rupture may result.[72]

Management

Prompt delivery, and control of the hypertension are required, in addition to correcting the factor deficiencies caused by the DIC. Corticosteroids have been used[73] as well as plasma exchange and plasmapheresis.[74] Maternal deaths, where these occur, are usually due to uncontrolled DIC.

Thrombocytopenia caused by massive blood transfusion

Massive transfusion whereby a patient's total blood volume is replaced over a short time period (24 h or less) may lead to thrombocytopenia, and although the degree of thrombocytopenia is largely related to the amount of blood transfused, the mechanism is not purely dilutional. In fact, there appears to be an element of platelet consumption. From previous studies, patients receiving 15 units of red cells within a 24-h period develop mild thrombocytopenia, with platelet counts between 47 and $100 \times 10^9/l$, whereas patients transfused with 20 units of red cells over the same period develop more pronounced thrombocytopenia $(25–61 \times 10^9/l)$.[75,76]

Management

Severe thrombocytopenia can be prevented by administering platelet concentrates prophylactically to patients receiving more than 20 units of red cells within a 24-h time period.

Liver disease

Thrombocytopenia secondary to alcohol

Thrombocytopenia occurring in alcoholic patients may be caused by a variety of mechanisms including cirrhosis, splenomegaly and folic acid deficiency. However, thrombocytopenia may be found in the absence of any or all of these pathologies, and is probably due to the direct toxic effects of alcohol on the bone marrow itself, since ethanol is a poison and can suppress the production of platelets by the marrow.[77,78] Examination of the bone marrow usually shows normal or slightly reduced numbers of megakaryocytes. Experimental studies have shown that alcohol is inhibitory to megakaryocytes,[12] and may even induce a mild reduction in platelet life span.[79]

Thrombocytopenia in hepatocellular failure

In addition to the other coagulopathies induced by liver failure, thrombocytopenia is often present and generally reflects the hypersplenism that occurs in portal hypertension. In fulminant hepatic failure, there are abnor-

malities of both platelet structure and function. On laboratory testing there may be evidence of mild DIC, although this is not generally of major clinical importance.[80] In addition, patients with chronic liver disease often have elevated levels of fibrin degradation products which interfere with platelet aggregation.

Thrombocytopenia caused by infection

There are numerous infections caused by a wide variety of pathogenic bacteria, fungi, viruses and protozoa that result in thrombocytopenia in humans. The mechanism underlying the thrombocytopenia is variable. In many cases there is suppression of marrow function, and this is particularly the case with viral infections and accounts for most cases of mild thrombocytopenia. Implicated viruses include mumps,[81] varicella,[82] EBV,[83] rubella[84] and many others. Viral infection is the commonest cause of mild transient thrombocytopenia.

Mechanism of thrombocytopenia

There is a variety of mechanisms involved in thrombocytopenia induced by infection. Following measles infection in children, there is a reduction in marrow megakaryocytes and by day 3 of the infection many of the megakaryocytes have vacuoles within the nucleus and cytoplasm.[85]

Thrombocytopenia induced by HIV infection

HIV infection probably induces thrombocytopenia through a variety of mechanisms, including immune-mediated thrombocytopenia with reduced platelet life span,[86–88] and through direct infection of megakaryocytes themselves. This may occur at any stage in the course of HIV infection, and 40% of HIV positive individuals develop thrombocytopenia at some point in the illness.[89–91] Unlike classical idiopathic thrombocytopenic purpura (ITP), males and females are affected equally and thrombocytopenia may be the presenting feature in 10% of HIV positive people.[92]

Management

Because of the risk of steroid-associated toxicity in patients infected with HIV, corticosteroids are used less often than in standard ITP. In addition, there is a suggestion that steroid administration may accelerate Kaposi's sarcoma.[93]

Splenectomy or intravenous immunoglobulin may be used to elevate the platelet count. Zidovudine may help elevate the count, and a positive response to zidovudine is seen in around 70% of patients treated.[94,95] Interferon-α may help some patients especially if the thrombocytopenia is recurrent and there has been a good response to the initial therapy.[96]

Thrombocytopenia due to hematinic deficiencies

Thrombocytopenia may be a feature of both vitamin B_{12} or folate deficiency, and mild thrombocytopenia is found in 20% of patients with megaloblastic anemia caused by vitamin B_{12} deficiency.[97] The underlying mechanism of thrombocytopenia is ineffective platelet production, possibly with an element of diminished platelet survival in a proportion of patients. Marrow examination will usually show normal or increased numbers of megakaryocytes.

Immunologic causes of thrombocytopenia

Here we have restricted our discussion to the more important immune-mediated causes of thrombocytopenia, namely neonatal alloimmune thrombocytopenia (NAIT), post-transfusion purpura (PTP), ITP, drug-induced thrombocytopenia and heparin-induced thrombocytopenia (HIT) (Table 26.6). Since the targets involved in several of these disorders are human platelet alloantigens we outline briefly their salient features.

Molecular basis of HPA antigens

Platelets have a variety of cell surface antigens, some of which are shared by other cells, such as HLA class I, and blood groups A and B. Others are platelet-specific and are not found on any other type of cell. To date there are 19 alloantigen systems described on platelets, all of which map to membrane proteins. Eleven of the 19 are carried on GPIIb/IIIa ($\alpha_{IIb}\beta_3$ integrin heterodimer), three are on GPIb/IX/V, two on GPIa/IIa ($\alpha_2\beta_1$), and one on each of GPIV, GPV and CD109. The molecular basis for most of these is now elucidated (see Chapter 30).[99]

Antibody response to non-self HPA antigens

The difference between self and non-self HPAs is determined by a single amino acid substitution, and for this reason HPAs are not particularly immunogenic, in comparison with, for example, Rhesus (D) and HLA class I antigens. The most clinically important HPAs are HPA-1a and HPA-5a, since antibodies to these antigens account for 95% of cases of NAIT. Alloantibodies to the other HPAs also occur but at much lower frequency.

Alloimmunization against platelet-specific antigens is associated with three major clinical syndromes: neonatal alloimmune thrombocytopenia, post-transfusion purpura and refractoriness to platelet transfusions. Only the first two are discussed here.

Alloantibody-mediated thrombocytopenia
Neonatal alloimmune thrombocytopenia

Antibodies to HPA occur in 1 in 365 pregnancies and cause severe thrombocytopenia in 1 in 1100 neonates at term, accounting for around 20% of cases of thrombocytopenia in neonates. NAIT occurs when there is feto-maternal incompatibility for HPA. The condition was first described by van Loghem *et al* in 1959.[100]

Table 26.6 Disorders associated with immune-mediated thrombocytopenia. From Chong[98]

Autoimmune	Idiopathic (ITP)
	Secondary immune
	Autoimmune disorders e.g. SLE, rheumatoid, thyroid disease
	Lymphoproliferative disorders e.g. CLL, NHL
	Cancer e.g. solid tumors
	Miscellaneous e.g. post-BMT, chemotherapy
	Viral infection
	e.g. HIV, measles, mumps, rubella, EBV, varicella
	Drug-induced
Alloimmune	Post-transfusion purpura
	Neonatal alloimmune thrombocytopenia

BMT, bone-marrow transfer, CLL, chronic lymphocytic leukemia; EBV, Epstein–Barr virus, HIV, human immunodeficiency virus; ITP, idiopathic thrombocytopenic purpura, SLE, systemic lupus erythematosus; NHL, Non-Hodgkin's lymphoma.

During pregnancy, or following a blood transfusion, the mother becomes sensitized and produces alloantibodies against HPA, most commonly HPA-1a. In a process analogous to hemolytic disease of the newborn, maternal IgG anti-HPA crosses the placenta resulting in premature destruction of fetal platelets.

Antigens involved in NAIT

In Caucasian females NAIT is most commonly due to anti-HPA-1a (98% of the population are HPA-1a$^+$). Other implicated antigens include HPA-1b,[101] HPA-2a,[102] HPA-3a,[103] HPA-3b,[104] HPA-4a,[105] HPA-4b,[106] HPA-5b[107] and HPA-5a.[108]

Diagnosis of NAIT

In contrast to maternal ITP, the mother in NAIT has a normal platelet count and is completely well. The neonate is generally asymptomatic at birth, apart from a low platelet count. In cases where neonates are symptomatic the platelet count is generally $< 30 \times 10^9/l$. If no treatment is given, the baby's platelet count may remain low for up to 2 weeks, and occasionally longer. The white cell count is usually normal and the hemoglobin is normal unless there has been significant bleeding. Bone-marrow aspirate will show normal numbers of megakaryocytes unless the mother's antibody has destroyed these in which case megakaryocytes may be low or even absent.

Modern serologic techniques may help confirm the diagnosis. Maternal serum is tested against the father's platelets in addition to normal control platelets. Occasionally, the maternal antibody titer is low at delivery and difficulty to detect using the above techniques. However, there are techniques available for the detection of low-titer maternal antibodies.[109]

Clinical features

Unlike hemolytic disease of the newborn where the firstborn child is unaffected, in NAIT the firstborn child is affected. Recurrence in subsequent pregnancies is common, if there is fetomaternal incompatibility. The newborn infant is usually normal at birth but most will have some degree of bleeding due to the marked thrombocytopenia. There may be generalized bruising, especially in severely affected neonates who are often born with petechial hemorrhages. Intracranial hemorrhage is the most serious complication, occurring around the time of birth or shortly afterwards. In neonates with platelet counts below $20 \times 10^9/l$ intracranial hemorrhage (ICH) may occur during the first few days of life.

Management

The NAIT may be very mild and require no therapy apart from close monitoring of the neonate's platelet count. If treatment is required there is a variety of options available including:

1. Corticosteroids, such as prednisolone 1–2 mg/kg/day, although it is uncertain whether corticosteroids reduce the period of thrombocytopenia.[110]
2. Platelet transfusions, which are useful if there is serious bleeding. These can be random donor platelets but more ideally should be antigen-negative (HPA-1a and HPA-5a negative). The mother's platelets may be used, but these should be washed to remove antibody which is present in the mother's plasma.[111]
3. Intravenous immunoglobulin at 0.4 g/kg/day for 5 days.[112]
4. Exchange transfusion, which removes antibody and reduces the period of thrombocytopenia.[113]

Future pregnancies

This depends on the father's genotype for the particular HPA. For example, if he is homozygous then each pregnancy will be affected. In cases where the father is heterozygous, 50% of pregnancies will be affected and the fetus can be typed using DNA obtained from chorionic villus sampling.[114] Where necessary, fetal platelet counts can be measured using umbilical vein sampling.[115,116] In terms of outlook for the neonate, some 15% of affected neonates die, usually of ICH,[117] and a proportion of infants who avoid ICH may still develop neurologic sequelae.[105,118] The overall outcome for neonates who do not develop ICH or other neurologic complications is good.[119]

Post-transfusion purpura (PTP)

This curious disorder occurs around 7–10 days following a red-cell transfusion in recipients who possess alloantibodies against platelet antigens of the donor. In addition to destroying the incoming platelets, the alloantibody also mediates destruction of the recipient's own platelets (i.e. lacking the target antigen). The disorder is uncommon but the exact prevalence is unknown.[120]

Pathogenetic basis

Platelet alloantibodies may be present in the recipient against any one of the six major platelet antigens: anti-HPA-1a,[121] anti-HPA-1b,[122] anti-HPA3a,[123] anti-bak-b,[124] anti-HPA-4a or anti-HPA-5b.[125] In most cases the antibody has specificity for HPA-1a.

Clinical features

PTP affects multiparous women, although it has been reported in males,[126] between the ages of 16 and 80 years. Patients have usually been exposed to platelet antigens through either pregnancy or transfusion or both. The platelet antigen most commonly involved is HPA-1a (2% of the population are HPA-1a⁻).[127]

Laboratory features

Patients usually have a platelet count less than $10 \times 10^9/l$ and the bone marrow will show normal or increased numbers of megakaryocytes. The coagulation screen is usually normal. A firm diagnosis of PTP requires the demonstration of the presence of platelet-specific alloantibodies in the serum of the affected patient. Most patients with PTP are HPA-1a⁻ and the presence of HPA-1a in the transfused blood boosts the primary response.[122–124,127,128] The antiplatelet antibodies produced are mainly of IgG1 and IgG3 class. Why patients destroy their own platelets which are HPA-1a⁻ is unclear but is believed to involve IgG3. Possibly HPA-1a⁺ platelets release HPA-1a which combines with the newly-formed anti-HPA-1a. This complex is absorbed on to the surface of the patient's HPA-1a⁻ platelets.

Management

Corticosteroids may help the purpura but do not appear to be effective in increasing the platelet count. Intravenous immunoglobulin (IVIg) at the standard dose of 0.4 g/kg/day is the mainstay of treatment.[120] Occasionally, plasma exchange may be required. If platelet are required these should be HPA-1a⁻; it is worth noting that most random donor platelets will be HPA-1a⁺ so are of limited value and are best avoided. Fatal intracranial hemorrhage occurs in 10% but most patients recover within 1–6 weeks.[120] There have been no controlled trials comparing different therapies.

Autoantibody-mediated thrombocytopenia

This includes acute and chronic ITP, in addition to thrombocytopenia secondary to other autoimmune disorders, lymphoproliferative diseases or drugs.

Idiopathic thrombocytopenic purpura (ITP)

In ITP platelets are opsonised with antiplatelet auto-antibodies and removed prematurely by the reticulo-endothelial system (RES) leading to a reduced peripheral blood platelet count. The etiology of ITP is obscure and the clinical course is variable and unpredictable. ITP has an incidence of 5.8–6.6 new cases per million population per year in the US[129] with a similar incidence in the UK. Childhood ITP is generally termed 'acute' since the illness is seasonal, typically follows a trivial viral infection or vaccination, and in most cases is transient, requiring no treatment with spontaneous recovery in 80% of cases. In the adult (chronic) form there is usually no obvious antecedent illness and most patients have chronic thrombocytopenia; spontaneous recovery is uncommon.[130] In most cases of adult ITP the platelet glycoprotein (GP) antigen targets are GPIIb/IIIa and GPIb/IX.[131]

Acute ITP

In 1951, Harrington showed that the plasma from patients with ITP could cause a reduction in the platelet counts in normal subjects,[132] thereby providing proof that there was something present in the plasma of ITP patients that was able to induce thrombocytopenia in non-ITP subjects. We have since learned that the factor is, in fact, antiplatelet antibody, most usually IgG.

Acute ITP is the most common form of ITP found in children, with an annual incidence of between 3 and 8 per 100 000 per year.[133,134]

Pathophysiology

It is believed that acute ITP is most likely due to an inappropriate immune response to an environmental trigger; the nature of this trigger is not yet identified.[135,136] The disorder may represent an abnormality of antigen-presenting cells, with an increase in the numbers of CD4⁺ and CD8⁺ cells. The platelets are rapidly destroyed by the immune complexes that bind to the Fc receptors on the platelets, or due to autoantibodies that bind to the antigenic site on the platelets. Platelets that are coated with antibody or immune complexes are rapidly cleared by the reticuloendothelial system.

Clinical features

The children affected by acute ITP are, in general, well. The disorder is commonest in children between the ages of 2 and 5 years of age and, unlike adult chronic ITP, there is no sex predominance. A viral illness predates the development of ITP in most cases of childhood ITP. Physical signs of thrombocytopenia usually take the form of bruising or petechial hemorrhage. Splenomegaly, hepatomegaly and lymphadenopathy are not features of acute ITP. A recent UK study reported that in some 76% of children with acute ITP the disorder was mild with bruising and occasional epistaxis.[134] Around 4% had no bleeding symptoms and only 3% had severe bleeding from the gastrointestinal tract, nose or vagina requiring hospitalization. In around 15% of children the disease persisted longer than 6 months and fell into the 'chronic ITP' group. The chronic form was found to be commoner in older children and in females.

Laboratory investigation

The blood count will show an isolated thrombocytopenia but should otherwise be normal. The platelet count is often less than $10 \times 10^9/l$.[134] Anemia may be present in cases in which there has been significant bleeding.

Antiplatelet antibody assays

These assays yield positive results in only 20–30% of patients with acute ITP, and the specificity, when tested, is usually against GPIb/IX. This contrasts with chronic ITP in which the antibody target is GPIIb/IIIa. Because of the low rate of positivity and the finding that antiplatelet IgG or IgM may be elevated in non-immune thrombocytopenia, there is little value in measuring these in patients with acute ITP.

Bone marrow aspirates

The need to carry out a bone marrow aspirate is debatable, but when this is carried out there tends to be normal or increased numbers of megakaryocytes confirming that the thrombocytopenia is due to peripheral destruction rather than a failure of production. However, since these children are well, and have no underlying disorder causing the thrombocytopenia such as acute leukemia, the bone marrow aspirate adds little to the management and is not routinely performed. However, if there is any suspicion regarding the presence of underlying disease accounting for the thrombocytopenia or the child has features not typical of acute ITP then performing a bone marrow aspiration may be indicated.

Thrombopoietin (TPO) levels

These are not measured routinely, but in cases where TPO has been assayed in acute ITP the levels tend not to be elevated.[137]

Management

The majority of children with acute ITP need no therapy and simple reassurance is all that is required. There is no set threshold for medical intervention and what constitutes a 'safe' platelet count is not known.[138] From studies of the natural history of patients with acute ITP, we know that patients with this disorder have far less bleeding problems than those patients with comparable platelet counts caused by other diseases, such as acute leukemia or aplastic anemia. This, in part, reflects the fact that platelet function in ITP is extremely good, with a large proportion of reticulated (young) platelets in the peripheral blood.[139] If therapy is required to elevate the platelet count then the options comprise oral corticosteroids, intravenous immunoglobulin and splenectomy.

Chronic ITP

Clinical features of ITP

This is the most common form of ITP in adults. Patients may be asymptomatic or may have purpura, bruising, or mucosal bleeding including gum bleeding, retinal haemorrhage, epistaxis, melaena or menorrhagia (see Fig. 26.10). The degree of bleeding is largely dependent on the platelet count, and patients with platelet counts below $10 \times 10^9/l$ are at greatest risk of bleeding.

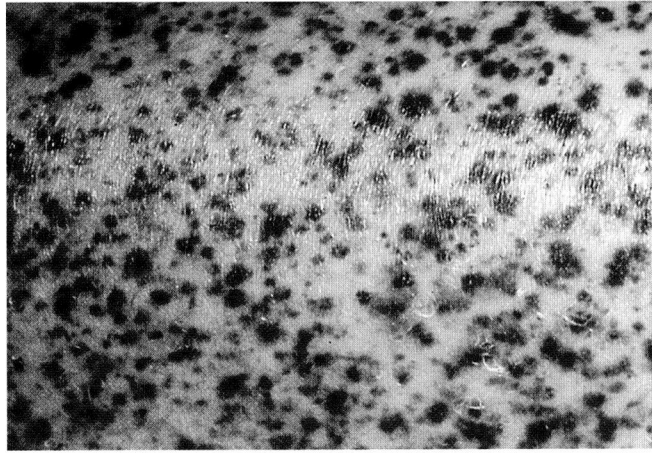

Fig. 26.10 Petechial hemorrhages on the shin of a patient with severe chronic ITP.

Splenomegaly is not a feature of ITP and if present, tends to suggest a diagnosis other than ITP.

Pathophysiology of ITP

ITP is an autoimmune disease characterized by increased platelet destruction due to the presence of antiplatelet antibodies. This results in increased platelet clearance by the RES. Several investigators have demonstrated specific autoantibodies against platelet membrane antigens, thus confirming the autoimmune nature of the disorder.[140,141] The cause is unknown but it appears likely that in a genetically predisposed individual, a trigger such as infection leads to loss of self-tolerance[142] (see Fig. 26.11).

Glycoprotein (GP)-specific autoantibodies may be important in the pathogenesis of chronic ITP;[143] from available data GPIIb/IIIa appear to play a major role in the development of chronic ITP in 30–40% of cases.[144,145] Figure 26.12 illustrates the structure of GPIIb/IIIa schematically. Previous investigators have looked for autoantigenic epitopes on the GPIIb/IIIa molecule using competitive binding between human autoantibodies and mouse monoclonal antibodies (MoAbs).[146–148] In addition, enzyme-cleaved IIb or IIIa fragments and synthesized peptides corresponding to different sequences of GPIIIa

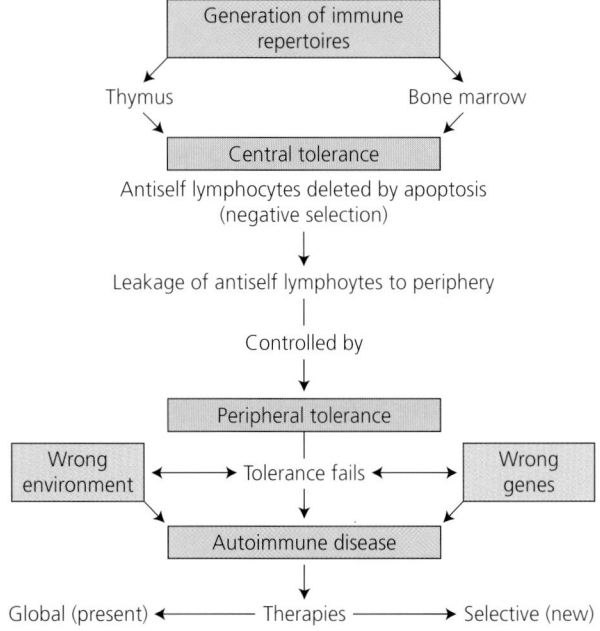

Fig. 26.11 Possible mechanism involved in the development of autoimmune disease such as ITP. Self-reactive lymphocytes are generated during B-cell development. These are normally eliminated but some may 'leak' into the periphery. This, by itself, is probably insufficient to lead to autoimmunity, and requires a specific genetic predisposition in addition to the 'wrong environment' (e.g. viral infection) to produce the autoimmune phenotype. From Mackay,[142] with permission.

have been used to localize epitopes on the respective glycoprotein.[149,150] The development of human monoclonal antibodies from ITP patients has aided the mapping of target antigens. Using an immunobead assay GPIIb/IIIa and GPIb/IX appear to be involved in 75% of cases.[151] GPIb/IX is the second most frequent target;[141] less frequent targets include Ia/IIa and IV. Recent reports suggest the possibility that 40% of autoantibodies are reactive to both GPIIb/IIIa and GPIb/IX,[152] possibly due to the serum in some patients with ITP containing two different IgG antibodies.

Implicated epitopes

Kekomaki *et al* have shown that the 33 kDa chymotryptic core fragment of IIIa is a frequent target in chronic ITP.[150] Fujisawa and colleagues have used synthetic peptides corresponding to IIIa sequences have shown that in five of 13 sera from patients with chronic ITP binding was to residues 721–744 or 742–762, corresponding to the carboxy terminal of IIIa.[153]

GP-specific human MoAbs have been developed as important tools in the search for GP autoepitopes in chronic ITP.[154,155] Some investigators have localized certain autoantigenic epitopes to regions of IIb or IIIa[148–150,156] but blocking experiments using murine MoAbs have produced contradictory data in terms of homogeneity of the IIb/IIIa antigenic repertoire.[146,147] Only a few cryptic epitopes on IIb/IIIa have been recognized using GP-specific human MoAbs.[154,155]

Antibody class

The autoantibodies involved in ITP are generally IgG, but IgA and IgM autoantibodies have also been reported.[157]

Diagnosis

Despite advances in serologic and other techniques the diagnosis of ITP remains largely clinical, and one of exclusion. Secondary causes include systemic lupus erythematosus (SLE), lymphoproliferative disease, HIV infection, and others. Standard investigative tests include full blood count which will confirm the presence of isolated thrombocytopenia, blood film to ensure there are no red-cell fragments or other diseases such as leukemia or parasitic infections, and an autoimmune profile, to exclude a secondary cause for the thrombocytopenia. A bone marrow aspirate is often carried out in adults, but not usually in children, and will usually show normal or increased numbers of megakaryocytes in an otherwise normal marrow (Fig. 26.13). Immunologic assays have

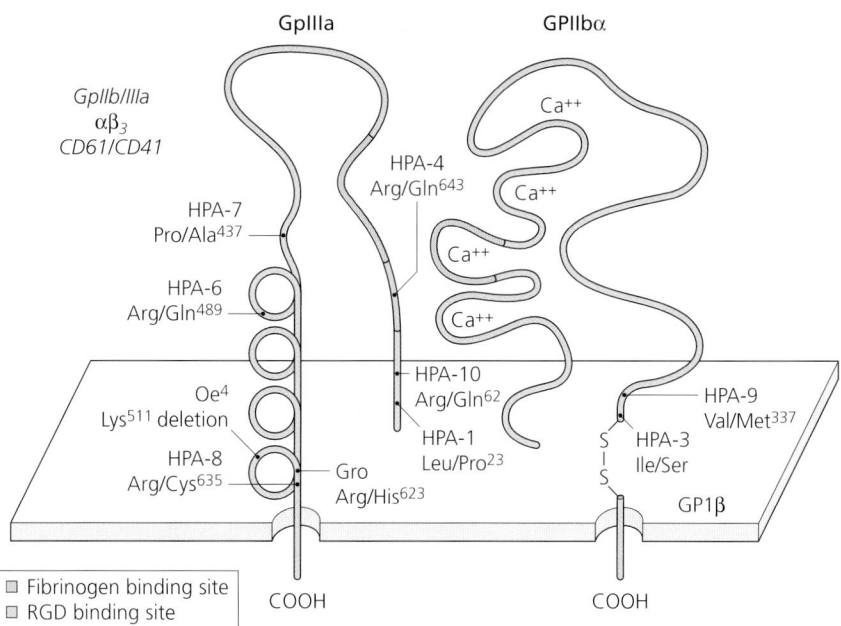

Fig. 26.12 Schematic representation of GPIIb/IIIa. From Provan D, Gribben JG 2000 (eds), Molecular haematology, Blackwell Science, Oxford, with permission.

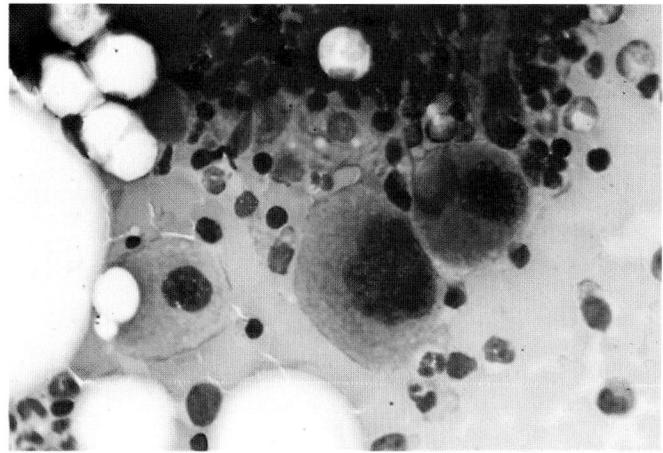

Fig. 26.13 Bone-marrow aspirate in patient with ITP showing increased numbers of megakaryocytes, some of which are young with fewer nuclei than mature megakaryocytes. Figure kindly provided by Dr John Amess, Barts & The London NHS Trust.

been devised including platelet-associated IgG or IgM, and monoclonal antibody immobilization of platelet antigens (MAIPA), but these do not alter the management and are of dubious value.

Standard first-line therapy

There are a lack of clinical trial data to help guide treatment and our energies should now be focused on constructing high-quality randomized trials in order to determine the most effective therapy in this disorder. Therapy is seldom necessary for patients whose platelet counts exceed $20\text{--}30 \times 10^9/l$ and in whom there are few spontaneous bleeding episodes[158] unless they are undergoing any procedure likely to induce blood loss.[159] Standard treatments including oral prednisolone,[130] intravenous immunoglobulin (IVIg),[130] and splenectomy will elevate the platelet count sufficiently in the majority of adults. However, some 20–25% of adults with ITP are refractory to first-line therapy.

Chronic refractory ITP

This defines those patients who fail to respond to first-line treatment or require unacceptably high doses of corticosteroids to maintain a safe platelet count. A number of agents have been used as second-line therapy for ITP including high-dose steroids, high-dose IVIg, intravenous anti-D, vinca alkaloids, danazol, azathioprine, combination chemotherapy and dapsone. An excellent summary is provided by McMillan.[129]

Experimental therapies

For those who fail to respond to standard first- and second-line therapy and who require treatment the options are limited and include: interferon-α,[130] cyclosporin A, CAMPATH 1H, and protein A columns.[160]

Secondary immune thrombocytopenia

Immune-mediated thrombocytopenia, similar to ITP, may occur in patients with other underlying autoimmune diseases such as systemic lupus erythematosus (SLE). Table 26.7 summarizes the main causes of immune-mediated thrombocytopenia caused by autoantibodies. Autoantibodies in SLE are highly complex and are directed against many target antigens including those of the plasma membrane in addition to nuclear and cytoplasmic antigens. Hematologic involvement is common in SLE and usually takes the form of anemia and cytopenias. In fact, immune cytopenias may be the presenting feature of SLE and provide a guide to disease activity. Three main forms of thrombocytopenia are recognized in SLE:[161] (1) rapid onset thrombocytopenia, with platelet counts falling to less than $10 \times 10^9/l$, and generally responsive to corticosteroid therapy; (2) progressive severe thrombocytopenia, generally resistant to corticosteroids alone, and often requiring other treatments such as IVIg, cytotoxics and possibly splenectomy; and (3) a chronic low-grade thrombocytopenia with platelet counts between 30 and $100 \times 10^9/l$.

Drug-induced thrombocytopenia

Drugs may induce thrombocytopenia through a variety of mechanisms, both immune and non-immune. Only drug-induced immune thrombocytopenia is discussed here; drug-induced qualitative abnormalities are discussed later in the chapter. In drug-induced immune-mediated thrombocytopenia, drug-dependent antibodies most commonly recognize epitopes of glycoproteins Ib-IX and IIb-IIIa.[162,163] Figure 26.14 shows the pathways involved in prostaglandin metabolism highlighting the sites of action of aspirin and non-steroidal anti-inflammatory drugs (NSAIDs).

Table 26.7 Causes of thrombocytopenia due to autoantibodies

Idiopathic	ITP (acute and chronic)
Secondary to other autoimmune or inflammatory disorders	SLE Other autoimmune disorders Lymphoproliferative disease e.g. CLL Post-BMT
Associated with viral infections	e.g. HIV
Drug-induced	e.g. quinine, quinidine, heparin, gold salts

BMT, bone-marrow transfer; CLL, chronic lymphocytic leukemia; HIV, human immunodeficiency virus; ITP, idiopathic thrombocytopenic purpura; SLE, systemic lupus erythematosus.

Clinical features

Thrombocytopenia is an uncommon drug-related side-effect. The predominant features are of bleeding or bruising. The number of drugs suspected of causing thrombocytopenia is quite large but strong evidence is only available for a few of these including: quinine,[164,165] quinidine,[166] sulfonamides,[167] trimethoprim and gold salts.[168]

The onset of thrombocytopenia is usually between 5 and 14 days after first exposure to the drug in cases of primary exposure, but only a few hours if it is a secondary exposure.

Patients present with petechial hemorrhages, bruising and in some cases bleeding from either the gastro-intestinal or genitourinary tracts. There may be associated hemolysis or neutropenia.

Investigations

Serologic tests may confirm the presence of drug-dependent antibodies. However, there are many patients in whom immune-mediated platelet destruction is believed to be occurring who have no detectable drug-dependent antibodies,[169] and the reverse is also true, whereby patients have drug-dependent antibodies in their plasma but with no accompanying thrombocytopenia.[170] Overall, therefore, the diagnosis of drug-induced thrombocytopenia through the action of drug-dependent antibodies remains largely clinical.

Management

The drug should be stopped and in most cases complete recovery will result in a few days. In cases of life-threatening bleeding therapeutic options include: plasma exchange, platelet transfusions, IVIg or corticosteroids.

Predictable (non-immune) thrombocytopenia

There are many drugs that will induce thrombocytopenia in a predictable fashion. These include anticancer (chemotherapy) drugs, which inhibit growth of stem cells, resulting in a reduction in all three cell lines (i.e. induce pancytopenia).

Drug-induced immune thrombocytopenia

Despite many reports of agents capable of inducing immune-mediated platelet destruction, there is good evidence for only a handful of these, namely heparin (see below), quin(id)ine, gold and trimethoprim-

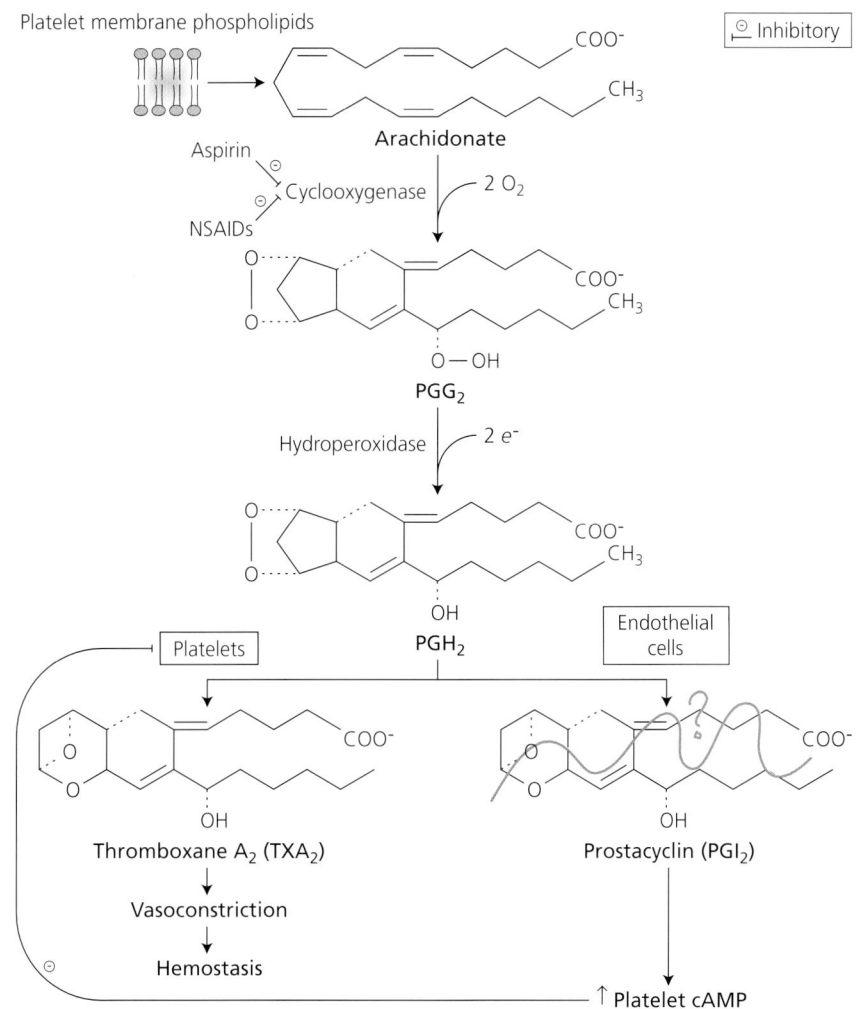

Fig. 26.14 Arachidonic acid metabolism and the generation of thromboxane A_2 and PGI_2. This is inhibited by aspirin and other NSAIDs leading to excessive bleeding.

sulfamethoxazole. Heparin-induced thrombocytopenia represents a serious drug-induced platelet disorder and is discussed in detail below.

Heparin-induced thrombocytopenia (HIT)

Variable degrees of thrombocytopenia in patients treated with heparin is fairly common, but in most cases is a benign observation with no serious adverse effects. This is termed HIT type I. Type II HIT is considerably more serious and represents the most severe adverse effect of heparin.[171]

Pathogenesis

In type I HIT there is platelet aggregation in the presence of heparin. HIT type I occurs predominantly with unfractionated heparin but can also occur with low-molecular-weight heparin,[172] and is induced by heparin-dependent antibodies, the target being heparin and platelet factor 4 (PF4).[173] There is usually no significant bleeding or thrombosis.

Type II HIT represents an immunologic reaction caused by antibodies directed against heparin–PF4 complexes that are able to activate platelets. Presentation is usually 5 or more days after the patient's first exposure to heparin.

Mechanism

Heparin binds to the platelets causing their activation.[174,175] Platelet proteins are then released and these bind to heparin which forms platelet protein–heparin complexes; PF4–heparin complexes are the most important (Fig. 26.15). The PF4-heparin complexes act as neoantigens, and induce an immune response in some patients treated

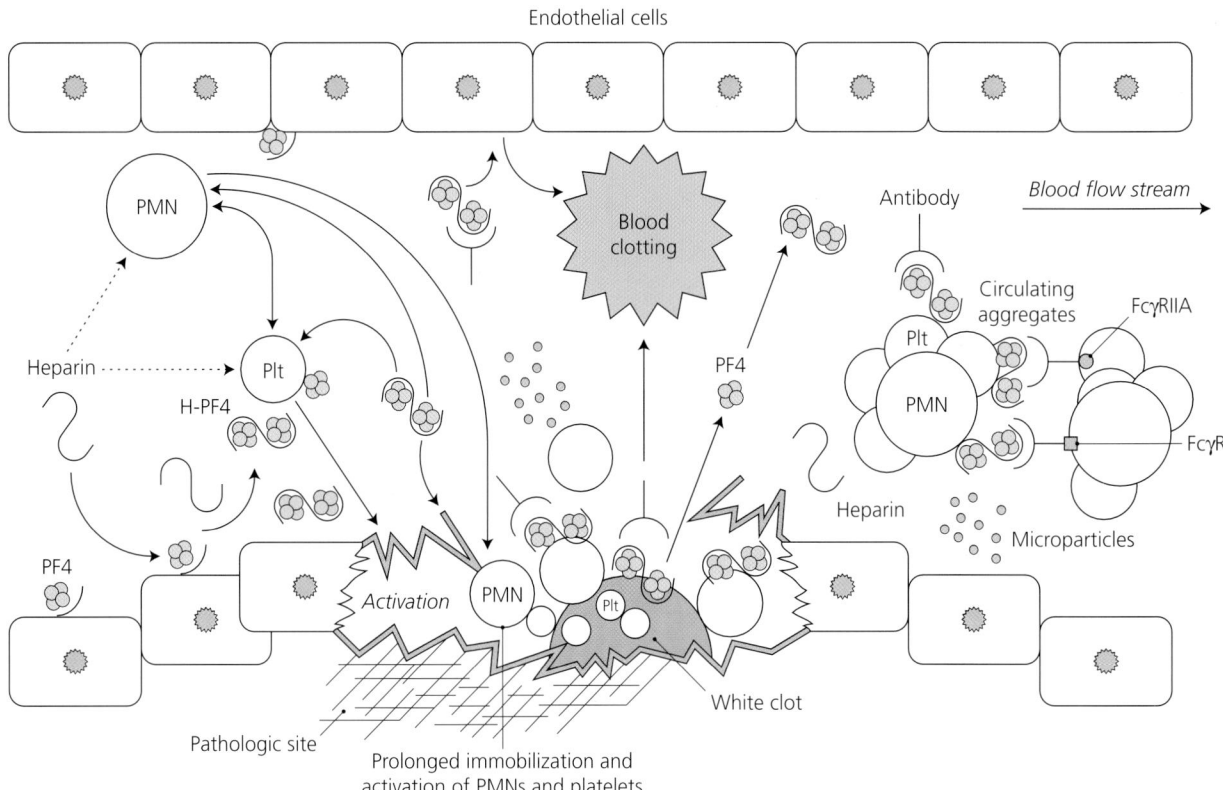

Fig. 26.15 Heparin-induced thrombocytopenia. Generation of heparin-platelet factor 4 complexes (H-PF4) in heparin-treated patients. Development of heparin-dependent antibodies which focus the immune response on to platelets and endothelial cells. Cell activation and cell–cell interactions, a phenomenon which is strongly enhanced at pathologic sites. Formation of a white clot, blood activation and clotting, and release of circulating aggregates and procoagulant microparticles in the blood circulation. PMN, polymorphonuclear cells (neutrophils). From Amiral & Meyer,[219] with permission.

with heparin. Immune complexes contain IgG molecules, which can link platelet FcγRIIa receptors, leading to FcγRIIa-dependent platelet activation.

Consequences

Platelets release granules after which activated platelets bind to fibrinogen and form a clot. Because platelet microparticles have phospholipid on the exterior surface there is enhanced thrombin generation. In effect, a process which starts as an immune-mediated platelet activation evolves into thrombin-induced coagulopathy with catastrophic consequences.

Clinical features

The associated thrombocytopenia may be moderate or severe. Although hemorrhage is uncommon, because of the enhanced thrombin generation as described above, there is a high rate of thrombotic events affecting major vessels. In patients treated with heparin for ischemic vascular disease, arterial thrombosis is common, and in

those receiving heparin for thrombotic diseases such as deep vein thrombosis (DVT), the associated thrombus is usually venous. Even in the presence of heparin there may be considerable extension of the DVT, which may prove fatal. The mortality rate from type II HIT is high at 30%.

Laboratory assessment

The blood count will show marked thrombocytopenia. A PF4–heparin complex ELISA is now available and can detect the presence of PF4–heparin complexes in patients with suspected HIT.[176] There are functional assays based on platelet aggregations tests,[177] and immunologic assays available.

Management

No treatment is required in type I HIT. However, in type II HIT the heparin should be stopped immediately and substituted for hirudin, heparinoids or ancrod. Although there is a lower incidence of type II HIT with low-molecular-weight heparins it is not recommended that patients are switched from unfractionated to low-molecular-weight heparin in suspected HIT. Platelet transfusions are contraindicated in HIT.

Other drugs causing immune-mediated platelet destruction

There are many drugs implicated in immune-mediated thrombocytopenia. The evidence is strongest for quinine, quinidine, heparin and gold salts,[111] as already discussed. Other implicated agents, though with fewer reports to date, include: α-methyldopa,[178] diclofenac,[179] rifampin,[180] carbamazepine[181] and sulfonamides. Readers are referred to George *et al* (1996) for an excellent review of the topic.[182]

Acquired functional abnormalities of platelets

Bleeding problems may arise through either inadequate numbers of platelets or functional abnormalities of the platelets themselves. This section discusses disorders in which there are abnormalities of platelet function along with their pathogenetic basis (Table 26.8).

Uremia in renal failure

Bleeding may be a feature of either acute or chronic renal failure,[183,184] with spontaneous bleeding into the skin, mucous membranes including the gastrointestinal or genitourinary tracts, central nervous system and other sites (also see Chapter 28).

Pathogenesis

Platelet function, in the presence of uremia, is abnormal,[183,185–187] and a variety of laboratory studies have shown that all aspects of platelet activity are affected, including platelet adhesion, aggregation and procoagulant activity.[188–190] Additional factors may play a role in the uremic bleeding diathesis including the presence of anemia, the degree of which correlates directly with the bleeding tendency. This tends to correct as the hematocrit is elevated to 30% or greater through the use of erythro-poietin or blood transfusion.[188] There is prolongation of the bleeding time in patients with anemia[191] and transfusion of red blood cells in patients who are uremic *and* anemic corrects the abnormal bleeding time in many, though not all, patients.

The normal process of platelet adhesion has been shown to involve contact of platelets to endothelial structures. This is dependent on the binding of vWF to GP lb/IX.[192] In the presence of uremia there may be a qualitative or quantitative abnormality of vWF or GPlb/IX itself. Measurement of vWF in patients with renal failure shows normal or increased levels but no evidence of any functional abnormality. But it has been shown that uremic plasma can inhibit platelet adhesion *in vitro*.

There are, of course, other factors contributing to the bleeding that occurs in patients with uremia, including the concomitant administration of drugs such as aspirin, and the presence of thrombocytopenia. The role of aspirin in this setting is not completely understood, since it does not simply reflect the inhibition of cyclooxygenase by aspirin, but rather correlates with the aspirin *level* in the peripheral blood.[193] Bleeding may become more severe during hemodialysis when heparin is introduced, which effectively compounds the other problems.

Management

The most important factor to consider is whether the patient is actively bleeding, rather than abnormalities detected using bleeding time, and other coagulation assays. Hemodialysis itself will help correct the bleeding induced by the uremia.[185] Desmopressin (DDAVP) which promotes the release of vWF from vascular endothelial cells may reduce the bleeding time in some uremic patients.[186] Red-cell transfusions ameliorate bleeding as the hematocrit rises.[186,194,195] Other treatments include estrogens which will reduce the bleeding time in most patients with uremia.[196] Cryoprecipitate has been used but with variable success; some authors have found it useful[197 198] whilst others report no benefit.[199]

Myeloproliferative disorders

The myeloproliferative diseases (MPDs) are neoplastic hematologic stem cell disorders and include essential

Table 26.8 Drugs and disorders interfering with platelet function

Systemic disorders	Uremia
	Cardiac by-pass surgery
Haematologic disorders	Myeloproliferative diseases
	Leukemia
	Myelodysplasia
	Paraproteinemias, including multiple myeloma
Drugs	Aspirin
	Antibiotics
	Anticoagulants
	Others

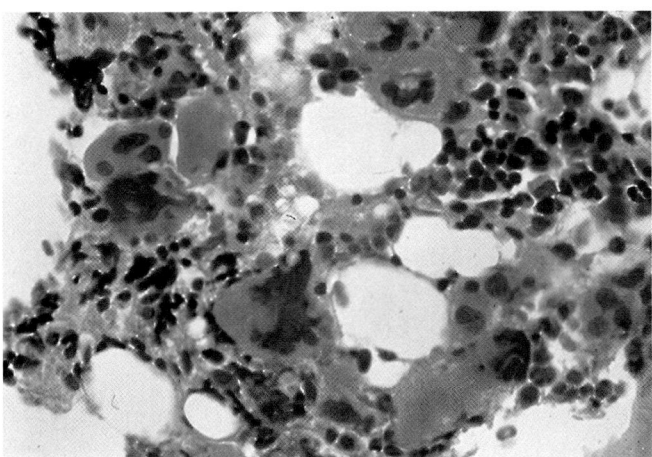

Fig. 26.16 Trephine biopsy in patient with essential thrombocythemia, one of the myeloproliferative disorders, showing greatly increased numbers of megakaryocytes with clustering. Figure kindly provided by Dr John Amess, Barts & The London NHS Trust.

thrombocythemia (ET) (see Fig. 26.16), polycythemia rubra vera (PRV), idiopathic myelofibrosis (IMF) and chronic myeloid leukemia (CML). These disorders are associated with both bleeding and thrombosis.

Pathophysiology

In PRV there is a rise in whole blood viscosity through elevation of the hematocrit which may contribute to thrombosis.[200] Abnormalities in platelet function have been reported in MPDs, and the bleeding time is prolonged in a minority of patients. However, bleeding may occur even if the template bleeding time is normal.[201] Thrombocytosis is a feature of all types of MPD but the actual contribution of a high platelet count to the development of thrombosis is uncertain.[202–205]

Platelet abnormalities in the myeloproliferative disorders

Platelets may be larger than normal, although in some cases they are smaller. Their survival may be reduced, especially in essential thrombocythemia. Platelet aggregation is abnormal with the standard aggregants including ADP and collagen,[201] though this is not a feature of thrombocytosis when the underlying cause is reactive, thereby excluding thrombocytosis *per se* as a cause of the abnormal aggregation.[206] It may, in fact, be a secondary consequence of the conversion of arachidonic acid to prostaglandin endoperoxides or lipooxygenase products,[207] or a decrease in platelet responsiveness to thromboxane A_2.[208]

Clinical features

Bleeding is common in the MPDs with bleeding reported in one form of another in one-third of patients. Thrombosis is equally common. The main clinical dilemma is the lack of ability to predict the likely risk of bleeding or thrombosis in patients who are asymptomatic.

Management

For PRV, a reduction in hematocrit, aiming for a level less than 0.45 (45%) is an approach adopted by most hematologists.[209] On-going clinical trials may help determine the optimal level of hematocrit. The bone marrow may be suppressed effectively using hydroxyurea or busulfan with an overall reduction in platelet count in patients with essential thrombocythemia.[204,210] However, even though the peripheral platelet count is lowered, this does not necessarily correct the associated platelet abnormalities. The management of the patient who is actively bleeding is more complex. Aspirin may be useful if thrombosis is present (e.g. in erythromelalgia or other ischemic event)[211] but is usually avoided in the asymptomatic patient.

Platelet abnormalities in leukemia and myelodysplastic syndromes

Bleeding is common in both types of disease, and is often due to thrombocytopenia. However, functional abnormalities of platelets are also recognized. In acute myeloid leukemia (AML) for example, platelets may be larger than usual, with abnormalities of shape and the appearance of their granules (Fig. 26.17). Functional assays show abnormalities of aggregation with ADP, adrenaline and collagen. In some instances the functional abnormalities may be secondary to acquired storage pool deficiency.[212–214] These functional defects most probably arise because the megakaryocytes in acute leukemia are derived from leukemic, rather than normal, blast cells that are, by definition, intrinsically abnormal.

Management

Patients with functional platelet abnormalities generally respond to platelet transfusion. Correction of the underlying malignancy with definitive therapy will also improve the acquired bleeding diathesis. Similar abnormalities are also seen in MDS and treatment generally consists of regular platelet transfusions.[213,215]

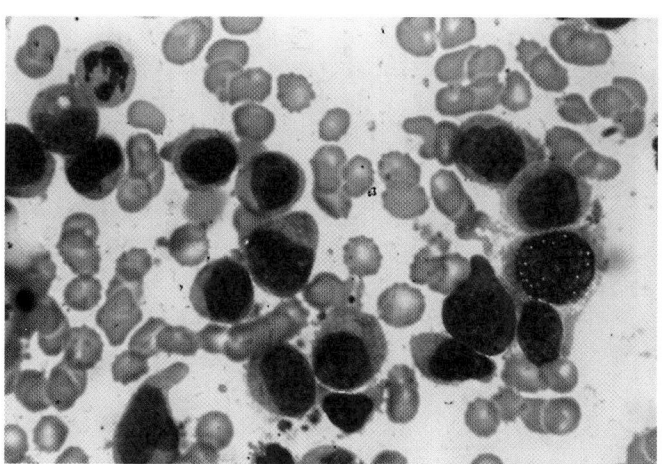

Fig. 26.17 Bone-marrow aspirate (high power) of AML M4 (acute myelomonocytic leukemia), showing large myeloblasts. Figure kindly provided by Dr John Amess, Barts & The London NHS Trust.

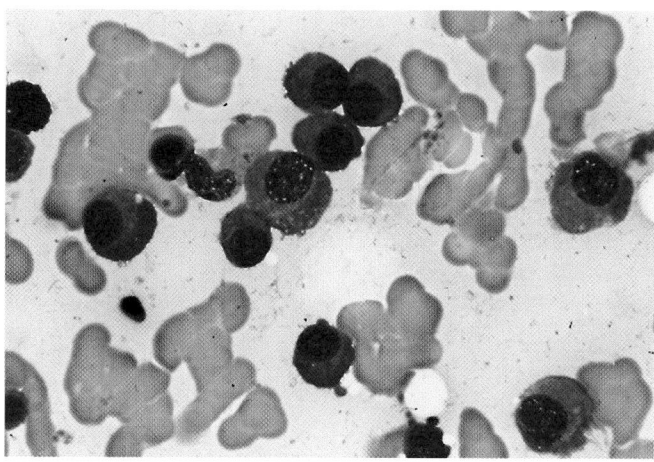

Fig. 26.18 Bone-marrow aspirate in multiple myeloma showing large numbers of plasma cells. The paraprotein may cause platelet dysfunction through a variety of mechanisms including hyperviscosity, development of uremia and other mechanisms. Figure kindly provided by Dr John Amess, Barts & The London NHS Trust.

Platelet dysfunction in patients with paraproteinemias

Abnormalities of platelet function are seen in one-third of all patients with IgA myeloma or Waldenström's macroglobulinemia, 15% of patients with IgG myeloma and occasionally in those with monoclonal gammopathy of undetermined significance[216,217] (Fig. 26.18). In addition to paraprotein-induced platelet function abnormalities there may also be hyperviscosity and thrombocytopenia associated with these diseases. Occasionally, amyloidosis may lead to an acquired factor X deficiency that may also lead to pathologic bleeding. The myeloma protein itself may interfere with laboratory tests of clotting through interference with fibrinogen polymerization.[216,217]

Pathogenesis

The template bleeding time may be prolonged even in the absence of active bleeding in patients with para-proteinemias. The paraprotein itself may interfere with the platelet surface, and interfere with platelet adhesion and stimulation.

Management

If the paraprotein interferes with platelet function sufficient to give rise to problematic bleeding problems then chemotherapy may reduce the plasma cell burden and ameliorate the symptoms. Occasionally, plasmapheresis may be used to reduce the quantity of paraprotein, and improve platelet function. Cryoprecipitate and DDAVP may be of value in some patients.[216]

Drugs that interfere with platelet function

In contrast with the many drugs that cause bleeding through the induction of profound thrombocytopenia, there are numerous agents that interfere with the normal function of platelets. Thus, although the platelet count may be entirely normal, the platelets are rendered functionally defective. Aspirin and non-steroidal anti-inflammatory agents (NSAIDs) are the most common cause of acquired platelet dysfunction (Table 26.9). Their effects are mediated through irreversibly inhibiting cyclo-oxygenase activity in the platelet resulting in impairment of the granule release reaction and defective aggregation. Aspirin, in particular, acetylates the serine residue at position 530 of prostaglandin synthase, the enzyme responsible for converting arachidonate to prostaglandin cyclic endoperoxides, and thereby inhibits the synthesis of prostacyclin and thromboxane A_2 (Fig. 26.19). These effects are seen in both the platelet and endothelium, but the effect of aspirin on platelet function is detectable for several days after the drug is stopped since there is a lag phase before new platelets lacking the drug enter the circulation. Endothelial cells, on the other hand, are able to generate prostaglandin synthase much more rapidly.

Table 26.9 Drugs interfering with platelet function

NSAIDs	Aspirin Diclofenac Mefenamic acid Others	Cyclooxygenase inhibitors
Antibiotics	Pencillins Cephalosporins Nitrofurantoin	In high doses, particularly in ill patients, many antibiotics may interfere with platelet aggregation
Anticoagulants	Heparin Epsilon aminocaproic acid	
Drugs that increase platelet cAMP	Dipyridamole Iloprost	Dipyridamole is a phosphodiesterase inhibitor
Cardiovascular system drugs	Diltiazem Isosorbide dinitrate Nifedipine Propranolol	
Psychotropics	Tricyclic antidepressants such as imipramine and amitryptiline Phenothiazines e.g. chlorpromazine, promethazine	
Anesthetics	Local and general anesthetics (e.g. halothane)	
Anticancer drugs	chemotherapeutic agents such as mithramycin, BCNU and daunorubicin	
Anticoagulants	Heparin and coumadin	
Miscellaneous	Dextrans Ticlopidine Lipid-lowering drugs e.g. clofibrate Quinidine Ethanol	

NSAIDs, non-steroid anti-inflammatory drugs. Modified from Rao AK, Carvalho ACA 1994. In: Colman RW et al (eds), In Hemostasis and thrombosis: principles and practice, 3rd edn. JB Lippincott, Philadelphia.

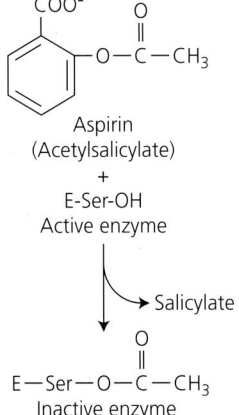

Fig. 26.19 Aspirin (acetylsalicylic acid) inhibits cyclooxygenase irreversibly by acetylation of a serine within the active site of the enzyme (E).

REFERENCES

1. Long MW, Gragowski LL, Heffner CH, Boxer LA 1985 Phorbol diesters stimulate the development of an early murine progenitor cell. The burst-forming unit-megakaryocyte. Journal of Clinical Investigation 76(2): 431–438
2. Jackson CW 1990 Megakaryocyte endomitosis: a review. International Journal of Cell Cloning 8(4): 224–226
3. Harker LA, Finch CA 1969 Thrombokinetics in man. Journal of Clinical Investigation 48(6): 963–974
4. Hynes RO 1987 Integrins: a family of cell surface receptors. Cell 48(4): 549–554
5. Kieffer N, Phillips DR 1990 Platelet membrane glycoproteins: functions in cellular interactions. Annual Review of Cell Biology 6: 329–357
6. Kunicki TJ, Newman PJ 1992 The molecular immunology of human platelet proteins. Blood 80(6): 1386–1404
7. Blockmans D, Deckmyn H, Vermylen J 1995 Platelet activation. Blood Reviews 9(3): 143–156
8. Waters AH 1999 The immune thrombocytopenias. In: Hoffbrand AV, Lewis SM, Tuddenham EGD (eds), Postgraduate haematology, 4th edn. Butterworth-Heinemann, Oxford, 597–611
9. Payne BA, Pierre RV 1984 Pseudothrombocytopenia: a laboratory artifact with potentially serious consequences. Mayo Clinic Proceedings 59(2): 123–125
10. Savage RA 1984 Pseudoleukocytosis due to EDTA-induced platelet clumping. American Journal of Clinical Pathology 81(3): 317–322
11. Aster RH 1966 Pooling of platelets in the spleen: role in the pathogenesis of 'hypersplenic' thrombocytopenia. Journal of Clinical Investigation 45(5): 645–657

12. Gewirtz AM, Hoffman R 1986 Transitory hypomegakaryocytic thrombocytopenia: aetiological association with ethanol abuse and implications regarding regulation of human megakaryocytopoiesis. British Journal of Haematology 62(2): 333–344

13. Boggs DR 1985 Amegakaryocytic thrombocytopenia. American Journal of Hematology 20(4): 413–416

14. Manoharan A, Williams NT, Sparrow R 1989 Acquired amegakaryocytic thrombocytopenia: report of a case and review of literature. Quarterly Journal of Medicine 70(263): 243–252

15. Mazur EM, Rosmarin AG, Sohl PA et al 1992 Analysis of the mechanism of anagrelide-induced thrombocytopenia in humans. Blood 79(8): 1931–1937

16. Wallerstein RO, Condit PK, Kasper CK et al 1969 Statewide study of chloramphenicol therapy and fatal aplastic anemia. Journal of the American Medical Association 208(11): 2045–2050

17. Kagan WA, Ascensao JA, Pahwa RN et al 1976 Aplastic anemia: presence in human bone marrow of cells that suppress myelopoiesis. Proceedings of the National Academy of Sciences USA 73(8): 2890–2894

18. Hoffman R, Zanjani ED, Lutton JD et al 1977 Suppression of erythroid-colony formation by lymphocytes from patients with aplastic anemia. New England Journal of Medicine 296(1): 10–13

19. Ascensao J, Pahwa R, Kagan W et al 1976 Aplastic anaemia: Evidence for an immunological mechanism. Lancet 1(7961): 669–671

20. Nissen C, Cornu P, Gratwohl A, Speck B 1980 Peripheral blood cells from patients wih aplastic anaemia in partial remission suppress growth of their own bone marrow precursors in culture. British Journal of Haematology 45(2): 233–243

21. Appelbaum FR, Fefer A 1981 The pathogenesis of aplastic anemia. Seminars in Hematology 18(4): 241–257

22. Camitta BM, Storb R, Thomas ED 1982 Aplastic anemia (first of two parts): pathogenesis, diagnosis, treatment, and prognosis. New England Journal of Medicine 306(11): 645–652

23. Kurnick JE, Robinson WA, Dickey CA 1971 *In vitro* granulocytic colony-forming potential of bone marrow from patients with granulocytopenia and aplastic anemia. Proceedings of the Society of Experimental Biology and Medicine 137(3): 917–920

24. Kern P, Heimpel H, Heit W, Kubanek B 1977 Granulocytic progenitor cells in aplastic anaemia. British Journal of Haematology 35(4): 613–623

25. Callera F, Garcia AB, Falcao RP 1998 Fas-mediated apoptosis with normal expression of bcl-2 and p53 in lymphocytes from aplastic anaemia. British Journal of Haematology 100(4): 698–703

26. Maciejewski JP, Selleri C, Sato T et al 1995 Increased expression of Fas antigen on bone marrow CD34+ cells of patients with aplastic anaemia. British Journal of Haematology 91(1): 245–252

27. Sanchez-Medal L, Castendo JP, Garcia-Rojas F 1963 Insecticides and aplastic anemia. New England Journal of Medicine 269: 1365

28. Darby SC, Doll R, Gill SK, Smith PG 1987 Long term mortality after a single treatment course with X-rays in patients treated for ankylosing spondylitis. British Journal of Cancer 55(2): 179–190

29. Ajlouni K, Doeblin TD 1974 The syndrome of hepatitis and aplastic anaemia. British Journal of Haematology 27(2): 345–355

30. Hagler L, Pastore RA, Bergin JJ, Wrensch MR 1975 Aplastic anemia following viral hepatitis: report of two fatal cases and literature review. Medicine (Baltimore) 54(2): 139–164

31. Shadduck RK, Winkelstein A, Zeigler Z et al 1979 Aplastic anemia following infectious mononucleosis: possible immune etiology. Experimental Hematology 7(5): 264–271

32. Marsh JC, Hows JM, Bryett KA et al 1987 Survival after antilymphocyte globulin therapy for aplastic anemia depends on disease severity. Blood 70(4): 1046–1052

33. Alexanian R 1973 Erythropoietin excretion in bone marrow failure and hemolytic anemia. Journal of Laboratory and Clinical Medicine 82(3): 438–445

34. Camitta BM, Thomas ED, Nathan DG et al 1979 A prospective study of androgens and bone marrow transplantation for treatment of severe aplastic anemia. Blood 53(3): 504–514

35. Bacigalupo A, Hows J, Gluckman E et al 1988 Bone marrow transplantation (BMT) versus immunosuppression for the treatment of severe aplastic anaemia (SAA): a report of the EBMT SAA working party. British Journal of Haematology 70(2): 177–182

36. Camitta BM, Thomas ED, Nathan DG et al 1976 Severe aplastic anemia: a prospective study of the effect of early marrow transplantation on acute mortality. Blood 48(1): 63–70

37. Young NS, Barrett AJ 1995 The treatment of severe acquired aplastic anemia. Blood 85(12): 3367–3377

38. Levi M, ten Cate H, van der Poll T, van Deventer SJ 1993 Pathogenesis of disseminated intravascular coagulation in sepsis. Journal of the American Medical Association 270(8): 975–979

39. Moschowitz E 1924 Hyaline thrombosis of the terminal arterioles and capillaries: a hitherto undescribed disease. Proceedings of the New York Pathological Society 24: 21–24

40. Mead PS, Griffin PM 1998 *Escherichia coli* O157:H7. Lancet 352(9135): 1207–1212

41. Siegler RL, Pavia AT, Hansen FL et al 1996 Atypical hemolytic–uremic syndrome: a comparison with postdiarrheal disease. Journal of Pediatrics 128(4): 505–511

42. Gordon LI, Kwaan HC 1999 Thrombotic microangiopathy manifesting as thrombotic thrombocytopenic purpura/hemolytic uremic syndrome in the cancer patient. Seminars in Thrombosis and Hemostasis 25(2): 217–221

43. Zarifian A, Meleg-Smith S, O'Donovan R et al 1999 Cyclosporine-associated thrombotic microangiopathy in renal allografts. Kidney International 55(6): 2457–2466

44. Gottschall JL, Neahring B, McFarland JG et al 1994 Quinine-induced immune thrombocytopenia with hemolytic uremic syndrome: clinical and serological findings in nine patients and review of literature. American Journal of Hematology 47(4): 283–289

45. Bennett CL, Davidson CJ, Raisch DW et al 1999 Thrombotic thrombocytopenic purpura associated with ticlopidine in the setting of coronary artery stents and stroke prevention. Archives of Internal Medicine 159(21): 2524–2528

46. George JN, El-Harake M 1995 Thrombocytopenia due to enhanced platelet destruction by non-immunologic mechanisms. In: Beutler E, Lichtman MA, Coller BS, Kipps TJ (eds), Williams hematology, 5th edn. McGraw-Hill, New York, 1290–1315

47. George JN 2000 How I treat patients with thrombotic thrombocytopenic purpura-hemolytic uremic syndrome. Blood 96(4): 1223–1229

48. Mitra D, Jaffe EA, Weksler B et al 1997 Thrombotic thrombocytopenic purpura and sporadic hemolytic–uremic syndrome plasmas induce apoptosis in restricted lineages of human microvascular endothelial cells. Blood 89(4): 1224–1234

49. Moake JL, Rudy CK, Troll JH et al 1982 Unusually large plasma factor VIII:von Willebrand factor multimers in chronic relapsing thrombotic thrombocytopenic purpura. New England Journal of Medicine 307(23): 1432–1435

50. Dent JA, Galbusera M, Ruggeri ZM 1991 Heterogeneity of plasma von Willebrand factor multimers resulting from proteolysis of the constituent subunit. Journal of Clinical Investigation 88(3): 774–782

51. Furlan M, Robles R, Solenthaler M et al 1997 Deficient activity of von Willebrand factor-cleaving protease in chronic relapsing thrombotic thrombocytopenic purpura. Blood 89(9): 3097–3103

52. Moake JL, Turner NA, Stathopoulos NA et al 1986 Involvement of large plasma von Willebrand factor (vWF) multimers and unusually large vWF forms derived from endothelial cells in shear stress-induced platelet aggregation. Journal of Clinical Investigation 78(6): 1456–1461

53. Rock GA, Shumak KH, Buskard NA et al 1991 Comparison of plasma exchange with plasma infusion in the treatment of thrombotic thrombocytopenic purpura. Canadian Apheresis Study Group. New England Journal of Medicine 325(6): 393–397

54. Bell WR, Braine HG, Ness PM, Kickler TS 1991 Improved survival in thrombotic thrombocytopenic purpura–hemolytic uremic syndrome. Clinical experience in 108 patients. New England Journal of Medicine 325(6): 398–403

55. Gasser C, Gautier E, Steck A et al 1955 Hamolytisch-uramische Syndrom: bilaterale Nierenrindennekrosen bei akuten erworbenen hamolytischen Anamien. Schweizerische Medíz Iní sche Wochenschrift 85: 905–909

56. Ashkenazi S 1993 Role of bacterial cytotoxins in hemolytic uremic syndrome and thrombotic thrombocytopenic purpura. Annual Review of Medicine 44: 11–18

57. Neill MA, Agosti J, Rosen H 1985 Hemorrhagic colitis with *Escherichia coli* 0157:H7 preceding adult hemolytic uremic syndrome. Archives of Internal Medicine 145(12): 2215–2217

58. White DJ, Yong F, McKendrick MW 1988 Haemolytic uraemic syndrome in adults. British Medical Journal (Clinical Research Edition) 296(6626): 899

59. Ostroff SM, Kobayashi JM, Lewis JH 1989 Infections with *Escherichia coli* O157:H7 in Washington State. The first year of statewide disease surveillance. Journal of the American Medical Association 262(3): 355–359

60. Martin DL, MacDonald KL, White KE et al 1990 The epidemiology and clinical aspects of the hemolytic uremic syndrome in Minnesota. New England Journal of Medicine 323(17): 1161–1167

61. Milford DV, Taylor CM, Guttridge B et al 1990 Haemolytic uraemic syndromes in the British Isles 1985–8: association with verocytotoxin producing *Escherichia coli*. Part 1: Clinical and epidemiological aspects. Archives of Diseases in Childhood 65(7): 716–721

62. Obrig TG 1992 Pathogenesis of Shiga toxin (verotoxin)-induced endothelial injury. In: Kaplan BS, Trompeter RS, Moake JL (eds), Hemolytic uremic syndrome and thrombotic thrombocytopenic purpura. Marcel-Dekker, New York, 405–419

63. Fitzpatrick MM, Shah V, Trompeter RS et al 1992 Interleukin-8 and polymorphoneutrophil leucocyte activation in hemolytic uremic syndrome of childhood. Kidney International 42(4): 951–956

64. Rowe PC, Orrbine E, Wells GA, McLaine PN 1991 Epidemiology of hemolytic–uremic syndrome in Canadian children from 1986 to 1988. The Canadian Pediatric Kidney Disease Reference Centre. Journal of Pediatrics 119(2): 218–224

65. Rizzoni G, Claris-Appiani A, Edefonti A et al 1988 Plasma infusion for hemolytic-uremic syndrome in children: results of a multicenter controlled trial. Journal of Pediatrics 112(2): 284–290

66. Brenner BM 1998 Vascular injury to the kidney. In: Fauci AS, Braunwald E, Isselbacher KJ (eds), Principles of internal medicine, 14th edn. McGraw-Hill, New York.

67. Ishibashi M, Ito N, Fujita M et al 1994 Endothelin-1 as an aggravating factor of disseminated intravascular coagulation associated with malignant neoplasms. Cancer 73(1): 191–195

68. Jones SL 1998 HELLP! A cry for laboratory assistance: a comprehensive review of the HELLP syndrome highlighting the role of the laboratory. Hematopathology and Molecular Hematology 11(3–4): 147–171

69. D'Anna R 1996 [The HELLP syndrome. Notes on its pathogenesis and treatment]. Minerva Ginecology 48(4): 147–154

70. Portis R, Jacobs MA, Skerman JH, Skerman EB 1997 HELLP syndrome (hemolysis, elevated liver enzymes, and low platelets) pathophysiology and anesthetic considerations. Journal of American Association of Nurse Anesthetists 65(1): 37–47

71. Stone JH 1998 HELLP syndrome: hemolysis, elevated liver enzymes, and low platelets. Journal of the American Medical Association 280(6): 559–562

72. Sheikh RA, Yasmeen S, Pauly MP, Riegler JL 1999 Spontaneous intrahepatic hemorrhage and hepatic rupture in the HELLP syndrome: four cases and a review. Journal of Clinical Gastroenterology 28: 323–328

73. Magann EF, Martin JN, Jr 1999 Twelve steps to optimal management of HELLP syndrome. Clinical Obstetrics and Gynecology 42(3): 532–550

74. Hamada K, Nakatomi Y, Shimada S 1992 Direct induction of tetraploids or homozygous diploids in the industrial yeast Saccharomyces cerevisiae by hydrostatic pressure. Current Genetics 22(5): 371–376

75. Leslie SD, Toy PT 1991 Laboratory hemostatic abnormalities in massively transfused patients given red blood cells and crystalloid. American Journal of Clinical Pathology 96(6): 770–773

76. Counts RB, Haisch C, Simon TL et al 1979 Hemostasis in massively transfused trauma patients. Annals of Surgery 190(1): 91–99

77. Lindenbaum J, Hargrove RL 1968 Thrombocytopenia in alcoholics. Annals of Internal Medicine 68(3): 526–532

78. Post RM, Desforges JF 1968 Thrombocytopenia and alcoholism. Annals of Internal Medicine 68(6): 1230–1236

79. Cowan DH 1973 Thrombokinetic studies in alcohol-related thrombocytopenia. Journal of Laboratory and Clinical Medicine 81(1): 64–76

80. Kelly DA, Summerfield JA 1987 Hemostasis in liver disease. Seminars in Liver Disease 7(3): 182–191

81. Ninomiya N, Maeda T, Matsuda I 1977 Thrombocytopenic purpura occurring during the early phase of a mumps infection. Helvetica Paediatrica Acta 32(1): 87–89

82. Espinoza C, Kuhn C 1974 Viral infection of megakaryocytes in varicella with purpura. American Journal of Clinical Pathology 61(2): 203–208

83. Angle RM, Alt HL. Thrombocytopenic purpura complicating infectious mononucleosis. Blood 1050 (5): 499

84. Bayer WL, Sherman FE, Michaels RH et al 1965 Purpura in congenital and acquired rubella. New England Journal of Medicine 273(25): 1362–1366

85. Oski FA, Naiman JL 1966 Effect of live measles vaccine on the platelet count. New England Journal of Medicine 275(7): 352–356

86. Walsh CM, Nardi MA, Karpatkin S 1984 On the mechanism of thrombocytopenic purpura in sexually active homosexual men. New England Journal of Medicine 311(10): 635–639

87. Ballem PJ, Belzberg A, Devine DV et al 1992 Kinetic studies of the mechanism of thrombocytopenia in patients with human immunodeficiency virus infection. New England Journal of Medicine 327(25): 1779–1784

88. Karpatkin S, Nardi M, Lennette ET et al 1988 Anti-human immunodeficiency virus type 1 antibody complexes on platelets of seropositive thrombocytopenic homosexuals and narcotic addicts. Proceedings of the National Academy of Sciences USA 85(24): 9763–9767

89. Treacy M, Lai L, Costello C, Clark A 1987 Peripheral blood and bone marrow abnormalities in patients with HIV related disease. British Journal of Haematology 65(3): 289–294

90. Frontiera M, Myers AM 1987 Peripheral blood and bone marrow abnormalities in the acquired immunodeficiency syndrome. Western Journal of Medicine 147(2): 157–160

91. Abrams DI, Chinn EK, Lewis BJ et al 1984 Hematologic manifestations in homosexual men with Kaposi's sarcoma. American Journal of Clinical Pathology 81(1): 13–18

92. Rossi G, Gorla R, Stellini R et al 1990 Prevalence, clinical, and laboratory features of thrombocytopenia among HIV-infected individuals. AIDS Research and Human Retroviruses 6(2): 261–269

93. Gill PS, Loureiro C, Bernstein-Singer M et al 1989 Clinical effect of glucocorticoids on Kaposi sarcoma related to the acquired immunodeficiency syndrome (AIDS). Annals of Internal Medicine 110(11): 937–940

94. Richman DD, Fischl MA, Grieco MH et al 1987 The toxicity of azidothymidine (AZT) in the treatment of patients with AIDS and AIDS-related complex. A double-blind, placebo-controlled trial. New England Journal of Medicine 317(4): 192–197

95. Fischl MA, Richman DD, Grieco MH et al 1987 The efficacy of azidothymidine (AZT) in the treatment of patients with AIDS and AIDS-related complex. A double-blind, placebo-controlled trial. New England Journal of Medicine 317(4): 185–191

96. Lever AM, Brook MG, Yap I, Thomas HC 1987 Treatment of thrombocytopenia with alfa interferon. British Medical Journal (Clinical Research Edition) (Clin Res Ed) 295(6612): 1519–1520

97. Stabler SP, Allen RH, Savage DG, Lindenbaum J 1990 Clinical spectrum and diagnosis of cobalamin deficiency. Blood 76(5): 871–881

98. Chong BH 1995 Diagnosis, treatment and pathophysiology of autoimmune thrombocytopenias. Critical Reviews in Oncology Hematology 20(3): 271–296

99. Ouwehand WH, Navarrete CV 2000 The molecular basis of blood cell alloantigens. In: Provan D, Gribben JG (eds), Molecular haematology. Blackwell Science, Oxford, 182–197

100. van Loghem JJ, Dorfmeyer H, van de Hart M, Schreuder F 1959 Serological and genetical studies on the platelet antigen (zw). Vox Sanguinis 4: 161–169

101. Mueller-Eckhardt C, Becker T, Weisheit M et al 1986 Neonatal alloimmune thrombocytopenia due to fetomaternal Zwb incompatibility. Vox Sanguinis 50(2): 94–96

102. Bizzaro N, Dianese G. 1988 Neonatal alloimmune amegakaryocytosis. Case report. Vox 54(2) 112–114

103. von dem Borne AE, von Riesz E, Verheugt FW et al 1980 Baka, a new platelet-specific antigen involved in neonatal allo-immune thrombocytopenia. Vox Sanguinis 39(2): 113–120

104. McGrath K, Minchinton R, Cunningham I, Ayberk H 1989 Platelet anti-Bakb antibody associated with neonatal alloimmune thrombocytopenia. Vox Sanguinis 57(3): 182–184

105. Friedman JM, Aster RH 1985 Neonatal alloimmune thrombocytopenic purpura and congenital porencephaly in two siblings associated with a 'new' maternal antiplatelet antibody. Blood 65(6): 1412–1415

106. Shibata Y, Matsuda I, Miyaji T, Ichikawa Y 1986 Yuka, a new platelet antigen involved in two cases of neonatal alloimmune thrombocytopenia. Vox Sanguinis 50(3): 177–180

107. Kaplan C, Morel-Kopp MC, Kroll H et al 1991 HPA-5b (Br(a)) neonatal alloimmune thrombocytopenia: clinical and immunological analysis of 39 cases. British Journal of Haematology 78(3): 425–429

108. Kiefel V, Shechter Y, Atias D et al 1991 Neonatal alloimmune thrombocytopenia due to anti-Brb (HPA-5a). Report of three cases in two families. Vox Sanguinis 60(4): 244–245
109. Mueller-Eckhardt C, Kayser W, Forster C et al 1982 Improved assay for detection of platelet-specific PIA1 antibodies in neonatal alloimmune thrombocytopenia. Vox Sanguinis 43(2): 76–81
110. Katz J, Hodder FS, Aster RS et al 1984 Neonatal isoimmune thrombocytopenia. The natural course and management and the detection of maternal antibody. Clinical Pediatrics (Philadelphia) 23(3): 159–162
111. Adner MM, Fisch GR, Starobin SG, Aster RH 1969 Use of 'compatible' platelet transfusions in treatment of congenital isoimmune thrombocytopenic purpura. New England Journal of Medicine 280(5): 244–247
112. Suarez CR, Anderson C 1987 High-dose intravenous gammaglobulin (IVG) in neonatal immune thrombocytopenia. American Journal of Hematology 26(3): 247–253
113. Pearson HA, Shulman NR, Marder VJ, Cone TE 1964 Isoimmune neonatal thrombocytopenic purpura: clinical and therapeutic considerations. Blood 23: 154
114. McFarland JG, Aster RH, Bussel JB et al 1991 Prenatal diagnosis of neonatal alloimmune thrombocytopenia using allelespecific oligonucleotide probes. Blood 78(9): 2276–2282
115. Bussel JB, Berkowitz RL, McFarland JG et al 1988 Antenatal treatment of neonatal alloimmune thrombocytopenia. New England Journal of Medicine 319(21): 1374–1378
116. Bussel J, Kaplan C, McFarland J 1991 Recommendations for the evaluation and treatment of neonatal autoimmune and alloimmune thrombocytopenia. The Working Party on Neonatal Immune Thrombocytopenia of the Neonatal Hemostasis Subcommittee of the Scientific and Standardization Committee of the ISTH. Thrombosis and Haemostasis 65(5): 631–634
117. Shulman NR, Jordan JV 1987 Platelet immunology. In: Colman RW, Hirsch J, Marder VJ, Salzman EW (eds), Hemostasis and thrombosis. Lippincott, Philadelphia, 452–529
118. Manson J, Speed I, Abbott K, Crompton J 1988 Congenital blindness, porencephaly, and neonatal thrombocytopenia: a report of four cases. Journal of Child Neurology 3(2): 120–124
119. Bussel JB, Tanli S, Peterson HC 1991 Favorable neurological outcome in 7 cases of perinatal intracranial hemorrhage due to immune thrombocytopenia. American Journal of Pediatric Hematology Oncology 13(2): 156–159
120. Mueller-Eckhardt C 1986 Post-transfusion purpura. British Journal of Haematology 64(3): 419–424
121. Chong BH, Burgess J, Ismail F 1993 The clinical usefulness of the platelet aggregation test for the diagnosis of heparin-induced thrombocytopenia. Thrombosis and Haemostasis 69(4): 344–350
122. Taaning E, Morling N, Ovesen H, Svejgaard A 1985 Post transfusion purpura and anti-Zwb (-P1A2). Tissue Antigens 26(2): 143–146
123. Keimowitz RM, Collins J, Davis K, Aster RH 1986 Post-transfusion purpura associated with alloimmunization against the platelet-specific antigen, Baka. American Journal of Hematology 21(1): 79–88
124. Kickler TS, Ness PM, Herman JH, Bell WR 1986 Studies on the pathophysiology of posttransfusion purpura. Blood 68(2): 347–350
125. Christie DJ, Pulkrabek S, Putnam JL et al 1991 Posttransfusion purpura due to an alloantibody reactive with glycoprotein Ia/IIa (anti-HPA-5b). Blood 77(12): 2785–2789
126. Seidenfeld AM, Owen J, Glynn MF 1978 Post-transfusion purpura cured by steroid therapy in a man. Canadian Medical Association Journal 118(10): 1285–1286
127. Simon T, Collins J, Kunicki T 1986 Post-transfusion purpura with antiplatelet antibody specific for the platelet antigen Penᵃ. Blood 68: 117a.
128. Waters AH 1989 Post-transfusion purpura. Blood Reviews 3(2): 83–87
129. McMillan R 1997 Therapy for adults with refractory chronic immune thrombocytopenic purpura. Annals of Internal Medicine 126(4): 307–314
130. George JN, Woolf SH, Raskob GE et al 1996 Idiopathic thrombocytopenic purpura: a practice guideline developed by explicit methods for the American Society of Hematology. Blood 88(1): 3–40
131. Warner MN, Moore JC, Warkentin TE et al 1999 A prospective study of protein-specific assays used to investigate idiopathic thrombocytopenic purpura. British Journal of Haematology 104(3): 442–447
132. Harrington WJ, Minnich V, Hollingsworth JW, Moore CV 1951 Demonstration of a thrombocytopenic factor in the blood of patients with thrombocytopenic purpura. Journal of Laboratory and Clinical Medicine 38: 1–10
133. Buchanan GR 1987 The nontreatment of childhood idiopathic thrombocytopenic purpura. European Journal of Pediatrics 146(2): 107–112
134. Bolton-Maggs PH, Moon I 1997 Assessment of UK practice for management of acute childhood idiopathic thrombocytopenic purpura against published guidelines. Lancet 350(9078): 620–623
135. Imbach P 1995 Immune thrombocytopenia in children: the immune character of destructive thrombocytopenia and the treatment of bleeding. Seminars in Thrombosis and Hemostasis 21(3): 305–312
136. Imbach PA, Kuhne T, Hollander G 1997 Immunologic aspects in the pathogenesis and treatment of immune thrombocytopenic purpura in children [published erratum appears in Curr Opin Pediatr 1997 Jun;9(3):298]. Current Opinion in Pediatrics 9(1): 35–40
137. Baatout S 1997 Thrombopoietin. A review. Haemostasis 27(1): 1–8
138. Lilleyman JS 1994 Intracranial haemorrhage in idiopathic thrombocytopenic purpura. Paediatric Haematology Forum of the British Society for Haematology. Archives of Diseases in Childhood 71(3): 251–253
139. Kienast J, Schmitz G 1990 Flow cytometric analysis of thiazole orange uptake by platelets: a diagnostic aid in the evaluation of thrombocytopenic disorders. Blood 75(1): 116–121
140. Woods VL, Oh EH, Mason D, McMillan R 1984 Autoantibodies against the platelet glycoprotein IIb/IIIa complex in patients with chronic ITP. Blood 63(2): 368–375
141. Woods VL, Jr., Kurata Y, Montgomery RR et al 1984 Autoantibodies against platelet glycoprotein Ib in patients with chronic immune thrombocytopenic purpura. Blood 64(1): 156–160
142. Mackay IR 2000 Tolerance and autoimmunity. British Medical Journal 321: 93–96
143. Hou M, Stockelberg D, Kutti J, Wadenvik H 1995 Glycoprotein IIb/IIIa autoantigenic repertoire in chronic idiopathic thrombocytopenic purpura. British Journal of Haematology 91(4): 971–975
144. McMillan R, Tani P, Millard F et al 1987 Platelet-associated and plasma anti-glycoprotein autoantibodies in chronic ITP. Blood 70(4): 1040–1045
145. Kiefel V, Santoso S, Kaufmann E, Mueller-Eckhardt C 1991 Autoantibodies against platelet glycoprotein Ib/IX: a frequent finding in autoimmune thrombocytopenic purpura. British Journal of Haematology 79(2): 256–262
146. Varon D, Karpatkin S 1983 A monoclonal anti-platelet antibody with decreased reactivity for autoimmune thrombocytopenic platelets. Proceedings of the National Academy of Sciences USA 80(22): 6992–6995
147. Tsubakio T, Tani P, Woods VL, McMillan R 1987 Autoantibodies against platelet GPIIb/IIIa in chronic ITP react with different epitopes. British Journal of Haematology 67(3): 345–348
148. Fujisawa K, Tani P, O'Toole TE et al 1992 Different specificities of platelet-associated and plasma autoantibodies to platelet GPIIb-IIIa in patients with chronic immune thrombocytopenic purpura. Blood 79(6): 1441–1446
149. Tomiyama Y, Kurata Y, Shibata Y et al 1989 Immunochemical characterization of an autoantigen on platelet glycoprotein IIb in chronic ITP: comparison with the Baka alloantigen. British Journal of Haematology 71(1): 77–83
150. Kekomaki R, Dawson B, McFarland J, Kunicki TJ 1991 Localization of human platelet autoantigens to the cysteine-rich region of glycoprotein IIIa. Journal of Clinical Investigation 88(3): 847–854
151. Berchtold P, Wenger M 1993 Autoantibodies against platelet glycoproteins in autoimmune thrombocytopenic purpura: their clinical significance and response to treatment. Blood 81(5): 1246–1250
152. Stockelberg D, Hou M, Jacobsson S et al 1995 Evidence for a light chain restriction of glycoprotein Ib/IX and IIb/IIIa reactive antibodies in chronic idiopathic thrombocytopenic purpura (ITP). British Journal of Haematology 90(1): 175–179
153. Fujisawa K, O'Toole TE, Tani P et al 1991 Autoantibodies to the presumptive cytoplasmic domain of platelet glycoprotein IIIa in patients with chronic immune thrombocytopenic purpura. Blood 77(10): 2207–2213
154. Nugent DJ, Kunicki TJ, Berglund C, Bernstein ID 1987 A human monoclonal autoantibody recognizes a neoantigen on glycoprotein IIIa expressed on stored and activated platelets. Blood 70(1): 16–22

155. Kunicki TJ, Plow EF, Kekomaki R, Nugent DJ 1991 Human monoclonal autoantibody 2E7 is specific for a peptide sequence of platelet glycoprotein IIb. Localization of the epitope to IIb231-238 with an immunodominant Trp235. Journal of Autoimmunity 4(3): 415–431

156. De Souza SJ, Sabbaga J, D'Amico E et al 1992 Anti-platelet autoantibodies from ITP patients recognize an epitope in GPIIb/IIIa deduced by complementary hydropathy. Immunology 75(1): 17–22

157. Kiefel V, Freitag E, Kroll H et al 1996 Platelet autoantibodies (IgG, IgM, IgA) against glycoproteins IIb/IIIa and Ib/IX in patients with thrombocytopenia. Annals of Hematology 72: 280–285

158. Karpatkin S 1985 Autoimmune thrombocytopenic purpura. Seminars in Hematology 22(4): 260–288

159. Yang R, Zhong CH 2000 Pathogenesis and management of chronic idiopathic thrombocytopenic purpura: an update. International Journal of Hematology 71: 18–24

160. Cahill MR, Macey MG, Cavenagh JD, Newland AC 1998 Protein A immunoadsorption in chronic refractory ITP reverses increased platelet activation but fails to achieve sustained clinical benefit. British Journal of Haematology 100(2): 358–364

161. Snaith ML, Isenberg DA 1996 Systemic lupus erythematosus and related disorders. In: Weatherall DJ, Ledingham JGG, Warrell DA (eds), Oxford textbook of medicine, 3rd edn. Oxford University Press, Oxford, 3017–3027

162. Ackroyd JF 1983 Drug-induced thrombocytopenia. An immunological phenomenon. Vox Sanguinis 45(3): 257–259

163. Garratty G 1993 Drug-induced immune cytopenia. Transfusion Medicine Reviews 7(4): 213–214

164. Kunicki TJ, Christie DJ, Aster RH 1983 The human platelet receptor(s) for quinine/quinidine-dependent antibodies. Blood Cells 9(2): 293–301

165. Connellan JM, Deacon S, Thurlow PJ 1991 Changes in platelet function and reactivity induced by quinine in relation to quinine (drug) induced immune thrombocytopenia. Thrombosis Research 61(5–6): 501–514

166. Salom IL 1991 Purpura due to inhaled quinidine. JAMA 266(9): 1220

167. Curtis BR, McFarland JG, Wu GG et al 1994 Antibodies in sulfonamide-induced immune thrombocytopenia recognize calcium-dependent epitopes on the glycoprotein IIb/IIIa complex. Blood 84(1): 176–183

168. Coblyn JS, Weinblatt M, Holdsworth D, Glass D 1981 Gold-induced thrombocytopenia. A clinical and immunogenetic study of twenty-three patients. Annals of Internal Medicine 95(2): 178–181

169. Christie DJ, Mullen PC, Aster RH 1987 Quinine- and quinidine-induced platelet antibodies can react with GPIIb/IIIa. British Journal of Haematology 67: 213–219

170. Warkentin TE, Chong BH, Greinacher A 1998 Heparin-induced thrombocytopenia: towards consensus. Thrombosis and Haemostasis 79(1): 1–7

171. Kelton J 1992 Pathophysiology of heparin-induced thrombocytopenia. British Journal of Haematology 82: 778–784

172. Visentin GP, Aster RH 1995 Heparin-induced thrombocytopenia and thrombosis. Current Opinion in Hematology 2(5): 351–357

173. Gruel Y, Boizard-Boval B, Wautier JL 1993 Further evidence that alpha-granule components such as platelet factor 4 are involved in platelet–IgG–heparin interactions during heparin-associated thrombocytopenia. Thrombosis and Haemostasis 70(2): 374–375

174. Greinacher A 1995 Antigen generation in heparin-associated thrombocytopenia: the nonimmunologic type and the immunologic type are closely linked in their pathogenesis. Seminars in Thrombosis and Hemostasis 21(1): 106–116

175. Warkentin TE 1996 Heparin-induced thrombocytopenia: IgG-mediated platelet activation, platelet microparticle generation, and altered procoagulant/anticoagulant balance in the pathogenesis of thrombosis and venous limb gangrene complicating heparin-induced thrombocytopenia. Transfusion Medicine Reviews 10(4): 249–258

176. Amiral J, Bridey F, Wolf M et al 1995 Antibodies to macromolecular platelet factor 4-heparin complexes in heparin-induced thrombocytopenia: a study of 44 cases. Thrombosis and Haemostasis 73(1): 21–28

177. Pouplard C, Amiral J, Borg JY 1997 Differences in specificity of heparin-dependent antibodies developed in heparin-induced thrombocytopenia and consequences on cross-reactivity with danaparoid sodium. British Journal of Haematology 99(2): 273–280

178. Manohitharajah SM, Jenkins WJ, Roberts PD, Clarke RC 1971 Methyldopa and associated thrombocytopenia. British Medical Journal 1(747): 494

179. Epstein M, Vickars L, Stein H 1990 Diclofenac induced immune thrombocytopenia. Journal of Rheumatology 17(10): 1403–1404

180. Burnette PK, Ameer B, Hoang V, Phifer W 1989 Rifampin-associated thrombocytopenia secondary to poor compliance. DICP – The Annals of Pharmacotherapy 23(5): 382–384

181. Casasin T, Allende A, Macia M, Guell R 1992 Two episodes of carbamazepine-induced severe thrombocytopenia in the same child. Annals of Pharmacotherapy 26(5): 715–716

182. George JN, El-Harake MA, Aster RH 1995 Thrombocytopenia due to enhanced platelet destruction by immunological mechanisms. In: Beutler E, Lichtman MA, Coller BS, Kipps TJ (eds), Williams hematology, 5th edn. McGraw-Hill, New York, 1315–1355

183. Rabiner SF 1972 Uremic bleeding. Progress in Hemostasis and Thrombosis 1: 233–250

184. Remuzzi G 1989 Bleeding disorders in uremia: pathophysiology and treatment. Advances in Nephrology Necker Hospital 00000000000000018: 171–186

185. Castaldi PA, Rozenberg MC, Stewart JH 1966 The bleeding disorder of uraemia. A qualitative platelet defect. Lancet 2(7454): 66–69

186. Livio M, Benigni A, Remuzzi G 1985 Coagulation abnormalities in uremia. Seminars in Nephrology 5(2): 82–90

187. Remuzzi G, Livio M, Marchiaro G et al 1978 Bleeding in renal failure: altered platelet function in chronic uraemia only partially corrected by haemodialysis. Nephron 22(4–6): 347–353

188. Castillo R, Lozano T, Escolar G et al 1986 Defective platelet adhesion on vessel subendothelium in uremic patients. Blood 68(2): 337–342

189. Zwaginga JJ, Ijsseldijk MJ, de Groot PG, Vos J et al 1991 Defects in platelet adhesion and aggregate formation in uremic bleeding disorder can be attributed to factors in plasma. Arteriosclerosis and Thrombosis 11(3): 733–744

190. Zwaginga JJ, Ijsseldijk MJ, Beeser-Visser N et al 1990 High von Willebrand factor concentration compensates a relative adhesion defect in uremic blood. Blood 75(7): 1498–1508

191. Small M, Lowe GD, Cameron E, Forbes CD 1983 Contribution of the haematocrit to the bleeding time. Haemostasis 13(6): 379–384

192. Weiss HJ, Turitto VT, Baumgartner HR 1978 Effect of shear rate on platelet interaction with subendothelium in citrated and native blood. I. Shear rate-dependent decrease of adhesion in von Willebrand's disease and the Bernard-Soulier syndrome. Journal of Laboratory and Clinical Medicine 92(5): 750–764

193. Gaspari F, Vigano G, Orisio S et al 1987 Aspirin prolongs bleeding time in uremia by a mechanism distinct from platelet cyclooxygenase inhibition. Journal of Clinical Investigation 79(6): 1788–1797

194. Fernandez F, Goudable C, Sie P et al 1985 Low haematocrit and prolonged bleeding time in uraemic patients: effect of red cell transfusions. British Journal of Haematology 59(1): 139–148

195. Moia M, Mannucci PM, Vizzotto L et al 1987 Improvement in the haemostatic defect of uraemia after treatment with recombinant human erythropoietin. Lancet 2(8570): 1227–1229

196. Livio M, Mannucci PM, Vigano G et al 1986 Conjugated estrogens for the management of bleeding associated with renal failure. New England Journal of Medicine 315(12): 731–735

197. Juhl A 1986 DDAVP, cryoprecipitate, and highly 'purified' factor VIII concentrate in uremia. Nephron 43(4): 305–306

198. Janson PA, Jubelirer SJ, Weinstein MJ, Deykin D 1980 Treatment of the bleeding tendency in uremia with cryoprecipitate. New England Journal of Medicine 303(23): 1318–1322

199. Triulzi DJ, Blumberg N 1990 Variability in response to cryoprecipitate treatment for hemostatic defects in uremia. Yale Journal of Biological Medicine 63(1): 1–7

200. Murphy S 1992 Polycythemia vera. Diseases Monthly 38(3): 153–212

201. Schafer AI 1991 Essential thrombocythemia. Progress in Hemostasis and Thrombosis 10: 69–96

202. Mitus AJ, Barbui T, Shulman LN et al 1990 Hemostatic complications in young patients with essential thrombocythemia. American Journal of Medicine 88(4): 371–375

203. Lahuerta-Palacios JJ, Bornstein R, Fernandez-Debora FJ et al 1988 Controlled and uncontrolled thrombocytosis. Its clinical role in essential thrombocythemia. Cancer 61(6): 1207–1212

204. Kessler CM, Klein HG, Havlik RJ 1982 Uncontrolled thrombocytosis in chronic myeloproliferative disorders. British Journal of Haematology 50(1): 157–167

205. McIntyre KJ, Hoagland HC, Silverstein MN, Petitt RM 1991 Essential thrombocythemia in young adults. Mayo Clinic Proceedings 66(2): 149–154

206. Ginsburg AD 1975 Platelet function in patients with high platelet counts. Annals of Internal Medicine 82(4): 506–511
207. Schafer AI 1982 Deficiency of platelet lipoxygenase activity in myeloproliferative disorders. New England Journal of Medicine 306(7): 381–386
208. Okuma M, Takayama H, Uchino H 1982 Subnormal platelet response to thromboxane A2 in a patient with chronic myeloid leukaemia. British Journal of Haematology 51(3): 469–477
209. Kaplan ME, Mack K, Goldberg JD et al 1986 Long-term management of polycythemia vera with hydroxyurea: a progress report. Seminars in Hematology 23(3): 167–171
210. Murphy S, Iland H, Rosenthal D, Laszlo J 1986 Essential thrombocythemia: an interim report from the Polycythemia Vera Study Group. Seminars in Hematology 23(3): 177–182
211. Preston FE 1983 Aspirin, prostaglandins, and peripheral gangrene. American Journal of Medicine 74(6A): 55–60
212. Sultan Y, Caen JP 1972 Platelet dysfunction in preleukemic states and in various types of leukemia. Annals of the New York Academy of Sciences 201: 300–306
213. Cowan DH, Haut MJ 1972 Platelet function in acute leukemia. Journal of Laboratory and Clinical Medicine 79(6): 893–905
214. Cowan DH, Graham RC, Jr., Baunach D 1975 The platelet defect in leukemia. Platelet ultrastructure, adenine nucleotide metabolism, and the release reaction. Journal of Clinical Investigation 56(1): 188–200
215. Meschengieser S, Blanco A, Maugeri N et al 1987 Platelet function and intraplatelet von Willebrand factor antigen and fibrinogen in myelodysplastic syndromes. Thrombosis Research 46(4): 601–606
216. Lackner H 1973 Hemostatic abnormalities associated with dysproteinemias. Seminars in Hematology 10(2): 125–133
217. Perkins HA, MacKenzie MR, Fudenberg HH 1970 Hemostatic defects in dysproteinemias. Blood 35(5): 695–707
218. Mackie IJ 2000 The biology of haemostasis and thrombosis. In: Ledingham JGG, Warrell DA (eds), Concise Oxford textbook of medicine. Oxford University Press, Oxford, 291–299
219. Amiral J, Meyer D 1998 Heparin-induced thrombocytopenia: diagnostic tests and biological mechanisms. Bailliere's Clinical Haematology 11: 447–460
220. Roth GJ 1991 Developing relationships: arterial platelet adhesion, glycoprotein Ib, and leucine-rich glycoproteins. Blood 77: 5–19

Inherited disorders of coagulation

27

CA Lee

Hemophilia A
Inheritance and diagnosis
The molecular basis of hemophilia A
Carrier detection

Hemophilia B
Inheritance and diagnosis

The clinical features of hemophilia A and hemophilia B

Treatment of hemophilia A – clotting factor concentrates

Recombinant clotting factors in the treatment of hemophilia
Recombinant FVIII
Recombinant FIX
The assay of recombinant clotting factors
Recombinant factor VIIa (FVIIa)

Therapeutic strategies

Treatment on demand

Prophylaxis

Inhibitors
The treatment of inhibitors
Desmopressin in the treatment of hemophilia A

Von Willebrand's disease (vWD)
Screening tests
vWF antigen

Ristocetin cofactor activity
Factor VIIIC (FVIIIC)
Ristocetin-induced platelet aggregation (RIPA)
vWF multimeric analysis
Platelet vWF
Factor VIII binding assay

The subtypes of VWD

Acquired vWD

Treatment of vWD
Desmopressin
Tranexamic acid
Clotting factor concentrates

The molecular basis of vWD

vWD in women
Pregnancy in women with vWD

Rare bleeding disorders

Fibrinogen

Prothrombin

Factor V deficiency

Factor VII

Factor X

Factor XI deficiency

Factor XIII deficiency

Hemophilia A

Inheritance and diagnosis

Hemophilia A is a deficiency of coagulation factor VIII (FVIII). A severe deficiency has a level of < 2 iu/dl (normal range 50–150). FVIII functions as a cofactor with activated factor IX (FIX) phospholipid and calcium for the activation of factor X (FX). Clinically, the factor VIII deficiency results in a life-threatening bleeding disorder with spontaneous bleeds into joints and muscles which without treatment can lead to crippling. In general, the level of FVIII correlates with the frequency and severity of bleeding. Hemophilia A is inherited as a sex-linked recessive disorder and carriers may have a reduced level of FVIII.

The molecular basis of hemophilia A

The cloning of the FVIII gene and the sequencing of the cDNA was reported in landmark papers in 1984.[1–3] It consists of 2332 amino acids with three identifiable domain types in the sequence A1-A2-B-A3-C1-C2. FVIII circulates in plasma with a heavy chain (A1,A2,B) and light (A3,C1,C2) chain in association with von Willebrand factor (vWF). The activation of FVIII occurs by cleavage at two specific sites and as well as resulting in the activation of the protein it also results in the dissociation of vWF.

The FVIII gene is 186 kilobases in length and is situated on the long arm of the X chromosome. It has 26 exons and includes the intron 22 which contains within itself the start points for two further genes, one entirely contained within the intron and apparently expressed in most tissues (F8A) and a second beginning within the intron and utilizing exons 23–26 of the FVIII gene itself (F8B).[4] Following cloning of the FVIII gene a number of mutations have been reported which are included in an internet database which is updated annually (*http://europiun.mrc.rpms.ac.uk/*). In almost 50% of cases with severe hemophilia A there is a defect within intron 22 which leads to failure of transcription across this intron. This is the result of an inversion of a section of the X chromosome at the tip of the long arm and this inversion results in the separation of the factor gene into two parts (Fig. 27.1).

Carrier detection

Hemophilia A is an X-linked disease and it is possible to precisely establish carrier status and offer prenatal diagnosis. It is thought that for each patient with hemophilia there averages 5–6 potential carriers. Obligate carriers are daughters of hemophilic individuals or mothers of a hemophilic child with a maternal history of the disease. The phenotypic assessment of carrier status in hemophilia can be made by measuring the level of plasma FVIII. However, this will only identify 80% of carriers and precise genetic mutational analysis may be necessary to establish carriership in others.

Hemophilia B

Inheritance and diagnosis

Hemophilia B is an X-linked deficiency of FIX and behaves clinically like hemophilia A. FIX is responsible for the activation of FX in the presence of activated FVIII, calcium and phospholipid. FIX is synthesized in the liver and is a vitamin-K-dependent serine protease comparable to prothrombin, FVII, FX and protein C. The FIX protein consists of 454 amino acids. The FIX gene is contained on the long arm of the X chromosome and contains eight exons. The complete sequence of the gene has been determined. Since the FIX gene is a simple gene it has been possible to perform detailed analysis using polymerase chain reaction (PCR)-based analysis. In this way, virtually all cases of hemophilia B genetic mutations have been established. A hemophilia B data base is also available on the internet at *http://www.unds.ac.uk/molgen/*).

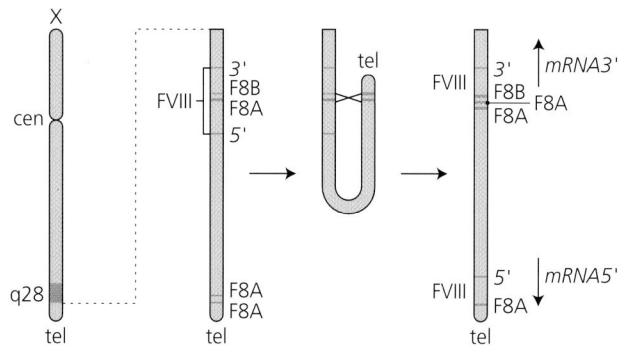

Fig. 27.1 How the tip flips: the mechanism of inversion through intron 22. cen, centromere; tel, telomere. Reproduced from Hoffbrand AV *et al* 1999. Postgraduate haematology. Tuddenham EGD (eds) 1999. Butterworth Heinemann, 625, with permission.

It is possible to perform mutational analysis to establish carriership because the complete DNA sequence of the gene is known.

The clinical features of hemophilia A and hemophilia B

There are approximately 6000 individuals registered with hemophilia in the UK. Hemophilia B is less common with approximately 1200 patients registered.[5] The clinical features of hemophilia A and B are similar. It is possible to differentiate three degrees of clinical severity:

1. Severe hemophilia where there is spontaneous hemorrhage into joints and muscles and the FVIII or FIX level is < 2 iu/dl (normal range 50–150).
2. Moderate hemophilia where bleeding occurs after minor trauma. FVIII or FIX levels lie between 2 and 5 iu/dl.
3. Mild hemophilia when prolonged bleeding only occurs with trauma or after operative procedure and the basal FVIII or FIX levels are between 5 and 50 iu/dl.

It is unusual for hemorrhagic symptoms to occur until the new-born child becomes active. However, rarely the first-born affected male may develop a large cephalohematoma and occasionally intracranial hemorrhage, particularly in cases of spontaneous hemophilia and where there is an instrumental delivery.

Spontaneous bleeding into joints is common in hemophilia A and hemophilia B. If such bleeding goes untreated these hemarthroses result in secondary crippling. The most common joints to be affected are the knee, elbow and ankle. Without treatment individuals with severe hemophilia can expect to sustain approximately 30 joint bleeds a year.

Bleeding into the muscles is also common and this can occasionally lead to pressure on underlying nerves. Thus, Volkman's contracture is a serious consequence of bleeding into the muscular compartment of the forearm. Retroperitoneal hemorrhage and bleeding into the iliopsoas muscle can result in femoral nerve compression and this can be life threatening. If there is inadequate treatment of hematomas a cystic collection of blood may form resulting in a 'pseudo tumor' and these are particularly common in patients in areas of the world where there is inadequate treatment of hemophilia. Bleeding into the central nervous system is particularly severe and next to acquired immunodeficiency syndrome is the most common cause of death.[6]

Treatment of hemophilia A – clotting factor concentrates

The discovery that factor VIII concentrate (FVIIIC) was concentrated in cryoprecipitate and the subsequent description of the production of antihemophilic globulin in a closed-bag system[7] made more specific replacement therapy for people with hemophilia possible. Home treatment for the majority of patients became feasible and with the advent of lyophilized concentrates prepared from the plasma from many thousands of donors the prospect of a normal life for the severely affected hemophilic individual was brought very close. Until virucidal methods were applied to such concentrates from 1985 onwards many individuals with hemophilia contracted hepatitis, chronic liver disease and AIDS. However, clotting factor concentrates are now virucidally treated and are very safe particularly with the advent of recombinant clotting factor concentrates. The plasma-derived clotting factor concentrates currently in use are high purity products with a high specific activity.[8,9] They are prepared by monoclonal immunoabsorption and other techniques which result in a pure final product of high specific activity. In the case of FVIII concentrate this may be purified using a monoclonal antibody specific for the von Willebrand protein or a monoclonal antibody specific to FVIIIC itself. Other techniques of fractionation use chromatographic purification.

Viral infections were a major complication of replacement therapy before adequate inactivation steps were applied. There are three main virucidal methods:

1. Terminal heating of the lyophilized product at 80°C (dry heating).
2. Heating in solution at 60°C (pasteurization) in the presence of stabilizers or in moisture with hot vapor under high pressure.
3. Adding a solvent detergent mixture during the manufacturing process.

Table 27.1 shows the main blood-borne viruses with their genomic and physicochemical characteristics. The safety of such procedures is summarized in Tables 27.2 and 27.3. It can be seen that the risk of HIV infection in virally inactivated concentrates is very small, probably as low as 1:200 000–1:300 000. The risk of transmission of hepatitis B and C has also been dramatically reduced. However, there remains the problem of transmission of hepatitis A and parvo virus which can break through solvent detergent sterilization and for this reason many

Table 27.1 Main blood-borne viruses transmitted by coagulation factor concentrates. From Mannucci 1996,[10] with permission

Virus	Genome	Lipid-enveloped	Size (nm)	Solvent/detergent resistant	Heat resistant
Human immunodeficiency virus, type I	RNA	Yes	80–100	No	No
Hepatitis A virus	RNA	No	27	Yes	No
Hepatitis B virus	DNA	Yes	42	No	No
Hepatitis C virus	RNA	Yes	35–65	No	No
Hepatitis D virus	RNA	Yes	35	No	No
B19 parvovirus	DNA	No	20	Yes	Yes

Table 27.2 Cumulative results of hepatitis B and C safety studies carried out in previously untreated hemophilic patients infused with currently available virally-inactivated concentrates. From Mannucci 1996,[10] with permission

Number of patients studied	Virucidal method	Number with hepatitis[a]	Confidence intervals of the hepatitis risk[b] (%)
153	Pasteurization	0/153	0–2
50	Vapour heating	0/50	0–6
51	Dry-heating	0/38	0–6
117	Solvent/detergent	0/117	0–3

[a] Some studies were carried out using elevations of transaminases as diagnostic criteria for non–A, non-B hepatitis, others using specific tests for antibodies to the hepatitis C virus.
[b] Expressed as one-sided 95% confidence intervals around the true risk of hepatitis, only for studies that resulted in no cases of hepatitis.

Table 27.3 Cumulative results of HIV safety studies carried out in anti-HIV negative hemophilic patients infused with currently available virally-inactivated concentrates. From Mannucci 1996,[10] with permission

Number of patients studied	Virucidal method	Number of seroconverters	Confidence intervals of the risk of seroconversion (%)[a]
210	Pasteurization	0/210	0–1.5
81	Vapor heating	0/81	0–3.7
245	Solvent/detergent	0/245	0–1.2

[a] Expressed as one-sided 95% confidence intervals around the true risk of anti-HIV seroconversion.

inactivation processes involve more than one virucidal method.[10] For FIX concentrate the process of nanofiltration has been used which can prevent transmission of hepatitis A and parvo virus.

Recombinant clotting factors in the treatment of hemophilia

Recombinant FVIII

The structure of the FVIII gene, the isolation of cDNA clones encoding the complete FVIII sequence in the *in vitro* expression of human FVIII in tissue culture were described in a single issue of *Nature* in 1984.[1–3] As a result it has been possible to develop a recombinant FVIII product: two full-length recombinant products, *Kogenate*

and *Recombinate,* and one which is B domainless known as rVIIISQ with the trade name of Refacto.[11]

Kogenate was made by transfecting cDNA for FVIII into an established mammalian cell line of baby hamster kidney. The secreted protein was purified by multiple purification steps including ion-exchange chromatography and immuno-affinity chromatography with murine monoclonal antibody. The first generation Kogenate requires albumin as a stabilizer but more recently this recombinant FVIII is stabilized using sucrose, avoiding the need for the addition of human albumin. Prelicensure clinical trials began in 1988. The previously treated patient (PTP) study showed an excellent effect with approximately three-quarters of the patients requiring only one treatment to treat bleeding episodes and the covering of surgical procedures was also very safe.[12] A previously untreated patient (PUP) study was begun in children in 1989 and it was this study that first showed the natural history of treatment in hemophilia with a high rate of inhibitor development.[13]

Recombinate was manufactured by introducing the human FVIII and the vWF DNA into Chinese hamster ovary cells. It was also shown to be very effective in PTPs and in the PUP study a similar rate of inhibitor development occurred.[11,14]

Refacto is a B-domain depleted recombinant FVIII: the B domain is dispensable for the hemostatic acitivity of FVIII. The B-domain depleted molecule is much more stable and albumin is not necessary for stabilization. The PTP and PUP studies have shown good safety and efficacy with a similar rate of inhibitor development to the full length recombinant FVIIIs.[14]

Recombinant FIX

Although the FIX gene was cloned in 1982[15] the development of recombinant FIX, Benefix, was more difficult because of the post-translational modification that is required. Clinical trials of the pharmacokinetics and treatment in PTPs and PUPs were begun in 1995. Although the clinical effect was good the recovery was only 72% of that observed with monoclonal plasma-derived FIX.[16]

The assay of recombinant clotting factors

Lusher *et al* have coined the phrase 'will the right FVIII level please stand up'.[17] It was found that pharmacokinetic studies showed that the chromogenic assay

produced considerably higher levels than one-stage assays. Mikaelsson *et al* studied the influence of phospholipids on these discrepancies.[18] It was found that when the activated partial thromboplastin time (APTT) reagent was replaced by platelets in the one-stage assays the results of the chromogenic assay and the one-stage assay were comparable (Figs 27.2 and 27.3). Furthermore, using the basic principle of 'like versus like' this discrepancy between chromogenic and one stage methods could be eliminated by using the recombinant product diluted in hemophilic plasma as a standard reference[19] (Fig. 27.4).

Recombinant factor VIIa (FVIIa)

Recombinant FVIIa was developed by scientists at Novo Nordis as a treatment for bleeding episodes in individuals with hemophilia complicated by inhibitor antibodies. Activated FVII is not proteolytically active itself and does not therefore produce systemic activation of coagulation when infused. The FVIIa complexes with tissue factor at the site of the injury and since it is not neutralized by circulating antithrombin, infused FVIIa can reach the site of injury where it complexes with tissue factor exposed at the site, inducing local hemostasis.[20] The process is independent of the presence of FVIII or FIX and is not affected by inhibitors to FVIII or FIX.

Human FVIIa was cloned in the mid 1980s and was expressed in baby hamster kidney cells. The baby hamster kidney cells are capable of γ-carboxylation and the FVII is secreted in the single chain form. The amino acid sequence has been shown to be identical to the human form.

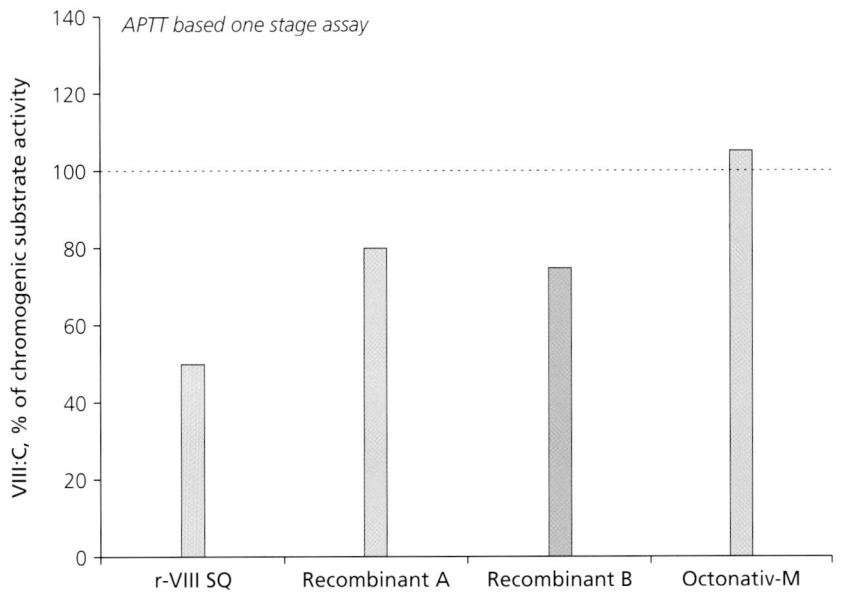

Fig. 27.2 APTT-based one-stage assays. From Mikaelsson M *et al* 1998,[18] with permission.

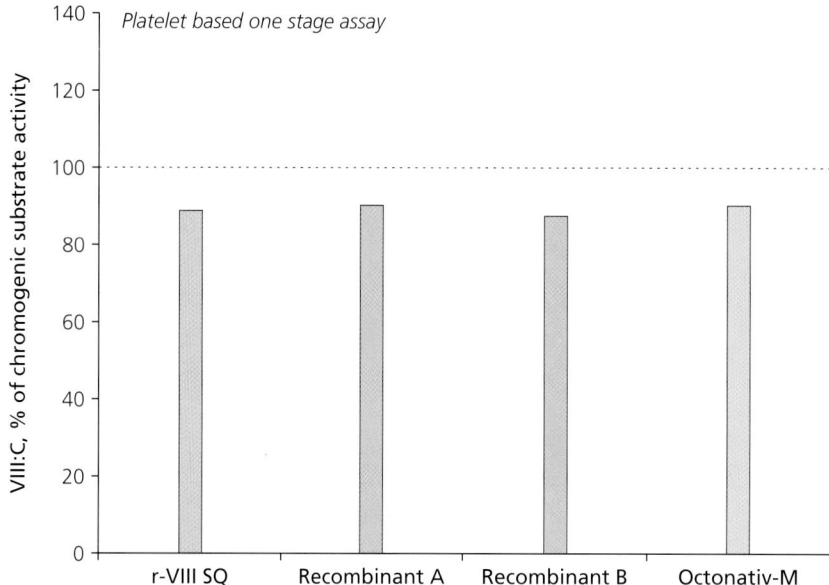

Fig. 27.3 Platelet-based one-stage assays. From Mikaelsson M, Oswaldison U, Sandberg H 1998,[18] with permission.

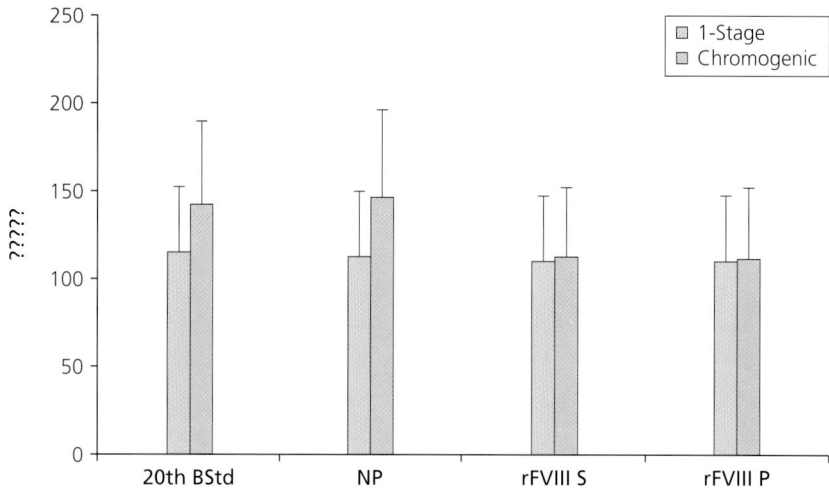

Fig. 27.4 FVIII recovery levels. Ratio of 1-stage APTT: Chromogenic. From Lee 1999,[11] with permission.

The advantages of recombinant FVIIa include viral safety, low systemic activation of coagulation, effectiveness independent of inhibitor titer and an excellent overall safety profile allowing for home use and ease of administration. The main disadvantage is the short half-life and therefore the need for frequent administration.

transmitted virus diseases have resulted in the development of very safe clotting factor concentrates. The challenges facing hemophilia treatment are the delivery of safe cost-effective therapy and a greater understanding of the most serious complications of treatment: the development of inhibitors.

Therapeutic strategies

There are now good therapeutic options for the treatment of hemophilia: advances in fractionation, molecular technology, and the past experience of transfusion-

Treatment on demand

In 1979, Allain published a remarkable paper entitled 'Dose requirement for replacement therapy in hemophilia A'.[21] It was shown that the relationship between plasma

FVIII levels or doses calculated in iu/kg body weight and clinical results followed an exponential curve. Thus, it was demonstrated in a group of boys with hemophilia that 100% clinical success could be achieved with one treatment for a bleeding episode if a dose of at least 30 iu/kg was used. This study was performed using cryoprecipitate which has a recovery of 1.5 iu/per kg infused. More recently, Aledort *et al* in 1994[22] have shown in the orthopedic outcome study that where treatment was given on 'demand' response to a bleed with a factor dose of over 25 iu/kg achieved the 'next best result after prophylaxis'. We now have the results from three large studies in PTPs using the recently licensed recombinant products. These give some guidance about optimal dosing. In the long-term study of *Kogenate* for treatment episodes requiring only one dose the mean dose was 25 iu/kg. The mean recovery for 885 infusions was 2.48%/unit/kg infused.[23] In the PTP study using *Recombinate* the recovery was 2.4%/unit/kg infused and the median dose used was 22.7 iu/kg.[14] For the B-domain depleted recombinant FVIII *Refacto* the recovery was 2.8%/unit/kg and the median dose used was 29.5 iu/kg.[24] Thus, using these recombinant products with recoveries of 2.7, 2.4 and 2.7 respectively, a dose of 20 iu/kg would achieve a level of 45 iu/dl which, historically, is equivalent to 30 iu/kg of intermediate purity concentrate. It is probable, however, that we should try and individualize the dose used. In the PTP study using *Recombinate* there was an enormous range of recoveries.[14] Also, Dutch workers have also shown a considerable individual variation in

half-life of infused FVIII.[25] It was also shown that the pharmacokinetics for FVIII were correlated with blood group(s): those with blood group 'O' had a shorter FVIII half-life than those with blood group 'A'. It has been speculated that anti-A antibodies in those with blood group 'O' may interact with the endogenous vWF thus affecting the half-life of the FVIII–vWF complex.

Prophylaxis

There is a long tradition of giving prophylaxis to young boys with hemophilia. This was begun in 1958 for boys with hemophilia A and in the late 1960s for those with hemophilia B.[26] The rationale for the prophylactic model was the observation that chronic arthropathy was seen less frequently and less severely in individuals for FVIII or FIX of 1–4 iu/dl. At the hemophilia center at Malmo, Sweden, based on the pharmacokinetic modeling, regular prophylactic treatment is begun at 1–1.5 years before the onset of joint bleeds. Ideally, FVIII is administered every second day at a dose of 20–40 iu/kg and FIX twice weekly or every third day. The goal is to achieve a trough level of > 1 iu/dl.[27] There is good evidence that the Malmo model is effective in preventing hemophilic arthropathy. For the youngest cohort of boys born in 1981–1990 who began prophylaxis between 1 and 2 years with 4000–9000 iu/kg annually both the orthopedic and radiologic scores were zero[26] (Fig. 27.5).

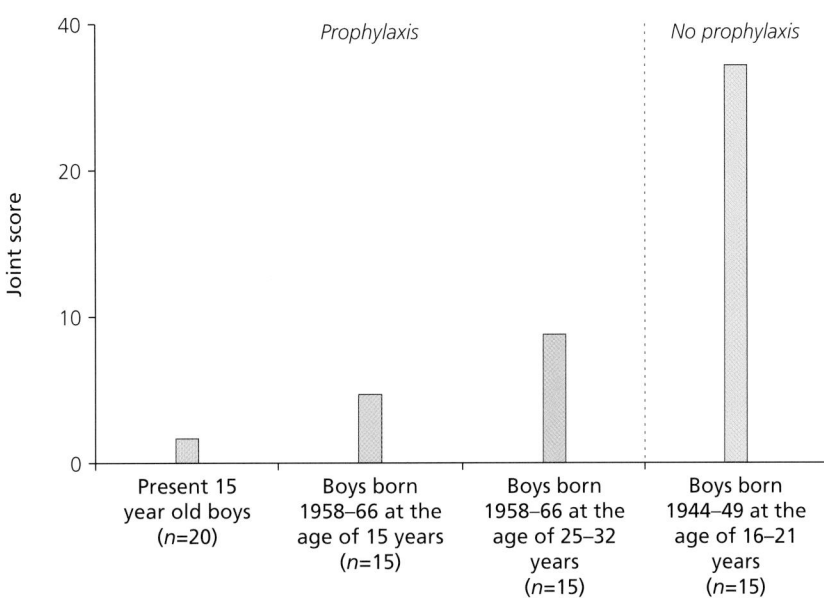

Fig. 27.5 Orthopedic joint scores for the present, intensively treated, 15-year-old group, compared with a less intensively treated group at different ages, and to patients not receiving prophylaxis (historical controls). From Nilson *et al* 1992,[26] with permission.

The use of the peripheral vein is the most preferable approach when beginning prophylactic treatment. However, if this is not possible then implantation of a portacath may be necessary. Substantial experience with portacaths has been published.[27-29] Although the advantages of such devices are recognized, septic complications remain a challenge. A number of studies have been published which show an infection rate ranging from 0.2 to 3.4 infections per 1000 catheter days.[30,31] The frequency of catheter access is likely to be an important factor in the incidence of infection and thus it is a particular problem for children on immune tolerance. Also, the subcutaneous bleeding which may occur at the site of insertion in children with inhibitors may result in an increased incidence of infection.

Inhibitors

One of the earliest references recording inhibitors was that of Davidson *et al* in 1949.[32] Inhibitors were not really recognized until patients with hemophilia A were exposed to FVIII or a blood product containing FVIII. In the UK, statistics before the HIV era showed an inhibitor incidence of 6% in hemophilia A of all severities between 1969 and 1980.[33] Between 1990 and 1997, 57 of 5100 patients with hemophilia A of all severities developed inhibitors.[34] However, there is a great difference in the reported rates of inhibitor formation in the literature.

The experience of the three recombinant PUP studies has demonstrated in prospective trials, which are carefully monitored with laboratory inhibitor assays with frequent intervals, that the incidence of inhibitor development in infants and children with severe hemophilia A is much higher than previously thought. Thus, in the *Kogenate* PUP study 20:101 (20%) developed an inhibitor but for severe hemophilia A 10:64 (16%) developed a high titer inhibitor (> 5 BU) (Bethesda units) and overall the cumulative probability of inhibitor development was 36% at 40 days treatment.[13] Similarly, in the *Recombinate* PUP studies the cumulative probability of developing an inhibitor was 38% at 25 days exposure and the overall incidence was 17:79 (24%) with five children who had titers > 10 BU.[11] In the B-domain depleted recombinant FVIII PUP studies the incidence was 29:101 (29%), 10:101 (10%) were > 5 BU and 5:101 (5%) were < 5 BU. At 40 exposure days the cumulative rate of inhibitor development was 35%.[11] The seemingly high incidence which began to emerge as these studies progressed stimulated a review of the previous experience using plasma-derived concentrate.

A review of treatment over 34 years (1964–1997) in London showed a frequency of inhibitors of 6.3%–27:431 (10%–24:239 for severe hemophilia A) among patients followed over a total of 5626 patient years in London.[35] This would be reduced to 3.6% in severe and 5.2% for all grades of severity if the 12 patients who were referred from elsewhere specifically to treat their inhibitors were excluded. Furthermore, there was an inhibitor-free period (1988–1995) when patients were exposed to a single intermediate purity plasma-derived concentrate.[36]

In contrast, there have been other reports of a high incidence of 20% and 30% following a variety of plasma-derived concentrates.[37,38] The highest reported incident was an alarming 52% in a variety of plasma-derived products.[39] These were similar to the finding as shown above where the cumulative incidence in the three recombinant PUP studies was 25%. Amongst reports of a much lower incidence following plasma-derived concentrate is a study by Peerlinck *et al*[40] reporting an incidence of 6%, a study by Guerois *et al*[41] reporting an incidence of 9% and that by Yee *et al* where only one transient inhibitor occurred over a 10-year period in 37 boys.[36]

Vermylen[42] has elegantly reviewed why some people develop inhibitors. Clearly it is multifactorial but there is substantial evidence that repeated switching from one FVIII product to another may facilitate an immune response. It is still unclear if there is a protective effect offered by plasma-derived concentrates particularly those that are of intermediate purity and contain vWF, which could block epitopes. There are reports of inhibitors occuring more frequently in African, American and Latino hemophilic patients.[43] More recently, attention has been drawn to the development of inhibitors with non-severe hemophilia. This may be related to dose, type and mode of delivery of concentrate.[44]

The development of inhibitors remains ill-understood. It is therefore important to maintain vigilance, practice surveillance and avoid unnecessary treatment, using 1D amino 8 arginine vasopressin (DDAVP) wherever possible in mild disease and avoiding repeated change of concentrates.

The treatment of inhibitors

The most serious complications of blood-product therapy in hemophilia is the development of FVIII antibodies which are usually IgG1 or IgG4. This means that treatment with FVIII concentrate is ineffective because of neutralization by the antibody. The majority of inhibitors develop within 9 and 15 exposure days and, thus, young children with severe hemophilia are at greatest risk. FVIII inhibitors are measured by the Bethesda assay and those with a titer of <5 BU/ml are defined as being low responding and those with >5 BU/ml as high responding. The classification into low responding and high responding is important as it provides the rationale for the treatment. The treatment of inhibitors is first to secure hemostasis alone and then to eradicate the antibody. Low-titer low-responding inhibitors can be treated with human or porcine FVIII concentrates at a dose and frequency in order to swamp the antibody and obtain therapeutic levels of FVIII. However, high-titer high-responding inhibitors are more resistant to treatment. Porcine FVIII or 'bypassing agents' may be used to treat acute hemorrhage. The most common available 'bypassing agents' are human recombinant FVIIa or plasma-derived concentrates which contain activated coagulation factors such as *FEIBA* and *Autoplex*. These work by activating the coagulation cascade at levels below the action of the inhibitor. It is also possible to use immuno depletion using staphylococcal protein A on a column. Immunotolerance regimes can be used for high-titer antibodies. It is best to allow the antibody titer to fall by using bypassing agents. FVIII can be used in varying dose regimes from 100 iu/kg bd to 25 iu/kg tds.[45]

Desmopressin in the treatment of hemophilia A

It was found in the mid 1970s that DDAVP increased the plasma concentration of FVIIIC, vWF and tissue plasminogen activator when infused into normal volunteers.[46,47] It is now an established treatment for mild hemophilia A and von Willebrand's disease (vWD).[48] DDAVP can be given intravenously, subcutaneously or intranasally. The dose for iv and sc administration is 0.3 μg/kg which results in a peak concentration of VIIIC and vWF at 30 min following an intravenous injection and in 1 h following subcutaneous injection. The increase of VIIIC is about 2–6 times and the increase in vWF about 2–4 times the baseline level. Lethagen *et al* have demonstrated the effectiveness of intranasal administration, which is an ideal choice for home administration;[49] 300 ug of DDAVP delivered by spray approximates to the effect obtained with the dosage of 0.3 μg/kg given intravenously or subcutaneously.[50] For mild hemophilia A the recommended dose of 0.3 μg/kg can be repeated at intervals of 8 and 12 h although there is some tachyphylaxis it was shown by Mannucci *et al* in 1998 that the response to a second dose is approximately 30% less than that obtained with the first dose.[51] It was also demonstrated that a full response is usually recovered within 3–4 days after a break in DDAVP treatment. Since DDAVP stimulates the

release of TPA the administration of fibrinolytic inhibitors such as tranexamic acid is usually given concomitantly. DDAVP is an antidiuretic and therefore water retention can be a problem. It is, therefore, best avoided in young children. It has also been suggested that it may have the risk of thromboembolism. However, this has not been substantiated.

von Willebrand's disease (vWD)

vWD is a bleeding disorder caused by quantitative or qualitative defect of vWF. vWF is a high-molecular-weight glycoprotein, which promotes platelet adhesion to the subendothelium and platelet aggregation under shéer conditions. vWF is also the carrier of FVIII (FVIIIC) in plasma. Thus, a deficiency of vWF will result in defects in both the primary phase of hemostasis and of blood coagulation. It is inherited in an autosomal dominant fashion, but an autosomal recessive pattern has also been described. Patients with vWD may have a mild, moderate or severe bleeding tendency, which is life-long and is usually proportional to the vWF level.

vWD is the most frequent inherited bleeding disorder. Rodeghiero *et al* performed during a large epidemiologic study in children and found the prevalence to be 0.82%. Further studies in America have shown the prevalence to be 1–2%.[52,53]

vWD has been divided into three types according to the pathophysiology. Type I and type 3 are respectively a partial, or a virtually complete, deficiency of vWF, whereas type 2 refers to a qualitative deficiency of vWF. Type I is the most frequent type, greater than 70%: type 2 vWD accounts for 15–20% and type 3 accounts for 2–5% of vWD patients[54] (Fig. 27.6).

The diagnosis of vWD should be suspected in any patient who has mucocutaneous bleeding, particularly if the family history suggests an autosomal pattern of inheritance. The most common bleeding symptoms are epistaxis, bleeding after dental extractions and menorrhagia. However, the bleeding tendency can be very variable and also depends on the type and the severity of the disease. Patients with type I and type 2 vWD can have a negative bleeding history, whereas patients with type 3 have a severe hemorrhagic tendency. Laboratory tests are very important in the diagnosis of vWD, because of the variable bleeding history.

Screening tests

The platelet count is usually normal but mild thrombocytopenia may occur in patients with type 2B vWD. The

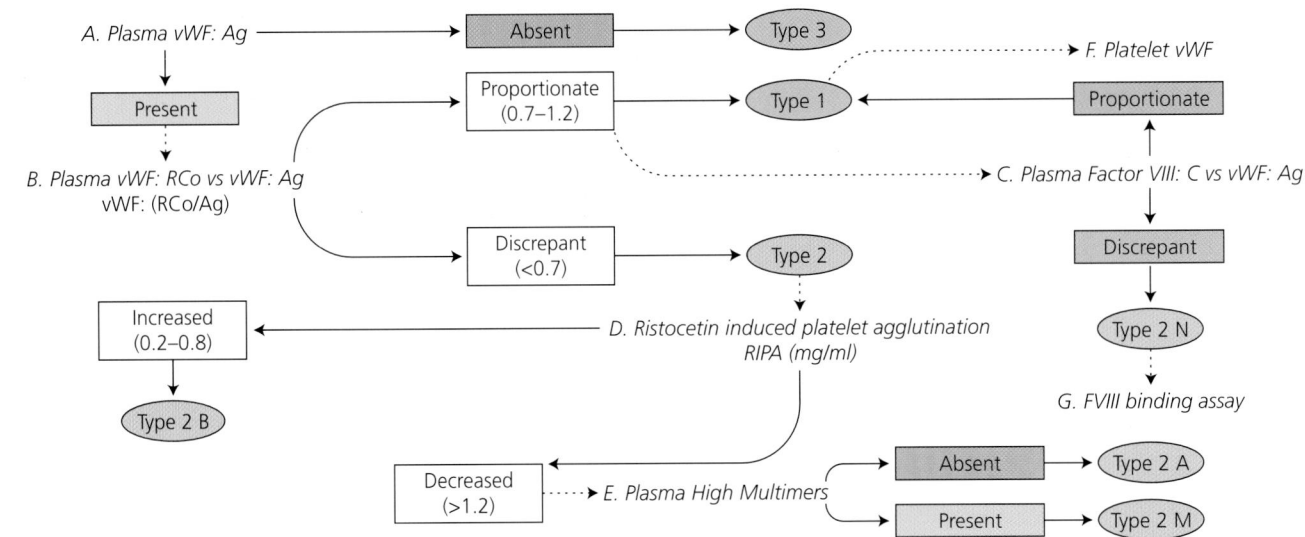

Fig. 27.6 Flow chart for the diagnosis of a patient with vWD. From Federici A B *et al* 1999. Haemophilia 5(suppl 2): 28–37, with permission.

bleeding time is usually prolonged, but it can be normal in patients with mild forms of vWD, particularly type I. The prothrombin time (PT) is normal, but the APPT may be prolonged, depending on the FVIIIC levels.

vWF antigen

This can be measured in plasma by electro-immuno assay, immuno-radiometric assay or a variety of enzyme-linked immunoadsorbent assays. It is unmeasurable in type 3 vWD, it may be low in type I and low, or normal in type 2.

Ristocetin cofactor activity

This measures the interaction of vWF with the platelet glycoprotein 1b/IX/V complex. It is based on the ability of the antibiotic ristocetin to agglutinate human platelets in the presence of vWF. In patients with a normal von Willebrand structure (type I vWD) values of vWF RiCof are similar to those of vWF antigen. Levels of vWF RiCof lower than those of vWF antigen are characteristic of type 2 vWD.

Factor VIIIC (FVIIIC)

FVIIIC plasma levels are very low (1–5 u/dl) in patients with type 3 vWD. In patients with type I or type 2, the FVIIIC may be normal, or mildly decreased.

Ristocetin-induced platelet agglutination (RIPA)

This is measured by mixing ristocetin with patient platelet-rich plasma. Most vWD types have a low response to ristocetin. However, patients with type 2B vWD are characterized by increased response to ristocetin, because in type 2B there is an increased affinity of vWF for the platelet GP1b/IX/V complex.

vWF multimeric analysis

This is performed on high-resolution agrosed gels, which will differentiate between type I and type 2 subtypes.

Platelet vWF

The platelet vWF plays an important role in primary hemostasis, when it is released from alpha granules at the site of vascular injury. On the basis of this measurement, patients can be differentiated into type I platelet normal, or type I platelet low.

Factor VIII binding assay

This measures the affinity of vWF for FVIIIC.

The subtypes of vWD

Type 1 vWD is the most frequent form and occurs in about 70% of patients. The inheritence is autosomal dominant. Patients with type I vWD have mild to moderate symptoms, with a normal or variably prolonged bleeding time and decreased levels of vWF antigen and vWF RiCof, and FVIII, but a normal multimeric structure. The vWF plasma levels are dependent on ABO blood group and vWF can be 25% lower in persons of blood type O. However, it has been found that when the range for vWF RiCof and vWF antigen are adjusted for this to two standard deviations below the population mean about half the individuals still have an abnormal family history and an abnormal bleeding history.[55,56] Thus, the diagnosis of type I vWD needs to take into account the clinical history. Depending on the platelet vWF content, three subtypes of type I vWD have been identified, paltelet normal, platelet low and platelet discordant.[57]

Type 2 vWD, type 2A is the most frequent subtype. It is mainly inherited as autosomal dominant, but recessive inheritance has also been described. Patients with type 2A vWD have normal to low vWF antigen levels and very low vWF RiCof with an abnormal multimer pattern, characterized by loss of high-molecular-weight multimers. More recently, two types of type 2A, based on the platelet and plasma von Willebrand structure have been differentiated. The reduction in high-molecular weight-multimers may be the result of abnormal biosynthesis of vWF or in some patients, may be due to increased proteolysis.[58]

Type 2B can be identified because of increased response to ristocetin and the absence of large multimers in the plasma. It is mostly inherited in an autosomal dominant way. There may be mild thrombocytopenia, with an increased platelet volume.

In type 2M the vWF multimeric distribution is normal, but the binding to platelets is impaired.

Type 2N (N for Normandy) is characterized by normal levels of vWF antigen and vWF RiCof, normal multimeric structure but low plasma FVIIIC levels. The inheritance is autosomal dominant, in contrast to hemophilia A, which is sex-linked recessive. It is due to a decreased plasma half-life of FVIII, which cannot bind to vWF.[59]

Type 3 vWD or severe vWD is caused by an impaired biosynthesis of vWF and unmeasurable levels of vWF in plasma and platelets are found. vWF is also the carrier of FVIIIC and therefore plasma levels of FVIIIC are also very low (1–5 u/dl). Thus, patients who have type 3 vWD as well as having mucocutaneous hemorrhages, also have hemarthroses and hematomas as found in severe hemophilia. The inheritance of type 3 vWD is autosomal recessive and its prevalence is 1–5/million population.[48–55]

Platelet type or pseudo vWD is a primary platelet disorder characterized by increased affinity of platelet GP1b/IX/V complex for normal vWF.[60] These patients have clinical and laboratory features similar to those of type 2B vWD. It can be distinguished by adding purified vWF to patient rich plasma (PRP) in an aggregometer. In the case of platelet or type pseudo vWF, normal vWF will induce platelet aggregation, but it will not in type 2B vWD.

Acquired vWD

Acquired vWD is similar to the congenital disease, in terms of the laboratory findings. It is characterized by prolonged bleeding time and low plasma levels of FVIIIC and vWF. It was originally described in relation to systemic lupus erythematosis.[61] It can occur in association with lymphomyeloproliferative disorders, immunologic disease and tumors. It is not always possible to identify an inhibitor to vWF. It is thought that vWF is normally synthesized, but rapidly removed from the plasma in four possible ways: (1) specific autoantibodies; (2) non-specific antibodies that form circulating immune complexes; (3) adsorption on to malignant clones; or (4) increased proteolytic breakdown. The severity varies from being mild to life-threatening.

Treatment of vWD

The aim of treatment is to correct the double abnormality of hemostasis – that is the prolonged bleeding time due to abnormal platelet adhesion and the abnormal intrinsic coagulation pathway due to the low factor VIII. There are two treatments of choice – DDAVP and clotting factor concentrate.

Desmopressin

Desmopressin (DDAVP) is a synthetic analog of vasopressin originally used for the treatment of diabetes insipidus. DDAVP increases the FVIIIC and vWF plasma concentration.[46] It is still not completely understood as to how DDAVP has its effect. The first clinical trial of DDAVP was performed in 1977 with mild hemophilia and vWD patients, who needed dental extraction and other surgical procedures.[47] The advantages of DDAVP are that it is relatively inexpensive and that it carries no risk of transmitting blood-borne viruses. It can be administered intravenously, or subcutaneously, or as a nasal spray. The normal dose is $0.3\,\mu/kg$.[49–50] When it is given intravenously, the FVIII and vWF levels are increased 3–5 times above basal levels within 30 min. When DDAVP is given subcutaneously, the peak level is obtained after approximately 1 h. Most patients treated repeatedly become less responsive to therapy – the phenomenon of tachyphylaxis.[51] Side-effects of DDAVP are usually mild tachycardia, headache and flushing. These are probably related to the vasomotor effects of the drug and can be reduced by slowing the rate of infusion when DDAVP is given intravenously. DDAVP can also cause volume overload, due to its antidiuretic effect, resulting in hyponatremia and a few cases have been described in young children, who have been given repeated infusions.[62] DDAVP should be used with caution in elderly patients with atherosclerotic disease, because of the risk of myocardial infarction or stroke.[63] DDAVP is most effective in type I vWD where there is a platelet normal type. DDAVP is contraindicated in type 2B because of the transient occurrence of thrombocyopenia.[64] Patients with type 3 vWD are usually unresponsive to DDAVP.

Tranexamic acid

Tranexamic acid is a synthetic drug which interferes with the lysis of newly formed clots by blocking the blinding site on plasminogen. Thus, plasminogen is unable to attach to fibrin. Tranexamic acid can be given orally, intravenously or topically, as a mouthwash. It is usually given in a dose of 25 mg/kg three times a day. It is contraindicated in patients with an underlying prothrombotic condition, because of the risk of thrombosis and it is also contraindicated in the management of urinary tract bleeding.

Clotting factor concentrates

For patients who are unresponsive to DDAVP, blood products containing FVIII and vWF are the treatment of choice. Cryoprecipitate was the mainstay of vWD treatment for many years. However, since virucidal methods cannot be applied to cryoprecipitate, this product has largely been replaced in the well-resourced world with plasma-derived clotting factor concentrate. These are intermediate-purity products, as those high-purity FVIII concentrates produced by immunoaffinity chromatography and monoclonal antibodies contain very little vWF and are therefore unsuitable for vWD management. A product rich in vWF with a low content of FVIII has been produced by chromatographic purification and is referred to as very high purity vWF concentrate.[65] The dosages of concentrates recommended for the control of bleeding are summarized in Table 27.4.[54] Since intermediate-purity purity FVIII vWF concentrates contain large amounts of FVIII and vWF, high post-infusion levels of both factors are obtained. There is a

Table 27.4 Management of different types and subtypes of vWD From Federici AB, Mannucci PM 1999,[54] with permission

	Treatment of choice	Alternative and adjunctive therapy
Type 1	Desmopressin	Antifibrinolytics, estrogens
Type 2 A	FVIII-vWF concentrates	Desmopressin
Type 2 B	FVIII-vWF concentrates	
Type 2 M	FVIII-vWF concentrates	Desmopressin
Type 2 N	Desmopressin	
Type 3	FVIII-vWF concentrate	Desmopressin, platelet concentrates
Type 3	Recombinant FVIII with alloantibodies	

sustained rise in FVIII, perhaps higher than predicted from the dose infused and this may last up to 24 h. This is because of the effect of the transfusion of vWF on endogenous FVIII, which is synthesized at the normal rate in patients with vWD. These intermediate-purity products are able to correct the FVIII deficiency. However, no plasma-derived clotting factor concentrate contains a completely functional vWF, as tested *in vitro* looking at the multimeric pattern. This is probably because vWF proteolysis occurs during the purification, due to the action of the platelet and leukocyte proteases contaminating the plasma use of fractionation.[66] Although FVIII vWF concentrates have a limited effect on the bleeding time, they are usually successful for the treatment of vWD patients who are unresponsive to DDAVP, particularly for the treatment of soft-tissue and post-operative bleeding.[67] Platelets, because they contain platelet vWF, may be useful in correcting the bleeding time and in some cases, it may be necessary to resort to cryoprecipitate.

The molecular basis of von Willebrand's disease

vWF cDNA was cloned in 1985 by four independent groups.[68–71] It was possible to deduce the structure of the von Willebrand protein and this was confirmed by direct amino acid sequence and shown schematically in Figure 27.7.[72] Figure 27.7 summarizes the specific functional domains within vWF. There is a large and complex vWF gene as well as a conserved partial pseudogene which was reported in 1991 by Sadler *et al*.[69] The vWF gene spans a 178 kb on the short arm of chromosome 12 and is composed of 52 exons. The FVIII-binding domain within vWF has been localized to an end-terminal 272 amino acid segment and the primary binding domain for the

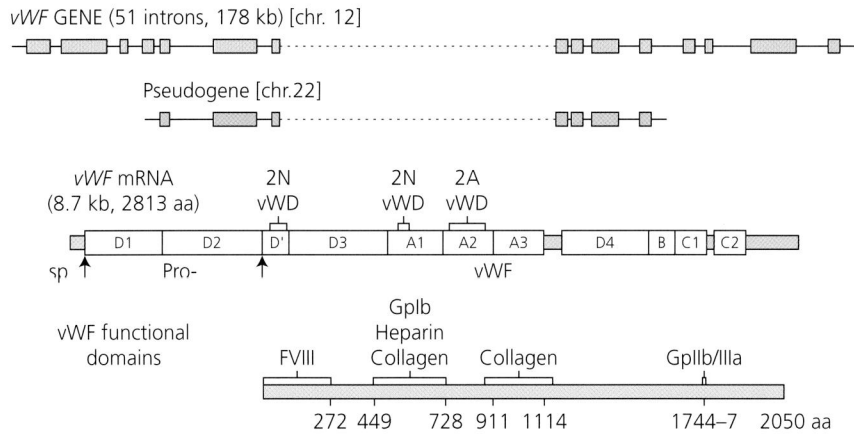

Fig. 27.7 The vWF gene, mRNA and protein. From Ginsburg D 1999 Haemophilia 5(suppl 2): 19–27, with permission.

platelet receptor like protein 1b has been mapped to the A1 repeat. The primary collagen-binding domain appears to lie within the A3 domain whereas the sequence recognized by intergrins such as the GPIIb/IIIa platelet receptor is near the C terminal of the protein.

The first genetic defects to be identified in patients with vWD were large gene deletions associated with type 3 vWD.[73] Following the introduction of the polymerase chain reaction it was possible to amplify and sequence small amounts of vWF mRNA from peripheral blood platelets and this led to the identification of the first point mutations in the vWF gene in type 2A vWD pedigrees.[74] A large number of mutations have now been identified accounting for most of the common qualitative type 2 variants of vWD. The mutations are held on an updated database on the world wide web and the address is HTTP: *mmg2.im.med.umich.edu\vWF*.

The identification of the genetic defect has enabled an understanding of the molecular basis of the different vWD subtypes. Thus, in type 3 von Willebrand deletions, nonsense, missense and frameshift mutations have been found throughout the gene and there have also been CIS-defects in the mRNA expression. In type 1 a few missense mutations have been reported presumably disrupting function and in some cases it is thought these represent a heterozygous form of type 3. In type 2A missense mutations clustered within the vWF A2 repeat have been described with two subgroups: group 1 where there is a defect in intracellular transport and group 2 where there is increased proteolysis in plasma after secretion. In type 2B there are missense mutations clustered in the vWF A1 repeat which results in increase of spontaneous binding to platelets. In type 2M there are missense mutations and small in frame deletions in the vWF A1 repeat.[75] In type 2N there are missense mutations within the end terminus of the mature vWF which interfere with FVIII binding.

vWD in women

In 1926, von Willebrand described a family in the Aland Island amongst whom he documented 16 of 35 women and 7 of 31 men who had the disease and he made the observation that 'the trait seemed especially to be seen among the women'[76] (Fig. 27.8).

In this family the index patient, Hjordis presented with epistaxis and subsequently died at the onset of her fourth menstrual period. Her mother had menorrhagia – her periods had always lasted 6 days or more and had always been copious; however, her deliveries had been normal without heavy bleeding. The maternal grand-mother had bled to death in childbirth.

The prevalence of vWD has been estimated at 1%.[51–53] Menorrhagia is a common complaint and it is thought that approximately 5% of women between the age of 30 and 49 years will consult their general practitioners about menorrhagia.[77] Menorrhagia has been defined subjectively as excessive or prolonged loss of blood on a regular cycle basis or objectively as menstrual blood loss of greater than 80 ml for the whole period.[78] Using an objective assessment of menorrhagia, the pictorial bleeding assessment chart,[79] where a score of > 100 defines menorrhagia as equivalent to 80 ml of blood it was possible to screen patients attending a routine gynecologic clinic.[80] It was found of 150 women tested that 15 had vWD of mild severity, and three of moderate severity. Thus, the frequency of vWD was 13%[80] compared to 1.3% in the general population.[53] The women with a bleeding disorder were more likely to suffer with easy bruising, bleeding after tooth extraction and postpartum and post-operative bleeding. However, the most significant finding in the history was menorrhagia since the menarche. It was concluded from the study that patients with menorrhagia and without obvious pelvic abnormalities

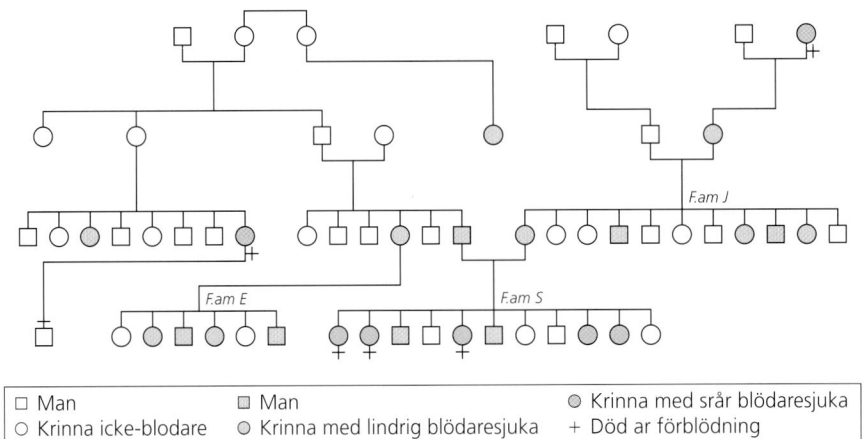

□ Man	■ Man	◉ Krinna med srår blödaresjuka
○ Krinna icke-blodare	◔ Krinna med lindrig blödaresjuka	+ Död ar förblödning

Fig. 27.8 From the original family described by von Willebrand in 1926. From Lee 1999 Haemophilia 5(suppl 2): 38–45, with permission.

should be tested for vWD. However, it is also important to test on more than one occasion and to sample 5–7 days in the menstrual cycle in order to reduce intra-individual variation.[81,82] When individuals with vWD were assessed using the pictorial bleeding assessment chart it is found that 73% of them have menorrhagia.[83] The quality of life was studied in 57 women with vWD using a questionnaire that included general health, health and daily activities, dysmenorrhea and the quality of life during the menstrual period. It was found that the quality of life scores were significantly lower in those with vWD.[84] Menorrhagia in vWD can be managed using tranexamic acid,[85] or DDAVP by intranasal spray[49] or subcutaneously.[50]

Pregnancy in women with vWD

FVIIIC and vWF antigen often increase in pregnancy.[86,87] However, for those with severe disease and low baseline levels the increase in absolute levels are limited. The spontaneous miscarriage rate in women is approximately 21%, which compares to the overall normal miscarriage rate of 16%.[87] However, the risk of both primary and secondary postpartum hemorrhage is increased – it has been reported as high as 28%,[87] 25%,[88] 28%.[89] The reason for postpartum hemorrhage is that the vWF level can fall rapidly after birth. This can be very variable as short as 24 h or it may take as long as a week. Thus, all patients should have their hemoglobin checked on discharge and encouraged to report excessive bleeding after discharge home.

For the management of women with vWD in child birth, those with type 1 disease should have the FVIIIC checked at the third trimester and it is usually unnecessary to give peripartum prophylaxis.[90] For individuals with type 2 and type 3 disease, vWF containing concentrates

should be used at the onset of labor and for 7 days subsequently if a Caesarean section is performed or 4–5 days for vaginal delivery.[91,92] There have been various concerns about the use of DDAVP antenatally although there are few firm data and this needs to be studied. Thus, the recommendation is that DDAVP should only be administered after the cord has been clamped.[92]

Rare bleeding disorders

Hemophilia A and B and vWD represent 85% of the inherited bleeding disorder and the other 15% are represented by the least common deficiencies which include deficiencies of fibrinogen, prothrombin, factor V, combined V/VIII, VII, X, XI and XIII.

Fibrinogen

Congenital afibrinogenemia can result in a mild to a severe bleeding disorder.[93] It is inherited as an autosomal recessive disorder and the incidence is one per two million individuals and it is common in countries where there is a practice of consanguinity. It can present early in life as umbilical stump bleeding but in older individuals bleeding can occur at any site and can be catastrophic – in particular there is a risk of spontaneous splenic rupture.[94] In women who have afibrinogenemia there is an increase rate of miscarriage in the first trimester.[95] Fibrinogen concentrates can be used as a replacement therapy and where these are not available cryoprecipitate can be used.

Prothrombin

Congenital prothrombin deficiency is extremely rare and is inherited as an autosomal recessive disorder. In the reported cases severe hemorrhage including intracerebral hemorrhage, mucus membrane bleeding and deep-tissue bleeding have been reported. Although heterozygous individuals are usually asymptomatic, bleeding following tooth extraction and tonsillectomy has been reported.[96] There have also been reports of a bleeding disorder with congenital dysprothrombinemia with a reduced level of prothrombin activity compared to antigen.[97] The treatment for prothrombin deficiency is to use prothrombin complex concentrates (PCCs). It may be necessary to do recovery studies as the dosing of PCCs is dependent on the FIX content.

Factor V deficiency

Factor V (FV) catalyses the conversion of prothrombin to thrombin by FXa. FV deficiency has a prevalence of 1 per million. FV deficiency is associated with mucus membrane bleeding and bruising and there are case reports of intracranial hemorrhage.[98] There are also reports of combined deficiencies of FV and FVIII.[99] The treatment for FV deficiency is the use of FFP in a dose of 20 ml/kg and ideally solvent detergent treated FFP should be used. The use of bovine thrombin has resulted in the appearance of FV inhibitors.[100]

Factor VII

FVII deficiency occurs at a rate of 1/500 000 individuals, Patients with less than 1 u/dl FVII activity have a severe bleeding disorder comparable to FVIII deficiency. Those individuals with more than 5 u/dl have relatively mild symptoms and the most common bleeding is mucus membrane bleeding and women may suffer menorrhagia.[101,102] Plasma-derived clotting factor concentrates of FVII are available and more recently the availability of recombinant VIIa for the treatment of hemophilia patients with inhibitors has provided a treatment for FVII deficiency. The dose required is less than that required for treating inhibitor patients.[103,104] Prothrombin complex concentrates can be used to correct FVII deficiency when FVII concentrate or recombinant VIIa is unavailable.

Factor X

FX is activated to Xa and as a component of the prothrombinase complex it converts prothrombin to thrombin. Congenital FX defecncy is a rare disorder and is transmitted as an autosomal recessive.[105] Acquired FX deficiency has been reported in relation to amyloidosis.[106]

In 32 Iranian patients with congenital FX deficiency the most common bleeding symptoms were epistaxis, menorrhagia, hemarthrosis and spontaneous hematomas.[105] Hematuria and umbilical cord bleeding were less common and the type of bleeding correlated with the degree of the factor deficiency. The treatment of FX deficiency is with prothrombin complex concentrates that contain FX. Where FX deficiency occurs in amyloidosis it is due to the affinity of FX to the particular amyloid fibril and treatment of the underlying amyloidosis or splenectomy has been shown to improve the circulating FX level.[106]

Factor XI deficiency

FXI deficiency was originally described in an American Jewish family in whom two sisters bled after dental extraction, and tonsillectomy and a maternal uncle also bled following dental extraction.[107] FXI deficiency is particularly common amongst Ashkenazi Jews where the gene frequency is 8%.[108] The inheritance is autosomal and severe deficiency of FXI level < 15–20 u/dl occurs in homozygous individuals and a partial deficiency occurs in heterozygous individuals with a FXI level between 20 u/dl and 70 u/dl, the lower limit of normal.[109] The severely affected individuals are at risk of bleeding after surgery, particularly in areas prone to fibrinolysis such as the oral cavity and the urogenital system. The bleeding is likely to occur after tonsillectomy, dental extractions and after prostatectomy. However, the bleeding may be unpredictable and some patients with severe deficiency have been reported as having no bleeding tendency. Homozygotes who have a low or undetectable FXI level more commonly have a type 2 mutation which produces a stop code on exon 5. In the type 3 mutation, where there is a point mutation in exon 9, this tends to be associated with a more mild bleeding disorder. Some heterozygotes may have excessive bleeding and women may experience bleeding with parturition and menorrhagia. An analysis of 247 bleeding histories in 50 kindreds showed that 30–50% of heterozygotes bled excessively including some with levels of 50–70 u/dl (normal range 70–150). Many of these women suffered with menorrhagia.[110] The treatment of FFP was used in one of the original patients described by Rosenthal *et al*[107] and more recently the use of FFP has been described in 38 procedures with excessive bleeding occurring in only one patient.[111] FFP has been made safer with the development of virally inactivated products using solvent detergent. FXI concentrates have also been produced made from pooled plasma. The FXI concentrate produced by BPL was shown to be hemostatically effective.[112] The mean FXI recovery was 91% of the

Table 27.5 Summary of treatment options for rare factor deficiencies. From Di Paola J, Nugent D, Young G 2001 Haemophilia 7 (1): 16–22, with permission

Deficiency	Hemostatic factor level	Treatment	Comments
Fibrinogen	800 mg/l	(a) Cryoprecipitate 1 bag/5 kg body weight, then 1 bag/15 kg body weight daily (b) Concentrates Fibrinogen HT (Japan Green Cross) Hemocomplettan (Aventis Behring, Germany) Fibrinogen Clottagen (LFB, France)	No reports of antifibrinogen antibodies in the last 40 years
Prothrombin	20–30% of normal level	(a) Fresh frozen plasma: loading dose 15–20 ml/kg, then 3 ml/kg every 12–24 h (b) PCCs (dose based on units of factor IX) Konyne 80 (Bayer, USA), Proplex T (Baxter, USA) Bebulin (Immuno, USA), Profilnine (Alpha, USA) Beriplex (Aventis Behring, Germany), Faktor IX HS (Aventis Behring, Germany) Hemofactor HT (Grifols, Spain), PTX-HT (CSL, Australia) HT Defix (SNBTS, Scotland), Kaskadil (LFB, France) Faktor IX-Komplex SRK (ZLB, SRK, Switzerland) Prothrombin Komplex NDS (BSD NSOB, Germany) Cofact (CLB, Netherlands), Factor IX comp (L.F.Bare, Brazil)	Risk of thromboembolic complications with PCCs if factor IX levels raised > 50% Monitor PT, aPTT, fibrinogen level, fibrin degradation products
Factor V	25% of normal	(a) Fresh frozen plasma: loading dose 15–20 ml/kg, then 5 mL/kg every 12–24 h	For acute bleeding, addition of platelet concentrates
Factor VII	10% of normal 15–25% for surgery	(a) Fresh frozen plasma: 10 ml/kg every 6–12 h [34] Surgery: loading dose 15–20 ml/kg, then 3–6 ml/kg every 12 h (b) PCCs (dose based on units of factor IX) (c) Concentrates Factor VII (Immuno, Austria) Factor VII (Bio Products Laboratory, UK) Factor VII LFB (LFB, France) Recombinant Factor VIIa (NovoSeven, Novo Nordisk, Denmark) (22–26 µg/kg)	Monitor prothrombin time as an indicator of FVII activity
Factor X	15–20%	(a) Fresh frozen plasma: loading dose 10–15 ml/kg, then 5–10 ml/kg every 24 h (b) PCCs that contain factor X: Proplex (Baxter, USA), Profiline HT (Alpha, USA) Konyne 80 (Bayer, USA), Bebulin VH (Immuno, USA)	Risk of thromboembolic complications with PCCs
Factor XI	> 30% of normal for for minor surgery > 45% of normal for for major surgery	(a) Fresh frozen plasma: loading dose 15 ml/kg, then 5 ml/kg every 24 h (b) Concentrates Factor XI (Bio Products Laboratory, UK), Hemoleven (LFB, France)	Factor levels do not necessarily correlate with bleeding Concentrates should be used with caution in patients at risk for thrombosis
Factor XIII	1–3% of normal	(a) Fresh frozen plasma: 3 ml/kg every 4–6 weeks (prophylaxis) (b) Cryoprecipitate: 1 bag × 10–20 kg every 3–4 weeks (prophylaxis) (c) Concentrates Factor XIII (Bio Products Laboratory, UK) Fibrogammin P (Aventis Behring, Germany): 10–20 U/kg every 4–6 weeks for prophylaxis 50–70 U/kg for hemorrhagic event	Factor XIII concentrates can be given every 21 days to affected individuals with history of spontaneous abortions

PCCs, prothrombin complex concentrates; PT, prothrombin time;

injected dose and the mean half-life was 52 h. However, both *in vitro* and *in vivo* there has been concerned about thrombogenicity.[113,114] This has been addressed by the addition of heparin to the concentrate and by the recommendation that the dose should be preferably controlled to maintain levels no greater than 70 u/dl. Such concentrate should be used with caution in individuals with pre-existing cardiovascular disease.[115]

Antifibrolytic drugs are an effective therapy and can often be used in place of clotting factor concentrate or FFP. One report showed that antifibrinolytic drugs alone are sufficient to cover dental extractions with patients with severe FXI deficiency.[116]

Inhibitors to FXI are rare but may occur in association with autoimmune disease. However, they can also occur in deficient patients and Schnall *et al* reviewed the literature in 1987 and reported four cases.[117] These patients can be treated successfully with prothrombin complex concentrates or recombinant FVIIa.[118]

Factor XIII deficiency

Congenital FXIII deficiency is a rare life-threatening disorder. It is inherited as an autosomal recessive condition and the prevalence is 1:5 000 000 individuals.[119] Homozygous individuals have a level of < 1 u/dl and heterozygous individuals may have levels of 50 u/dl but normally do not have bleeding. The most common presentation is bleeding of the umbilical stump.[120] Other bleeding symptoms include intracranial hemorrhage, hemarthrosis, menorrhagia, bleeding following trauma,[121,122] delayed wound healing and spontaneous abortion may also result from FXIII deficiency.[122] Replacement therapy as FXIII concentrate or cryoprecipitate can be used. FXIII has a very long half life of 8–12 days and the levels required to maintain hemostasis are 1:3%. Factor concentrate can be used on a prophylactic basis.[123]

REFERENCES

1. Gitschier J, Wood WI, Goralka TM et al 1984 Characterization of the human factor vrn gene. Nature 312: 326–330
2. Vehar GA, Keyt B, Eaton D et al 1984 Structure of human factor vrn. Nature 312: 337–342
3. Toole JT, Knopf JL, Wozney JM et al 1984 Molecular cloning of a cDNA encoding human antihaemophilic factor. Nature 312: 342–347
4. Tuddenham EGD, Laffan MA 1999 Inherited bleeding disorders. In: Hoffbrand A V, Mitchell Lewis S, Tuddenham EGD (eds), Postgraduate haematology. Butterworth Heinemann
5. UKHCDO Report on the annual returns for 1998
6. Rizza CR, Spooner RJD, Giangrande PLF 2001 Treatment of haemophilia in the United Kingdom 1981–1996. Haemophilia (in press)
7. Pool JG, Shannon AE 1965 Production of high-potency concentrates of antihaemophilic globulin in a closed-bag system. New England Journal of Medicine 273: 1443–1447
8. Lee CA 1992 Coagulation factor replacement therapy. In Recent advances in haematology. Churchill Livingstone
9. UKHCDO 1997 Guidelines on therapeutic products to treat haemophilia and other hereditary coagulation disorders. Haemophilia 3: 63–77
10. Mannucci P. The choice of plasma-derived clotting factor concentrates. Baillière's clinical haematology – Vol. 9. No. 2, June 1996 Ch 5
11. Lee C 1999 Recombinant clotting factors in the treatment of hemophilia. Thrombosis and Haemostasis 82(2): 516–524
12. Schwartz RS, Abildgaard CF, Aledort LM et al 1990 Human recombinant DNA-derived antihemophilic factor (factor VIII) in the treatment of hemophilia A. New England Journal of Medicine 323: 1800–1805
13. Lusher IM, Arkin S, Abildgaard CF, Schwartz RS 1993. Recombinant factor VIII for the treatment of previously untreated patients with hemophilia A. New England Journal of Medicine 328: 453–459
14. White GC, Courter S, Bray GL et al 1997 A multi-center study of recombinant factor VIII (RecombinateTM) in previously treated patients with hemophilia A. Thrombosis and Haemostasis 77: 660–667
15. Choo GH, Gould KG, Rees DJ, Brownlee GG 1982 Molecular cloning of the gene for human anti-haemophilic factor IX. Nature 299: 178–180
16. White GC, Beebe A, Niejsen B 1997 Recombinant factor IX. Thrombosis and Haemostasis 78: 261–265
17. Lusher IM, Hillman-Wiseman C, Hurst D 1998 *In vivo* recovery with products of very high purity assay discrepancies. Haemophilia 4: 641–645
18. Mikaelsson M, Oswaldsson U, Sandberg H 1998 Influence of phospholipids on the assessment of factor VIII activity. Haemophilia 4: 646–650
19. Lee C, Owens D, Giangrande P et al 1998 Assay discrepancies in recovery levels of rFVIII 'Recombinate' Blood 92(10 suppl): 354a
20. Hedner U, Glazer S 1992 Management of hemophilia patients with inhibitors. Hematology-Oncology Clinics of North America 6: 1035–1036
21. Allain JP 1979 Dose requirement for replacement therapy in hemophilia A. Thrombosis and Haemostasis (Stuttg) 42: 825–831
22. Aledort LM, Haschmeyer RH, Petersson H and The Orthopaedic Outcome Study Group 1994 A longitudinal study of orthopaedic outcomes for severe factor VIII-deficient haemophiliacs
23. Seremetis S, Lusher JM, Abildgaard CF et al and The Kogenate ® Study Group 1999 Human recombinant DNA-derived antihaemophilic factor (factor VIII) in the treatment of haemophilia A: conclusions of a 5-year study of home therapy. Haemophilia 5: 9–16
24. Kessler CM, Spira J, Magill M 1998 Safety and efficacy of a second generation B-domain deleted recombinant factor VIII 9r- VIII SQ in previously treated patients (PTPs). A four year update. Blood 92(sO suppl): 555a
25. Vlot AJ, Mauser-Bunschoten EP, Zarkova AG et al 2000 The half-life of infused factor VIII is shorter in hemophiliac patients with blood group O than in those with blood group A. Thrombosis Haemostasis 83(1): 65–69
26. Nilsson IM, Berntorp E, Lofqvist T, Pettersson H 1992 Twenty-five years' experience of prophylactic treatment in severe haemophilia A and B. Journal of International Medicine 232: 25–32
27. Ljung R, Petrini P, Lindgren AK, Berntorp E 1992 Implantable central venous catheters facilitate prophylactic treatment in children with heamophilia. Acta Paediatrica 81: 918–920
28. Liesner RJ, Khair K, Hann IM 1996 The impact of prophylactic treatment on children with severe haemophilia. British Journal of Haematology 92: 973–978
29. Bollard CM, Teague LR, Berry EW, Ockelford PA 2000 The use of central venous catheters (portacaths) in children with haemophilia. Haemophilia 6: 6670
30. Warrier I, Baird-Cox K, Luscher JM 1997 Use of central venous catheters on children with haemophilia: one haemophilia treatment centre experience. Haemophilia 3: 194–198
31. Santagostino E, Gringeri A, Muca-Perja M, Mannucci PM 1998 A prospective clinical trial of implantable central venous access in children with haemophilia. British Journal of Haematology 102:79: 762–766, 1224–1228
32. Davidson Cs, Epstein RD, Miller G F, Taylor FHL 1949 Hemophilia: a clinical study of forty patients. Blood 4: 97–119
33. Rizza CR, Spooner RD 1983 Treatment of haemophilia and related disorders in Britain and Northern Ireland during 1976–80: report on behalf of the directors of haemophilia centres in the United Kingdom. British Medical Journal 286(1): 29–932
34. Hay CR, Colvin BT, Ludlam CA et al 1996 Recommendations for the treatment of factor VIII inhibitors: from the UK Haemophilia Centre Directors' Organisation Inhibitor Working Party. Blood Coagulation and Fibrinolysis 7 (2): 134–138
35. Yee TT, Pasi KJ, Lilley PA, Lee CA 1999 Factor VIII inhibitors in haemophiliacs: a single centre experience over 34 years, 1964–97. British Journal of Haematology 104: 909–914
36. Yee TT, Williams MD, Hill FGH et al 1997 Absence of inhibitors in previously untreated patients with severe haemophilia A after exposure to a single intermediate purity factor VIII product. Thrombosis and Haemostasis 78: 1027–1029

37. Addiego J, Kasper C, Abildgaard C et al 1993 Frequency of inhibitor development in haemophiliacs treated with low-purity factor VIII. Lancet 342: 462–464

38. Schwaab R, Brackmann I, Meyer C et al 1995 Haemophilia A: mutation type determines risk of inhibitor formation. Thrombosis and Haemostasis 74: 1402–1406

39. Ehrenforth S, Kreutz W, Scharrer I et al 1992 Incidence of development of factor VIII and factor IX inhibitors in haemophiliacs. Lancet 339: 549–598

40. Peerlinck K, Rosendaal FR, Vermylen J 1993 Incidence of inhibitor development in a group of young hemophilia A patients treated exclusively with lyophilized cryoprecipitate. Blood 81: 3332–3335

41. Guerois C, Laurian Y, Rothschild C et al 1995 Incidence of factor VIII inhibitor development in severe hemophilia A patients treated only with one brand of highly purified plasma derived concentrate. Thrombosis and Haemostasis 73: 215–218

42. Vermylen J 1998 How do some haemophiliacs develop inhibitors? Haemophilia 4: 538–542

43. Aledort LM, Dimichele DM 1998 Inhibitors occur more frequently in African–American and Latine haemophiliacs. (Letter) Haemophilia 598 (4): 68

44. Hay CRM, Ludlam CA, Colvin BT et al 1998 Factor VIII inhibitors in mild and moderate severity haemophilia A. Thrombosis and Haemostasis 79: 762–766

45. De Michele DM 1998 Immune tolerance: a synopsis of the intenational experience. Haemophilia 4: 568–573

46. Cash JD, Garder, AMA, Da Costa J 1974 The release of plasminogen activator and factor VIII by LVP, AVP, DDAVP, ATII and OT in man. British Journal of Haematology 27: 363–364

47. Mannucci PM, Ruggeri ZM, Pareti FI, Captanio A 1977 A new pharmacological approach to the management of haemophilia and von Willebrand disease. Lancet i: 869–872

48. UK von Willebrand Working Party 1997 Guidelines for the diagnosis and management of von Willebrand disease. Haemophilia 3 (suppl 2): 1–25

49. Lethagen S, Ragnarson Tennvall G 1993 Self-treatment with desmopressin intranasal spray in patients with bleeding disorders: effect on bleeding symptoms and socioeconomic factors. Annals of Hematology 66: 257–260

50. Rodeghiero F, Castaman G, Manucci PM 1996 Prospective multicentre study on subcutaneous concentrated desmopressin for home treatment of patients with von Willebrand disease and mild or moderate haemophilia A. Thrombosis and Haemostasis 76: 692–696

51. Mannucci PM, Bettega D, Cattaneo M 1992 Consistency of responses to repeated DDAVP infusions in patients with von Willebrand disease and haemophilia A. British Journal of Haematology

52. Miller CH, Lenzi R, Breen C 1987 Prevalence of von Willebrand's disease among US adults. Blood 70: 377–383

53. Werner EI, Broxson EH, Tucker EI et al 1991 Prevalence of von Willebrand disease in children: a multiethnic study. Blood 78: 68a

54. Federici AB, Mannucci PM 1999 Diagnosis and management of von Willebrand disease. Haemophilia 5(2): 28–37

55. Sadler JE 1994 A revised classification of von Willebrand disease. Thiombosis and Haemostasis 71: 520–525

56. Nitu-Whalley IC, Lee CA, Griffioen A et al 2000 Type I von Willebrand disease – a clinical retrospective study of the diagnosis, the influence of the ABO blood group and the role of the bleeding history. British Journal of Haematology 108: 259–264

57. Weiss HI, Meyer D, Rabinowitz R et al 1982 Pseudo-von Willebrand disease. An intrinsic platelet defect with aggregation by unmodified human factor VIII–von Willebrand factor and enchanced absorption of its high-molecular-weight multimers. New England Journal of Medicine

58. Lyons SE, Bruck ME, Bowie EJW, Ginsburg D 1992 Impaired intracellular transport produced by a subset of type 2A vWD mutations. Journal of Biological Chemistry 267: 4424–4430

59. Mazurier C, Dieval J, Joneux S et al 1990 A new vWF defect in a patient with FVIII deficiency but with normal level and multimeric patterns of both plasma and platelet vWF. Characterization of abnormal vWF/FVIII interaction. Blood 75: 20–26

60. Miller JL, Castella A 1982 Platelet4yBc von Willebrand disease characterization of a new bleeding disorder. Blood 60: 790–794

61. Simone JV, Cornet JA, Abildgaard CF 1968 Acquired von Willebrand syndrome in systemic lupus erythematosus. Blood 31: 806–812

62. Smith TL, Gill JL, Ambrose DR, Hathaway WE 1989 Hyponatremia and seizures in young children given DDAVP. American Journal of Hematology 31: 199–202

63. Bond L, Bevin D 1988 Myocardial infarction in a patient with hemophilia A treated with DDAVP. New England Journal of Medicine 318: 121

64. Holmberg L, Nilsson N, Borge L et al 1983 Platelet aggregation induced by I-desamino-8-D-arginine vasopressin (DDAVP) in type 2B von Willebrand disease. New England Journal of Medicine 309: 816–821

65. Burnouf-Radosevich M, Burnouf T 1992 Chromatographic preparation of a therapeutic highly purified von Willebrand factor concentrate from human cryoprecipitate. Vox Sanguinis 62: 1–11

66. Mannucci PM, Lattuada A, Ruggeri ZM 1994 Proteolysis of von Willebrand factor in therapeutic plasma concentrates. Blood 83: 3018–3027

67. Nitu-Whalley IC, Griffioen A, Harrington C, Lee CA 2001 Retrospective review of the management of elective surgery with desmopressin and clotting factor concentrates in patients with von Willebrand disease. American Journal of Haematology 66: 280–284

68. Ginsburg D, Handin RI, Bonthron DT et al 1985 Human von Willebrand factor (vWF): isolation of complementary DNA (cDNA) clones and chromosomal localization. Science 228: 1401

69. Sadler JE, Shelton-Inloes BB, Sorace JM et al 1985 Cloning and characterization of two cDNAs coding for human von Willebrand factor. Proceedings of the National Academy of Sciences, USA 82: 6394

70. Verweij CL, de Vries CN, Distel B et al 1985 Construction of cDNA coding for human von Willebrand factor using antibody probes for colony-screening and mapping of the chromosomal gene. Nucleic Acids Research 13: 4699

71. Lynch DC, Zimmerman TS, Collins CI et al 1985 Molecular cloning of cDNA for human von Willebrand factor: authentication by a new method. Cell 41: 49

72. Titani K, Kumar S, Takio K et al 1986 Amino acid sequence of human von Willebrand factor. Biochemistry 25: 3171

73. Shelton-Inloes BB, Chehab FF, Mannucci PM et al 1987 Gene deletions correlate with the development of alloantibodies in von Willebrand Disease. Journal of Clinical Investigation 79: 1459

74. Ginsburg D, Konkle BA, Gill IC et al 1989 Molecular basis of human von Willebrand disease analysis of platelet von Willebrand factor mRNA. Proceedings of the National Academy of Sciences USA 86: 3723–3727

75. Ioana C, Nitu-Whalley AR et al 2000 Identification of Type 2 von Willebrand disease in previously diagnosed type 1 patients: a reappraisal using phenotypes, genotypes and molecular modelling. Thrombosis and Haemostasis 84: 998–1004

76. Von Willebrand EA 1926 Hereditir pseudohemofili. Finska Lakaresallskapets Handlinger Band LXVII (2): 7–111

77. Royal College of General Practitioners, Office of Population Censuses and Surveys, Department of Health and Social Security 1986 Morbidity statistics from general practice. Third national study 1981–82. Series MBS No 1, London, HMSO

78. Hallberg L, Nilsson L 1964 Determination of menstrual blood loss. Scandinavian Journal of Clinical and Laboratory Investigation 16: 244–248

79. Higham JM, O'Brien PMS, Shaw RW 1990 Assessment of menstrual blood loss using a pictorial chart. British Journal of Obstetrics and Gynaecology 97 734–739

80. Kadir RA, Economides DL, Sabin CA et al 1998 Frequency of inherited bleeding disorders in women with menorrhagia. Lancet 351: 485–489

81. Nilsson IM 1997 Von Willebrand's disease-fifty years old. Acta Medical Scandinavica 201: 97–508

82. Kadir RA, Economides DL, Sabin CA et al 1999 Variations in coagulation factors in women: effects of age, ethnicity, menstrual cycle and combined oral contraceptive. Thrombosis and Haemostasis 82: 1456–1461

83. Kadir RA, Economides DL, Sabin CA et al 1999 Assessment of menstrual blood loss and gynaecological problems in patients with inherited bleeding disorders. Haemophilia 5: 40–48

84. Kadir RA, Sabin CA, Pollard D et al 1998 Quality of life during menstruation in patients with inherited bleeding disorders. Haemophilia 4: 836–841

85. Bonnar J, Sheppard BL 1996 Treatment of menorrhagia during menstruation: randomised controlled trial of ethamsylate, mefanamic acid and tranexamic acid. British Medical Journal 131: 579–582

86. Stirling Y, Woolf L, North WRS 1984 Haemostasis in normal pregnancy. Thrombosis and Haemostasis 52: 17–82

87. Kadir RA, Sabin CA, Pollard D et al 1998 Pregnancy in women with von Willebrand's disease or factor XI deficiency. British Journal of Obstetrics and Gynaecology 105: 314–321

88. Ramsahoye BH, Davies SV, Dasani H, Pearson JF 1995 Obstetric management in von Willebrand's disease: a report of 24 pregnancies and a review of the literature. Haemophilia 1: 140–144

89. Greer IA, Lowe GDO, Walker JJ, Forbes CD 1991 Haemorrhagic problems in Obstetrics and Gynaecology in patients with congenital coagulopathies. British Journal of Obstetrics and Gynaecology 98: 908–918

90. Conti M, Mori D, Conti E et al 1986 Pregnancy in women with different types of von Willebrand's disease. Obstetrics and Gynecology 68: 282–285

91. Chediak JR, Alban G, Maxey B 1986 von Willebrand disease in pregnancy. Management during delivery and outcome of offspring 155: 618–624

92. Walker ID, Walker ID, Colvin BT et al 1994 Investigation and management of haemorrhagic disorders in pregnancy. Haemostasis and Thrombosis Task Force. Journal of Clinical Pathology 100–108

93. AI-Mondhiry H, Ehmann WC 1994 Congenital afibrinogenemia. American Journal of Hematology 46: 343–347

94. Shima M, Tanaka I, Sawamoto Y et al 1997 Successful treatment of two brothers with congenital afibrinogenemia for splenic rupture using heat- and solvent detergent-treated fibrinogen concentrates. Journal of Paediatric Hematology/Oncology 19: 462–465

95. Evron S, Anteby SO, Brzezinsky A *et al* 1985 Congenital afibrinogenemia and recurrent early abortion: a case report. European Journal of Obstetrics Gynecology and Reproductive Biology 19: 307–311

96. Girolami A, Scarano L, Saggiorato G et al 1998 Congenital deficiencies and abnormalities of Prothrombin. Blood Coagulation and Fibrinolysis 9: 557–569

97. Poort SR, Michels JJ, Reitsma PH, Bertina RM 1994 Homozygosity for a novel missense mutation in the prothrombin gene causing a severe bleeding disorder. Thrombosis and Haemostasis 72: 819–824

98. Salooja N, Martin P, Khair K et al 2000 Severe factor V deficiency and neonatal intracranial haemorrhage: a case report. Haemophilia 6: 44–46

99. Peyvandi F, Tuddenham EGD, Akhtari AM et al 1998 Bleeding symptoms in 27 Iranian patients with the combined deficiency of factor V and factor VIII. British Journal of Haematology 100: 773–776

100. Rappaport SI, Zivelin A, Minow RA et al 1992 Clinical significance of antibodies to bovine and human thrombin and factor V after surgical use of bovine thrombin. American Journal of Clinical Pathology 97: 84–91

101. Roberts HR, Lefkowitz JB 1994 Inherited disorders of prothrombin conversion. In: Colman RW, Hirsh J, Marder VJ, Salzman EW (eds), Haemostasis and thrombosis, 3rd edn. JB Lipincott, Philadelphia, 206–208

102. Peyvandi F, Mannucci PM, Asti D et al Clinical manifestations in 28 Iranian and Italian patients with severe factor VII deficiency

103. Scharrer I 1999 Recombinant factor VIIa for patients with inhibitors to factor VIII or IX or factor VII deficiency. Haemophilia 5: 253–259

104. Mariani G, Testa MG, Di Paolantonia T et al 1999 Use of recombinant, activated factor VII in the treatment of congenital factor VII deficiencies. Vox Sanguinis 77: 131–136

105. Peyvandi F, Mannucci PM, Lak M et al 1998 Congenital factor X deficiency: Spectrum of bleeding symptoms in 32 Iranian patients. British Journal of Haematology 102: 626–628

106. Furie B, Voo L, McAdam KPWJ, Furie BC 1981 Mechanism of factor X deficiency in systemic amyloidosis. New England Journal of Medicine 304: 827–830

107. Rosenthal RL, Dreskin OH, Rosenthal N 1998 Plasma thromboplastin antecedent (PTA) deficiency: clinical, coagulation. Haemophilia 4: 683–688

108. Seligsohn U 1993 Factor XI deficiency. Thrombosis and Haemostasis 70: 68–71

109. Bolton-Maggs PHB, Young Wan Yin B, McCraw AH et al 1988 Inheritance and bleeding in factor XI deficiency. British Journal of Haematology 69: 521–528

110. Bolton-Maggs PHB, Patterson DA, Wensley RT, Tuddenham EGD 1995 Definition of the bleeding tendency in factor XI kindreds – a clinical and laboratory study. Thrombosis and Haemostasis 73: 194–202

111. Collins PW, Goldman E, Lilley P et al 1995 Clinical experience of factor XI deficiency: the role of fresh frozen plasma and factor XI concentrate. Haemophilia 1: 227–231

112. Bolton-Maggs PHB, Wensley RT, Kernoff PBA et al 1992 Production and therapeutic use of a factor XI concentrate from human plasma. Thrombosis and Haemostasis 67: 314–319

113. Winkelman L, McLaughlin LF, Gray E, Thomas S 1993 Heat-treated factor XI concentrate: evaluation of *in vivo* thrombogenecity in two animals models. Thrombosis and Haemostasis 69: 1286

114. Bolton-Maggs PHB, Colvin BT, Satchi G 1994 Thrombogenic potential of factor XI concentrate. Lancet 344: 748

115. UKHCDO 1994 Guidelines for the management of factor XI deficiency. Revised 1998.

116. Berliner S, Horowitz I, Martinowitz U et al 1992 Dental surgery in patients with severe factor XI deficiency without plasma replacement. Blood Coagulation and Fibrinolysis 3: 465–474

117. Schnall SF, Duffy TP, Clyne LP 1987 Acquired factor XI inhibitors in congenitally deficient patients. American Journal of Hematology 26: 323–328

118. Hedner U 1990 Factor VIIa in the treatment of haemophilia. Blood Coagulation and Fibrinolysis 1: 307–317

119. Berliner S, Lusky A, Zivelin A, Modan M 1984 Hereditary factor XIII deficiency: Report of four families and definition of the carrier state. British Journal of Haematology 56: 495–505

120. Kitchens CS, Newcomb TF 1979 Factor XIII. Medicine (Baltimore) 58: 413–429

121. Abbondanzo SL, Gootenberg JE, Lofts RS, McPherson RA 1988 Intracranial haemorrhage in congenital deficiency of factor XIII. American Journal of Pediatric Hematology/Oncology 10: 65–68

122. Rodeghiero R, Castaman GC, DiBona E et al 1987 Sucessful pregnancy in a woman with congenital factor XIII deficiency treated with substitute therapy. Blut 55: 45–48

123. Brackmann HE, Edbring R, Ferster A et al 1995 Pharmacokinetics and tolerability of factor XIII concentrates prepared from human placenta or plasma: a crossover randomized study. Thrombosis and Haemostasis 74: 622–625

Acquired bleeding disorders 28

DJ Perry

Indroduction

Physiologic deficiencies
Neonates

Drug-induced bleeding disorders

Heparin
Laboratory monitoring

Hirudin
Laboratory monitoring

Warfarin
Laboratory monitoring

Thrombolytic agents
Laboratory monitoring

Antiplatelet drugs
Laboratory monitoring

Hemostatic defects associated with vitamin K deficiency

Vitamin K and vitamin K deficiency
Vitamin K deficiency in neonates and young infants
Vitamin K deficiency in adults
Clinical features of vitamin K deficiency
Laboratory findings
Management of vitamin K deficiency

Hemostatic defects in liver disease
Laboratory findings in liver disease
Management of the coagulopathy of liver disease

Hemostatic defects associated with renal disease and uremia
Laboratory diagnosis
Treatment

Hemostatic defects associated with 'massive' blood transfusion
Laboratory diagnosis
Treatment

Hemostatic defects associated with the use of extracorporal circuits
Clotting factor abnormalities
Quantitative platelet abnormalities
Platelet activation
Fibrinolytic activity
Drugs
Acquired inhibitors
Disseminated intravascular coagulation (DIC)
Laboratory monitoring
Treatment

Disseminated intravascular coagulation (DIC)
Laboratory diagnosis of DIC
Clinical evaluation of patients with acute DIC
Management of acute DIC

Chronic DIC

Acquired hyperfibrinolysis
Laboratory investigation of systemic hyperfibrinolysis
Management of systemic hyperfibrinolysis

Bleeding and malignancy
Acute leukemias
Myeloproliferative disorders
Paraproteinemias

Acquired inhibitors of coagulation
Laboratory findings in acquired inhibitors
Management of acquired inhibitors
Toxic coagulopathies

Introduction

Acquired disorders of hemostasis are significantly more common than inherited disorders of hemostasis and as such are frequently encountered in routine clinical practice. Acquired disorders of coagulation may be physiologic such as those that are seen in pregnancy, the new-born and old age or they may be pathologic. The latter often arise as a complication of multisystem disease and are associated with multiple clotting abnormalities.

The common and some of the less common causes of an acquired hemostatic defect are summarized in Table 28.1.

Physiologic deficiencies

Neonates

The coagulation system of the new-born infant is complex and fragile and reflects in part hepatic immaturity. Most

Table 28.1 Disorders associated with an acquired hemostatic defect

Physiologic deficiencies
Neonates

Liver disease

Drug-induced bleeding
Anticoagulants
Thrombolytic agents
Antiplatelet agents
Miscellaneous e.g. dextran

Massive blood transfusion

Acquired inhibitors of coagulation
Factor VIII inhibitors
Other factor inhibitors
Antiphospholipid antibodies

Vitamin K deficiency
Neonates
Gastrointestinal disease
Vitamin K antagonists
Biliary obstruction
Liver disease
Miscellaneous e.g. cephalosporins, TPN (total parenteral nutrition), tropical sprue

Disseminated intravascular coagulation

Renal disease and renal failure

Cardiopulmonary bypass and extracorporeal circuits

Miscellaneous
Snake venoms and other toxic agents
Myeloproliferative disorders
Malignancy
Paraproteinemias

of the clotting factors are present in reduced concentration in the new-born infant apart from factors V, VIII and fibrinogen.[1,2] These physiologic deficiencies in clotting factors result in prolongation of the prothrombin time (PT) and activated partial thromboplastin time (APTT) and as a consequence of this, reference ranges reflecting both gestational and neonatal age must be used to assess coagulation in the neonate.[1,2]

The platelet count is normal in the neonate and although there is often a qualitative platelet abnormality, the bleeding time is usually normal. Fibrinolysis in the neonate is normal.

The pattern of bleeding seen in neonates – umbilical bleeding, cepalohematomas, bleeding after circumcision, oozing after venepuncture and bleeding into the skin – is different from that seen in adults. Children seem to be particularly susceptible to intracranial bleeds in the neonatal period.

Drug-induced bleeding disorders

Drugs are a common cause of an acquired bleeding disorder. In many cases the drug may be quite obvious, for example an anticoagulant such as warfarin. However, in other cases it may be less clear, for example the inhibitory effect on vitamin K metabolism observed with some cephalosporins.[3] In any patient wilth an apparent acquired bleeding disorder, an accurate and comprehensive drug history must be obtained. Such a history must include not only prescription drugs but also non-proprietary agents.

Heparin

Unfractionated heparin (UFH) and the low molecular weight heparins (LMWHs) are anticoagulants that potentiate the action of antithrombin, accelerating its inhibitory activity several thousand-fold.[4] The inhibitory activity of UFH is directed against both thrombin (IIa) and factor Xa whereas that of the LMWH is almost exclusively directed against factor Xa.[4] Heparin is metabolized by the liver and excreted by the kidneys. Bleeding in patients receiving heparin is usually secondary to excessive anticoagulation but may occasionally occur as a result of heparin-induced thrombocytopenia (HIT).[5,6] Heparin also has an effect upon platelet function and capillary permeability and these effects can contribute to the bleeding tendency. LMWHs may accumulate in patients with renal failure as the main route for excretion is through the kidneys.[7]

In patients receiving unfractionated heparin intravenously the risk of serious hemorrhage is about 5%.[8] The risk of hemorrhage is significantly increased if there is concomitant use of other anticoagulants, particularly antiplatelet agents such as aspirin. In individuals who are actively bleeding, unfractionated heparin can be effectively neutralized by protamine sulfate, a strongly basic drug that binds to the heparin. One milligram of protamine sulfate will neutralize approximately 100 units of heparin. In overdose, protamine sulfate can function as an anticoagulant and for these reasons no more than 50 mg of protamine sulfate should be administered at any one time. Protamine sulfate neutralizes only 60% of the anti-Xa activity of the LMWHs and is, therefore, less effective in correcting the bleeding problems associated with their use.[9]

Laboratory monitoring

Therapeutic anticoagulation with unfractionated heparin is monitored by means of the APTT aiming to maintain the APTT at 1.5–2 times the mid-point of the normal range. In patients in whom the APTT is prolonged prior to the initiation of anticoagulation therapy, for example factor XII deficiency or some patients with a lupus anticoagulant, the measurement of plasma anti-Xa levels may be necessary. LMWHs have primarily anti-Xa activity and have little effect upon the APTT unless given in overdose. For patients receiving LMWHs therapeutically, routine monitoring is not usually indicated. However, the thrombin time, APTT and the plasma anti-Xa levels should be measured if there are concerns that a LMWH may be responsible for a bleeding problem. In patients receiving prophylactic anticoagulation with either unfractionated heparin or a LMWH, routine monitoring is not necessary but may be of value if a patient is actively bleeding.

Hirudin

Hirudin is a direct and specific inhibitor of thrombin, which does not require antithrombin for its action.[10,11] Originally isolated from leeches (*Hirudo medicinalis*) the protein is now available in a recombinant form – r-hirudin. Hirudin not only inhibits the conversion of fibrinogen to fibrin but also other thrombin-catalyzed reactions such as the activation of clotting factors and thrombin-induced platelet aggregation. Hirudin is a potent anticoagulant but has a very narrow therapeutic window and plasma levels of hirudin show high levels of interindividual variability even when the dose is adjusted for body weight. Over-anticoagulation with hirudin can

lead to severe bleeding problems. Hirudin has a short half-life and its natural clearance through the kidneys may be sufficiently rapid such that in cases of overdose, specific neutralization is not required. It may be possible to antagonize the effects of hirudin by increasing endogenous thrombin generation through the use of agents such as rVIIa or prothrombin complex concentrates. Alternatively, plasmaphoresis or exchange transfusion may remove hirudin from the circulation.

Laboratory monitoring

Therapeutic anticoagulation with hirudin is commonly monitored by the APTT or thrombin time. However, there is considerable interindividual variability in the degree of prolongation of the APTT at identical plasma levels of hirudin. For these reasons the 'ecarin' clotting time has been suggested as a more accurate means for monitoring individuals receiving hirudin.[12]

Warfarin

Warfarin is a 4-hydroxycoumarin derivative that exerts its action by blocking the regeneration of vitamin from its epoxide. The major complication of all oral anticoagulants is bleeding and this risk increases as the intensity of treatment (i.e. the international normalized ratio (INR)) increases.[13,14] Major bleeding is also increased by other diseases that may be present in an individual, for example malignancy, cerebrovascular disease. Independent risk factors for bleeding during long-term warfarin therapy include age greater than 65 years, a history of past gastrointestinal bleeding, stroke, atrial fibrillation and one or more of three comorbid conditions – myocardial infarction, renal insufficiency and severe anemia.[15] For any individual the risk of bleeding is related to the duration of anticoagulant therapy, although the risk may be higher in the early phase of treatment than later. Most studies in unselected groups of patients suggest that the risk of major bleeding is approximately 3% per annum and that CNS hemorrhage occurs at a rate of 0.1% per annum.[16]

The anticoagulant action of warfarin is potentiated by many drugs and these include:

- Drugs that displace warfarin from its plasma protein binding sites (e.g. phenylbutazone, the statins, clofibrate).
- Drugs that inhibit the metabolic clearance of warfarin (e.g. cimetidine, omeprazole, amiodarone, allopurinol).
- Drugs that interfere with vitamin K metabolism (e.g. cephalosporins, high-dose salicylates).

- Drugs that independently increase the anticoagulant action (e.g. clofibrate, anabolic steroids, erythromycin).

Minor bleeding episodes in patients receiving oral anticoagulants may be treated with local measures and withdrawal of the drug. In cases of severe or life-threatening hemorrhage, rapid reversal of anticoagulation is required and this is most effectively achieved by the use of a combination of vitamin K and clotting-factor concentrates (containing factors II, VII, IX and X) and less effectively by vitamin K and fresh-frozen plasma.[17]

Laboratory monitoring

Warfarin is monitored by measuring the INR, which takes into account the differing sensitivities of the tissue factors (thromboplastins) used in the assay. The INR is derived from the formula:

$$\left[\frac{\text{Patient prothrombin time in seconds}}{\text{Normal mean prothrombin time of a donor plasma pool}}\right]^{ISI}$$

where the ISI (international sensitivity index) is a value derived by calibrating the tissue factor used in the assay against an international WHO standard, the ISI of which is 1.0.

Thrombolytic agents

Thrombolytic drugs act by stimulating endogenous fibrinolysis and thereby dissolving thrombi. Of the activators currently available, recombinant tissue plasminogen activator (rt-PA) and urokinase (U-PA) produce their pharmacologic actions by converting plasminogen to plasmin at the site of fibrin deposition. In contrast, staphylokinase, streptokinase and its anisoylated derivative APSAC (acylated plasminogen streptokinase activator complex) become activators after binding to plasminogen.[18]

Bleeding occurs in between 3 and 40% of patients receiving thrombolytic therapy and this risk is greatly increased in patients who are also receiving antiplatelet drugs or other anticoagulants.[18] Thrombolytic therapy predisposes to bleeding by depleting the plasma concentration of procoagulant proteins and by the generation of anticoagulant fibrin(ogen) degradation products. Thrombolytic therapy cannot distinguish between a pathologic thrombus occluding some critical vessel (e.g. coronary artery) and a physiologic thrombus that is preventing bleeding from a critical site (e.g. cerebral circulation). Platelet function in patients receiving thrombolytic therapy is also impaired because of inhibition of platelet aggregation by high levels of fibrin – fibrinogen degra-

dation products (FDPs) and also by impaired platelet adhesion by plasmin-induced proteolysis of glycoprotein lb (Gplb) and von Willebrand factor.[19]

For minor bleeding episodes the thrombolytic agent together with any concomitant anticoagulant or antiplatelet agent must be stopped. For life-threatening bleeding episodes in addition to the above, a fibrinolytic inhibitor should be given, for example tranexamic acid or aprotinin. In addition, fresh-frozen plasma and/or cryoprecipitate should be given to restore depleted clotting factors.[18]

Laboratory monitoring

Laboratory monitoring of thrombolytic therapy is often unnecessary when its administration is short-term. However, during a more prolonged infusion (greater than 24 h) sequential monitoring is of value. Blood for monitoring of patients receiving thrombolytic therapy should be collected into citrate containing a fibrinolytic inhibitor such as aprotinin or EACA (ε-aminocaproic acid) to prevent continued lysis occurring *in vivo*. Fibrinolytic therapy alters most laboratory tests of coagulation but few tests predict either the efficacy of thrombolysis or the risks of bleeding. The APTT is prolonged in patients receiving thrombolytic therapy because of depletion of fibrinogen, factors V and VIII and the generation of high levels of fibrin(ogen) degradation products. An APTT ratio of 1.5 indicates significant systemic fibrinolysis.[18] Plasma fibrinogen concentration falls during thrombolytic therapy reflecting the presence of free plasminogen activator within the circulation. The actual fibrinolytic activity of the plasma can be measured by means of the euglobulin clot lysis time (ELT), which is shortened in patients receiving thrombolytic therapy, or the fibrin plate lysis test (demonstrating increased zones of lysis) but these are not routinely used. The thromboelastogram (TEG) can also be of value in monitoring patients undergoing thrombolytic therapy and is considerably easier to perform than either the ELT or the fibrin plate lysis test. In patients receiving thrombolytic therapy, tests that measure the levels of FDPs are markedly elevated whereas those that detect only fibrin degradation products (D dimers) are usually normal or slightly raised.

Antiplatelet drugs

A wide variety of drugs are in common use that have potent antiplatelet actions and such drugs are often used in combination (e.g. aspirin and ticlopidine). The risk of hemorrhage is significantly increased when antiplatelet drugs are used in combination with other anticoagulants (e.g. warfarin and aspirin).

Aspirin and non-steroidal anti-inflammatory drugs inhibit platelet function by inhibiting preferentially platelet cyclooxygenase activity whilst maintaining the activity of the enzyme within the endothelial cells.[20] In this way, there is a reduction in the production of platelet thromboxane A_2 (TxA$_2$), a potent inducer of platelet aggregation, but a preservation in prostacyclin (PGI$_2$) synthesis by the endothelial cell. Omega-3 fatty acids can substitute for arachadonic acid in prostaglandin synthesis resulting in the synthesis of thromboxane A_3 (TxA$_3$), which has little effect upon platelet aggregation. However, within the endothelial cell, synthesis of a novel prostaglandin occurs (PGI$_3$) which has potent antiplatelet activity.

Several drugs such as dipyridamole result in a decrease in platelet intracellular calcium concentration by inhibiting cAMP degradation. Elevated levels of cAMP favor movement of Ca^{2+} into the dense bodies where it is inert and so effectively decreases intracellular Ca^{2+} levels.[21] Similar, but less marked, effects are observed with caffeine and theophylline.

Drugs such as ticlopidine and clopidogrel are thienopyridine derivatives which selectively inhibit platelet aggregation by blocking ADP-inducted aggregation.[22,23] Reopro is a monoclonal antibody that selectively binds to and blocks the GpIIb/IIIa complex resulting in a complete loss of platelet activity. The major side-effect of Reopro is bleeding and in a small number of patients it can also result in profound thrombocytopenia which can further exacerbate the bleeding tendency.[24] Platelet-function abnormalities can be induced by certain antibiotics particularly the β-lactam antibiotics.[25,26] Penicillin, particularly penicillin G, ticarcillin and carbenicillin have been reported to inhibit platelet function and to cause a clinically significant bleeding tendency particularly when administered in high doses.[25,26]

Cephalosporins such as moxalactam, nitfofurantoin and hydroxychloroquine can similarly interfere with platelet function.[3] Some cephalosporins also appear to interfere with vitamin K metabolism resulting in an additional and additive increased risk of bleeding.[27]

Finally, a variety of drugs appear to have non-specific effects upon platelet function. B-adrenergic agents have a weak but inconsistent effect on platelet function *in vitro* but rarely if at all are associated with a clinical bleeding tendency. Sodium valproate can result not only in thrombocytopenia but can also result in qualitative platelet abnormalities.[28] Dextrans have suppressive effects upon normal coagulation but in addition can also inhibit platelet aggregation resulting in prolongation of the bleeding time.[29]

Laboratory monitoring

In general, laboratory monitoring in patients receiving antiplatelet agents in not required. In occasional patients, it may be of value to establish whether specific drugs are having their desired effect or not. In such cases, platelet aggregation or the use of the platelet function analyser 100 (PFA100) may be of value.[30–32] The bleeding time is commonly prolonged in patients taking antiplatelet therapy.

Hemostatic defects associated with vitamin K deficiency

Vitamin K and vitamin K deficiency

Vitamin K_1 is a fat-soluble vitamin obtained primarily from green leafy vegetables. It is absorbed in the upper part of the small intestine and its absorption is dependant upon the presence of pancreatic lipases and bile. Most of the vitamin K absorbed from the gut is stored in the liver although the stores of vitamin K are only a few days. The normal daily requirement of vitamin K is 0.5–1.0 μg/kg. Vitamin K_2 is synthesized by the gut flora but cannot compensate for a total deficiency of vitamin K_1. Vitamin K_3 is a synthetic form of vitamin K. Vitamin K oxidation to its epoxide form is essential for the posttranslational gamma-carboxylation of the glutamic acid residues present in the N-terminal region of factors II, VII, IX, X, protein C and S. Efficient gamma-carboxylation allows the modified glutamic acid residues to bind calcium and subsequently to the phospholipid receptors on cell membranes allowing coagulation to proceed. In the absence of efficient gamma-carboxylation, partially carboxylated forms of the clotting factors are released into the circulation, so-called 'PIVKAS'. During carboxylation, vitamin K is oxidized to vitamin K epoxide and recycled to its active form by reductases. Oral anticoagulants such as warfarin inhibit vitamin K epoxide reduction and prevent recycling of vitamin K to its active form, thereby limiting the activity of the carboxylase.

Vitamin K deficiency in neonates and young infants

Three types of vitamin K deficiency are seen in the newborn child and young infant.

- Early form. An early form of hemorrhagic disease in the new born infant, occurring within the first 24 h of life, is most commonly seen in infants whose mothers have received anticonvulsant therapy during pregnancy. This condition is prevented by the administration of daily vitamin K to the mother, for the 2 weeks prior to delivery.
- Hemorrhagic disease of the new-born (HDN). HDN is the classic hemorrhagic diathesis associated with a deficiency of vitamin K and arises because of: (1) the limited transplacental passage of vitamin K during development; (2) hepatic immaturity particularly in premature infants; (3) the sterile gut of the new-born infant; and (4) the poor intake of nutrients in the first few days of life and because human breast milk in comparison to cows milk contains little vitamin K. In such cases, bleeding usually occurs between the second and fifth days of life and commonly presents with intracranial hemorrhage which may be fatal in up to 20% of cases. To prevent this potentially fatal hemorrhagic disorder, new-born infants are routinely given 1 mg intramuscular vitamin K_1 at birth.[33,34]
- Late form. Infants who are not given vitamin K_1 at birth and who are exclusively breast fed may develop a later form of the disorder at between 3 and 8 weeks of age. Again, such infants frequently present with intracranial bleeds. Infants who do not receive intramuscular vitamin K should receive oral vitamin K within the first 24 h of birth, again at 1 week and again at 4 weeks of life. Oral vitamin K is ineffective in infants who have liver disease or malabsorption problems and these children should receive regular doses of parenteral vitamin K.

Vitamin K deficiency in adults

Vitamin K deficiency in adults can occur in a variety of situations including malabsorption, fasting, alcoholism and in association with various drugs particularly coumarins, some antibiotics and salicylates. Vitamin K deficiency may also be seen in patients receiving parenteral nutrition and for these reasons such patients should receive prophylactic vitamin K.

Clinical features of vitamin K deficiency

Neonates with vitamin K deficiency may present with a variety of clinical problems including massive intracranial hemorrhage, gastrointestinal bleeding, bleeding at the time of circumcision and skin bleeding. Adults with vitamin K deficiency may also present with a wide variety of clinical hemorrhagic problems but particularly gastrointestinal bleeding and recurrent epistaxes.

Laboratory findings

Adults and children with vitamin K deficiency both show a normal platelet count (unless there is an associated pathology such as liver disease or disseminated intravascular coagulation (DIC) which may result in thrombocytopenia), a prolonged PT, a prolonged APTT but a normal thrombin time and fibrinogen level (Table 28.2). The functional activity of the vitamin K dependent clotting factors are reduced and dysfunctional forms – PIVKAs can be detected in the presence of affected individuals.[35] These dysfunctional clotting factors appeared to be cleared more rapidly from the plasma than the fully carboxylated forms and this results in a shorter half-life and so the immunologic levels of these proteins are also reduced.

Management of vitamin K deficiency

The principles of treatment involve treating the underlying cause, the administration of vitamin K and in cases of severe hemorrhage, transfusion with fresh-frozen plasma. The use of clotting factor concentrates provides a rapid means for correcting the coagulation abnormalities in vitamin K deficiency but may be contraindicated particularly in patients with coexisting liver disease in which there is a risk of precipitating a thrombosis.[36]

There have been some concerns that the use of parenteral vitamin K, but not oral vitamin K, in the new-born infant may be associated with an increased risk of childhood cancers. However, such subsequent studies have not confirmed these early findings.[33,37]

Hemostatic defects in liver disease

The liver is responsible for the synthesis of all the coagulation factors apart from von Willebrand Factor (vWF).[38] The liver also synthesizes either completely or in part many of the proteins involved in the regulation of coagulation – antithrombin, protein C, protein S, heparin cofactor II, and those involved in fibrinolysis – plasminogen and α_2-antiplasmin. The liver is also responsible for the clearance of activated clotting factors that are generated by the clotting cascade and during fibrinolysis. Liver disease is, therefore, associated with a major disruption of the clotting system resulting in an increased

Table 28.2 Summary of coagulation abnormalities in acquired coagulation disorders

	Platelet count	PT	APTT	TT	Fibrinogen	Comments
Vitamin K deficiency	Normal	↑	↑	N	N	All vitamin K dependent clotting factors reduced
Liver disease	Normal reduced secondary to hypersplenism + impaired platelet function	↑	↑	↑	↓ + acquired dysfibrinogenemia	Reduced synthesis of coagulation factors both vitamin K dependent and vitamin K independent Increased fibrinolysis
Renal disease	Normal/reduced	N	N	N/↑	N[+ acquired dysfibrinogenemia]	Acquired qualitative platelet defect Loss of high molecular weight vWF multimers ↑ Reptilase time in some patients secondary to acquired dysfibrinogenemia ↑ NO production ↑ Half-life of many drugs
Massive blood transfusion	↓	↑	↑	↑	↓	Hypocalcemia and hypothermia may also be seen with the rapid infusion of large volumes of cold blood
DIC	↓	↑	↑	↑	↓	Increased FDPs which have an inhibitory action on both platelets and fibrin polymerization Red-cell fragmentation may be present Increased fibrinolysis
Cardiopulmonary bypass	↓	↑	↑	↑	↓	Bleeding time is prolonged Acquired qualitative platelet defect Increased fibrinolysis Heparin used in CPB may also contribute to the bleeding tendency DIC is a recognized complication of CPB Acquired factor V inhibitors are a rare complication
Acquired factor inhibitor	Usually normal	↑ or ↓	↑ or ↓	N	N	The pattern of abnormalities is dependant upon the specificity of the inhibitor e.g. FVIII, FV, FXIII
Malignancy	↑ or ↓	↑ or ↓	↑ or ↓	↑ or ↓	↑ or ↓	The pattern of test results is very variable reflecting the variety of abnormalities that may occur DIC may be a feature Acquired inhibitors may occur Thrombocytopenia may be secondary to the disease or its treatment Heparin-like anticoagulants have been reported
Paraproteinemias	↑ or ↓	↑ or ↓	↑ or ↓	↑ or ↓	↑ or ↓	The pattern of test results is very variable reflecting the variety of abnormalities that may occur Acquired inhibitors may occur Thrombocytopenia may be secondary to the disease or its treatment Heparin-like anticoagulants have been reported
Snake venoms	↑ or ↓	↑ or ↓	↑ or ↓	↑ or ↓	↑ or ↓	The pattern of test results is very variable reflecting the nature of the venom DIC may be a feature

N-normal; ↓-decreased; ↑-increased. APTT, activated partial thromboplastin time; CBP, cardiopulmonary bypass; DIC, disseminated intravascular coagulation; FDPs, fibrin–fibrinogen degradation products; PT, prothrombin time; TT, thrombin time.

risk of hemorrhage which may be severe. Factors V and VII are sensitive markers of hepatic function and may be used as an index of severity.[39,40]

Defective production of clotting factors arises because of a failure in hepatic synthetic function including gamma-carboxylation of the vitamin K dependent clotting factors although there may also be reduced absorption of the fat-soluble vitamins, including vitamin K, as a result of cholestasis. vWF is often raised in patients with liver failure, reflecting its extrahepatic site of synthesis (endothelial cells and megakaryocytes) and its acute phase nature. Thrombobocytopenia is a common finding in liver disease and is often due to sequestration of platelets within the spleen – hypersplenism. Thrombocytopenia may also be seen in association with alcohol abuse, folate deficiency, DIC and in some cases of viral hepatitis where the causative virus may have a direct effect upon megakaryopoiesis or accelerate peripheral destruction.[41] A qualitative platelet abnormality is often seen in patients with liver failure which further exacerbates the bleeding tendency.

Fibrinogen is relatively well maintained in liver disease until the terminal stages when the levels may drop dramatically. In addition, as a result of an increased sialic acid content of fibrinogen, patients with liver failure may develop an acquired dysfibrinogenemia resulting in slow fibrin polymerization and a relatively unstable fibrin clot.[42,43] Abnormal fibrinogens and non-carboxylated prothrombin are also synthesized by patients with primary hepatocellular carcinoma and have been used as markers of these disorders.[44] Many patients with liver disease have evidence of systemic fibrinolysis secondary to reduced synthesis of α_2-antiplasmin, reduced clearance of t-PA and by low-grade DIC.[45,46] Primary fibrinolysis may result in severe bleeding problems following surgery in patients with liver disease where tissue damage results in the release of large amounts of plasminogen activators which swamp the impaired protective mechanisms of the liver resulting in systemic fibrinolysis.

Chronic low-grade DIC is a common feature of liver disease. This occurs secondary to release of tissue thromboplastin from the damaged hepatocytes, reduced synthesis of the inhibitors of coagulation – antithrombin, protein C and protein S- and reduced clearance of activated clotting factors. Ascitic fluid appears to contain a potent thromboplastin-like material and may result in severe DIC following creation of a peritovenous shunt in which large amounts of ascitic fluid are infused directly into the circulation.[47,48]

Laboratory findings in liver disease

Individuals with liver disease show reduced synthesis of both the vitamin K dependent and independent clotting factors resulting in prolongation of the prothrombin time and activated partial thrombosplastin time. vWF and protein S may be normal to high, reflecting their extra-hepatic sites of synthesis. Features of DIC, including raised D-dimers and FDPs, are common in liver disease and this may contribute to the thrombocytopenia observed in such patients although hypersplenism may also result in thrombocytopenia. An acquired qualitative defect

platelet may also be present. Fibrinogen levels are often well maintained but patients may show an acquired dys-fibrinogenemia resulting in a prolonged thrombin time and reptilase time. Finally, there is evidence of systemic fibrinolysis with a shortened euglobulin clot lysis time.

Management of the coagulopathy of liver disease

Patients with liver disease may require no active management in terms of their coagulopathy unless actively bleeding or about to undergo an invasive procedure. In such cases, patients may require vitamin K, fresh-frozen plasma and occasionally cryoprecipitate or fibrinogen concentrates to correct the clotting factor deficiencies and platelet transfusions to maintain the platelet count about $50 \times 10^9/l$. Prothrombin complex concentrates should be avoided in patients with liver disease as they contain significant amounts of activated clotting factors and may precipitate a thrombotic event.[49,50] Similarly, inhibitors of fibrinolysis such as tranexamic acid should also be avoided for the same reason.

Antithrombin concentrates may be of value in some patients with liver disease as they may serve to correct the DIC. Finally, DDAVP (Desmopressin) has been shown to be of some value in some patients with cirrhosis who are actively bleeding.[51]

Hemostatic defects associated with renal disease and uremia

The coagulopathy associated with renal disease is complex, rarely due to deficiency of a single clotting factor and may be difficult to treat.

Recognized causes of a coagulopathy in patients with renal disease include:

- Anemia. The anemia that is often associated with renal disease disrupts normal platelet function. There is an inverse relationship between the template bleeding time and the hematocrit. This arises because of a decrease in the interaction of platelets with the vascular endothelium due to changes in axial blood flow with cells moving from the periphery to the center of the flowing blood. In addition red cells also contain enzymes that augment platelet function.
- Thrombocytopenia. Individuals with uremia often have a mild thrombocytopenia.[52,53] This may arise because of a suppressive effect of the uremic state on megakaryopoiesis.

- Decreased platelet adhesion. Patients with uremia often display reduced platelet adhesion. In part, this may reflect disordered platelet function particularly of the GpIb receptor which is important in the binding of vWF,[54] but it may also be secondary to a reduction in the levels of the high molecular weight vWF multimers.[55] These high molecular forms of vWF are critical for the interaction of platelets with the vascular endothelium.

- Qualitative platelet defect. The toxins that accumulate in renal failure may also impair platelet function in a non-specific manner. Some patients may show an acquired storage-pool-like defect with reduced platelet 5-HT and ADP content.[56] In addition, there may be abnormal intracellular calcium mobilization and increased intracellular levels of both cAMP and cGMP.[57] Finally, there may be decreased thromboxane A_2 production – a potent inducer of platelet aggregation.[58]

- Endothelial cells may show alterations in prostacyclin (PGI_2) release.[59]

- Increased nitric oxide (NO) production by endothelial cells which leads to platelet dysfunction.[60]

- Increased fibrinolysis. Antiplasmin complexes, fibrinogen and fibrin degradation products are significantly increased in patients with renal failure and the activity of plasminogen activator inhibitor is slightly reduced, denoting an activation of fibrinolysis.[56]

- Drugs. The half-life of heparin is increased in patients with renal failure and its effects following hemodialysis may persist for some time. It should be remembered that patients with renal disease are often on a number of drugs that may interfere with coagulation and this emphasizes the careful drug history that should be taken in any patient with a bleeding history.

The cause of many of these problems is unclear but may in part be related to the failure to remove so called 'middle molecules' (0.5–3 kDa)' which accumulate in renal failure (e.g. guanidinosuccinic acid, phenols). Such molecules are more efficiently removed by peritoneal dialysis than hemodialysis and this may explain the reduced incidence of bleeding problems observed in patients undergoing peritoneal dialysis. However, dialysis may only partially correct the prolonged bleeding time and abnormal platelet function seen in uremia and even these partial corrections may not be achieved in some patients. Recent work has shown that the breakdown products of fibrinogen containing the RGD (Arg-Gly-Asp) amino acid sequence accumulate in the plasma of patients with renal failure. These low molecular weight products can inhibit platelet aggregation by binding to the GpIIb/IIIa receptors on the platelet membrane.[61]

Laboratory diagnosis

The bleeding time is frequently prolonged in patients with renal disease and uremia. Platelet aggregation tests are often abnormal but there is a poor correlation between the abnormality and the risk of bleeding. vWF multimer analysis may show a loss of the high molecular weight forms although the latter is not always a consistent finding. There is usually no specific clotting factor deficiency in renal disease unless there is some other coexisting disease process. However, the thrombin times and reptilase times may be prolonged in patients with renal disease due to an acquired dysfibrinogenemia arising from a low serum albumin.[62] However, these patients do not seem to be at risk of bleeding because of this and may actually be at increased risk of thrombosis due to increased platelet activation.

Treatment

Increasing the frequency of dialysis tends to shorten the bleeding time and reduce the bleeding symptoms in some, but not all, patients with renal failure. Correction of the anemia and raising the hematocrit by approximately 30% by transfusion of red cells or by the use of erythropoietin results in a reduction in the bleeding time and reduces the symptoms of bleeding.[63,64] Increasing the hematocrit by more than 30% may be associated with an increased risk of thrombosis.

The administration of cryoprecipitate which contains large amounts of the high molecular forms of vWF may correct the bleeding time and may be of value in patients with renal disease who are actively bleeding. The synthetic vasopressin derivative desmopressin or DDAVP has also been shown to be of value in patients with renal disease and works probably by increasing the release of high molecular weight vWF multimers from the Weible Pallade bodies.[65] The effects are rapid and usually persist for 3–4 h and sometimes as long as 8 h. However, patients exhibit tachyphylaxis with a reduction in the response to treatment. Finally, the use of conjugated estrogens has been shown to be of benefit in reducing the bleeding time and decreasing bleeding symptoms in patients with chronic renal disease. Intravenous estrogens given for 4–5 days cause detectable improvement in the bleeding time of most patients after 6 h, with the maximal improvement seen between the first and second week of treatment and with the effects persisting for 10–14 days.[66]

Similar effects have been observed with oral conjugated estrogens and with transdermal 17β-estradiol patches.[67]

Hemostatic defects associated with 'massive' blood transfusion

Massive blood transfusion is usually defined as the replacement of more than one blood volume in less than 24 h. However, most healthy individuals can cope with the replacement of up to 80% of their circulating blood volume with stored blood and suffer no hemostatic defects. Hemostatic defects usually arise when more than one blood volume is lost and replaced within 2 h. Blood is commonly separated into its component parts shortly after collection and only concentrated red cells are then available for transfusion. Transfusion of large amounts of concentated red cells without adequate replacement of clotting factors or platelets is likely to result in disordered hemostasis.

Similar problems occur when large amounts of colloid are infused. *In vitro* hemodilution with hydroxyethyl starch, gelatin or albumin leads to significant effects changes in coagulation when assessed by thrombo-elastography, with the most pronounced effects seen with hydroxyethyl starch.[68,69]

However, even when whole blood is administered there are a number of hemostatic defects that arise. Stored blood undergoes a progressive loss in factors V and VIII. After 24 h at 4°C there is a 50% loss in factor VIII activity and after 14 days there is a 50% loss in the activity of factor V. Platelets stored at 4°C rapidly lose activity and after 48 h they show virtually no activity. Massive hemorrhage particularly if associated with an underlying disease process such liver disease, sepsis or placental abruption may be associated with DIC, which exacerbates the bleeding tendency. Furthermore, the transfusion of large amounts of red cells in itself may precipitate DIC. Hemorrhage in advanced liver disease is common and such individuals often show increased systemic fibrinolysis. Bleeding secondary to the use of thrombolytic therapy is also well recognized and may occasionally be catastrophic. Finally, both hypothermia and hypocalcemia can occur as a complication of the rapid infusion of large amounts of cold blood that contains citrate as an anticoagulant.

Laboratory diagnosis

A prolongation of the prothrombin time, activated partial thromboplastin time and thrombin time, a reduction in circulating fibrinogen and a reduction in the platelet count are common features of massive blood transfusion.

FDPs and D-dimer may be raised and there may be other evidence of systemic fibrinolysis, for example shortened ELT. The TEG is very useful in monitoring patients who receive large amounts of blood as it allows a relatively rapid global and dynamic assessment of blood coagulation.

Treatment

The treatment of the coagulopathy arising from massive blood transfusion is dictated by the results of laboratory tests. Individuals with a prolonged PT and APTT (usually greater than 1.5 × control values) but only a borderline reduction in fibrinogen benefit from the use of fresh-frozen plasma. If there is a significant fall in fibrinogen (< 0.5 g/l) then fibrinogen replacement is indicated most frequently with cryoprecipitate but occasionally with fibrinogen concentrates. If the platelet count falls below $75 \times 10^9/l$, then platelet concentrates should be given to restore levels.

A unit of fresh frozen plasma takes 15–20 min to thaw and its infusion results in an increase in each of the coagulation factors of about 5%. A unit of cryoprecipitate takes 10–15 min to thaw and an infusion of 10–15 bags will raise the fibrinogen level in the plasma by approximately 0.5–1 g/l in a 70-kg adult.

Guidelines have been developed that suggest for every 8–10 units of red cells transfused, one pool of platelets (from five to six donors) and two units of fresh-frozen plasma should be administered. However, such empirical approaches whilst of value should not remove the necessity for regular clotting tests.

In some individuals, hemorrhage cannot be arrested despite adequate clotting factor replacement. In some cases there may a surgical cause for this and this should be pursued. The use of DDAVP is probably of little value as such patients are already stressed and as a result have elevated vWF levels. The use of prothrombin complex concentrates are best avoided in this group of patients because of the potential thrombotic risks associated with their use. In individuals in whom the bleeding cannot be arrested, there have been some encouraging reports of successful treatment with recombinant factor VIIa (rVIIa).[70]

Hemostatic defects associated with the use of extracorporal circuits

Patients undergoing cardiopulmonary bypass (CPB) develop a complex coagulopathy in part related to the bypass machine, in part to the various drugs that patients may receive during bypass and finally to their underlying illness. In some cases bleeding may be due to defective surgical hemostasis and such patients may require surgical re-exploration.

Clotting factor abnormalities

During CPB there is generation of kallikrein and depletion of kallikrein and factor XIIa inhibitors.[71] There are also some data that suggest activation of the XII-plasma kallikrein pathway occurs during CPB.[71] In addition, there is also some evidence to support thrombin generation via the tissue factor-factor VIIa route.[72]

Quantitative platelet abnormalities

The platelet count falls during CPB often as early as 5 min after institution of bypass. The platelet count may remain depressed for several days after the procedure. Hemodilution and platelet adhesion to synthetic surfaces are two primary contributors to CPB-induced thrombocytopenia. During CPB, blood dilution results from priming the circuit with either crystalloid or colloid solutions. The bleeding time is markedly prolonged in patients undergoing hypothermic CPB although it usually normalizes within 24 h following cessation of bypass.[73] The prolonged bleeding time does not correlate with the fall in platelet count suggesting that it is secondary to impaired platelet function.

Platelet activation

Circulation through an extracorporeal circuit causes transient morphologic changes in platelets that are consistent with primary aggregation and activation.[74] Hypothermia exacerbates this acquired platelet function defect. Platelets have been shown by scanning electron microscopy to adhere to the synthetic surfaces of the circuits. Fibrinogen, a potent cofactor in platelet aggregation, is readily adsorbed on to synthetic surfaces and together with small amounts of thrombin also present on such surfaces induces platelet aggregation. When platelets adhere to synthetic surfaces they are activated and the contents of the α-granules are released into the circulation. Plasma levels of β-TG (β-thromboglobulin) and platelet factor 4 (PF-4) are increased both during and immediately after CPB but return to normal with 24-h following cessation of bypass.[75]

Assays of thromboxane B_2 (TxB_2), the major metabolites of thromboxane A_2, in blood shed from the site of surgery are markedly increased soon after institution of CPB in contrast to plasma levels that show a decrease.[76] Changes in 6-keto-prostaglandin F1α, the major metabolite of prostacyclin (PGI_2) are generally the opposite from TxB_2 and probably reflect changes in plasma 6-keto-prostaglandin F1α.[75]

There is a loss of platelet membrane glycoproteins during CPB that can be demonstrated by the use of specific monoclonal antibodies.[77] This may occur because of receptor occupancy, or loss of receptors either by internalization or proteolysis. Platelets are also subject to significant physical trauma during CPB that can strip the glycoproteins from the surface of the platelet. A loss of platelet membrane glycoproteins results in decreased platelet adhesion and impaired fibrinogen binding.

Fibrinolytic activity

Fibrinolytic activity increases significantly both during and after CPB and this contributes to the increased risk of bleeding.[78] Increased fibrinolytic activity is observed shortly after heparinization and before the patient is started on bypass. Heparin appears to induce a risk of systemic plasmin activity that only improves after completion of CPB. The effect is induced by a fall in $α_2$-antiplasmin that is caused both by heparin and CPB.[78] Systemic plasmin levels return to normal immediately after cessation of CPB but $α_2$-antiplasmin may take several days before returning to normal values.

Levels of tissue plasminogen activator (t-PA) are increased during CPB and this suggests that CPB is a stimulus to the release of t-PA from the vascular bed. It is probable that tissue damage may also contribute to this effect.[79] Plasminogen and antithrombin (III) also fall during CPB and remain depressed for 2–3 days postoperatively.[80] Increased fibrinolysis in patients undergoing CPB may also contribute to the acquired platelet abnormality.[81]

Hypothermia has also been shown in animal experiments to induce activation of the fibrinolytic pathway and may, therefore, increase the systemic fibrinolytic activity associated with CPB.[82]

Drugs

Anticoagulation with heparin is fundamental to CPB. Heparin is administered before CPB is commenced as an IV bolus dose usually 250–300 U/kg and its effect during bypass is monitored by means of the activated clotting time (ACT). At the end of CPB, the heparin is reversed with protamine, given in incremental doses until the ACT returns to normal. Protamine must be administered slowly because of its frequent adverse hemodynamic effects, including severe pulmonary hypertension and peripheral vascular collapse.[83,84] This seems to be particularly common in patients who have been previously exposed to protamine, for example diabetics treated with protamine-containing insulin and who subsequently develop IgG or IgE antiprotamine antibodies.

Protamine has been shown to induce complement activation and the severity of this activation correlates with subsequent hemodynamic disturbance. Whilst the anticoagulant effect of heparin mediated through its action on antithrombin may be reversed by protamine, its effects upon fibrinolysis and platelets is not and this may contribute to the bleeding observed following CPB. In addition, increased bleeding after CPB may occur due to 'heparin rebound'.[85–87] This arises for a variety of reasons including: (1) release of heparin from protamine–heparin complexes; (2) the movement of cold heparin-containing extracellular fluid into the periphery following post-operative rewarming; and (3) replacement of antithrombin in plasma, which facilities the anticoagulant action of heparin. Heparin may also bind to the synthetic surfaces of the CPB circuit, activating platelets on the surface and contributing to the platelet dysfunction.

Acquired inhibitors

The use of topical bovine thrombin in patients undergoing cardiothoracic surgery is common and the use of such agents has been associated with the development of factor V inhibitors.[88–90] The mechanism is believed to be the development of an antibody directed against the bovine factor V molecule but which is capable of cross-reacting with human factor V resulting in its rapid clearance from the plasma.

Disseminated intravascular coagulation (DIC)

DIC may occasionally complicate patients undergoing CPB. Its pathophysiology is complex and likely to reflect both the release of various procoagulant proteins during the actual surgery and the activation of coagulation by its passage through the bypass machine

Laboratory monitoring

Preoperative screening tests suggestive of a previously undiagnosed bleeding disorder are of little value in predicting those patients who are likely to develop significant postoperative bleeding. A personal and family history of a bleeding disorder and a comprehensive drug history are essential before any form of major surgery. Almost all laboratory tests are abnormal both during and immediately after CPB due to the effects of CPB on coagulation and platelets and the use of heparin to anticoagulate the patient. In the bleeding patient, laboratory tests including the PT, APTT, fibrinogen and platelet count should be performed. However, there is often a delay in obtaining the results of these tests and a more global assessment of hemostasis such as that obtained with the TEG may be of value.[91] The TEG also provides a rapid method for screening for the presence of heparin (by the use of heparinase-treated cups) and also provides a relatively simple method for assessing fibrinolysis, something that is otherwise difficult to perform.

Treatment

Platelet transfusions are often empirically given to patients during or at the end of CPB on the basis of the thrombocytopenia and acquired platelet defects that are seen in such patients. Aprotinin, a basic polypeptide of bovine origin is a broad-spectrum serine protease inhibitor that inhibits trypsin, kallikrein and plasmin. A regime employing aprotinin has been shown to reduce blood loss in patients undergoing cardiac surgery by 80%, in addition to shortening operating times.[92,93] Although aprotinin appears to relatively safe, there are theoretical concerns that it may increase the risk of thrombosis and it should, therefore, be used with caution and perhaps be reserved for patients undergoing high-risk cardiac surgery where excessive blood loss might be expected. Fresh-frozen plasma and cryoprecipitate should be used to correct prolongation of the PT, APTT and reductions in fibrinogen concentration. Finally, in patients in whom the presence of heparin is demonstrated the use of small amounts of protamine to neutralize the heparin may be appropriate. Similarly, where excessive fibrinolysis is demonstrated the use of aprotinin may be of value in suppressing this and controlling excessive bleeding.[93]

Disseminated intravascular coagulation (DIC)

DIC is a pathologic process in which there is systemic activation of coagulation through a number of triggering processes resulting in widespread fibrin deposition within the vascular tree. The activation of coagulation can result in the formation of microthrombi and the consumption of both platelets and clotting factors. Whilst the hemorrhage complications of DIC may be treatable, it is often the irreversible end-organ damage secondary to the microvascular thrombosis that leads to the morbidity and mortality. DIC is always secondary to some process although the disorders that may be associated with DIC are diverse (Table 28.3).

Four major pathways can lead to the development of DIC:

1. Tissue injury. Tissue damage following, for example, trauma surgery, malignancy or some obstetric complication[94–97] results in the release of procoagulant material into the circulation which results in the direct activation of the coagulation cascade.
2. Endothelial cell damage. Damage to endothelial cells changes the physiologic properties of the endothelium, exposing collagen and making it intensely procoagulant. Such damage is commonly seen in immune-mediated causes of DIC, in association with various infections and some metabolic disorders.
3. Platelet/monocyte activation. Direct platelet activation leading to intravascular platelet microaggregates can lead to the development of DIC. This is seen in association with some infections[98–101] and in some patients with circulating immune complexes.
4. Abnormal activators of coagulation. These are found in association with malignant disease,[102–104] pancreatitis[105] and some snake venoms.[106,107]

Activation of coagulation through any of the above trigger mechanisms leads to excess thrombin generation, platelet activation and the formation of microthrombi within the circulation. However, post-mortem data show microthrombi in only 65–75% of patients with documented DIC. It is probable these microthrombi are removed by the fibrinolytic system or that their formation is limited particularly in patients with hypofibrinogenemia as a consequence of their DIC. In patients who develop microthrombi these occulude the microcirculation leading to organ and tissue damage.

In the later stages of DIC, consumption of clotting factors and platelets as well as the effects of fibrinolysis may result in uncontrolled bleeding. Increased fibrinolytic activity is an inevitable consequence of intravascular thrombin formation. Continued activation of the coagulation cascade results in increased thrombomodulin expression on the surface of endothelial cells which, together with thrombin, leads to the activation of protein C. Activated protein C leads to inactivation of factor Va

Table 28.3 Disorders associated with the development of disseminated intravascular coagulation (DIC)

Infections
Bacterial
Viral
Protozoal
Toxic shock syndrome

Malignancies
Solid tumors
Acute leukemias (M3)
Tumor lysis syndrome

Tissue damage
Physical trauma
Burns
Surgery
Hepatic necrosis
Snake bites
Ischemia/Infarction
Rhabdomyolysis

Vascular/circulatory disorders
Giant hemangiomas/vascular tumors
Major vascular surgery
Malignant hypertension
Cardiopulmonary bypass
Vasculitis

Immunological disorders
Anaphylaxis
Allergic reactions
Transfusion reactions
Heparin-associated thrombocytopenia
Transplant rejection

Direct activation of coagulation
Snake bites
Pancreatitis

Pregnancy-related complications
Placental abruption
Amniotic fluid embolism
Pre-eclampsia/eclampsia
Hydatidiform mole
Dead fetus
Missed abortion
Septic abortion

Miscellaneous
Prothrombin complex concentrates
Hemolytic uremic syndrome
Homozygous protein C or S deficiency
Adult respiratory distress syndrome

and VIIIa, further increasing the bleeding tendency. Activated protein C also leads to inhibition of PAI-1 (Plasminogen Activator Inhibitor Type 1), the major intravascular inhibitor of t-PA, thereby stimulating fibrinolysis. Damage to endothelial cells results in increased release of t-PA, further stimulating fibrinolysis. In the latter stages of DIC, the natural anticoagulants including antithrombin and protein C are depleted. Depletion of protein C seems particularly severe in patients with DIC secondary to meningococcal septicemia.[108]

Laboratory diagnosis of DIC

The diagnosis of DIC is usually made using laboratory tests that measure platelet consumption, the consumption of various clotting factors and increased fibrinolysis. The tests that are most frequently abnormal in DIC are:

- platelet count
- fibrin(ogen) degradation products (FDPs)
- prothrombin time
- activated partial thromboplastin time
- thrombin time
- fibrinogen concentration.

The precise pattern of abnormalities is dependent upon the triggering mechanism responsible for the development of DIC. The platelet count is frequently reduced in DIC and is particularly low in patients with DIC secondary to sepsis. Examination of the blood film in cases of DIC may show the presence of fragmented red cells although if these are present in high concentration, then the possibility of a microangiopathic hemolytic anemia (MAHA) should be considered. Increased fibrinolytic activity results in an increase in the levels of circulating fibrin complexes and FDPs. However, some patients with severe DIC have no elevation in FDPs and such patients tend to have a poor prognosis.

In the early stages of DIC and before the consumptive coagulopathy is established, sensitive markers of coagulation or of fibrinolysis, for example activation peptides or enzyme-inhibitor complexes, may be useful. However, such tests are not widely available, are time-consuming to perform and are often performed retrospectively and so fail to provide the clinician with potentially useful information.

Clinical evaluation of patients with acute DIC

Patients with established DIC have features reflecting the tissue/organ damage secondary to the formation of microvascular thrombi and a severe bleeding diathesis secondary to the consumption of clotting factors and platelets.

Signs of thrombi in the microcirculation include: (1) the development of digital ischemia and gangrene; (2) adult respiratory distress syndrome (ARDS); (3) neurological signs including confusion, fits and coma; (4) intravascular hemolysis; and (5) deteriorating renal function and renal failure. Signs of bleeding include oozing from venepuncture sites, the development of petechiae, purpura and hematomas, hematuria, intracranial bleeding, gastrointestinal hemorrhage, pulmonary hemorrhage and epistaxes.

Management of acute DIC

The management of acute DIC is controversial. The aims of therapy are to treat the underlying trigger mechanism and to control the coagulation defect to arrest hemorrhage. In patients who are actively bleeding, rapid infusion of fluid is required to maintain the intravascular volume. Specific clotting factors should be administered to correct the clotting defect. Fresh frozen plasma contains all the coagulation factors and the inhibitiors of coagulation but in individuals who are severely deficient in fibrinogen (<0.5 g/l) the administration of fibrinogen concentrates or cryoprecipitate may be required. Platelet infusions should be administered to correct the thrombocytopenia. Some cases of DIC are associated with dramatic falls in protein C and/or antithrombin. In such situations supplementation with protein C or antithrombin concentrates may be beneficial.[108–110] The use of heparin in DIC is controversial and should probably be reserved for cases in which there is a poor clinical response to conventional treatment. The use of prothrombin complex concentrates that contain factors II, VII, IX and X is contraindicated in DIC because such concentrates contain activated clotting factors which may potentate the intravascular thrombosis.[49] The use of antifibrinolytic agents again is unwise in the majority of patients with DIC but may be of value in patients with primary hyperfibrinolysis.

Chronic DIC

This condition is occasionally seen in women in whom there has been an intrauterine death and there is tissue injury/necrosis with the release of tissue factor into the circulation. The disorder is also seen in patients with an underlying malignancy and this probably accounts for the majority of cases of chronic DIC. Liver disease may also be associated with the development of chronic DIC. Some patients with vascular malformations, for example Kasabach Merrit syndrome, a benign tumor in which there is a convoluted mass of vascular channels which consumes platelets and clotting factors, may also develop chronic DIC.[111–113] In some patients with aortic aneurysms,[114,115] or renal disease and some cases of ARDS there may also be chronic localized DIC in which consumption of clotting factors is strictly defined.

Laboratory tests in cases of chronic, localized DIC show a reduction in the platelet count, a normal or prolonged PT and APTT and a reduction in fibrinogen concentration. D-dimer levels and FDPs are usually raised. Clinically, the management of patients with chronic DIC involves treatment of the underlying disorder. This may be removal of a dead fetus in cases of intrauterine death, or the surgical repair of an aortic aneurysm. Some benign vascular malformations respond to treatment with anti-coagulants such as heparin or occasionally steroids.

Acquired hyperfibrinolysis

This unusual disorder occurs as a consequence of in-appropriate of excessive activation of fibrinolysis or a decrease in the inhibitors of fibrinolysis and results in an increased risk of hemorrhage. Acquired hyperfibrinolysis can arise for a number of reasons:

- increased release into the circulation of plasminogen activators, e.g. in prostatic carcinoma[116]
- defective clearance of activators, e.g. liver disease[117]
- secondary to thrombolytic therapy[18]
- localized systemic release of activator, e.g. prostatectomy[116]
- defective inhibition of fibrinolysis, e.g. liver disease, DIC, congenital or acquired α_2-antiplasmin deficiency[118]

Laboratory investigation of systemic hyperfibrinolysis

The platelet count in acquired hyperfibrinolysis is usually normal unless this is accompanied by DIC, in which cases the platelet count may be low. The D-dimer level is frequently normal because the lysis is primarily of fibrinogen rather that cross-linked fibrin. However, the D-dimers may be elevated if the hyperfibrinolysis is secondary to DIC. Markers of fibrinolysis such as the ELT, the fibrin plate lysis test and the TEG are abnormal, reflecting the underlying hyperfibrinolytic state. Alpha 2-antiplasmin levels are often reduced.

Management of systemic hyperfibrinolysis

Patients with hyperfibrinolysis and who are bleeding should be managed by correcting the underlying disorder wherever possible. Correction of the depleted inhibitors, for example PAI-1 and α_2-antiplasmin, requires the ad-ministration of fresh-frozen plasma and cryoprecipitate. In cases in which there is no evidence of DIC, the admin-istration of fibrinolytic inhibitors may be of value.

Bleeding and malignancy

In general, bleeding associated with malignancy is often secondary to DIC, liver disease, the effects of treatment and very occasionally to the development of specific clotting factor inhibitors.[103,119–122] Many tumors can activate coagulation and fibrinolysis to facilitate their spread.[103] Tumors also appear to stimulate the release of various cytokines including IL-1 and tumor necrosis factor (TNF), stimulating monocytes and macrophages to increase the expression of tissue factor and thereby initiating coagulation. Hemorrhage as a consequence of DIC in patients with malignancy is rarely a problem unless the platelet count is less that $50 \times 10^9/l$ or the fibrinogen concentration less than 0.5 g/l. High concen-trations of fibrin degradation products may impair platelet function and fibrin polymerization.

Hyperfibrinolysis in patients with malignancy is uncommon although it has been reported in patients with prostatic carcinoma. However, several studies have shown that hyperfibrinolysis is not a consistent feature of prostatic carcinoma.[123–125]

Acute leukemias

DIC can complicate many types of acute leukemia both lymphoblastic and myeloblastic[126] although it is particu-larly well described with acute promyelocytic leukemia – the FAB M3 variant. Some recent data have shown that in acute promyelocytic leukemia the leukemic cells express abnormally high levels of annexin II.[127] Such cells expressing annexin II appear to stimulate the generation of cell-surface t-PA dependent plasmin twice as efficiently as non-leukemic cells. Over-expression of annexin II leading to hyperfibrinolysis may be a mechanism for the hemorrhagic complications of acute promyelocytic leukemia. Replacement of clotting factors with fresh-frozen plasma and cryoprecipitate and the transfusion of platelets is of value and there are some reports of the successful use of low-dose heparin in such patients.

L-aspariginase is commonly used in the treatment of acute lymphoblastic leukemia (ALL) and whilst it more frequently is associated with thrombotic complications (through its effects on antithrombin, protein C and S) it can occasionally cause a bleeding tendency by inhibiting the synthesis of various clotting factors.[128,129]

Myeloproliferative disorders

The myeloproliferative disorders are a group of diseases that include polycythemia rubra vera (PRV), chronic myeloid leukemia (CML), essential thrombocythemia (ET) and myelofibrosis. Thrombocytopenia may occur in such patients either as a consequence of bone marrow replacement/failure or secondary to chemotherapy. A wide variety of acquired platelet defects have been described in patients with myeloproliferative disorders.[130-136] However, the results of platelet aggregation studies are variable, although there is often a lack of aggregation in response to adrenaline.[135] A number of studies have shown specific loss of platelet membrane glycoproteins – llb/llla and occasionally Gplb.[137,138] Myeloproliferative disorders can also be associated with an acquired platelet storage-pool deficiency and both dense body and α-granule deficiency have been reported.[139] Acquired von Willebrand's disease (vWD) has also been associated with the myeloproliferative disorders. Multimeric analysis in such patients usually shows a loss of the high molecular weight forms of the protein and there is a disproportionate decrease in ristocetin cofactor activity resembling type 2A vWD.[140]

Despite these many abnormalities it is difficult to predict or to identify which patients with a myeloproliferative disorder are at risk of bleeding and which are at risk of thrombosis.

Paraproteinemias

Patients with paraproteinemias such as myeloma or Waldenström's macroglobulinemia often have an abnormal clotting profile although bleeding is relatively uncommon. A variety of abnormalities have been described and these usually reflect the effect the abnormal paraprotein has on platelet and/or clotting factor function.[141-143] Occasionally, patients with myeloma can develop a circulating heparin-like anticoagulant which can result in a severe, unrelenting bleeding that is often fatal.[144-146] Chemotherapy to reduce the tumor mass, plasmaphoresis to remove the anticoagulant and protamine sulfate to neutralize the anticoagulant have all been used with varying success.

Amyloidosis may on occasion be associated with the development of selective factor X deficiency.[147-151] The mechanisms for this are unclear but it is believed that the factor X is adsorbed from plasma on to the amyloid deposits. Such patients, particularly when the factor X levels is low (< 10%), can be difficult to treat and show a poor response to treatment. The administration of factor X is of little benefit as the protein is rapidly removed from the circulation. Splenectomy may be of value in some cases.[152]

Acquired inhibitors of coagulation

Acquired inhibitors of coagulation are antibodies directed against various coagulation factors which rapidly neutralize their procoagulant activity and result in a bleeding diathesis or an increase in severity of a pre-existing coagulation disorder. Such antibodies may occur in response to treatment in patients with an inherited coagulation disorder, for example hemophilia A or B (alloantibodies) or develop as autoantibodies in individuals with or without an underlying immune disorder.

The most frequent spontaneous inhibitors or antibodies are directed against the factor VIII molecule, have an equal sex incidence and occur primarily in the elderly (after the seventh decade of life). Less frequently, they develop in post-partum women.[153-155] Other conditions that are associated with an increase risk of inhibitor formation include solid tumors, lymphoproliferative disorders, systemic lupus erythematosus (SLE) and rheumatoid arthritis.

The frequency of inhibitors directed against other clotting factors is much less. Factor V inhibitors are rare but occasionally seen following the use of bovine clotting factors or the use of β-lactam antibiotics.[88,156-158] In the case of factor V inhibitors that arise following the use of bovine clotting factors it is believed that an antibody develops to the bovine factor V that cross-reacts with the human factor V. Inhibitors directed against factor II (prothrombin) have been reported in association with SLE, liver cirrhosis and some patients with prosthetic cardiac valves. Factor VII inhibitors in the absence of factor VII deficiency are rare but occasionally seen in patients with an underlying tumor, in some patients with myeloma, chronic lymphocytic leukemia and non-Hodgkin's lymphoma.[159,160] In myeloma the inhibitors frequently resolve as the disease is treated. Inhibitors to factor XIII have been reported in SLE, in association with monoclonal gammopathies and in some patients receiving Isoniazid.

Acquired heparin-like anticoagulants have been described in some patients with myeloma and various solid tumors.[144] The inhibitors behave as glycosaminoglycans and may be neutralized by protamine sulfate or heparinase.

Laboratory findings in acquired inhibitors

The laboratory findings in patients with an acquired inhibitor depend upon which clotting factor the antibody is directed against. In patients with an acquired factor VIII inhibitor, the prothrombin time is normal but the APTT is grossly prolonged and fails to correct in a mix with normal plasma. Assay of factor VIII coagulant activity is reduced and factor VIII inhibitors are present.

The inhibitor in a patient with an acquired factor VIII deficiency is complex and the linear relationship between inhibitor concentration and the amount of factor VIII inhibited observed in hemophilia A patients who develop inhibitors is not seen.

Management of acquired inhibitors

The management of patients who develop an acquired coagulation factor inhibitor is complex. In patients who are not actively bleeding no treatment may be required. However, any potential cause for the development of the inhibitor should be sought and wherever possible treated.

In patients who develop acquired factor VIII inhibitors and who show no cross-reactivity with porcine-derived factor VIII then treatment with porcine clotting factor concentrates may be life-saving. However, many patients show significant cross-reacting antibodies and in such cases the use of FEIBA (Factor Eight Inhibitor Bypassing Activity) or other activated prothrombin complex concentrates (APCCs) may be of value. More recently, the use of a recombinant form of activated factor VII (rVIIA) has proved to be very useful in such cases. Treatment is often combined with immunosuppressive therapy including steroids, intravenous IgG and in some cases cyclophosphamide. In life-threatening cases that do not improve with other treatment modalities, removal of the inhibitor by means of a protein A separose column may be of value.

Toxic coagulopathies

A number of agents may be associated with acquired hemostatic defect leading to a bleeding disorder (see Table 28.4).[161] Frequently, these agents manifest their effects by a DIC-like syndrome.

- Snake venoms. A number of snake venoms cause activation of the coagulation cascade and indeed some of these venoms are routinely used in hemostasis laboratories. Russell's viper (*Vipera russeli*) activates factor X directly and results in defibrination and secondary fibrinolysis. The venom from this snake forms the basis of one of the screening tests for a lupus anticoagulant. The venom from the saw-scaled viper (*Echis carinatus*) activates prothrombin directly and is used both in monitoring of patients receiving hirudin but also as a screening test for lupus anticoagulants.

Table 28.4 Toxin-induced coagulopathies

Animal/toxin	Mechanism of action
Snake	
Bothrops jararaca	Factor X activation
Vipera russelli	Activation of factor X
	Defibrination
	Hyperfibrinolysis
Crotalus atrox	Fibrinogenase
Echis carinatus	Prothrombin activator
Crotalus adamanteus	Cleavage and release of FpA
	(Fibrinopeptide A)
	Secondary fibrinolysis
Caterpillar	
Lonoma achelous	Hypofibrinogenemia
	Low factors XIII and V
Miscellaneous	
IL-2	DIC-like syndrome with
	systemic hyperfibrinolysis

DIC, disseminated intravascular coagulation.

- Caterpillar. *Lonoma achelous* is a caterpillar with a particular toxic saliva that induces hypofibrinogenemia together with low levels of factors V and XIII. Fibrin degradation products are increased and plasminogen is decreased.[162–164]
- Pharmacologic agents, for example interleukin-2 (IL-2) when used at high concentration can induce a DIC-like syndrome with systemic hyperfibrinolysis.[165]

REFERENCES

1. Andrew M, Paes B, Milner R et al 1988 Development of the human coagulation system in the healthy premature infant. Blood 72(5): 1651–1657
2. Andrew M, Vegh P, Johnston M et al 1992 Maturation of the hemostatic system during childhood. Blood 80(8): 1998–2005
3. Sattler FR, Weitekamp MR, Sayegh A, Ballard JO 1988 Impaired hemostasis caused by beta-lactam antibiotics. American Journal of Surgery 155(5A): 30–39
4. Perry DJ 1994 Antithrombin and its inherited deficiencies. Blood Reviews 8: 37–55
5. Amiral J, Meyer D 1998 Heparin-induced thrombocytopenia: diagnostic tests and biological mechanisms. Baillière's Clinical Haematology 11(2): 447–460
6. Greinacher A 1998 Heparin-induced thrombocytopenia: pathophysiology and clinical concerns. Baillière's Clinical Haematology 11(2): 461–474
7. Barrowcliffe TW 1995 Low molecular weight heparin(s). British Journal of Haematology 90(1): 1–7
8. Thomas DP 1997 Does low molecular weight heparin cause less bleeding? Thrombosis and Haemostasis 78(6): 1422–1425
9. Hubbard AR, Jennings CA 1985 Neutralisation of heparan sulphate and low molecular weight heparin by protamine. Thrombosis and Haemostasis 53(1): 86–89
10. Kaiser B 1991 Anticoagulant and antithrombotic actions of recombinant hirudin. Seminars in Thrombosis and Haemostasis 17(2): 130–136
11. Bichler J, Fritz H 1991 Hirudin, a new therapeutic tool? Annals of Hematology 63(2): 67–76
12. Potzsch B, Hund S, Madlener K et al 1997 Monitoring of recombinant hirudin: assessment of a plasma-based ecarin clotting time assay. Thrombosis Research 86(5): 373–383
13. Hull R, Hirsh J, Jay R et al 1982 Different intensities of oral anticoagulant therapy in the treatment of proximal-vein thrombosis. New England Journal of Medicine 307(27): 1676–1681

14. Panneerselvam S, Baglin C, Lefort W, Baglin T 1998 Analysis of risk factors for over-anticoagulation in patients receiving long-term warfarin. British Journal of Haematology 103(2): 422–424

15. Landefeld CS, Goldman L 1989 Major bleeding in outpatients treated with warfarin. American Journal of Medicine 87: 144–152

16. Palareti G, Leali N, Coccheri S et al 1996 Bleeding complications of oral anticoagulant treatment: an inception-cohort, prospective collaborative study (ISCOAT). Italian Study on Complications of Oral Anticoagulant Therapy. Lancet 348(9025): 423–428

17. Makris M, Greaves M, Phillips WS et al 1997 Emergency oral anticoagulant reversal: the relative efficacy of infusions of fresh frozen plasma and clotting factor concentrate on correction of the coagulopathy. Thrombosis and Haemostasis 77(3): 477–480

18. Ludlam CA, Bennett B, Fox KA 1995 Guidelines for the use of thrombolytic therapy. Haemostasis and Thrombosis Task Force of the British Committee for Standards in Haematology. Blood Coagulation and Fibrinolysis 6(3): 273–285

19. Bonnefoy A, Legrand C 2000 Proteolysis of subendothelial adhesive glycoproteins (fibronectin, thrombospondin, and von Willebrand factor) by plasmin, leukocyte cathepsin G, and elastase. Thrombosis Research 98(4): 323–332

20. Vane JR, Botting RM 1998 Anti-inflammatory drugs and their mechanism of action. Inflammatory Research 47(suppl 2): S78–87

21. Fitzgerald G 1987 Dipyridamole. The New England Journal of Medicine 316: 1247–1257

22. Easton JD 1999 Clinical aspects of the use of clopidogrel, a new antiplatelet agent. Circulation 100(15): 1667–1672

23. Quinn MJ, Fitzgerald DJ 1999 Clopidogrel and ticlopidine – improvements on aspirin Drugs and Therapeutic Bulletin 37(8): 59–61

24. Nurden AT, Poujol C, Durrieu-Jais C, Nurden P 1999 Platelet glycoprotein llb/llla inhibitors: basic and clinical aspects. Arteriosclerosis, Thrombosis and Vascular Biology 19(12): 2835–2840

25. Brown CH, Natelson EA, Bradshaw MW 1974 The haemostatic defect produced by carbenicillin. The New England Journal of Medicine 291: 265–270

26. Burroughs SF, Johnbson GJ 1990 β-lactam antibiotic-induced platelet dysfunction: evidence for irreversible inhibition on platelet activation *in vitro* and *in vivo* are prolonged exposure to penicillin. Blood 75: 1473–1480

27. Shearer MJ 1988 Mechanism of cephalosporin-induced hypoprothrombinemia: Relation of cephalosporin side chain, vitamin K metabolism and vitamin K status. Journal of Clinical Pharmacology 28: 88–95

28. Loiseau P 1981 Sodium valproate, platelet dysfunction, and bleeding. Epilepsia 22(2): 141–146

29. Weiss HJ 1967 The effect of clinical dextran on platelet aggregation, adhesion and ADP release in man: *in vivo* and *in vitro* studies. Journal of Laboratory and Clinical Medicine 69: 37–46

30. Kerenyi A, Schlammadinger A, Ajzner E et al 1999 Comparison of PFA-100 closure time and template bleeding time of patients with inherited disorders causing defective platelet function. Thrombosis Research 96(6): 487–492

31. Mammen EF, Comp PC, Gosselin R et al 1998 PFA-100 system: a new method for assessment of platelet dysfunction. Seminars in Thrombosis and Haemostasis 24(2): 195–202

32. Harrison P, Robinson MS, Mackie IJ et al 1999 Performance of the platelet function analyser PFA-100 in testing abnormalities of primary haemostasis. Blood Coagulation and Fibrinolysis 10(1): 25–31

33. Zipursky A 1999 Prevention of vitamin K deficiency bleeding in newborns. British Journal of Haematology 104(3): 430–437

34. von Kries R 1999 Oral versus intramuscular phytomenadione: safety and efficacy compared. Drug Safety 21(1): 1–6

35. Fujimura Y, Okubo Y, Sakai T et al 1984 Studies on precursor proteins PIVKA-II, -IX, and -X in the plasma of patients with 'hemorrhagic disease of the newborn'. Haemostasis 14(2): 211–217

36. Kohler M 1999 Thrombogenicity of prothrombin co plex concentrates. Thrombosis Research 95(4 suppl 1): S13–17

37. McKinney PA, Juszczak E, Findlay E, Smith K 1998 Which vitamin K preparation for the newborn? Case-control study of childhood leukaemia and cancer in Scotland: findings for neonatal intramuscular vitamin K. Drugs and Therapeutic Bulletin 36(3): 17–19

38. Jaffe EA 1973 Synthesis of antihemophilic factor antigen by cultured human endothelial cells. Journal of Clinical Investigation 52: 2757–2764

39. Dymock IW, Tucker JS, Woolf IL et al 1975 Coagulation studies as a prognostic index in acute liver failure. British Journal of Haematology 29(3): 385–395

40. Green G, Poller L, Thomson JM, Dymock IW 1976 Factor VII as a marker of hepatocellular synthetic function in liver disease. Journal of Clinical Pathology 29(11): 971–975

41. Nagamine T, Ohtuka T, Takehara K et al 1996 Thrombocytopenia associated with hepatitis C viral infection. Journal of Hepatology 24(2): 135–140

42. Martinez J, Palascak JE, Kwasniak D 1978 Abnormal sialic acid content of the dysfibrinogenemia associated with liver disease. Journal of Clinical Investigation 61(2): 535–538

43. Green G, Thomson JM, Dymock IW, Poller L 1976 Abnormal fibrin polymerization in liver disease. British Journal of Haematology 34(3): 427–439

44. Nakao A, Virji A, Iwaki Y et al 1991 Abnormal prothrombin (DES-gamma-carboxy prothrombin) in hepatocellular carcinoma. Hepatology and Gastroenterology 38(5): 450–453

45. Pernambuco JR, Langley PG, Hughes RD et al 1993 Activation of the fibrinolytic system in patients with fulminant liver failure. Hepatology 18(6): 1350–1356

46. Paramo JA, Rifon J, Fernandez J et al 1991 Thrombin activation and increased fibrinolysis in patients with chronic liver disease. Blood Coagulation and Fibrinolysis 2(2): 227–230

47. Patrassi GM, Sartori MT, Sgarabotto D et al 1988 A DIC-like picture on plasma and ascitic fluid of cirrhotic patients. Research in Experimental Medicine (Berlin) 188(5): 351–356

48. Tempero MA, Davis RB, Reed E, Edney J 1985 Thrombocytopenia and laboratory evidence of disseminated intravascular coagulation after shunts for ascites in malignant disease. Cancer 55(11): 2718–2721

49. Kohler M 1999 Thrombogenicity of prothrombin complex concentrates. Thrombosis Research 95(4 suppl 1): S13–17

50. Marassi A, Manzullo V, di Carlo V, Mannucci PM 1978 Thromboembolism following prothrombin complex concentrates and major surgery in severe liver disease. Thrombosis and Haemostasis 39(3): 787–788

51. Cattaneo M, Tenconi PM, Alberca I et al 1990 Subcutaneous desmopressin (DDAVP) shortens the prolonged bleeding time in patients with liver cirrhosis. Thrombosis and Haemostasis 64(3): 358–360

52. Michalak E, Walkowiak B, Paradowski M, Cierniewski CS 1991 The decreased circulating platelet mass and its relation to bleeding time in chronic renal failure. Thrombosis and Haemostasis 65(1): 11–14

53. Zachée P, Vermylen J, Boogaerts MA 1994 Hematological aspects of end-stage renal failure. Annals of Hematology 69: 33–40

54. Sloand EM, Sloand JA, Prodouz K et al 1991 Reduction of platelet glycoprotein Ib in uraemia. British Journal of Haematology 77(3): 375–381

55. Gralnick HR, McKeown LP, Williams SB et al 1988 Plasma and platelet von Willebrand factor defects in uremia. American Journal of Medicine 85(6): 806–810

56. Mezzano D, Tagle R, Panes O et al 1996 Hemostatic disorder of uremia: the platelet defect, main determinant of the prolonged bleeding time, is correlated with indices of activation of coagulation and fibrinolysis. Thrombosis and Haemostasis 76(3): 312–321

57. Vlachoyannis J, Schoeppe W 1982 Adenylate cyclase activity and cAMP content of human platelets in uraemia. European Journal of Clinical Investigation 12(5): 379–381

58. Smith MC, Dunn MJ 1981 Impaired platelet thromboxane production in renal failure. Nephron 29(3–4): 133–137

59. Remuzzi G, Cavenaghi AE, Mecca G 1977 Prostacyclin-like activity and bleeding in renal failure. Lancet 2: 1195–1197

60. Noris M, Benigni A, Boccardo P et al 1993 Enhanced nitric oxide synthesis in uremia: implications for platelet dysfunction and dialysis hypotension. Kidney International 44(2): 445–450

61. Walkowiak B, Michalak E, Borkowska E 1994 Concentration of RGDS-containing degradation products in uremic plasma is correlated with progression in renal failure. Thrombosis Research 76: 133–144

62. Gandrille S, Jouvin MH, Toulon P et al 1988 A study of fibrinogen and fibrinolysis in 10 adults with nephrotic syndrome. Thrombosis and Haemostasis 59(3): 445–450

63. Fabris F, Cordiano I, Randi ML et al 1991 Effect of human recombinant erythropoietin on bleeding time, platelet number and function in children with end-stage renal disease maintained by haemodialysis. Pediatric Nephrology 5(2): 225–228

64. Vigano G, Benigni A, Mendogni D et al 1991 Recombinant human erythropoietin to correct uremic bleeding. Acta anaesthesiologica Scandinavica 18(1): 44–49

65. Mannucci PM, Remuzzi G, Pusineri F et al 1983 Deamino-8-D-arginine vasopressin shortens the bleeding time in uremia. New England Journal of Medicine 308(1): 8–12

66. Livio M, Mannucci PM, Vigano G et al 1986 Conjugated estrogens for the management of bleeding associated with renal failure. New England Journal of Medicine 315(12): 731–735

67. Sloand JA, Schiff MJ 1995 Beneficial effect of low-dose transdermal estrogen on bleeding time and clinical bleeding in uremia. American Journal of Kidney Disease 26(1): 22–26

68. Petroianu GA, Liu J, Maleck WH et al 2000 The effect of *in vitro* hemodilution with gelatin, dextran, hydroxyethyl starch, or Ringer's solution on thrombelastograph. Anaesthesia and Analgesia 90(4): 795–800

69. Niemi TT, Kuitunen AH 1998 Hydroxyethyl starch impairs *in vitro* coagulation. Acta Anaesthesiologica Scandinavica 42(9): 1104–1109

70. Kenet G, Walden R, Eldad A, Martinowitz U 1999 Treatment of traumatic bleeding with recombinant factor VIIa. Lancet 354(9193): 1879

71. Wendel HP, Jones DW, Gallimore MJ 1999 FXII levels, FXIIa-like activities and kallikrein activities in normal subjects and patients undergoing cardiac surgery. Immunopharmacology 45(1–3): 141–144

72. Boisclair MD, Lane DA, Philippou H et al 1993 Mechanisms of thrombin generation during surgery and cardiopulmonary bypass. Blood 82(11): 3350–3357

73. Harker LA, Malpass TW, Branson HE 1980 Mechanism of abnormal bleeding in individuals undergoing cardiopulmonary bypass: acquired transient platelet dysfunction associated with selective α-granule release. Blood 56: 824–834

74. Rinder CS, Bohnert J, Rinder HM et al 1991 Platelet activation and aggregation during cardiopulmonary bypass. Anesthesiology 75(3): 388–393

75. Khuri SF, Wolfe JA, Josa M 1993 Hematologic changes during and after cardiopulmonary bypass and their relationship to the bleeding time and nonsurgical blood loss. Journal of Thoracic and Cardiovascular Surgery 104: 94–107

76. Kestin AS, Valeri CR, Khuri SF et al 1993 The platelet function defect of cardiopulmonary bypass. Blood 82(1): 107–117

77. Kondo C, Tanaka K, Takagi K et al 1993 Platelet dysfunction during cardiopulmonary bypass surgery. With special reference to platelet membrane glycoproteins. American Society for Artificial Internal Organs Journal 39(3): M550–553

78. Ray MJ, Marsh NA, Hawson GA 1994 Relationship of fibrinolysis and platelet function to bleeding after cardiopulmonary bypass. Blood Coagulation and Fibrinolysis 5(5): 679–685

79. Valen G, Eriksson E, Risberg B, Vaage J 1994 Fibrinolysis during cardiac surgery. Release of tissue plasminogen activator in arterial and coronary sinus blood. European Journal of Cardiothoracic Surgery 8(6): 324–330

80. Despotis GJ, Levine V, Joist JH et al 1997 Antithrombin III during cardiac surgery: effect on response of activated clotting time to heparin and relationship to markers of hemostatic activation. Anaesthesia and Analgesia 85(3): 498–506

81. de Haan J, Schonberger J, Haan J et al 1993 Tissue-type plasminogen activator and fibrin monomers synergistically cause platelet dysfunction during retransfusion of shed blood after cardiopulmonary bypass. Journal of Thoracic and Cardiovascular Surgery 106(6): 1017–1023

82. Yoshihara H, Yamamoto T, Mihara H 1985 Changes in coagulation and fibrinolysis occurring in dogs during hypothermia. Thrombosis Research 37(4): 503–512

83. Weiss ME, Adkinson NF 1991 Allergy to protamine. Clinical Reviews in Allergy 9(3–4): 339–355

84. Kimmel SE, Sekeres MA, Berlin JA et al 1998 Adverse events after protamine administration in patients undergoing cardiopulmonary bypass: risks and predictors of under-reporting. Journal of Clinical Epidemiology 51(1): 1–10

85. Teoh KH, Young E, Bradley CA, Hirsh J 1993 Heparin binding proteins. Contribution to heparin rebound after cardiopulmonary bypass. Circulation 88(5 pt 2): 11420–11425

86. Martin P, Horkay F, Gupta NK et al 1992 Heparin rebound phenomenon – much ado about nothing? Blood Coagulation and Fibrinolysis 3(2): 187–191

87. Pifarre R, Babka R, Sullivan HJ et al 1981 Management of postoperative heparin rebound following cardiopulmonary bypass. Journal of Thoracic and Cardiovascular Surgery 81(3): 378–381

88. Zumberg MS, Waples JM, Kao KJ, Lottenberg R 2000 Management of a patient with a mechanical aortic value and antibodies to both thrombin and factor V after repeat exposure to fibrin sealant. American Journal of Hematology 64(1): 59–63

89. Berruyer M, Amiral J, Ffrench P et al 1993 Immunization by bovine thrombin used with fibrin glue during cardiovascular operations. Development of thrombin and factor V inhibitors. Journal of Thoracic and Cardiovascular Surgery 105(5): 892–897

90. Zehnder JL, Leung LL 1990 Development of antibodies to thrombin and factor V with recurrent bleeding in a patient exposed to topical bovine thrombin. Blood 76(10): 2011–2016

91. Tuman KJ, Spiess BD, McCarthy RJ, Ivankovich AD 1989 Comparison of viscoelastic measures of coagulation after cardiopulmonary bypass. Anaesthesia and Analgesia 69(1): 69–75

92. Lu H, Du Buit C, Soria J et al 1994 Postoperative hemostasis and fibrinolysis in patients undergoing cardiopulmonary bypass with or without aprotinin therapy. Thrombosis and Haemostasis 72(3): 438–443

93. Orchard MA, Goodchild CS, Prentice CR et al 1993 Aprotinin reduces cardiopulmonary bypass-induced blood loss and inhibits fibrinolysis without influencing platelets. British Journal of Haematology 85(3): 533–541

94. Steiner PE, Lushbaugh CC 1986 Maternal pulmonary embolism by amniotic fluid as a cause of obstetric shock and unexpected deaths in obstetrics. Journal of the American Medical Association 255(16): 2187–2203

95. Graeff H, Kuhn W 1980 Coagulation disorders in obstetrics. Major Problems in Obstetrics and Gynecology 13(1): 1–157

96. Graeff H, Hafter R, von Hugo R 1977 Molecular aspects of defibrination in a case of amniotic fluid embolism. Thrombosis and Haemostasis 38(3): 724–727

97. Bonnar J, McNicol GP, Douglas AS 1971 Coagulation and fibrinolytic systems in pre-eclampsia and eclampsia. British Medical Journal 2(752): 12–16

98. Abildgaard CF, Corrigan JJ, Seeler RA et al 1967 Meningococcemia associated with intravascular coagulation. Pediatrics 40(1): 78–83

99. Yoshikawa T, Tanaka KR, Guze LB 1971 Infection and disseminated intravascular coagulation. Medicine (Baltimore) 50(4): 237–258

100. Faust SN, Heyderman RS, Levin M 2000 Disseminated intravascular coagulation and purpura fulminans secondary to infection. Baillières Best Practice and Research Clinical Haematology 13(2): 179–197

101. Gikas A, Samonis G, Christidou A et al 1998 Gram-negative bacteremia in non-neutropenic patients: a 3-year review. Infection 26(3): 155–159

102. Higuchi T, Shimizu T, Mori H et al 1997 Coagulation patterns of disseminated intravascular coagulation in acute promyelocytic leukemia. Hematology Oncology 15(4): 209–217

103. Francis JL, Biggerstaff J, Amirkhosravi A 1998 Hemostasis and malignancy. Seminars in Thrombosis and Haemostasis 24(2): 93–109

104. Francis JL, Elbaruni K, Roath OS, Taylor I 1988 Factor x-activating activity in normal and malignant colorectal tissue. Thrombosis Research 52: 207–217

105. Lasson A, Ohlsson K 1986 Consumptive coagulopathy, fibrinolysis and protease-antiprotease interactions during acute human pancreatitis. Thrombosis Research 41(2): 167–83

106. Than T, Hutton RA, Myint L et al 1988 Haemostatic disturbances in patients bitten by Russell's viper (*Vipera russelli siamensis*) in Burma. British Journal of Haematology 69(4): 513–520

107. Hasiba U, Rosenbach LM, Rockwell D, Lewis JH 1975 DiC-like syndrome after envenomation by the snake, *Crotalus horridus horridus*. New England Journal of Medicine 292(10): 505–507

108. Smith OP, White B, Vaughan D et al 1997 Use of protein-C concentrate, heparin, and haemodiafiltration in meningococcus-induced purpura fulminans. Lancet 350(9091): 1590–1593

109. van Beek EJ, von der Mohlen MA, ten Cate JW et al 1994 Antithrombin III concentrate in the treatment of DIC: a retrospective follow-up study. Netherlands Journal of Medicine 45(5): 206–210

110. Balk R, Emerson T, Fourrier F et al 1998 Therapeutic use of antithrombin concentrate in sepsis. Seminars in Thrombosis and Haemostasis 24(2): 183–194

111. Hoak JC, Warner ED, Cheng HF et al 1971 Hemangioma with thrombocytopenia and microangiopathic anemia (Kasabach–Merritt syndrome): an animal model. Journal of Laboratory and Clinical Medicine 77(6): 941–950

112. Watzke HH, Linkesch W, Hay U 1989 Giant hemangioma of the liver (Kasabach–Merritt syndrome): successful suppression of intravascular coagulation permitting surgical removal. Journal of Clinical Gastroenterology 11(3): 347–350

113. White CW 1990 Treatment of hemangiomatosis with recombinant interferon alfa. Seminars in Hematology 27(3 Suppl 4): 15–22

114. Micallef EP, Ludlam CA 1991 Aortic aneurysms and consumptive coagulopathy. Blood Coagulation and Fibrinolysis 2(3): 477–481

115. Gibney EJ, Bouchier HD 1990 Coagulopathy and abdominal aortic paneurysm. European Journal of Vascular Surgery 4(6): 557–562

116. Okajima K, Kohno I, Tsuruta J et al 1992 Direct evidence for systemic fibrinogenolysis in a patient with metastatic prostatic cancer. Thrombosis Research 66(6): 717–727

117. Grosse H, Lobbes W, Frambach M et al 1991 The use of high dose aprotinin in liver transplantation: the influence on fibrinolysis and blood loss. Thrombosis Research 63(3): 287–297

118. Cofrancesco E, Pogliani E, Salvatore M et al 1989 Alpha-2 antiplasmin in acute nonlymphoblastic leukemia. Acta Haematologica 81(3): 122–125

119. Colman RW, Rubin RN 1990 Disseminated intravascular coagulation due to malignancy. Seminars in Oncology 17(2): 172–186

120. Bick RL 1992 Coagulation abnormalities in malignancy: a review. Seminars in Thrombosis and Haemostasis 18(4): 353–372

121. Kunkel LA 1992 Acquired circulating anticoagulants in malignancy. [Review]. Seminars in Thrombosis and Hemostasis 18(4): 416–423

122. Zacharski LR, Wojtukiewicz MZ, Costantini V et al 1992 Pathways of coagulation/fibrinolysis activation in malignancy. Seminars in Thrombosis and Haemostasis 18(1): 104–116

123. Geenen RW, Delaere KP, van Wersch JW 1997 Coagulation and fibrinolysis activation markers in prostatic carcinoma patients. European Journal of Clinical Chemistry and Clininical Biochemistry 35(2): 69–72

124. Bell CR, Cox DJ, Murdock PJ et al 1996 Thrombelastographic evaluation of coagulation in transurethral prostatectomy. British Journal of Urology 78(5): 737–741

125. de Campos Freire G, de Campos Pachelli L, Cordeiro P et al 1986 Blood loss during and following transurethral resection. Prostate 8(1): 87–92

126. Sletnes KE, Godal HC, Wisloff F 1995 Disseminated intravascular coagulation (DIC) in adult patients with acute leukaemia. European Journal of Haematology 54(1): 34–38

127. Menell JS, Cesarman GM, Jacovina AT et al 1999 Annexin II and bleeding in acute promyelocytic leukemia. New England Journal of Medicine 340(13): 994–1004

128. Priest JR, Ramsay NK, Latchaw RE et al 1980 Thrombotic and hemorrhagic strokes complicating early therapy for childhood acute lymphoblastic leukemia. Cancer 46(7): 1548–1554

129. Ramsay NK, Coccia PF, Krivit W et al 1977 The effect of L-asparaginase on plasma coagulation factors in acute lymphoblastic leukemia. Cancer 40(4): 1398–1401

130. Baker RI, Manoharan A 1988 Platelet function in myeloproliferative disorders: characterization and sequential studies show multiple platelet abnormalities, and change with time. European Journal of Haematology 40(3): 267–272

131. Boneu B, Nouvel C, Sie P et al 1980 Platelets in myeloproliferative disorders. I. A comparative evaluation with certain platelet function tests. Scandinavian Journal of Haematology 25(3): 214–220

132. Ginsburg AD 1975 Platelet function in patients with high platelet counts. Annals of Internal Medicine 82(4): 506–511

133. Holme S, Murphy S 1990 Platelet abnormalities in myeloproliferative disorders. Clinical and Laboratory Medicine 10(4): 873–888

134. Wehmeier A, Sudhoff T, Meierkord F 1997 Relation of platelet abnormalities to thrombosis and hemorrhage in chronic myeloproliferative disorders. Seminars in Thrombosis and Haemostasis 23(4): 391–402

135. Waddell CC, Brown JA, Repinecz YA 1981 Abnormal platelet function in myeloproliferative disorders. Archives of Pathology and Laboratory Medicine 105(8): 432–435

136. Vignal CV, Lourenco DM, Noguti MA et al 1997 Hemorrhagic and thrombotic complications in patients with myeloproliferative diseases. Revista Paulista de Medicina 115(6): 1575–1579

137. Jensen MK, de Nully Brown P, Lund BV et al 2000 Increased platelet activation and abnormal membrane glycoprotein content and redistribution in myeloproliferative disorders. British Journal of Haematology 110(1): 116–124

138. Mazzucato M, De Marco L, De Angelis V et al 1989 Platelet membrane abnormalities in myeloproliferative disorders: decrease in glycoproteins Ib and IIb/IIIa complex is associated with deficient receptor function. British Journal of Haematology 73(3): 369–374

139. Yamamoto K, Sekiguchi E, Takatani O 1984 Abnormalities of epinephrine-induced platelet aggregation and adenine nucleotides in myeloproliferative disorders. Thrombosis and Haemostasis 52(3): 292–296

140. Budde U, Dent JA, Berkowitz SD et al 1986 Subunit composition of plasma von Willebrand factor in patients with the myeloproliferative syndrome. Blood 68(6): 1213–1217

141. Silberstein LE, Abrahm J, Shattil SJ 1987 The efficacy of intensive plasma exchange in acquired von Willebrand's disease. Transfusion 27(3): 234–237

142. Endo T, Yatomi Y, Amemiya N et al 2000 Antibody studies of factor VIII inhibitor in a case with Waldenstrom's macroglobulinemia. American Journal of Hematology 63(3): 145–148

143. Krumdieck R, Shaw DR, Huang ST et al 1991 Hemorrhagic disorder due to an isoniazid-associated acquired factor XIII inhibitor in a patient with Waldenstrom's macroglobulinemia. American Journal of Medicine 90(5): 639–645

144. Tefferi A, Nichols WL, Bowie EJ 1990 Circulating heparin-like anticoagulants: report of five consecutive cases and a review. American Journal of Medicine 88(2): 184–188

145. Chapman GS, George CB, Danley DL 1985 Heparin-like anticoagulant associated with plasma cell myeloma. American Journal of Clinical Pathology 83(6): 764–766

146. Palmer RN, Rick ME, Rick PD et al 1984 Circulating heparan sulfate anticoagulant in a patient with a fatal bleeding disorder. New England Journal of Medicine 310(26): 1696–1699

147. Furie B, Greene E, Furie BC 1977 Syndrome of acquired factor X deficiency and systemic amyloidosis *in vivo* studies of the metabolic fate of factor X. New England Journal of Medicine 297(2): 81–85

148. Furie B, Voo L, McAdam K, Furie BC 1981 Mechanism of factor X deficiency in systemic amyloidosis. New England Journal of Medicine 304: 827–830

149. Girmann G, Wilker D, Stadie H, Scheurlen PG 1980 Acquired isolated factor X deficiency associated with systemic amyloidosis. Case report and review of literature. Klinische Wochenschrift 58: 859–862

150. Greipp PR, Kyle RA, Bowie EJ 1981 Factor-X deficiency in amyloidosis: a critical review. American Journal of Hematology 11(4): 443–450

151. Zeitler KD, Blatt PM 1982 Amyloidosis and factor X deficiency. South Medical Journal 75(3): 306–308

152. Greipp PR, Kyle RA, Bowie EW 1979 Factor X deficiency in primary amyloidosis. Resolution after splenectomy. New England Journal of Medicine 302: 1050–1051

153. Yee TT, Taher A, Pasi KJ, Lee CA 2000 A survey of patients with acquired haemophilia in a haemophilia centre over a 28-year period. Clinical and Laboratory Haematology 22(5): 275–278

154. Saxena R, Mishra DK, Kashyap R et al 2000 Acquired haemophilia – a study of ten cases. Haemophilia 6(2): 78–83

155. Michiels JJ 2000 Acquired hemophilia A in women postpartum: clinical manifestations, diagnosis, and treatment. Clinical and Applied Thrombosis and Hemostasis 6(2): 82–86

156. Shastri KA, Ho C, Logue G 1999 An acquired factor V inhibitor: clinical and laboratory features. Journal of Medicine 30(5–6): 357–366

157. Knobl P, Lechner K 1998 Acquired factor V inhibitors. Baillière's Clinical Haematology 11(2): 305–318

158. Feinstein DI 1978 Acquired inhibitors of factor V. Thrombosis and Haemostasis 39(3): 663–674

159. Delmer A, Andreu G, Horellou MH et al 1988 Acquired factor VII inhibitor: treatment using high-dose immunoglobulins, corticotherapy and plasma exchange. Annales de Medicine Interne (Paris) 139 suppl 1(4): 48–50

160. Ndimbie OK, Raman BK, Saeed SM 1989 Lupus anticoagulant associated with specific inhibition of factor VII in a patient with AIDS. American Journal of Clinical Pathology 91(4): 491–493

161. Hutton RA, Warrell DA 1993 Action of snake venom components on the haemostatic system. Blood Reviews 7(3): 176–189

162. Guerrero BA, Arocha-Pinango CL, Gil San Juan A 1997 Degradation of human factor XIII by lonomin V, a purified fraction of Lonomia achelous caterpillar venom. Thrombosis Research 87(2): 171–181

163. Guerrero BA, Arocha-Pinango CL, Gil San Juan A 1997 Lonomia achelous caterpillar venom (LACV) selectively inactivates blood clotting factor XIII. Thrombosis Research 87(1): 83–93

164. Guerrero B, Arocha-Pinango CL 1992 Activation of human prothrombin by the venom of *Lonomia achelous* (Cramer) caterpillars. Thrombosis Research 66(2–3): 169–177

165. Richard V, Bernier M, Themelin L et al 1991 Blood coagulation abnormalities during adoptive immunotherapy with interleukin-2 (r-Met Hu IL-2 [ala 125]). Annals of Oncology 2(1): 67–68

Natural anticoagulants and thrombophilia

29

MA Laffan

Introduction

Normal coagulation

Tissue factor pathway inhibitor (TFPI)

Antithrombin (AT)

The protein C – protein S
(PC–PS syndrome)

Overview

Thrombomodulin

The endothelial protein C receptor (EPCR)

Protein C

Protein S

Other anticoagulant factors

Protein Z-ZPI

Heparin cofactor II (HCII)

Histidine-rich glycoprotein

Alpha 2 macroglobulin

Alpha-1-antitrypsin

C1 esterase inhibitor

Thrombophilia

Deficiency of anticoagulant factors

Antithrombin deficiency

Protein C (PC)

Protein S (PS)

Factor V Leiden and APCR

Excess procoagulant activity

Fibrinogen

Fibrinolysis

Factor XII

Factor XIII

Acquired thrombophilic states
Lupus anticoagulant and
the antiphospholipid syndrome
Hematologic, inflammatory and
metabolic disorders
Hyperhomocystinemia

Thrombophilia as a multifactorial
disorder

Measuring thrombophilia and
procoagulant states

Factor VIIa

Thrombophilia and clinical management

Introduction

The evolution of a powerful coagulation system is an essential consequence of a fluid circulation and it is equally essential that a corresponding regulatory or anti-coagulant system should also have evolved. If it were not for this system of regulation we would rapidly die from thrombosis soon after the coagulation system was first triggered. It is also understandable that a fibrinolytic system has evolved to remove the clot once it has fulfilled its initial purpose and healing has been established. These systems must coexist in an appropriate balance or pathologic states will arise. The need for an appropriate balance between these opposing systems has probably been an important evolutionary pressure which at present is vividly seen in studies of maternal mortality where thrombosis and hemorrhage are both prominent. Just as deficiencies or abnormalities of the procoagulant system have been found to cause a tendency to bleeding, so corresponding deficiencies of the anticoagulant system result in abnormal or inappropriate coagulation, which we call thrombosis. Some individuals appear to have an unusually high tendency to thrombosis and develop the problem spontaneously and at an unusually young age. This increased tendency to thrombosis is termed thrombophilia and can arise in many different ways. This chapter begins with a description of the natural anticoagulant systems followed by a discussion of the clinical and laboratory manifestations of thrombophilia.

Normal coagulation

In vivo coagulation is triggered by the exposure of tissue factor (TF) which is present on virtually all extravascular tissues. TF is then able to bind the small circulating amounts of activated factor VII (FVIIa). FVIIa is enzymatically inactive until it binds to tissue factor but is thereafter able to cleave and activate factors X and IX into their active forms IXa and Xa. Thus VIIA-TF provides the initial stimulus for coagulation as Xa is able to convert a small amount of prothrombin to thrombin. Then route of activation is rapidly terminated by the action of tissue factor pathway inhibitor (TFPI; see below). Once the TF pathway has been blocked, the progression of coagulation is dependent on the small amount of thrombin that has been generated. Thrombin activates factors VIII and V which are cofactors for IXa and Xa respectively, increasing their activity many thousand-fold. Thus VIIIa augments the activity of the IXa generated by TF-VIIa and converts more X to Xa. This is in turn augmented in its action on prothrombin by the presence of Va. The assembly and activity of these coagulation factor complexes is facilitated by activated platelets which provide specific receptors and an appropriate phospholipid surface. The result of this positive feedback loop is an explosive burst of thrombin generation.[1] The propagation and extent of this burst is limited by the natural anti-coagulant mechanisms described below.

Tissue factor pathway inhibitor (TFPI)

TFPI has previously been known as extrinsic factor pathway inhibitor and lipoprotein-associated coagulation inhibitor. It is a Kunitz-type inhibitor comprising an acidic amino terminus, three Kunitz-type domains and a basic carboxy terminus of molecular weight 34–40 kD. The gene has been cloned and lies on chromosome 2, it gives rise to mRNAs of 1.4 and 4.0 kb; the result of alternative polyadenylation sites. It seems likely that the major site of TFPI synthesis is the vessel wall although it was originally isolated from human hepatoma cells. The effective plasma concentration of TFPI is difficult to determine and of dubious significance because a large portion (> 80%) of TFPI is bound either to lipoprotein or to the vessel wall. Release of TFPI from the endothelial binding sites accounts for some of heparin's anticoagulant activity, but it is not known which of these pools is normally active in coagulation.

Although patients with abetalipoproteinemia have very low (< 20%) plasma levels of TFPI they do not suffer from an increased risk of thrombosis. Approximately 10% of the blood TFPI is present in platelets which appear to release it at sites of platelet activation.

TFPI inhibits the FVIIa – TF complex by forming a quaternary complex with it and factor Xa, which is thus also inactivated. The first Kunitz domain binds VIIa-TF and the second binds Xa; the function of the third Kunitz domain is unknown and directed mutagenesis of this region does not appear to alter function. Physiologically, the action of TFPI is to damp the initial procoagulant stimulus to thrombin generation. After this occurs, the progression of coagulation depends on the feedback effect of thrombin in generating Va and VIIIa and the small amount of IXa that has been generated. It is the inability to sustain this secondary burst that results in bleeding in hemophilia. In some circumstances the factor IXa initially generated may be insufficient and effective coagulation depends on XIa generated by the action of thrombin.

So far there are no established disease associations with abnormal levels of TFPI, or with mutation of its gene.

Antithrombin (AT)

Antithrombin, a member of the serpin group of protease inhibitors, is synthesized primarily in the liver and circulates as a plasma glycoprotein of 52.8 kD, concentration 1.5–3.5 µmol/l. The gene is composed of 7 exons located at chromosome 1q23–25. Plasma AT is heterogeneous with respect to glycosylation and an important fraction called beta antithrombin lacks glycosylation at Asn 135, which results in a greater affinity for heparin and greater anticoagulant activity. AT is the principal physiologic inhibitor of the enzymes of coagulation, in particular thrombin and Xa, although it also acts against IXa and XIa. It is also active against the TF–VIIa complex but not against free VIIa.[2] AT acts by engaging the serine protease but behaves as a pseudosubstrate so that instead of cleavage a conformational change takes place trapping the enzyme and AT in a stable complex that is later cleared by the liver.

The antithrombin molecule also contains a binding site for heparin and other related compounds that contain a specific pentasaccharide sequence. Binding causes a conformational change in the AT which accelerates its interaction with the enzymes > 1000-fold. Whilst this is utilized therapeutically with heparin, this function is probably performed *in vivo* by the heparans present on the vascular endothelium. Binding by the polysaccharide is sufficient to accelerate neutralization of Xa, IXa and XIa but for thrombin, an additional effect of 'approximation' is required. This is effected by long (18 residue) chains of saccharide which bind thrombin and bring it close to the antithrombin molecule. After the AT–enzyme complex has formed the heparin molecule is released and can interact with further AT or thrombin molecules. The importance of the heparin cofactor effect is illustrated by the severity of thrombotic problems seen in individuals with variant AT molecules lacking this site (i.e. homozygous for Type II HBS mutations – see below).

The protein C – protein S (PC–PS) system

Overview

The enzymes of the procoagulant system are inhibited largely and most importantly by antithrombin whereas the principal cofactors VIIIa and Va are neutralized by the PC–PS system. The interaction of this system with coagulation is more complex, however, as it also interferes directly with assembly of prothrombinase and tenase complexes, interacts with the fibrinolytic system and is able to convert factor V into an anticoagulant form. The principal components of the PC–PS system are protein C, protein S, thrombomodulin, endothelial protein C receptor and factor V.

Thrombomodulin

Thrombomodulin is a transmembrane protein found on normal endothelium and possibly also on mononuclear cells. The extracellular amino terminus comprises a lectin-type domain followed by six epidermal growth factor (EGF)-like domains, a serine–threonine rich domain, a single transmembrane domain and a short cytoplasmic tail. The gene is without introns and is on chromosome 20. Thrombomodulin (TM) binds thrombin (or its active precursors) and alters the substrate specificity of the enzyme. Thrombin binds to the two EGF domains closest to the cell surface and in doing so its ability to convert fibrinogen to fibrin and activate factor V or platelets is diminished. Instead its ability to convert PC to activated protein C (APC) is increased several thousand-fold over that in fluid phase. It is this conversion from a pro- to anticoagulant molecule that gave rise to thrombomodulin's name. It has subsequently become apparent that binding to TM produces a similar increase in the rate at which thrombin can activate the carboxypeptidase TAFI (thrombin activated fibrinolysis inhibitor) as well as making thrombin more susceptible to neutralization by antithrombin. It is difficult to imagine the benefit that may arise from inhibiting both coagulation and fibrinolysis in this way. A number of mutations have been described in thrombomodulin which may result in an increased risk of arterial and venous thrombosis but this relationship is not yet entirely clear although there is some evidence for an interaction with other risk factors such as smoking.[3] However, none of the changes is of polymorphic frequency. Soluble thrombomodulin, which is cleaved from the endothelial cell (EC), can be measured in plasma but has an uncertain relationship to thrombotic risk.[4] It may provide a measure of endothelial damage. Soluble TM retains its ability to bind thrombin and potentiate PC activation.

The endothelial protein C receptor (EPCR)

Although TM is widely expressed in small and large blood vessels, the fact that it is membrane bound means that its effective concentration in large vessels is very much reduced. Recently, a 43 kd transmembrane endothelial protein C receptor (EPCR) was identified which binds protein C via the glutamic acid (GLA) domain and appears to increase its effective concentration on the membrane surface in the vicinity of TM.[5] EPCR is expressed principally in large vessels where it tends to offset the relative reduction in TM concentration. It is not yet clear whether mutations in EPCR are a significant contributor to thrombosis although this is theoretically feasible. An effective null mutation (insertion of 23bp in exon 3) has been reported to have an association with increased risk of thrombosis.[6] Similarly to TM a proteolytically cleaved[7] soluble form of EPCR can be detected in plasma, although its significance is unknown.

Protein C

Protein C is a vitamin K dependant plasma glycoprotein of 62 kd molecular weight and the zymogen circulates at a plasma concentration of approximately 4 μg/ml. The 12 kb gene is on chromosome 2 and yields a 1.7 kb mRNA. The protein appears to be transcribed as a single polypeptide but some cleavage occurs so that both single and two chain forms circulate. Like other proteins of this group it has a modular structure comprising, a signal peptide, GLA domain, aromatic stack, EGF-like domains and serine protease domain. After activation via cleavage by thrombomodulin-bound thrombin it acquires serine protease activity. In concert with its cofactor protein S (see below), activated protein C (APC) cleaves the active forms of factor V and factor VIII thus inactivating them. It also cleaves unactivated factor V into a form called Vi which no longer has procoagulant activity but which acts as a cofactor in the APC–PS mediated degradation of factor VIIIa. APC is neutralized in plasma by a serpin called APC inhibitor but also identified as PA1–3 because APC is reported to have some profibrinolytic activity.

Protein S

Protein S is a curious and enigmatic protein that interacts with numerous other proteins and has several anticoagulant properties, the relative importance of which are not fully understood. It is a vitamin K dependent glycoprotein of 70 kd molecular weight which circulates at a concentration of 20–25 μg/ml. The functional (PSα or PROS1) gene consists of 15 exons located on chromosome 3p11. A non-functional pseudogene is nearby but lacks the first exon and has a number of inactivating mutations. Unlike protein C it is synthesized in megakaryocytes, endothelial, bone and Leydig cells as well as hepatocytes.

The significance of this is not known but may contribute to a significance in arterial as well as venous thrombosis. The amino terminal portion of protein S is familiar; signal peptide, GLA domain, aromatic stack and four EGF-like domains. However at the carboxy terminus, in place of the serine protease module, there is a region closely homologous to sex-hormone binding globulin (SHBG), which none the less does not bind sex hormones and has no enzymic activity. The SHBG region is responsible for the ability of PS to bind to C4b-binding protein (C4bBP), a regulatory protein of the complement pathway.

Although PS has been shown to function as a cofactor for APC in the degradation of factors (F) Va and VIIIa it seems unlikely that its anticoagulant role is restricted to this effect. In purified human systems including phospholipid vesicles, its ability to potentiate APC degradation of FVa is only 2–3-fold. Additional actions of PS, which may also be important in its anticoagulant effect, are to abrogate the protective effect of FXa on APC-mediated degradation of FVa and to inhibit directly the enzymatic activity of FXa, to which it also binds. PS also binds directly to FV and competes with prothrombin for binding to FVa. Most recently, PS has been shown to have a further action, impeding the activation of FX by an interaction with FVIII. These actions are independent of APC and have the net result of inhibiting both tenase and prothrombinase activity. The relative contributions of these numerous properties to the overall anticoagulant effect of PS are not known and recent work has produced only conflicting data. van't Veer and colleagues found that thrombin formation in a continuous flow model was 5–25-fold increased in PS-deficient plasma compared to normal, independent of protein C. In contrast, Arnljots and Dahlback, using cross species differences to dissect out function in a rabbit artery model of thrombosis, found that PS alone had no antithrombotic effect but significantly enhanced the antithrombotic effect of APC. At present there is no satisfactory explanation for the discrepancy in these findings.[8,9]

In human plasma, approximately 60% of PS circulates in non-covalent combination with C4bBP. Although PS is able to bind to APC in this complex it is not able to function as its cofactor. C4bBP binding also inhibits the binding of PS to factor and Va but not to Xa. Hence C4bBP inhibits some, but not all, of PS activities. This again complicates interpretation of plasma assay results. C4bBP's other physiologic function is to downregulate the complement system by acting as a cofactor for the cleavage of C4b by factor I. The significance of the interaction between the PS–PC pathway and the C' system is not clear, but C4bBP function is not impaired by PS binding.

Other anticoagulant factors

Protein Z–ZPI

Protein Z is a vitamin K dependent plasma protein of molecular weight 62 kD plasma concentration 2.9 ± 1.0 µg/ml and half-life 2.5 days. It is similar in structure to the vitamin K dependant serine proteases but has no reactive site and no catalytic activity. It has recently been found to participate in an anticoagulant mechanism neutralizing factor Xa. It does this in concert with a PZ dependent protease inhibitor ZPI (molecular weight 72 kD and plasma concentration 1.0–1.6 µg/ml) on phospholipid surfaces. The overall effect of PZ–ZPI is not clear as it also impairs neutralization of Xa by antithrombin, but studies in mice suggest that its net effect is anticoagulant although complete deficiency does not produce a severe phenotype in mice.[10]

Heparin cofactor II (HCII)

HCII is a serine protease inhibitor molecular weight 65 kD and plasma concentration 1.2 µmol/l which neutralizes only thrombin. This is potentiated by heparin (> 18 residues), chondroitin sulfate and dermatan sulfate. Heparin binding does not utilize the pentasaccharide required by AT and its affinity for HCII is 5–10 times lower. Low levels of HCII compatible with a heterozygous deficiency state are found in 1% of the general population but are not found more commonly in patients with thrombosis.

Histidine-rich glycoprotein

Histidine-rich glycoprotein (HRG) forms a 1:1 complex in plasma which has previously been thought to have a neutralizing effect. However, other workers have demonstrated that it can enhance plasminogen activation.[11] Although high levels of HRG have been identified in some patients with thrombosis as well as some with deficiency, a causal relationship is not established.

Alpha 2 macroglobulin

Alpha 2 macroglobulin (α2MG) is a large glycoprotein which non-specifically inhibits a number of plasma proteases. It does this by binding to lysyl residues in the protease distant from the reactive site. Inhibition of enzymic activity is by steric hindrance so that some enzymic acitivty against small (e.g. chromogenic) substrates is retained. It contributes approximately 50%, 20% and 10% of the plasma inhibitory activity against kallikerin, thrombin and Xa respectively. The importance of α2MG inhibitory activity is not such that deficiency results in a prothrombotic state but it is postulated that the high levels found in children may be responsible for the rarity of thrombotic episodes before puberty.[12]

Alpha-1-antitrypsin

Alpha-1-antitrypsin is another serpin which has activity against enzymes of the coagulation system, in particular factors XIa and Xa (70% and 35% of plasma-neutralizing activity respectively) although its principal targets are pancreatic and leukocyte elastases.

C1 esterase inhibitor

C1 esterase inhibitor is the principal plasma inhibitor of FXIIa (90% of plasma activity) and also provides 50% of plasma activity against kallikrein as well as minor activity against XIa. Deficiency results in a characteristic syndrome of angioneurotic edema due to excessive complement activity but does not have any thrombotic features.

Thrombophilia[13,14]

Deficiency of anticoagulant factors

Deficiency of the anticoagulant factors, antithrombin, protein C or protein S is associated with an increased tendency to thrombosis that fulfills the classical description of thrombophilia given in the introduction. Homozygosity or compound heterozygosity for deficient alleles of PC or PS leading to levels of less than 0.1–0.2 iu/ml leads shortly after birth to an extremely severe thrombotic syndrome called purpura fulminans, which is frequently fatal. Complete deficiency of antithrombin is probably not compatible with life and is lethal to mouse embyos at 14.5 days.[15] In general AT, PC or PS deficiency refers to a relative deficiency of 50% normal levels associated with inheritance of single deficient allele and therefore inherited as an autosomal dominant trait. However, some kindreds have demonstrated what appears to be a recessive pattern of inheritance.[16] The explanation appears to be that frequently the thrombophilic phenotype is exposed by the coinheritance and interaction of additional traits: for example 20% of families with thrombophilia and protein C deficiency also have factor V Leiden (FVL) segregating within them.[17] Family studies suggest that further factors, as yet identified, may also modify the phenotype.[18]

The mutations responsible for PC, PS and AT deficiency are essentially sporadic and do not reach polymorphic frequency either singly or collectively so that accurate assessment of the associated thrombotic risk is difficult. Analysis of affected families members shows that by the age of 50 years, approximately 85% of affected members have had a thrombotic episode,[19] corresponding to a relative risk of 10–20-fold over the general population. This analysis probably over-estimates slightly the risk attributable solely to the factor deficiency because the thrombotic rate in unaffected members of the kindreds is also slightly higher than population controls, indicating that other genetic factors are also operating. However, it retains utility because it corresponds to the most frequent clinical situation in which the information is required. Databases of identified mutations are maintained. Although deficiencies of AT, PC and PS are potent causes of thrombophilia, they are infrequent and together are found in only approximately 8% of patients presenting with their first venous thromboembolic event.[20] A retrospective analysis suggests that they do not have any significant impact on overall mortality.[21]

Antithrombin deficiency

AT deficiency can be divided into types I and II. In type I there is a concordantly low level of AT antigen and function. In type II the functional activity of the AT is low whilst the antigenic level is higher and may be normal. Type II AT variants are divided into those affecting the reactive site (RS), those affecting the heparin-binding site (HBS) and those affecting both functional centers (pleiotropic effect: PE).[22] The population frequency of type 1 antithrombin deficiency is estimated at 0.2 per 1000 though it may be higher for the type 2 HBS variants which are not, in the heterozygous state, associated with thrombosis.[23]

Protein C (PC)

PC deficiency is also divided into types I and II on the same basis. Of note is that some type II variants have mutations affecting the gamma carboxylation of the molecule, which produces low functional activity in coagulation – but not in chromogenic – assays. A number of polymorphisms in the promoter region of the gene have been identified which further modify the PC levels

Table 29.1 Classification of protein S deficiency

Category	Total protein S	Free protein S	Functional protein S
Type I	Low	Low	Low
Type II	Normal	Normal	Low
Type III	Normal	Low	Low

of the patient. PC deficiency causing thrombophilia is most frequently found in association with other thrombophilic traits (see below).

Protein S (PS)

As a result of its interaction with C4bBP, deficiency of PS presents a complex picture and is sometimes difficult to diagnose. There is also uncertainty regarding the significance of functional assays for PS which have been difficult to standardize and which are falsely low in the presence of factor V Leiden sometimes leading to the erroneous diagnosis of type II PS deficiency. The most widely used classification of PS deficiency is that shown in Table 29.1.

Recent studies have shown that type I and type III PS deficiency can coexist in the same family implying that they arise from the same PS mutation.[24] Further work showed that this may be an effect of age so that as C4bBP rises with age so does the total PS, but the free PS remains low.[25]

Low levels of PS may be an acquired phenomenon during pregnancy, oral anticoagulation, nephrotic syndrome, use of oral contraceptives and with systemic lupus erythematosus or liver disease. Catastrophically low levels have been reported in children after varicella infection.[26] It is important to note that the normal range for premenopausal women is significantly lower than in other groups and local normal ranges should be determined to avoid misinterpretation, paying attention to the additional effects of hormonal therapy and artifactual reduction in PS as described above.[27, 28] Although C4bBP is elevated during an acute phase reaction, the amount of PS binding β chain does not rise and as a result free PS does not fall.[29] All the above problems with protein S have made assessing the true frequency of deficiency in the population and hence the associated relative risk of thrombosis very difficult.

Factor V Leiden and APCR

In 1993, Dahlback and colleagues described an inherited tendency to thrombosis characterized by a defective plasma response to APC.[30] This became known as APC resistance (APCR) and was subsequently shown in > 90% of cases to result from a mutation Arg506Gln in factor V (factor V Leiden; FVL).[31] This mutation destroys a cleavage site for APC which greatly slows APC-mediated inactivation of factor Va. It also blocks the conversion by APC of FV into FVi which acts as a cofactor for APC degradation of FVIIIa. APCR is found in approximately 20% of patients with a first episode of venous thrombosis and confers a seven-fold increase in risk of thrombosis.[32] Very rarely, a similar effect may be produced by a mutation at another APC cleavage site at Arg306.[33] Curiously, the relative risk for pulmonary embolism associated with FVL appears to be rather less,[34] possibly because leg thrombi associated with FVL tend to be more distal.[35] In keeping with this, studies have not been able to demonstrate an effect of FVL on mortality.[36]

FVL is found predominantly in white Caucasian populations where the frequency of heterozygotes ranges from 2 to 10%. It is found less frequently in neighboring populations in North Africa and the Middle East and appears to have arisen as a single new mutation approximately 20 000–30 000 years ago. It is extremely rare in African, Far Eastern and Amerindian populations.[37] The propensity of FVL heterozygotes to thrombosis and their measured APCR appear to be increased by the co-inheritance of the HR2 factor V haplotype.[38] The means by which this effect is mediated are not clear but may be via altered glycosylation of factor V.[39] A small number of individuals have a poor response to APC but do not have the FVL mutation and it has recently been shown that this too is associated with an increased risk of thrombosis[40] albeit less than that of APCR associated with FVL. Numerous factors in plasma will contribute to the APC responsiveness of plasma, including factor VIII and lupus anticoagulants.[41] However, the increased risk of FVL negative APCR persists after adjustment for these variables, giving an odds ratio for thrombosis of 2.5 for the lowest quartile APCR.[40]

Excess procoagulant activity

Although neglected until recently, it is not surprising from the 'balance' view of thrombophilia that an excess procoagulant activity should be a risk factor for thrombosis in the same way as a deficiency of anticoagulant activity. Indeed, a later finding from the Leiden thrombophilia survey was that elevated levels of prothrombin were significantly associated with thrombosis. The majority of elevated levels were themselves associated with a mutation in the 3′ untranslated region of the gene (G20210A). The frequency of heterozygotes for this polymorphism

was 2.35% in the control group and 6.2% in those with first episode thrombosis, corresponding to an odds ratio (OR) of 2.8 (95%CI 1.4–5.6) after correction for other factors. The OR for prothrombin levels > 1.15 iu/ml was similar and 87% of G20210A heterozygotes fell into this group compared to 23% of wild type.[42] It is not clear how (if) the polymorphism causes an elevated level of FII but it is also associated with higher levels of FII mRNA. Like FVL the G20210 mutation is found predominantly in the white Caucasian population.[43]

An elevated level of factor VIII (> 1.5 iu/ml) was associated with a crude odds ratio for thrombosis of 6.8 in the Leiden study and several other studies have confirmed an incidence of approximately 24% in patients with first episode thrombosis.[44, 45] The OR was reduced slightly to 4.8 after adjustment for ABO blood group. The cause of this elevation is obscure but it does not appear to be related to an acute phase reaction as may be suspected.[46] Family studies of women heterozygous for hemophilia showed familial clustering of FVIII levels with a suggestion that a locus on the X chromosome was involved.[47] However a preliminary search for a genetic polymorphism in the FVIII gene was negative.[48]

Subsequently, elevated levels of other factors including FXI[49] and FIX[50] have been shown to have an association with thrombosis. The cause of these elevations is equally obscure but they all show a dose response relationship suggesting they are real if not yet proven to be independant. In contrast, levels of factor V[47] and factor X were not found to have any association with thrombosis.

Fibrinogen

Abnormal fibrinogen molecules (dysfibrinogens) are an unusual but well-recognized cause of thrombophilia and are found in approximately 1% of patients presenting with venous thromboembolism (VTE). Dysfibrinogens are usually detected as a result of a prolonged thrombin time, following which further investigation reveals a discrepancy between functional and total fibrinogen assays. Roughly 25% of dysfibrinogens are associated with thrombosis, 25% with bleeding and the remainder have no associated problems.[51] The relationship between the molecular abnormality and the phenotype is in most cases poorly understood. High levels of fibrinogen have been found to confer a slightly increased risk of thrombosis.

Fibrinolysis

The investigation of fibrinolysis has an uncertain place in thrombosis. It seems well established that uncontrolled

Table 29.2 The prevalence and associated thrombotic risk of some thrombophilic traits

Trait	Frequency in population (%)	Frequency in 1st episode VTE (%)	Odds ratio for thrombosis (95%CI)
Antithrombin deficiency	0.05–0.1	1–2	~10–20
Protein C deficiency	0.3	3	~10–20
Protein S deficiency	?	1–2	~10–20
Factor V Leiden[a]	3–10	20	6.6 (3.6–12.0)
Prothrombin G20210A	2	6	2.8 (1.4–5.6)[42]
Elevated FVIII (>1.5 u/ml)	12	24	4.8 (2.3–10)[44]
Elevated FIX (>1.29 u/ml)	9.7	20.2	2.5 (1.6–3.9)[50]
Elevated FXI (>1.21 u/ml)	9.9	19.5	2.2 (1.5–3.2)[49]
Dysfibrinogen	?	1	?
Hyperhomocysteinemia	4.8	10	2.5 (1.2–5.2)

[a] This figure is for all abnormal activated protein C resistance (APCR). VTE, venous thromboembolism.

fibrinolytic capacity due to antiplasmin or plasminogen activator inhibitor (PAI)-1 deficiency can, although rare, lead to a hemorrhagic tendency.[52, 53] In contrast, there is no good evidence that an impaired fibrinolytic capacity results in a tendency to venous thrombosis. This may be attributed in part to the poor reproducibility of the global tests such as euglobulin clot lysis or fibrin plate lysis, but the uncertainty has not been removed by use of either specific assays or polymorphic genetic markers.[54] Complete deficiency of plasminogen does not lead to an increased tendency to thrombosis[55] (although abnormal fibrin deposition results in ligneous conjunctivitis) and family studies provide no further support for an association.[56] Whilst reduced fibrinolysis is a common finding in patients who have had a venous thrombosis it appears to have no prospective value. Similarly, high (*sic*) levels of tissue plasminogen activator (tPA) were shown to be predictive of myocardial infarction (MI) in the ECAT study but it seems likely that in both cases the association can be best interpreted as demonstrating an abnormality of endothelial function rather than a problem with fibrinolysis *per se*.[57–60]

Fibrinolysis shows considerable diurnal variation as well as interference from plasma lipids and stress. It is therefore generally preferred to perform these tests in the morning after an overnight fast, no smoking and after the subject has lain resting for ≥15 min (the plasma half life of tPA is approximately 5 min). Fibrinolytic activity is at its lowest around 5 a.m., which interestingly is also the peak time for MI.

Factor XII

A small amount (~15%) of the fibrinolytic potential of plasma is dependant on factor XII activation. It has therefore been suggested that deficiency of factor XII may result in an increased tendency to thrombosis. However, there is very little evidence to support this and no association between factor XII level and thrombosis was found in the Leiden thrombophilia survey.[61]

Factor XIII

Factor XIII is a transglutamidase which, following activation by thrombin, acts to cross-link fibrin monomers to produce shear- and fibrinolysis- resistant fibrin. A Val 34 Leu polymorphism has been identified which results in an increased activation by thrombin and an increase in cross-linking reactivity. Paradoxically, there have been suggestions that this is associated with a protective effect against thrombosis, in a case control study,[62] and in a second study the Leu–Leu genotype was associated with a relative risk (RR) of 0.16 (0.05–0.5) for thrombosis.[63] However, this association requires confirmation.

The Leiden thrombophilia survey found that the level of thrombin-activated fibrinolysis inhibitor (TAFI) had a weak effect on risk of thrombosis (RR 2 for TAFI >90th centile) and may interact with factor VIII levels but not factor V Leiden.[64] A summary of the prevalence and associated risks of these abnormalities is given in Table 29.2.

Acquired thrombophilic states

Lupus anticoagulant and the antiphospholipid syndrome[65]

The antiphospholipid syndrome (APLS) describes the clustering of a number of clinical phenomena; principally arterial and venous thrombosis or recurrent pregnancy loss in association with antibodies against a number of protein–phospholipid complexes, particularly cardiolipin. The antibodies may be detected directly in ELISA-based assays or indirectly as a lupus anticoagulant in a coagulation-based test. The term lupus anticoagulant is clearly somewhat misleading because although the effect of the antibodies *in vitro* is anticoagulant their effect *in vivo* is thrombotic. The syndrome may occur in association with systemic lupus erythematosus or other disorder when it is called secondary APLS, or without, in which case it is called primary APLS. In both cases the relationship between the antibodies, the laboratory abnormalities and the clinical problems remains enigmatic.

The antibodies found in the antiphospholipid syndrome are heterogeneous and bind to combinations of certain proteins with negatively charged phospholipids. The best characterized of these proteins are β2 glycoprotein I and prothrombin but many others such as annexin V and protein C have been described. It is not yet clear whether the antibody binds to a protein neo-epitope produced by binding to phospholipid, a compound protein–phospholipid epitope or whether phospholipid enhances binding by increasing the effective concentration of epitopes facilitating cross-linking by the antibody. There are also limited *in vitro* data that some of these effects may be pathogenic but this is largely circumstantial. The specificity with the closest correlation to thrombosis and with evidence for pathogenicity in a mouse model is against β2 glycoprotein I.

The lupus anticoagulant effect of these antibodies is detected *in vitro* using coagulation tests that are phospholipid dependent and with greatest sensitivity when the amount of phospholipid is reduced to a limiting extent. Criteria for determining the presence of a lupus anticoagulant have been proposed[66] as have international guidelines. In general, the detection of a lupus anticoagulant has been found to be a more powerful predictor of thrombosis than the detection of antiphospholipid antibodies *per se*, reflecting our lack of understanding of their pathophysiology.

The relationship of these antibodies to the observed thrombosis remains obscure and it is still not clear that they are pathogenic rather than an epiphenomenon reflecting some other underlying thrombotic process. Lupus anticoagulant (LAC) are associated with both venous and arterial thrombosis (particularly stroke). Placental thrombosis and infarction appear to largely explain the association of these antibodies with fetal loss and intrauterine growth restriction. A number of putative prothrombotic mechanisms have been proposed involving inhibition of the protein C–protein S system and of fibrinolysis. An alternative hypothesis suggests that they may operate by triggering platelet activation in a manner analogous to the antibodies in heparin-induced thrombocytopenia and thrombosis. Not infrequently, the antibodies arise in association with an infection, including HIV or with drug use, in which cases they are less likely to be associated with thrombosis. Because these transient antibodies may cause confusion, the diagnosis of APLS requires demonstration that the antibodies are persistent and are still present on repeat testing 8 weeks later.

Hematologic, inflammatory and metabolic disorders

An increased tendency to thrombosis is a feature of many acquired disorders and which in most cases is only partially understood. A summary of these conditions and their possible mechanisms of action is given in Table 29.3. The best characterized are the myeloproliferative disorders, particularly primary proliferative polycythemia (PPP) and essential thrombocythemia in which arterial and venous thrombosis are seen. The mechanism appears to be an alteration in platelet function, exacerbated in the case of PPP by increased whole blood viscosity. An increase in the activation of circulating platelets can be demonstrated by flow cytometry.[67] In paroxysmal nocturnal hemoglobinuria (PNH) the increased sensitivity of the abnormal clone to complement again results in platelet activation and consequent thrombosis. Curiously, both disorders are associated with the otherwise rare Budd–Chiari syndrome in which thrombosis occurs in the hepatic veins.

Table 29.3 Acquired causes of an increased tendency to thrombosis

Disorder	Postulated mechanisms
Myeloproliferative disorders	Platelet activation Blood viscosity
PNH	Platelet activation
Malignancy	Inflammatory response Tissue factor production by tumor Increased monocyte TF expression
Pregnancy	Increased procoagulant factors Reduced anticoagulant factors Impaired fibrinolysis Impaired flow in pelvic veins
Behcet's syndrome	Vessel wall activation Impaired fibrinolysis
Nephrotic syndrome	Increased fibrinogen and lipid synthesis Hemoconcentration Loss of some proteins (e.g. AT) in urine
Diabetes	Endotheliopathy, increased factor VIII
Renal failure	Endotheliopathy, increased factor VIII
Estrogen therapy	Complex changes in coagulation factors plus some effects on endothelium
Paraproteinemia	Hyperviscosity Specific property of antibody

AT, antithrombin; PNH, paroxysmal nocturnal hemoglobinuria; TF, tissue factor.

The acute phase reaction results in elevation of several procoagulant proteins such as fibrinogen and factor VIII as well as increased tissue factor expression. Thus, any condition in which there is an acute phase reaction, often combined with relative immobility, is likely to result in thrombosis which is consequently common among general medical inpatients and among which pulmonary embolism a major cause of mortality. These inflammatory mechanisms account in large part for the increased rate of thrombosis among patients with cancer. Although approximately 10% of patients presenting with VTE will be found to have malignancy in the subsequent year;[68, 69] this is usually apparent from simple tests and an extensive search for malignancy is not warranted.[70] A similar increase in procoagulant factors coupled with an increased hematocrit is seen in the nephrotic syndrome which is also associated with thrombosis. The contribution of low levels of AT, which leak via the kidney, is uncertain. Diabetes and chronic renal failure are associated with a chronic endotheliopathy, which also increases the rate of thrombosis.

Hyperhomocystinemia

Homocystinuria is a rare autosomal recessive condition which is characterized by very high levels of homocysteine (HCy) and amongst other problems a very high rate of venous and arterial thrombosis. Many individuals have levels of HCy which, although not as high as those seen in homocystinuria, are none the less higher than those in normal healthy populations. It has therefore been a matter of some interest to know whether these individuals also have an increased rate of thrombosis. This condition is referred to as hyperhomocysteinemia (HHCy) and studies have established that levels > 18.5 µmol are found in 5–10% of the population and have an associate relative risk for venous and arterial thrombosis of 2.[71, 72] However, there are no prospective studies and so a causal assoiation has not been conclusively established and the high levels may reflect endothelial damage from some other cause. Plasma levels of HCy are affected by food intake and HCy measurement is therefore standardized by performing either fasting or after intake of a methionine load.

Homocystinuria results from complete deficiency of one of the enzymes in the methionine–homocysteine cycle, but interest in HHCy has been fuelled greatly by the identification of a polymorphic variant of the enzyme methylene tetrahydrofolate reductase (MTHFR), which participates in the homocysteine–methionine cycle. The polymorphism results in a thermolabile form of the enzyme which has reduced activity. Approximately 12%

of the population are homozygous for this thermolabile variant and tend to have higher levels of HCy. However, attempts to show an association between the thermolablie variant and thrombosis have been difficult, largely due to the confounding effect of folate status which is another important determinant of Hcy levels. The introduction of folate supplements in grain products in the USA (140 µg per 100 g) introduced in 1996 has resulted in a significant fall in plasma homocysteine levels.[73]

Thrombophilia as a multifactorial disorder

In the above sections the thrombophilic states have been considered in isolation. However, there is much evidence that in most instances the thrombophilic state arises from the interaction of a number of different factors. The high prevalence of FVL has allowed this to be studied directly and its combination with AT, PC or PS deficiency clearly results in increased rate of thrombosis above those seen with the individual traits alone.[17, 74–76] Moreover, the FVL and prothrombin polymorphisms interact powerfully with exogenous agents such as oral contraceptives in increasing the risk of thrombosis.[77–79]

Measuring thrombophilia and procoagulant states

The conversion of several coagulation zymogens into their active form is by proteolytic cleavage and liberation of a small peptide: an activation peptide. These can be assayed in plasma and give an estimation of the rate at which the conversion is taking place and thus of coagulation activation. The best studied of these is prothrombin fragment F1+2 which is released when prothrombin is converted to thrombin and has a half-life of approximately 45 min allowing measurable amounts to accumulate and indicating the rate of thrombin generation. Conversely, once generated, thrombin is neutralized by antithrombin with the formation of thrombin–antithrombin (TAT) complexes. These might also be expected to give a measure of thrombin generation and correlate well with F1+2. Similar principles underlie the measurement of other activation peptides and complexes, including fibrinopeptide A, plasmin–antiplasmin complexes and even cross-linked fibrin degradation products (D-dimers).[80]

Whilst these are attractive measures they have unfortunately not proved to be good indicators of prothrombotic states nor predictors of thrombosis,[81] indicating that the prothrombotic state is more complex than simply an increased background rate of coagulation activation.

Factor VIIa

Unlike other coagulation enzymes, the conversion of factor VII to its active form does not result in the generation of an activation peptide. However, the production of recombinant soluble tissue factor allowed the development of coagulation-based assay to measure the small amounts of VIIa in plasma.[82] The interest in VIIa arose largely from the results of the Northwick Park Heart Study which suggested that elevated VIIc may be an important predictor of ischemic heart events and that this may reflect higher VIIa levels. However, this finding has not been confirmed in subsequent studies and measurement of FVIIa remains a research rather than a clinical tool.

Thrombophilia and clinical management

The identification of a prothrombotic state usually takes place after a thrombosis has taken place. When it is identified in an asymptomatic individual, usually as a result of a family study, it is rarely sufficient to warrant continuous anticoagulant prophylaxis. This represents largely an inability of current laboratory tests to predict thrombosis on an individual basis. Clearly, these individuals should receive prophylaxis at times of high risk but because many events are spontaneous (without clear precipitant) this will not be entirely effective. It has been more difficult to develop tests that are good predictors of recurrent thrombosis after a first event. Those patients with deficiencies of AT, PS and PC have high recurrence rates and should receive long-term anticoagulation but they constitute only a small minority of patients. The more common genetic polymorphisms FVL and prothrombin have been shown in some, but not all, studies to have a modest effect on recurrence rates and in one study, to increase recurrence when present together.[83–86] Recently, increased levels of factor VIII were shown to have a strong predictive value for recurrence.[87] The influence of these factors on rates of recurrence is of crucial clinical importance because it is principally in this circumstance that they may influence management.

REFERENCES

1. Butenas S, van't Veer C, Mann KG 1999 'Normal' thrombin generation. Blood 94: 2169–2178
2. Rao LV, Rapaport SI, Hoang AD 1993 Binding of factor VIIa to tissue factor permits rapid antithrombin III/heparin inhibition of factor VIIa. Blood 81: 2600–2607
3. Doggen CJ, Kunz G, Rosendaal FR et al 1998 A mutation in the thrombomodulin gene, 127G to A coding for Ala25Thr, and the risk of myocardial infarction in men. Thrombosis and Haemostasis 80: 743–748
4. Salomaa V, Matei C, Aleksic N et al 1999 Soluble thrombomodulin as a predictor of incident coronary heart disease and symptomless carotid artery atherosclerosis in the Atherosclerosis Risk in Communities (ARIC) Study: a case-cohort study. Lancet 353: 1729–1734
5. Esmon CT 2000 The endothelial cell protein C receptor. Thrombosis and Haemostasis 83: 639–643
6. Merati G, Biguzzi E, Oganesyan N et al 1999 A 23bp Insertion in the endothelial protein C receptor (EPCR) gene in patients with myocardial infarction and deep vein thrombosis. Thrombosis and Haemostasis 82 (suppl): 507
7. Liaw PC, Neuenschwander PF, Smirnov MD, Esmon CT 2000 Mechanisms by which soluble endothelial cell protein C receptor modulates protein C and activated protein C function. Journal of Biological Chemistry 275: 5447–5452
8. van 't Veer C, Butenas S, Golden NJ, Mann KG 1999 Regulation of prothrombinase activity by protein S. Thrombosis and Haemostasis 82: 80–7
9. Arnljots B, Dahlback B 1995 Antithrombotic effects of activated protein C and protein S in a rabbit model of microarterial thrombosis. Arteriosclerosis Thrombosis and Vascular Biology 15: 937–941
10. Yin ZF, Huang ZF, Cui J et al 2000 Prothrombotic phenotype of protein Z deficiency. Proceedings of the National Academy of Sciences USA 97: 6734–8
11. Borza DB, Morgan WT 1997 Acceleration of plasminogen activation by tissue plasminogen activator on surface-bound histidine-proline-rich glycoprotein. Journal of Biological Chemistry 272: 5718–5726
12. Mitchell L, Piovella F, Ofosu F, Andrew M 1991 Alpha-2-macroglobulin may provide protection from thromboembolic events in antithrombin III-deficient children. Blood 78: 2299–2304
13. Lane DA, Mannucci P, Bauer K et al 1996 Inherited thrombophilia: part 1. Thrombosis and Haemostasis 76: 651–662
14. Lane DA, Mannucci P, Bauer K et al 1996 Inherited thrombophilia: part 2. Thrombosis and Haemostasis 76: 824–834
15. Ishiguro K, Kojima T, Kadomatsu K et al 2000 Complete antithrombin deficiency in mice results in embryonic lethality. Journal of Clinical Investigation 106: 873–878
16. Miletich J, Sherman L, Broze G, Jr 1987 Absence of thrombosis in subjects with heterozygous protein C deficiency. New England Journal of Medicine 317: 991–996
17. Koeleman BP, Reitsma PH, Allaart CF, Bertina RM 1994 Activated protein C resistance as an additional risk factor for thrombosis in protein C-deficient families. Blood 84: 1031–1035
18. Hasstedt SJ, Bovill EG, Callas PW, Long GL 1998 An unknown genetic defect increases venous thrombosis risk, through interaction with protein C deficiency. American Journal of Human Genetics 63: 569–576
19. Pabinger I, Schneider B et al 1996 Thrombotic risk in hereditary antithrombin III, protein C or protein S deficiency. Ateriosclerosis Thrombosis and Vascular Biology 16: 742–748
20. Heijboer H, Brandjes DP, Buller HR et al 1990 Deficiencies of coagulation-inhibiting and fibrinolytic proteins in outpatients with deep-vein thrombosis. New England Journal of Medicine 323: 1512–1516
21. Rosendaal FR, Heijboer H, Briet E et al 1991 Mortality in hereditary antithrombin-III deficiency—1830 to 1989. Lancet 337: 260–262
22. Lane DA, Olds RJ, Conard J et al 1992 Pleiotropic effects of antithrombin strand 1C substitution mutations. Journal of Clinical Investigation 90: 2422–2433
23. Tait RC, Walker ID, Perry DJ et al 1994 Prevalence of antithrombin deficiency in the healthy population. British Journal of Haematology 87: 106–12
24. Zoller B, Garcia dFP, Dahlback B 1995 Evaluation of the relationship between protein S and C4b-binding protein isoforms in hereditary protein S deficiency demonstrating type I and type III deficiencies to be phenotypic variants of the same genetic disease. Blood 85: 3524–31
25. Simmons RE, Zoller B, Irland H et al 1997 Genetic and phenotypic analysis of a large (122 member) protein S deficient kindred provides an explanation for the co-existence of type I and type III plasma phenotypes. Blood 89: 4364–4370
26. Levin M, Eley BS, Louis J et al 1995 Postinfectious purpura fulminans caused by an autoantibody directed against protein S. Journal of Pediatrics 127: 355–363
27. Faioni EM, Valsecchi C, Palla A et al 1997 Free protein S deficiency is a risk factor for venous thrombosis. Thrombosis and Haemostasis 8: 1343–1346

28. Gari M, Falkon L, Urrutia T et al 1994 The influence of low protein S plasma levels in young women, on the definition of normal range. Thrombosis Research 73: 149–152

29. Garcia de Frutos P, Alim RI, Hardig Y et al 1994 Differential regulation of alpha and beta chains of C4b-binding protein during acute-phase response resulting in stable plasma levels of free anticoagulant protein S. Blood 84: 815–822

30. Dahlback B, Carlsson M, Svensson PJ 1993 Familial thrombophilia due to a previously unrecognized mechanism characterized by poor anticoagulant response to activated protein C: prediction of a cofactor to activated protein C. Proceedings of the National Academy of Sciences USA 90: 1004–1008

31. Bertina RM, Koeleman BP, Koster T et al 1994 Mutation in blood coagulation factor V associated with resistance to activated protein C. Nature 369: 64–67

32. Koster T, Rosendaal FR, de RH et al 1993 Venous thrombosis due to poor anticoagulant response to activated protein C: Leiden thrombophilia study. Lancet 342: 1503–1506

33. Williamson D, Brown K, Luddington R et al 1998 Factor V Cambridge: a new mutation (Arg306—>Thr) associated with resistance to activated protein C. Blood 91: 1140–4

34. Turkstra F, Karemaker R, Kuijer PM et al 1999 Is the prevalence of the factor V Leiden mutation in patients with pulmonary embolism and deep vein thrombosis really different? Thrombosis and Haemostasis 81: 345–8

35. Bounameaux H 2000 Factor V Leiden paradox: risk of deep-vein thrombosis but not of pulmonary embolism. Lancet 356: 182–183

36. Hille ET, Westendorp RG, Vandenbroucke JP, Rosendaal FR 1997 Mortality and causes of death in families with the factor V Leiden mutation (resistance to activated protein C). Blood 89: 1963–1967

37. Rees DC 1996 The population genetics of factor V Leiden (Arg506Gln). British Journal of Haematology 95: 579–586

38. Faioni EM, Franchi F, Bucciarelli P et al 1999 Coinheritance of the HR2 haplotype in the factor V gene confers an increased risk of venous thromboembolism to carriers of factor V R506Q (factor V Leiden). Blood 94: 3062–3066

39. Hoekema L, Castoldi E, Tans G et al 1999 Characterization of blood coagulation factor V (a) encoded by the R2-gene. Thrombosis and Haemostasis 82 (suppl): 11

40. de Visser MCH, Rosendaal FR, Bertina RM 1999 A reduced sensitivity for activated protein C in the absence of factor V Leiden increases the risk of venous thrombosis. Blood 93: 1271–1276

41. Laffan MA, Manning R 1996 The influence of factor VIII on measurement of activated protein C resistance. Blood Coagulation and Fibrinolysis 7: 761–765

42. Poort S, Rosendaal F, Reitsma P, Bertina R 1996 A common genetic variation in the 3' untranslated region of the prothrombin gene is associated with elevated plasma prothrombin levels and an increase in venous thrombosis. Blood 88: 3698–3703

43. Franco RF, Santos SE, Elion J et al 1998 Prevalence of the G20210A polymorphism in the 3'-untranslated region of the prothrombin gene in different human populations. Acta Haematologica 100: 9–12

44. Koster T, Blann A, Briet E et al 1995 Role of clotting factor VIII in effect of von Willebrand factor on occurrence of deep vein thrombosis. Lancet 345: 152–155

45. O'Donnell J, Tuddenham EGD, Manning R et al 1997 High prevalence of elevated factor VIIIc levels in patients referred for thrombophilia screening: role of increased synthesis and relationship with the acute phase reaction. Thrombosis and Haemostasis 77: 825–828

46. O'Donnell J, Mumford AD, Manning RA, Laffan M 2000 Elevation of FVIII: C in venous thromboembolism is persistent and independent of the acute phase response. Thrombosis and Haemostasis 83: 10–3

47. Kamphuisen PW, Houwing Duistermaat JJ, van Houwelingen HC et al 1998 Familial clustering of factor VIII and von Willebrand factor levels. Thrombosis and Haemostasis 79: 323–327

48. Mansveldt E, Laffan M, McVey J, Tuddenham E. 1998 Analysis of the F8 gene in individuals with high plasma FVII:C levels and associated venous thrombosis. Thrombosis and Haemostasis 80: 561–565

49. Meijers JC, Tekelenburg WL, Bouma BN et al 2000 High levels of coagulation factor XI as a risk factor for venous thrombosis. New England Journal of Medicine 342: 696–701

50. van Hylckama Vlieg A, van der Linden IK, Bertina RM, Rosendaal FR 2000 High levels of factor IX increase the risk of venous thrombosis. Blood 95: 3678–82

51. Haverkate F, Samama M 1995 Familial dysfibrinogenemia and thrombophilia. Report on a study of the SSC Subcommittee on Fibrinogen. Thrombosis and Haemostasis 73: 151–161

52. Fay WP, Parker AC, Condrey LR, Shapiro AD 1997 Human plasminogen activator inhibitor-1 (PAI-1) deficiency: characterization of a large kindred with a null mutation in the PAI-1 gene. Blood 90: 204–208

53. Lind B, Thorsen S 1999 A novel missense mutation in the human plasmin inhibitor (alpha2-antiplasmin) gene associated with a bleeding tendency. British Journal of Haematology 107: 317–322

54. Lane D, Grant P 2000 Role of hemostatic gene polymorphisms in venous and arterial thrombotic disease. Blood 95: 1517–1532

55. Schuster V, Mingers AM, Seidenspinner S et al 1997 Homozygous mutations in the plasminogen gene of two unrelated girls with ligneous conjunctivitis. Blood 90: 958–966

56. Dolan G, Greaves M, Cooper P, Preston FE 1988 Thrombovascular disease and familial plasminogen deficiency: a report of three kindreds. British Journal of Haematology 70: 417–421

57. Juhan VI, Pyke SD, Alessi MC et al 1996 Fibrinolytic factors and the risk of myocardial infarction or sudden death in patients with angina pectoris. ECAT Study Group. European Concerted Action on Thrombosis and Disabilities. Circulation 94: 2057–2063

58. Pyke SD, Thompson SG, Buchwalsky R, Kienast J 1993 Variability over time of haemostatic and other cardiovascular risk factors in patients suffering from angina pectoris. ECAT Angina Pectoris Study Group. Thrombosis and Haemostasis 70: 743–746

59. Ridker PM, Vaughan DE, Stampfer MJ et al 1993 Endogenous tissue-type plasminogen activator and risk of myocardial infarction. Lancet 341: 1165–1168

60. Thompson SG, Kienast J, Pyke SD et al 1995 Hemostatic factors and the risk of myocardial infarction or sudden death in patients with angina pectoris. European Concerted Action on Thrombosis and Disabilities Angina Pectoris Study Group. New England Journal of Medicine 332: 635–41

61. Koster T, Rosendaal FR, Briet E, Vandenbroucke JP 1994 John Hageman's factor and deep-vein thrombosis: Leiden thrombophilia study. British Journal of Haematology 87: 422–424

62. Catto AJ, Kohler HP, Coore J et al 1999 Association of a common polymorphism in the factor XIII gene with venous thrombosis. Blood 93: 906–908

63. Franco RF, Reitsma PH, Lourenco D et al 1999 Factor XIII Val34Leu is a genetic factor involved in the etiology of venous thrombosis. Thrombosis and Haemostasis 81: 676–679

64. van Tilburg NH, Rosendaal FR, Bertina RM 2000 Thrombin activatable fibrinolysis inhibitor and the risk for deep vein thrombosis. Blood 95: 2855–9

65. Greaves M 1999 Antiphospholipid antibodies and thrombosis. Lancet 353: 1348–1353

66. Haematology BCfSi 2000 Guidelines on the investigation and management of the antiphospholipid syndrome. British Journal of Haematology 109: 704–1715

67. Wehmeier A, Tschope D, Esser J et al 1991 Circulating activated platelets in myeloproliferative disorders. Thrombosis Research 61: 271–8

68. Prandoni P, Lensing AW, Buller HR et al 1992 Deep-vein thrombosis and the incidence of subsequent symptomatic cancer. New England Journal of Medicine 327: 1128–1133

69. Sorensen HT, Mellemkjaer L, Steffensen FH et al 1998 The risk of a diagnosis of cancer after primary deep venous thrombosis or pulmonary embolism. New England Journal of Medicine 338: 1169–1173

70. Cornuz J, Pearson SD, Creager MA et al 1996 Importance of findings on the initial evaluation for cancer in patients with symptomatic idiopathic deep venous thrombosis. Annals of Internal Medicine 125: 785–793

71. de Heijer M, Koster T, Blom HJ et al 1996 Hyperhomocysteinemia as a risk factor for deep-vein thrombosis. New England Journal of Medicine 334: 759–762

72. Simioni P, Prandoni P, Burlina A et al 1996 Hyperhomocysteinemia and deep-vein thrombosis. A case-control study. Thrombosis and Haemostasis 76: 883–886

73. Jacques PF, Selhub J, Bostom AG et al 1999 The effect of folic acid fortification on plasma folate and total homocysteine concentrations. New England Journal of Medicine 340: 1449–54

74. Mandel H, Brenner B, Berant M et al 1996 Coexistence of hereditary homocystinuria and factor V Leiden – effect on thrombosis. New England Journal of Medicine 334: 763–768

75. Zoller B, Berntsdotter A, Garcia dFP, Dahlback B 1995 Resistance to activated protein C as an additional genetic risk factor in hereditary deficiency of protein S. Blood 85: 3518–23

76. van Boven HA, Reitsma PH, Rosendaal FR et al 1996 Factor V Leiden (FVR506Q) in families with inherited antithrombin deficiency. Thrombosis and Haemostasis 75: 417–21

77. Vandenbroucke JP, Koster T, Briet E et al 1994 Increased risk of venous thrombosis in oral-contraceptive users who are carriers of factor V Leiden mutation. Lancet 344: 1453–7

78. Martinelli I, Sacchi E, Landi G et al 1998 High risk of cerebral-vein thrombosis in carriers of a prothrombin-gene mutation and in users of oral contraceptives. New England Journal of Medicine 338: 1793–1797

79. Martinelli I, Taioli E, Bucciarelli P et al 1999 Interaction between the G20210A mutation of the prothrombin gene and oral contraceptive use in deep vein thrombosis. Arteriosclerosis, Thrombosis and Vascular Biology 19: 700–703

80. Bauer KA, Rosenberg RD 1994 Activation markers of coagulation. Baillière's Clinical Haematology 7: 523–540

81. Kyrle PA, Eichinger S, Pabinger I et al 1997 Prothrombin fragment F1+2 is not predictive for recurrent venous thromboembolism. Thrombosis and Haemostasis 77: 829–833

82. Morrissey JH, Macik BG, Neuenschwander PF, Comp PC 1993 Quantitation of activated factor VII levels in plasma using a tissue factor mutant selectively deficient in promoting factor VII activation. Blood 81: 734–744

83. Simioni P, Prandoni P, Lensing A et al 1997 The risk of recurrent venous thromboembolism in patients with an Arg^{506}-Gln mutation in the gene for factor V (factor V Leiden). New England Journal of Medicine 336: 399–403

84. De Stefano V, Martinelli I, Mannucci PM et al 1999 The risk of recurrent deep venous thrombosis among heterozygous carriers of both factor V Leiden and the G20210A prothrombin mutation. New England Journal of Medicine 341: 801–806

85. Ridker PM, Miletich JP, Stampfer MJ et al 1995 Factor V Leiden and risks of recurrent idiopathic venous thromboembolism. Circulation 92: 2800–2802

86. van den Belt AG, Sanson BJ, Simioni P et al 1997 Recurrence of venous thromboembolism in patients with familial thrombophilia. Archives of Internal Medicine 157: 2227–32

87. Kyrle PA, Minar E, Hirschl M et al 2000 High plasma levels of factor VIII and the risk of recurrent venous thromboembolism. New England Journal of Medicine 343: 457–462

Immunohematology

Blood groups on red cells, platelets and neutrophils   615

Transfusion medicine for pathologists   637

Histocompatibility: HLA and other systems   665

Blood groups on red cells, platelets and neutrophils

30

G Daniels   A Hadley

Introduction

Red cell surface antigens

The ABO and H histo-blood-group systems and other carbohydrate antigens
The ABO and H antigens
HDN caused by ABO antibodies
Altered expression of ABO antigens in leukemia
Lewis antigens
ABH and Lewis antigens on tumors

The Rh blood-group system
Rh-deficiency syndrome, Rh_{null} and Rh_{mod}
HDN caused by Rh antibodies

The Kell system and Kx
Anti-K and HDN
The Kell–Kx complex and McLeod syndrome

Blood groups on red cell transporters

Receptors and adhesion molecules
The Duffy antigen receptor for chemokines
Glycoproteins of the immunoglobulin superfamily
Other putative receptor or adhesion molecules with blood-group activity

Complement regulatory glycoproteins

Red cell glycoproteins that anchor the membrane to its skeleton

Associations with infectious disease

Platelet antigens

Structure and function
Antigens on the glycoprotein IIb/IIIa complex
Antigens on the glycoprotein Ib/IX/V complex
Antigens on the glycoprotein Ia/IIa complex
Antigens on CD109

Neonatal alloimmune thrombocytopenia
Pathophysiology
Clinical features

Alloantigenic platelet glycoprotein polymorphisms and hemostasis
HPA-1
HPA-2
HPA-3
HPA-4 and other platelet antigens

Granulocyte antigens

Structure and function
Antigens on Fcγ receptor III
Antigens on CD11/CD18
Granulocyte antigens on other glycoproteins

Neonatal alloimmune neutropenia
Pathophysiology
Clinical features

Autoimmune neutropenia of infancy

Granulocyte antigenic polymorphisms and disease

Introduction

Blood groups can be defined as inherited allogeneic variation detected on the surface of blood cells. Although the term is often considered to refer exclusively to erythrocytes, it is equally applicable to other blood cells. In this chapter red cell, platelet and neutrophil groups are described. This is approached, first, from the direction of the structures of these antigens and how they relate to their functions and, second, from their associations with disease, including alloimmune disease.

Red cell surface antigens

Red cell blood groups have been recognized for over a century, since Landsteiner's discovery of the ABO system in 1900. Red cell surface antigens are validated and classified by the International Society of Blood Transfusion (ISBT), which currently recognizes 267 antigens, 221 belonging to one of 25 blood-group systems. Each system consists of between one and 45 antigens encoded either by a single gene or by two or three closely linked homologous genes.[1,2] The 25 blood group systems are listed in Table 30.1.

Blood-group antigens may be carbohydrate structures on red cell surface glycoproteins or glycolipids, or they may be determined primarily by the amino acid sequence of polypeptides or glycoproteins. At least 23 red cell surface proteins express blood-group polymorphism. The functions of some of these structures are reasonably well understood, such as transport of biologically important molecules in and out of the cell, protection of the cell from autologous complement, and anchoring the membrane to the membrane skeleton. Functions of many, however, can only be speculated on from structural similarity to proteins and glycoprotein of known function.[3]

Pathology associated with blood-group polymorphism is usually the result of alloimmune destruction of red cells. This might be a hemolytic transfusion reaction following transfusion of red cells to a patient with an alloantibody directed against a determinant present on donor red cells, or hemolytic disease of the fetus and newborn (HDN), following placental transfer of maternal IgG antibodies into the fetal circulation. Most blood group systems contain a null-phenotype in which the antigens of that system are not expressed. This usually results from an inactivating mutation in the gene encoding the antigen, yet in most cases null-phenotypes are not associated with any pathology, probably due to functional redundancy of cell surface proteins. For reviews on red cell groups see Daniels[4] and Issitt and Anstee.[5]

Table 30.1 The blood group systems, the genes that encode them, and their chromosomal location

No.	System name	System symbol	Gene name(s)	Chromosome	No. of antigens
001	ABO	ABO	ABO	9	4
002	MNS	MNS	GYPA, GYPB, GYPE	4	43
003	P	P1	P1	22	1
004	Rh	RH	RHD, RHCE	1	45
005	Lutheran	LU	LU	19	18
006	Kell	KEL	KEL	7	23
007	Lewis	LE	FUT3	19	6
008	Duffy	FY	FY	1	6
009	Kidd	JK	SLC14A1	18	3
010	Diego	DI	SLC4AI	17	18
011	Yt	YT	ACHE	7	2
012	Xg	XG	XG	X	1
013	Scianna	SC	SC	1	3
014	Dombrock	DO	DO	12	5
015	Colton	CO	AQP1	7	3
016	Landsteiner-Wiener	LW	LW	19	3
017	Chido/Rodgers	CH/RG	C4A, C4B	6	9
018	Hh	H	FUT1	19	1
019	Kx	XK	XK	X	1
020	Gerbich	GE	GYPC	2	7
021	Cromer	CROM	DAF	1	10
022	Knops	KN	CR1	1	5
023	Indian	IN	CD44	11	2
024	Ok	OK	CD147	19	1
025	Raph	RAPH	MER2	11	1

The ABO and H histo-blood-group systems and other carbohydrate antigens

ABO and H antigens

ABO is the most important blood-group system from the perspective of clinical blood transfusion. The ABO histo-blood-group antigens, are present in many tissues throughout the body and, in soluble form, in body fluids.

At its most basic level, there are two ABO antigens, A and B, and four phenotypes, A, B, AB and O. O is a null phenotype in which neither A nor B is expressed. The A and B determinants are carbohydrate structures, present on red cell membrane glycoproteins and glycolipids. The major carriers of A and B on red cells are the abundant N-glycosylated glycoproteins, the anion exchanger (band 3) and the glucose transporter. Carbohydrate chains are synthesized by the action of glycosyltransferases, enzymes that catalyse the transfer of specific monosaccharides from a nucleotide donor substrate to an acceptor substrate. The acceptor substrate for A- and B-transferases, products of the *A* and *B* alleles, is a terminally fucosylated structure called H antigen (Fig. 30.1). The *A* gene product is an N-acetylgalactosaminyltransferase that transfers N-acetylgalactosamine from a uridine diphosphate (UDP)-N-acetylgalactosamine donor substrate to the fucosylated galactosyl residue of the H antigen, to produce an A-active structure (Fig. 30.1). *B* gene product is a galactosyltransferase that transfers galactose from UDP-galactose to the fucosylated galactose of H, to produce B-active structure (Fig. 30.1). The *O* allele produces no active enzyme, so on group O red cells the H antigen remains unconverted. N-acetylgalactosamine and galactose are the immunodominant sugars of A and B blood groups, respectively.

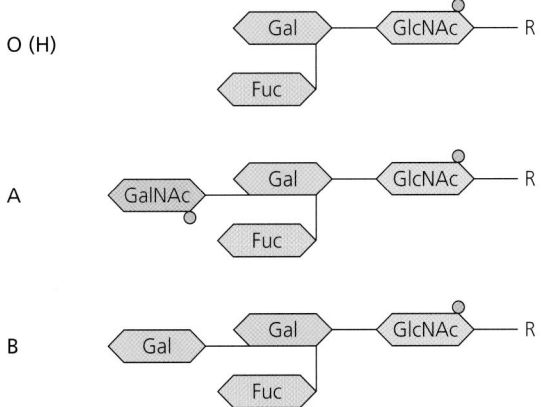

Fig. 30.1 A and B tetrasaccharides and the precursor trisaccharide that expresses H and is abundant on group O cells. R represents the remainder of the molecule.

A- and B-transferases are encoded by a single gene on chromosome 9, cloned by Yamamoto *et al*[6] in 1990. The *ABO* gene spans about 18–20 kb organized into seven exons of coding sequence. Exons 6 and 7, the two largest, include 77% of the full coding region and encodes all of the catalytic domain. The products of the *A* and *B* alleles differ by four amino acid substitutions at residues 176, 235, 266 and 268. Leu266Met and Gly268Ala substitutions are most important in determining whether the gene product has predominantly N-acetylgalactosaminyltransferase (A) or galactosyltransferase (B) activity. The sequence of the most common *O* allele (O^1) is identical to the *A* sequence, apart from a single nucleotide deletion that is responsible for a reading frame shift after codon 86 and the generation of a translation stop signal at codon 117. This allele encodes a truncated protein lacking the catalytic site. There are two other common *O* alleles: O^{1v}, that, like O^1, has the single nucleotide deletion, but differs from O^1 by nine nucleotide changes within the coding sequence and O^2, that does not have the single nucleotide deletion, but is inactivated by a missense mutation encoding a Gly268Arg substitution (reviewed in Ref 7).

A antigen is divided into two main subgroups, A_1 and A_2. Red cells of the A_1 and A_2 (and A_1B and A_2B) phenotypes react with anti-A, A_1 cells reacting more strongly than A_2 cells. A_1 cells also react with anti-A_1, an antibody present in the serum of some A_2 and A_2B individuals, so the A antigens of A_1 and A_2 cells differ quantitatively and qualitatively. A_2-transferase is substantially less efficient than A_1-transferase. A^2 DNA has a single base deletion in the codon before the usual translation stop codon, resulting in a reading frameshift and loss of the stop codon. The protein product has an extra 21 amino acid residues at the C-terminus, presumed to be responsible for reduction in enzyme activity.

About 80% of group A and B people have soluble A and B antigens in their body secretions. The remaining 20% do not secrete A or B substance because their secretions contain no H antigen, the substrate for the A- and B-transferases. This H-deficiency results from inactivity of the fucosyltransferase that is crucial for biosynthesis of H, due to mutations within the fucosyltransferase gene, *FUT2*, active in endodermally-derived tissues. These ABH 'non-secretors' have H and A or B antigens on their red cells because a different fucosyltransferase gene (*FUT1*) is responsible for synthesis of H antigen on mesodermally-derived tissues, including red cells. In the very rare Bombay phenotype mutations in *FUT1* and *FUT2* result in no H, and consequently no A or B, on red cells or in secretions, regardless of ABO genotype. Bombay phenotype individuals usually make a potent anti-H.

HDN caused by ABO antibodies

Anti-A and -B are predominantly IgM, but may be IgG. Anti-A,B, which reacts with both A and B antigens, is present in the sera of most group O people and is often partly IgG. ABO HDN is restricted almost exclusively to fetuses of group A mothers and IgG anti-A,B is generally considered culpable.[8] Issitt and Combs,[9] however, claim that anti-A and -B in group O women cause HDN more often and in more severe form than anti-A,B.

About 15% of pregnancies in women of European origin involve a group O mother with a group A or B fetus. This figure does not vary greatly in most other major ethnic groups, yet ABO HDN requiring clinical intervention is rare, though minor symptoms involving a small degree of red cell destruction may be relatively common. Hydrops due to ABO HDN is exceedingly rare, but very occasionally exchange transfusion for the prevention of kernicterus is indicated.[8] The main explanation for the low prevalence of clinically significant ABO HDN is that A and B antigens are present in many tissues. Any antibody crossing the placenta is likely to become bound to placental tissue, reducing the quantity available for destruction of red cells. In addition, A and B red cell antigens are not fully developed in the fetus or neonate.

Altered expression of ABO antigens in leukemia

The association of weak A antigen expression with acute leukemia is well documented and changes in B and H antigens are also recorded.[4,5] In some cases all red cells show weakness of the A antigen, whereas in others two populations of red cells are clearly apparent. In a patient with acute monoblastic leukemia, initially only 2% were agglutinated with anti-A, but in remission the proportion of agglutinable cells rose to 65% before falling again shortly before death.[10] Between 17 and 37% of patients with leukemia have significantly lower A, B or H antigenic expression compared with healthy controls.[4] In all cases the changes represent a loss or diminution of antigen strength and never the expression of a new red cell antigen.

Although modifications of ABH antigens are usually associated with acute leukemia, they are also often manifested before diagnosis of malignancy and therefore indicate preleukemic states.[11] Loss of an ABH antigen in a patient with a haematologic disorder is generally prognostic of acute leukemia.[12]

Depression of A or B antigens in acute myeloid leukemia (AML) and in preleukemic states is usually associated with a severe reduction in red cell A- or B-transferase

activity, but little or no reduction in red cell H-transferase activity.[13] In patients with separable populations of red cells, A- or B-transferase activity was greatly reduced in the membranes of those cells that had lost their A or B antigens, but were normal in those that had not.[13] The loss of A or B antigen expression in acute leukemia results from a defect or deficiency of the *A* or *B* gene products and not a defect in membrane precursors. The *ABO* locus is close to the *ABL1* oncogene locus on chromosome 9q34. *ABL1* is at the breakpoint of the Philadelphia-chromosome, a leukemia-specific reciprocal translocation involving paternal chromosome 9 and maternal chromosome 22.[14]

Lewis antigens

The Lewis antigens, Le[a] and Le[b], are not synthesized by erythroid cells, but become incorporated into the red cell membrane from the plasma. Their synthesis from H antigen and from its precursor is catalyzed by an α1,4-fucosyltransferase, the product of *FUT3*, a gene on chromosome 19. This fucosyltransferase competes with the H-(*FUT2*), A-, and B-transferases in endodermal tissue for acceptor substrate. The antigens known as Le[x] and Le[y], which are not detected on red cells, are isomers of Le[a] and Le[b], respectively.[15]

ABH and lewis antigens on tumors

ABH antigens are often absent from malignant tissue despite being present in the surrounding epithelium. In a study of many cases of carcinoma of the gastrointestinal tract, uterine cervix, lung and bladder, with very few exceptions, loss of ABH antigens preceded formation of distant metastases and hence a poor prognosis.[7] Loss of A or B antigens is generally due to a disappearance of A- or B-transferase activity and results in an accumulation of H, Le[b] or Le[y]. This results from downregulated transcription of the *ABO* gene, as no A or B mRNA can be detected in high-grade tumors.[7,16] Presence or absence of N-acetylgalactosamine (A) or galactose (B) from integrin receptors on tumor cells may affect motility and proliferation and, consequently, their ability to form metastases.[7]

ABH structures and Le[b], Le[x] and Le[y] antigens are present on fetal distal colon; they are not present in healthy adult distal colon, but are often re-expressed in adults in carcinoma of the distal colon.[17] Malignancy in the distal colon is associated with increased α1,2-fucosyltransferase activity (*FUT1* and *FUT2* products), so α1,2-fucosyltransferases probably control, at least partially, oncodevelopmental expression of ABH and related antigens in the colon.[18]

Upregulation of glycosyltransferases in tumors may result in increased levels of certain carbohydrate structures in the plasma.[19] The quantity of circulating sialylated-Le[a] (sLe[a]), otherwise known as the CA 19–9 antigen, is widely used as a marker to support diagnosis of colorectal, pancreatic and gastric cancer, and as an aid to prognosis after potential curative surgery.[20,21] A marker for cancerous regions of colon of Le(a–b–) patients, who have no circulating CA 19-9, is sialyl-Le[c] (DU-PAN-2), a precursor of sialyl-Le[a].[21]

Another phenomenon associated with malignancy is the incompatible A antigen occasionally expressed on tumors of group O or B people. About 10% of colonic tumors from group O patients, shown to be homozygous for the O^1 allele, express A antigen and contain active A-transferase activity.[22,23] The molecular basis of this O to A conversion is not known, but alternative splicing of *ABO* RNA, resulting in loss of exons 5 and 6, would introduce no frameshift or translation-termination codons, but would eliminate the single nucleotide deletion in exon 6 of O^1 and the putative gene product would be a truncated glycosyltransferase with a potential for A-transferase activity.[7] The higher incidence of gastric and ovarian adenocarcinomas in group A people could be due to a suppression of development of tumors bearing an A antigen by the anti-A naturally present in group O and B, but not A, patients.[24]

The Rh blood-group system

Rh is the most complex of the human blood-group systems. It has 45 well-defined antigens, the most immunogenic of which is D (RH1). Between 82% and 88% of Caucasians, about 95% of black Africans, and almost 100% of people from the Far East are D-positive. The other main Rh polymorphisms are C/c and E/e, two pairs of antithetical antigens. C has a frequency of 70% and c a frequency of 80% in Europeans. In black Africans the frequency of c is much higher and the frequency of C much lower, whereas in Eastern Asia the opposite is the case, with C approaching 100%. In most populations E has a frequency of about 30% and e about 98%.[4,5]

The antigens of the Rh system are encoded by two genes, *RHD* and *RHCE* (reviewed in Refs 25 and 26). They are highly homologous and have very similar genomic organization, each containing 10 coding exons arranged in opposite orientation on chromosome 1 (Fig. 30.2).[27,28] *RHCE* encodes the C/c and E/e antigens, plus many others such as C[w], C[x] and VS. *RHD* encodes the many epitopes of the D antigen. In Caucasians the D-negative phenotype almost always results from homozygosity for a deletion of *RHD*, whereas about 66% of D-negative Africans, have an *RHD* pseudogene.[29] The products of the Rh genes are polypeptides that are palmitoylated but, unlike most cell surface proteins, not glycosylated. The D and CcEe proteins differ by only 32–35 amino acids, depending on CcEe phenotype. Hydropathy analysis of the amino acid sequences of the Rh proteins together with immunologic evidence suggests that the Rh proteins span the red cell surface membrane 12 times, with internal termini and six extracellular loops (Fig. 30.2).

In the D-negative phenotype no D protein is present in the membrane, explaining the high immunogenicity of D compared with other Rh antigens. The C/c and E/e polymorphisms represent amino acid substitutions at different positions in the CcEe protein. Rh epitopes are conformational and may be discontinuous; that is, they are very dependent on the shape of the whole molecule and may involve more than one extracellular loop. Studies with monoclonal antibodies have shown that the D antigen consists of numerous epitopes. There are many variant phenotypes in which some D epitopes are missing, making it possible for a D-like antibody to be produced. Some of these partial D antigens result from

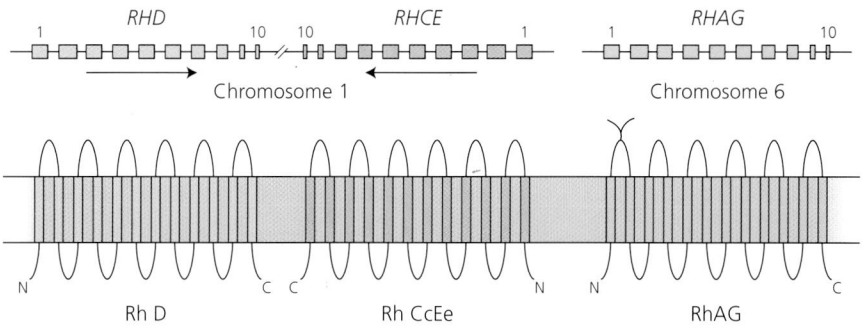

Fig. 30.2 Diagrammatic representation of the 10 exons of the *RHD* and *RHCE* genes and the encoded RhD and RhCcEe proteins, and the 10 exons of *RHAG* and the encoded glycoprotein with its single N-glycan (**Y**).

missense mutations in *RHD*, others because a section of *RHD*, ranging from part of an exon to several exons, has been replaced by the equivalent region of *RHCE*. These hybrid genes are probably the products of gene misalignment and intergenic recombination during meiosis. In addition to the *RHD-CE-D* hybrid genes responsible for partial D, *RHCE-D-CE* hybrid genes are responsible for some CcEe variants.[25,26]

The non-glycosylated Rh proteins are closely associated in the red cell membrane with a glycoprotein, the Rh-associated glycoprotein (RhAG), which has sequence and conformational similarities to the Rh proteins, but has a single N-glycan (Fig. 30.2). RhAG is encoded by a gene (*RHAG*) on chromosome 6.[30]

The functions of the Rh proteins and associated glycoprotein are not known.

Rh-deficiency syndrome, Rh$_{null}$ and Rh$_{mod}$

Red cells with the very rare Rh$_{null}$ phenotype have no Rh antigens and lack the Rh proteins. The most usual cause of Rh$_{null}$ is homozygosity for inactivating mutations in *RHAG*. In the absence of RhAG, no Rh protein is expressed at the red cell surface. Missense mutations in *RHAG* may result in reduced expression of the Rh proteins in the membrane and reduced Rh antigen expression, a phenotype called Rh$_{mod}$. Very rarely, Rh$_{null}$ occurs in the presence of RhAG, but with a deletion of *RHD* and an inactivating mutation in *RHCE*.[25,26]

Rh$_{null}$ and Rh$_{mod}$ red cells are morphologically and functionally abnormal. Most Rh$_{null}$ individuals have some degree of hemolytic anemia associated with stomatocytosis and spherocytosis, which has been referred to as Rh-deficiency syndrome. Rh$_{null}$ red cells have abnormal organization of their membrane phospholipids, and other anomalies associated with Rh$_{null}$ include increased cation permeability partially compensated by an increase in the number of K^+Na^+ pumps, reduced cation and water contents, and reduced membrane cholesterol content.[25]

HDN caused by Rh antibodies

The most common form of HDN results from IgG anti-D crossing the placenta and facilitating the immune destruction of D+ fetal red cells. The severity of anti-D HDN is highly variable: the most severely affected fetuses die *in utero* from about the 17th week of gestation onwards; in less severe cases, hydrops fetalis may occur. In those severely affected infants born alive, jaundice

may develop rapidly and lead to kernicterus. About 70% of infants who develop kernicterus die within a few days; of those who survive, many have permanent cerebral damage.[8]

Prior to the late 1960s, HDN caused by anti-D was a relatively common cause of fetal and neonatal mortality and morbidity. Since then the prevalence of severe anti-D HDN has been dramatically reduced by anti-D immuno-globulin prophylaxis, in which D− women receive an injection of anti-D IgG within 72 h of delivery of a D+ baby. This prevents immunization of the mother by D+ fetal cells, protecting D+ fetuses in subsequent pregnancies. Despite anti-D immune prophylaxis, HDN due to anti-D still occurs. D− women may become immunized because no or insufficient immunoglobulin is given or because of transplacental hemorrhage during the pregnancy. In England in 1992 there were still over 1000 cases of HDN per year, many requiring intrauterine transfusion and up to 160 resulting in fetal or neonatal death.[31] In an attempt to reduce the occurrence of D immunization during pregnancy, antenatal administration of anti-D immunoglobulin is being introduced in many countries.

In Caucasians, approximately 50% of fetuses of D− women are D−. When a D− pregnant woman has anti-D, it is beneficial to be able to determine the D phenotype of her fetus in order to determine whether there is any risk from HDN. Fetal D phenotype can be predicted by polymerase chain reaction-based tests performed on fetal DNA obtained by amniocentesis or chorionic villus sampling. Basically, the tests determine the presence or absence of *RHD* in order to predict whether the fetus is D+ or D−, respectively. Modifications of the technology prevent the potential errors that would arise from the presence of certain rare variant genes in Caucasians and the relatively common *RHD*-pseudogene in Africans.[25,29,32]

All antibodies to Rh-system antigens should be considered capable of causing HDN, but the only Rh antibody other than anti-D that regularly causes severe HDN is anti-c. Anti-C, -E, -e, and -G have all caused HDN, but the occurrence is rare and the outcome seldom severe.

The Kell system and Kx

The Kell blood group system comprises 23 determinants, almost all of which represent single amino acid substitutions in the Kell glycoprotein.[23] The Kell-null phenotype, K_0, in which no Kell glycoprotein is present in the red cell membrane, is heterogeneous in its molecular background. Kell glycoprotein is a type 2 integral membrane protein with an N-terminal cytoplasmic domain, a single transmembrane domain, and a large C-terminal extracellular domain, containing six potential N-glycosylation sites and 15 cysteine residues (Fig. 30.3).[33] One of these cysteine residues, Cys72, is linked by a disulfide bond to Cys347 of Kx, a multiple membrane spanning protein[34] (see below).

The Kell glycoprotein is an enzyme. It shares a pentameric zinc-binding motif, HEXXH, with a large family of zinc-dependent endopeptidases, and particular homology with two enzymes, neutral endopeptidase 24.11 (NEP or CD10) and endothelium-converting enzyme (ECE).[35] The Kell glycoprotein is able to cleave big endothelin-3, a biologically inactive 40-amino acid peptide, to endothelin-3, a 21-amino acid peptide with vasoconstrictor activity.[36] It is not known, however, whether the Kell glycoprotein serves this function *in vivo* and people with the Kell-null phenotype are apparently healthy.

Anti-K and HDN

Kell-system antibodies cause severe HDN. In Caucasian populations anti-K is often the most common immune red cell antibody outside of the ABO and Rh systems.[8] Most anti-K appear to be induced by blood transfusion and it is becoming common practice for girls and women of childbearing age to be transfused only with K– red cells.

The pathogenesis of HDN caused by anti-K differs from that due to anti-RhD. The severity of the anti-K disease is harder to predict than the anti-D disease. This is because there is very little correlation between anti-K titer and severity of disease and because anti-K HDN is associated with lower concentrations of amniotic fluid bilirubin than in anti-D HDN. Postnatal hyper-bilirubinemia is not prominent in babies with anemia caused by anti-K. There is also reduced reticulocytosis and erythroblastosis in the anti-K disease, compared with

anti-D HDN. These characteristics suggest that there is less hemolysis in HDN caused by anti-K, compared with HDN of comparable severity due to anti-D. This has led to speculation that fetal anemia in anti-K HDN results predominantly from a suppression of erythropoiesis.[37,38] Kell glycoprotein is one of the first erythroid-specific antigens to appear on erythroid progenitors during erythropoiesis, whereas the Rh proteins appear much later.[39–41] Vaughan *et al*[42] found that *in vitro* proliferation of K+ erythroid blast-forming units (BFU-E) and colony-forming units (CFU-E) was specifically inhibited by monoclonal and polyclonal anti-K. They speculated that the Kell glycoprotein might be involved in regulating the growth and differentiation of erythroid progenitors, possibly by enzymatically modulating peptide growth factors on the cell surface. Consequently, binding of anti-K could block the enzymatic activity of the Kell glyco-protein and suppress erythropoiesis. This theory, however, does not take into account the K_0 phenotype, in which no Kell glycoprotein is present on the surface of erythroid cells, yet erythropoiesis is apparently normal. It is more likely, therefore, that anti-K suppresses erythropoiesis through the immune destruction of early erythroid progenitors in the fetal liver. Daniels *et al*[41] have used a functional assay to demonstrate that K+ erythroid progenitors cultured from neonatal K+ Rh D+ CD34+ cells elicited a strong response from monocytes; no response was obtained with anti-D because Rh antigens do not appear on erythroid cells before they become hemoglobinized erythroblasts.

The Kell–Kx complex and McLeod syndrome

Kx is a protein with the structural appearance of a membrane transporter, but its function is not known. The 444 amino acid polypeptide is unglycosylated and probably spans the membrane 10 times, with internal N-

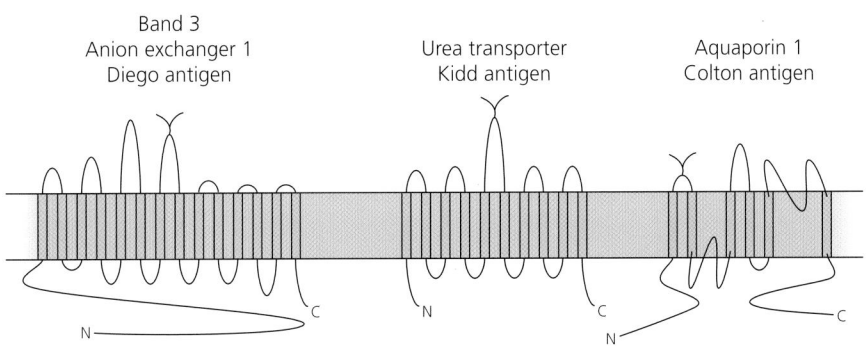

Fig. 30.3 Proposed conformations of the membrane transporters band 3, the Kidd glycoprotein, and aquaporin-1. Each has a single N-glycan (**Y**).

and C-termini.[43] The predicted topographic arrangement is identical to that of members of a family of proteins that cotransport a neurotransmitter together with Na+ and Cl− ions, the amino acid sequence bearing closest resemblance to a Na+-dependent glutamate transporter.[43]

Kx protein is associated with the Kell glycoprotein as a disulfide-bonded complex in the red cell membrane.[34] Kx is encoded by an X-linked gene, *XK*. The rare absence of Kx gives rise to McLeod syndrome, a multisystem disorder that results from either a gene deletion or from various inactivating mutations within *XK*.[33,43] McLeod syndrome is characterized by weakness of Kell-system antigens and by acanthocytic red cells. Late-onset muscular and neurological defects, including muscle wasting, diminished deep tendon reflex, choreiform movements, and cardiomyopathy are common symptoms; elevated serum creatine kinase is a constant feature. The reason for the association between Kx deficiency and neuroacanthocytosis is unknown.

A small minority of patients with X-linked chronic granulomatous disease (CGD) has the McLeod phenotype. CGD, an inherited disorder that may be either autosomal or X-linked, impairs the functioning of phagocytes resulting in severe susceptibility to infection. X-linked CGD results from deletion of the gene (*CYBB*) for the beta subunit of cytochrome b_{558}, or from mutations within that gene.[44] The locus for X-linked CGD and the *XK* locus are discrete and the association of McLeod phenotype with CGD is due to deletions of part of the X-chromosome that encompass both genes.[4] Three of 46 patients with X-linked CGD had McLeod phenotype; all three had large interstitial deletions of Xp21.1, whereas the other 40 had simple mutations within *CYBB*.[45]

Blood groups on red cell transporters

Membrane transporters facilitate the transport of biologically important molecules in or out of cells. They are typically polytopic, with an even number of α-helical membrane spanning domains of about 21 amino acids each, and have both termini inside the cytosol (see Fig. 30.3). Three red cell membrane transporters have blood group activity: band 3, the anion exchanger is the Diego system antigen; aquaporin 1, a water channel, is the Colton antigen; and HUT11, a urea transporter, is the Kidd antigen. The Rh proteins and associated glycoprotein and the Kx protein also resemble transporters structurally, although no function has been demonstrated.

Band 3, the Diego blood-group antigen, has a very important function in red cells. It acts as an anion

exchanger, an antiporter that permits bicarbonate (HCO_3^-) ions to cross the membrane in exchange for Cl− ions, rapidly reversing the accumulation of HCO_3^- in the red cells that would occur when CO_2 in the blood is hydrated to HCO_3^- by carbonic anhydrase located in the red cell cytoplasm. This facilitates transport of HCO_3^- in the plasma, greatly increasing the quantity of CO_2 that the blood can convey to the lungs.[46]

Unlike most blood-group systems, no Diego-null phenotype has been reported, probably reflecting its functional importance. There is one report, however, of a child homozygous for a band 3 mutation, whose red cells had no band 3, and no band 4.2, a glycoprotein of the membrane skeleton associated with band 3. The severely hydropic, anemic baby, was delivered by emergency Cesarean section and resuscitated and kept alive by blood transfusion.[47] A cord blood smear revealed dramatic erythroblastosis and poikilocytosis. At 8 months the baby was still thriving on regular blood transfusions and daily supplements of sodium bicarbonate. So, absence of band 3 is compatible with life, but only with extreme medical intervention. Band 3 'knockout' mice and cattle with a band 3 nonsense mutation were able to survive, despite spherocytosis, hemolytic anemia, and growth retardation.[48–50]

The Kidd glycoprotein (Fig. 30.3) is a urea transporter (HUT11 or UT3).[51] In addition to red cells, the Kidd urea transporter is present in endothelial cells of the vasa recta, the vascular supply of the renal medulla, but is not present in renal tubules.[52] A urea transporter in red cells has two main functions: (1) transporting urea rapidly in and out the cells to prevent shrinkage as they pass through the high urea concentration of the renal medulla and subsequent swelling as they leave; and (2) to prevent the red cells from carrying urea away from the renal medulla, which would decrease the urea concentrating efficacy of the kidney.[53] Despite this, a Kidd-null phenotype, resulting from homozygosity for a splice site mutation and exon skipping,[54,55] is relatively common in Polynesians, with an incidence of about 1 in 400.[56] This phenotype results in absence of the Kidd glycoprotein from the red cells and a gross reduction in transport of urea in and out of the cells. Yet no clinical syndrome has been associated with Kidd-null phenotype possibly because a homologous urea transporter compensates for the absence of the Kidd urea transporter in the kidney and because maximal urea concentrating ability is rarely required under normal conditions.

The Colton system antigen is aquaporin-1 (AQP-1), a member of a family water channel glycoproteins (see Fig. 30.3).[57,58] In addition to red cells, AQP-1 is strongly expressed in the kidney, where it functions to form water-selective channels in the plasma membrane that enhance osmotically driven water transport and plays a role in reabsorption of water from the glomerular filtrate in the proximal tubule and thin descending loop of Henle.[57] AQP-1 might also enable red cells to rehydrate rapidly after their shrinkage in the hypertonic environment of the renal medulla[59] and may play a part in CO_2 transport in the peripheral blood.[60] AQP-1 has been detected in several other organs and tissues: lung, where it may be involved in maintaining water balance; brain, where it may play a part in regulation of cerebral-spinal fluid; and eye, where it may have a role in secretion and uptake of the aqueous humor.[57] The Colton-null phenotype is extremely rare and associated with homozygosity for different inactivating mutations in each propositus.[61] No pathology is associated with the Colton-null phenotypes, probably because other cell surface proteins are capable of functioning as water channels.

Receptors and adhesion molecules

There are some red cell surface proteins that resemble receptor or adhesion molecules. Their precise functions, at least on red cells, are not clear. Cell surface receptors bind specific ligands, often hormones, and then activate an effector that produces an intracellular signal. In addition to functioning as receptors, adhesion molecules are involved in the adhesion of cells to other cells and to the extracellular matrix.[62] It is far from obvious why red cells should display adhesion molecules at their surface and these glycoproteins could be vestigial, having served their function during erythropoiesis.

The Duffy antigen receptor for chemokines

The Duffy blood group antigen is a member of the seven-transmembrane-segment class of the G protein-coupled superfamily of receptors, which bind many ligands including chemokines.[63] The Duffy glycoprotein crosses the plasma membrane seven times and has a glycosylated extracellular domain, which carries Fy[a] or Fy[b] blood group activity. It is also known as the Duffy antigen receptor for chemokines (DARC), as it is a receptor for a variety of chemokines, pro-inflammatory cytokines that motivate recruitment of leukocytes, as well as being involved in other cellular processes. The function of DARC is not known. It has been suggested that it may act as a clearance receptor for inflammatory mediators and that Duffy-positive red cells function as scavengers for the removal of unwanted chemokines.[64] DARC is also

present on endothelial cells lining postcapillary venules throughout the body, other vascular endothelial cells, epithelial cells of renal collecting ducts and pulmonary alveoli, and Purkinje neurones of the cerebellum.[63]

DARC is exploited by *Plasmodium vivax* as a receptor and is essential for invasion of the red cells by the parasite. *P. vivax* is responsible for tertian malaria, a form of malaria prevalent in Africa, but less severe than that caused by *P. falciparum*.[65] A Duffy-null phenotype, Fy(a–b–), in which the DARC is absent from red cells, is common in Africans, the frequency reaching 100% in some regions of West Africa.[4] Fy(a–b–) red cells are refractory to invasion by *P. vivax* merozoites and individuals with the Fy(a–b–) phenotype are resistant to vivax malaria. Fy(a–b–) phenotype in Africans results from homozygosity for a single nucleotide substitution in a GATA-1 transcription factor binding site in the promoter region of the Duffy gene.[66] This mutation abolishes binding of the erythroid-specific GATA-1 transcription factor and prevents expression of DARC on erythroid cells, although it is still present in other tissues.[67] No adverse effect of the Fy(a–b–) phenotype in Africans is apparent, whereas the evolutionary advantages are obvious. DARC may have an important function in other tissues, but in a few Caucasians and a family of native Americans an Fy(a–b–) phenotype has been found that arises from homozygosity for inactivating mutations in the Duffy gene.[68,69] In these individuals, therefore, DARC is unlikely to be present in any tissues, yet all are apparently healthy.

Glycoproteins of the immunoglobulin superfamily

The immunoglobulin superfamily (IgSF) is a large collection of glycoproteins, abundant on leukocytes, but also present on some other cells. IgSF glycoproteins contain repeating extracellular domains with sequence homology to immunoglobulin domains (Fig. 30.4). Each IgSF domain consists of approximately 100 amino acids and is structured into two β-sheets stabilized by a conserved disulfide bond. IgSF glycoproteins mostly function as receptors and adhesion molecules, and may be involved in signal transduction.[70]

At least five IgSF glycoproteins are present in the red cell surface membrane. Three – the Lutheran glycoproteins,[71] LW glycoprotein[72] and CD147 (Ok glycoprotein)[73] – carry blood group determinants; two – CD47 and CD58 (LFA-3) – are non-polymorphic. The functions of these structures on red cells are unknown, but they may play roles in erythropoiesis. Lutheran

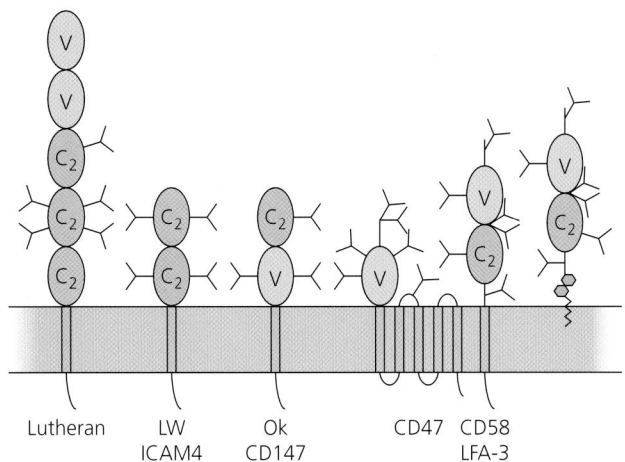

Lutheran   LW   Ok   CD47   CD58
         ICAM4   CD147   LFA-3

Fig. 30.4 Diagrammatic representation of the five members of the immunoglobulin superfamily (IgSF) detected in the red cell membrane, including the Lutheran, LW, and Ok blood group antigens. IgSF domains are shown as V or C_2. CD58 is present both as membrane-spanning and glycosylphosphatidylinositol-anchored forms. **Y** represents N-glycosylation.

glycoproteins bind laminin, an extracellular matrix glycoprotein of basement membranes.[74,75] LW glycoprotein (ICAM-4) binds integrins on hemopoietic and non-hemopoietic cells.[72] It is likely that these structures play a role in erythropoiesis, as such adhesion molecules would not be expected to be required on mature erythrocytes. Both appear in the later stages of erythropoiesis. Adhesive interactions between LW and integrins on other erythroblasts and on macrophages might assist in the stability of the erythroblastic islands.[76] Interactions between Lutheran and laminin could be involved in facilitating movement of the erythroblasts from the erythroblastic islands to the sinus endothelium.[39] No apparent pathology is associated with rare null phenotypes resulting from inactivating mutations in both the Lutheran and LW systems.[77,78] Putative functions for CD147 are even less clear, though no null-phenotype has been detected.

Other putative receptor or adhesion molecules with blood-group activity

CD44 is a widely distributed glycoprotein that has a variety of functions, many of which involve binding proteins of the extracellular matrix, in particular hyaluronan. CD44 carries the Indian (In^a/In^b) blood group polymorphism. Two glycoproteins, Xg and CD99, encoded by genes on the X- and Y-chromosomes, may also be adhesion molecules. The functions of CD44, Xg and CD99 on red cells are not known.[3]

Complement regulatory glycoproteins

Three red cell surface glycoproteins protect the cell from destruction by autologous complement. Two, decay-accelerating factor (DAF, CD55) and complement receptor-1 (CR1, CD35), are polymorphic; CD59 (membrane inhibitor of reactive lysis), is not.[3]

DAF expresses the Cromer blood group antigens. The extracellular domain contains four complement control protein domains (CCPs), regions of marked homology of about 60 amino acid residues each held in a double loop formation by two disulfide bonds. DAF protects cells from complement-mediated damage by inhibiting the amplification stage of complement activation. DAF inhibits association and accelerates dissociation of C4b2a and C3bBb, the C3 convertases of the classical and alternative pathways, respectively.[79] CD59, a member of the Ly-6 superfamily that does not have blood-group activity, inhibits complement-mediated hemolysis by binding to C8 and C9 and preventing assembly of the membrane-attack complex.[80]

DAF and CD59 have no membrane-spanning domain, but are anchored to cell membranes by means of a glycophospholipid called glycosylphosphatidylinositol (GPI).[81] Paroxysmal nocturnal hemoglobinuria (PNH), a disease characterized by intravascular hemolysis, is caused by multifarious somatic mutations in *PIG-A*, an X-linked gene essential for the biosynthesis of the GPI anchor.[82] The affected red cells in PNH patients (PNHIII cells) are deficient in all GPI-linked proteins, including DAF and CD59, and can be lysed, *in vitro*, by acidified human serum, a process that involves the activation of the alternative complement pathway. Despite DAF deficiency, red cells of the Cromer-null phenotype show no evidence of hemolysis and none of the six individuals with this phenotype had any symptoms of hematologic disease.[83–86] A patient with red cell CD59 deficiency due to homozygosity for single base deletion within the CD59 gene, but with normal levels of DAF and other GPI-linked glycoproteins, had a mild PNH-like hemolytic anemia.[87] CD59, therefore, appears to be more important than DAF, from the point of view of protecting red cells from hemolysis by autologous lysis.

Antigens of the Knops blood-group systems are expressed on CR1, a large glycoprotein with an extracellular domain composed of about 30 CCP domains.[88,89] The major function of red cell CR1 is to bind and process C3b/C4b coated immune complexes and to transport them to the liver and spleen for removal from the peripheral blood. CR1 has decay accelerating activity for the C3-convertase complexes of the classical and alternative pathways and acts as a cofactor for the factor I-mediated cleavage of C3b and C4b.[90] CR1 also enhances phagocytosis of C3b and C4b coated particles by neutrophils and monocytes. No true Knops-null phenotype has been found, but red cells of some individuals have such low red cell CR1 copy numbers that the Knops-system antigens cannot be detected by conventional serologic techniques.[91] No diseases are associated with this phenotype, but low CR1 copy number might play a part in the deposition of immune complexes on blood vessel walls leading to inflammatory damage. Acquired deficiencies of red cell CR1 have been reported in some malignant tumors, AIDS, systemic lupus erythematosus (SLE), and other autoimmune diseases.[92] Red cells lose CR1 during physiologic aging, the rate of loss being accelerated in SLE and HIV infection.[93]

Red cell glycoproteins that anchor the membrane to its skeleton

Band 3, the Diego blood-group antigen, is the red cell anion exchanger, but also has an important structural function. Band 3 has a long N-terminal domain, which interacts with the red cell membrane skeleton, a sub-membranous matrix of glycoproteins that is responsible for maintaining the shape and integrity of the red cell. Band 3 interacts with the membrane skeleton through the glycoproteins ankyrin, band 4.2 and band 4.1.[46] Heterozygosity for a 27 basepair deletion in the band 3 gene, encoding a nine amino acid deletion, is responsible for Southeast Asian ovalocytosis (SAO), a condition common in the southern Pacific region and among Melanesians and characterized by ovalocytic red cells. Homozygosity for this mutation has not been found, suggesting that it is lethal. About 20% of cases of hereditary spherocytosis, a common, familial hemolytic anemia characterized by small spheroid red cells, result from a variety of mutations within the band 3 gene and an absence or decrease of the mutant protein from the red cell membrane.[46,94]

The Gerbich blood-group antigens are located on two red cell glycoproteins, glycophorins C and D (GPC and GPD), encoded by a single gene (*GYPC*) by initiation of translation at two sites.[4,5] The C-terminal cytoplasmic domains of GPC and GPD form a complex with protein 4.1, which links them to the spectrin/actin network. Another glycoprotein, p55, may function as an adapter protein to stabilize this interaction.[95,96] Between 20% and 60% of the GPC- and GPD-deficient red cells of individuals with the rare Gerbich-null phenotype (Leach phenotype) are elliptocytes, but no hemolytic anemia is associated with this phenotype.[97] Patients with hereditary elliptocytosis due to protein 4.1 deficiency have a 70% to 90% reduction of GPC and GPD, are p55 deficient, and have complete elliptocytosis.[98]

Associations with infectious disease

Cell surface antigens may be exploited by pathogenic micro-organisms for attachment to the cells and their subsequent invasion. Many such associations have been reported involving antigens present on red cells, although the targets for the pathogens are often cells other than erythroid cells. Examples of these are associations are Le[b] and *Helicobacter pylori*, P antigen and the Dr[a] antigen of CD55 and *Escherichia coli*, CD35 (Knops antigen) and *Mycobacterium leprae*, and AnWj (an antigen associated with CD44) and *Haemophilus influenzae* (reviewed in Refs 99 and 100). It is probable that pathogenic micro-organisms have played the major role in the evolution of blood-group polymorphism. The only pathogens that invade red cells and their precursors are, however, malarial parasites and B19 parvovirus.

The association between the malarial parasite *Plasmodium vivax* and the Duffy antigen is described in a previous section of this chapter. *P. falciparum* is a far more virulent pathogen, responsible for over a million deaths annually. Glycophorins, and particularly the most abundant glycophorin, GPA, are important ligands for the attachment and invasion of *P. falciparum* merozoites. Red cells with rare GPA-deficiency phenotypes [En(a−) and M[k]] are substantially less susceptible to invasion than normal cells, and the deficiency phenotype for GPB (S−s−U−), which is relatively common in people of African origin, also appears to afford some resistance.[4] Both sialic acid on the O-glycans of GPA and the amino acid backbone appear to be essential for the binding of GPA to the *P. falciparum* ligand, EBA-175.[101] Cryptic regions around external loops 3 and 7 of band 3, the Diego antigen, only become exposed when the red cells are infected with *P. falciparum* and may be adhesive receptors, involved in the sequestration of infected red cells.[102] CD35, the Knops antigen, appears to be involved in the rosetting of *P. falciparum*-infected red cells with uninfected cells, a characteristic associated with severe disease. Red cells with low levels of CD35 and those with the Sl(a−) variant of CD35, common in black people, show reduced levels of rosetting with infected red cells.[103]

P antigen (globoside) is a cellular receptor for parvovirus B19, a human pathogen that replicates in erythroid progenitor cells, the only nucleated cells expressing P. B19 is the cause of fifth disease, a common childhood illness, and occasionally more severe disorders of erythropoiesis, particularly in immunocompromised patients.[104] Individuals with P deficiency (p phenotype) appear to be naturally resistant to parvovirus B19 infection.

Platelet antigens

The normal hemostatic function of platelets involves membrane glycoproteins, which function as receptors during platelet adhesion and aggregation. Several of the key platelet glycoproteins are polymorphic. Many of these polymorphisms are alloantigenic and were first recognized because of their potential to cause feto-maternal incompatibility characterized by the production of platelet-specific alloantibodies in the mother and a condition termed neonatal alloimmune thrombocytopenia (NAITP) in the fetus and newborn. In addition to the well-established role of platelet antigens in the pathogenesis of NAITP, there is evidence that some alloantigenic polymorphisms may affect platelet function and the predisposition to thrombotic disease.

Structure and function

Platelet alloantigens have been identified by many groups around the world and this has resulted in the evolution of several different terminologies. Since 1990, the Human Platelet Antigen (HPA) nomenclature has been almost universally adopted.[105] Currently, five systems (HPA-1 to HPA-5) and eight low-frequency alloantigens (HPA-6bw to HPA-13bw) have been assigned (Table 30.2). Alleles of genes encoding five platelet membrane glycoproteins result in the expression of alloantigens on the cell surface. Three antigens are expressed on glycoprotein Ia, four on glycoprotein Ib, three on glycoprotein IIb, and 10 on glycoprotein IIIa. Two antigens are expressed on CD109.

Table 30.2 Platelet antigens

System	Antigen	Alternative names	Glycoprotein	Nucleotide change	Amino acid change	References
HPA-1	HPA-1a	Zw^a, Pl^{A1}	GPIIIa	T196	Leu33	106
	HPA-1b	Zw^b, Pl^{A2}		C196	Pro33	
HPA-2	HPA-2a	Ko^b	GPIb	C524	Thr145	107
	HPA-2b	Ko^a, Sib^a		T524	Met145	
HPA-3	HPA-3a	Bak^a, Lek^a	GPIIb	T2622	Iso843	108
	HPA-3b	Bak^b		G2622	Ser843	
HPA-4	HPA-4a	Yuk^b, Pen^a	GPIIIa	G526	Arg143	109
	HPA-4b	Yuk^a, Pen^b		A526	Gln143	
HPA-5	HPA-5a	Br^b, Zav^b	GPIa	G1648	Glu505	110,111
	HPA-5b	Br^a, Zav^a, Hc^a		A1648	Lys505	
HPA-6w	HPA-6bw	Ca^a, Tu^a	GPIIIa	G1564	Arg489	112
				A1564	Gln489	
HPA-7w	HPA-7bw	Mo	GPIIIa	C1267	Pro407	113
				G1267	Ala407	
HPA-8w	HPA-8bw	Sr^a	GPIIIa	T2004	Arg636	114
				C2004	Cys636	
HPA-9w	HPA-9bw	Max^a	GPIIb	G2603	Val837	115
				A2603	Met837	
HPA-10w	HPA10bw	La^a	GPIIIa	G281	Arg62	116
				A281	Gln62	
HPA-11w	HPA11bw	Gro^a	GPIIIa	G1996	Arg633	117
				A1996	His633	
HPA-12w	HPA12bw	Iy^a	GPIb	G141	Gly15	118
				A141	Glu15	
HPA-13w	HPA13bw	Sit^a	GPIa	C2531	Thr799	119
				T2531	Met799	
		Oe^a	GPIIIa	AAG1929–1931 deletion	Lys611 deletion	120
		Va^a	GPIIb/IIIa			121
		Gov^a	CD109			122
		Gov^b				
		Pe^a	GPIb			123
		Dy^a	38kD GP			124

In addition, there are several reports describing less well-characterized antigens.

Antigens on the glycoprotein IIb/IIIa complex

Glycoprotein IIb/IIIa (CD41/CD61 or $\beta_3\alpha_{IIb}$) is the major platelet integrin, present at approximately 50 000 copies per platelet. Glycoprotein IIIa has a molecular weight of 90 kDa and consists of three domains: a large extracellular region that is cross-linked by 28 disulfide bonds, a transmembrane domain, and a short cytoplasmic region. Glycoprotein IIb is cleaved intracellularly before being expressed on the cell surface as a 116 kDa heavy chain disulfide-linked to a 22 kDa transmembrane protein. Upon platelet activation, glycoprotein IIb/IIIa is involved in platelet aggregation by binding adhesive proteins such as fibrinogen, fibronectin, vitronectin and von Willebrand factor (vWF).[125] A bleeding disorder called Glanzmann's thrombasthenia results when glycoprotein IIb/IIIa is absent or dysfunctional.

Three alloantigenic forms of glycoprotein IIb have been identified (HPA-3a, -3b, -9bw). Carbohydrate residues that are added post-translationally to glycoprotein IIb appear to contribute to the binding site of HPA-3 antibodies.[126]

Glycoprotein IIIa is the most polymorphic molecule on the platelet surface apart from HLA class I. The molecular bases of 10 of the antigens on glycoprotein IIIa have been determined (Table 30.2). Seven of the antigens (HPA-1b, -4b, -6w, -7w, -8w, -10w and -11w) are encoded by relatively rare single nucleotide substitutions in the common ancestral or wild-type form of glycoprotein IIIa (see Table 30.2 for references). The exception to date is the Oe[a] antigen, which results from the deletion of three nucleotides from the gene encoding the HPA-1b form of the glycoprotein.

The HPA-1a antigen is the most frequent cause of maternal alloimmunization to fetal platelets and is responsible for most cases of NAITP in Caucasians (discussed below). The gene frequencies for HPA-1a and HPA-1b in Caucasians are 85% and 15%, respectively. The immune response to HPA-1a is under genetic control and has been characterized at a molecular level. Although only 5–10% of HPA-1a-negative women with HPA-1a-positive fetuses produce anti-HPA-1a, the presence of the *HLA-DRB3*0101* allele increases the risk of alloimmunization by a factor of 140.[127] HPA-1b is caused by a Leu33Pro substitution. The immune response to HPA-1b does not appear to be HLA restricted.[128] An explanation for this observation was provided when Wu

et al[129] used an *in vitro* peptide-binding assay to show that leucine, but not proline, at position 33 anchors the peptide to the *HLA DRB3*0101*-encoded molecule. This also explains the rarity of anti-HPA-1b.

Antigens on the glycoprotein Ib/IX/V complex

Glycoprotein Ib/IX/V (CD42) binds vWF and mediates the adhesion of platelets to exposed vascular subendothelium under conditions of high shear stress. Glycoprotein Ib comprises two disulfide-bonded subunits called glycoprotein Ibα (CD42b) and glycoprotein Ibβ (CD42c). Glycoprotein Ib is non-covalently associated with glycoprotein IX (CD42a) and glycoprotein V (CD42d). There are approximately 25 000 glycoprotein Ib/IX molecules and 12 000 glycoprotein V molecules per platelet. The absence of the complex results in an inherited bleeding disorder called Bernard–Soulier syndrome.

Four antigens (HPA-2a, -2b -12w and Pe[a]) on glycoprotein Ib have been described (see Table 30.2). The frequencies of the genes encoding HPA-2a and HPA-2b are 93% and 7%, respectively, in Caucasians. In addition to these antigenic variations, there are four size variants of glycoprotein Ibα termed A, B, C and D (from largest to smallest). The differences are due to the number of 13 amino acid tandem repeats within the Ibα polypeptide (A = 4, B = 3, C = 2, D = 1).[130] Only the relatively rare A and B forms of glycoprotein Ibα contain Met145, which is required for the expression of the HPA-2b epitope.[131]

Antigens on the glycoprotein Ia/IIa complex

Glycoprotein Ia/IIa (CD49/CD29 or $\alpha_2\beta_1$), also known as VLA-2 (very late antigen), is an integrin expressed at relatively low density on platelets as well as on activated T-lymphocytes. The glycoprotein Ia/IIa heterodimer comprises a 167 kDa α_2 polypeptide and a 130 kDa β_1 polypeptide. It is a receptor for collagen and laminin and a mild bleeding disorder may result when the complex is absent.[132]

The three alloantigens (HPA-5a, -5b and -13w) that reside on glycoprotein Ia result from single nucleotide substitutions (see Table 30.2). Alloimmunization to the HPA-5b antigen could be responsible for approximately 15% of cases of NAITP in Caucasians (described below). In addition to these antigenic variations, there is silent dimorphism at nucleotide 807 within the gene encoding glycoprotein Ia, which results in variable expression of the Ia/IIa complex. Individuals with a C807 allele have relatively low receptor density.[133]

Antigens on CD109

CD109 is a 175 kDa GPI-anchored glycoprotein expressed on platelets, activated T-lymphocytes, cultured endothelial cells, and several tumor cell lines.[122] CD109 expresses two alloantigens, Gov[a] and Gov[b], with gene frequencies of 53% and 47%, respectively. Antibodies to both antigens may cause NAITP but they are encountered rarely. This might be due to the difficulty in detecting the antibodies because CD109 is expressed at low density on platelets.

Neonatal alloimmune thrombocytopenia

Neonatal alloimmune thrombocytopenia (NAITP), sometimes called fetomaternal alloimmune thrombocytopenia, is a syndrome characterized by thrombocytopenia in a fetus or neonate. It is caused by maternal antibodies that cross the placenta and bring about the immune destruction of fetal platelets. NAITP is, therefore, analogous to HDN.

Pathophysiology

In Caucasians, NAITP occurs in about 1 in 1500 births.[127] The natural history of NAITP differs from HDN in that maternal sensitization to fetal platelet antigens can occur in the first pregnancy; approximately 40% of cases occur in primiparae.[134] Platelet antigens might be more immunogenic than red cell antigens. For example, glycoprotein IIIa is found on syncytiotrophoblasts of the placental brush border[135] and might be released into the maternal circulation as the cells undergo apoptosis, perhaps during invasion of the endometrium.

All the well-characterized platelet-specific alloantigens have been associated with NAITP. In a study of 415 cases of NAITP in a Caucasian population, alloimmunization to HPA-1a was implicated in 73% of cases and anti-HPA-5b in 19% of cases. Antibodies of other specificities were each implicated in less than 1% of cases.[136] Although antibodies to HPA-1a are most commonly implicated in alloimmune thrombocytopenia in Caucasians, HPA-1b is very rare among blacks and Orientals and so anti-HPA-1a antibodies are also rare.[137,138] Among Orientals, anti-HPA-4a and -HPA-4b cause alloimmune thrombocytopenia more frequently than other platelet antibodies.

Maternal HPA antibodies are predominantly IgG1[139] and are, therefore, transported across the placenta to the fetus. There are few data on the cellular interactions involved in the alloimmune destruction of platelets in the fetus. However, studies of autoimmune thrombocytopenia in adults suggest that antibody-mediated platelet destruction involves the sequestration of platelets by splenic macrophages in a manner analogous to the extravascular destruction of IgG-sensitized red cells.[140] Fcγ receptor III (FcγRIII) might be involved in the recognition of sensitized platelets: administration of monoclonal anti-FcγRIII to a patient with autoimmune thrombocytopenia was associated with a rise in platelet count.[141]

In addition to causing the immune destruction of platelets, anti-HPA-1a from some cases of NAITP are able to inhibit fibrinogen binding to glycoprotein IIb/IIIa.[142] The HPA-1a polymorphism is located near the Arg-Gly-Asp fibrinogen binding motif. However, the ability of sera from patients with NAITP to inhibit fibrinogen binding is probably exceptional and is unlikely to be a major risk factor for fetal hemorrhage.[143]

Clinical features

Fetal thrombocytopenia may start early in pregnancy; almost 50% of affected fetuses have a platelet count of less than $20 \times 10^9/l$.[144] There is no spontaneous remission of the thrombocytopenia *in utero* and, in the absence of therapy, platelet counts usually fall as gestation progresses. In the absence of screening programs, alloimmune thrombocytopenia is usually recognized at birth when the majority of affected cases have petechiae, purpura or overt bleeding. Up to 28% of these affected cases show evidence of central nervous system hemorrhage and up to one-half of these hemorrhages occur prenatally.[145] *In utero* intracranial hemorrhages may be associated with severe neurological sequelae, porencephaly and optic hypoplasia.[146]

Clinically, alloimmune thrombocytopenia is a diagnosis of exclusion. Infants have no signs of disseminated intravascular coagulation, infection, or congenital anomalies that may be associated with thrombocytopenia. The mother has no history of autoimmune disease, thrombocytopenia, or ingestion of drugs that may cause thrombocytopenia. At delivery, standard laboratory tests show that neonatal platelet counts are low. Fetal hemoglobin concentration may be low if bleeding has occurred. Bone marrow biopsy usually reveals normal levels of megakaryocytes. Cranial ultrasound and computerized tomographic scans may reveal dilated cerebral ventricles and evidence of intraventricular hemorrhage.[147] Once suspected on clinical grounds, a provisional diagnosis of NAITP should be confirmed by establishing the presence of platelet-specific alloantibodies in the maternal serum that react with fetal platelets.

Alloantigenic platelet glycoprotein polymorphisms and hemostasis

HPA-1

Evidence that alloantigenic polymorphisms in glycoprotein IIb/IIIa affect platelet function is conflicting; when compared to platelets from *HPA-1a* homozygous individuals, HPA-1b platelets have been reported to exhibit increased,[148] decreased,[149] and similar[150] levels of binding to fibrinogen. Similarly, there is conflicting evidence on the association of HPA-1b with the predisposition to thrombotic disease. In 1996, Weiss *et al*[151] reported a relatively small study of 71 patients in which the *HPA-1b* allele was over-represented in subjects with coronary artery disease compared to normal controls (39.4% vs 19.1%, respectively); the *HPA-1b* allele was associated with a 2.8-fold increased risk of disease. Shortly thereafter, several much larger studies failed to confirm the association.[152,153] Similarly, four large studies on a total of 1140 patients failed to demonstrate an association with cerebrovascular disease.[154] Although HPA-1b may not represent a risk factor for coronary artery disease in the general population, it may represent a significant risk factor in patients with pre-existing coronary artery disease.[155]

HPA-2

The HPA-2 polymorphism does not appear to affect ristocetin-mediated platelet agglutination[156] or the binding of vWF to immobilized recombinant GPIbα.[157] Nevertheless, two studies of patients with coronary heart disease and cerebral vascular disease have found an increased frequency of the *HPA-2b* allele, suggesting that the mutation may have a functional effect.[158,159]

HPA-3

The HPA-3 polymorphism on glycoprotein IIb does not appear to affect susceptibility to developing thrombosis and restenosis after coronary stent placement.[160] Therefore, unlike the well-characterized association between the many antigenically-silent mutations in glycoprotein IIb/IIIa and Glanzmann's thrombasthenia, there is no consistent evidence for an association between the HPA-1 and HPA-3 polymorphisms and disease.

HPA-4 and other platelet antigens

The affinity of interaction between fibrinogen and glycoprotein IIb/IIIa does not appear to be affected by HPA-4 status, suggesting that polymorphism has little or no effect on integrin function.[161] Santoso *et al*[119] reported that the collagen-induced aggregation responses of platelets from Sit^a(+) individuals were diminished compared to Sit^a(−) individuals, indicating that the mutation affects the function of the GPIa/IIa complex. None of the individuals studied, however, had signs of an altered hemostasis.

Granulocyte antigens

Granulocyte-specific polymorphisms are less well characterized than those on red cells and platelets. Nevertheless, it is well established that some polymorphisms are antigenic and capable of eliciting alloimmune responses resulting in, for example, neonatal alloimmune neutropenia (NAIN). Most granulocyte antigens are expressed on membrane receptors involved in inflammation and the clearance of immune complexes and there is some evidence that these polymorphisms might affect cell function and the risk of some infectious or autoimmune diseases.

Structure and function

Some granulocyte antigens have been localized to FcγRIIIb (CD16), CD11a or CD11b. Granulocytes also express antigens with a wide tissue distribution. These include the I and P1 blood group antigens, Le^x and sialyl-Le^x (CD15), and HLA class I, and are not discussed further.

A human neutrophil antigen (HNA) nomenclature system has recently been adopted to include neutrophil-specific, granulocyte-specific, and some more widely distributed antigens.[162] Some antigens have not been incorporated into the system because they are insufficiently characterized. A list of granulocyte antigens is given in Table 30.3, which includes old names still in common usage.

Antigens on Fcγ receptor III

FcγRIIIb is a low-affinity receptor for complexed IgG, which is selectively expressed on neutrophils.[177] FcγRIIIb has an extracellular region consisting of two disulfide-bonded immunoglobulin-like domains and is linked to the plasma membrane via a GPI-anchor. Five alloantigenic polymorphisms have been located on Fcγ RIII: HNA-1a,

Table 30.3 Granulocyte antigens

System	Antigen	Alternative names	Glycoprotein	Nucleotide change	Amino acid change	References
HNA-1	HNA-1a	NA1	FcγRIIIb	G108 C114 A197 G247G319	Arg36, Asp65, Asp82, Val106	163
	HNA-1b	NA2 or NC1		C108 T114 G197A247A319	Ser36, Ser65, Asp82, Ile106	163
	HNA-1c	SH		A266	Asp78	164
HNA-2	HNA-2a	NB1	56–64 kDa	nk	nk	165,166
HNA-3	HNA-3a	5b	70–95 kDa	nk	nk	167
HNA-4	HNA-4a	Mart^a	CD11b	G302	Arg61	168
HNA-5	HNA-5a	Ond^a	CD11a	G2466	Arg766	168
–		NB2	45–56 kDa	nk	nk	169
ND		ND1	nk	nk	nk	170
NE		NE1	nk	nk	nk	171
LAN		LAN^a	FcγRIIIb	nk	nk	172
SAR		SAR^a	FcγRIIIb	nk	nk	173
9		9a	nk	nk	nk	174
5		5a	nk	nk	nk	175
SL		SL^a	nk	nk	nk	176

nk, not known.

-1b, -1c, LAN and SAR. When subjected to polyacrylamide gel electrophoresis, Fcγ RIIIb migrates as a broad band with a molecular weight between 50 kDa and 80 kDa. The differences in electrophoretic migration arise from amino acid differences between HNA-1a and HNA-1b at positions 65 and 82, which result in two additional glycosylation sites in HNA-1b.[163] At the DNA level, there are five nucleotide differences between the *HNA-1a* and *HNA-1b* genes, but only four of these substitutions give rise to amino acids changes (Table 30.3).

The HNA-1c antigen is associated with a nucleotide sequence identical to the *HNA-1b* gene, except for a C266A substitution.[164] Gene duplication appears to have led to many HNA-1c(+) individuals having three rather than two *Fcγ RIIIB* genes and expressing proportionately greater amounts of Fcγ RIIIb.[178] LAN and SAR are high frequency antigens on Fcγ RIIIb, but their molecular genetic bases are unknown.

Approximately 0.1% of Caucasians do not express FcγRIIIb as a result of *Fcγ RIII* gene deficiency. Women with this HNA-1 null phenotype can form isoantibodies causing severe neonatal neutropenia.[179]

Antigens on CD11/CD18

The HNA-4a (Mart^a) and HNA-5a (Ond^a) antigens are located on the CD11b and CD11a chains of the β2-integrins CD11b/18 (C3bi receptor, Mac1) and CD11a/CD18 (lymphocyte function-associated antigen 1, LFA-1), respectively. CD11a is expressed on all leukocytes while CD11b is expressed on granulocytes, monocytes and natural killer cells. HNA-4a and HNA-5a are both encoded by single nucleotide substitutions.[168]

Granulocyte antigens on other glycoproteins

The HNA-2a (NB1) antigen is expressed on granulocytes from 97% of the population.[180] Antibodies to HNA-2a (NB1) recognize a 56–64 kDa GPI-linked glycoprotein.[165] Anti-NB2 appears to recognize a smaller 46–56 kDa glycoprotein and so an antithetical relationship between the two antigens is doubtful.[181] The HNA-3a antigen (5b) is carried on a 70–95 kDa glycoprotein, which is probably expressed only on granulocytes.[167]

Neonatal alloimmune neutropenia

Pathophysiology

NAIN occurs in approximately 1 in 1500 births.[182,183] It is characterized by neutropenia in a fetus or infant caused by placental transfer of granulocyte antibodies. Granulocyte antigens are well expressed from before birth and the condition may occur in the first born infant.[183,184] Neutrophil destruction is probably mediated by macrophages in the fetal spleen; macrophages containing ingested neutrophils have been isolated from the spleens of patients with autoimmune neutropenia.[185]

Clinical features

NAIN usually has a relatively benign course with infants developing mild infections, predominantly of the skin and mucous membranes. Occasionally, more serous infections resulting in pneumonia and meningitis develop. Hematologic investigation reveals a severe neutropenia, which may persist for up to 6 months.[183] The bone marrow picture may be normal or hypercellular with the appearance of maturation arrest. NAIN is probably under-diagnosed as infants are usually asymptomatic at birth and white cell counts might not be performed routinely. Diagnosis is largely one of exclusion. In the absence of disease processes, drugs and environmental factors that can cause neutropenia or impairment of neutrophil function, a provisional diagnosis of NAIN should be confirmed by demonstrating the presence of antibodies in the maternal plasma that react with the infant's granulocytes.

Autoimmune neutropenia of infancy

In addition to their role in the pathogenesis of NAIN, some alloantigenic polymorphisms on granulocytes are also the target of autoantibodies implicated in autoimmune neutropenia of infancy (AIN). Disease onset usually occurs between 4 months and 2 years with spontaneous remission in 95% of patients within 7–24 months.[186,187] AIN is a relatively benign condition associated with infections of the skin, middle ear, throat, and respiratory and digestive tracts. The incidence of AIN is approximately 1 in 100 000.[188] Pathogenesis may involve a deficiency of suppresser T-lymphocytes, which results in the production of granulocyte-specific IgG or IgM autoantibodies, usually specific for HNA-1a.[187]

Granulocyte antigenic polymorphisms and disease

Several different receptors on granulocytes express non-alloantigenic polymorphisms, associated with altered cell function. Allogeneic forms of FcγRIIa for example, exhibit different affinities for human IgG2 and C-reactive protein and are associated with different risks for a range of infectious and autoimmune diseases.[189,190] In contrast, there are relatively few reports on the relationship between the alloantigenic polymorphisms and disease processes. Granulocytes from HNA-1a individuals have been reported to exhibit relatively enhanced phagocytosis of IgG-sensitized red cells and of IgG1-sensitized *Staphylococcus aureus, Haemophilus influenzae* and *Neisseria meningitidis*.[191,192] Homozygosity for *HNA-1a* has also been reported to predispose patients with myasthenia gravis to relatively severe disease and patients with multiple sclerosis to a relatively benign course.[193,194]

REFERENCES

1. Daniels GL, Anstee DJ, Cartron JP et al 1995 Blood group terminology 1995. From the ISBT Working Party on Terminology for Red Cell Surface Antigens. Vox Sanguinis 69: 265–279
2. Daniels GL, Anstee DJ, Cartron JP et al 1999 Terminology for red cell surface antigens. ISBT Working Party Oslo report. Vox Sanguinis 77: 52–57. Also see online:http//www.iccbba.com/page25.htm
3. Daniels G 1999 Functional aspects of red cell antigens. Blood Reviews 13: 14–35
4. Daniels G 1995 Human blood groups. Blackwell Science, Oxford
5. Issitt PD, Anstee DJ 1998 Applied blood group serology, 4th edn. Montgomery Scientific Publications, Durham, NC
6. Yamamoto F, Clausen H, White T et al 1990 Molecular genetic basis of the histo-blood group ABO system. Nature 345: 229–233
7. Hakomori S 1999 Antigen structure and genetic basis of histo blood groups A, B and O: their changes associated with human cancer. Biochimica et Biophysica Acta 1473: 246–266
8. Mollison PL, Engelfriet CP, Contreras M 1997 Blood transfusion in clinical medicine, 10th edn. Blackwell Science, Oxford
9. Issitt PD, Combs MR 1996 The specificity of antibodies causative of ABO HDN [abstract]. Transfusion 36(suppl): 23S
10. Gold ER, Tovey GH, Benney WE et al 1959 Changes in the group A antigen in a case of leukaemia. Nature 183: 892–893
11. Salmon C 1976 Blood groups changes in preleukemic states. Blood Cells 2: 211–220
12. Kolins J, Holland PV, McGinniss MH 1978 Multiple red cell antigen loss in acute granulocytic leukemia. Cancer 42: 2248–2253
13. Salmon C, Cartron JP, Lopez M et al 1984 Level of the A, B and H blood group glycosyltransferases in red cell membranes from patients with malignant hemopathies. Revue Française de Transfusion et Immuno-Hématologie 27: 625–637
14. Haas OA, Argyriou-Tirita A, Lion T 1992 Parental origin of chromosomes involved in the translocation t(9;22). Nature 359: 414–416
15. Henry S, Oriol R, Samuelsson B 1995 Lewis histo-blood group system and associated secretory phenotypes. Vox Sanguinis 69: 166–182
16. Ørntoft TF, Meldgaard P, Pedersen B et al 1996 The blood group ABO gene transcript is down-regulated in human bladder tumors and growth-stimulated urothelial cell lines. Cancer Research 56: 1031–1036
17. Yuan M, Itzkowitz SH, Palekar A et al 1985 Distribution of blood group antigens A, B, H, Lewis^a, and Lewis^b in human normal, fetal, and malignant colonic tissue. Cancer Research 45: 4499–4511
18. Ørntoft TF, Greenwell P, Clausen H et al 1991 Regulation of the oncodevelopmental expression of type 1 chain ABH and Lewis^b blood group antigens in human colon by α-2-L-fucosylation. Gut 32: 287–293
19. Ørntoft TF, Bech E 1995 Circulating blood group related carbohydrate antigens as tumour markers. Glygoconjugate Journal 12: 200–205
20. Steinberg W 1990 The clinical utility of the CA 19 9 tumor associated antigen. American Journal of Gastroenterology 85: 350–355
21. Narimatsu H, Iwasaki H, Nakayama F et al 1998 *Lewis* and *Secretor* gene dosages affect CA19–9 and DU-PAN-2 serum levels in normal individuals and colorectal cancer patients. Cancer Research 58: 512–518
22. Clausen H, Hakomori S, Graem N et al 1986 Incompatible A antigen expressed in tumors of blood group O individuals: immunochemical, immunohistologic, and enzymatic characterization. Journal of Immunology 136: 326–330
23. David L, Leitao D, Sobrinho-Simoes M et al 1993 Biosynthetic basis of incompatible histo-blood group A antigen expression: anti-A transferase antibodies reactive with gastric cancer tissue of type O individuals. Cancer Research 53: 5494–5500
24. Hakomori S 1991 Immunochemical and molecular genetic basis of the histo-blood group ABO(H) and related antigen system. Baillière's Clinical Haematology 4: 957–974
25. Avent ND, Reid ME 2000 The Rh blood group system: a review. Blood 95: 375–387
26. Huang C-H, Liu PZ, Cheng JG 2000 Molecular biology and genetics of the Rh blood group system. Seminars in Hematology 37: 150–165
27. Suto Y, Ishikawa Y, Hyodo H et al 2000 Gene organization and rearrangements at the human Rhesus blood group locus revealed by fiber-FISH analysis. Human Genetics 106: 164–171
28. Wagner FF, Flegel WA 2000 The *RHD* gene deletion occurred in the Rhesus box. Blood 95: 3662–3668

29. Singleton BK, Green CA, Avent ND et al 2000 The presence of an *RHD* pseudogene containing a 37 base pair duplication and a nonsense mutation in most Africans with the Rh D-negative blood group phenotype. Blood 95: 12–18

30. Ridgwell K, Spurr NK, Laguda B et al 1992 Isolation of cDNA clones for a 50 kDa glycoprotein of the human erythrocyte membrane associated with Rh (Rhesus) blood-group antigen expression. Biochemical Journal 287: 223–228

31. MacKenzie IZ, Bowell PJ, Selinger M 1992 Deaths from haemolytic disease of the newborn. British Medical Journal 304: 1175–1176

32. Flegel WA, Wagner FF, Müller TH et al 1998 Rh phenotype prediction by DNA typing and its application to practice. Transfusion Medicine 8: 281–302

33. Lee S, Russo D, Redman C 2000 Functional and structural aspects of the Kell blood group system. Transfusion Medicine Reviews 14: 93–103

34. Russo D, Redman C, Lee S 1998 Association of XK and Kell blood group proteins. Journal of Biological Chemistry 273: 13950–13956

35. Turner AJ, Tanzawa K 1997 Mammalian membrane metallopeptidases. NEP, ECE, KELL, and PEX. FASEB Journal 11: 355–364

36. Lee S, Lin M, Mele A et al 1999 Proteolytic processing of big endothelin-3 by the Kell blood group protein. Blood 94: 1440–1450

37. Vaughan JI, Warwick R, Letsky E et al 1994 Erythropoietic suppression in fetal anemia because of Kell alloimmunization. American Journal of Obstetrics and Gynecology 171: 247–252

38. Weiner CP, Widness JA 1996 Decreased fetal erythropoiesis and hemolysis in Kell hemolytic anemia. American Journal of Obstetrics and Gynecology 174: 547–551

39. Southcott MJG, Tanner MJA, Anstee DJ 1999 The expression of human blood group antigens during erythropoiesis in a cell culture system. Blood 93: 4425–4435

40. Bony V, Gane P, Bailly P et al 1999 Time-course expression of polypeptides carrying blood group antigens during human erythroid differentiation. British Journal of Haematology 107: 263–274

41. Daniels GL, Hadley AG, Green CA 1999 Fetal anaemia due to anti-K may result from immune destruction of early erythroid progenitors [abstract]. Transfusion Medicine 9(suppl): 16.

42. Vaughan JI, Manning M, Warwick RM et al 1998 Inhibition of erythroid progenitor cells by anti-Kell antibodies in fetal alloimmune anemia. New England Journal of Medicine 338: 798–803

43. Ho M, Chelly J, Carter N et al 1994 Isolation of the gene for McLeod syndrome that encodes a novel membrane transport protein. Cell 77: 869–880

44. Roos D, de Boer M, Kuribayashi F et al 1996 Mutations in the X-linked and autosomal recessive forms of chronic granulomatous disease. Blood 87: 1663–1681

45. Curnutte J, Bemiller L 1995 Chronic granulomatous disease with McLeod phenotype: an uncommon occurrence [abstract]. Transfusion 35(suppl): 60S.

46. Tanner MJA 1997 The structure and function of band 3 (AE1): recent developments (review). Molecular and Membrane Biology 14: 155–165

47. Ribeiro ML, Alloisio N, Almeida H et al 1997 Hereditary spherocytosis with total absence of band 3 in a baby with mutation Coimbra (V488M) in the homozygous state [abstract]. Blood 90(suppl 1): 265a.

48. Peters LL, Shivdasani RA, Lui SC et al 1996 Anion exchanger 1 (band 3) is required to prevent erythrocyte membrane surface loss but not to form the membrane skeleton. Cell 86: 917–927

49. Southgate CD, Chisti AH, Mitchell B et al 1996 Targeted disruption of the murine erythroid band 3 gene results in spherocytosis and severe haemolytic anaemia despite a normal membrane skeleton. Nature Genetics 14: 227–230

50. Inaba M, Yawata A, Koshino I et al 1996 Defective anion transport and marked spherocytosis and membrane instability caused by hereditary total deficiency of red cell band 3 in cattle due to a nonsense mutation. Journal of Clinical Investigation 97: 1804–1817

51. Olivès B, Mattei M-G, Huet M et al 1995 Kidd blood group and urea transport function of human erythrocytes are carried by the same protein. Journal of Biological Chemistry 270: 15607–15610

52. Xu Y, Olivès B, Bailly P et al 1997 Endothelial cells of the kidney vasa recta express the urea transporter HUT11. Kidney International 51: 138–146

53. Macey RI, Yousef LW 1988 Osmotic stability of red cells in renal circulation required rapid urea transport. American Journal of Physiology 254: C669–C674

54. Lucien N, Sidoux-Walter F, Olivès B et al 1998 Characterization of the gene encoding the human Kidd blood group/urea transporter protein. Evidence for splice site mutations in Jk$_{null}$ individuals. Journal of Biological Chemistry 273: 12973–12980

55. Irshaid NM, Henry SM, Olsson ML 2000 Genomic characterization of the Kidd blood group gene: different molecular basis of the Jk(a–b–) phenotype in Polynesians and Finns. Transfusion 40: 69–74

56. Henry S, Woodfield G 1995 Frequencies of the Jk(a–b–) phenotype in Polynesian ethnic groups. Transfusion 35: 277

57. King LS, Agre P 1996 Pathophysiology of the aquaporin water channels. Annual Review of Physiology 58: 619–648

58. Preston GM, Agre P 1991 Isolation of the cDNA for erythrocyte integral membrane protein of 28 kilodaltons: member of an ancient channel family. Proceedings of the National Academy of Sciences USA 88: 11110–11114

59. Smith BL, Baumgarten R, Nielsen S et al 1993 Concurrent expression of erythroid and renal aquaporin CHIP and appearance of water channel activity in perinatal rats. Journal of Clinical Investigation 92: 2035–2041

60. Nakhoul NL, Davis BA, Romero MF et al 1998 Effect of expressing the water channel aquaporin-1 on the CO_2 permeability of *Xenopus* oocytes. American Journal of Physiology 274: C543–C548

61. Preston GM, Smith BL, Zeidel ML et al 1994 Mutations in aquaporin-1 in phenotypically normal humans without functional CHIP water channels. Science 265: 1585–1587

62. Telen MJ 2000 Red blood cell adhesion molecules: their possible roles in normal human physiology and disease. Seminars in Hematology 37: 130–142

63. Murdoch C, Finn A 2000 Chemokine receptors and their role in inflammation and infectious diseases. Blood 95: 3032–3043

64. Darbonne WC, Rice GC, Mohler MA et al 1991 Red blood cells are a sink for interleukin 8, a leukocyte chemotaxin. Journal of Clinical Investigation 88: 1362–1369

65. Hadley TJ, Peiper SC 1997 From malaria to chemokine receptor: the emerging physiologic role of the Duffy blood group antigen. Blood 89: 3077–3091

66. Tournamille C, Colin Y, Cartron JP et al 1995 Disruption of a GATA motif in the *Duffy* gene promoter abolishes erythroid gene expression in Duffy-negative individuals. Nature Genetics 10: 224–228

67. Peiper SC, Wang Z, Neote K et al 1995 The Duffy antigen/receptor for chemokines (DARC) is expressed in endothelial cells of Duffy-negative individuals who lack the erythrocyte receptor. Journal of Experimental Medicine 181: 1311–1317

68. Mallinson G, Soo KS, Schall TJ et al 1995 Mutations in the erythrocyte chemokine receptor (Duffy) gene: The molecular basis of the Fy^a/Fy^b antigens and identification of a deletion in the Duffy gene of an apparently healthy individual with the Fy(a–b–) phenotype. British Journal of Haematology 90: 823–829

69. Rios M, Chaudhuri A, Mallinson G et al 2000 New genotypes in Fy(a–b–) individuals: nonsense mutations (Trp to stop) in the coding sequence of either *FY A* or *FY B*. British Journal of Haematology 108: 448–454

70. Wang J, Springer TA 1998 Structural specializations of immunoglobulin superfamily members for adhesion to integrins and viruses. Immunological Reviews 163: 197–215

71. Parsons SF, Mallinson G, Holmes CH et al 1995 The Lutheran blood group glycoprotein, another member of the immunoglobulin superfamily, is widely expressed in human tissues and is developmentally regulated in human liver. Proceedings of the National Academy of Sciences USA 92: 5496–5500

72. Bailly P, Hermand P, Callebaut I et al 1994 The LW blood group glycoprotein is homologous to intercellular adhesion molecules. Proceedings of the National Academy of Sciences USA 91: 5306–5310

73. Spring FA, Homes CH, Simpson KL et al 1997 The Ok^a blood group antigen is a marker for the M6 leukocyte activation antigen, the human homolog of OX-47 antigen, basigin and neurothelin, an immunoglobulin superfamily molecule that is widely expressed in human cells and tissues. European Journal of Immunology 27: 891–897

74. Udani M, Zen Q, Cottman M et al 1998 Basal cell adhesion molecule/Lutheran protein. The receptor critical for sickle cell adhesion to laminin. Journal of Clinical Investigation 101: 2550–2558

75. Nemer WE, Gane P, Colin Y et al 1998 The Lutheran blood group glycoproteins, the erythroid receptors for laminin, are adhesion molecules. Journal of Biological Chemistry 273: 16686–16693

76. Parsons SF, Spring FA, Chasis JA et al 1999 Erythroid cell adhesion molecules Lutheran and LW in health and disease. Baillière's Clinical Haematology 12: 729–745

77. Mallinson G, Green CA, Okubo Y et al 1997 The molecular background of recessive Lu(a–b–) phenotype in a Japanese family [abstract]. Transfusion Medicine 7(suppl 1): 18

78. Hermand P, Le Pennec PY, Rouger P et al 1996 Characterization of the gene encoding the human LW blood group protein in LW+ and LW– phenotypes. Blood 87: 2962–2967

79. Lublin DM, Atkinson JP 1989 Decay-accelerating factor: biochemistry, molecular biology, and function. Annual Revue of Immunology 7: 35–58

80. Lachmann PJ 1991 The control of homologous lysis. Immunology Today 12: 312–315

81. Rosse WF, Ware RE 1995 The molecular basis of paroxysmal nocturnal hemoglobinuria. Blood 86: 3277–3286

82. Tomita M 1999 Biochemical background of paroxysmal nocturnal hemoglobinuria. Biochimica et Biophysica Acta 1455: 269–286

83. Telen MJ, Green AM 1989 The Inab phenotype: characterization of the membrane protein and complement regulatory defect. Blood 74: 437–441

84. Merry AH, Rawlinson VI, Uchikawa M et al 1989 Studies on the sensitivity to complement-mediated lysis of erythrocytes (Inab phenotype) with a deficiency of DAF (decay accelerating factor). British Journal of Haematology 73: 248–253

85. Wang L, Uchikawa M, Tsuneyama H et al 1998 Molecular cloning and characterization of decay-accelerating factor deficiency in Cromer blood group Inab phenotype. Blood 91: 680–684

86. Daniels GL, Green CA, Mallinson G et al 1998 Decay-accelerating factor (CD55) deficiency in Japanese. Transfusion Medicine 8: 141–147

87. Motoyama N, Okada N, Yamashina M et al 1992 Paroxysmal nocturnal hemoglobinuria due to hereditary nucleotide deletion in the HRF20 (CD59) gene. European Journal of Immunology 22: 2669–2673

88. Rao N, Ferguson DJ, Lee S-F et al 1991 Identification of human erythrocyte blood group antigens on the C3b/C4b receptor. Journal of Immunology 146: 3502–3507

89. Moulds JM, Nickells MW, Moulds JJ et al 1991 The C3b/C4b receptor is recognized by the Knops, McCoy, Swain-Langley, and York blood group antisera. Journal of Experimental Medicine 173: 1159–1163

90. Ahearn JM Fearon DT 1989 Structure and function of the complement receptors, CR1 (CD35) and CR2 (CD21). Advances in Immunology 46: 183–219

91. Moulds JM, Moulds JJ, Brown M, Atkinson JP 1992 Antiglobulin testing for CR1-related (Knops/McCoy/Swain-Langley/York) blood group antigens: negative and weak reactions are caused by variable expression of CR1. Vox Sanguinis 62: 230–235

92. Moulds JM 1994 Association of blood group antigens with immunologically important proteins. In: Garratty G (ed), Immunobiology of transfusion medicine. Dekker, New York, 273–297

93. Lach-Trifilieff E, Mafurt J, Schwarz S et al 1999 Complement receptor 1 (CD35) on human reticulocytes: normal expression in systemic lupus erythematosus and HIV-infected patients. Journal of Immunology 162: 7549–7554

94. Jarolim P, Murray JL, Rubin HL et al 1996 Characterization of 13 novel band 3 gene defects in hereditary spherocytosis with band 3 deficiency. Blood 88: 4366–4374

95. Marfatia SM, Morais-Chabral JH, Kim AC et al 1997 The PDZ domain of human erythrocyte p55 mediates its binding to the cytoplasmic carboxyl terminus of glycophorin C. Analysis of the binding interface by *in vitro* mutagenesis. Journal of Biological Chemistry 272: 24191–24197

96. Workman RF, Low PS 1998 Biochemical analysis of potential sites for protein 4.1-mediated anchoring of the spectrin-actin skeleton to the erythrocyte membrane. Journal of Biological Chemistry 273: 6171–6176

97. Daniels GL, Shaw M-A, Judson PA et al 1986 A family demonstrating inheritance of the Leach phenotype: a Gerbich-negative phenotype associated with elliptocytosis. Vox Sanguinis 50: 117–121

98. Alloisio N, Venezia ND, Rana A et al 1993 Evidence that red blood cell protein p55 may participate in the skeleton-membrane linkage that involves protein 4.1 and glycophorin C. Blood 82: 1323–1327

99. Eder AF, Spitalnik SL 1997 Blood group antigens as receptors for pathogens. In: Blancher A, Klein J, Socha WW (eds), Molecular biology and evolution of blood group and MHC antigens in primates. Springer, Berlin 268–304

100. Rios M, Bianco C 2000 The role of blood group antigens in infectious diseases. Seminars in Hematology 37: 177–185

101. DeLuca GM, Donnell ME, Carrigan DJ et al 1996 *Plasmodium falciparum* merozoite adhesion is mediated by sialic acid. Biochemical and Biophysical Research Communications 225: 726–732

102. Oh SS, Chisti AH, Palek J et al 1997 Erythrocyte membrane alterations in *Plasmodium falciparum* malaria sequestration. Current Opinion in Hematology 4: 148–154

103. Rowe JA, Moulds JM, Newbold CI et al 1997 *P. falciparum* rosetting mediated by a parasite-variant erythrocyte membrane protein and complement-receptor 1. Nature 388: 292–295

104. Brown KE, Young NS 1995 Parvovirus B19 infection and hematopoiesis. Blood Reviews 9: 176–182

105. von dem Borne AEG Kr, Decary F 1990 Nomenclature of platelet specific antigens. British Journal of Haematology 74: 239–240

106. Newman PJ, Derbes RS, Aster RH 1989 The human platelet alloantigens, P1A1 and P1A2, are associated with a leucine33/proline33 amino acid polymorphism in membrane glycoprotein IIIa, and are distinguishable by DNA typing. Journal of Clinical Investigation 83: 1778–1781

107. Kuijpers RW, Faber NM, Cuypers HT et al 1992 NH2-terminal globular domain of human platelet glycoprotein Ib alpha has a methionine 145/threonine145 amino acid polymorphism, which is associated with the HPA-2 (Ko) alloantigens. Journal of Clinical Investigation 89: 381–384

108. Lyman S, Aster RH, Visentin GP et al 1990 Polymorphism of human platelet membrane glycoprotein IIb associated with the Baka/Bakb alloantigen system. Blood 75: 2343–2348

109. Wang R, Furihata K, McFarland JG et al 1992 An amino acid polymorphism within the RGD binding domain of platelet membrane glycoprotein IIIa is responsible for the formation of the Pena/Penb alloantigen system. Journal of Clinical Investigation 90: 2038–2043

110. Santoso S, Kalb R, Walka M et al 1993 The human platelet alloantigens Br(a) and Brb are associated with a single amino acid polymorphism on glycoprotein Ia (integrin subunit alpha 2). Journal of Clinical Investigation 92: 2427–2432

111. Simsek S, Gallardo D, Ribera A et al 1994 The human platelet alloantigens, HPA-5(a+, b–) and HPA-5(a–, b+), are associated with a Glu505/Lys505 polymorphism of glycoprotein Ia (the alpha 2 subunit of VLA-2). British Journal of Haematology 86: 671–674

112. Wang R, McFarland JG, Kekomaki R et al 1993 Amino acid 489 is encoded by a mutational 'hot spot' on the beta 3 integrin chain: the CA/TU human platelet alloantigen system. Blood 82: 3386–3391

113. Kuijpers RW, Simsek S, Faber NM et al 1993 Single point mutation in human glycoprotein IIIa is associated with a new platelet-specific alloantigen (Mo) involved in neonatal alloimmune thrombocytopenia. Blood 81: 70–76

114. Santoso S, Kalb R, Kroll H et al 1994 A point mutation leads to an unpaired cysteine residue and a molecular weight polymorphism of a functional platelet beta 3 integrin subunit. The Sra alloantigen system of GPIIIa. Journal of Biological Chemistry 18: 8439–8444

115. Noris P, Simsek S, de Bruijne-Admiraal LG et al 1995 Max(a), a new low-frequency platelet-specific antigen localized on glycoprotein IIb, is associated with neonatal alloimmune thrombocytopenia. Blood 86: 1019–1026

116. Peyruchaud O, Bourre F, Morel-Kopp MC et al 1997 HPA-10w(b) (La(a)): genetic determination of a new platelet-specific alloantigen on glycoprotein IIIa and its expression in COS-7 cells. Blood 89: 2422–2428

117. Simsek S, Folman C, van der Schoot CE et al 1997 The Arg633His substitution responsible for the private platelet antigen Gro(a) unravelled by SSCP analysis and direct sequencing. British Journal of Haematology 97: 330–335

118. Sachs UJ, Kiefel V, Bohringer M et al 2000 Single amino acid substitution in human platelet glycoprotein Ibbeta is responsible for the formation of the platelet-specific alloantigen Iy(a). Blood 95: 1849–1855

119. Santoso S, Amrhein J, Hofmann HA et al 1999 A point mutation Thr(799)Met on the alpha(2) integrin leads to the formation of new human platelet alloantigen Sit(a) and affects collagen-induced aggregation. Blood 94: 4103–4111

120. Santoso, S. Pylypiw R, Wilke IG et al 1998 One amino acid deletion of the PlA2 allelic form of GPIIIa leads to the formation of the new platelet alloantigen, Oe(a). Transfusion Medicine 8: 257a

121. Kekomäki R, Raivio P, Kero P 1992 A new low-frequency platelet alloantigen, Va^a, on glycoprotein IIbIIIa associated with neonatal alloimmune thrombocytopenia. Transfusion Medicine 2: 27–33

122. Smith JW, Hayward CP, Horsewood P et al 1995 Characterization and localization of the Gova/b alloantigens to the glycosylphosphatidylinositol-anchored protein CDw109 on human platelets. Blood 86: 2807–2814

123. Kekomäki R, Partanen J, Pitkänen S et al 1993 Glycoprotein Ib/IX-specific alloimmunization in an HPA-2b-homozygous mother in association with neonatal thrombocytopenia. Thrombosis and Haemostasis 69:99

124. Smith JW, Horsewood P, McCusker PJ et al 1998 Severe neonatal alloimmune thrombocytopenia due to a novel low-frequency alloantigen Dy^a. Blood 92(suppl 1): 180a

125. Calvete JJ 1999 Platelet integrin GPIIb/IIIa: structure-function correlations. An update and lessons from other integrins. Proceedings of the Society of Experimental Biology and Medicine 222: 29–38

126. Calvete JJ, Muniz-Diaz E 1993 Localization of an O-glycosylation site in the alpha-subunit of the human platelet integrin GPIIb/IIIa involved in Bak^a (HPA-3a) alloantigen expression. FEBS Letters 328: 30–34

127. Williamson LM, Hackett G, Rennie J et al 1998 The natural history of fetomaternal alloimmunization to the platelet-specific antigen HPA-1a (PL^{A1}, Zw^a) as determined by antenatal screening. Blood 92: 2280–2287

128. Kuijpers RWAM, von dem Borne AEG, Kiefel V et al 1992 Leucine³³-proline³³ substitution in human platelet glycoprotein IIIa determines HLA-DR52a (Dw24) association of the immune response against HPA-1a (Zw^a/PI^{A1}) and HPA-1b (Zw^b/PI^{A2}). Human Immunology 34: 253–356

129. Wu S, Maslanka K, Gorski J 1997 An integrin polymorphism that defines reactivity with alloantibodies generates an anchor for MHC class II peptide binding: a model for unidirectional alloimmune responses. Journal of Immunology 158: 3221–3226

130. Lopez JA, Ludwig EH, McCarthy BJ (1992) Polymorphism of human glycoprotein Ib alpha results from a variable number of tandem repeats of a 13-amino acid sequence in the mucin-like macroglycopeptide region. Structure/function implications. Journal of Biological Chemistry 267: 10055–10061

131. Simsek S, Bleeker PM, van der Schoot CE et al 1994 Association of a variable number of tandem repeats (VNTR) in glycoprotein Ib alpha and HPA-2 alloantigens. Thrombosis and Haemostasis 72: 757–761

132. Nieuwenhuis HK, Akkerman JW, Houdijk WP et al 1985 Human blood platelets showing no response to collagen fail to express surface glycoprotein Ia. Nature 318: 470–472

133. Kunicki TJ, Kritzik M, Annis DS et al 1997 Hereditary variation in platelet integrin alpha 2 beta 1 density is associated with two silent polymorphisms in the alpha 2 gene coding sequence. Blood 89: 1939–1943

134. Mueller-Eckhardt C, Kiefel V, Grubert A et al 1989 348 cases of suspected neonatal alloimmune neonatal thrombocytopenia. Lancet 1: 363–366

135. Vanderpuye OA, Labarrere CA, McIntyre JA 1991 A vitronectin-receptor-related molecule in human placental brush border membranes. Biochem J 280: 9–17

136. Kroll H, Kiefel V, Santoso S 1998 Clinical aspects and typing of platelet alloantigens. Vox Sanguinis 74(suppl 2): 345–354

137. Ramsey G, Salamon DJ 1986 Frequency of PI^{A1} in blacks. Transfusion 26: 531–532

138. Shibata Y, Matsuda I, Miyaji T et al 1986 Yuk^a, a new platelet antigen involved in two cases of neonatal alloimmune thrombocytopenia. Vox Sanguinis 50: 177–180

139. Proulx C, Filion M, Goldman M et al 1994 Analysis of immunoglobulin class, IgG subclass and titre of HPA-1a antibodies in alloimmunized mothers giving birth to babies with or without neonatal alloimmune thrombocytopenia. British Journal of Haematology 87: 813–817

140. McMillan R, Longmire RL, Tavassoli M et al 1974 In vitro platelet phagocytosis by splenic leukocytes in idiopathic thrombocytopenic purpura. New England Journal of Medicine 290: 249–251

141. Clarkson SB, Bussel JB, Kimberley RP et al 1986 Treatment of refractory immune thrombocytopenic purpura with an anti-Fcγ-receptor antibody. New England Journal of Medicine 314: 1236–1239

142. van Leeuwen EF, Leeksma OC, van Mourik JA et al 1984 Effect of the binding of anti-Zw^a antibodies on platelet function. Vox Sanguinis 47: 280–289

143. Beadling WV, Herman JH, Stuart MJ et al 1995 Fetal bleeding in neonatal alloimmune thrombocytopenia mediated by anti-PI^{A1} is not associated with inhibition of fibrinogen binding to platelet GPIIb/IIIa. American Journal of Clinical Pathology 103: 636–641

144. Bussel JB, Zabusky MR, Berkowitz RL et al 1997 Fetal alloimmune thrombocytopenia. New England Journal of Medicine 337: 22–26

145. Herman JH, Jumbelic ML, Ancona RJ et al 1986 In utero cerebral hemorrhage in alloimmune thrombocytopenia. American Journal of Pediatric Hematology and Oncology 8: 312–317

146. Sitarz AL, Driscoll JM Jr, Wolff JA 1976 Management of isoimmune neonatal thrombocytopenia. American Journal of Obstetrics and Gynecology 124: 39–42

147. Burrows RF, Caco CC, Kelton JG 1988 Neonatal alloimmune thrombocytopenia: spontaneous in utero intracranial hemorrhage. American Journal of Hematology 28: 98–102

148. Goodall AH, Curzen N, Panesar M et al 1999 Increased binding of fibrinogen to glycoprotein IIIa-proline 33 (HPA-1b, PI^{A2}, Zw^b) positive platelets in patients with cardiovascular disease. European Heart Journal 20: 742–747

149. Goldschmidt-Clermont PJ, Weiss EJ, Shear WS et al 1996 Platelets from PI^{A2}(–) individuals bind more exogenous fibrinogen than platelets from PI^{A2}(+) individuals. Blood 88: 26a

150. Meiklejohn DJ, Urbaniak SJ, Greaves M 1999 Platelet glycoprotein IIIa polymorphism HPA 1b (PI^{A2}): no association with platelet fibrinogen binding. British Journal of Haematology 105: 664–666

151. Weiss EJ, Bray PF, Tayback M et al 1996 A polymorphism of a platelet glycoprotein receptor as an inherited risk factor for coronary thrombosis. New England Journal of Medicine 334: 1090–1094

152. Ridker PM, Hennekens CH, Schmitz C et al 1997 PI^{A1}/PI^{A2} polymorphism of platelet glycoprotein IIIa and risks of myocardial infarction, stroke, and venous thrombosis. Lancet 349: 385–388

153. Herrmann SM, Poirier O, Marques-Vidal P et al 1997 The Leu33/Pro polymorphism (PI^{A1}/PI^{A2}) of the glycoprotein IIIa (GPIIIa) receptor is not related to myocardial infarction in the ECTIM Study. Etude Cas-Temoins de l'Infarctus du Myocarde. Thrombosis and Haemostasis 77: 1179–1181

154. Lane DA, Grant PJ 2000 Role of hemostatic gene polymorphisms in venous and arterial thrombotic disease. Blood 95: 1517–1532

155. Zotz RB, Klein M, Dauben HP et al 2000 Prospective analysis after coronary-artery bypass grafting: platelet GP IIIa polymorphism (HPA-1b/PI^{A2}) is a risk factor for bypass occlusion, myocardial infarction, and death. Thrombosis and Haemostasis 83: 404–407

156. Mazzucato M, Pradella P, de Angelis V et al 1996 Frequency and functional relevance of genetic threonine¹⁴⁵/methionine¹⁴⁵ dimorphism in platelet glycoprotein Ibα in an Italian population. Transfusion 36: 891–894

157. Li CQ, Garner SF, Davies J et al 2000 Threonine-145/methionine-145 variants of baculovirus produced recombinant ligand binding domain of GPIbalpha express HPA-2 epitopes and show equal binding of von Willebrand factor. Blood 95: 205–211

158. Murata M, Matsubara Y, Kawano K et al 1997 Coronary artery disease and polymorphisms in a receptor mediating shear stress-dependent platelet activation. Circulation 96: 3281–3286

159. Gonzalez-Conejero R, Lozano ML, Rivera J et al 1998 Polymorphisms of platelet membrane glycoprotein Ib associated with arterial thrombotic disease. Blood 92: 2771–2776

160. Bottiger C, Kastrati A, Koch W et al 1999 Polymorphism of platelet glycoprotein IIb and risk of thrombosis and restenosis after coronary stent placement. American Journal of Cardiology 84: 987–991

161. Wang R, Newman PJ 1998 Adhesive and signaling properties of a naturally occurring allele of glycoprotein IIIa with an amino acid substitution within the ligand binding domain-the Pen^a/Pen^b platelet alloantigenic epitopes. Blood 92: 3260–3267

162. Bux J 1999 Nomenclature of granulocyte alloantigens. Transfusion 39: 662–663

163. Ory PA, Clark MR, Kwoh EE et al 1989 Sequences of complementary DNAs that encode the NA1 and NA2 forms of Fc receptor III on human neutrophils. Journal of Clinical Investigation 84: 1688–1691

164. Bux J, Stein E-L, Bierling P et al 1997 Characterization of a new alloantigen (SH) on the human neutrophil Fcγ receptor IIIb. Blood 89: 1027–1034

165. Stroncek DF, Skubitz KM, McCullough JJ 1990 Biochemical characterization of the neutrophil-specific antigen NB1. Blood 75: 744–755

166. Goldschmeding R, van Dalen CM, Faber N et al 1992 Further characterization of the NB1 antigen as a variably expressed 56–62 kD GPI-linked glycoprotein of plasma membranes and specific granules of neutrophils. British Journal of Haematology 81: 336–345

167. de Haas M, Muniz-Diaz E, Alonso LG et al 2000 Neutrophil antigen 5b is carried by a protein, migrating from 70 to 95 kDa, and may be involved in neonatal alloimmune neutropenia. Transfusion 40: 222–227

168. Simsek S, van der Schoot CE, Daams M et al 1996 Molecular characterization of antigenic polymorphisms (Onda and Marta) of the beta 2 family recognized by human leukocyte alloantisera. Blood 88: 1350–1358

169. Wu GG. Curtis BR, Shao YL et al 1993 Investigation of human neutrophil antigens with a new nonradioactive technique: characterization of NB1 and NB2 antigenic targets. Transfusion 33: 78S

170. Verhuegt FWA, von dem Borne AEG Kr, van Noord-Bokhorst JC et al 1978 ND1, a new neutrophil granulocyte antigen. Vox Sanguinis 35: 13–17

171. Class JHJ, Langerak, J, Sabbe LJM et al 1979 NE1: a new neutrophil specific antigen. Tissue Antigens 13: 129–134

172. Metcalfe P, Waters AH 1993 Location of the granulocyte-specific antigen LAN on the Fc-receptor III. Transfusion Medicine 2: 283–287

173. Bux J, Hartmann C, Mueller-Eckhardt C 1994 Alloimmune neonatal neutropenia resulting from immunization to a high frequency antigen on the granulocyte Fcγ receptor III. Transfusion 34: 608–611

174. Jager MJ, Claas FHJ, Witvvliet M et al 1986 Correspondence of the monocyte antigen HMA-1 to the non-HLA antigen 9a. Immunogenetics 23: 71–77

175. van Leeuwen A, Eernnisse JG, van Rood JJ 1964 A new leucocyte group with two alleles: Leucocyte group five. Vox Sanguinis 9: 431–446

176. Stroncek DF, Ramsey G, Herr GP et al 1994 Identification of a new white cell antigen. Transfusion 34: 706–711

177. van de Winkel JGJ, Capel PJA 1993 Human IgG Fc receptor heterogeneity: molecular aspects and clinical implications. Immunology Today 14: 215–221

178. Koene HR, Kleijer M, Roos D et al 1998 FcγRIIIB genes in NA(1+,2+)SH(+)individuals. Blood 91: 673–679

179. de Haas M, Kleijer M, van Zwieten R et al 1995 Neutrophil FcγRIII deficiency, nature and clinical consequences: a studt of 21 individuals from 14 families. Blood 86: 2403–2413

180. Lalezari P, Murphy GB, Allen FH 1971 NB1, a new neutrophil-specific antigen involved in the pathogenesis of neonatal neutropenia. Journal of Clinical Investigation 50: 1108–1115

181. Stroncek DF, Shankar RA, Plachta LB et al 1993 Polyclonal antibodies against the NB1-bearing 58- to 64-kDa glycoprotein of human neutrophils do not identify an NB2-bearing molecule. Transfusion 33: 399–404

182. Levine DH, Madyastha P, Wade TR et al 1982 Neonatal isoimmune neutropenia. Pediatric Research 16: 296A

183. Bux J, Jung D, Kauth T et al 1992 Serological and clinical aspects of granulocyte antibodies leading to alloimmune neonatal alloimmune neutropenia. Transfusion Medicine 2: 143–149

184. Madyastha PR, Glassman AB, Levine DH 1984 Incidence of neutrophil antigens on human cord neutrophils. American Journal of Reproductive Immunology 6: 124–127

185. Blaschke J, Goeken NE, Thompson JS et al 1979 Acquired agranulocytosis with granulocyte-specific cytotoxic autoantibody. American Journal of Medicine 66: 862–866

186. Lalezari P, Jiang AF, Yegen L et al 1975 Chronic autoimmune neutropenia due to anti-NA2 antibody. New England Journal of Medicine 293: 744–747

187. Bux J, Behrens G, Jaeger G et al 1998 Diagnosis and clinical course of autoimmune neutropenia in infancy: analysis of 240 cases. Blood 91: 181–186

188. Lyall EGH, Lucas GF, Eden OB 1992 Autoimmune neutropenia of infancy. Journal of Clinical Pathology 45: 431–434

189. van der Pol W, van der Winkel JG 1998 IgG receptor polymorphisms: risk factors for disease. Immunogenetics 48: 222–232

190. Stein MP, Edberg JC, Kimberly RP et al 2000 C-reactive protein binding to FcgammaRIIa on human monocytes and neutrophils is allele-specific. Journal of Clinical Investigation 105: 369–376

191. Salmon JE, Edberg JC, Brogle NL et al 1992 Allelic polymorphisms of human Fc gamma receptor IIA and Fc gamma receptor IIIB. Independent mechanisms for differences in human phagocyte function. Journal of Clinical Investigation 89: 1274–1281

192. Bredius RG, Fijen CA, De Haas M et al 1994 Role of neutrophil Fc gamma RIIa (CD32) and Fc gamma RIIIb (CD16) polymorphic forms in phagocytosis of human IgG1 – and IgG3-opsonized bacteria and erythrocytes. Immunology 83: 624–630

193. Raknes G, Skeie GO, Gilhus NE et al 1998 FcgammaRIIA and FcgammaRIIIB polymorphisms in myasthenia gravis. Journal of Neuroimmunology 81: 173–176

194. Myhr KM, Raknes G, Nyland H et al 1999 Immunoglobulin G Fc-receptor (FcgammaR) IIA and IIIB polymorphisms related to disability in MS. Neurology 52: 1771–1776

Transfusion medicine for pathologists

31

J McCullough

Introduction

Blood supply systems throughout the world

Whole blood

Blood donor recruitment

Plasma

Impact of AIDS epidemic

Whole blood
Medical history
Physical and laboratory examination of the blood donor
Collection of whole blood
Venipuncture and blood collection
Adverse reaction to blood donation

Special blood donations
Autologous blood donation
Directed donor blood
Therapeutic bleeding

Preparations, storage and characteristics of blood components

Red blood cells

Fresh frozen plasma

Plasma and source plasma

Cryoprecipitate

Random-donor platelet concentrates – platelet-rich plasma method

Random-donor platelet concentrates – buffy coat method

Granulocytes

Collection and production of blood components by apheresis

Platelet concentrates

Granulocyte concentrates

Mononuclear cell concentrates

Plasma

Peripheral blood stem cells (PBSCs)

Selection of apheresis donors

Reactions in apheresis donors

Laboratory testing of donated blood

Compatibility testing (cross-matching)

Transfusion therapy

Transfusion of components containing red blood cells
Clinical indications
Whole blood
Red blood cells
Leukoreduced red cells
Washed red cells
Frozen deglycerolized red blood cells

Effects of red blood cell transfusion

Transfusion of products containing coagulation factors
Fresh frozen plasma
Coagulation factor concentrates
Cryoprecipitate

Transfusion of platelets
Indications for platelet transfusion

Granulocyte transfusion

Blood derivatives

Transfusion of cytomegalovirus
(CMV)-negative blood products

Irradiated blood components

Transfusion of neocytes

Fibrin glue

Transfusion in special situations

Massive transfusion

Cardiovascular surgery

Transplantation

Neonates

Hemophilia

Provision of red cells in urgent situations

Exchange transfusion of the neonate

Autoimmune hemolytic anemia

Pregnant women

Autoimmune thrombocytopenia

Neonatal alloimmune thrombocytopenia

Neonatal alloimmune neutropenia

Rare blood types

Techniques of blood transfusion

Complications of transfusion:
recognition and management

Transfusion reactions
Hemolytic transfusion reactions
Febrile reactions
Allergic reactions
Pulmonary reactions
Anaphylactic reactions

Reactions to platelets

Graft-versus-host disease (GVHD)

Other complications of blood transfusion

Transfusion-transmitted diseases

Post-transfusion hepatitis

HIV infection and AIDS

Other transfusion-transmitted
infectious diseases

Role of hematopoietic growth factors
in transfusion medicine

Erythropoietin

Granulocyte-macrophage colony
stimulating factor (GM-CSF)

Platelet growth factor

Blood substitutes

Introduction

Blood transfusion and transfusion medicine at the beginning of the 20th century is a discipline involving complex, structured, standardized, and regulated production processes along with sophisticated hemotherapy. The laboratory techniques are far different from those of Landsteiner who discovered the ABO blood group system by observing clumps of red cells or hemolysis when the cells from some of his laboratory workers were mixed with the serum from others. Other chapters in this book beautifully describe the extensive knowledge of the structure and function of blood groups[1] and immune hemolytic anemias.[2] In developed countries, virtually all whole blood is collected from non-paid volunteer donors by either regional, community-based or individual, hospital-based blood banks. The whole blood is separated into its components shortly following donation; thus each component is available for use for the most appropriate specific clinical condition. This approach, called blood-component therapy, places responsibility on the clinician to identify the specific blood deficit of the patient and to choose a specific blood component. In this chapter, we describe the approaches used to obtain blood, the medical uses of blood components and the complications of transfusion.

Blood supply systems throughout the world

Whole blood

Approximately 75 000 000 units of whole blood are collected worldwide, but this almost certainly does not meet worldwide needs. The organizations and systems that collect and provide blood vary greatly throughout the world. Most developed countries, except the United States, have some form of a national blood program.[3] The program may be operated by that country's Red Cross or by the Government. The extent to which this program is structured, the mechanisms of funding, and the effectiveness of the national blood program in meeting the total blood needs for that country also vary greatly throughout the world. In many third world (undeveloped) countries, the blood supply may be inadequate to meet the needs and the blood that is available has a high likelihood of transmitting infectious disease.[4]

The United States does not have a national blood system.[5] In the United States, approximately 13.5 million units of whole blood are collected each year primarily in regional or community blood centers.[6] Hospitals collect less than 10% of the United States' blood supply and in the past approximately 250 000 units were imported from Western Europe, although this practice is ending. The American Red Cross is the largest blood collecting organization in the United States, accounting for about 45% of the blood supply. Other regional or community blood centers are non-profit organizations governed by local volunteer Boards of Directors.

It is policy of the International Society for Blood Transfusion and at the World Health Organization that blood should be donated voluntarily. The reason for advocating volunteerism in blood donation is not only based on the morale principle of not selling body parts or tissues but also has a very practical basis. It has been well established that blood from paid donors has a much higher risk of disease transmission.[7] When a financial payment is involved, there is an incentive for the potential donor to be dishonest about his or her medical history. Despite the increased sophistication of laboratory testing of donated blood, some infectious units of blood will not be detected by present tests.[8] Thus, if the donor is dishonest about his or her medical history, there is more likelihood that the unit may be infectious.

In developed countries, the collection, processing, testing and preparation of blood components is subject to some form of regulation. Although blood is biological, and thus different from a pharmaceutical, some form of pharmaceutical-type regulation is applied. Thus, there are requirements for donor eligibility, laboratory testing of donated blood, blood preservation, and the minimum content of various blood components. Usually these requirements define procedures, records, staff proficiency, specific testing, and donor medical requirements that blood banks must follow, In the United States, additional standards have been promulgated by the American Association of Blood Banks – a voluntary organization that accredits blood banks as a way of assuring high quality and providing continued education for blood-bank professionals.[9–11]

Blood donor recruitment

In developed countries, whether or not there is a national blood program, blood is collected from volunteer donors. The costs that are incurred in collection, testing, production and distribution of blood components are covered in a variety of ways depending on the method of financing healthcare in each country. In some countries, these costs are part of the national health service budget and the funds may be provided to the hospitals to purchase blood from the national blood program or the Red Cross. In other countries, the funds may be provided directly to the national blood program or the Red Cross and the blood is then provided without charge to the hospitals. In the past in the United States, it was sometimes possible for patients to partially reduce the cost of blood by arranging for replacement of the blood they used. This practice also served as an effective donor-recruitment system, but the practice has been almost eliminated because of the pressures it places on the family of the patient at particularly stressful times. However, in many parts of the world, especially in areas without a structured blood system and where individual hospitals must attempt to meet their own blood requirements, this practice is still widely used. In those situations, patients and their families may be required to obtain a certain number of donors or of units of blood before procedures involving blood loss will be undertaken. This requirement may even lead to families paying individuals to donate blood on their behalf. The payment then creates the difficulties of a paid-donor system described earlier.

In developed countries, most people will require a blood transfusion at some time in their lives, yet less than 5% of the total population has ever donated blood.[12] The blood supply comes from a small group of dedicated donors, and of those who donate, most donate only once per year or infrequently. In the United States, blood donors differ from the general population in that they are more likely to be male, age 30–50 years, more highly educated, employed and Caucasian.[12] Although there have been some studies of the social psychology and motivation of blood donors the process is not well understood and is likely to vary for different ethnic or cultural groups or countries.[13] A recent developing concern is that with the increasingly stringent donor requirements resulting from the AIDS epidemic, a larger portion of the population is being excluded as potential donors. In addition, as the population in many developed countries ages, there is a decreasing portion of the population available for blood donation.

Plasma

A large number of therapeutic products such as albumin, intramuscular and intravenous immune globulin, and coagulation factor concentrates are prepared from plasma by using large-scale manufacturing processes. The plasma to serve as raw material may be obtained from individual units of whole blood or by plasmapheresis. Worldwide, the demand for these plasma derivatives exceeds that provided from plasma obtained from whole blood donations. Thus, a large amount of the plasma that

serves as raw material for the production of derivatives is obtained by plasmapheresis. Plasmapheresis donation requires more time than whole blood donation, and because red cells are returned to the donor, the donor can donate plasma more frequently than whole blood; in some countries, plasmapheresis donors are paid. Because of the ramifications of the AIDS epidemic, some developed countries have an objective to become self-sufficient in generating an adequate amount of plasma to produce the number of derivatives needed in that country.

In the United States, the plasmapheresis collection and plasma fractionation system is separate from the whole blood collection system. This system is operated by large commercial companies that pay donors and produce plasma derivatives for profit. Thus, it differs in many ways from the whole blood collection system in the United States, which relies on volunteer donors and is operated by non-profit organizations. In most other developed countries, the plasma system is operated as a not-for-profit system, often as part of the regular, whole blood collection system. Some countries operate their own plasma fractionation plant while others contract with plants operated in other countries. Plasma fractionation involves the processing of up to 10 000 l of plasma, which may be pooled from as many as 50 000 donors. Thus, the potential for infectivity is substantial. Since the AIDS epidemic, the plasma fractionation industry has moved much more rapidly to introduce pathogen inactivation systems and today most, if not all, plasma derivatives are free of transmission of most viral diseases.

Impact of AIDS epidemic

The AIDS epidemic has had a major impact on blood banking and transfusion medicine. Although blood-bank professionals believe they acted properly, with reasonable speed, and with the public's interest in mind to balance blood safety and blood availability, in many countries the public was not satisfied with this response. The plasma industry was subjected to even more severe criticism, particularly from the hemophilia community. Because plasma derivatives, including coagulation-factor concentrates, are prepared from large pools of plasma containing plasma from many donors, a large proportion of these derivatives was contaminated with HIV and many hemophiliacs were infected. Although the plasma industry moved expeditiously to introduce pathogen-inactivation steps into the manufacturing process, there was a widely held belief that these companies should have implemented these steps sooner. In addition, in some countries, particularly France and Japan, criminal actions were taken successfully against leaders of the blood programs for failure to take certain actions that might have helped to mitigate the impact of the AIDS epidemic on transfusion recipients. As a result of the AIDS epidemic, there has been a substantial increase in the eligibility requirements for blood donors and an increase in the number and specificity of questions about donor's medical history and activities that might place them at risk of being infected with transfusion-transmitted diseases. In addition, the number of tests performed on donated blood has increased substantially.[5,13] There has also been a fundamental shift in the regulatory philosophy. Particularly in the United States, but in most developed countries, the expectation developed that blood donor screening, collection, processing and component production would be carried out much like a pharmaceutical manufacturing process.[5,14,15] This in turn required extensive and fundamental changes in the administrative structure and style or culture of organizations collecting blood. In addition to the enormous impact of the AIDS epidemic on the blood collection process and organizations, the use of blood products also changed dramatically. Physicians became much more conservative in prescribing blood and more extensive use of guidelines and monitoring of transfusions has occurred in developed countries.

Whole blood

Medical history

Selection of blood donors involves ensuring the safety of the donor and obtaining a blood component that is high in quality and has the least possible chance of transmitting disease. This is accomplished by using volunteer blood donors, questioning the donors about their general health and medical history, carrying out a brief physical examination of the donor, and laboratory testing the donated blood.

Since the AIDS epidemic has heightened concerns about transfusion-transmitted diseases, the number and type of donor questions have changed extensively. Questions related to sexual behavior especially have become very specific. These examples of questions are based on those used in the United States. The questions used in each country will differ to reflect the kinds of disease exposure donors are most likely to encounter. The general principles will apply however – questions intended to protect the donor from risks of blood donation and questions (primarily related to infectious diseases) intended to protect the recipient by identifying and excluding donors whose blood might be infectious.

Examples of questions in the medical history designed to protect the donor include whether the donor is under the care of a physician and has a history of cardiovascular or lung disease, seizures, present or recent pregnancy, recent donation of blood or plasma, recent major illness or surgery, unexplained weight loss, unusual bleeding or is taking medications.

Questions about medications help to identify any diseases or illnesses that might make blood donation a risk for the donor. Most of the questions designed to protect the recipient deal with exposure to infectious diseases. Examples of these questions are: (1) the occurrence of or exposure to hepatitis or other liver disease, HIV (or symptoms of AIDS), Chagas' disease or babesiosis; (2) use of injected drugs; (3) receipt of growth hormone, coagulation factor concentrates, blood transfusion, recent immunizations, tattoo, acupuncture, ear piercing or an organ or tissue transplant; (4) travel to areas endemic for malaria; (5) presence of a major illness or surgery; or (6) previous notice of a positive test for a transmissible disease. Examples of questions related to HIV-risk behavior include whether the potential donor has had sex with anyone with AIDS, has given or received money or drugs for sex, (for males) has had sex with another male, (for females) has had sex with a male who has had sex with another male.

Physical and laboratory examination of the blood donor

The donor's general appearance is assessed for any signs of illness or the influence of drugs or alcohol. The skin is examined for signs of intravenous drug abuse, lesions suggestive of Kaposi's sarcoma, and local lesions that might make it difficult to sterilize the skin and, thus, lead to contamination of the blood unit during venipuncture. Physical examination of the potential donor usually includes the temperature, pulse, blood pressure, weight and blood hemoglobin concentration. The specific requirements for these measures are established by the regulatory agency of each country.

Collection of whole blood

Blood is collected into plastic bags, each of which is sterile and can be used only once. Often combinations of bags are used so that whole blood can be separated into its components in a closed system, thus minimizing the chance of bacterial contamination while making storage of the components for days or weeks possible. The venipuncture site is an area free of skin lesions; it is scrubbed with a soap solution, followed by an iodine solution. Because bacterial contamination of blood can be a serious or even fatal complication of transfusion,[16,17] it is important to minimize bacterial contamination by selecting a good venipuncture site and sterilizing it properly. The needle is an integral part of the tubing and bag system. If the first venipuncture attempt fails, a new needle and bag set should be used.

Venipuncture and blood collection

The blood must flow freely and be mixed with anti-coagulant frequently as the blood fills the container to avoid the development of small clots. The actual time for phlebotomy and bleeding is usually about 7 min and almost always less than 10 min. In much of the world it has been customary to collect 450 ml of blood, although some blood banks are now collecting 500 ml and in some parts of the world less than 450 ml is collected routinely. The anticoagulant is composed of citrate, phosphate and dextrose (CPD) in a ratio of approximately 1:15 with whole blood. The amount of blood withdrawn must be within prescribed limits in order to maintain the proper ratio with the anticoagulant; otherwise the blood cells may be damaged and/or anticoagulation may not be satisfactory. The red cells can be stored in the citrate anti-coagulant; although in many countries, the anticoagulated plasma is removed and the red cells are resuspended in a solution that allows extended red cell storage.

Adverse reactions to blood donation

Donors have a reaction following approximately 4% of blood donations, but serious reactions are rare. Reactions are more likely to occur in younger, first-time, single donors who have a higher predonation heart rate and lower diastolic blood pressure.[20] The most common reactions include mild weakness, cool skin, diaphoresis, lightheadedness and/or nausea. More extensive reactions involve dizziness, pallor, hypertension, nausea and vomiting, bradycardia and/or hyperventilation which sometimes leads to twitching or muscle spasms. Bradycardia indicates a vasovagal reaction rather than hypotensive or cardiovascular shock, where tachycardia would be expected. Other complications of blood donation include hematoma at the venipuncture site and injury to the bracheal nerve and resulting pain and/or paresthesia due to needle puncture of the nerve or compression from a hematoma.[21–23] Rare but severe donor reactions involve loss of consciousness, convulsions, serious cardiac difficulties and/or involuntary passage of urine or stool.[18,19,24]

Donors are advised to drink extra fluids to replace lost blood volume and minimize the chance of fainting and to avoid strenuous exercise for the remainder of the day of donation in order to minimize the possibility that a hematoma will develop at the venipuncture site. Because some donors are subject to lightheadedness or even fainting if they change position quickly, donors are usually advised not to return to work for the remainder of the day in an occupation where fainting would be hazardous to themselves or others.

Special blood donations

Most blood is collected for placement in a 'bank' to provide for the general community and, thus, may be used by any patient. However, some blood donations are made intentionally to be used by a specific patient. Examples of these include autologous donation, directed donation and patient-specific donation. In some of these situations the usual regulations for blood donation may not apply.

Autologous blood donation

Much interest developed in autologous blood donation as a result of the AIDS epidemic. Autologous blood donation can be done in several ways. Individuals may donate blood for their own use if the need for blood can be anticipated, such as with elective surgery. Autologous blood for transfusion can be obtained by preoperative donation, acute normovolemic hemodilution also known as perioperative hemodilution, intraoperative salvage and/or postoperative salvage.

Preoperative donation

If an elective procedure is scheduled and there is a high likelihood of blood transfusion, the patient can donate blood for his/her own use. Since the donor is actually a patient, they usually do not meet the regulatory requirements for normal blood donation and, thus, the blood is usually not transferred to the general blood inventory and used for someone else if it is not needed by the original donor/patient. Thus, it is important that autologous blood be collected only for procedures in which there is substantial likelihood that it will be used.[25] Without this type of planning, there is a very high rate of wastage of autologous blood (estimated at 52.4% in the United States in 1994).[6] This amount of waste also means that the costs of autologous blood are quite high.[26]

Although there are some contraindications for preoperative autologous blood donation such as bacteremia, symptomatic angina, recent seizures and symptomatic valvular heart lesions, the usual donor requirements do not apply and the final decision whether to withdraw blood from an autologous donor rests with the medical director of the blood bank. This decision may necessitate consultation between the donor/patient's physician and the blood-bank physician.

In most countries, autologous blood must be typed for ABO and D antigen, and at least the first unit must be tested for transmissible diseases. If any of the transmissible disease tests are positive, it may be necessary to label the unit(s) as biohazard in order to alert healthcare personnel to the hazard presented by the potentially infectious blood.

There are no age or weight restrictions for autologous donation. Pregnant women may donate, but donation is not recommended routinely because these patients rarely require transfusion. The autologous donor's hemoglobin may be lower than that required for routine donors, and autologous donors may donate several times within a few weeks prior to the planned surgery. However, usually it is only possible to obtain two to four units of blood before the hemoglobin falls to unacceptably low levels.

With the discovery of erythropoietin, there was great hope that it could be given to autologous blood donors to increase the number of units they could donate and substantially reduce the use of the general blood supply. Unfortunately this has not occurred. Except for a few specific situations,[27] erthropoietin does not result in a meaningful increase in autologous blood units obtained from each patient and does not reduce the patient's use of allogeneic blood.

In the early 1990s, there was great excitement about the potential of autologous blood and it was estimated that in the United States autologous blood could account for 20% of all blood used. This has not occurred because much of the autologous blood was collected from patients undergoing procedures with little likelihood of needing blood, surgeons became more skilled at minimizing blood loss, and anesthesiologists became more skilled at managing fluid administration and maintaining patients with lower hemoglobin levels. Thus, blood use decreased, especially for many elective procedures. Recently a much more conservative view of the use of autologous blood has emerged.[28]

Perioperative hemodilution (acute normovolemic hemodilution)

Perioperative hemodilution is carried out in the operating room usually after the patient has undergone general anesthesia. One to two units of whole blood are collected and replaced with an electrolyte solution at three times the volume of blood collected. The patient's hematocrit is maintained at least at 30%. This procedure does not pose unusual risks to patients who are stable and undergoing elective surgery. If it is carried out prior to surgical procedures in which substantial expected blood loss is expected, the two units of freshly collected blood are kept in the operating room and can be transfused to the patient during surgery. Theoretical advantages of perioperative hemodilution in addition to having the blood available are that blood loss during surgery occurs at a lower hematocrit and thus there is less red cell loss, that surgery is carried out at lower hematocrit which improves blood viscosity and possibly provides better tissue oxygenation, and that the blood that is available for transfusion is fresh. Perioperative hemodilution must be carried out by a committed, knowledgeable anesthesia staff and it appears to have limited but definite value.

Intraoperative blood salvage

In either elective, urgent or trauma surgery when substantial blood loss is expected, some of the shed blood can be recovered and returned to the patient. Several devices that combine suction, centrifugation and washing are available for this purpose. Because of the cost of operating these devices, intraoperative blood salvage is usually reserved for situations in which the blood loss is expected to exceed 1000 ml. The device suctions or aspirates blood from the operative site. The collected blood is centrifuged, and, in some cases, a wash solution is added. After processing, the blood is pumped out of the device into a plastic bag so it can be used for transfusion. Contraindications to intraoperative blood salvage are bacterial contamination of the operative site and surgery for malignancy. In both of these situations, transfusion of blood containing bacteria or malignant cells would be undesirable. Examples of situations in which intraoperative blood salvage is used most commonly are vascular surgery, cardiovascular surgery and some major orthopedics procedures.

Postoperative blood salvage

In some situations such as cardiovascular or orthopedic surgery, if there is extensive postoperative bleeding or draining from the surgical site, devices can be used to collect this drainage so that the shed blood can be used for transfusion. This use of postoperative blood salvage has not gained widespread acceptance because the volume of red cells that can be obtained is usually small; if substantial surgical site drainage is occurring, this often indicates a surgical problem that requires intervention. The shed blood usually contains activated coagulation factors, fibrin strands, cellular aggregates, and other debris which make transfusion of this material undesirable.

Directed donor blood

Directed donors are friends or relatives who wish to give blood for a specific patient. Usually this is done because the patient hopes those donors will be 'safer' than regular blood donors. In some parts of the world, however, directed donation is a necessity because the general blood supply is not adequate. In the United States, data do not indicate that directed donors have a lower incidence of transmissible disease markers,[28,29] and there may not be a factual rationale for these donations. Directed donors must meet all of the regulatory requirements for routine blood donation. Their blood becomes part of the community's general blood supply if it is not used for the originally intended patient.

Therapeutic bleeding

Blood may be collected as part of the therapy for diseases such as polycythemia vera or hemochromatosis. Often the patient or the physician asks that the blood be used for transfusion. Such blood is not usually used for transfusion since the cause of the disease is not known and the donors do not meet the FDA (Food and Drugs Administration) requirements. Recently, in the United States, efforts have begun to gain approval for the use of blood obtained from patients with hemochromatosis.[30,31]

Preparation, storage and characteristics of blood components

In developed countries, almost all blood collected is separated into red cells, platelets and plasma. Each component is stored under conditions optimum for that component so that valuable platelets and coagulation factors are recovered and maintained. Plastic bag systems are used for this blood separation, and thus bacterial contamination is avoided. In many parts of the world, blood is not separated into components but is stored as whole blood.

Red blood cells

If whole blood is centrifuged and most of the platelets and plasma are removed, the resulting packed red cells

or red cell concentrate is resuspended in a solution to optimize red cell preservation and allow storage of red cells for 42 days at 1–6°C. During the 42 days of storage, there is some loss of viability, adenosine triphosphate, membrane lipid and 2,3-diphosphoglycerate (2,3-DPG) (causing increased affinity of hemoglobin for oxygen), reduced transmembrane transport of sodium and potassium, and accumulation of metabolites. Each unit of red cells has a volume of approximately 300 ml and contains about 200 ml of red cells. Red cells are used to provide oxygen-carrying capacity in anemic patients. The number of units given depends on the degree of anemia or blood loss.

Fresh frozen plasma

In the United States, when the unit of whole blood is centrifuged, platelet-rich plasma results. The platelet-rich plasma is then centrifuged, and the plasma and platelets are separated resulting in a unit of plasma and a platelet concentrate. If this plasma is placed at –18°C or colder within 6 h of collection it is called fresh frozen plasma. Fresh frozen plasma can be stored for up to 1 year at –18°C or colder. The unit of fresh frozen plasma has a volume of approximately 185 ml and contains all the constituents of citrated normal plasma such as the coagulation factors, the components of the complement and fibrinolytic systems, and the plasma proteins that maintain osmotic pressure and modulate immunity.

For transfusion, fresh frozen plasma is thawed in a 37°C water bath for approximately 30 min. Microwave ovens usually are not used to thaw fresh frozen plasma because they create hot spots that damage the plasma proteins. Thawed plasma should be transfused as soon as possible, but at the latest within 24 h.

Plasma and source plasma

Plasma can also be removed from whole blood more than 6 h and less than 5 days after collection and stored either at –18°C or less (plasma) or at 1–6°C (liquid plasma). Source plasma is collected by plasmapheresis and is intended to serve as the raw material for further manufacture into blood derivatives.

Cryoprecipitate

When previously frozen plasma is thawed at 1–6°C, an insoluble material called cryoprecipitate remains. Each bag of cryoprecipitate contains about 100 units of factor VIII and 200 mg of fibrinogen and has a volume of about 10 ml. It can be stored for up to 1 year at –18°C or lower.

Cryoprecipitate is thawed in a 37°C water bath, and cryoprecipitate from multiple bags is usually pooled into a single container that is dispensed by the blood bank. Cryoprecipitate is usually given in the same ABO type as the recipient. If there is a shortage, small amounts of ABO-incompatible cryoprecipitate can be given. There is usually little risk of hemolysis from small volumes of ABO-incompatible plasma because the volume of plasma from any individual donor who might have a high-titer antibody is only 10 ml. Because cryoprecipitate contains few red cells, it can be given without regard to Rh type.

Cryoprecipitate was developed originally as a source of factor VIII and was the first concentrated form of this coagulation factor available to treat hemophilia. With the development of coagulation factor concentrates that have undergone viral inactivation, the major use of cryoprecipitate currently is as a source of fibrinogen or as fibrin glue.

Random-donor platelet concentrates – platelet-rich plasma method

Platelets can be produced from units of whole blood or by plateletpheresis. In the United States, when platelets are prepared from whole blood, the unit of whole blood is maintained at room temperature and centrifuged, and the platelet-rich plasma is passed into a satellite bag. The platelet-rich plasma is centrifuged again, and the platelet-poor plasma is passed into another satellite bag leaving the platelet concentrate, which has a volume of proximately 50 ml. At least 75% of random donor-platelet concentrates contain at least 5.5×10^{10} platelets. Four to six units of random-donor platelet are pooled to provide a therapeutic dose for transfusion. These random-donor platelet concentrates may then be stored for up to 5 days at room temperature (20–24°C). The variables known to be important in platelet preservation are: temperature, method of agitation, volume of suspending plasma and type of storage container.[32] At the end of the storage period, the intravascular recovery and half-life of the stored platelets are approximately 51% and 3.1 days,[33] and the platelets effectively correct the bleeding time in thrombocytopenic patients.[33,34]

Random-donor platelet concentrates – buffy coat method

In Western Europe, the whole blood is centrifuged and the buffy coat containing leukocytes and platelets is removed.[35] Buffy coats from several units are pooled, the pooled buffy coats are centrifuged, and the platelets are separated from the leukocytes to provide a random-donor platelet concentrate. This method provides a therapeutic dose of platelets and no further pooling is necessary. It is thought that this method of preparation provides better platelet function,[35] although it has not been adopted in the United States.

Granulocytes

Granulocytes are not usually isolated from fresh units of whole blood because the very small number of granulocytes then isolated would provide a dose suitable only for small patients. Instead, granulocyte concentrates for transfusion are usually produced by apheresis.

Collection and production of blood components by apheresis

Many blood components are prepared from whole blood, but they also can be obtained by apheresis. Apheresis is derived from the Greek word meaning to take away and thus refers to the blood donation process in which one component is removed while the remainder of the donor blood is returned. This process enables a larger number of cells to be obtained than would be available in one unit of whole blood. Usually whole blood is pumped out of one arm, anticoagulant is added, and the blood is passed through an instrument in which it is centrifuged and separated into red cells, plasma and a leukocyte/platelet fraction. One of the components is removed and the remainder of the blood is returned via the other arm. Several semi-automated instruments are available for the collection of platelets, granulocytes, peripheral blood stem cells (PBSCs), mononuclear cells, plasma or red cells.[36,37] Some newer instruments allow collection of different combinations of components, such as plasma and platelets.

Platelet concentrates

Plateletpheresis usually takes about 90 min during which about 4000–5000 l of the donor's blood are processed through the blood cell separator. These platelet concentrates have a volume of about 200 ml and contain about 3.5×10^{11} platelets and less than 0.5 ml of red cells. This provides a therapeutic dose of platelets for transfusion. Plateletpheresis has been used increasingly so that in the United States more than half of platelets are produced by plateletpheresis.

Granulocyte concentrates

Because of the small number of circulating granulocytes, it is not practical to prepare granulocyte concentrates from whole blood donations. Instead, leukapheresis can be used to process 6.5–8.0 ml of donor blood during about 3 h[37] and obtain a granulocyte concentrate. Hydroxyethyl starch is added to the blood cell separator flow system to sediment the red cells and improve the separation of granulocytes from other blood components.[37] To increase the donor's peripheral blood granulocyte count and, thus, increase the yield of granulocytes, dexamethazone and recently, granulocyte colony-stimulating factor (G-CSF) has been administered to granulocyte donors.[38–40]

Mononuclear cell concentrates

Mononuclear cell collection is also done by cytapheresis. This produces a component containing approximately 1×10^{10} mononuclear cells, which are a mixture of lymphocytes and monocytes. These mononuclear cell concentrates may be used for direct transfusion such as in adoptive immunotherapy to prevent relapse of chronic myeloid leukemia (CML) following stem cell transplantation[41–43] or as the starting material for further processing as part of gene therapy[44] or adoptive immunotherapy.[45–48]

Plasma

Plasmapheresis can be done using sets of multiple, attached bags, but this is time consuming, cumbersome and involves disconnecting the blood bags from the donor to centrifuge and separate the plasma from the red cells. This creates the chance of returning the blood to the wrong donor. During the past decade, semiautomated instruments have become available that require less operator involvement than the bag systems, while producing up to 750 ml of plasma in about 30 min depending on the size of the donor. Because few red cells are removed, the procedure can be repeated frequently so that a donor could provide large amounts of plasma.

Peripheral blood stem cells (PBSCs)

The observation that hematopoietic stem cells are present in the peripheral blood[38] and that these cells are capable of providing complete hematopoietic reconstitution in humans[49–51] stimulated the development of methods to collect peripheral blood stem cells by cytapheresis.[38,52,53]

The number of PBSCs circulating under usual conditions is low but following chemotherapy there is a rebound and a large number of PBSCs can be obtained. G-CSF is also given to patients or normal donors to increase the number of circulating PBSCs and provide an adequate dose of cells for successful reconstitution of hematopoiesis.[38,49–53] Usually approximately 1×10^{10} mononuclear cells and $2–6 \times 10^7$ CD34$^+$ cells are obtained after processing up to 15 l of the donor's blood during 4–5 h. The concentrate has a volume of about 200 ml.

Selection of apheresis donors

The criteria and requirements for donors of whole blood apply to the selection of donors for apheresis;[36,37] however, there are some additional requirements. These may vary in different countries, but they generally define the volume of blood that can be extracorporeal during apheresis, the volume of red cells or plasma that can be removed in a given time, the frequency of donation, and any laboratory tests in addition to those performed for whole blood donation. The laboratory testing of donors for transmissible diseases is the same as that for whole blood donation. Thus, the likelihood of disease transmission from apheresis components is the same as that from whole blood.

Reactions in apheresis donors

In general, the types of adverse reactions that occur following cytapheresis are similar to those following whole blood donation. However, some side-effects or reactions unique to cytapheresis occur. These include paresthesias due to the infusion of the citrate used to anticoagulate the donor's blood while it is in the cell separator; myalgia, arthralgia, headache or flu-like symptoms due to G-CSF in granulocyte donors;[38,49–53] or headache and/or hypertension[37] from blood volume expansion due to the sedimenting agent hydroxyethyl starch used in the cell separator to improve the granulocyte yield.

Laboratory testing of donated blood

Since the beginning of the AIDS epidemic, concern about transfusion-transmitted diseases has increased and new diseases have been identified. As a result, testing of donated blood has become much more extensive.[5] In addition to transmissible disease testing, blood is tested for the ABO and Rh type, and red cell antibody screening (detection) is performed. Tests for cytomegalovirus, HLA antibodies, or rare red cell antigens may be done depending on the needs of the blood bank and the patients it serves. Because of the large amount of laboratory and donor data, today's blood center uses pharmaceutical-type manufacturing processes and quality control systems in order to ensure accuracy and safety.[5,14,15,36]

Compatibility testing (cross-matching)

Compatibility testing includes all the steps and procedures involved in providing blood cells that will have an acceptable *in vivo* survival. The cross-match is only one part of compatibility testing. Other steps in compatibility testing include ABO Rh typing of donor red cells, acquiring a proper sample from the patient, ABO Rh testing of the patient, testing the patient's serum for red cell antibodies, selecting the proper blood component, carrying out the cross-match, labeling the component with the identity of the recipient and appropriate release from the blood bank. The antibody-detection test has become increasingly important during the last few years as it has been established that for patients with no antibodies detectable in this test, cross-match can be abbreviated to one that will detect ABO incompatibility. This can be done with a simple saline suspension of red cells and an incubation of approximately 5 min at room temperature. Thus, the approach that has developed during the last decade involves a careful, thorough, sensitive antibody-detection test and then the exact method used for the cross-match depends on the results of the antibody-detection test. If no antibodies are found, the simple rapid test to detect ABO incompatibility is used for the cross-match.[55] If antibodies are detected in the detection test, then the cross-match uses the longer, more complex methodology used in the antibody-detection test.

In the antibody-detection test, the patient's serum is reacted with blood cells specially selected from two normal individuals whose cells contain antigens reactive with all of the common clinically significant antibodies. The conditions of this test usually involve incubation of the patient's serum and test red cells suspended either in saline or albumin followed by the anti-human globulin test. Other methods to enhance antibody-detection that might be used include treating the red cells with enzymes, changing the serum cell ratio, suspending red cells in low ionic strength solution or the use of chemicals such as polybrene to enhance agglutination

Transfusion therapy

Transfusion of components containing red blood cells

Clinical indications

Red cells are transfused to improve oxygen-carrying capacity or for restoration of blood volume following blood loss. There is no specific hemoglobin value above which patients have a better outcome, feel better, or have improved wound healing. Thus, in making a decision to transfuse a patient to improve oxygen capacity, the patient's overall condition must be considered. For instance, when anemia has developed over a long period of time, the patient adjusts to lower hemoglobin levels and may not require transfusion despite very low hemoglobin levels. The few studies that deal with the physiology of blood loss and the indications for red cell transfusion have been done in normal animals or essentially healthy humans. Thus, the indications for transfusion in patients with cardiac disease, coronary atherosclerosis or other vascular insufficiency are not known.

Many anesthesiologists and surgeons transfuse patients to achieve a hemoglobin level of 10 g/dl prior to surgery. However, there is no scientific basis or clinical data to support this practice. Many patients would not be at risk if a transfusion was withheld until the hemoglobin level was approximately 7 g/dl.

Transfusion for restoration of blood volume should not be initiated too rapidly because it is clear that in most 'normal' patients the loss of approximately 1000 ml of blood can be replaced by colloid or crystalloid solutions alone. The hemoglobin level may not be of value in this situation because if blood loss has been acute, the patient may have a normal or nearly normal hemoglobin level until equilibration between the intravascular and extravascular space occurs.

Whole blood

Whole blood is rarely used in the developed countries. Instead, it is converted into components to take advantage of the need for plasma and platelets. Acute blood loss is managed by transfusion of red cells and crystalloid or colloid solutions.

Red blood cells

Patients with severe anemia usually do not need intravascular volume replacement, and thus, red cells are the component of choice. In patients with acute massive hemorrhage, who may need both intravascular volume and red cell replacement, crystalloid or colloid solutions, not human plasma, are used with red cells. Crystalloid and colloid solutions have few adverse effects, and their use allows the plasma from the original unit of whole blood to be used for the production of coagulation factor concentrate.

Leukoreduced red cells

Leukoreduced red cells are being used increasingly throughout the world. In the past, these red cells were used to prevent febrile non-hemolytic transfusion reactions in patients who received multiple transfusions. Leukocyte-depleted red cells reduce the likelihood of HLA alloimmunization and platelet refractoriness.[56–58] Methods that have been used to prepare leukocyte-depleted red cells include centrifugation, washing, freezing and deglycerolization, or filtration. The availability of filters that remove about > 99% of the leukocytes have made this the common method presently.

Washed red cells

When red cells are washed and resuspended in an electrolyte solution, most of the plasma, platelets and leukocytes have been removed. Thus, washed red cells are indicated for patients who have reactions caused by plasma. For instance, patients with IgA deficiency can have severe, often fatal, anaphylactic reactions when exposed to plasma containing IgA. Although washed red cells have been used to prevent febrile reactions due to transfused leukocytes, the availability of filters for leukocyte removal should eliminate the use of washed red cells for this purpose.

Frozen deglycerolized red blood cells

Red cells can be protected from injury during freezing by the addition of glycerol. They can then be stored for 10 years or more.[59] Because most of the plasma, platelets and leukocytes have been removed and after thawing and washing these red cells are suspended in an electrolyte solution, they can be used similarly as washed red cells. However, the main advantage of frozen red cells is that they can be stored for years, thus allowing development of a depot of red cells of rare types or of autologous red cells. Frozen deglycerolized red cells do not have a reduced likelihood of disease transmission.

Effects of red blood cell transfusion

The effects of red blood cell transfusion on the recipient's hemoglobin and hematocrit levels will be affected by the recipient's blood volume, pretransfusion hemoglobin level, clinical condition (stable, bleeding, etc.) and the hemoglobin content of the donor unit. In general one unit of red cells will increase the hemoglobin value 1 g/dl in an average-size adult.

Transfusion of products containing coagulation factors

Blood components that can be used to replace coagulation factors are fresh frozen plasma and cryoprecipitate. Several plasma derivatives including factor VIII, factor IX, antithrombin III and von Willebrand factor concentrates are available for various coagulation disorders. The plasma derivatives are most useful for single or isolated coagulation factor deficiencies and discussion of this therapy is not within the scope of this book.

Fresh frozen plasma

The most common combined coagulation factor deficiency involves the vitamin K dependant factors. This deficiency is best managed by treating the underlying condition with or without vitamin K administration. However, if rapid reversal is necessary, fresh frozen plasma or plasma of any age can be used since these coagulation factors do not deteriorate during storage of whole blood at 1–6°C.

Recommended indications for use of fresh frozen plasma are:[60]

1. Replacement of isolated coagulation factor deficiencies when specific components are not available. Examples of this are factors V, VIII, IX, X and XI.
2. Reversal of warfarin effect in patients actively bleeding or who require emergency surgery.
3. Antithrombin III deficiency in patients undergoing surgery or who require heparin for treatment of thrombosis.
4. Treatment of thrombotic thrombocytopenic purpura usually as part of plasma exchange.
5. Replacement of immunoglobulins in the treatment of immunodeficiency, such as in patients with protein-losing enteropathy or children or adults with immunodeficiency. The availability of intravenous

immunoglobulin preparations has almost eliminated this as an indication for fresh frozen plasma.

6. Replacement of coagulation factors in massive transfusion is a questionable indication. Usually the bleeding diathesis in massive transfusion is due to depletion of platelets rather than coagulation factors. There is no evidence that the empiric use of fresh frozen plasma in some ratio with units of red cells is necessary. Fresh frozen plasma should be used in massive transfusion only when there is evidence that lack of coagulation factors is a major contributor to the bleeding diathesis.

7. Replacement of coagulation factors in patients who have depletion of multiple coagulation factors usually due to liver disease and are bleeding or about to undergo surgery. Fresh frozen plasma is not indicated for blood volume replacement or as a nutritional source.

Because fresh frozen plasma is usually given to replace multiple plasma proteins, the dose is difficult to determine. The desired level of each protein may be different although for many coagulation factors, a level of 30% is considered adequate to provide hemostasis. In an average-size adult, five units of fresh frozen plasma would be necessary to reach this level. This would involve transfusion of about 1000 ml of plasma; the patient's blood volume and cardiovascular status must be considered.

Coagulation factor concentrates

Deficiency of isolated factor VIII or IX is usually treated with the appropriate factor concentrate. This allows larger doses to be given and the dose can be accurately calculated because each vial of concentrate is assayed for its content of factor.

Cryoprecipitate

Hypofibrinogenemia may occur as an isolated inherited deficiency or it may be in obstetrical complications, disseminated intravascular coagulation and some forms of cancer. In acquired hypofibrinogenemia, treatment should be directed toward the underlying cause of the disease rather than toward replacement of fibrinogen; however, when the fibrinogen level reaches 50 mg/ml or less, fibrinogen replacement may be necessary.[61–63] Cryoprecipitate is usually used as the source of fibrinogen. The dose of fibrinogen for an adult is 6000–8000 mg, although this varies depending on the patient's fibrinogen level. Usually about 30 bags of cryoprecipitate would be used. If cryoprecipitate is used as a source of fibrinogen,

a quality-control program should be established by the blood bank so the fibrinogen content of the cryoprecipitate will be known.

Transfusion of platelets
Indications for platelet transfusion

Platelet transfusion has increased more than that of other blood components during the past decade.[6] The most common reason for platelet transfusion is to prevent bleeding (prophylactic)[64,65] and prophylactic platelet transfusions are usually given to patients with transient thrombocytopenia due to chemotherapy for malignancy including bone marrow transplantation. Platelets can also be transfused to treat active bleeding, but this accounts for fewer transfusions. As with red cell transfusion, there is not a specific laboratory value that is an indication for transfusion. The decision whether to transfuse platelets depends upon the clinical condition of the patient, the cause of the thrombocytopenia, the a platelet count, and the functional ability of the patient's own platelets.

In the early days of platelet transfusion, only a few controlled studies of prophylactic platelet transfusion were done.[66–68] These and other studies established that there is little risk of spontaneous hemorrhage when the platelet count is more than $20\,000/\mu l$, but the risk increases with lower platelet counts.[69] As a result, it became common practice to transfuse platelets to prevent serious bleeding when the platelet count was less than $20\,000/\mu l$. More recent studies have established that prophylactic transfusion can be initiated at a platelet count of $10\,000/\mu l$ without increased bleeding[70–72] and this is the current practice.

The usual dose of platelets in a prophylactic platelet transfusion is 1 unit/10 kg patient weight/day. It has been suggested that frequent transfusions of smaller doses will result in less total platelet usage[73] while others believe that larger doses of platelets are preferable.[74] These proposals have not yet altered practice.

The optimum platelet count to achieve in a bleeding patient is not known. The bleeding time increases when the platelet count is less than $100\,000/\mu l$,[75] which suggests that this number could be the goal of transfusion in actively bleeding patients. However, few studies are available to assist in this decision. It appears that bleeding may be more related to the severity of the surgical procedure than the platelet count[76] and no excess bleeding was observed in patients undergoing lumbar puncture at very low platelet counts.[77] In actively bleeding patients, an attempt to achieve a platelet count of greater than $50\,000/\mu l$ is recommended.

In patients with autoimmune thrombocytopenic purpura or drug-induced immune thrombocytopenia, platelet antibodies cause shortened survival of transfused platelets, and thus transfusion is recommended only for treatment of severe thrombocytopenia with active hemorrhage.

There is a dose–response effect from platelet transfusion. One to three hours after transfusion, the usual dose of platelets transfused should cause a platelet count increase of 5000–10 000/μl in an average-sized adult.[78,79] Some patients do not attain the expected post-transfusion increment in platelet count because they are alloimmunized to platelet or leukocyte antigens.[78,80] In addition, platelet survival can be affected by many clinical factors in the patient,[80] such as (1) disseminated intravascular coagulopathy; (2) amphotericin B administration; (3) palpable spleen; (4) presence of HLA antibody, platelet antibody, and fever; and (5) status after marrow transplantation. Prevention of alloimmunization has been accomplished using single-donor (apheresis) platelets,[56] leukocyte-depleted blood components,[81] and UV irradiation.[82]

Because refractoriness is often associated with bleeding and with a poor outcome, this is a major clinical problem in transfusion medicine. Refractoriness is managed by treating clinical factors that might cause refractoriness, the use of ABO-compatible platelets,[83–85] and the use of platelets less than 24 h old.[86] If these measures fail, an improved response may be obtained by selecting a platelet donor whose HLA type matches that of the recipient,[87–89] although about 30% of HLA-matched transfusions do not provide a satisfactory response.[87–90] Another approach is to cross-match the patient's serum with platelets and to select compatible donors based on this laboratory test. This approach is about as effective as the use of HLA-matched donors.[90,91]

Granulocyte transfusion

Many chemotherapy and stem cell transplant regimens cause severe and prolonged granulocytopenia. These patients are at increased risk of infection,[92,93] which is a major cause of death. The availability of blood cell separators and of donor-stimulation techniques has made it possible to collect large numbers of granulocytes for transfusion. Previous studies have shown that granulocyte transfusion provides improved survival in patients with documented Gram-negative sepsis who remained granulocytopenic for at least 10 days,[94–96] but granulocyte transfusion is not helpful in patients with fever of unknown origin[96] or as prophylaxis in newly diagnosed acute leukemia patients.[97] Today, most patients

respond to antibiotics and granulocyte transfusion is rarely used for bacterial infections. Fungal infections, however, continue to be a major problem,[98–100] and granulocyte transfusions are being used in this setting. No clinical trials have documented the effectiveness of granulocyte transfusion for fungal infections, although animal and clinical studies support their use, and granulocytes do kill fungi *in vitro*.

Blood derivatives

During the late 1930s, the technique was developed for the separation of different plasma proteins. This technique is now used to process thousands of liters of plasma in large batches to produce many plasma proteins, termed plasma derivatives, for therapeutic use (Table 31.1). Some of the plasma for production of derivatives is obtained from units of voluntarily donated whole blood separated into components, but most of the plasma is obtained by plasmapheresis of paid donors. This aspect of the blood supply has been extremely effective in producing large amounts of important therapeutic proteins such as albumin, coagulation factor concentrates and immune globulins. However, the risk of disease transmission from paid donors was high[7,101] and this fact was tragically demonstrated with the onset of the AIDS epidemic.[102] Improvements in the manufacturing technique have now made these products free of transmission of most viruses[103,104] and some are now being produced by recombinant DNA methods. In some parts of the world, virtually all of the factor VIII and much of the factor IX are recombinant products. The demand for the intravenous form of immune serum globulin is very great because of its use in many situations in addition to the FDA-licensed indications of primary congenital immune deficiency and autoimmune thrombocytopenia. A discussion of the use of plasma derivatives is beyond the scope of this chapter.

Transfusion of cytomegalovirus (CMV)-negative blood products

CMV can be transmitted by blood transfusion with a severe, even fatal, result. Transfusion-transmitted CMV occurs in immunosuppressed patients and can be prevented by using CMV antibody-negative blood components or blood components filtered to remove the leukocytes that are thought to be the source of latent CMV. These CMV-safe blood components are indicated in neonates,[105] pregnant women,[106] patients undergoing bone marrow transplantation,[107–109] patients with AIDS or

Table 31.1 Plasma derivative products and their uses

Albumin	Restoration of plasma volume subsequent to shock, trauma, surgery and burns
Alpha-1 proteinase inhibitor	Treatment of emphysema caused by a genetic deficiency
Anti-hemophilic factor	Treatment or prevention of bleeding in patients with hemophilia A
Anti-inhibitor coagulant complex	Treatment of bleeding episodes in the presence of factor VIII inhibitor
Antithrombin III	Treatment of bleeding episodes associated with liver disease, antithrombin III deficiency and thromboembolism
Cytomegalovirus immune globulin	Passive immunization subsequent to exposure to cytomegalovirus
Factor IX complex	Prophylaxis and treatment of hemophilia B bleeding episodes and other bleeding disorders
Factor XIII	Treatment of bleeding and disorders of wound healing due to factor XIII deficiency
Fibrinogen	Treatment of hemorrhagic diathesis in hypofibrinogenemia, dysfibrinogenemia and afibrinogenemia
Fibrinolysin	Dissolution of intravascular clots
Haptoglobin	Supportive therapy in viral hepatitis and pernicious anemia
Hepatitis B immune globulin	Passive immunization subsequent to exposure to hepatitis B
IgM-enriched immune globulin	Treatment and prevention of septicemia and septic shock due to toxin liberation in the course of antibiotic treatment
Immune globulin (intravenous and intramuscular)	Treatment of agammaglobulinemia and hypogammaglobulinemia; passive immunization for hepatitis A and measles
Plasma protein fraction	Restoration of plasma volume subsequent to shock, trauma, surgery and burns
Rabies immune globulin	Passive immunization subsequent to exposure to rabies
$Rh_O(D)$ immune globulin	Treatment and prevention of hemolytic disease of fetus and newborn resulting from Rh incompatibility and incompatible blood transfusions
Rubella immune globulin	Passive immunization subsequent to exposure to German measles
Serum cholinesterase	Treatment of prolonged apnea after administration of succinylcholine chloride
Tetanus immune globulin	Passive immunization subsequent to exposure to tetanus
Vaccinia immune globulin	Passive immunization subsequent to exposure to smallpox
Varicella-zoster immune globulin	Passive immunization subsequent to exposure to chicken pox

Source: from information provided by the American Blood Resources Association.

severe combined immune deficiency, and patients receiving extensive chemotherapy. There is little information available about the value of CMV-safe blood components in patients who receive solid organ transplants. Most, if not virtually all, of the CMV disease in these patients is due to reactivation of a previous infection, thus CMV-safe blood components are not usually provided to these patients.

Irradiated blood components

Viable lymphocytes contained in blood components can cause fatal graft-versus-host disease (GVHD) in immuno-compromised patients.[110] Transfusion-induced GVHD can be prevented by using blood components that have been gamma irradiated. Irradiation with 1500–5000 Gy interferes with the ability of lymphocytes to proliferate without damaging the cell function.[111] Doses of up to 5000 Gy do not have an adverse effect on red cells, platelets or granulocytes. As the use of irradiated blood components has increased, often it is not possible to transfuse them immediately after they are irradiated. Doses of 2000 or 3000 rads to units of red cells result in potassium levels two and three times normal after storage for 4–5 days, which suggests that there is some irradiation damage to

the red cell membrane or the sodium–potassium pump. However, the amount of potassium in the supernatant is not considered dangerous, and the normal survival of these cells *in vivo* is the basis for allowing storage of irradiated red cells for the original expiration date or 28 days after irradiation, whichever comes first.[112]

It is difficult to determine which patients should receive irradiated blood components because there are no *in vitro* assays of immunodeficiency that satisfactorily predict which patients are susceptible to transfusion-associated GVHD. However, several kinds of patients are so severely immunocompromised that transfusion-associated GVHD is very likely unless blood components are irradiated. These include fetuses undergoing intra-uterine or exchange transfusion, patients with severe combined immunodeficiency syndrome or Wiskott–Aldrich syndrome, and patients undergoing allogeneic or autologous hematopoietic stem cell transplantation.

Occasionally, blood is irradiated for patients who are not immunocompromised. In immunocompetent patients, some cases of transfusion-associated GVHD occurred after transfusion of blood from relatives or unrelated donors who were partially HLA-matched with the patient.[113] Apparent transfusion-associated GVHD has been reported due to fresh blood transfused to two immunocompetent children who underwent cardiac surgery and received blood from donors who were homozygous for an HLA class I antigen haplotype shared with the recipient. In these cases, the recipient would not have recognized the HLA class I antigens on the transfused cells as foreign, but lymphocytes in the donated blood would have recognized the recipient's cells as foreign. Because of additional reports of transfusion-associated GVHD in other immunocompetent patients,[114,115] irradiation of the blood components donated by first-degree relatives of the patient has been instituted. Because of the high frequency of certain HLA antigens in the Japanese population and the resulting likelihood that a random, unrelated-donor may be partially HLA-matched with the recipient, irradiation may be used more commonly there.

There are several other clinical situations in which isolated cases of transfusion-associated GVHD have been reported and for which a few medical centers use irradiated blood components, but there is no consensus on recommended practice. These include: (1) neonates, although there is no evidence that newborns who do not have a congenital immunodeficiency are at increased risk of developing transfusion-associated GVHD; (2) patients with hematologic malignancies especially those receiving very severe chemotherapy regimens often with radiation; (3) patients with aplastic anemia, although these patients usually do not have defective cellular immunity and there have not been documented cases of transfusion-associated GVHD due to transfusion of normal cells; (4) patients with solid tumors such as neuroblastoma or glioblastoma; and (5) patients with AIDS, although no cases of transfusion-associated GVHD have been reported.

Although irradiation of fresh frozen plasma and cryoprecipitate is probably not necessary, transfusion-associated GVHD has occurred in patients with congenital immune deficiency after transfusion of fresh, liquid plasma. Because previously frozen components contain fragments of leukocytes, but few viable lymphocytes, these components would not be expected to cause transfusion-associated GVHD. Still many blood banks irradiate these plasma components to avoid clerical errors in which a cellular blood component might not be irradiated when necessary.

Transfusion of neocytes

Neocytes are units of red cells that are enriched with younger cells with the hope that the transfusion requirements would be reduced for patients who require chronic transfusion therapy such as those with hemoglobinopathies.[116,117] This approach has had limited success but it is very complex and costly and has not gained wide use.

Fibrin glue

Fibrin glue refers to the use of fibrinogen (in some form) and thrombin as a topical adhesive to control bleeding.[118] Fibrin glue is used predominantly by surgeons to stop microvascular bleeding in cardiovascular surgery and to reduce mediastinal drainage, to seal synthetic vascular grafts and bleeding surfaces of the liver or spleen, and in maxillofacial surgery to seal dura and repair peripheral nerves. During the past few years, commercial preparations of fibrin glue have become available.

Transfusion in special situations

Transfusion of blood components in many specific situations is complex hemotherapy and involves considerations that are not appropriate for detailed discussion in this book. Brief examples of a few of these situations are summarized here.

Massive transfusion

Massive transfusion is transfusion equivalent to the patient's blood volume during a 24-h interval. The effects of massive transfusion upon the recipient are due to the biochemical and functional characteristics of stored blood and include hypothermia, acidosis, hypocalcemia, hyperkalemia, coagulopathy and thrombocytopenia.[119] In patients undergoing acute blood loss and/or massive transfusion, the issues faced are the type of replacement fluid, the kind of blood component to use, the necessity to replace coagulation factors or platelets, the speed with which red cells can be made available, and the blood bank's ability to respond urgently.

Cardiovascular surgery

For patients undergoing cardiovascular surgery, fresh blood and routine platelet transfusions are not necessary. Patients undergoing cardiopulmonary bypass often develop thrombocytopenia and platelet function abnormalities.[20] However, most patients do not experience unusual bleeding and the extent of bleeding is not associated with these hemostatic abnormalities.[120] Patients who bleed excessively should be managed like any other surgical patients.

Transplantation

In patients undergoing hematopoietic stem cell transplantation consideration must be given to transfusion strategies before and after transplantation and in ABO- and Rh-incompatible transplants.[121] In solid organ transplantation, routine blood components are usually used for patients receiving kidney and heart transplants, but liver transplant recipients are treated more like patients undergoing massive transfusion.

Neonates

Neonates have special transfusion requirements including pretransfusion testing, need for CMV-negative blood, and/or irradiated blood components and exchange transfusion. Larger pediatric patients are usually managed similarly to adults. Smaller pediatric patients may require special infusion devices and adjusted doses of components.[122]

Hemophilia

The management of hemophilia patients is a complex subject and is not covered here.

Provision of red cells in urgent situations

The speed and methods of making blood available are crucial in several of these above-mentioned situations. Where transfusion is or may be urgent, a blood specimen should be obtained and sent to the blood bank for emergency type and cross-match. An ABO and Rh type can be performed in about 5 min and blood of the same type as the patient selected for transfusion. This blood can be released without a full cross-match. The cross-match procedure can be shortened to detect only ABO incompatibility since that is usually the most disastrous kind of transfusion reaction. Partially cross-matched blood of the patient's ABO type can be available usually in about 15 min. Usually Rh-positive blood would be chosen, but Rh-negative blood may be used if the patient is a young female. When the patient's ABO type is not known, group O red cells are used. This practice has led to the designation of group O, Rh-negative individuals as universal donors because group O, Rh-negative red cells would not be hemolyzed by either anti-A, anti-B, or anti-D if present and would not immunize recipients to D. Group O, Rh-negative (universal donor) red cells do not avoid the potential risk that the recipient may have a red cell antibody other than anti-D or a red cell autoantibody, and hemolysis or transfusion reactions can occur after transfusion. Stocking group O, Rh-negative red cells routinely in emergency departments is inappropriate.

The red cells may not be stored properly, and there may not be a system of checks for release of the units; these are practices that can lead to serious problems. Techniques of fluid management and resuscitation are so highly developed today that patients can be maintained for the time required to obtain red cells from the blood bank. Blood-bank personnel are well aware that there may be situations in which there is an urgent need for blood and each blood bank should have a procedure for the rapid release of red cells.

Exchange transfusion of the neonate

The indications for exchange transfusion in the neonate are: hyperbilirubinemia, sepsis, disseminated intravascular coagulopathy, polycythemia, respiratory distress syndrome, hyperamonemia, anemia, toxin removal, thrombocytopenia, and sickle cell disease. The exchange transfusion can be done via the umbilical vein for newborns or a peripheral vein. Exchange of one blood volume should remove about 65% of the original intravascular constituent, and an exchange of two blood volumes should remove about 85%.[38] Exchange transfusion is usually done with red cells that are only a few days old. If necessary, because of coagulopathy, fresh frozen plasma can be used with the red cells to provide coagulation factors during the exchange transfusion. The potential complications of exchange transfusion are: infection, rebound hypoglycemia, hypocalcemia (due to citrate anticoagulant in the transfused blood), hyperkalemia (if older red cells are used), late-onset alkalosis, volume overload, hemolysis, thrombocytopenia, neutropenia, coagulopathy, GVHD and hypothermia. These complications can be avoided or minimized by careful technique and good general patient care, although because many of these patients are quite ill and unstable, exchange transfusion can be a risky procedure.

Autoimmune hemolytic anemia

Patients with autoimmune hemolytic anemia present a special problem for the blood bank because the patient's serum usually reacts with red cells from all donors because of the presence and broad spectrum of reactivity of the autoantibody. This autoantibody reactivity may obscure alloantibodies present in the patient's serum and it may not be possible to obtain red cells for transfusion that are serologically compatible (negative cross-match). The decision to transfuse a patient with autoimmune hemolytic anemia should be based on the severity of the anemia, whether the anemia is rapidly progressive, and the associated clinical findings. In newly diagnosed patients with autoimmune hemolytic anemia, the hemoglobin should be measured frequently to determine whether the anemia is stable or progressing. Transfusion is not recommended unless the hemoglobin is in the 5–8 g/dl range. Many of these patients will compensate for their anemia, especially on bed rest in the hospital, and transfusion is not necessary. Although autoimmune hemolytic anemia patients are experiencing hemolysis, they usually do not experience signs or symptoms of an acute hemolytic transfusion reaction. In addition to the usual complications associated with transfusion, patients with autoimmune hemolytic anemia may experience increased hemolysis and/or congestive heart failure.

If transfusion is necessary, the two goals of compatibility testing are to select red cells that will survive at least as long as the patient's own cells and to avoid transfusing red cells that are incompatible with any clinically significant alloantibodies the patient may have. There are several serologic strategies to accomplish and these can be found in immunohematology reference texts.

The autoantibodies usually cause the red cells from all donors to have shortened post-transfusion survival. Despite this ongoing hemolysis, patients with autoimmune hemolytic anemia do not require special red cell components. It is advisable to choose units which are in the first week or two of their storage life to obtain the maximum benefit from the transfusion. Packed red cells are satisfactory although leukocyte-depleted red cells are preferable to avoid a possible febrile transfusion reaction, which might be confused with a hemolytic transfusion reaction. There is no reason to use frozen deglycerolized red cells for autoimmune anemia patients.

Pregnant women

Anemia is common during pregnancy; however, transfusion is rarely necessary. If so, it is usually because of some other complicating factor and the choice of blood components should be based on the specific reason for the transfusion (i.e. acute blood loss, sickle cell disease). Pregnant patients receive CMV-safe blood components to prevent acute CMV infection that might cause birth defects in the child.

Autoimmune thrombocytopenia

Most patients with autoimmune thrombocytopenia do not require platelet transfusion despite very low platelet counts.[75,123] These patients have platelet autoantibodies

that severely shorten the intravascular survival of transfused platelets. The transfused platelets survive for only a few minutes or hours[124] and a beneficial effect may not be obtained. If autoimmune thrombocytopenic patients do experience serious hemorrhage, platelet transfusions should be given.

Neonatal alloimmune thrombocytopenia

Neonatal alloimmune thrombocytopenia is the platelet analog of hemolytic disease of the newborn. That is, the mother becomes immunized to an antigen that she lacks but that the fetus has inherited from the father. Maternal IgG platelet antibodies then cross the placenta and cause thrombocytopenia in the fetus. The antibodies can be detected in the mother;[125] HPA-1 (formerly known as Pl[A1]) is the most common. If the neonate requires transfusion, platelets lacking the offending antigen should be used. Alternatively, an exchange transfusion can be done to remove the offending antibody. Platelets lacking the antigen can be obtained from the mother, although the plasma containing the antibody should be removed before transfusion, and the platelets should be resuspended in saline or group AB plasma. If the mother is not available or cannot donate platelets, most large blood banks have a few HPA-1 negative donors available to provide compatible platelets. The half-life of IgG is approximately 21 days; therefore, more than one platelet transfusion may be necessary in severely affected infants.

Neonatal alloimmune neutropenia

This is the neutrophil analog of hemolytic disease of the newborn and of neonatal alloimmune thrombocytopenia. Patients usually are discovered because they develop an infection at the circumcision site or in the perineal area. Cases due to several different neutrophil-specific antibodies have been reported.[126] Although these infants can be given granulocytes attained from a whole blood donation by the mother, the very short half-life of granulocytes limits the effectiveness of this approach. Thus, exchange transfusion is the recommended for these patients.

Rare blood types

There is no universal definition of a rare blood type. This term usually refers to an individual who lacks a blood-group antigen that is present in a very high frequency in the normal population. This means that the individual will almost certainly be exposed to the antigen if they are pregnant or receive a transfusion. First, it is necessary to determine whether the antibody is clinically significant and likely to cause accelerated destruction of red cells. If the antibody is clinically significant, efforts should be made to obtain red cells that lack the antigen. Most countries have a rare donor registry that can be consulted. Considerable planning may be necessary to obtain the red cells, especially if the donors live in other cities or if the transfusion is to replace blood loss during elective surgery. Red cells from most rare donors may be available only in the frozen state which may create additional problems if the transfusion is for anticipated but uncertain blood loss. If transfusion is needed urgently, close communication is necessary between the blood-bank physician and the patient's attending physician to determine a course of action. For instance, if the antibody may cause shortened red cell survival but little or no acute hemolysis, the decision might be made to use incompatible red cells while the search continues for red cells that lack the antigen.

Techniques of blood transfusion

Because complications of transfusion can be caused by improper handling or administration of blood components[127–129] or the administration of the incorrect component to the patient, it is essential the blood transfusions be adminstered according to clearly defined procedures that are well understood and carried out by qualified personnel. Blood components should be administered only on the written order of a physician. The issues important in administering a transfusion are: (1) obtaining consent for transfusion;[130] (2) obtaining the blood sample for compatibility testing; (3) use of blood administration sets and filters; (4) use of venipuncture, procedures for starting the transfusion; (5) use of infusion solutions,[131] (6) identification of the patient and blood component; (7) determination of rate of transfusion; (8) warming of blood; (9) and nursing care of patients receiving a transfusion.

Complications of transfusion: recognition and management

Despite its life-saving role, there are risks associated with blood transfusion. Immunologic complications involve various forms of transfusion reactions while non-immunologic complications are due to the physical effects of the blood component or to transmission of disease. Complications occur during or shortly after about 1–3% of transfusions, although it has been estimated that almost 20% of transfusions result in some kind of adverse effect,[132] and the fatality rate is about 1.0–1.2/100 000 patients who receive a transfusion.[133] This is approximately 35 transfusion-related deaths/year in the United States.

Transfusion reactions

Hemolytic transfusion reactions

The most dangerous immunologic complication of transfusion is an ABO-incompatible hemolytic transfusion reaction. About 41% of transfusion fatalities in the United States are due to ABO-incompatible transfusions.[133] This means that in the United States, about 16 patients/year die, giving an apparent incidence of fatal ABO-incompatible transfusion of 1/200 000 patients transfused.

ABO incompatibility causes severe hemolytic transfusion reactions because the patient has IgM ABO antibodies that bind complement and cause activation of the complement system, release of cytokines and red cell lysis. The signs and symptoms of a hemolytic transfusion reaction are due to complement activation and also to the effects of cytokines.[134,135] The severity of the symptoms does not correlate with the volume of ABO-incompatible red cells transfused or the ultimate outcome of the transfusion reaction.[136,137] The signs of a hemolytic transfusion reaction are well known and include fever, chills, flushing, low back pain, hypotension, dyspnea, abdominal pain, vomiting, diarrhea, chest pain or unexpected bleeding. The most common signs and symptoms are fever, chest pain and hypotension. In a hemolytic transfusion reaction, the coagulation system may be activated and these patients may develop a coagulopathy and/or disseminated intravascular coagulation. Oliguria and renal failure may also be part of a hemolytic transfusion reaction because a variety of factors such as kinens, intravascular coagulation, and microthrombi lead to reduced renal blood flow and damage.

There is a classic pattern of alteration in laboratory tests in a hemolytic transfusion reaction. In an acute hemolytic transfusion reaction, the common findings are hemoglobinemia and/or hemoglobinuria, reduced serum haptoglobin, elevated serum bilirubin, a postive direct antiglobulin test, and the presence of unexpected red cell antibodies.[136] Laboratory testing should make the diagnosis of hemolysis and identify the red cell antibody involved.

Febrile reactions

These reactions occur in association with about 0.5–1.0% of transfusions. They are due to the patient's leukocyte antibodies, which react with leukocytes present in the transfused components[138] or cytokines contained in the donor blood component.[139] The severity of the reaction is directly related to the number of leukocytes in the blood component.[138] These febrile reactions can be prevented by removing leukocytes from the blood components. Many febrile reactions can be prevented by the administration of antipyretics such as acetaminophen. However, the use of antipyretics should be reserved for patients who have experienced a febrile reaction. With the increasing use of leukoreduced components, the problem of febrile transfusion reactions should decrease to very low levels.

Allergic reactions

Allergic reactions manifested by hives but with no other symptoms occur following 1–2% of transfusions. When this occurs, the transfusion should be stopped; if it is then established that hemolysis is not occurring and there are no other signs or symptoms, the patient can be given an antihistamine and after about 30 min the transfusion can be restarted.

Pulmonary reactions

The occurrence of pulmonary reactions to transfusions, also called transfusion-related acute lung injury (TRALI), has been known for years, and these reactions are similar to adult respiratory distress syndrome. These reactions are acute, sometimes fatal, occur usually within 1–2 h of the transfusion, and are characterized by acute respiratory distress, severe hypoxemia, bilateral pulmonary edema, hypotension, fever, and diffuse bilateral infiltrates on chest X-ray.[140] Cyanosis may or may not be present. The frequency of these reactions is estimated between 1/300 and 1/5000 transfusions of plasma-containing components.[141] They may be more common than previously believed. The reactions are thought to be due to transfusion of HLA- or granulocyte-specific antibodies in the donor unit that react with the patient's leukocytes and the transfusion of inflammatory mediators.[140] In either situation, it is likely that leukocytes, endothelial cells, and lipid and protein inflammatory mediators are involved and lead to endothelial damage, increased cell membrane permeability, increased neutrophil adhesion to endothelium, and release of cytokines. These patients can be successfully managed if there is prompt recognition of the reaction and initiation of supportive treatment.

Anaphylactic reactions

Patients who are IgA-deficient and who have IgA antibodies may experience dramatic and rapidly fatal anaphylactic reaction if they receive blood components containing IgA.[142] The treatment is the same as for any anaphylactic reaction. The reactions can be prevented by using red cells or platelet concentrates washed to remove plasma IgA and by using plasma components prepared from IgA-deficient donors.

Reactions to platelets

Transfusion reactions can occur during platelet transfusion. These reactions present as chills and fever similar to those seen in a non-hemolytic febrile transfusion reaction. Platelet transfusion reactions are caused by cytokines that accumulate in the platelet concentrate during storage[139,143] or by the patient's platelet or HLA antibodies that react with leukocytes contained in the platelet concentrates. These reactions can be prevented by removing the leukocytes before storage of platelets.[143]

The most common signs and symptoms of a transfusion reaction to platelets are chills, fever and urticaria. The cause, severity and outcome of a transfusion reaction are difficult to predict from the presenting signs and symptoms. Therefore, all patients who exhibit signs or symptoms during or within several hours after platelet transfusion should be managed initially as if a transfusion reaction was occurring. When a transfusion reaction is suspected, the transfusion should be stopped immediately, the needle should be left in the vein, and normal saline should be infused while vital signs are obtained and a brief physical examination is carried out. A new blood sample should be obtained for repeat red blood cell compatibility testing and inspection of the plasma for evidence of hemolysis, and a urine sample should be obtained if the patient can void. If pulmonary symptoms are prominent, a chest X-ray should be obtained. Based on these actions, a preliminary assessment of the situation can be made and definitive treatment initiated.

Graft-versus-host disease (GVHD)

Blood components contain viable lymphocytes and can cause GVHD in patients who are severely immunocompromised. Transfusion-associated GVHD can also occur in immunocompetent patients if they receive blood from an HLA-matched (usually homozygous) donor.[113–115]

The syndrome characterized by fever, liver dysfunction, skin rash, diarrhea and marrow hypoplasia begins less than 30 days following transfusions and is fatal in approximately 90% of patients.[110] Transfusion-associated GVHD can be prevented by irradiating the blood components prior to transfusions.[110]

Other complications of blood transfusion

Immunization to blood-group antigens, iron overload, microemboli, citrate toxicity, hypocalcemia, hyperkalemia, acidosis, alkalosis, and cardiac arrhythmias due to cold blood can occur following transfusion.

Transfusion-transmitted diseases

In developed countries, since the AIDS epidemic, the blood supply is safer than ever, but the epidemic and the growing awareness of post-transfusion hepatitis have heightened the public's fears of blood transfusion. In response, physicians have developed more conservative transfusion practices. This has led to several actions or changes that have improved blood safety. These changes include new donor screening criteria, increased laboratory tests, reduced use of blood because of more conservative transfusion practices, increased use of autologous blood, and the use of pharmacologic agents to reduce transfusion requirements. The single action that had the largest impact on improving blood safety was the conversion to an all volunteer donor system in the United States.[143] The major transfusion-transmitted diseases are described below.

Post-transfusion hepatitis

Post-transfusion hepatitis is the most common disease transmitted by blood transfusion and it has a major health impact. Post-transfusion hepatitis can be due to hepatitis C virus, hepatitis B virus, hepatitis A virus, CMV, or Epstein–Barr virus. The incidence varies in different parts of the world. During the 1970s, in the United States, rates of post-transfusion hepatitis ranged from 5.9 to 21% of patients;[144] but the present estimate for hepatitis C is 1/unit and for hepatitis B is 1/unit.[144] Thus, in the United States there are about 90–111 cases of post-transfusion hepatitis C and 66–153 of post-transfusion hepatitis B annually per million units of antibody negative blood.[145–150]

Hepatitis A usually has a short period of viremia and generally does not involve a carrier state. Thus, post-transfusion hepatitis A is rare, although it can occur if an individual donates blood during the short period of viremia before symptoms develop.[151–152] Donated blood is not tested for hepatitis A because hepatitis A antibodies are not present at this early stage of infection, there is no practical test for the virus itself, and post-transfusion hepatitis A is rare.

Because most individuals infected with the hepatitis B virus are asymptomatic and because about 10% of patients develop persistent viremia and chronic hepatitis B, an infectious, but apparently healthy, individual may meet all of the donor medical history criteria and donate a unit of infectious blood. Routine screening of blood donors for hepatitis B surface antigen has reduced the previous high incidence of post-transfusion hepatitis B. Because many cases of post-transfusion hepatitis were not due to hepatitis A or B, 'surrogate' testing for non-A, non-B hepatitis was introduced in the United States during the 1980s. There was an association between either elevated alanine aminotransferase (ALT) level hepatitis antibody to hepatitis B core antigen or the presence of and post-transfusion non-A non-B hepatitis.[153–155] It was projected that discarding blood units with either an elevated ALT or a positive test for antibody to hepatitis B core antigen would eliminate about 40% of post-transfusion hepatitis.[153–159]

In the late 1980s, the hepatitis C virus was discovered[158–159] and this virus accounts for almost all cases of non-A, non-B hepatitis. Testing for antibodies to hepatitis C virus was introduced in the early 1990s and has greatly reduced post-transfusion hepatitis C. Because the screening test for hepatitis C detects antibody to the virus, there is a 'window' period during which the individual has viremia and is infectious, but during which the test for antibodies to hepatitis C virus is negative. Blood donation by asymptomatic individuals during this window period accounts for much of the remaining post-transfusion hepatitis. This delay in antibody production had led to the development of tests to screen donated blood by detection of viral DNA or RNA. This method has been referred to as nucleic acid amplification testing (NAT) and is discussed later.

HIV infection and AIDS

When the epidemiology of HIV infection became known and when it was clear that transfusion-transmitted AIDS did occur, blood banks altered their medical screening practices to defer potential donors from AIDS risk groups, and when the HIV-1 virus was shown to be the cause of AIDS, initiated routine testing of all donated blood for antibodies to HIV-1 (anti-HIV-1). These two steps greatly improved blood safety and reduced the risk of acquiring HIV infection following transfusion from up to 91% to very low levels. The HIV-1 antibody test is an excellent test with a specificity of up to 99.9994%.[160] When a blood donor is found to be anti-HIV-1 positive on the initial screening test, confirmatory testing is done by the Western blot method.

Despite the effectiveness of the medical history questioning and laboratory testing of donated blood, there is a remaining risk of acquiring HIV-1 by transfusion. This risk has decreased from 1/33 000 units[161] to the current estimate of more than 5/10,000,000 units[149,150] may be up to 20 units. This would still mean that 5–10 persons could become infected with HIV-1 annually by transfusion of donated blood which was negative for anti-HIV-1 antibodies.

The reasons for the continued risk of transfusion-transmitted HIV-1 are: (1) failure of some infected individuals to developed antibody; (2) lack of representation of variant viral strains of test reagents; (3) laboratory testing errors; and (4) the window phase of infection.[162] Because the window phase accounts for almost all transfusion-transmitted HIV in developed countries, efforts have been made to overcome this problem. Testing for the HIV antigen itself was adopted and, although it was predicted to shorten the window period and further reduce the likelihood of HIV-1 transmission, the method was not sufficiently sensitive to detect many infectious HIV-1 seronegative donors.[163,164] More recently, methods that amplify HIV-1 DNA sequences are being applied to blood donor testing, thus making it possible to detect minute amounts of viral DNA or RNA. This nucleic acid amplification testing (NAT) is being implemented in the United States and many developed countries.

Because of the complexity and cost of NAT, sera from multiple donors are tested in a pool, which somewhat limits the sensitivity of the test. Methods in use at the time of this writing detect a level of Hepatitis C Virus or HIV viral particles/ml near to the levels that occur during the window phase of infection. During the first year of testing the rate of NAT-positive, antibody-negative samples was 1:210 000 to 1:321 000 for HCV and 1:800 000 to 1:4 600 000 for HIV depending on the NAT method used.[165] Thus, it is projected in the United States that NAT will reduce the HIV-1 window phase period from 22 to 10–15 days and the hepatitis C window phase period from 70 to 41–60 days.[165] This reduction should prevent approximately 2–15 cases of transfusion-transmitted HIV-1 and 40–60 cases of hepatitis C annually in the United States.[166]

Other transfusion-transmitted infectious diseases

Malaria can be transmitted by transfusion. This is rare in North America and Western Europe. Most cases involve *Plasmodium malariae*. Donors who might transmit malaria undergo screening by medical history, although this screening method is becoming increasingly difficult as worldwide travel increases. Laboratory testing of donors for malaria is not practical or cost effective in the United States but is often done in parts of the world where malaria is endemic. Transmission of syphilis by blood transfusion was common years ago but now it is extremely rare.[167] The treponema that causes syphilis can survive in refrigerated blood for 48 h[168] at room temperature and, thus, can be transmitted from red cell components stored for only a few days or from platelet concentrates stored at room temperature. Although all blood donors are tested for syphilis, this is not a very effective method of preventing transfusion-transmitted syphilis because the serologic tests do not closely coincide with periods of infectivity.

CMV is a herpes virus that is common in the general population and can be transmitted by blood transfusion to both immunocompetent or immunodeficient patients. A large proportion of blood donors have been infected with CMV. There is no practical laboratory test to determine which patients previously infected with CMV but presently healthy enough to donate blood may transmit the virus. Transfusion-transmitted CMV can be prevented by using blood that lacks antibody to CMV or by removing the leukocytes from cellular components.

Transmission of HTLV-I via blood transfusion does occur,[169] although no cases of transfusion-transmitted adult T-cell leukemia or tropical spastic paraperesis have been identifed in the United States. All donated blood in the United States is tested for antibodies to HTLV-I. *Trypanosoma cruzi*, the organism that causes Chagas' disease, can survive in refrigerated blood and can be transmitted by transfusion.[170,171] Cases of transfusion-transmitted Chagas' disease are rare in the United States. No laboratory tests or screening procedures are used in the United States or Western Europe to detect carriers of *T. cruzi*. Attempts to identify donors potentially infectious for *T. cruzi* by medical history have not been effective. *Babesia microti* can be transmitted by blood donated by asymptomatic infected donors.[172] The ticks that carry this parasite are prevalent in the Northeast, Mid Atlantic, and Upper Midwest. There is no suitable laboratory screening test for *B. microti*. Some blood banks defer individuals from heavily tick-infested areas during the summer months.

Borrelia burgdorferi, a spirochete transmitted by ticks to humans, can survive in stored blood for up to 45 days.[173] Although transmission of *B. burgdorferi* by transfusion is theoretically possible, it has not been reported. A serologic test is available, but it is not suitable for donor screening. The widespread prevalence of the host tick makes it impractical to defer donors from endemic areas. Parvovirus B19 has been transmitted by blood transfusion.[174,175] No steps are taken to prevent transfusion-transmission of parvovirus B19, but a recent case of transmission by pooled, solvent/detergent-treated plasma[175] led to the screening of lots of this plasma to minimize the likelihood of infection. Theoretically, any disease in which microbes circulate in the blood and survive for a few days in stored blood components could be transmitted by transfusion. However, the diseases of most concern have been discussed. A few other diseases that almost never occur due to transfusions in the United States are toxoplasmosis, leishmaniasis, microfilaria and African trypanosomiasis.

Role of hematopoietic growth factors in transfusion medicine

Erythropoietin

The availability of hematopoietic growth factors opens a new era in transfusion medicine. The first of these, erythropoietin, has eliminated the need for red cell transfusions in most patients with end-stage renal failure.[176] It has been estimated nationally that this may eliminate as many as 50 000 transfusions in the United States. The use of erythropietin would make these red cell units available for other patients and yet allow patients with renal failure to maintain higher hemoglobin levels and improved quality of life[177] and to avoid the complications of transfusions. Erythropoietin is being used in forms of anemia not due to erythropoietin deficiency, but the benefits are limited.[178–182] Erythropoietin is also being used to increase autologous blood donation or reduce the homologous blood requirements of patients undergoing elective surgery.[183] This exciting drug has now taken its place in red cell transfusion practice.

Granulocyte-macrophage colony stimulating factor (GM-CSF)

It appears that G or GM-CSF may decrease the period of chemotherapy-induced leukopenia in patients with

malignancy or in those undergoing bone marrow transplantation. Although this reduction may reduce the morbidity and mortality of these procedures, it probably will not greatly alter transfusion therapy in the near future because leukocyte replacement is not widely practiced. However, reducing the incidence and/or severity of infection could modify transfusion therapy if sepsis and disseminated intravascular coagulopathy are avoided with a resulting decline in the use of platelets and fresh frozen plasma.

Platelet growth factor

Development and use of the platelet growth factors thrombopoietin and megakaryocyte growth and development factor could have a major impact on transfusion medicine. Platelet transfusions have increased more rapidly than other blood components[6] and their use presently constitutes a very large part of the activity of most large blood banks. The ability to shorten the duration of thrombocytopenia, reduce the risk of hemorrhage, and reduce the need for platelet transfusion has a very great potential benefit.

Platelet growth factors shorten the period of thrombocytopenia and elevate the platelet nadir in patients with solid tumors, but these patients do not require many platelet transfusions and so there is little impact on platelet demand. No beneficial effect on platelet recovery has been found in patients undergoing hematopoietic stem cell transplantation. Thus, despite the exciting development of the availability of platelet growth factors, they have had little impact on transfusion medicine.

Blood substitutes

The functions of blood can be grouped generally as: (1) maintenance of intravascular volume; (2) delivery of oxygen to the tissues; (3) provision of coagulation factors, and some defense mechanisms; and (4) transportation of metabolic waste products. A blood substitute, or artificial blood, substitutes only for the oxygen-delivery function. Thus, more appropriate terms for blood substitutes are hemoglobin or red cell substitute.

For years there has been considerable interest in the use of a red cell substitute that would effectively transport oxygen from the lungs to the tissues. The ideal acellular red cell substitute would not require cross-matching or blood typing, could be stored, preferably at room temperature, for a long period, would have a reasonable intravascular life span and thereafter be exited promptly, and would be free of toxicity or disease transmission. The two compounds which have undergone most study are hemoglobin solutions and perfluorocarbons. Hemoglobin chemically binds oxygen whereas perfluorocarbons have a solubility for oxygen 20 times greater than that of water but even so do not carry as much oxygen as hemoglobin. During the 1980s, a specific perfluorocarbon product underwent clinical trials in patients who required urgent medical care and who refused to receive blood components. The amount of oxygen that can be delivered by perfluorocarbons is based on the oxygen content of inspired air. At ambient oxygen tension, the tested perfluorocarbon product was not effective, but when patients breathed 100% oxygen, perfluorocarbon provided increased oxygen consumption, increased mixed venous oxygen tension, and increased mixed venous hemoglobin saturation.[184]

In a separate study, eight severely anemic patients (hemoglobin 1.2–4.5 g/dl) who received the perfluorocarbon product were compared with 15 who did not.[185] All patients refused blood transfusion. The amount of perfluorocarbon product that could be given to patients and the oxygen tension, even when 100% oxygen was inspired, were such that the perfluorocarbon product contributed only about half the oxygen-carrying capacity of the patient's plasma. The amount of oxygen delivered by the perfluorocarbon product was not clinically significant and the patients did not benefit. The major observation in this study was the ability of all the patients to tolerate remarkably low hemoglobin levels and the lack of need for increased arterial oxygen content in the 15 control patients who had hemoglobin levels of approximately 7 g/dl.

Work with hemoglobin solutions has progressed steadily. Hemoglobin can be prepared in solution by lysis of red cells. If the remaining cell stroma is removed, the stroma-free hemoglobin is relatively non-toxic and non-antigenic. However, stroma-free hemoglobin in solution has a short intravascular life span and has a low P^{50} (the point at which 50% is saturated). Thus, research has focused on modifying the structure of the hemoglobin molecule and/or binding the hemoglobin molecule to other molecules to overcome these two problems.[186] At least one stroma-free hemoglobin product has undergone extensive *in vitro* and animal trials and is being used experimentally in humans.[186] It seems possible that a hemoglobin substitute may become available in the future.

It is likely that hemoglobin substitutes will supplement, not replace, most red cell transfusions. Since the intravascular life span of the hemoglobin substitutes would be a few days, their major use is expected to be in the treatment of acute blood loss. Since blood typing and crossmatching would not be necessary, hemoglobin substitutes might be stocked in ambulances and used by paramedics outside of healthcare facilities. Other potential uses of hemoglobin substitutes include organ perfusion and preservation prior to transplantation and improving oxygen delivery to tissues that have an impaired blood supply. If the use of hemoglobin solutions follows this course, the need for donated blood might increase instead of decline as might have been expected.

REFERENCES

1. Daniels G, Hadley A 2002 Blood groups on red cells, platelets, and neutrophils. In: Wickramasinghe S, McCullough J (eds), Blood and bone marrow pathology. Churchill Livingstone, Edinburgh.
2. Kelton J 2002 Acquired hemolytic anemias. In: Wickramasinghe SN, McCullough J (eds), Blood and bone marrow pathology. Churchill Livingstone, Edinburgh.
3. McCullough J 1996 National blood programs in developed countries. Transfusion 36: 1019–1032
4. Leikola J 1988 How much blood for the world? Vox Sanguinus 54: 1–5
5. McCullough J 1993 The nation's changing blood supply system. Journal of the American Medical Association 269: 2239
6. Wallance EL, Churchill WH, Surgenor DM et al 1998 Collection and transfusion of blood and blood components in the United States, 1994. Transfusion 38: 625–636
7. Eastlund T 1998 Monetary blood donation incentives and the risk of transfusion-transmitted infection. Transfusion 38: 881–884
8. Busch M, Garratty G 1997 Applications of molecular biology to blood transfusion medicine. American Association of Blood Banks; Bethesda, MD, 123–176
9. McCullough J 1993 The nation's changing blood supply system. Journal of the American Medical Association 269: 2239
10. McCullough J 1996 The continuing evolution of the nation's blood supply system. American Journal of Clinical Pathology 105: 689–695
11. Zuck TF 1995 Current good manufacturing practices. Transfusion 35: 95–66
12. McCullough J 1998 Transfusion medicine. McGraw Hill, New York
13. Piliavin JA, Callero PL (eds) 1991 Giving blood. The development of an altruistic identify. The Johns Hopkins University Press, Baltimore
14. McCullough J 1996 The continuing evolution of the nation's blood supply system. American Journal of Clinical Pathology 105 :689–695
15. Zuck TF 1995 Current good manufacturing practices. Transfusion 35: 95–66
16. Morduchowicz G, Pitlik SD, Huminer D et al 1991 Transfusion reactions due to bacterial contamination of blood and blood products. Reviews of infectious Diseases 13: 307
17. Sazama K: 1990 Reports of 355 transfusion-associated deaths: 1976 through 1985. Transfusion 30: 583
18. Kasprisin DO, Glynn SH, Taylor F, Miller KA 1992 Moderate and severe reactions in blood donors. Transfusion 32: 23–26
19. Ogata H, Iinuma N, Nagashima K, Akabane T 1980 Vasovagal reactions in blood donors. Transfusion 679–683
20. Callahan R, Edelman EB, Smith MS, Smith JJ: 1963 Study of the incidence and characteristics of blood donor 'reactors'. Transfusion 3: 76
21. Newman BH, Waxman DA 1996 Blood donation-related neurologic needle injury: evaluation of 2 years' worth of data from a large blood center. Transfusion 36: 213–215
22. Berry PR, Wallis WE 1997 Venipuncture nerve injuries. Lancet 1: 1236–1237
23. Horowitz SH 2000 Venipuncture-induced causalgia: anatomic relations of upper extremity superficial veins and nerves, and clinical considerations. Transfusion 40: 1036–1040
24. Popovsky MA, Whitaker B, Arnold NL 1995 Severe outcomes of allogeneic and autologous blood donation: frequency and characterization. Transfusion 35: 734–737
25. Axelrod FB, Pepkowitz SH, Goldfinger D 1989 Establishment of a schedule of optimal preoperative collection and autologous blood. Transfusion 29: 677

26. Birkmeyer JD, Goodnough LT, AuBuchon JP et al 1993 The cost-effectiveness of preoperative autologous blood donation for total hip and knee replacement. Transfusion 33: 544

27. Goodnough LT, Rednick S, Price TH et al 1989 Increased preoperative collection of autologous blood with recombinant human erythropoietin therapy. New England Journal of Medicine 321: 1163

28. Anonymous 1996 Royal College of Physicians of Edinburgh consensus conference on autologous transfusion. Edinburgh 4–6 October 1995. Transfusion 36: 625–667

29. Williams AE, Kleinman S, Gilcher RO et al 1992 The prevalence of infectious disease markers in directed versus homologous blood donations (abstract). Transfusion 32: 45S

30. Barton JC, Grindon AJ, Baron NH, Bertoli LF 1999 Hemochromatosis probands as blood donors. Transfusion 39: 578–585

31. Tan L, Khan MK, Hawk JC 1999 Use of blood therapeutically drawn from hemochromatosis patients. Transfusion 39: 1018–1026

32. Slichter SJ, Harker LA 1976 Preparation and storage of platelet concentrates. II. Storage and variables influence platelet viability and function. British Journal of Haematology 34: 403

33. Filip DJ, Aster RH 1978 Relative hemostatic effectiveness of human platelet stored at 4°C and 22°C. Journal of Laboratory and Clinical Medicine 91: 618

34. Kunicki TJ, Tuccelli M, Becker GA, Aster RH 1975 A study of variables affecting the quality of platelets stored at 'room temperature'. Transfusion 15: 414

35. Murphy S, Heaton WA. Rebulla P 1996 Platelet production in the old world – and the new Transfusion 36: 751–754

36. McCullough J 1998 Transfusion medicine. McGraw Hill, New York

37. McLeod BC, Price TH, Drew MI (eds) 1997 Apheresis: principles and practice. Bethesda, AABB Press, Bethesda, 27–65

38. Bensinger WI, Price TH, Dale DC et al 1993 The effects of daily recombinant human granulocyte-colony-stimulating factor administration on normal granulocyte donors undergoing leukopheresis. Blood 81: 1883–1888

39. Dale DC, Liles WC, Llewellyn C et al 1998 Neutrophil transfusions: kinetics and functions of neutrophils mobilized with granulocyte colony-stimulating factor (G-CSF) and dexamethasone. Transfusion 38: 713–721

40. McCullough J, Clay M, Herr G et al 1999 Effects of granulocyte colony stimulating factor (G-CSF) on potential normal granulocyte donors. Transfusion 39: 1136–1140

41. Porter D, Roth M, McGarigle C et al 1993 Adoptive immunotherapy induces molecular remission in relapsed CML following allogeneic bone marrow transplantation (BMT). Proceedings of the American Society of Clinical Oncologists 12: 303

42. Drobyski WR, Keever CA, Roth MS et al 1993 Salvage immunotherapy using donor leukocyte infusions as treatment for relapsed chronic myelogenous leukemia after allogeneic bone marrow transplantation: Efficacy and toxicity of a defined T cell dose. Blood 82: 2310

43. Van Rhee F, Lin F, Cullis JO et al 1994 Relapse of chronic myeloid leukemia after allogeneic bone marrow transplant: the case for giving donor leukocyte transfusions before the onset of hematologic relapse. Blood 83: 3377–3383

44. Stroneck DF, Hubel A, Shankar RA et al 1999 Retroviral transduction and expansion of peripheral blood lymphocytes for the treatment of mucopolysaccharidosis II, Hunter syndrome. Transfusion 39: 343–350

45. Murphy G, Tjoa B, Ragde H et al 1996 Phase I clinical trial: T-cell therapy for prostate cancer using autologous dendritic cells pulsed with HLA-A0201-specific peptides from prostate-specific membrane antigen. Prostate 29: 371

46. Nestle FO, Gilliet M, Alljagic S et al 1997 Vaccination of melanoma patients with peptide-pulsed dendritic cells. Melanoma Research 7: S14

47. Choudhury A, Gajewski JL, Liang J et al 1997 Use of leukemic dendritic cells for the generation of antileukemic cellular cytotoxicity against Philadelphia chromosome-positive chronic myelogenous leukemia. Blood 89: 1133–1142

48. Troy AJ, Hart DNJ 1997 Dendritic cells and cancer: progress toward a new cellular therapy. Journal of Hematotherapy 6: 523–533

49. Pettengell R, Morgenstern GR, Woll PJ et al 1993 Peripheral blood progenitor cell transplantation in lymphoma and leukemia using a single apheresis. Transfusion 82: 3770–3777

50. Ottinger HD, Beelen DW, Scheulen B et al 1996 Improved immune reconstitution after allotransplantation of peripheral blood stem cells instead of bone marrow. Blood 88: 2775–2779

51. Bensinger WI, Clift R, Martin P et al 1996 Allogeneic peripheral blood stem cell transplantation in patients with advanced hematologic malignancies: a retrospective comparison with marrow transplantation. Blood 88: 2794–2800

52. Anderlini P, Przepiorka D, Champlin R, Korbling M et al 1996 Biologic and clinical effects of granulocyte colony-stimulating factor in normal individuals. Blood 88: 2819–2825

53. Stroncek DF, Clay ME, Petzoldt ML et al 1996 Treatment of normal individuals with granulocyte-colony-stimulating factor: donor experiences and the effects on peripheral blood CD34+ cell counts and on the collection of peripheral blood stem cells. Transfusion 36: 601–610

54. Office of Medical Applications of Research, National Institutes of Health 1988 Perioperative red cell transfusion. Journal of the American Medical Association 260: 2700

55. Heddle NM, O'Hoski P, Singer J et al 1992 A prospective study to determine the safety of omitting the antiglobulin crossmatch from pretransfusion testing. British Journal of Haematology 81: 579–584

56. Gmur J, von Felten A, Osterwalder B et al 1983 Delayed alloimmunization using random single donor platelet transfusions: a prospective study in thrombocytopenic patients with acute leukemia. Blood 62: 473

57. Sniecinski I, O'Donnell MR, Nowicki B, Hill LR et al 1988 Prevention of refractoriness and HLA- alloimmunization using filtered blood products. Blood 71: 1402

58. Kao KJ, Mickel M, Braine HG et al 1995 White cell reduction in platelet concentrates and packed red cells by filtration: a multicenter clinical trial. Transfusion 35: 13–19

59. Valeri CR, Pivacek LE, Gray AD, Cassidy GP, Leavy ME, Dennis RC, Melaragno AJ, Niehoff J, Yeston N, and Emerson CP 1989 The safety and therapeutic effectiveness of human red cells stored at – 80 degrees C for as long as 21 years. Transfusion 29: 429–437

60. National Institutes of Health Consensus Conference 1985 Fresh frozen plasma: indications and risks. Journal of the American Medical Association 253: 546

61. Counts RB, Haisch C, Simon TL et al 1979 Hemostasis in massively transfused trauma patients. Annals in Surgery 190: 91

62. Mannucci PM, Federici AB, Sirchia G et al 1982 Hemostasis testing during massive blood replacement: a study of 172 cases. Vox Sanguinus 42: 113

63. Ness PM, Perkins HA 1979 Cryoprecipitate as a reliable source of fibrinogen replacement. Journal of the American Medical Association 241: 1690

64. McCullough J, Steeper TA, Connelly DP et al 1988 Platelet utilization in a university hospital. Journal of the American Medical Association JAMA 259: 2414

65. Baer MR, Bloomfield CD 1992 Controversies in transfusion medicine. Prophylactic platelet transfusion therapy: pro. Transfusion 32: 377

66. Roy AJ, Jaffe N, Djerassi I 1973 Prophylactic platelet transfusions in children with acute leukemia: a dose-response study. Transfusion 13: 283

67. Higby DJ, Cohen E, Holland JF, Sinks L et al 1974 The prophylactic treatment of thrombocytopenic leukemia patients with platelets: a double blind study. Transfusion 14: 440

68. Soloman J, Bokefkamp T, Fahey JL et al 1978 Platelet prophylaxis in acute non-lymphocytic leukemia. Lancet 1: 267

69. Gaydos LA, Freireich EJ, Mantel N et al 1962 The quantitative relation between platelet count and hemorrhage in patients with acute leukemia. New England Journal of Medicine 266: 905

70. Heckman KD, Weiner GJ, Davis CS et al 1997 Randomized study of prophylactic platelet transfusion threshold during induction therapy for adult acute leukemia: 10,000/µL versus 20,000/µL. Journal of Clinical Oncology 15: 1143–1149

71. Rebulla P, Finazzi G, Marangoni F et al 1997 The Gruppo Italiano Malattie Ematologiche Maligne dell'Adulto: The threshold for prophylactic platelet transfusions in adults with acute myeloid leukemia. New England Journal of Medicine 337: 1870–1875

72. Wandt H, Frank M, Ehninger G et al 1988 Safety and cost effectiveness of a 10×10^9/L trigger for prophylactic platelet transfusions compared with the traditional 20×10^9/L trigger: a prospective comparative trial in 105 patients with acute myeloid leukemia. Blood 91: 3601–6

73. Hersh JK, Hom EG, Brecher ME et al 1998 Mathematical modeling of platelet survival with implications for optimal transfusion practice in the chronically platelet transfusion-dependent patient. Transfusion 38: 637–644

74. Klumpp TR, Herman JH, Gaughan JP et al 1999 Clinical consequences of alterations in platelet transfusion dose: a prospective, randomized, double-blind trial. Transfusion 37: 674–681

75. Harker LA, Slichter SJ 1972 The bleeding time as a screening test for evaluation of platelet function. New England Journal of Medicine 287: 155

76. Bishop JF, Schiffer CA, Aisner J, Matthews JP, Wiernik PH et al 1987 Surgery in acute leukemia: a review of 167 operations in thrombocytopenic patients. American Journal of Hematology 26: 147

77. Howard SC, Gajjar A, Ribeiro RC et al 2000 Safety of lumbar puncture for children with acute lymphoblastic leukemia and thrombocytopenia. Journal of the American Medical Association 284: 2222–2224

78. Freireich EJ, Kliman A, Gaydos LA et al 1963 Response to repeated platelet transfusion from the same donor. Annals of Internal Medicine 50: 277

79. Daly PA, Schiffer CA, Aisner J, Wiernik PH 1980 Platelet transfusion therapy: one-hour posttransfusion increments are valuable in predicting the need for HLA-matched preparations. Journal of the American Medical Association 243: 435

80. Bishop JF, McGrath K, Wolf MM et al 1988 Clinical factors influencing the efficacy of pooled platelet transfusions. Blood 71: 383

81. Class FHJ, Smeenk RJT, Schmidt R et al 1981 Alloimmunization against the MHC antigens after platelet transfusions is due to contaminating leukocytes in the platelet suspension. Experimental Hematology 9: 84

82. Deeg HJ 1989 Transfusions with a tan: prevention of allosensitization by ultraviolet irradiation. Transfusion 29: 450

83. Lee EJ, Schiffer CA 1989 ABO compatibility can influence the results of platelet transfusion: results of a randomized trial. Transfusion 29: 384

84. Heal JM, Blumberg N, Masel D et al An evaluation of crossmatching, HLA, and ABO matching for platelet transfusions to refractory patients. Blood 70: 23

85. Murphy S 1988 ABO blood groups and platelet transfusion. Transfusion 28: 401

86. Lazarus HM, Herzig RH, Warm SE, Fishman DJ et al 1982 Transfusion experience with platelet concentrates stored for 24 to 72 hours at 22°C. Transfusion 22: 39

87. Duquesnoy RJ, Filip DJ, Rodey GE et al 1977 Successful transfusion of platelets 'mismatched' for HLA antigens to alloimmunized thrombocytopenic patients. American Journal of Hematology 2: 219

88. Duquesnoy RJ, Vieira J, Aster RH et al 1977 Donor availability for platelet transfusion support of alloimmunized thrombocytopenic patients. Transplantation Proceedings 9: 519

89. Yankee RA, Grumet FC, Rogentine GN et al 1969 Platelet transfusion therapy: the selection of compatible platelet donors for refractory patients by lymphocyte HLA typing. New England Journal of Medicine 281: 1208

90. Moroff G, Garratty G, Heal JM et al 1992 Selection of platelets for refractory patients by HLA matching and prospective crossmatching. Transfusion 32: 633

91. Heal JM, Blumberg N, Masel D 1987 An evaluation of crossmatching, HLA, and ABO matching for platelet transfusions to refractory patients. Blood 70: 23

92. Bodey GP, Buckley M, Sath YS, Freireich EJ 1966 Quantitative relationships between circulating leukocytes and infection in patients with acute leukemia. Annals of internal medicine 64: 328

93. Gurwith MJ, Brunton JL, Lank BA et al 1978 Granulocytopenia in hospitalized patients. I. Prognostic factors and etiology of fever. American Journal of Medicine 61: 121

94. Graw RH Jr, Herzig G, Perry S, Henderson ES 1972 Normal granulocyte transfusion therapy. Treatment of septicemia due to gram-negative bacteria. New England Journal of Medicine 287: 367

95. Herzig GP, Graw RG Jr 1975 Granulocyte transfusions for bacterial infections. In: Brown EB (ed), Progress in hematology, vol 9. Grune & Stratton, New York 207

96. Alavi JB, Roat RK, Djerassi I et al 1977 A randomized clinical trial of granulocyte transfusions for infection of acute leukemia. New England Journal of Medicine 296: 706

97. Strauss RG, Connett JE, Gale RP et al 1981 A controlled trial of prophylactic granulocyte transfusion during initial induction. New England Journal of Medicine 305: 597

98. Ruthe RC, Ansersen BR, Cunningham BL, Epstein RB 1978 Efficacy of granulocyte transfusions in the control of systemic candidiasis in leukopenic host. Blood 52: 493

99. Raubitschek AA, Levin AS, Stites DP et al 1973 Normal granulocyte infusion therapy for aspergillosis in chronic granulomatous disease. Pediatrics 51: 230

100. Bhatia S, McCullough JJ, Perry EH et al 1994 Granulocyte transfusions: efficacy in fungal infections in neutropenic patients following bone marrow transplantation. Transfusion 34: 226–232

101. Walsh JH, Purcell RH, Morrow AG et al 1970 Post-transfusion hepatitis after open-heart operations: incidence after administration of blood from commercial and volunteer donor populations. Journal of the American Medical Association 211: 261

102. Evatt B, Gompaerts E, McDougal J, Ramsey R 1985 Coincidental appearance of LAV/HTLV antibodies in hemophiliacs and the onset of the AIDS epidemic. New England Journal of Medicine 312: 483

103. Prince AM, Horowitz B, Brotman B 1986 Sterilization of hepatitis and HTLV-III viruses by exposure to try (n-butyl) phosphate and sodium cholate. Lancet 1: 706

104. Aronson, DL 1990 The development of the technology and capacity for the production of factor VIII for the treatment of hemophilia A. Transfusion 30: 748

105. Yaeger AS, Grumet FC, Hafleigh EB et al 1981 Prevention of transfusion-acquired cytomegalovirus infections in newborn infants. Journal of pediatrics 98: 281

106. Stagno S, Pass RF, Dworsky ME et al 1982 Congenital cytomegalovirus infection: the relative importance of primary and recurrent maternal infection. New England Journal of Medicine 306: 945

107. Miller W, Flynn P, McCullough J et al 1986 Cytomegalovirus infection after bone marrow transplantation: an association with acute graft-vs-host disease. Blood 67: 1162

108. Bowden RA, Sayers M, Flournoy N et al 1986 Cytomegalovirus immune globulin and seronegative blood products prevent primary cytomegalovirus infection after marrow transplantation. New England Journal of Medicine 314: 1006

109. Miller WJ, McCullough J, Balfour HH et al 1991 Prevention of CMV infection following bone marrow transplantation: a randomized trial of blood product screening. Bone Marrow Transplant 7 : 227–234

110. Leitman SF, Holland PV 1985 Irradiation of blood products: indications and guidelines. Transfusion 25: 293

111. Button LN, DeWolf WC, Newburger PE et al 1981 The effects of irradiation on blood components. Transfusion 21: 419

112. Strauss RG 1990 Routinely washing irradiated red cells before transfusion seems unwarranted. Transfusion 30: 675–677

113. Thaler M, Shamiss A, Orgad S et al 1989 The role of blood from HLA-homozygous donors in fatal transfusion-associated graft-versus-host disease after open-heart surgery. New England Journal of Medicine 321: 25

114. Arsura EL, Bertelle A, Minkowitz S et al 1988 Transfusion-associated graft-versus-host disease in a presumed immunocompetent patient. Archives in Internal Medicine 148: 1941

115. Otsuka S, Kunieda K, Hirose M et al 1989 Fatal erythroderma (suspected graft-versus-host disease) after cholecystectomy. Transfusion 29: 544

116. Propper RD, Button LN, Nathan DG 1980 New approaches to the transfusion management of thalassemia. Blood 55: 55

117. Bracey AW, Klein HG, Chambers S, Corash L 1983 *Ex vivo* selective isolation of young red blood cells using the IBM-2991 cell washer. Blood 61: 1068

118. Gibble JW, Ness PM. Fibrin glue 1990 the perfect operative sealant? Transfusion

119. Collins JA 1974 Problems associated with the massive transfusion of stored blood. Surgery 75: 274

120. Bick RL 1980 Hemostasis defects associated with cardiac surgery, prosthetic devices, and other extracorporeal circuits. Seminars in Thrombosis and Hemostasis 11: 249

121. McCullough J 1999 Principles of transfusion support before and after hematopoietic cell transplantation. In: Thomas ED, Blume KG, Forman SJ (eds), Hematopoetic cell transplantation. Blackwell Science, Massachusetts 685–703

122. Sacher RA, Luban NLC, Strauss RG 1989 Current practice and guidelines for the transfusion of cellular blood components in the newborn. Transfusion Medicine Reviews 3: 39

123. Schwartz SI, Bernard RP, Adams JT, Bauman AW 1970 Splenectomy for hematologic disorders. Archives in Surgery 101: 338
124. Aster RH, Jandl JH 1964 Platelet sequestration in man. II. Immunological and clinical studies. Journal of Clinical Investigation 43: 856
125. McFarland JG, Frenzke M, Aster RH 1989 Testing of maternal sera in pregnancies at risk for neonatal alloimmune thrombocytopenia. Transfusion 29: 128
126. Lalezari P 1984 Alloimmune neonatal neutropenia. In: Engelfriet CP, von Loghem JJ, von dem Borne AEGKr (eds), Immunohematology. Elsevier Science, Amsterdam 178
127. Linden JV, Paul B, Dressler KP 1992 A report of 104 transfusion errors in New York State. Transfusion 32: 601–606
128. Iserson KV, Huestis DW 1991 Blood warming: current applications and techniques. Transfusion 31: 558–571
129. Mercuriali F, Inghilleri G, Colotti MT et al 1996 Bedside transfusion errors: analysis of 2 years' use of a system to monitor and prevent transfusion errors. Vox Sanguinus 70: 16–20
130. Sazama K 1997 Practical issues in informed consent for transfusion. American Journal of Clinical Pathology 107: S72–S74
131. Ryden SE, Oberman HA 1975 Compatibility of common intravenous solutions with CPD blood. Transfusion 15: 250
132. Walker RH 1987 Special report: transfusion risks. American Journal of Clinical Pathology 88: 374
133. Sazama K 1990 355 reports of transfusion-associated deaths. Transfusion 30: 583
134. Davenport RD, Strieter RM, Kunkel SL 1991 Red cell ABO incompatibility and production of tumour necrosis factor-alpha. British Journal of Haematology 78: 540–544
135. Davenport RD, Burdick MD, Strieter RM, Kunkel SL 1994 *In vitro* production of interleukin-1 receptor antagonist in IgG-mediated red cell incompatibility. Transfusion 34: 297–303
136. Pineda AA, Brzica SM, Taswell HF 1978 Hemolytic transfusion reaction: recent experience in a large blood bank. Mayo Clinic Proceedings 53: 378
137. Honing CL, Bove JR 1980 Transfusion-associated fatalities: review of burea of biologics reports, 1976–1978. Transfusion 20: 653
138. Perkins HA, Payne R, Ferguson J et al 1966 Nonhemolytic febrile transfusion reactions: quantitative effects of blood components with emphasis on isoantigenic incompatibility of leukocytes. Vox Sanguinus 11: 578
139. Heddle NM, O'Hoski P, Singer J et al 1992 A prospective study to determine the safety of omitting the antiglobulin crossmatch from pretransfusion testing. British Journal of Haematology 81: 579–584
140. Popovsky MA, Davenport RD 2001 Transfusion-related acute lung injury: femme fatale? Transfusion 41: 312–315 (editorial)
141. Popovsky MA, Chaplin HC, Moore SB 1992 Transfusion-related acute lung injury: a neglected, serious complication of hemotherapy. Transfusion 32: 589
142. Vyas GN, Holmdahl L, Perkins HA, Fundenberg HH 1969 Serologic specificity of human anti-IgA and its significance in transfusion. Blood 34: 573
143. Alter HJ, Holland PV, Purcell RH et al 1972 Posttransfusion hepatitis after exclusion of commercial and hepatitis-B antigen-positive donors. Annals in Internal Medicine 77: 691
144. Bove JR. Transfusion-associated hepatitis and AIDS: What is the risk? New England Journal of Medicine 1987; 317: 242
145. Dodd RY 1992 The risk of transfusion-transmitted infection. New England Journal of Medicine 327: 419
146. Kleinman S, Alter H, Busch M et al 1992 Increased detection of hepatitis C virus (HCV)-infected blood donors by a multiple-antigen HCV enzyme immunoassay. Transfusion 32: 805
147. Williams AE, Thomson RA, Schreiber GB et al 1997 Estimates of infectious disease risk factors in US blood donors. Journal of the American Medical Association 277: 967–72
148. Sloand EM, Pitt E, Klein HG 1995 Safety of the blood supply. JAMA 274: 1368–73
149. Lackritz EM, Satten GA, Aberle-Grasse J et al 1995 Estimated risk of transmission of the human immunodeficiency virus by screened blood in the United States. New England Journal of Medicine 333: 1721–25
150. Schreiber GB, Busch MP, Kleinman SH 1996 The risk of transfusion-transmitted viral infections. New England Journal of Medicine 334: 1685–90
151. Hollinger FB, Khan NC, Oefinger PA et al 1983 Posttransfusion hepatitis type A. Journal of the American Medical Association 250: 2313
152. Noble RC, Kane MA, Reeves SA, Roeckel I 1984 Posttransfusion hepatitis A in a neonatal intensive care unit. Journal of the American Medical Association 252: 2711
153. Aach RD, Szmuness W, Mosley JW 1981 Serum alanine aminotransferase of donors in relation to the risk of non-A, non-B hepatitis in recipients. New England Journal of Medicine 304: 989
154. Stevens CE, Aach RD, Hollinger FB 1984 Hepatitis B virus antibody in blood donors and the occurence of non-A, non-B hepatitis in transfusion recipients: an analysis of the transfusion-transmitted viruses study. Annals of Internal Medicine 101: 733
155. Koziol DE, Holland PV, Alling DW et al 1986 Antibody to hepatitis B core antigen as a paradoxial marker for non-A, non-B hepatitis agents in donated blood. Annals of Internal Medicine 104: 488
156. Alter HJ, Purcell RH, Holland PV et al 1981 Donor transaminase and recipient hepatitis: impact on blood transfusion services. Journal of the American Medical Association JAMA 246: 630
157. Blajchman MA, Bull SB, Feinman SV 1995 Post-transfusion hepatitis: impact of non-A, non-B hepatitis surrogate tests. Lancet 345: 21–25
158. Choo QL, Kuo G, Weiner AJ et al 1989 Isolation of a cDNA derived from a blood-borne non-A, non-B viral hepatitis genome. Science 244: 359
159. Alter HJ, Purcell RH, Shih JW et al 1989 Detection of antibody to hepatitis C virus in prospectively followed transfusion recipients with acute and chronic non-A, non-B hepatitis. New England Journal of Medicine 321: 1494
160. MacDonald KL, Jackson JB, Bowman RJ et al 1989 Performance characteristics of serologic tests for human immunodeficiency virus type I (HIV-1) antibody among Minnesota blood donors. Annals of Internal Medicine 110: 617
161. Cohen ND, Munoz A, Reitz BA et al 1989 Transmission of retroviruses by transfusion of screened blood in patients undergoing cardiac surgery. New England Journal of Medicine 320: 1172
162. Busch M, Garratty G 1997 Applications of molecular biology to blood transfusion medicine. American Association of Blood Banks; Bethesda, MD, 123–176
163. Busch MP, Taylor PE, Lenes BA et al 1990 Screening of selected male blood donors for p24 antigen of human immunodeficiency type 1. Transfusion Safety Study Group. New England Journal of Medicine 323: 1308–1312
164. Alter HJ, Epstein JS, Swenson SG et al 1990 Prevalence of human immunodeficiency virus type 1 p24 antigen in US blood donors – an assessment of the efficacy of testing in donor screening. HIV-antigen study group. New England Journal of Medicine 323: 1312–1317
165. Busch MP, Kleinman SH, Stramer SL 2000 In: Molecular biology in blood transfusion Smit Sibinga CTh, Klein HG, (eds), Nucleic acid amplification testing of blood donations. Kluwer Academic, Dordrecht 81–103
166. Report of the Interorganizational Task Force on Nucleic Acid Amplification Testing of Blood Donors 2000 Nucleic acid amplification testing of blood donors for transfusion-transmitted infectious disease. Transfusion 40: 143–159
167. Greenwalt TJ, Rios JA 2001 To test or not to test for syphilis: a global problem. Transfusion 41: 976
168. Turner TB, Diseker TH 1941 Duration of infectivity of *Treponema pallidum* in citrated blood stored under conditions obtaining in blood banks. Bulletin of Johns Hopkins Hospital 68: 269
169. Okochi K, Sato H 1985 Adult T-cell leukemia virus, blood donors and transfusion: experience in Japan. Progress in Clinical and Biological Research 182: 245
170. Grant IH, Gold JWM, Wittner M et al 1989 Transfusion-associated acute Chagas disease acquired in the United States. Annals of Internal Medicine 111: 849–851
171. Galel S, Kirchhoff LV 1996 Risk factors for *Trypanosoma cruzi* infection in California blood donors. Transfusion 36: 227–231
172. Smith RP, Evans AT, Popovsky M et al 1986 Transfusion-acquired babesiosis and failure of antibiotic treatment Journal of the American Medical Association 256: 2726
173. Badon SJ, Fister RD, Cable RG 1989 Survival of *Borrelia burgdorferi* in blood products. Transfusion 29: 581
174. Mortimer PP, Luban NL, Kelleher JF, Cohen BJ 1983 Transmission of serum parvovirus-like agent by clotting factor concentrates. Lancet 2: 482
175. Koenigbauer UF, Eastlund T, Day JW 2000 Clinical illness due to parvovirus B19 infection after infusion of solvent/detergent-treated pooled plasma. Transfusion 40: 1203–1206

176. Eschbach JW, Abdulhadi MH, Browne JK et al 1989 Recombinant human erythropoietin in anemic patients with end-stage renal disease: results of a phase III multicenter clinical trial. Annals in Internal Medicine 1989; 111: 992–1000

177. Evans R, Rader B, Manninen D 1990 Cooperative multicenter EPO clinical trial group: the quality of life of hemodialysis recipients treated with recombinant human erythropoietin. Journal of the American Medical Association 263: 825–830

178. Spivak JL 1994 Recombinant human erythropoietin and the anemia of cancer. Blood 84: 997–1004

179. Pincus T, Olsen NJ, Russell IJ et al 1990 Multicenter study of recombinant human erythropoietin in correction of anemia in rheumatoid arthritis. American Journal of Medicine 89: 161–168

180. Schreiber S, Howaldt S, Schnoor M et al 1996 Recombinant erythropoietin for the treatment of anemia in inflammatory bowel disease. New England Journal of Medicine 334: 619–623

181. Henry D, Beall G, Benson C et al 1992 Recombinant human erythropoietin in the treatment of anemia associated with human immunodificiency virus (HIV) infection and zidovudine therapy: overview of four clinical trials. Annals in Internal Medicine 117: 739–748

182. Strauss RG 1995 Erythropoietin in the pathogenesis and treatment of neonatal anemia. Transfusion 35: 68–73

183. Fullerton DA, Campbell DN, Whitman GJ 1991 Use of human recombinant erythropoietin to correct severe preoperative anemia. Annals in Thoracic Surgery 51: 825–826

184. Tremper KK, Friedman AE, Levine EM 1982 The preoperative treatment of severely anemia patients with a perfluorochemical oxygen-transport fluid, fluosol-DA. New England Journal of Medicine 307: 277

185. Gould SA, Rosen AL, Sehgal R et al 1986 Fluosol-DA as a red cell substitute in acute anemia. New England Journal of Medicine 314: 1653

186. Stowell CP, Levin J, Spiess BD, Windlow RM 2001 Progress in the development of RBC substitutes. Transfusion 41: 287–299

Histocompatibility: HLA and other systems

32

PE Posch   RJ Hartzman   CK Hurley

Introduction

The human major histocompatibility complex

History

Genomic organization

The human leukocyte antigens

Genomic organization

Diversity

Expression

Structure of class I and class II molecules

Function
Peptide processing and binding
T-lymphocyte recognition of HLA molecules
Allorecognition and transplantation

Non-classical MHC class I molecules
HLA-E
HLA-F
HLA-G

Other potential histocompatibility molecules

MHC class I chain-related molecules (MIC)

CD1 molecules

Minor histocompatibility antigens

Other immune system receptors that recognize histocompatibility molecules as their ligands

Killer-cell inhibitory receptors

CD94/NKG2

Immunoglobulin-like transcripts

Techniques for the identification of HLA polymorphism

Serologic detection of class I and class II molecules

Cellular detection of HLA disparity

DNA-based identification of class I and class II alleles
Sequence-specific priming (SSP)
Sequence-specific oligonucleotide probe hybridization (SSOPH)
Gel-mobility assays of DNA strands
Nucleic acid sequence-based typing (SBT)

Measurement of sensitization to histocompatibility differences

HLA assignments

Serologic specificities

Cellular specificities

DNA-based allele designations

National Marrow Donor Program (NMDP) DNA nomenclature

Limitations in the assignment of HLA alleles

Correlation between serologic specificities and DNA-based allele assignments

Identification of HLA in clinical situations

Autoimmunity

Identity

Cell, tissue and organ transplantation
Solid organ transplantation
Platelets
HSC transplantation

Summary

Introduction

The classical human leukocyte antigens (HLA-A, HLA-B, HLA-C, HLA-DR, HLA-DQ and HLA-DP) are an integral part of the maintenance of self integrity and of the specific immune response to microbial pathogens and malignancies. Encoded within the human major histocompatibility complex, the HLA molecules display extensive variability (polymorphism) among their gene and protein sequences. HLA polymorphism is important to survival of the species, threatened with a large number of diverse pathogens with the potential to rapidly mutate to avoid the immune response.

The same diversity of HLA molecules that helps preserve the human species from pathogens impedes successful transplantation of tissues from one individual to another, especially transplantation of hematopoietic stem cells (HSC). Theoretically, HSC transplantation requires that the donor and recipient be identical (matched) for all classical HLA molecules in order to avoid immune recognition. Any disparity might cause graft rejection, where the donor's cells are destroyed by the recipient's immune system, or graft-versus-host disease (GVHD), where the donor's cells recognize the recipient's tissues as foreign and react to them. However, even in cases where the donor and recipient are HLA matched, GVHD can occur. Thus, despite the progress made in our understanding of histocompatibility, it is evident that there are histocompatibility antigens which likely have a role in maintaining self integrity and in transplant outcome, in addition to the classical HLA molecules. We are now beginning to broaden our knowledge of what constitutes a histocompatibility antigen and of the immune system receptors that recognize these molecules.

The human major histocompatibility complex

History

What has become known as the major histocompatibility complex (MHC) was initially identified in the early 1900s, but it was not until the late 1930s that studies began to focus on graft acceptance (histocompatibility) and antigen response phenotypes (H-2) in different stains of mice.[1,2] In the 1950s, Dausset detected the first histocompatibility antigens in humans, the MHC class I antigens, with antibodies from multiply transfused patients.[3,4] These antibodies revealed in the human population differing patterns of binding to white blood cells (leukocytes) and each pattern of binding came to define a human leukocyte antigen (HLA) specificity.[5,6] These HLA specificities were later determined to be encoded by three distinct polymorphic loci, HLA-A, HLA-B and HLA-C. The human MHC class II antigens were initially described via their ability to stimulate the proliferation of T-cells from one individual when mixed with lymphocytes from a second individual.[7] Each pattern of T-cell reactivity (allorecognition) to a panel of homozygous typing cells (HTC) was assigned an HLA-D phenotype.[8] It is now known that the HLA-D phenotypes are due to T-cell allorecognition of the products of the MHC class II loci, primarily HLA-DR. HLA-DQ and HLA-DP make minor contributions to these phenotypes. The genes specifying both class I and class II antigens are tightly clustered in a single chromosomal region, the MHC.

Genomic organization

The human MHC is a genetic region located on the short arm of chromosome 6 (6p21.3) extending approximately 4 megabases (Mb) (Fig. 32.1). The MHC was assigned to chromosome 6 based on cytogenetic studies of aberrant chromosomes. Family segregation analysis of recombination between the genes in the MHC and genomic DNA sequencing of large DNA fragments have produced an exquisite genetic map of this region. The MHC encodes over 225 genes and pseudogenes of which at least 148 are expressed as proteins.[9,10] This genetic complex is divided into three regions: (centromere) class II, class III and class I (telomere). Although the proteins encoded within the MHC participate in a variety of functions, approximately 40% are devoted to immune system functions.

The class II region (~1.2 Mb) contains at least 34 expressed genes and 16 pseudogenes and spans from SynGAP (Ras-GTPase-activating protein, centromeric) to TSBP (testis-specific basic protein, telomeric).[11] This region includes the genes that encode for the classical class II molecules (HLA-DR, -DQ and -DP). In addition, gene products involved in MHC class I antigen processing (LMP2 and LMP7, the large multifunctional proteosome genes), peptide transport (TAP1 and TAP2, the transporter associated with antigen-processing genes) and complex assembly (tapasin) and gene products involved in MHC class II complex assembly (HLA-DM and HLA-DO) are encoded in this region (see section on Peptide Processing and Binding).

The class III region (~1 Mb) extends from NOTCH4 (transmembrane receptor involved in cell differentiation, centromeric) to BAT1 (RNA helicase, telomeric).[9,10] This

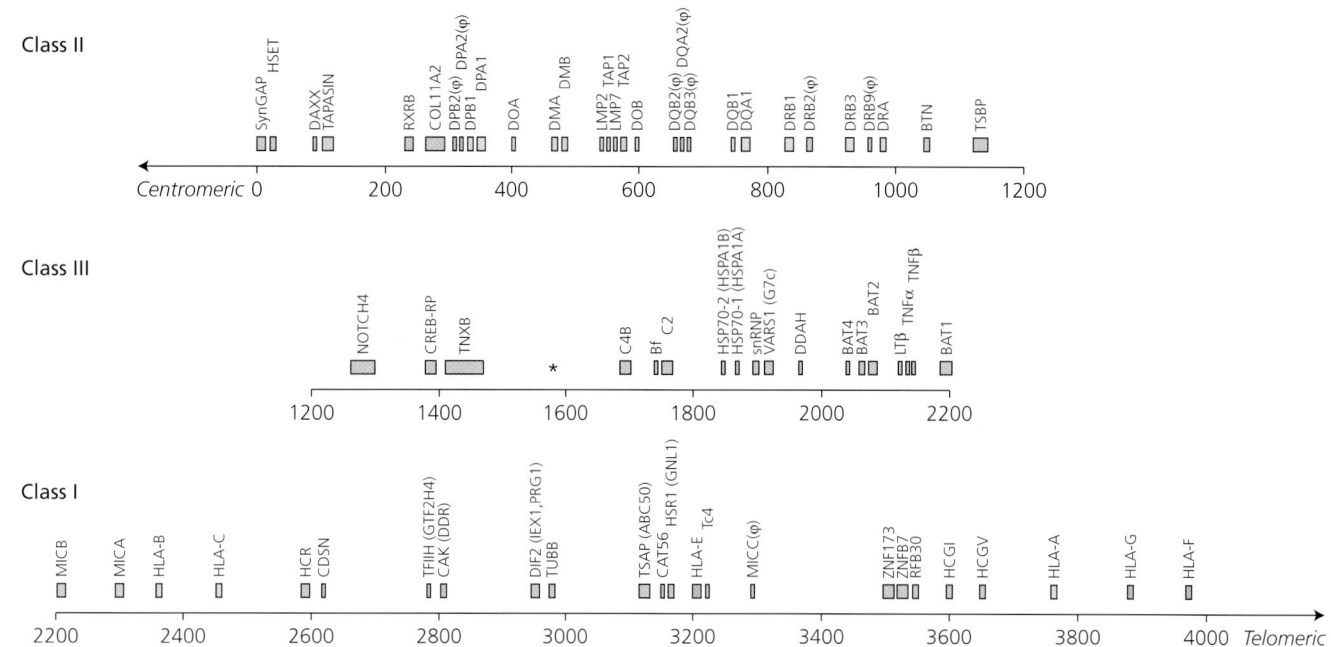

Fig. 32.1 Map of the human major histocompatibility complex (MHC) located on the short arm of chromosome 6. The map (drawn closely to scale) is divided into the three regions (class II, class III and class I) and shows the relative positions of various MHC-encoded genes and pseudogenes (Ψ). Not all MHC-encoded genes and pseudogenes are shown. The class II region contains the genes encoding the expressed classical HLA class II molecules (yellow). The number of HLA-DRB (DRB) genes and pseudogenes present differs for different haplotypes (DR52 haplotype group shown; see Fig. 32.3). Genes encoding protein products intimately involved in MHC class I and class II molecule assembly and in peptide processing and binding (green) also are found in the class II region. The class III region contains several immune system relevant genes and varies in length among individual chromosomes due to duplications in the area encoding C4B (asterisk). The class I region contains the genes encoding the classical HLA class I heavy chain polypeptides (yellow). This region also encodes the expressed non-classical HLA class I genes (red) and MHC class I chain-related genes (blue). The figure was generated from data contained in References 9–12.

region encodes at least 57 expressed genes including complement components (e.g. C2 and C4B), heat shock proteins (e.g. Hsp70-1 and Hsp70-2) and cytokines of the tumor necrosis factor family (e.g. TNFα and TNFβ). Some individuals have duplications in the area encoding C4B. Thus, this area varies in length and may contain many pseudogenes.

The class I region (~1.8 Mb) from MICB (centromeric) to HLA-F (telomeric) encodes at least 118 genes; 57 expressed genes and 61 pseudogenes.[12] This region includes the classical class I genes (HLA-A, -B and -C) and the non-classical class I genes (HLA-E, -F and -G). This region also encodes the MHC class I chain-related (MIC) genes (MICA and MICB) and genes that encode proteins which regulate gene transcription (transcription factors) such as zinc finger DNA binding proteins (e.g. ZNF173 and ZNFB7) and the p52 subunit of transcription factor IIH (TFIIH). The focus of this chapter is on the MHC-encoded gene products involved in histocompatibility, primarily the classical human leukocyte antigens. Other MHC and non-MHC encoded genes that participate in histocompatibility are also covered.

The human leukocyte antigens

The classical human leukocyte antigens (HLA molecules) include the MHC class I molecules (HLA-A, -B and -C) and the MHC class II molecules (HLA-DR, -DQ and -DP). The primary function of the classical class I and class II molecules is to bind small fragments of proteins (peptides) and present them on the surface of cells for immune system surveillance. The principal player in recognition of these HLA molecule + peptide complexes is the T-cell receptor (TCR) expressed by T-lymphocytes (T-cells). Recognition of these complexes by specific T-cells can lead to a plethora of immunologic outcomes including inflammation, antibody production and cellular cytotoxicity. At least two of the non-classical class I molecules perform functions similar to the classical class I molecules, but are more specialized antigen presentation molecules. The following sections discuss the genetics and structures of the classical HLA molecules, their function with respect to recognition by TCR and their identification, nomenclature and importance in HSC transplantation. Also included are brief sections on the non-classical

MHC class I molecules, additional MHC and non-MHC encoded histocompatibility antigens and on the receptors, other than the TCR, that recognize histocompatibility molecules as ligands.

Genomic organization

The heavy chains of the classical MHC class I (class Ia) molecules are encoded in the class I region of the MHC. The class I heavy chain associates with beta 2 microglobulin (encoded on chromosome 15; see section on Structure) to form the mature class I molecule. The gene order within the MHC is shown in Figure 32.1. Each of the classical MHC class I heavy chains is encoded by a single gene that is divided into eight exons (Fig. 32.2(a)).[13] Exon 1 encodes the 5' untranslated region (UTR) and the hydrophobic leader sequence. The leader sequence directs insertion of the protein into the membrane of the cell and is cleaved from the mature protein. The extracellular portion of the class I heavy chain is encoded by exons 2–4. Exon 5 encodes the transmembrane region and exons 6

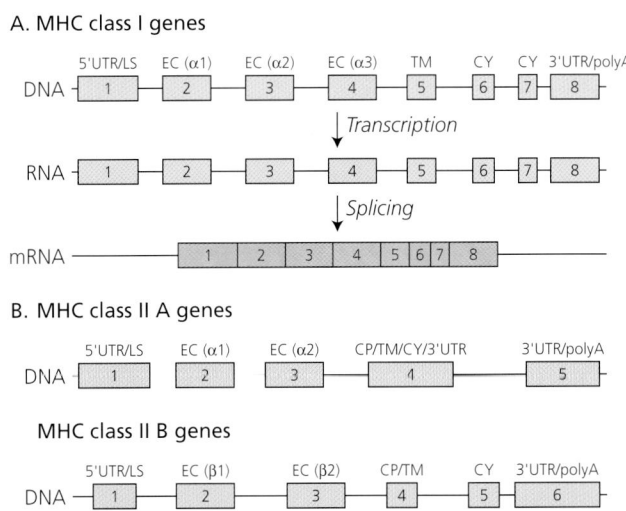

Fig. 32.2 Exon–intron organization of the classical HLA genes. (A) The classical MHC class I heavy chain gene organization with exons denoted by numbered blocks. Exon 1 encodes the 5' untranslated region (UTR) and leader sequence (LS). Exons 2–4 encode the extracellular domains (EC), α1–α3, respectively. Exon 5 encodes the transmembrane region (TM) and exons 6 and 7 encode the cytoplasmic tail (CY). Exon 8 encodes the 3'UTR and polyadenylation signal (polyA). Both exons and introns are transcribed into RNA. The RNA is processed by splicing to remove introns yielding mRNA which is translated into the HLA class I heavy chain polypeptide. (B) MHC class II A and B gene organization with exons denoted as numbered blocks. Unlike the class I heavy chain genes, the extracellular domains of each gene are followed by a connecting peptide (CP) encoded as part of exon 4. Both class II A and B genes are transcribed and processed similarly to the class I heavy chain genes. The map only depicts relative gene organization and the exon and intron sizes are not drawn to scale.

and 7 encode the intracellular cytoplasmic tail. The 3' UTR and the polyadenylation [poly(A)] site are encoded by exon 8. The mRNA, which is translated into protein, includes all eight exons after removal by splicing of the intervening sequences (introns) from the class I RNA.

The class II region of the MHC contains three sub-regions (centromere) HLA-DP, -DQ and -DR (telomere), each of which encodes at least one cell surface class II molecule (Fig. 32.1). The class II molecules are non-covalently associated heterodimers that consist of an α chain and a β chain.[13,14] Each chain is encoded by a separate gene, an A gene for the α chain and a B gene for the β chain. The expressed HLA-DP heterodimer is encoded by the DPA1 and DPB1 genes. The HLA-DP sub-region contains two DP pseudogenes, DPA2 and DPB2. The HLA-DQ subregion contains two A (DQA1 and DQA2) and three B (DQB1, DQB2 and DQB3) genes. The expressed HLA-DQ heterodimer is encoded by the DQA1 and DQB1 genes, while the remaining DQ genes are pseudogenes. Each individual has two copies of chromosome 6 and, thus, two copies of each of the expressed HLA-DP and HLA-DQ genes. These genes are polymorphic (see section on Diversity) and, consequently, an individual can have two different expressed A genes and two different expressed B genes for HLA-DP and for HLA-DQ. While not all combinations form,[15] the products of some of these genes can associate in several αβ combinations, regardless of chromosomal origin. Therefore, an individual could express up to four different HLA-DP and up to four different HLA-DQ molecules.

The HLA-DR subregion is more complex.[16] A HLA-DR molecule composed of a conserved α chain encoded by the DRA gene and a polymorphic β chain encoded by the DRB1 gene is almost always present. This is the major class II molecule expressed on the cell surface. An additional eight DRB genes and pseudogenes have been identified in the HLA-DR subregion. The number of DRB genes present and the number of expressed DRB gene products is characteristic of each chromosome (haplotype) a person inherits (Fig. 32.3). For example, the DR1 haplotype carries two DRB genes, the expressed DRB1 gene and a DRB6 pseudogene. The DR8 haplotype carries only one DRB gene, the expressed DRB1 gene. Other DR subregion haplotypes can encode a second expressed HLA-DR molecule composed of the DRA gene product associated with a DRB3 gene product (DR52 molecule), a DRB4 gene product (DR53 molecule) or a DRB5 gene product (DR51 molecule) and can contain one to three DRB pseudogenes encoded by the DRB2, DRB6, DRB7, DRB8 or DRB9 genes. The designations DR51, DR52 and DR53 are antibody (serologically) defined (see section on HLA Assignments).

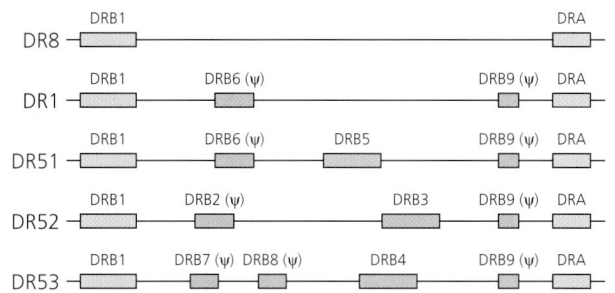

Fig. 32.3 Relative gene organization of DR subregion of different DR haplotype groups. The protein products of the DRA and DRB1 genes (yellow) combine to form the primary expressed HLA-DR molecule. The protein products of the expressed DRB5 (green), DRB3 (blue) and DRB4 (red) genes encoded by the DR51, DR52 and DR53 haplotype groups, respectively, also are expressed on the surface of cells in combination with the DRA polypeptide to form functional DR molecules. The DRB pseudogenes (Ψ) encoded by each haplotype group are shown in gray. Table 32.4 lists the alleles associated with each haplotype.

Table 32.1 HLA class I alleles[a,b]

HLA-A	HLA-B	HLA-C
A*0101-*0104N	B*07021-*0713	Cw*0102-*0103[c]
A*02011-*0230	B*0801-*0806	Cw*02021-*0203
A*03011-*0304	B*1301-*1304	Cw*0302-*0309
A*1101-*1105	B*1401-*1405	Cw*04011-*0406
A*2301	B*1501101-*1549	Cw*0501-*0502
A*2402101-*2420	B*1801-*1807	Cw*0602-*0604
A*2501-*2502	B*2701-*2715	Cw*0701-*0712
A*2601-*2612	B*3501-*3527	Cw*0801-*0806
A*2901-*2904	B*3701-*3702	Cw*12021-*1206
A*3001-*3007	B*3801-*3803	Cw*1301
A*31012-*3104	B*39011-*3916	Cw*14021-*1404
A*3201-*3203	B*40011-*4020	Cw*1502-*1508
A*3301-*3304	B*4101-*4103	Cw*1601-*16041
A*3401-*3402	B*4201-*4202	Cw*1701-*1702
A*3601	B*4402-*4411	Cw*1801-*1802
A*4301	B*4501-*4502	
A*6601-*6603	B*4601	
A*68011-*6809	B*4701-*4703	
A*6901	B*4801-*4805	
A*7401-*7403	B*4901	
A*8001	B*5001-*5002	
	B*51011-*5116	
	B*52011-*52012	
	B*5301-*5303	
	B*5401	
	B*5501-*5508	
	B*5601-*5605	
	B*5701-*5705	
	B*5801-*5802	
	B*5901	
	B*67011-*67012	
	B*7301	
	B*7801-*7803	
	B*8101	
	B*8201	

[a] Reprinted with permission of Munksgaard and Anthony Nolan Research Institute.[17,18] It is likely that the number of HLA class I alleles will increase as more individuals are studied. Alleles are defined by DNA sequencing.

[b] Each column is independent. Each row lists the names of one to several alleles. For example, A*0101-A*0104N includes alleles, A*0101, A*0102, A*0103 and A*0104N. The number of alleles included depends on the number and characteristics of the alleles described. The names of alleles are discarded if the nucleotide sequences are found to be in error. B*0701 is one example of an allele which was deleted by the nomenclature committee so today, the alleles in this group include B*07021, *07022, 0703, 0704 etc. An expanded table has been published.[18]

[c] 'w' is added to avoid confusion with the complement genes.

The A genes, which encode the α chains of class II molecules, contain five exons (Fig. 32.2(B)).[13,14] The 5′UTR and hydrophobic leader sequence are encoded by exon 1, like the class I genes. Exons 2 and 3 encode the extracellular domains. Exon 4 encodes the connecting peptide, the transmembrane region, the intracellular cytoplasmic tail and a portion of the 3′ UTR. The remainder of the 3′ UTR and the poly(A) signal are encoded by exon 5. Each class II β chain is encoded by a B gene divided into 6 exons (Fig. 32.2(B)). Exons 1–3 are similar to that of the A genes. Exon 4 encodes the connecting peptide and transmembrane region, while exon 5 encodes the cytoplasmic tail. The 3′ UTR and poly(A) signal are encoded by exon 6. All exons and introns are transcribed into RNA for the class II A and B genes. Again, introns are removed by splicing to form the mRNA which is translated into protein.

Diversity

The nucleotide sequences of many of the HLA genes differ among individuals. These sequence variants are termed alleles; genes with many alleles are termed polymorphic. Alleles of a locus may differ by a single nucleotide to many nucleotides potentially resulting in changes in the amino acid sequence of the protein specified by that gene. The classical HLA class I and class II loci are the most polymorphic loci in humans. The HLA-B heavy chain and HLA-DRB1 loci have over 240 known alleles (Tables 32.1 and 32.2).[17,18] In contrast to non-HLA genes, the nucleotide differences found among HLA alleles are usually non-synonymous (alter the amino acid sequence) and are focused in the exon(s) encoding the most functionally important region of the HLA

molecule, the antigen binding site[16] (described under Structure). It is thought that this diversity has been maintained to provide the human population with the capacity to recognize a diverse repertoire of pathogenic peptides.[19,20] Unfortunately, the allelic differences in HLA molecules expressed on the cells of different individuals can be recognized as foreign when tissue is grafted from one individual to another.

Based on the characteristics of the HLA allelic differences, several mechanisms are hypothesized to have generated this HLA diversity over evolutionary time. The majority of the polymorphism is hypothesized to have

Table 32.2 HLA class II alleles[a,b]

DR	DQ	DP
DRA*0101-*0102[c]	DQA1*0101-0105[h]	DPA1*01031-*0106[j]
DRB1*0101-*0106[d]	DQA1*0201	DPA1*02011-*0203
DRB1*15011-*1508	DQA1*03011-*0303	DPA1*0301-*0302
DRB1*16011-*1608	DQA1*0401	DPA1*0401
DRB1*03011-*0313	DQA1*05011-*0505	DPB1*01011-*8101[k]
DRB1*04011-*0432	DQA1*06011-*06012	
DRB1*11011-*1135	DQB1*0501-*0504[i]	
DRB1*1201-*1206	DQB1*06011-*0615	
DRB1*1301-*1334	DQB1*0201-*0203	
DRB1*1401-*1433	DQB1*03011-*0309	
DRB1*0701-*0704	DQB1*0401-*0402	
DRB1*0801-*0821		
DRB1*09012		
DRB1*1001		
DRB3*01011-*0105[e]		
DRB3*0201-*0208		
DRB3*0301-*0303		
DRB4*0101101-*0105[f]		
DRB4*0201N		
DRB4*0301N		
DRB5*01011-*0110N[g]		
DRB5*0202-*0204		

[a] Reprinted with permission of Munksgaard and Anthony Nolan Research Institute.[17,18] It is likely that the number of HLA class II alleles will increase as more individuals are studied. Alleles are defined by DNA sequencing. A description of the nomenclature in this table can be found in Table 32.1.

[b] Each column is independent.

[c] Alleles of the DRA locus. The differences between these DR alpha chain alleles are not considered important for transplantation matching.

[d] Alleles of the DRB1 locus. Most haplotypes contain a DRB1 locus.

[e] Alleles of the DRB3 locus, the second expressed DR molecule in haplotypes carrying DRB1*03, *11, *12, *13, *14 alleles.

[f] Alleles of the DRB4 locus, the second expressed DR molecule in haplotypes carrying DRB1*04, *07, *09 alleles.

[g] Alleles of the DRB5 locus, the second expressed DR molecule in haplotypes carrying DRB1*15, *16 alleles.

[h] Alleles of the DQA1 locus. DQA1 allelic products pair with DQB1 allelic products to form the DQ molecule.

[i] Alleles of the DQB1 locus.

[j] Alleles of the DPA1 locus. DPA1 allelic products pair with DPB1 allelic products to form the DP molecule.

[k] Alleles of the DPB1 locus. The approach to naming of DPB1 alleles was slightly different than that used for other loci because of the lack of serologic information. Most DPB1 alleles have a unique number forming the first two digits of their name. There are at least 89 DPB1 alleles.

arisen by the non-reciprocal exchange of short polymorphic regions or cassettes among alleles, a process referred to as gene conversion. As a result, the HLA alleles are patchworks of polymorphic cassettes, each cassette shared by some of the other alleles at the locus, embedded in a conserved framework (Fig. 32.4). Exchange of cassettes among alleles at different loci, reciprocal recombination involving the exchange of entire exons, and mutation also have contributed to the HLA diversity.[16,21] The number of alleles identified at each locus varies from the over 240 at HLA-B and HLA-DRB1 to the approximately 25 alleles at HLA-DRB3 to the two alleles at HLA-DRA.

Each individual inherits two copies of the chromosome carrying the MHC, one from each parent, and thus has two copies of each gene in the MHC. Individuals who carry two identical alleles at a locus are homozygous; individuals with two different alleles at a locus are heterozygous. Because the HLA genes are located within a small genetic distance, they are usually inherited as a block unless separated by recombination. The block, a specific set of alleles at the multiple HLA loci inherited together from a parent, is termed a HLA haplotype. Figure 32.5 illustrates the inheritance of HLA-A, -B and -DRB1 alleles within a family. By convention, the paternal haplotypes are generally designated a and b and the maternal haplotypes, c and d. Thus, there are four possible MHC genotypes in the offspring: ac, ad, bc and bd. Because the chances of inheriting a given genotype are random, the probability of occurrence of any one of the four genotypes is one in four in a mating. In a family with five children, at least two of the children will be MHC identical unless recombination has occurred.

The alleles in the MHC complex can be reshuffled by crossing over between homologous chromosomes during the generation of sperm or eggs. The frequency of recombination across the MHC from HLA-A to HLA-DPB1 is 2–2.5%.[22,23] Studies in humans suggest that there are several sites at which recombination preferentially occurs within the MHC. The frequency of recombination between HLA-A and HLA-B is 0.7%, between HLA-B and HLA-DRB1 is 1.0%, and between DQB1 and DPB1 is 0.8%. Recombinations between DQA1 and DRB1 loci and between B and C loci are very rare.

The HLA alleles and haplotypes found in individuals depend on their ethnic backgrounds (e.g. References 24–27). For example, the alleles DRB1*0302 and DRB1*1117 are found in African Americans, but are only rarely observed in individuals of Northern European or Asian descent.[28] Likewise, the frequency of a combination of alleles on a single copy of chromosome 6 can differ among population groups. Table 32.3 lists the 10 most common haplotypes identified in several US populations found in the unrelated bone marrow volunteer donor registry maintained by the National Marrow Donor Program (NMDP).[26,29] For example, the most common haplotype in Asians is A33,B58,DR3 found at a frequency of 1.5859%. This haplotype was ranked 743rd in caucasoids, 350th in African Americans and 743rd in Latinos.

There are, however, some alleles and haplotypes that are found in many populations. For example, the alleles A*0201 and DRB1*1301 are common alleles in many US populations.[30,31] The most common haplotype in caucasoids, A1,B8,DR3, is the second most frequent haplotype in African Americans and the third most frequent

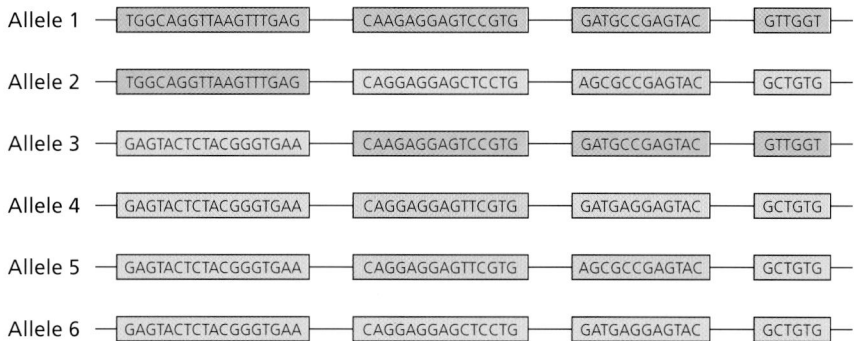

Fig. 32.4 Representation of a polymorphic exon of several HLA alleles. Each allele is a combination of conserved (solid line, nucleotides not shown) and polymorphic (colored blocks) nucleotide sequences. The polymorphic nucleotides form 'cassettes' which are shared among HLA alleles. The combination of cassettes within an HLA gene characterizes a specific allele. To identify the exact HLA alleles present in an individual, DNA-based typing must be able to identify these multiple cassettes and to link the cassettes to one another.

Table 32.3 Ten most common haplotypes in US registry[a,b]

	Caucasian	African American	Latino	Asian/Pacific Islander
1	A1,B8,DR3[c]	A30,B42,DR3	A2,B35,DR8	A33,B58,DR3
2	A3,B7,DR2	A1,B8,DR3	A29,B44,DR7	A33,B44,DR6
3	A2,B44,DR4	A3,B7,DR2	A1,B8,DR3	A24,B52,DR2
4	A2,B7,DR2	A2,B44,DR4	A2,B35,DR4	A2,B46,DR9
5	A29,B44,DR7	A33,B53,DR8	A3,B7,DR2	A33,B44,DR7
6	A2,B62,DR4	A2,B7,DR2	A28,B39,DR4	A30,B13,DR7
7	A3,B35,DR1	A28,B58,DR12	A2,B39,DR4	A24,B7,DR1
8	A1,B57,DR7	A2,B45,DR6	A24,B39,DR6	A33,B58,DR6
9	A2,B60,DR6	A30,B42,DR8	A33,B14,DR1	A11,B62,DR4
10	A2,B8,DR2	A34,B44,DR2	A24,B35,DR4	A1,B57,DR7

[a] Printed with permission of Lippincott, Williams and Wilkins.[26] An expanded list of haplotypes has been provided on a web site.[29]

[b] Only serologically defined HLA types were analyzed.

[c] Underline indicates a haplotype that is also found in the 10 most frequent haplotypes of another ethnic group.

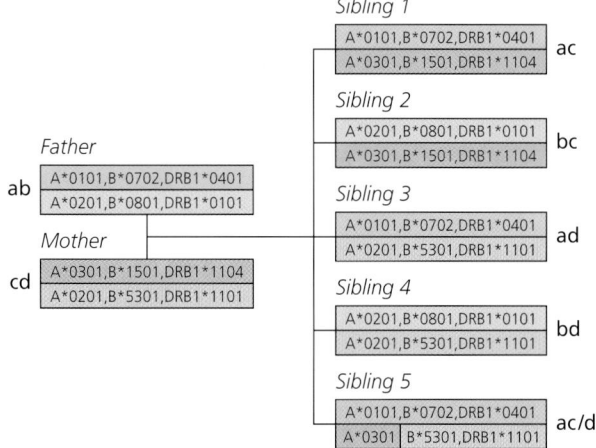

Fig. 32.5 The inheritance of HLA alleles and haplotypes within a family. Paternal haplotypes are labeled a,b; maternal haplotypes, c,d. Sibling 5 inherits a recombinant chromosome from the mother. Not all HLA genes are shown.

haplotype in Latinos, although it is the 54th most frequent haplotype in Asians. Information on the distribution of alleles and haplotypes can be used to assist in searches for HLA-matched tissue donors. For this reason, information on the ethnic background of the volunteer donors is often provided in HSC registries and umbilical cord blood banks.

When large databases of HLA-typed individuals are analyzed, only a small per cent of potential HLA phenotypes are found. (Phenotype is defined as the observed characteristics determined by the HLA genes and is identified by HLA typing.) Using serologic assignments from the NMDP, of the predicted 19 536 660 HLA-A,-B, -DR phenotypes, only 1.6% were observed.[26] This suggests that not all HLA allele combinations will be found. Indeed, some HLA haplotypes appear more frequently than expected. Linkage disequilibrium measures the degree of

Table 32.4 DR haplotypes[a]

DR molecules encoded	Expressed DR loci included in haplotype	DRB1 alleles associated with haplotype
DR, DR51	DRA, DRB1, DRB5	DRB1*15, *16
DR, DR52	DRA, DRB1, DRB3	DRB1*03, *11, *12, *13, *14
DR, DR53	DRA, DRB1, DRB4	DRB1*04, *07, *09
DR	DRA, DRB1	DRB1*01, *08, *10

[a] It should be noted that there are exceptions to these associations. For examples, DRB1*15 haplotypes have been observed which lack a DRB5 locus and some DRB5 positive haplotypes lack a DRB1 locus. In addition, some DRB1*01 haplotypes carry a DRB5 locus.

non-random association between alleles of separate loci. Apparently high disequilibrium across the DR–DQ sub-region coupled with a lack of recombination have resulted in specific associations between DQA1 and DQB1 alleles and between DRB1 and DQ alleles although a single allele such as DQB1 may be associated with one of several partner alleles. For example, the DQB1 allele, DQB1*0602, is found on the same chromosome as the DQA1 alleles DQA1*0101, *0102 or *0103, but has never been observed with DQA1*0201, *0301, *0401 or *0501.[32,33] These associations may differ among individuals of different ethnic backgrounds. For example, DRB1*0901 is associated with DQB1*0201 in African Americans but with DQB1*0303 in individuals of Northern European descent. Within the DR subregion, specific allele combinations at the several DRB loci are associated with families of DR haplotypes (Fig.32.3).[16] For example, the DRB3 locus is found in haplotypes carrying specific DRB1 alleles including DRB1*0301, *1101, *1201, *1301 and *1401 alleles (Table 32.4). In the class I region, associations between HLA-B and -C alleles have also been noted.[34]

Extension of linkage disequilibrium across longer regions of the MHC has resulted in associations between specific class I and class II alleles. The associations of multiple alleles result in extended haplotypes.[35] The best known extended haplotype is HLA-A1,B8,DR3 which is common in Northern Europe appearing at a frequency of approximately 5–15%.[26,27] It has been hypothesized that these associations may have been maintained in the population by selection; that is, associations between DR and DQ as well as associations within an extended haplotype might represent optimal combinations of immune response molecules. It is also likely that features of the genome structure limiting recombination or changes in the structure of the population, such as through admixture of different ethnic groups, have caused the linkage disequilibrium. Because alleles at various HLA loci are non-randomly associated, these associations enhance the frequency with which individuals share alleles across multiple HLA loci facilitating the selection of HLA identical individuals as tissue donors.

Expression

Classical MHC class I proteins are expressed by most nucleated cells, but the level of expression on the cell surface varies for different cell types. *Cis*-acting sequence blocks (enhancer A, interferon-stimulated response element (ISRE), site α and enhancer B) in the regulatory (promoter) region upstream of each class I gene control gene expression (Fig. 32.6(A).[36] Each promoter sequence block binds numerous proteins (transcription factors) that regulate the level of transcription of the gene and ultimately the amount of protein at the cell surface. For example, enhancer A binds the SP1 transcription factor and various members of the NF-κB/rel family (p50, p52, RelA, RelB and c-Rel) of transcription factors. Collectively, the complex is termed NF-κB. Normal class I gene expression requires the coordinated action of each of these regulatory elements; however, disruption of any one sequences block reduces, but does not appear to ablate MHC class I expression.

The amounts of HLA-A, -B and -C molecules expressed at the surface of a cell are not equal.[36] HLA-A and -B are abundant with HLA-A expressed at somewhat higher levels than HLA-B, in many instances. HLA-C is expressed at very low levels in comparison accounting for about 10% of cell surface class I molecules. This is due to sequence variations in the regulatory blocks of each class I locus (Fig. 32.6(B)) which alter the type and affinity of transcription factor binding. For example, only NF-κB/rel family members bind to enhancer A in the HLA-A promoter, while enhancer A in the HLA-B promoter binds SP1 in addition to NF-κB/rel family members. The inclusion of SP1 in the NF-κB complex bound to enhancer A leads to less efficient expression of the HLA-B gene. There are also allele-specific differences in the nucleotide sequence of these regulatory elements such that, for example, different HLA-B alleles are expressed at different levels.

MHC class I gene expression can be up-regulated by various cytokines.[36] Interferon-γ (IFN-γ) performs a fundamental role in enhancing MHC class I expression by inducing increased gene transcription via transactivation of the ISRE. Again, locus and allele specific sequence differences in the ISRE result in different levels of transcriptional enhancement for each of the class I genes. Other cytokines, such as tumor necrosis factor α (TNF-α), can enhance the stimulatory effect of INF-γ on MHC class I gene expression.

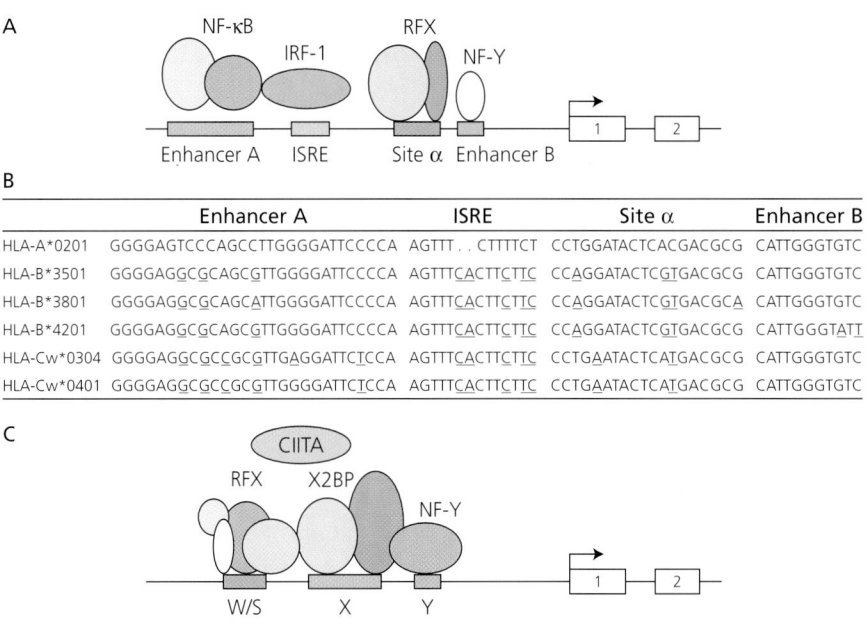

Fig. 32.6 The promoter regions of the classical MHC class I and class II genes. (A) MHC class I gene expression is regulated by four blocks of sequences; enhancer A (green), interferon-stimulated response element (ISRE) (yellow), site α (red) and enhancer B (blue), located in its promoter region. Each block binds a specific transcription factor complex termed nuclear factor kappa B (NF-κB), interferon response factor 1 (IRF-1), regulatory factor X (RFX) and nuclear factor Y (NF-Y), respectively. (B) Nucleotide sequences of each regulatory block of several MHC class I alleles. The sequences are compared to that of HLA-A*0201 with nucleotide variations underlined. Variations in the nucleotide sequence of each regulatory sequence block between different MHC class I alleles dictate the set of individual transcription factors that comprise each complex and the affinity of binding of the complex to the regulatory block. These differences lead to variations in the level of transcription of each class I gene and ultimately to differences in the level of specific MHC class I molecules expressed at the cell surface. (C) MHC class II gene expression is regulated by three blocks of sequences; W/S box (red), X box (green) and Y box (blue), located in its promoter region. Each of these also bind a specific transcription factor complex termed regulatory factor X (RFX), X2 binding protein (X2BP) and nuclear factor Y (NF-Y), respectively. Like MHC class I, many individual transcription factor proteins can participate in the formation of each complex. Unlike MHC class I gene expression, MHC class II gene expression is dependant on a coactivator, the class II transactivator (CIITA) (yellow). Similar to regulation of MHC class I gene expression, there are differences in the nucleotide sequence of MHC class II allele regulatory sequence blocks (examples not shown) that ultimately affect the level of specific MHC class II molecules expressed at the cell surface. Transcription start site in (A) and (C) denoted with an arrow.

MHC class II protein expression is more limited than that of MHC class I proteins. Cell surface HLA-DR, -DQ and -DP molecules are found primarily on professional antigen presenting cells (APC) and on other immune system cells such as T-lymphocytes.[36,37] Professional APC are bone marrow-derived cells dedicated to the task of peptide presentation by MHC molecules and include B-lymphocytes, macrophages, dendritic cells, thymic epithelial cells and Kupffer cells. IFN-γ can induce class II expression in other cell types. Like the class I genes, the promoter regions of the class II genes contain *cis*-acting sequence blocks (termed W/S box, X box and Y box) that bind numerous transcription factors and regulate gene expression (Fig. 32.6(C). In contrast to the class I regula-

tory elements, the class II regulatory elements act in concert in the formation of a large multiprotein transcription complex in the promoter region of the class II genes and coordinated occupancy of all three regulatory elements is absolutely required for expression and IFN-γ induction of class II gene expression.

Occupancy of the class II gene regulatory elements by the transcription factor complex is not adequate for expression of the A and B genes of HLA-DR, -DQ and -DP. Another protein called the class II transactivator (CIITA), which binds to the transcription factor complex and coactivates class II gene expression, is also required.[36,37] Cell type specific and IFN-γ induction of class II expression is the direct result of CIITA expression patterns. Expression of CIITA occurs normally only in professional APC and other immune system cells and can be induced by IFN-γ in other cell types, paralleling expression of MHC class II. All of the other transcription factors that regulate class II gene transcription are ubiquitously expressed and constitutively occupy the regulatory sequence blocks in the MHC class II gene promoters. Of interest, patients with bare lymphocyte syndrome (MHC class II deficiency) can have a defect in any one of a number of the transcription factors that bind to the regulatory sequence blocks or in CIITA.

HLA-DR, -DQ and -DP are not expressed at the same levels on cell surfaces, similar to expression of the different MHC class I molecules. HLA-DR is the most abundant MHC class II molecule expressed by cells. HLA-DQ is expressed at reduced levels and HLA-DP is the least abundant cell surface class II molecule. Like the regulatory elements in the promoters of class I genes, there are both locus and allele specific sequence differences in the regulatory elements of the class II genes.[36] These sequence differences account for the dissimilar levels of class II molecule expression in two ways: (1) alter the binding affinity of the transcription factors; and (2) allow binding of proteins that repress gene transcription of specific class II loci. For example, the X box in the HLA-DPA1 gene promoter region specifically binds the X box repressor protein which diminishes transcription of the HLA-DPA1 gene and reduces the overall level of HLA-DP on the cell surface.

Some pathogenic microorganisms and many malignant cells downregulate HLA gene expression to avoid recognition by the immune system.[38,39] For example, human cytomegalovirus (CMV) interferes with IFN-γ induction of MHC class I and class II gene expression. To avoid detection by T-cells, many carcinomas and lymphomas lack cell surface HLA-A and HLA-B molecules due to defects in the expression or the binding of specific transcription factors to the promoter regulatory blocks of these genes. In many instances, expression of HLA-C in these malignant cells is unaffected, allowing the cell also to avoid recognition by natural killer (NK) cells (see section on Other Immune System Receptors).

There are haplotypes which retain at least remnants of a normally expressed HLA locus but have lost the ability to express this locus.[40] Some of these non-expressed alleles contain nucleotide insertions (e.g HLA allele A*0104N), deletions (e.g. A*0303N), or substitutions (e.g. A*0215N) which alter the reading frame of the mRNA causing a termination in polypeptide synthesis. Still other alleles (e.g. DRB4*0103102N) contain defects in regulatory regions such as the mRNA splice junction which prevent the generation of a functional mRNA. Furthermore, some haplotypes appear to completely lack specific loci. For example, individuals have been identified who appear to lack either the DRB1*15 associated DRB1 locus or the DRB5 locus. The frequency of these null alleles is not yet known although many are expected to be uncommon.

Structure of class I and class II molecules

The classical class I molecules (HLA-A, -B and-C) are expressed on cell surfaces as a trimolecular complex. This complex is composed of the HLA class I polypeptide (heavy chain), beta 2 microglobulin (β_2m) and a peptide. The MHC encoded class I heavy chains are glycosylated transmembrane proteins of approximately 340 amino acids (~ 44 kD) that belong to the immunoglobulin (Ig) superfamily of proteins.[13,41] The extracellular portion of the class I heavy chain is composed of the amino-terminal 275 amino acids. The following 40 amino acids make up the hydrophobic transmembrane region and the carboxy-terminal 25 amino acids comprise the intracellular cytoplasmic tail.

The extracellular portion of the class I heavy chain is divided into three domains, termed α1, α2 and α3 (Fig. 32.7(A)). Each domain is encoded by a separate exon (exons 2–4, respectively; see Fig. 32.2(A) and is approximately 90 amino acids long. The 3D structures of the extracellular portion of several class I molecules were resolved by X-ray crystallography.[42,43] The α1 and α2 domains fold together to form a groove (termed the antigen-binding groove) distal to the cell membrane that consists of a floor of eight antiparallel beta pleated strands topped by two alpha helices fashioned into the walls. The membrane proximal α3 domain folds into a structure which is similar to that of the constant region domains of immunoglobulins (antibodies). This domain is composed of two antiparallel beta sheets, one with four strands and one with three strands. The sheets are linked by a disulfide bond. β_2m (~12 kD) is non-covalently associated with the α3 domain of the class I heavy chain and is required for cell surface expression. Its 3D structure is identical to that of the α3 domain of the heavy chain. Unlike the MHC encoded genes for class I heavy chains (chromosome 6), the gene that encodes β_2m is located on chromosome 15 and is non-polymorphic.

The peptide, the third component of the trimolecular complex, is generally 8–10 amino acids in length and non-covalently bound to the class I heavy chain.[42,43] It lays in the groove formed by the α1 and α2 domains (Fig. 32.7(C)). The peptide is anchored at its amino- and carboxy-terminal ends by non-covalent bonds to amino acid residues in the class I heavy chain. There are pockets

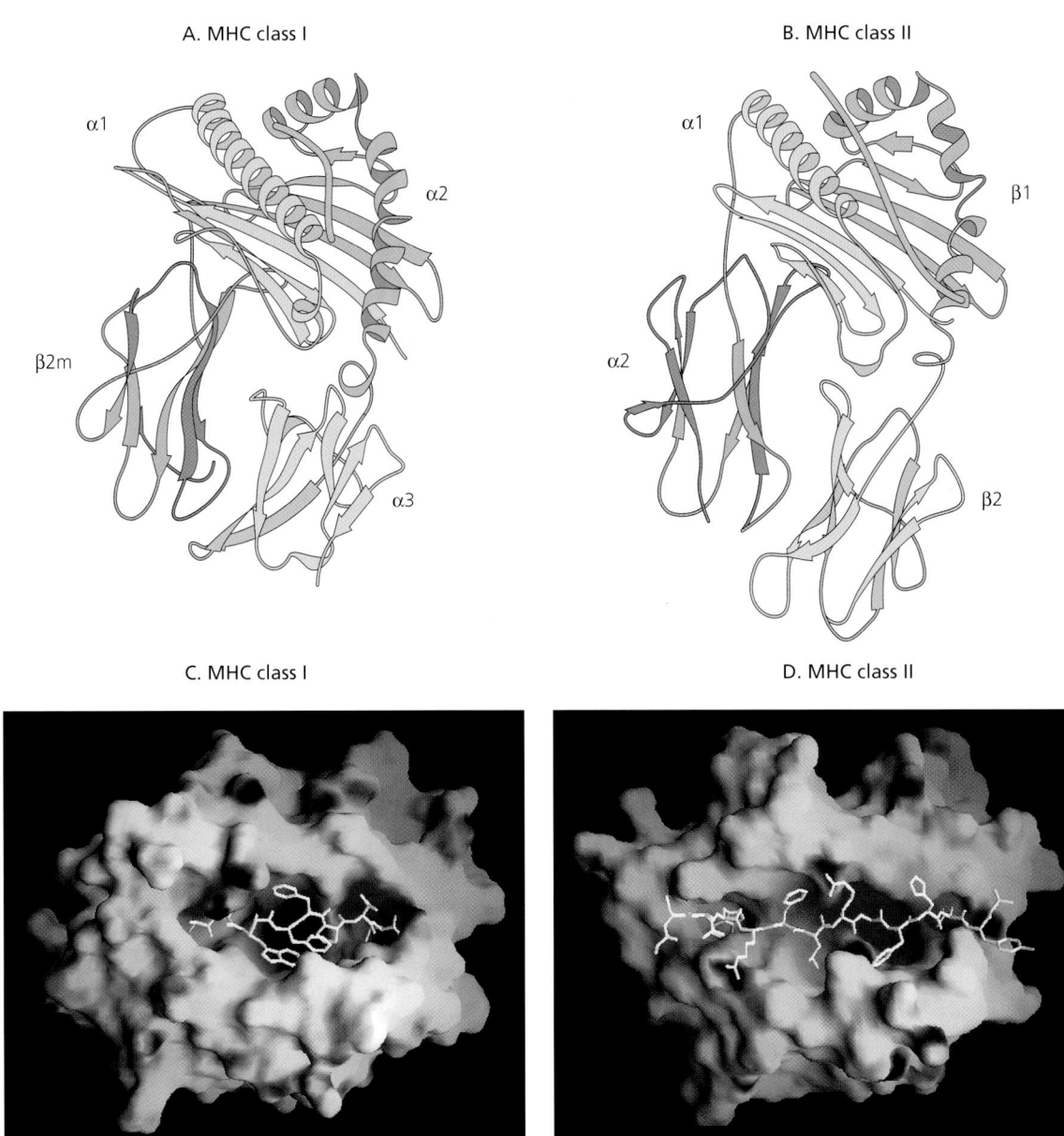

A. MHC class I

α1

α2

β2m

α3

B. MHC class II

α1

β1

α2

β2

C. MHC class I

D. MHC class II

Fig. 32.7 Classical MHC class I and class II structures. (a) Ribbon diagram of the extracellular portion of a MHC class I molecule, HLA-A*0201. The antigen-binding groove is formed by the α1 (green) and α2 (blue) domains of the class I heavy chain. An eight-stranded β pleated sheet (broad arrows) forms the floor of the groove which is overlaid on two sides by α helical walls (twists). The backbone of human peptide p1049 (pink) is seen within the groove. The α3 domain (yellow) of the class I heavy chain non-covalently associates with beta 2 microglobulin (β2m; red). The transmembrane region and cytoplasmic tail (not visualized) would extend toward the bottom of the figure. X-ray crystallographic studies have shown that several other MHC class I molecules have identical overall structures. (b) Ribbon diagram of the extracellular portion of a MHC class II molecule, HLA-DR1; DR(α,β1*0101). The antigen binding groove of the class II molecule is formed by first domains of the α chain (α1; green) and β chain (β1; blue) and has an overall structure similar to the binding groove of MHC class I. The backbone of influenza hemaglutinin peptide 306–318 (pink) is shown in the groove. The class II α chain α2 domain (red) and class II β chain β2 domain (yellow) form structures similar to β2m and the class I heavy chain α3 domain, respectively. The transmembrane region and cytoplasmic tail (not visualized) would extend toward the bottom of the figure. Top view of the electrostatic surface of the antigen binding grooves of the (c) class I molecule and (d) class II molecule shown in (a) and (b), respectively. Negatively and positively charged surfaces are denoted by red and blue, respectively. The respective peptides (yellow) are depicted as stick models showing the carbon backbone and side chains. Pockets binding amino acid side chains of each peptide are clearly visible in each figure. Ribbon diagrams were generated with the program Molescript and electrostatic surface models were generated with the program Grasp on a Silicon Graphics workstation from Protein Data Bank accession codes 1b0g (MHC class I) and 1aqd (MHC class II).

along the groove which accommodate amino acid side chains at various positions along the peptide. The pockets are unique for each class I molecule because polymorphic residues from the α1 and α2 domains participate in their formation. Each pocket has specific physical and chemical characteristics that are determined by the conserved and polymorphic class I residues that form the pocket. These characteristics, in turn, dictate which amino acid side chains are accommodated at the corresponding peptide position. This defines the peptide-binding motif of each class I molecule and defines the overall character of the set of peptides bound (Table 32.5).[44–47] For example, the protein encoded by A*1101 will accommodate a variety of 'small' amino acids at peptide postions 2, 3 and 6 and prefers basic amino acids at peptide position 9. However, each pocket does not make an equal contribution to peptide binding. Certain pockets, specific to each class I molecule, play a more predominant role and the corresponding peptide position is termed an anchor position.

The preferred amino acids at an anchor position are termed anchor residues. Using the protein encoded by A*1101 again as an example, although peptide positions 2, 3 and 6 contribute to peptide binding, it is peptide position 9 that is the anchor position. Lysine and arginine are the anchor residues at this position with lysine preferred over arginine. It is of note that not all peptides that bind to an HLA molecule fully adhere to the defined peptide-binding motif and that amino acids other than anchor residues can be found at anchor positions in these peptides (refer to Table 32.6). In the end, each class I molecule does bind a unique, large set of peptides and the peptide set shares particular sequence characteristics which are dictated by the amino acid residues that make up the groove of the HLA class I heavy chain.

There are benefits to determining the peptide binding motif for HLA molecules. For example, these motifs can be used to identify antigenic peptides from pathogen proteins as candidates for use in peptide-based vaccines.

Table 32.5 MHC class I and class II peptide-binding motifs[a]

Allele	\multicolumn{9}{c}{Relative amino acid position in peptide}

Allele	1	2	3	4	5	6	7	8	9
A*0201		LMIVAT[b,c]		EPDG		LVI			VLIAM
A*0204		L		EP		LIV			LFV
A*0206		VQIL	ILPV	EPDG		LIVF			VLI
A*0207		LV	DP	EDGP		IFVYDL			LFV
A*0101		TSM	DEAS						Y
A*1101		small[d]	small			small			KR
B*2705	RKGA	R	Ho[e]						RK/Ho
B*3701		DE			VI			FML	ILMF
Cw*0301		A	VIY	PE		FY			L
Cw*0401		YP	DH						LFM
DRB1*0101	YFWIL			LMAIV		AG			LMAV
DRB1*0301	FILV			DNQT		RK			FYII
DRB1*1501	LVI			FYI			ILVMF		RK
DRB5*0101	FYLM			QVIM					RK
DQA1*0102[f] DQB1*0602						LIV			AGST
DQA1*0501[f] DQB1*0201	FW			DELVIH		PDEH	ED		FYWVILM
DPA1*0103[f] DPB1*0201	YLFV			STQD		YFWV			LVI
DPA1*0201[f] DPB1*0901	RK					AGL			LV

[a] References 44–47.
[b] Amino acids denoted by single letter designation.
[c] Bold indicates amino acids that are optimal anchor residues. Normal face type indicates amino acids that can also serve as anchor residues. Strike through indicates that the amino acid is not allowed at that relative peptide position.
[d] 'Small' amino acids include: A, G, S, T, L, M, I, V, N.
[e] Ho = hydrophobic amino acids which include: L, I, V, G, F, Y, W, M.
[f] The alleles specifying both chains of the DQ and DP molecules contribute to the HLA antigen-binding site and the characteristics of the bound peptides.

As another example, expression of specific HLA allelic products is associated with an increased risk of developing many autoimmune diseases.[48] In most cases, this is thought to be the result of the differential binding capacity of HLA molecules for particular peptides. Thus, knowing the binding motif for an HLA molecule aids in the identification of the culprit peptide and allows the potential for the design of synthetic peptides that mimic disease-associated peptides for use in blocking autoimmune responses.

The class II molecules are expressed on cell surfaces as a trimolecular complex, structurally analogous to the class I molecules, and consist of the class II α chain, the class II β chain and a peptide. Both the class II α (34 kD) and β (28 kD) chains are transmembrane glycoproteins and are Ig superfamily members, comparable to the class I heavy chain.[13,14,49] The extracellular portion of the α and β chains are divided into two domains, the membrane distal α1 and β1 domains and the membrane proximal α2 and β2 domains. Similar to the class I heavy chains, each domain is encoded by a separate exon (exons 2 and 3, respectively; see Fig. 32. 2(B) and is about 90 amino acids in length. Three additional regions complete each chain of the class II molecule; a connecting peptide of 12 amino acids which is highly hydrophilic and links the membrane proximal domain to the transmembrane region, a 23 amino acid hydrophobic transmembrane region and an intracellular cytoplasmic tail that consists of the carboxy terminal 8–15 amino acids. As an aside, soluble isoforms of the classical HLA molecules are produced and may have immuno-regulatory roles.[50]

The 3D structures of the extracellular portion of several HLA-DR molecules have been determined by X-ray crystallography.[42,43] These structures are strikingly similar to that of class I molecules. The α1 and β1 domains fold together to form a peptide-binding groove like the groove formed by the class I heavy chain α1 and β2 domains (Fig. 32.7(B). The α2 and β2 domains of the class II chains fold to form Ig constant region domain like structures similar to that of the class I α3 domain and β2m. The 3D structures of HLA-DQ and HLA-DP molecules are expected to be analogous to HLA-DR.

The peptides that bind to class II molecules are anchored to the class II antigen-binding groove by non-covalent bonds to the peptide backbone and by binding of peptide amino acid side chains into pockets along the groove (Fig. 32.7(D), similar to the class I molecules.[43,51,52] Because of the polymorphic nature of the MHC class II proteins, each class II molecule, like each class I molecule, also binds a large set of peptides which share a peptide-binding motif specific to that class II molecule (Table 32.5). The peptides that bind to class II molecules are heterogenous in length and generally 13–25 amino acids long (Table 32.6). The low and open ends of the class II groove allow peptides of varying lengths to bind in an extended conformation with the ends of the peptide overhanging the ends of the groove. This is in contrast to the class I molecules which bind peptides of 8–10 amino acids. The ends of the class I groove are high and closed; thus, MHC class I molecules optimally accommodate shorter peptides whose ends are tucked into the groove (compare Fig. 32.7(B) and 32.7(D).

Table 32.6 Naturally processed peptides bound to HLA-A and HLA-DR molecules[a]

	Peptide sequence[b]	Peptide length	Source protein
HLA-A*0101	Y **T** D Y G G L I F N S **Y**	12	cytochrome c oxidase
	Y L **D** D P D L K **Y**	9	cytosine methyl transferase
	S **T** D H I P I L **Y**	9	fructose-6-p-amino transferase
	D S **D** G S F F L **Y**	9	Ig gamma-4
	A **T** D F K F A M **Y**	9	cyclin protein D type
	Y **T** N P Q F N V **Y**	9	unknown
HLA-DRBI*0101	I P A D L R I I **S** A N G C K V D N S	18	(Na+ + K+) ATPase
	S D **W** R F **L** R **G** Y H Q Y A	13	HLA-A2
	K M R M **A** T P L L **M** Q A L P	14	invariant chain
	R V E **Y** H F **L** S P Y V S P K E S P	17	transferrin receptor
	Y K H T L N Q **I** D S V K **V** W P R R P	18	bovine fetuin
HLA-DRB1*1501	E A E Q L R A **Y** L D G T G V E	15	HLA-A3
	L E E F G R **F** A S F E A Q G	14	HLA-DRα
	A I L E F R A **M** A Q F S R K T D	16	SP3
	P V V H F F K N I V T	11	myelin basic protein
	G T L S K I F K **L** G G R D S R S G	17	myelin basic protein

[a] Table compiled from data in publication.[44]
[b] Sequences aligned by relative motif positions. Anchor residues that correspond to the binding motif for each HLA molecule are in bold (see *Table 32.5*). Note that an optimal amino acid residue need not be present at all anchor positions for a peptide to bind to a HLA molecule.

Function

Peptide processing and binding

Mature cell surface class I molecules are formed in the endoplasmic reticulum (ER) with the aid of several resident ER proteins including tapasin, calnexin and calreticulin.[53] Initially, the class I heavy chain and β_2m fold and associate facilitated by calnexin and calreticulin (Fig. 32.8). This complex then transiently associates with the transporter associated with antigen processing (TAP) where a peptide is loaded into the groove of the class I heavy chain. Finally, the trimolecular complex is dispatched to the cell surface.

Peptides, derived from both self (normal cellular) proteins (potential autoantigens) or foreign proteins (antigens), are generated in the cytosol by the proteosome.[53–55] The proteosome is a macromolecular structure that proteo-lytically cleaves proteins into peptides (a process termed antigen processing) and consists of members of the large multifunctional proteosome (LMP) family. Two LMP family members (LMP2 and LMP7) are encoded in the class II region of the MHC. The proteosome is tightly associated with the TAP molecule which shuttles the peptides into the lumen of the ER.[53,55] TAP is the complex formed by the association of the products of the TAP1 and TAP2 genes also encoded in the MHC class II region. Another MHC-encoded gene product, tapasin, links the class I heavy chain to TAP for peptide loading. Once a suitable peptide is bound, the stable complex routes to the surface of the cell.

The class II α and β chains fold and associate in the ER with the assistance of resident ER chaperones such as calnexin (Fig. 32.8),[56] similar to class I molecules. Unlike class I, full maturation of the class II molecule does not

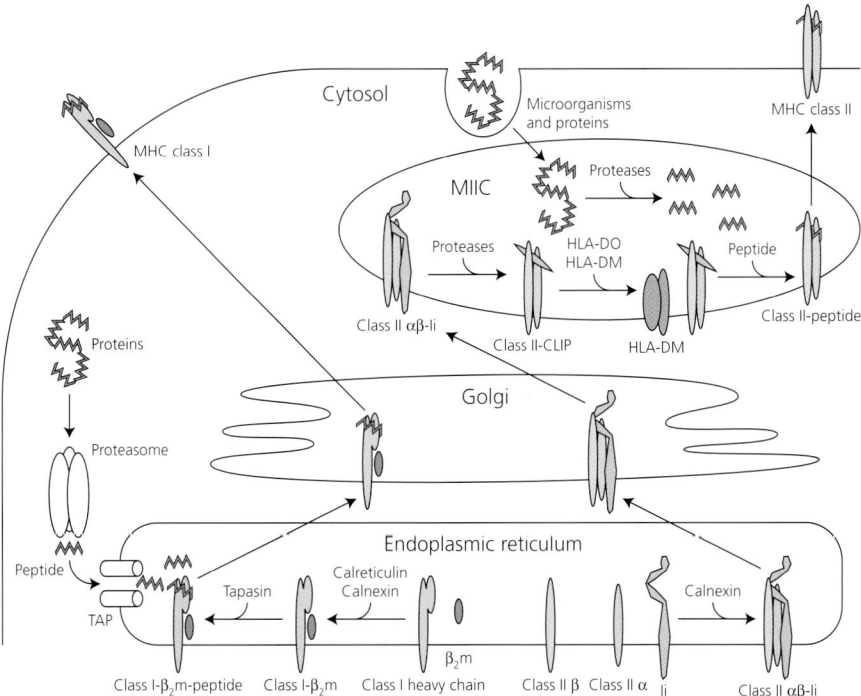

Fig. 32.8 MHC class I and class II peptide processing and binding. MHC class I peptide processing and binding is depicted in the left portion of the figure. Class I heavy chain (blue) and beta 2 microglobulin (β_2m) (lavender) fold and associate in the endoplasmic reticulum (ER) aided by resident ER proteins. Cytosolic-derived proteins are converted into peptides (red) by the proteosome and shuttled into the ER by the transporter associated with antigen processing (TAP) where they bind to the class I antigen binding groove. Stable class I + β_2m + peptide complexes are transported from the ER to the Golgi where the class I polypeptide is glycosylated. Mature MHC class I molecules then are shuttled to the cell surface. MHC class II peptide processing and binding is depicted in the right portion of the figure. Like MHC class I and aided by resident ER proteins, the class II α (green) and β (yellow) chains associate in the ER along with the invariant chain (Ii) (light gray). The class II $\alpha\beta$ + Ii complex is glycosylated as it is transported through the Golgi to the MHC class II compartment (MIIC). Here, proteases cleave Ii leaving only the Ii derived peptide CLIP bound to the class II binding groove (class II – CLIP). HLA-DM (dark gray) catalyzes the exchange of CLIP for peptides (red) derived by proteolytic degradation from internalized microorganisms and proteins. Stable class II + peptide complexes then traffic to the cell surface and represent mature MHC class II molecules.

take place in the ER. Instead, class II heterodimers are directed to specialized endosomal compartments (MHC class II compartments, MIIC). In the MIIC, peptides are loaded into the antigen-binding groove and mature class II molecules are dispatched to the cell surface.

MHC class II molecules bind peptides derived from endocytosed microorganisms and from self and foreign proteins degraded by proteases in the endocytic pathway.[55,56] This is in contrast, yet complementary, to the peptides bound by MHC class I molecules. In general, class II molecules bind peptides from cell surface and extracellular sources, while class I molecules bind peptides from intracellular sources. Thus, proteins from the whole environment of a cell can be surveyed by the immune system. Invariant chain (Ii), a non-MHC-encoded glycoprotein, plays a key role in facilitating this division of function.

Ii performs several functions in assuring proper antigen presentation by class II molecules. Ii chain serves as a chaperone in the folding and assembly of class II αβ heterodimers and protects the class II peptide-binding groove from binding peptide in the ER via a 25 residue internal peptide segment termed CLIP (class II associated invariant chain peptide).[55,56] Ii also provides the intracellular targeting signals that direct the complex to the MIIC. Under the acidic conditions of the MIIC, Ii is proteolytically cleaved and dissociates from the class II molecule, while CLIP remains bound to the class II antigen-binding groove. CLIP is exchanged for antigenic peptides in a reaction catalyzed by HLA-DM, a resident MIIC protein that tightly associates with the class II heterodimer.[57–59] HLA-DM also appears to retain class II molecules in the MIIC until a stable, high-affinity complex between the class II molecule and a peptide is formed. Another resident MIIC protein, HLA-DO, negatively regulates the actions of HLA-DM.[60] Once a peptide has bound to the groove and HLA-DM has been released, the class II molecule moves to the cell surface.

Analogous to the MHC class II molecules, both HLA-DM and HLA-DO are class II related Ig superfamily members expressed as heterodimers that consist of an α chain and a β chain.[57–60] The HLA-DM and HLA-DO α and β chains are encoded by A and B genes, respectively, in the MHC class II region and regulation of these genes is identical to that of the MHC class II genes.[61] The 3D structure of HLA-DM resembles that of the MHC class II molecules except that its peptide-binding groove is almost entirely obscured.[42]

Components of the peptide processing and binding pathways of MHC class I and class II molecules are a favorite target of disruption by many pathogens and malignant cells to avoid detection by the immune system.[38,39,62] For example, two proteins (US3 and US6) encoded by human CMV block cell surface expression of MHC class I molecules and thus, detection of the infected cell by cytotoxic T-cells (see section on T-lymphocyte recognition of HLA molecules). US3 binds to MHC class I molecules and retains them in the ER and US6 inhibits peptide transport into the ER by TAP. Lack of cell surface MHC class I, however, renders the CMV-infected cell susceptible to lysis by NK cells. To circumvent NK cell recognition, CMV encodes a class I like decoy termed UL18 which is recognized by NK cells and inhibits their function. As a second example, some malignant cells have severely reduced levels or complete loss of MHC class I cell surface expression because these cells lack expression of functional LMP or TAP proteins due to deletion of or mutations in their genes. Other pathogens and malignant cells employ a variety of unique strategies to block MHC expression.

T-lymphocyte recognition of HLA molecules

As stated earlier, the predominant function of classical MHC class I and class II molecules is to bind peptides from the cell's environment and present these peptides on the surface of the cell for inspection by the immune system. The archetypical receptor involved in the inspection process is the T-cell receptor (TCR) on T-lymphocytes (Fig. 32.9). There are two types of TCR (αβ and γδ) both of which are multiprotein complexes that consist of a TCR α chain covalently paired with a TCR β chain or of a TCR γ chain covalently paired with a TCR δ chain tightly, but non-covalently, associated with several chains of the CD3 family (γ, δ, ε, ζ, η).[63,64] The TCR chains are involved in the direct recognition of the HLA molecule and of the peptide bound to the HLA molecule.[42,63,65] CD3 is involved in the signaling process which activates the T-cell after recognition of the ligand by the TCR chains.[66] CD3 does not interact directly with the ligand.

T-lymphocytes are classically divided into two groups based on expression of coreceptors (CD4 and CD8), which are intimately involved in recognition of the HLA molecule.[63,67–69] CD4 expressing (CD4+) T-cells are usually MHC class II restricted; that is, their TCR recognizes either an HLA-DR, -DQ or -DP molecule which all have a CD4-binding site (Fig. 32.9). CD8 expressing (CD8+) T-cells are generally MHC class I restricted recognizing either an HLA-A, -B or -C molecule which all have a CD8-binding site. CD4 and CD8 enhance the interaction between the TCR and HLA molecule and provide signals, in addition to the CD3 chains, to activate the T-cell.

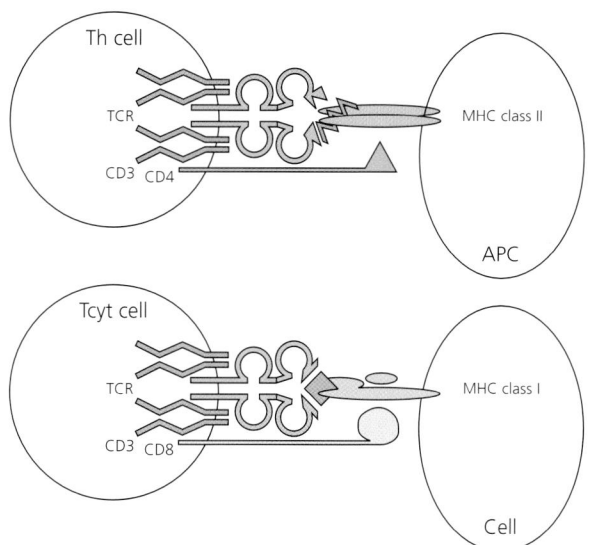

Fig. 32.9 CD4⁺ versus CD8⁺ T-cells. T-cells are classically divided into two groups based on their expression of either CD4 (top, dark gray) or CD8 (bottom, light gray). Both types of T-cells express the T-cell receptor (TCR) (blue) and CD3 complex (CD3) (lavender). CD4 expressing T-cells are primarily of the helper phenotype (Th) and CD8 expressing T-cells are generally of the cytotoxic phenotype (Tcyt). The TCR expressed by CD4⁺ Th cells is usually restricted to MHC class II molecules (green), while the TCR expressed by CD8⁺ Tcyt cells is generally restricted to MHC class I molecules (yellow). Each T-cell expresses a unique TCR (see Fig. 32.10) that recognizes a specific peptide (red) in complex with a particular MHC class I or class II molecule.

The CD4/CD8 division in MHC restriction, for the most part, also extends to the general phenotypic function of the T-cell. CD4⁺ T-cells are mostly of the helper phenotype (helper T-lymphocyte; Th-cell). Th-cells are dedicated to the initiation and generation of immune responses to specific antigens, including antibody production by B-lymphocytes and cytotoxic cellular responses. CD8⁺ T-cells are usually of the cytotoxic phenotype (cytotoxic T-lymphocyte; Tcyt-cell) and are the principal component of the cytotoxic cellular response to specific antigens. Tcyt-cell recognition of a foreign peptide bound to a MHC class I molecule leads to killing of the abnormal or infected cell.

The CD4/CD8 division is not absolute with regard to restriction or function. First, there are CD4⁺ and CD8⁺ T-cells which are restricted by histocompatibility molecules other than the classical MHC class I or class II molecules (see section on Other Histocompatibility Molecules). Second, some CD4⁺ T-cells are cytotoxic in nature. In addition, there are T-cells that do not express either CD4 or CD8 (double negative; DN T-cells). DN T-cells are primarily restricted by other histocompatibility molecules, such as CD1 molecules, and can be either helper or cytotoxic in phenotype.

The TCR chains are highly variable members of the Ig superfamily. Each chain is encoded by a novel gene formed by the combining of gene segments termed variable, diversity, joining and constant.[70,71] There are multiple, different copies of each gene segment encoded in the genome. For example, there are approximately 46 functional TCR β chain variable gene segments. Additional diversity in the amino acid sequence of these proteins is generated by several mechanisms collectively at the level of the gene. The outcome of this diversity is the generation of a large pool of T-cells expressing a wide range of TCR that, in turn, can recognize a wide variety of antigenic peptides. Simplistically, each T-cell, through its TCR, recognizes a specific HLA molecule (MHC restriction) in combination with a distinct peptide (antigen-specific recognition) (Fig. 32.10). In actuality, the TCR of each T-cell can recognize with different affinities many different MHC/peptide complexes that share common structural features.[72]

MHC class I and class II molecules are essential to the creation of the T-cell pool available for immune surveillance. T-cell maturation and selection occurs in the thymus in a process called thymic education.[73–75] In the thymus, T-cells are in contact with MHC class I and class II molecules that are complexed with a variety of self peptides. The TCR on a T-cell must be able to interact with a self HLA molecule complexed with a self peptide. T-cells whose TCR has a high affinity for and are reactive to (autoreactive) these complexes are deleted (negative selection) from the T-cell pool via the generation of a variety of intracellular signals.[74] Many T-cells have a TCR that is unable to bind to self HLA plus self peptide complexes. These T-cells just die in the thymus. T-cells whose TCR has a low-affinity interaction with and are partially activated by self HLA plus self peptide complexes (positive selection) are self tolerant and leave the thymus for peripheral tissues. These T-cells, which maintain some degree of partial autoreactivity, constitute the pool available for immune responses to foreign peptides.

The diversity of HLA molecule + self peptide complexes is central not only to the selection of a diverse repertoire of T-cells in the thymus, but also to the maintenance of the multiplicity of available T-cells in peripheral tissues.[73,75] Disruptions in this process can result in autoreactivity and autoimmune diseases. Other histocompatibility antigens (non-classical MHC class I molecules, MHC class I related chains and CD1 molecules) are expressed in the thymus and by other tissues and likely help to select and maintain the available T-cell pool. In a HSC transplant, amino acid sequence differences (mismatches) between any of the HLA molecules expressed by the cells of the donor and of the recipient, theoretically, can cause T-cell

Antigen-specific T-cell recognition

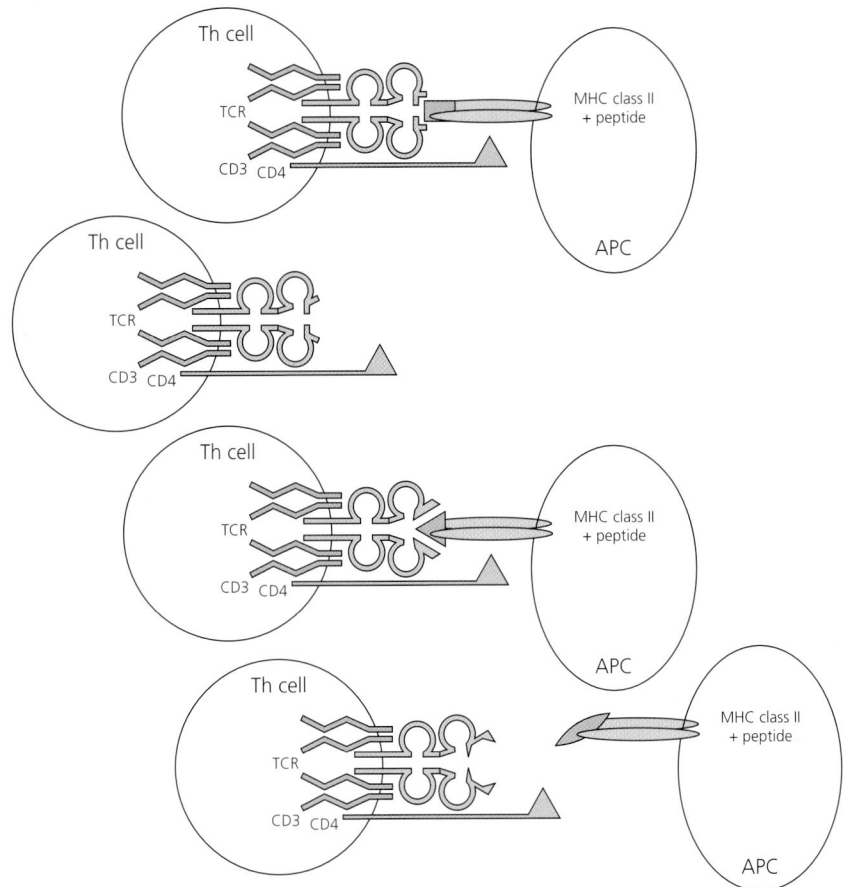

Fig. 32.10 T-cell recognition is antigen specific. The T-cell receptors (TCR; blue) expressed by different individual T-cells differ and, thus, each recognizes a specific peptide bound to a specific MHC molecule. In the example shown, the four CD4⁺ (gray) Th-cells have differing specificities for particular peptides (red) due to variations in the sequence of their TCR. However, each recognizes their respective peptide bound to the same MHC class II molecule (green). The CD3 complex (CD3) is depicted in lavender.

reactivity (see section on Allorecognition) to the foreign HLA molecule. This reactivity can manifest itself as either GVHD or graft rejection and results because the T-cells were not educated for tolerance to the disparate HLA molecule.

The TCR is not the only receptor that binds HLA molecules as its ligand. Members of the killer cell inhibitory receptor (KIR) and immunoglobulin-like transcript (ILT) receptor families interact with groups of HLA molecules as their ligands (see section on Other Immune System Receptors). These interactions regulate a variety of functions by immune system cells.

Allorecognition and transplantation

Allorecognition results when T-cells of one individual react to foreign (allogeneic) HLA molecules of another individual.[76,77] There are two distinct types of allo-

recognition termed direct and indirect (Fig. 32.11). Direct allorecognition occurs when T-cells recognize as foreign a variant determinant on an intact allogeneic HLA molecule. The foreign HLA + self peptide complexes recognized by these alloreactive T-cells are varied. Some alloreactive T-cells react directly to the differences of the foreign HLA molecule without regard for the bound self peptides.[78] Other alloreactive T-cells recognize the foreign HLA molecule complexed with a specific self peptide.[79,80] In this instance, the amino acid disparities of the foreign HLA molecule combined with a specific self peptide likely result in a tertiary structure that is dissimilar from that of the same self peptide bound to a self HLA molecule. The change in tertiary structure of the complex is then recognized as foreign by T-cells.

Indirect allorecognition occurs when T-cells recognize a self HLA molecule that has bound a peptide derived from the foreign HLA molecule which contains the amino

Direct allorecognition

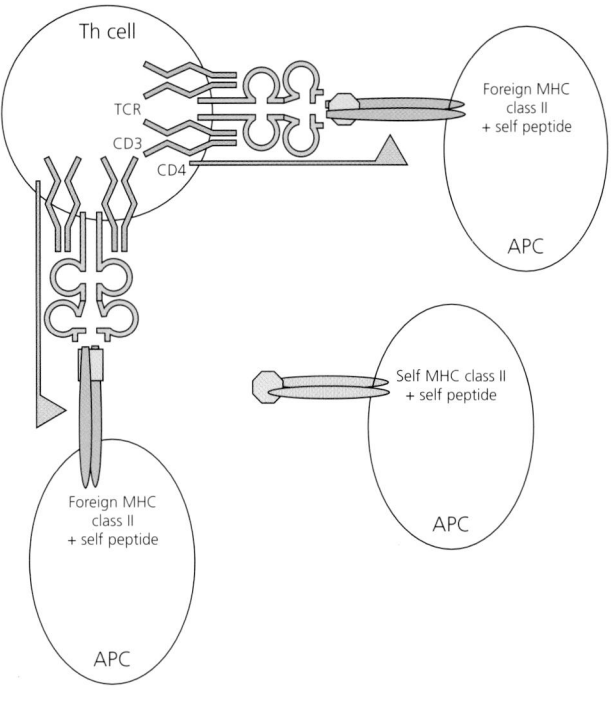

Indirect allorecognition

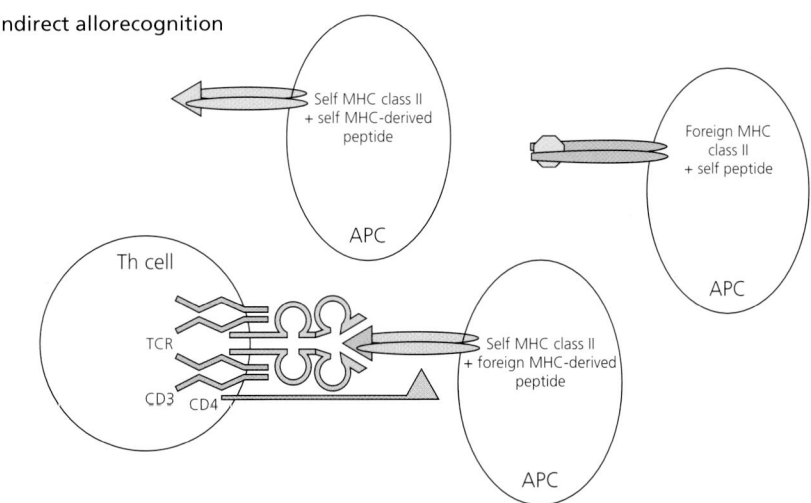

Fig. 32.11 Allorecognition is the recognition of and reaction to determinants of foreign MHC molecules by T-cells. There are two types of allorecognition, direct (top) and indirect (bottom). In the example depicted of direct allorecognition (top), the T-cell receptor (TCR; blue) expressed by a CD4⁺ (gray) Th-cell is recognizing directly the differences of the foreign MHC class II molecule (red). The foreign class II molecules are complexed with self peptides (yellow) which may or may not play a direct role in recognition of the complex. An identical self peptide bound to a self MHC class II molecule (green) is not recognized by the Th-cell. In the example of indirect allorecognition (bottom), the TCR expressed by a CD4⁺ Th cell is recognizing a peptide (red) derived from the foreign MHC class II molecule in complex with a self MHC class II molecule (green). This peptide contains one or more amino acids that differ from the comparable peptide (green) derived from the self MHC class II molecule. The foreign MHC molecule (red) is not recognized directly by the Th-cell and neither is a self MHC class II molecule complexed with the equivalent peptide derived from a self class II molecule. The CD3 complex (CD3) is depicted in lavender.

acid difference(s).[76,77,81] This type of allorecognition is identical to antigen-specific T-cell recognition of any foreign peptide. It involves the uptake of grafted cellular material, from which the foreign HLA molecules are processed into peptides and bound to self HLA molecules via the normal MHC class I and class II peptide processing and binding pathways.

Allorecognition is purely a transplantation phenomenon. Successful transplantation of tissues, especially HSC grafts, relies heavily on the HLA identity of the donor and the recipient.[82] Unfortunately, HLA mismatches between a donor and recipient are often unavoidable. Any HLA disparity between a donor and recipient has the potential to cause allorecognition which increases the risk of graft rejection or GVHD. However, not all HLA disparity leads to destructive alloreactive T-cell responses.

The frequency of T-cells of any individual that respond to allogeneic HLA can be as high as 1 in 10^2, which is substantially greater than the frequency of T-cells that respond to a specific foreign antigen (estimated to be between 1 in 10^5–10^6).[76] The high frequency of potentially alloreactive T-cells is most likely due to the fact that the available T-cell pool consists of T-cells that are inherently partially reactive to self HLA molecules complexed with self peptides.[73,75,76] Additionally, a normal and substantial proportion of the self peptides bound to self HLA molecules are derived from self HLA molecules (see Table 32.6).[83] Thus, many T-cells also are inherently partially reactive to self HLA derived peptides. While these complexes make a significant contribution to thymic education of T-cells and maintenance of the available T-cell pool, changes to these complexes in the form of intact allogeneic HLA and allogeneic HLA derived peptides are readily recognized by many T-cells as foreign.

Non-classical MHC class I molecules

The non-classical MHC class I (class Ib) molecules, HLA-E, HLA-F and HLA-G, have been the focus of intense research in recent years. Much has been learned of their structure, expression and function. Each of the non-classical class I heavy chain genes is encoded in the class I region of the MHC (see Fig. 32.1) and the proteins expressed by these genes are structurally similar to the classical class I molecules (class Ia). However, the class Ib molecules, in general, are noticeably less polymorphic and expressed at lower levels on cell surfaces than the class Ia molecules. These glycoproteins also display unique tissue distribution patterns and participate in specialized immune system functions. The impact of the

class Ib molecules on immune responses directed toward foreign tissue is not yet known.

HLA-E

HLA-E shares many features with the classical class I molecules. Its gene is organized and regulated in a manner identical to that of the class Ia genes and is highly transcribed in most nucleated cells.[36] In fact, HLA-E protein expression parallels the expression of the classical class I molecules.[84,85] HLA-E is expressed on cell surfaces as a trimolecular complex that includes the HLA-E heavy chain, β_2m and peptide and has a similar overall 3D conformation.[42,86,87] Assembly of the HLA-E molecule and binding of peptides requires all of the same ER components. Like the class Ia molecules, the peptides that bind to HLA-E are optimal at nine amino acids in length.

In contrast to classical MHC class I genes, HLA-E is the least polymorphic of the MHC class I genes. Although high levels of HLA-E gene transcripts and intracellular protein are found in most cells, very little HLA-E protein is detected at cell surfaces. These observations are likely the consequence of the unique function of HLA-E, which has been well conserved across species. The peptide-binding groove of HLA-E is highly hydrophobic and specializes in the binding of hydrophobic peptides primarily derived from the leader sequences of many of the classical class I molecules and HLA-G. These HLA-E + leader sequence complexes serve as the ligand recognized by some members of the CD94/NKG2 family of natural killer (NK) cell receptors (see section on Other Immune System Receptors). Recognition of HLA-E by CD94/NKG2 family members regulates NK-cell mediated lysis of a potential target cell. The coordinate expression of HLA-E with classical MHC class I molecules and the binding of peptides derived from their leader sequences provides a means for NK cells to monitor the efficacy of expression and translation of the classical class I genes which is often disrupted in malignant and virally infected cells. Although there is limited experimental evidence that HLA-E can bind peptides derived from other sources, such as viral proteins, a role outside of NK-cell recognition is yet to be determined.

HLA-F

HLA-F remains the most mysterious of the class Ib molecules, Like HLA-E, HLA-F also shares properties associated with the classical MHC class I molecules. The organization and regulation of the HLA-F gene is identical to that of the class Ia genes.[36] Its gene is highly transcribed in a variety of cell types, but not as ubiquitously as expression of the classical MHC class I genes.[87,88] The HLA-F heavy chain associates with β_2m, as well as several of the ER components, including TAP, involved in class Ia molecule assembly.

Contrary to the class Ia genes, polymorphisms reported in the HLA-F gene are very limited, The HLA-F heavy chain (42 kD) is smaller than the classical class I molecules and HLA-E (44 kD) because of a shorter cytoplasmic tail (exon 7 is absent in the mRNA; refer to Fig 32.2(A)). Although its gene is transcribed in many cell types, the HLA-F protein has only been detected intracellularly in B-cells, B-cell lines and tissues containing B-cells. In these cells, HLA-F was found associated with β_2m, but with no bound peptides, although 3D models suggest that the HLA-F antigen-binding groove could accommodate peptides. Only one report has possibly detected HLA-F on a cell surface, interestingly on a B-cell line. Whether HLA-F is non-functional, performs a specialized role intracellularly, or is a highly specialized antigen presentation molecule remains to be determined.

HLA-G

HLA-G is more analogous to the classical class I molecules than HLA-E and HLA-F. Its gene has the typical class Ia gene exon/intron organization and is transcribed in a variety of tissues.[89] HLA-G is the most polymorphic of the class Ib genes.[90,91] Although less polymorphic than the classical class I genes, the number of reported polymorphisms in the HLA-G gene is rapidly expanding. Assembly and expression of the HLA-G trimolecular complex (HLA-G heavy chain, β_2m and peptide) is identical to classical MHC class I molecules.[92,93] The 3D structure of HLA-G is expected to be akin to class Ia molecules since it has 86% homology with the classical MHC class I consensus protein sequence. HLA-G binds a large set of peptides with a defined motif that are optimal between 8 and 10 amino acids in length.

HLA-G has unique features. The HLA-G heavy chain is smaller than the classical class I heavy chains due to an in-frame stop codon in exon 6 (refer to Fig. 32.2 (a)) which yields a shortened cytoplasmic tail.[92,93] In addition, six different HLA-G proteins (isoforms) are expressed as a result of alternative splicing of its mRNA. HLA-G1 is the full length isoform that is membrane bound and associated with β_2m. There are three other membrane-bound isoforms of HLA-G (HLA-G2, -G3 and -G4) that lack various extracellular domains. Each of these membrane-bound isoforms appears to be expressed as a homodimer at the cell surface and not associated with β_2m. Alternative mRNA that includes intron 4 produces the two soluble isoforms of HLA-G, HLA-G1sol and HLA-G2sol.

These isoforms are comparable to HLA-G1 and -G2 and include 21 amino acids encoded by intron 4, but lack exons 5–8 due to an in-frame stop codon in intron 4 (refer to Fig 32.2(A)). All isoforms appear to bind peptides and, thus, may be functional. The HLA-G promoter lacks all of the regulatory sequence blocks, except for a modified enhancer A, typical of the classical MHC class I genes, HLA-E and HLA-F.[89] Identification of HLA-G regulatory sequence blocks has been problematic.

HLA-G is unique in that it is the primary histocompatibility molecule expressed during pregnancy in placental tissues.[92,93] HLA-E is also expressed, but classical class I molecules are not expressed in these tissues. HLA-G likely presents foreign peptides on the surface of infected cells to TCR maintaining the well being of fetal tissue. HLA-G also has a dual role in maternal tolerance of the fetus. First, HLA-G provides a leader sequence peptide for expression of HLA-E which, in turn, regulates maternal NK cell recognition of fetal tissue. Second, HLA-G regulates the functional interaction of a variety of immune system cells with fetal tissue by serving directly as the ligand for members of the ILT family of receptors (see section on Other Immmune System Receptors) which are expressed by professional APC of myeloid lineage and by some lymphocytes. HLA-G is also expressed in several other tissue types including thymic epithelial cells, T-cells and B-cells suggesting that it may participate in immune system functions outside of fetal development and tolerance.

Other potential histocompatibility molecules

MHC class I chain-related molecules (MIC)

The genes encoding the MHC class I chain-related molecules (MIC) are located in the class I region of the MHC. The expressed MIC genes (MICA and MICB) are located centromeric to HLA-B (see Fig. 32.1). There are several MIC pseudogenes dispersed throughout the MHC class I region. The MICA and MICB genes are encoded by six exons. Exons 1–5 are similar to the classical MHC class I genes (see Fig. 32.2(A). Exon 6 encodes the cytoplasmic tail, 3'UTR and polyadenylation signal.[94] MICA and MICB are relatively polymorphic.[18,95,96] For example, 40 alleles of MICA have been described. The MICA and MICB proteins are heavily glycosylated members of the Ig superfamily that share a low level of homology (up to 30%) with MHC class I molecules.[86,94]

Several features are unique to MICA and MICB. Expression of MICA and MICB is upregulated in response to stress because of a heat shock response element in the promoter region of their genes.[86,97] In fact, the promoter regions of the MICA and MICB genes do not contain any of the classical MHC class I regulatory elements (see Fig. 32.6). Instead, their promoters share homologies with the heat shock protein 70 promoter. MICA and MICB protein expression is limited to epithelial cells primarily in the gastrointestinal tract and thymus and does not require association with β2m, peptide or TAP.[94,97] The 3D structure of the extracellular domains of MICA revealed that the folding resembles that of the class Ia molecules, but that the overall orientation of these domains is dissimilar.[98] In comparison to the classical class I peptide-binding groove, the MICA α1 and α2 domains are tilted with respect to the α3 domain such that the α1 domain is distal to the membrane and the α2 domain is tilted toward the α3 domain. This exposes a portion of the underside of the groove, as well as the groove itself to interactions with receptors. The peptide-binding groove is mostly obscured leaving only a reduced area that might bind small antigens.

The function of these molecules remains obscure. However, there is evidence to suggest that MICA and MICB may function in the presentation of tumor specific, viral and bacterial antigens to γδ Tcyt-cells.[99,100] Current research suggests that MICA is the ligand for NKG2D, an activating NK-cell receptor.[101] The interaction of NKG2D and MICA leads to NK-cell mediated lysis of the epithelial cell. The importance of MICA and MICB to transplantation, if any, is also undefined. Whatever their immune system function, it is increasingly apparent that these molecules participate extensively in maintaining the integrity of mucosal tissue.

CD1 molecules

CD1 is a family of proteins whose genes are encoded on an MHC paralogous region on chromosome 1.[102] The CD1 molecules are members of the Ig superfamily with homology equidistant from MHC class I and MHC class II molecules.[103,104] Similar to MHC class I molecules, CD1 molecules associate with β2m; similar to MHC class II molecules, CD1 molecules associate with invariant chain and appear to follow the class II antigen presentation pathway. Like both MHC class I and class II molecules, CD1 molecules appear to present antigens to T-lymphocytes for immune recognition.

In contrast to classical MHC class I and class II, the CD1 genes appear to be non-polymorphic and assembly of the CD1 molecules is TAP and HLA-DM independant.[103,104] Five CD1 molecules (CD1a, -b, -c, -d, -e) have been described which are classified into two groups based on sequence homology and tissue distribution. Members of group I (CD1a, -b, -c, -e) are expressed primarily on professional APC, while members of group II (CD1d) are expressed mainly on intestinal epithelium. The antigen-binding grooves of the CD1 molecules are very hydrophobic. In addition to peptides, the group I CD1 molecules have been shown to bind lipid (mycolic acid) and glycolipid (lipoarabinomannan), the principal components of mycobacteria cell walls, and are ligands for double negative (DN) and CD8+ T-cells that express γδ TCR or αβ TCR. The group II CD1 molecules bind glycophospholipids and hydrophobic peptides. These CD1 molecules are ligands for DN and CD4+ T-cells expressing either γδ TCR or αβ TCR. Both groups of CD1 molecules appear to help broaden antigen presentation to the immune system during bacterial infections. It remains to be determined whether these molecules have an impact on transplantation.

Minor histocompatibility antigens

Clinically significant GVHD is observed in HLA identical sibling transplants of HSC implicating histcompatibility antigens specified by genes other than the classical HLA genes in the allorecognition of foreign tissue.[105] These so called minor histocompatibility antigens (mHag) were identified coincident with the major histocompatibility antigens, but not until recently have we had an understanding of what constituted a mHag. mHag are peptides derived from self proteins, other than HLA, whose sequence differs among individuals in the population. Theoretically, any polymorphic protein that differs between the tissue donor and recipient has the potential to provide a peptide which functions as a mHag. Over 50 mHag loci have been described in humans utilizing mHag-specific T-cell clones in cytotoxicity assays. However, only a handful of peptides derived from these loci have been identified (Table 32.7).[106–112] The peptides containing the variant amino acid(s) are processed through the normal MHC class I and class II antigen presentation pathways, are bound to an HLA molecule and are recognized as foreign by T-cells.

The HLA alleles expressed by a donor and recipient determine whether a mHag might contribute to allorecognition in transplantation. Furthermore, the contribution of a mHag on transplant outcome might be contingent on the genders of the donor and recipient and on the type of tissue transplanted (Table 32.7). HLA alleles are important

Table 32.7 Examples of human minor histocompatibility antigens[a]

Minor antigen	Sequence[b]	Source protein	Tissue distribution	HLA restriction[c]	Characterization of antigenicity
HA-1	VLHDDLLEA VLRDDLLEA	Gene locus KIAA0223	Hematopoietic cells	A*0201	HA-1 R variant does not bind to A*0201 encoded molecule
HA-2	YIGSVLISV	Class IC myosin family member	Hematopoietic cells	A*0201	nd
H-Y	SPSVDKARAEL SPAVDKAQAEL	SMCY SMCX	Ubiquitous	B*0702	Females do not carry a Y chromosome and react to variant male SMCY peptide
H-Y	FKDSICQV FKDSIC(-C)QV[d]	SMCY	Ubiquitous	A*0201	Both bind A*0201 encoded molecule, but peptide with modified cysteine preferentially recognized by T-cells
H-Y	IVDSLTEMY IVDC(-C)LTEMY[d]	DFFRX DFFRY	Ubiquitous	A*0101	Both bind A*0101 encoded molecule, but male peptide DFFRY with modified cysteine preferentially recognized by T-cells
HB-1	EEKRGSLHVW EEKRGSLYVW	HB-1 gene	Transformed B cells[e]	B*4402 B*4403	Both bind B*44 encoded molecule, but HB-1 Y variant not recognized by T-cells

[a] References 106–112.
[b] Bold denotes variant amino acid residues in peptides.
[c] HLA molecules other than those listed may bind each mHag, but studies have not been performed.
[d] (-C) indicates a disulfide bonded cysteine.
[e] High levels of expression in B-cell acute lymphoblastic leukemia and in small percentage of B-cell lymphomas and undifferentiated B-cell leukemias. Also high expression levels in EBV transformed B-cells. Very low levels of expression detected in normal B-cells and in testis.

because each HLA allelic product binds peptides that fit a specific binding motif and, thus, each mHag is only bound by certain HLA molecules. Therefore, the mHag(s) of significance differ widely depending on which HLA alleles are carried by the tissue donor and recipient (transplant pair). For example, mHag HA-1 could have an impact if the donor or recipient expresses HLA-A*0201 and there is HA-1 disparity between the transplant pair.[106,107] Recognition of the H allelic form of the HA-1 peptide bound to the A*0201 encoded molecule stimulates allorecognition. HA-1 would be of no consequence to the graft when, for instance, both donor and recipient are homozygous for HLA-A*0101, as HA-1 H is not able to bind to this HLA-A molecule and consequently is never presented to T-cells. To date, the HA-1 R peptide does not appear to be recognized by the immune response. HA-1 also can be used to demonstrate the importance of the type of tissue involved in the transplant. HA-1 is expressed only on cells of hematopoietic origin. Therefore, HA-1 most likely would not be pertinent in the case of a kidney transplant, even if the transplant pair expresses HLA-A*0201, since HA–1 would not be expressed by the transplanted kidney.

Because some mHags may have a major impact on graft outcome in HLA-matched transplants,[113] research efforts are now focused on the identification of the amino acid sequence, the source protein, the HLA restriction, and the tissue expression patterns of specific mHags and on the evaluation of their impact on graft outcome. Once characterized, mHags can be included in matching protocols when they are pertinent to transplantation of tissue.[114]

Other immune system receptors that recognize histocompatibility molecules as their ligands

Several families of receptors that interact with histocompatibility molecules, supplemental to the TCR, were identified and characterized in the 1990s. The quest to find a receptor(s) involved in NK-cell discrimination of normal cells from malignant and infected cells led to the identification and characterization of the first two receptor families (killer cell inhibitory receptors and CD94/NKG2). Members of these two families were found to recognize specific groups of MHC class I molecules and regulate NK-cell function. Since these initial findings, another family of receptors (immunoglobulin-like transcripts) were identified and characterized. These receptors are expressed by many immune system cell types and appear to regulate a variety of immune cell functions. Their role in transplantation is not yet defined.

Killer-cell inhibitory receptors

The killer-cell inhibitory receptors (KIR) are, at least, a 12-member family of proteins whose genes are encoded on chromosome 19.[115,116] The KIR, like the HLA molecules and TCR, belong to the Ig protein superfamily and possess either two (KIR2D) or three (KIR3D) glycosylated extracellular Ig-like domains (Fig. 32.12). KIR are expressed

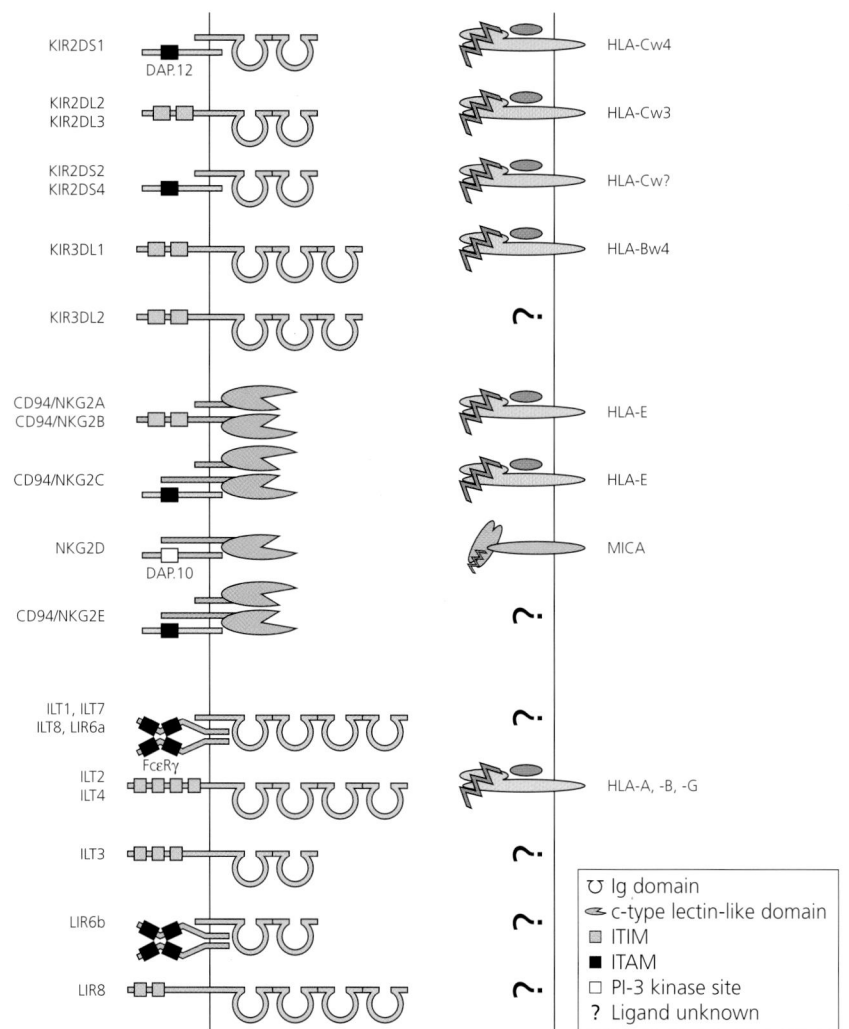

Fig. 32.12 Examples of the three receptor families that recognize HLA molecules as their ligands. The killer cell inhibitory receptors (KIR, blue, top) have either two or three extracellular Ig-like domains. Inhibitory KIR have long cytoplasmic tails and signal via immunoreceptor tyrosine based inhibitory motifs (ITIM, gray box). Activating KIR with short cytoplasmic tails associate with a signaling protein called DAP. 12 (yellow) that has an immunoreceptor tyrosine-based activation motif (ITAM) (black box) in its cytoplasmic tail. The ligands for many of the KIR are groups of class I HLA molecules (heavy chain, green; β_2m, lavender; peptide, red). For example, KIR2DS1 recognizes HLA-C class I molecules that possess the HLA-Cw4 public epitope such as those specified by HLA-Cw*0403, *0707 and *1205. Other two domain KIR (e.g. KIR2DL3) recognize HLA-C class I molecules that possess the HLA-Cw3 public epitope such as molecules encoded by Cw*0302 and *0702. Some three domain KIR recognize all HLA-B class I molecules that possess the HLA-Bw4 public epitope (see Table 32.11). Some KIR recognize groups of HLA-C or -B molecules, but the specific group has not been definitively determined (denoted by HLA-Cw?). The ligand for other KIR is unknown (denoted by question mark). The CD94 and NKG2 family of receptors (orange, center) are members of the c-type lectin superfamily. NKG2A, -B, -C and -E are expressed as heterodimers with CD94. NKG2D is expressed as a monomer. Like the KIR, inhibitory members contain ITIM in their cytoplasmic tails, while activating members associate with DAP.12. The exception is NKG2D, an activating receptor, which associates with another signaling protein called DAP.10 (gray) that is similar to DAP.12, but possesses a phosphatidylinositol-3 (PI-3) kinase binding site (open box) instead of an ITAM. The ligand for CD94/NKG2A, -B and -C is the non-classical MHC class I molecule, HLA-E (green; β_2m, lavender; peptide, red). NKG2D recognizes the MHC class I chain-related A (MICA) molecule (lavender; antigen, red). The ligand for CD94/NKG2E has not been identified. The immunoglobulin-like transcript (ILT)/leukocyte immunoglobulin-like transcripts (LIR) family of receptors have either two or four extracellular Ig-like domains (cyan, bottom). Again, inhibitory members possess ITIM in their cytoplasmic tails. Activating members associate with Fc epsilon receptor gamma chains (FcεRγ, magenta) that contain ITAM in their cytoplasmic tails. The ligand recognized by two family members (ILT2 and ILT4) is encoded by several alleles of HLA-A, -B and -G. The ligand(s) recognized by the remaining family members remains to be determined.

primarily by NK cells, but also are expressed on a subset of T-cells and regulate (inhibit or activate) the function of these cells. The signal generated by a KIR is dictated by the cytoplasmic tail it encodes. Members that generate inhibitory signals have a long cytoplasmic tail (e.g. KIR3DL1 and KIR2DL2) which contains immunoreceptor tyrosine-based inhibitory motifs (ITIM). Binding of the inhibitory KIR to its ligand leads to phosphorylation of the tyrosine residue in each ITIM and ultimately to inhibition of NK and T-cell functions. Activating KIR family members have a short cytoplasmic tail without ITIM (e.g. KIR2DS1 and KIR2DS4). Instead, these members associate via a conserved positively charged residue in their transmembrane regions with a protein, called DAP.12, that contains immunoreceptor tyrosine-based activation motifs (ITAM) in its cytoplasmic tail. Interaction of an activating KIR with its ligand causes phosphorylation of the ITAM in DAP.12 which ultimately results in activation of NK and T-cell functions. DAP.12 has almost no extracellular region and does not interact with the ligands.

Classical MHC class I molecules serve as the ligand for several of the KIR family members (Fig. 32.12). Some KIR with two extracellular Ig-like domains interact with groups of HLA-C molecules. Almost all HLA-C molecules can be divided into one of two groups (Cw3-like and Cw4-like) based on the presence of a shared (public) epitope determined by amino acid residues 77 and 80 in the α1 domain of the HLA-C molecule. HLA-C molecules that belong to the Cw3 group have a serine at residue 77 and an asparagine at residue 80 and those that belong to the Cw4 group have an asparagine at residue 77 and a lysine at residue 80. HLA-Cw3 group molecules are ligands for KIR2DL2 and KIR2DL3, while HLA-Cw4 group molecules are ligands for KIR2DL1 and KIR2DS1. Some KIR with three extracellular Ig-like domains interact with groups of HLA-B molecules. The interaction is dependent on the Bw4 and Bw6 public epitope split which is determined by the amino acid sequence between residues 77 and 83 of the α1 domain of the HLA-B molecules. For example, HLA-B molecules with the Bw4 public epitope are ligands for KIR3DL1. To date, no three domain KIR have been found to interact with HLA-B molecules containing the Bw6 public epitope. Some HLA-A molecules also share the Bw4 and Bw6 public epitopes, but are not recognized as ligands for KIR. Thus, other residues not shared between HLA-B and HLA-A molecules are likely involved in the interaction with KIR. Peptide also can influence the KIR/HLA interaction. It recently was shown that certain amino acid residues when present at two positions in the HLA-bound peptide can disrupt the interaction between the KIR and the HLA molecules.[117] Ligands for some KIR have not been identified.

KIR may have an impact on transplantation outcome. First, there appears to be allelic variants of the KIR genes[118] and possibly different haplotypes in the human population,[119,120] similar to HLA molecules. Thus, the repertoire of KIR expressed by different individuals may vary. Second, each KIR recognizes a different set of HLA molecules. These observations suggest that differences in KIR or in the HLA molecules expressed by a transplant pair could impact NK and T-cell recognition of donor and recipient tissues and, ultimately, transplant outcome. In HSC transplantation, this is important not only to GVHD, but also to graft rejection since NK cells are relatively radioresistant and may not be destroyed during the pre-transplant conditioning regimens.

CD94/NKG2

CD94 and the NKG2 family (NKG2A-NKG2F) are transmembrane glycoproteins with homology to the c-type lectin superfamily and their genes are encoded in the NK complex on chromosome 12.[84,115,116] NKG2A, NKG2C and NKG2E share greater than 90% protein sequence homology and each are expressed as covalently linked heterodimers with CD94. NKG2B is an alternative mRNA splice product of the NKG2A gene and also is expressed as a heterodimer covalently linked to CD94. NKG2D is the renegade member of the NKG2 family. NKG2D shares only ~20% protein identity with other NKG2 family members and does not form a heterodimer with CD94. Instead, NKG2D is expressed as a monomer on the cell surface.[121] It is not known whether NKG2F is expressed.

Like the KIR, CD94/NKG2 and NKG2D receptors are expressed by NK cells and some T-cells and can either inhibit or activate cellular functions.[84,115,116] The action of the CD94/NKG2 heterodimeric receptors is determined by the NKG2 family member, as CD94 has a short cytoplasmic tail of eight amino acids with no known signaling motifs. CD94/NKG2A and CD94/NKG2B are inhibitory as a result of the two ITIM in the NKG2A and NKG2B cytoplasmic tails. NKG2C and NKG2E lack ITIM in their cytoplasmic tails and, like activating KIR, are associated non-covalently with DAP.12 and are activating receptors. NKG2D also activates NK and T-cells.[101] Signaling is achieved by association with DAP.10 which contains a phosphatidylinositol-3 kinase binding site in its cytoplasmic tail.[121]

CD94/NKG2A, CD94/NKG2B and CD94/NKG2C recognize the non-classical class I molecule HLA-E as their ligand. Polymorphism has not been demonstrated in these receptors, nor is it likely that extensive polymorphism will be demonstrated, since their ligand, HLA-E, is highly conserved in the population. On the other hand, it has been demonstrated that the HLA-bound peptide can affect CD94/NKG2A recognition of HLA-E.[122] This could have consequences on the regulation of NK and T-cell recognition of tissues in transplantation, especially since there is polymorphism in the HLA class I leader sequences bound by HLA-E. NKG2D was recently shown to interact with MICA.[101] Although NKG2D polymorphisms have not been described, differences in NKG2D may exist between individuals since MICA, its ligand, is highly polymorphic. Regardless, it is possible that NKG2D might have aberrant interactions with some MICA allelic products and, ergo, affect NK and T-cell responses to grafts. The ligand for CD94/NKG2E has not been identified and its immune function awaits definition.

Immunoglobulin-like transcripts

The immunoglobulin-like transcripts (ILT) or leukocyte immunoglobulin-like receptors (LIR) are a multigene family located on the long arm of chromosome 19 closely linked to the KIR genes.[123,124] Ten ILT members have been identified, nine of which are glycosylated transmembrane proteins and one being a glycosylated soluble molecule. The ILT, like the KIR, belong to the Ig superfamily and have either two or four Ig-like extracellular domains (see Fig. 32.12). There are inhibitory and activating ILT receptors, similar to the KIR and CD94/NKG2 receptor families. Inhibitory ILT have long cytoplasmic tails that contain 2–4 ITIM and activating ILT have short cytoplasmic tails devoid of known signaling motifs. Activating ILT do not associate with DAP.12 or DAP.10. Instead, these receptors associate with the Fc epsilon receptor γ chain which contains an ITAM in its cytoplasmic tail.

Distinct to the NK cell receptor families, the ILT receptors are expressed primarily on myeloid cells such as monocytes, macrophages and dendritic cells.[123] Some ILT family members, however, are also expressed on B-cells and on subsets of NK and T-cells. Two of the inhibitory ILT, ILT4 and ILT2, interact with several allelic products of HLA-A -B and -G genes. ILT4 appears to regulate cytokine production by dendritic cells and inflammatory responses by monocytes and macrophages. ILT2 has been shown to inhibit NK cell mediated lysis and increase the antigenic threshold required to activate B-cells and CD8+ T-cells. The ligands recognized by other members of the ILT receptor family remain elusive.

There appears to be a fair degree of polymorphism in the ILT receptor genes which clusters in several discrete areas of the extracellular domains.[123] The functional significance of these polymorphisms is not known, but they could alter the allelic specificity of the HLA-A,-B

and -G molecules recognized by these receptors which could have consequences in transplantation outcome.

Techniques for the identification of HLA polymorphism

Since differences in HLA proteins may stimulate allorecognition during transplantation of human tissues, selection of individuals expressing the same HLA molecules (an HLA identical or matched donor) has been used to decrease the detrimental immune response. HLA alleles and differences in the HLA proteins specified by different alleles are identified through a variety of testing methods including serology, cellular assays, and DNA-based detection methods. This process is termed tissue or HLA typing. The methods and quality control for typing have been described.[125,126] HLA-testing laboratories are accredited through the American Society for Histocompatibility and Immunogenetics (ASHI), the European Foundation for Immunogenetics (EFI) and other organizations.

Serologic detection of class I and class II molecules

Lymphocyte microcytotoxicity testing has been used for HLA typing since the 1960s. This assay is still fairly widely used to detect HLA-A and-B polymorphism, but has been replaced by DNA-based testing for detecting HLA-C and class II (HLA-DR,-DQ,-DP) polymorphism. It is likely that DNA-based testing for HLA-A and-B will replace serologic testing over the next few years (Table 32.8).

The HLA phenotype is determined by testing unseparated lymphocyte preparations or T-lymphocytes (for HLA-A,-B,-C) or enriched B-lymphocytes (for HLA-DR, -DQ) for the presence of specific HLA molecules as detected by a panel of well-characterized HLA antibody preparations (alloantisera or monoclonal antibodies).[125,127] Cells are distributed into multiple wells of a multiwell plate (typing tray). Each well contains a specific antibody preparation. In the first step of the procedure, the lymphocytes are incubated with the antibody reagents. In the second step, complement is added in excess and the lymphocytes are incubated for an additional time period. If the lymphocytes carry a cell surface HLA molecule recognized by a complement-fixing antibody, the antibody binds to the cells and the cells are subsequently lysed following addition of complement. Following termination of the reaction and staining, the percent lysis of the cells is determined for each antibody reagent using a micro-

Table 32.8 Comparison of HLA testing methods

Criteria	Method	
	Serology	DNA-based (SSP/SSOPH)
Reagents	Human alloantisera or monoclonal antibodies	Synthetic oligonucleotides
Reagent supply	Limited	Unlimited
Reagent specificity	Complex alloantisera polyspecific and crossreactive; monoclonal antibody availability limited	Defined by nucleotide sequence; reagents can be synthesized to detect new polymorphisms
Ability to distinguish alleles	Specificity of lots may alter over time; not available to distinguish all alleles	Alleles defined although test may require several steps and alleles may be missed if not known at time of testing
Identification of relevant polymorphisms	Alloantisera contain antibodies produced by sensitized individuals potentially targeting 'relevant' polymorphisms	Polymorphisms detected may be of unknown relevance
Test substrate	Viable peripheral blood lymphocytes; requires 10–20 ml blood	Any nucleated cell; 0.2–1 ml blood often sufficient; less susceptible to poor cell viability
Use in clinical laboratory	Used for many years; commercial typing trays available	More recent technology; typing kits commercially available, but issues still to be addressed
Use in large-scale testing	Has been used, but reagents often suboptimal due to cost considerations	Robust in large-scale screening

SSOPH, sequence – specific oligonucleotide probe hybridization; SSP, sequence – specific priming.

scope and a numerical grade is assigned (e.g. 1 = 0–10% lysis, 6 = 51–80%, 8 = 81–100%). Scores of 6–8 indicate that the specific HLA molecules detected by the antibody reagent are present.

The antibodies used to detect specific HLA molecules (or 'specificities') are derived primarily from the sera of alloimmunized individuals including multiparous women, transplant recipients, and multi-transfused patients. Most HLA alloantisera preparations react with more than one HLA allelic product. This phenomenon results from the presence in a single alloantiserum of multiple antibodies with distinct specificities which detect different HLA molecules. The phenomenon can also result when a single antibody detects more than one HLA allelic product (cross-reactivity). The latter occurs because polymorphic sequence cassettes are shared among HLA molecules. Because of the complex reactivity patterns of alloantisera, several alloantisera are used to define each specificity. To address this complexity, monoclonal antibodies detecting HLA specificities have been generated; however, the availability of these reagents is limited.

Cellular detection of HLA disparity

The response of one cell (responder) in tissue culture to the foreign histocompatibility molecules on the surface of a second cell (stimulator) is called the mixed leukocyte culture (MLC) or mixed lymphocyte reaction (MLR).[128] The response is made unidirectional by preventing cells from one of the two individuals from replicating by treating those cells with radiation or an alkylating agent, such as mitomycin-C, prior to addition to the culture. The MLC represents a summation response of a responder cell to differences in the HLA class II molecules (HLA-DR, -DQ, and -DP) encoded by the irradiated stimulator cell haplotypes. The response to DR molecules predominates. When reference cells which are homozygous for genes in the MHC region (homozygous typing cells or HTC) are used as stimulators, the MLC response is used to define HLA-D specificities (Dw1–Dw26). Responder cells showing a weak or no response to a given HTC are assumed to express the same HLA class II alleles as the HTC. Other cellular assays related to the MLC rely on primed T-lymphocytes or T-cell clones. Both assays utilize isolated populations of T-lymphocytes primed to recognize differences in class II molecules expressed by another individual. The use of cellular assays to determine the similarity between two individuals has declined significantly because DNA-based testing procedures can now be used to identify class II disparity between individuals and because the MLC can be influenced by a variety of factors including the health of the individuals contributing the cells, the patient's disease, and the history of prior transfusion.[129]

Other cellular assays measure the frequency of cytotoxic or helper T-lymphocytes in the potential HSC donor. Limiting dilution is used to isolate and measure the frequency of T-lymphocyte precursors which respond to recipient cells. The differences stimulating these responses are thought to be HLA class I differences or minor histocompatibility antigens for cytotoxic precursors and HLA class II differences for helper precursors. The correlation between the precursor frequency and transplantation outcome is controversial.[130,131]

DNA-based identification of class I and class II alleles

With the advent of rapid and reliable methods for the isolation and characterization of class I and II genes and the determination of the nucleotide sequences of class I and II alleles, it has become possible to use DNA-based methods that target differences in the nucleotide sequences of alleles for HLA typing.[132] Commercial kits employing all of the methodologies described below are available although some laboratories design their own reagents.[133]

Any cell with a nucleus can be used as a source of DNA; however, DNA is usually prepared from a small quantity (0.2–1 ml) of whole blood. The sensitivity of detection of HLA alleles is enhanced greatly by the amplification of DNA encoding HLA genes using the polymerase chain reaction (PCR).[134] Two synthetic single-stranded DNA molecules (oligonucleotides) of approximately 21 nucleotides in length containing sequences found flanking a specific HLA gene are used as primers to initiate synthesis of millions of copies of that gene for use in the HLA-typing reaction (Fig. 32.13). Cycling of the synthesis reaction through the steps of denaturation of double stranded DNA, annealing (or hybridization) of the primers, and DNA synthesis results in the amplified product. Many typing reactions utilize primer sequences that are broadly specific and are shared by all alleles at an HLA locus. Other typing procedures utilize primer sets that are narrowly specific and are shared by only a subset of alleles at a locus. In this way, the laboratory can isolate large quantities of specific HLA alleles for identification as described below.

Sequence-specific priming (SSP)

One method of typing uses a large panel of pairs of amplification primers.[135,136] Each pair of primers anneals to a limited number of potential alleles. In the subsequent PCR, only certain primer pairs will amplify the DNA from a given individual. Amplification is detected by electrophoresis in an agarose gel or, if the DNA is labeled with a dye during amplification, by fluorescence. The HLA alleles carried by an individual are then determined by the pattern of positive and negative amplifications

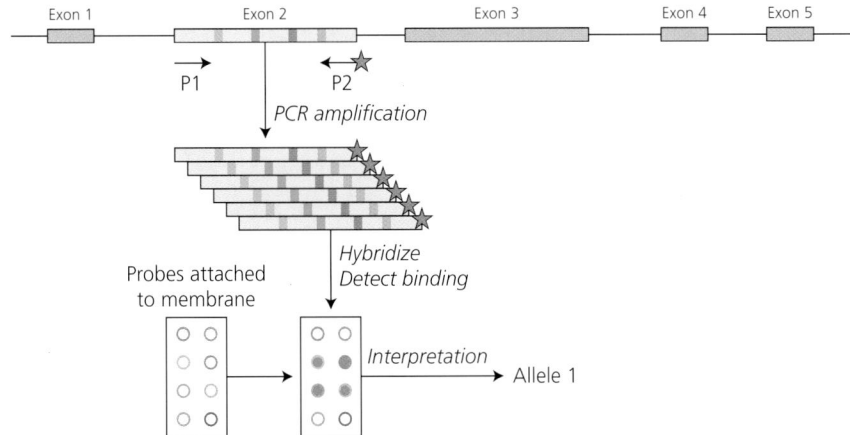

Fig. 32.13 One procedure used for DNA-based typing is sequence specific oligonucleotide probe hybridization. An HLA gene is amplified by the polymerase chain reaction using primers (P1, P2) which flank the polymorphic exon (in this example, exon 2 of DRB1). The DNA is labeled (indicated by a star) during amplification. The labeled DNA is hybridized to a series of oligonucleotide probes which are fixed to a solid support (a membrane or plate). Each probe detects a polymorphic region of exon 2 (indicated by colored blocks). The denatured DNA binds to those probes which contain sequences complementary to HLA allele sequences contained within the amplified DNA. Binding of the labeled DNA is detected by a variety of methods. The positive and negative probe hybridization results are interpreted by comparison of the nucleotide sequences of the probes with the sequences of known HLA alleles to determine those present in the sample.

with the primer panel using a knowledge of which alleles amplify with which primer pairs.

Sequence-specific oligonucleotide probe hybridization (SSOPH)

It is possible to use the binding of synthetic single-stranded DNA molecules approximately 18 nucleotides in length (probes) to identify HLA alleles (e.g. see refs 133 and 137). A panel of probes, each capable of identifying a short polymorphic region of a group of HLA alleles, is hybridized to denatured PCR-amplified DNA. Because each allele has a unique combination of polymorphic sequence cassettes (see section on Diversity), specific alleles are identified through the use of several probes and/or the use of SSP followed by hybridization with several probes. In one format, as an example, the oligonucleotide probes are bound to a solid support (Fig. 32.13). DNA from the sample to be tested is amplified by PCR using primers labeled, for example, with biotin. The biotin, which binds to avidin, is incorporated into the amplified DNA. Following denaturation, the labeled DNA is incubated with the immobilized probes and will hybridize to any complementary probes. After visualization (using an avidin-linked detection system), the pattern of hybridization, including which probes bound and which did not, can be read to determine the nucleotide polymorphisms present or absent. Comparison of this result with the known sequences of alleles at the locus will predict the HLA alleles present or absent.

Gel mobility assays of DNA strands

Other, although little used, methods of identification of HLA alleles analyze the electrophoretic mobility of amplified DNA, either as denatured single stranded DNA (sequence-specific conformational polymorphism or SSCP) or as renatured double-stranded DNA (heteroduplex analysis). The techniques are based on the premise that each allele (characterized by a unique sequence of nucleotides) will have a unique mobility upon electrophoresis. For instance, in heteroduplex analysis, the PCR-amplified DNA strands are denatured and allowed to reanneal under non-stringent conditions. In a heterozygote (with two alleles present), this results in two homoduplexes containing the original DNA duplexes present before denaturation and two heteroduplexes containing the strand of one allele hybridized with the complementary but mismatched strand of the second allele. The mobility of the four DNA duplexes is compared to the mobility of amplified DNA from known HLA alleles to identify which alleles are present. A variant of

the heteroduplex approach, termed reference strand conformational analysis (RSCA), introduces a reference allele into the hybridization mixture.[138] Labeling of one strand of this reference allele results only in the labeling of the heteroduplexes which incorporate this strand. Visualization of the label simplifies the electrophoretic pattern which facilitates interpretation. These procedures are primarily useful in comparisons of specific individuals, such as the comparison of the HLA alleles of a patient to those of several selected donors.

Nucleic acid sequence-based typing (SBT)

A final method of identification of HLA alleles involves the direct determination of the DNA sequences of the HLA alleles carried by an individual (e.g. see Refs 139 and 140). Alleles are identified following PCR amplication. The choice of PCR primers determines whether the alleles will be isolated separately based on sequence polymorphisms (SSP) or whether the two alleles of a locus will be characterized as a mixture. Dideoxynucleotide terminators are used in the synthesis of DNA fragments.[141] If the dideoxynucleotide is labeled, for example, fluorescent DNA fragments are generated by the synthesis reaction. These fragments are identified by mobility during gel electrophoresis. Automated instruments equipped with lasers detect the unique fluorescent tags associated with each dideoxynucleotide (A,T,C,G) and interpret results using software programs. The presence of two alleles in the sequencing reaction is indicated by the presence of two half-height peaks at each polymorphic nucleotide position.[142] Sequencing is labor intensive and highly complex, but is the most powerful approach to determine if two individuals share the same HLA alleles.

Measurement of sensitization to histocompatibility differences

Individuals may become sensitized to foreign histocompatibility molecules through transfusion, pregnancy or prior transplantation. This sensitization may result in the presence of HLA-specific antibodies and/or significant numbers of cytotoxic T-cells which may cause lysis of cells expressing foreign HLA molecules. If a presensitized patient, such as a patient with severe aplastic anemia or a prospective kidney transplant patient who has received prior blood transfusions, undergoes transplantation, these pre-existing antibodies or T-cells may cause destruction of the graft. In solid organ (kidney) transplantation, antibodies are detected prospectively by incubation of serum from the putatively sensitized individual with a panel of cells expressing a variety of HLA molecules.[125,127] This test is a measurement of panel reactive antibodies (PRA). Once a potential tissue donor has been selected, patient antibodies specific for cells of the donor are detected in a donor-specific cross-match. There are several approaches used to measure alloreactive antibodies which vary in sensitivity and in the level of information provided on the specificity of the antibodies.[125,127] In some centers, an HLA mismatch between a patient and donor with a positive donor directed cross-match would be considered a high risk for graft failure after HSC transplantation.[143]

HLA assignments

HLA terminology is assigned by a World Health Organization (WHO) committee for HLA nomenclature. Several different naming systems are in use, each the result of the technology used to identify HLA diversity: serologic (Table 32.9), cellular, or DNA based (Tables 32.1 and 32.2). The nomenclature is described in reports of the HLA nomenclature committee[17,144] and on a web site.[18] Since not all techiques identify specific HLA alleles, the assignments are called HLA 'types'. Individuals who differ at the level of resolution of each test are assigned different HLA 'types'. For example, an individual tested by serology might express HLA types, HLA-A1 and -A2 (heterozygous) while another individual might express HLA-A2 and -A74. Within the limits of resolution of the serologic technique, the two individuals in this example share one HLA-A type (A2) but differ for the second (A1 vs A74). Within the limits of DNA-based testing, however, these individuals may differ in the A2 allele carried by each individual, for example A*0201 and A*0206.

Serologic specificities

Historically, serologic and cellular reagents were used to define HLA types. These reagents defined specificities (or determinants) localized to one or several HLA molecules; these specificities were used as surrogates of alleles. The specificities identified through these methods were defined and standardized during international workshops in which typing reagents and cells were exchanged among participating laboratories and a consensus reached on the definition of each specificity.[6] Serologic specificities have been used to define diversity in the HLA-A, -B, -C, -DR and -DQ molecules (Table 32.9). These specificities were named by the HLA molecule and by a numerical designation based on the order of discovery. As additional

Table 32.9 HLA class I and class II specificities defined by serology[a,b]

A	B		C	DR	DQ
A1	B5	B50(21)	Cw1[e]	DR1	DQ1
A2	B7	B51(5)	Cw2	DR103	DQ2
A203	B703	B5102	Cw3	DR2	DQ3
A210	B8	B5103	Cw4	DR3	DQ4
A3	B12	B52(5)	Cw5	DR4	DQ5(1)
A9	B13	B53	Cw6	DR5	DQ6(1)
A10	B14	B54(22)	Cw7	DR6	DQ7(3)
A11	B15	B55(22)	Cw8	DR7	DQ8(3)
A19	B16	B56(22)	Cw9(w3)	DR8	DQ9(3)
A23(9)[c]	B17	B57(17)	Cw10(w3)	DR9	
A24(9)	B18	B58(17)		DR10	
A2403	B21	B59		DR11(5)	
A25(10)	B22	B60(40)		DR12(5)	
A26(10)	B27	B61(40)		DR13(6)	
A28	B2708	B62(15)		DR14(6)	
A29(19)	B35	B63(15)		DR1403	
A30(19)	B37	B64(14)		DR1404	
A31(19)	B38(16)	B65(14)		DR15(2)	
A32(19)	B39(16)	B67		DR16(2)	
A33(19)	B3901	B70		DR17(3)	
A34(10)	B3902	B71(70)		DR18(3)	
A36	B40	B72(70)		DR51[f]	
A43	B4005	B73		DR52[f]	
A66(10)	B41	B75(15)		DR53[f]	
A68(28)	B42	B76(15)			
A69(28)	B44(12)	B77(15)			
A74(19)	B45(12)	B78			
A80	B46	B81			
	B47	Bw4[d]			
	B48	Bw6[d]			
	B49(21)				

[a] Reprinted with permission of Munksgaard.[144] DP is difficult to define by serology.
[b] Each column of the table is independent and unrelated to the other columns.
[c] () indicates the broad serologic specificity as described in Table 32.10. The serologic type may be listed without the broad specificity. For example, both A23(9) and A23 are correct designations.
[d] Bw4 and Bw6 are serologic specificities found on multiple HLA-B and -A molecules.
[e] 'w' is added to avoid confusion with the complement genes.
[f] DR51, DR52 and DR53 are serologic specificities associated with a number of DR serologic types as described in Table 32.4.

reagents were identified, serologically defined specificities were often subdivided (i.e. 'split'). For example, the serologic specificity HLA-B5 defined in the 1967 international workshop was subdivided into HLA-B51 and -B52 as a result of the reagents tested in the 1975 workshop. Table 32.10 lists the broader, shared (supertypic) specificities for the current 'split' (subtypic) specificities.

The numbering system used to define HLA 'types' is based on the date of assignment so that the relationships among various types is not immediately clear. Thus, for example, subdivisions of B5 were assigned as B51 and B52 since they were the 51st and 52nd serologic specificities to be assigned. Their relationship to B5 is not immediately clear unless their more complete nomenclature, B51(5) and B52(5), is provided. The assignments associated with

Table 32.10 Serologic splits and associated antigens[a,b]

Original broad specificities	Splits	Associated antigens[c]
A2		A203, A210
A9	A23, A24	A2403
A10	A25, A26, A34, A66	
A19	A29, A30, A31, A32, A33, A74	
A28	A68, A69	
B5	B51, B52	B5102, B5103
B7		B703
B12	B44, B45	
B14	B64, B65	
B15	B62, B63, B75, B76, B77	
B16	B38, B39	B3901, B3902
B17	B57, B58	
B21	B49, B50	B4005
B22	B54, B55, B56	
B27		B2708
B40	B60, B61	
B70	B71, B72	
Cw3	Cw9, Cw10	
DR1		DR103
DR2	DR15, DR16	
DR3	DR17, DR18	
DR5	DR11, DR12	
DR6	DR13, DR14	DR1403, DR1404
DQ1	DQ5, DQ6	
DQ3	DQ7, DQ8, DQ9	

[a] Reprinted with permission of Munksgaard.[144]

[b] Each row of the table lists a broad specificity and its associated splits and antigens. For example, A203 and A210 antigens are variants of A2; A68 and A69 are 'splits' of A28.

[c] The associated antigens can be considered variants of the broad serologic specificity. These serologic specificities were thought to detect the product of a specific HLA allele. For example, the A203 serologic specificity was thought to be located on a molecule encoded by an allele in the A2 family, A*0203. It is now thought that it is unlikely that a serologic reagent will detect the product of only a single allele and the serologic designations of associated antigens, like A203 or DR103, may be discontinued.

Table 32.11 HLA class I cross-reactive epitope groups (CREGs)[a]

CREG	Associated private specificities
1C	A1, 3, 36, 23, 24, 25, 26, 11, 28, 29, 30, 31, 32, 33, 34
2C	A2, 28, 23, 24, B57, 58
5C	B51, 52, 62, 63, 57, 58, 18, 35, 53, 71, 72
7C	B7, 13, 27, 54, 55, 56, 60, 61, 41, 42, 47, 48
8C	B8, 63, 64, 18, 38, 39
12C	B44, 45, 49, 50, 13, 60, 61, 41
4C (Bw4)	A23, 24, 25, 32, B13, 27, 37, 38, 44, 47, 49, 51, 52, 53, 57, 58, 59, 63, 77
6C (Bw6)	B7, 8, 18, 35, 39, 41, 42, 45, 46, 48, 50, 54, 55, 56, 60, 61, 62, 64, 65, 71, 72, 73

[a] Printed with permission of Human Immunology.[147] The inclusion of HLA specificities within a CREG is not standard (i.e. CREG nomenclature has not been assigned by consensus of the HLA community). There is considerable overlap between the various groupings reported in the literature.[148,149]

the HLA-A and HLA-B serologic specificities are further complicated because it was not initially appreciated that these were carried by two allelic series (two different loci).

Thus, the naming system is based on a single numerical series. The names were derived from the fact that the LA 1,2,3 allelic series (HLA-A) was described by Payne in 1967 and the 4a,4b allelic series (HLA-B) was described by van Rood in 1969.[5,6] Thus, numerical designations of HLA-A include HLA-A1, -A2, -A3, -A9, -A10, -A11, etc., while the HLA-B designations include the remaining numbers in the series, HLA-Bw4, -B5, -Bw6, -B7, -B8, -B12, etc.

The HLA-Bw4 and -Bw6 serologic specificities are broad, supertypic determinants which reside on the same molecule as the B locus subtypic specificities. HLA-B locus molecules (and some HLA-A locus molecules) characteristically carry either Bw4 or Bw6 specificities. The 'w' in the name indicates the preliminary or workshop designation for a specificity. In the case of Bw4 and Bw6, the 'w' designation has been retained because of the shared nature of the determinant. The region of the HLA-B molecule carrying the Bw4/Bw6 specificities has been identified to lie in the α1 alpha helix between amino acid residues 77 and 83 (see Fig. 32.7).[145]

Antibody reactivity patterns have been used to group HLA-A and HLA-B molecules into cross-reactive epitope groups (CREG).[146,147] Examples of CREGs are listed in Table 32.11. An antigenic determinant (epitope) shared among members of a CREG is called a public specificity. Class I molecules within a CREG share one or more determinants that are not shared by molecules in another CREG. These groupings have been used as the basis for matching schemes for selection of solid organ donors[148,149] and to predict the reactivity of HLA-specific antibodies in sensitized patients.[147]

Limitations in serologic testing reagents have resulted in inconsistent assignments of some HLA types. This can complicate the selection of HLA-matched donors from HSC donor registries and umbilical cord blood banks. The assignment of a specificity is dependent on the antibody reagents used and on the HLA molecules expressed by an individual. The presence of two similar HLA allelic products, for example B35 and B53 in a heterozygote, can produce typing results that are difficult to interpret. This may result in an individual receiving different assignments in different typing laboratories. Likewise, the presence of a homozygous allele can be over-interpreted by some laboratories resulting in two antigen assignments instead of one. Other assignments might be missed if reagents are suboptimal or not available. For example, the HLA-A74 antigen has been frequently missed by serologic testing because robust sera defining this type were not routinely available. A search for a patient with an HLA-A type, HLA-A1,-A74, might require the selection of donors typed as only A1 and performance of additional testing to determine if any of these donors might also express A74. Because time and funding is limited for most searches, the ability to accurately predict which donors to select for further testing is important. In these cases, access to experts in histocompatibility testing and to tools such as a software program to predict the combinations of alleles previously observed as haplotypes[150] are essential. With the increased use of DNA-based HLA typing and its increased resolution and consistency, these difficulties are expected to disappear as the number of DNA-typed donors increases.

Cellular specificities

There are 26 HLA-D specificities (Dw1, Dw2, Dw3, etc.) which were identified by mixed leukocyte culture. All of the HLA-D specificities retain the 'w' designation because these specificities are only defined functionally. HLA-DP molecules are not adequately defined serologically although six HLA-DP types (DPw1–DPw6) were originally defined by primed lymphocyte typing. Cellular testing to define HLA specificities has largely been replaced by DNA based testing.

DNA-based allele designations

Nucleotide sequencing has been used to identify the many alleles encoding the HLA molecules. Tables 32.1 and 32.2 list the HLA class I and class II alleles which were current when this chapter was written. Each HLA allele is designated by the name of the gene followed by an asterisk and a 4–7 digit number indicating the allele.[17] Additional and optional letters added to the end of the numerical designation relate to the expression of the allele at the protein level. The nomenclature system is summarized in Table 32.12 and is described below.

The most confusing feature of the allele name is related to the *first two numbers* in the numerical designation of each allele. Initially, the intention of the HLA nomenclature committee was to select these numbers based on the serologic type of the resultant molecule. Thus, the first HLA-A allele characterized from a cell bearing the HLA-A1

Table 32.12 Examples of allele nomenclature and their meaning[a]

Example	Interpretation
Four digit designation: A*0101 B*0703 Cw*1702 DRB1*0101 DQA1*0502	The four digits are based on the serologic assignment or structural similarity (digits 1–2) and on the order in which the allele was described (digits 3–4). The digits are preceded by letters and/or numbers that indicate the HLA locus. An asterisk always separates the name of the locus from the numerical allele designation
Five digit designation: A*02011 vs A*02012 B*51011 vs B*51012 DRB1*11011 vs DRB1*11012 vs DRB1*11013	Alleles that share digits 1–4 differ by silent (synonymous) substitution in the nucleotide sequence of the coding region. These alleles encode the same amino acid sequence
Seven digit designation: B*1501101 vs B*1501102N DRB4*0103101 vs DRB4*0103102N	Alleles differ only by nucleotide sequence outside of the coding region which results in a change in expression i.e. B*1501102N is not expressed as a protein product
Null or N designation: A*0104N (or A*0104) B*1526N (or B*1526) DRB5*0110N (or DRB5*0110)	Allele is not expressed at the protein level. The N indicates a 'null' allele, but its inclusion in the designation is not required i.e. A*0104N = A*0104
Shortened name: A*01 B*08 DRB1*04 A*0201 B*5101 DRB4*0103	An assignment that has narrowed down the possible identity of the HLA alleles carried by an individual to a group of alleles that can be summarized by the use of truncated digits (i.e. A*01 = A*0101 or A*0102 or A*0103 or A*0104; A*0201 = A*02011 or A*02012; DRB4*0103 = DRB4*0103101 or DRB4*0103102N)
Shortened name (related to a serologic broad assignment): A*09 B*05 DRB1*02	An assignment that has narrowed down the possible identity of the HLA alleles carried by an individual to a group of alleles that reflect the DNA equivalent of a broad serologic assignment (see Table 32.10). In the case of A*09, the allele lies within the A*23 or A*24 allele group. Since these alleles encode A23(9) and A24(9) antigens, the nomenclature is based on the serologic broad specificity A9

[a] Reference 17.

serologic specificity was assigned as A*0101 and the first HLA-B allele characterized from a cell bearing the HLA-B8 serologic specificity was assigned as B*0801. Identification of new alleles from other A1 or B8 positive cells led to the assignment of alleles A*0102 and B*0802. Alleles which share the first two digits of their name share extensive sequence homology with other alleles in the group. This sequence similarity is also a criteria for nomenclature assignment and may take precedence over the serologic association in assigning an allele name.

Individuals who carry different alleles usually express HLA molecules with different amino acid sequences. Since most differences lie within the antigen-binding groove of the HLA molecule, it is theoretically possible that these differences will stimulate allorecognition. There are two exceptions in which different allele names may not indicate different HLA molecules: (1) Alleles which differ in the DNA sequence of their protein coding regions but which do not differ in their encoded polypeptides are assigned a five digit designation. The first four digits are shared among these alleles and each allele is distinguished by the addition of a fifth digit (e.g. B*39011 and B*39013). The differences among alleles in these clusters are not important to consider in transplantation matching since these alleles encode the same HLA proteins; however, the differences are important to consider in DNA-based HLA typing if they affect the hybridization of primers and probes. (2) Alleles which have identical nucleotide sequences in their coding regions but which differ in the nucleotide sequences outside of the coding region (e.g. in the sequences of 5′ regulatory regions or in the sequences of introns) have been assigned a seven digit designation (e.g. DRB4*0103101 and DRB4*0103102). The first four digits are shared and each allele is designated by a unique three digit extension (digits 5–7). The differences among alleles in these clusters may or may not be important to consider in transplantation matching depending on the effect of the sequence difference. Allelic differences that result in loss of protein expression are an important consideration in matching, while a difference which has no impact on the expression of the allele is not important to consider in the selection of a donor.

Alleles which are not expressed as proteins at the cell surface may have an 'N' added to their names (e.g. A*0215N; DRB4*0103102N) to indicate 'null'. Since each allele has a unique numerical designation, the 'N' designation is not always written (A*0215 and A*0215N are the same allele). Null alleles are important to consider in transplantation since individuals who carry a null allele are functional homozygotes. For example, an individual who carries A*0101, A*0215N alleles would be serologically typed as A1 only compared to an individual who carries A*0101,A*02011 who would be serologically typed as A1,A2.

National Marrow Donor Program (NMDP) DNA nomenclature

The ability to distinguish among alleles (the level of resolution) by DNA-based typing methods is controlled by the choice and number of reagents used and the typing technique. Large-scale volunteer donor typing for a HSC registry or umbilical cord blood bank is usually carried out at low to intermediate resolution in which the choice of alleles at each HLA locus is narrowed down to a few possibilities. This level of resolution represents a balance between the need for high volume, low cost testing and the need of a physician to rapidly find a HLA-matched donor for their patient. For example, the HLA-DRB1 test results of a volunteer might narrow the possible alleles at this locus to DRB1*1301 or 1320 encoded by one copy of the MHC and DRB1*0403 or *0406 or *0407 or *0411 or *0417 encoded by the second copy of the MHC. In order to include these possibilities within their database, the NMDP has developed a coding system for these multiple allele combinations. Thus, the combination DRB1*1301 or 1320 has been condensed to DRB1*13VS where VS means 01 or 20 and DRB1*0403 or *0406 or *0407 or *0411 or *0417 has been condensed to DRB1*04DZ in which DZ means 03 or 06 or 07 or 11 or 17. The letter codes are purely descriptive, with codes being created only for allele combinations which have been observed during HLA testing. A listing of codes can be found on the NMDP web sites.[151] In contrast, typing of a specific patient who requires a HSC graft and of a specific donor selected for that patient will often identify the specific alleles carried by the two individuals (high or allele level resolution). Table 32.13 provides examples.

Limitations in the assignment of HLA alleles

Since identification of HLA alleles may often be based on partial nucleotide sequence information obtained through the use of a small set of primers and probes, it is possible that the interpretation of the assay results will miss alleles which were unknown at the time of the typing.[152] For example, the identification of the DNA sequence GGTAAGTATAAG encompassing codons 11–14 in the DRB1 gene was once interpreted to mean that the individual carried the allele DRB1*0701 since only DRB1*0701 was known to carry that polymorphic sequence cassette. In 1998, two new alleles were described which also carry

Table 32.13 Patient and potential donor HLA assignments and level of match

	HLA assignment[a]	Method of testing (locus)	Level of match with patient
Patient	A*01,*68; B*07,*08; DRB1*0301,*0701	DNA (HLA-A) DNA (HLA-B) DNA (HLA-DRB1)	HLA-A: Alleles encode A1 and A68 antigens[a] HLA-B: Alleles encode B7 and B8 antigens HLA-DRB1: Alleles encode DR3 and DR7 antigens
Donor 1	A1,68; B7,8; DRB1*0301,*0701	Serology Serology DNA	HLA-A: Identical at split antigen level HLA-B: Identical at split antigen level HLA-DRB1: Identical at allele level
Donor 2	A1,28; B7,8; DRB1*03ASX[b],*0701	Serology Serology DNA	HLA-A: Potentially identical at broad antigen level since A28 may be either A68 or A69 HLA-B: Identical at split antigen level HLA-DRB1: Potentially identical at allele level since DRB1*03ASX may be DRB1*0301 or *0304 or *0306 or *0311
Donor 3	A1,2; B7,8; DRB1*03,*07	Serology Serology DNA	HLA-A: Single antigen mismatch since patient has A68 and donor has a different antigen, A2 HLA-B: Identical at split antigen level HLA-DRB1: Potentially identical at allele level since it is not known which of the many DRB1*03 and DRB1*07 alleles are carried by the donor
Donor 4	A*01,*02; B*07,*08; DRB1*0302,*0701	DNA DNA DNA	HLA-A: Single antigen mismatch since patient has A68 and donor has A2 encoded by A*02 HLA-B: Identical at split antigen level HLA-DRB1: Single allele mismatch since patient and donor carry two different DRB1*03 alleles

[a] Reference 153.
[b] A listing of the letter codes can be found on the NMDP web site.[151] In the NMDP registry, a typing such as A*01 will be listed A*01XX where XX indicates that any allele which begins with A*01 (such as A*0101, A*0102, A*0103, or A*0104N) is potentially present. Likewise, ASX is an NMDP code that indicates multiple allele possibilities.

this sequence, DRB1*0703 and DRB1*0704. Thus, individuals tested prior to 1998 and characterized as carrying DRB1*0701 might alternatively carry DRB1*0703 or DRB1*0704. The continued discovery of new HLA alleles has significant implications for the HLA assignments since HLA types of some individuals are stored and used for many years (e.g. in HSC registries or cord blood banks). For this reason, the NMDP is initiating procedures to collect the raw typing data (i.e. which primers and probes were positive and negative) so that the HLA assignments of volunteer donors can be reinterpreted if new alleles are described. Similarly, an unrelated donor search can take several years and a clinical laboratory, which might type a patient at the start of a search, should also maintain its primary data and update the HLA assignments for that patient as new alleles are described.

Correlation between serologic specificities and DNA-based allele assignments

Today, patients requiring HSC transplants are often typed by DNA-based technologies while registries and banks of potential donors are predominantly composed of serologically typed volunteers or cord blood units. Thus, it is important to understand which HLA alleles correspond to which serologic types. Table 32.14 provides some examples of the association between HLA types. In many cases, the first two numbers assigned to each HLA allele are based on the serologic assignment of the HLA molecule so, for example, alleles such as A*0201, B*2701, and DRB1*0401 correspond to A2, B27, and DR4, respectively. In addition, several alleles may encode the same serologic type such as B*2701, *2702, *2703, and *2704 which all encode a HLA-B molecule carrying a B27 serologic specificity.

It is important to note, however, the many examples where the associations between an allele and the serologic type of the HLA molecule encoded by that allele are not known or are apparently different. For example, even though B*2708 encoded a molecule which bore a B7 serologic determinant, it was found to have a closer structural relationship to alleles in the B*27 group which took precedence in the assignment of the allele name. In this case, the name of the allele can not be used to predict the serologic type of its allelic product.

Still other alleles, like B*8201, have unique serologic reactivity patterns which have not yet received a serologic designation by the HLA nomenclature committee.

Table 32.14 Association between HLA-B*27 alleles and serologic specificities[a]

Allele	Serologic specificity[b]
B*2701	B27
B*2702	B27
B*2703	B27
B*2704	B27
B*2705	B27
B*2706	B27
B*2707	B27
B*2708	B2708 (B7Qui, sera detecting B7 positive and most of B27 sera are negative)
B*2709	B27
B*2710	B27
B*2711	B27 variant (B27 sera positive and some B40 sera positive)
B*2712	B27 variant (most B27 sera negative, sera detecting both B7 and B27 positive, some B40 sera positive)
B*2713	B27
B*2714	Not defined
B*2715	B"X" (B27 sera negative)

[a] Reference 153.
[b] Serologic typing of specific B*27 allelic products.

Furthermore, since many individuals are tested by only DNA-based methods, the HLA molecules encoded by many new HLA alleles have not been characterized by serology. In these cases, the nomenclature assigned to these alleles is based on their structural similarity or dissimilarity to other alleles. This means that some HLA alleles may not have an associated serologic asssignment (see B*2714 in Table 32.14) or that the assignment might consist of a pattern of specificities (see B*2712 in Table 32.14).

At present, the HLA nomenclature committee suggests that each allele name be considered nothing more than a unique identifier for the allele. In many cases, the name may also carry other information regarding the serologic assignment or the structural similarity but, because this is not uniformly true, it is best to include an HLA expert in the interpretation of any test results. A more detailed discussion of this topic including a table of known serology-allele associations has been published.[153,154]

Identification of HLA in clinical situations

Autoimmunity

Autoimmune diseases are characterized by an abnormal immune response to self antigens. Many of these diseases are associated with the presence of specific HLA types.[48,155] The association of HLA-B27 with ankylosing spondylitis is one of the best known examples. This disease is likely caused by a response of the immune system to antigens on tissues in the affected joints of the back.[156] Approximately 94% of patients with ankylosing spondylitis express B27 compared to 9% of the general population. Yet, since only a fraction of individuals with B27 develop ankylosing spondylitis, B27 is most likely one out of several genetic and/or environmental factors that combine to cause susceptibility to the disease.

A variety of mechanisms involving the HLA molecule have been evoked to explain the observed HLA associations.[48,51,155] One hypothesis suggests that a peptide from a pathogen which mimics a self peptide binds to the HLA molecule associated with the disease to initially stimulate autoreactive T-cells. A second hypothesis suggests that disease occurs as the result of altered thymic selection in which self reactive T-cells escape selection in the thymus as a result of poor self peptide binding properties of the disease associated HLA molecules. Still another hypothesis suggests that it is not the HLA molecule itself, but the product of another as yet unknown gene within the MHC which affects susceptibility. It is likely that the immune mechanisms resulting in a loss of tolerance to self antigens will vary among autoimmune diseases; thus, elucidation of the role that HLA plays will await the unraveling of each complex disease.

Identity

Because of the extraordinary polymorphism of HLA genes and haplotypes, HLA testing has been used to establish a level of certainty about the identity of an individual. Thus, HLA testing has been used to establish paternity, to determine the presence of an individual at a crime scene, and to identify human remains where physical identification is difficult. HLA has also been used to establish chimerism; that is, the presence of tissue from more than a single individual. For example, following a HSC transplant, the blood and marrow of the recipient will contain donor cells along with some fraction of the patient's orginal cells. The analysis of HLA has been used to monitor the extent of engraftment of foreign tissue. Today, other highly polymorphic regions of the human genome (e.g. variable tandem repeats (VNTR) and short tandem repeats (STR)) are more commonly used to establish identity.[157]

Cell, tissue and organ transplantation

Allogeneic grafts of HSC (primarily bone marrow), organs and other tissues have become everyday life-saving procedures over the last 30 years.[4] During 1999, there were approximately 5000 marrow transplants, 22 000 solid organ transplants and innumerable transplants of non-viable tissues such as skin and bone in the United States.[158,159]

The necessity for HLA matching of donor and recipient differs for each type of graft. For HSC transplantation, close matching for HLA is required for successful outcome. For kidney transplantation, close matching increases the likelihood of long-term organ survival, but survival of grafts in mismatched donor – recipient pairs is also good. For logistic reasons, HLA matching plays a small role in transplants of organs other than HSC and kidney and outcome relies on management of graft rejection using immune suppression. Grafts of non-viable tissues rarely take HLA matching into consideration, as these non-viable tissues generally are used temporarily (skin) or are used primarily as 'scaffolding' for replacement with autologous tissue.

Solid organ transplantation

According to data reported by the United Network for Organ Sharing (UNOS) Scientific Registry,[158] there were approximately 22 000 transplants of organs in 1999 in the United States. Of these, 12 517 were kidney transplants, 4500 liver, 364 pancreas, 1157 combined kidney and pancreas, 71 intestine, 2185 heart, 48 heart and lung, and 899 lung transplants. Included in this number are 4153 kidney transplants from living donors. All of the other reported transplants were from cadaveric donors.

In the US, there is a nationwide organ sharing system run by UNOS.[158] One of the primary purposes for nationwide organ sharing is to provide an opportunity for matching of kidney recipient and donor for HLA. Organs are allocated based on the best opportunity for successful outcome both for patients local to the organization that obtained the cadaveric organ and for patients located nationwide. Matching for HLA has evolved since the 1960s when the technology for kidney transplantation was first developed. Initially, HLA-matched siblings were commonly the donor for kidneys. When cadaveric grafts were introduced, the number of available organs was limited and matching for HLA was difficult; however, the national system has improved this process. As technical success with both the surgical procedure and immune suppressive technology improved, it has been questioned whether matching for HLA significantly improved outcome. Recently, results at 5 years post-transplantation obtained by the Collaborative Transplant Study in Europe showed that the degree of HLA matching had a statistically significant effect on long-term

survival of the transplanted kidney.[160,161] UNOS data also showed the influence of HLA matching.[158]

Platelets

Platelet transfusions are required for clinical conditions where bleeding occurs or is threatened and there is a low platelet count. The clinical decision to transfuse platelets is made more difficult because patients can become refractory to platelet transfusion due to allosensitization to HLA antigens and platelet specific antigens expressed on the transfused platelets.[162,163] Platelets express significant amounts of HLA class I antigens (but not class II antigens) and can be readily destroyed by platelet-directed antibodies. Immune sensitization can be reduced by removing leukocytes from the transfused product; however, the patients may be allosensitized prior to platelet transfusions because of pregnancies or prior transfusion of blood products.[164,165]

For patients who do become sensitized, transfusions from donors who express the same HLA antigens as the patient can be life saving. Practically, this is accomplished by finding donors who share the HLA-A, -B types of the patient or who have fewer types (e.g. patient: A1,A2,B7,B8 and donor: A1,B8). In addition to HLA matching, lymphocytes or platelets from the prospective donor can be tested with serum from the patient to detect sensitization.[166] Donors can also be screened for platelet alloantigens.[163]

HSC transplantation

The requirement for HLA matching for HSC transplantation and, to a lesser extent, solid organ transplantation has been the greatest impetus to identify HLA genes and their alleles. Successful HSC grafts could not be achieved until donors adequately matched for HLA could be identified. The first successful grafts in the United States were performed in 1968 using HLA-matched sibling donors to treat patients with immune deficiency disease.[4,167] By the mid 1970s, it was established that marrow transplants from sibling donors could save the lives of people with a number of diseases. Unfortunately, only 30% of patients needing a transplant had HLA-matched siblings. Transplant physicians and families began to seek ways to identify alternate donors. Two approaches were initiated. First, a small percentage (1–5%) of patients had parents, children, siblings, or other relatives who did not precisely match them, but were incompatible by only a limited number of HLA types. Transplantation survival following donation from a single antigen (HLA-A, or-B or -DR) mismatch were nearly identical to outcomes where the donor was perfectly matched. However, survival following transplantation with donors mismatched for two or more types was lower than matched donor transplants.[168]

A second way donors were sought for patients who did not have matched sibling donors was from unrelated individuals. The first successful transplant from an unrelated donor was in 1975, for a patient with severe combined immunodeficiency.[169] In 1979, a patient with leukemia was successfully transplanted in Seattle.[170] This patient, although they did not have a sibling donor, had two of the most common HLA haplotypes in the United States population. A perfectly matched donor was found from a modest file of volunteers. Following this, many families attempted to find unrelated donors for their children where there was no matched sibling. This approach was successful at identifying a few matched donors from files of volunteers who had been typed for HLA as platelet pheresis donors. Several parents then asked members of their local communities to volunteer to be tested for HLA for their children. However this approach did not identify adequate numbers of matched donors for the patient needing the transplant, but these growing files did find donors for over 100 patients over the next 10 years.[171]

Unrelated donor registries and umbilical cord blood banks

Today, over 43 registries of HLA typed potential adult HSC donors and 19 umbilical cord blood banks have been established in 36 countries.[172] In the United States, the National Marrow Donor Program (NMDP) lists over 4 million donors in its database and has facilitated over 9000 transplants.[151,173] At any given time, there is an average of 3000 patients searching the NMDP registry. While a donor search usually begins within the country of origin of the patient, searches failing to identify a donor can extend to foreign registries and banks. Many registries have established cooperative relationships with one another to facilitate searches of these international resources. For example, the NMDP has independent and cooperative agreements with 14 registries outside of the United States so that searches of these registries can be handled through the NMDP office. Of the approximately 9500 transplants facilitated by the NMDP as of May, 2000, 1283 have utilized bone marrow from a donor in another country. US donors of marrow have facilitated 1173 transplants in other countries. An international voluntary organization of registries and banks worldwide, the World Marrow Donor Association (WMDA), has published policies and procedures for these international exchanges.[126,154,174,175]

Testing of unrelated donors is conducted in stages. Initially, 10 ml blood samples from adult volunteers are obtained at HSC donor drives following informed consent. Samples collected for the NMDP are sent to a repository for aliquoting and distribution. One of the aliquots is sent to an HLA testing laboratory for identification of the key HLA types, HLA-A,-B and sometimes -DR, using low to intermediate resolution DNA-based or serologic testing. The majority of the sample is retained in the repository for future additional testing. A similar process is used for umbilical cord blood, although the initial resolution of HLA typing may be higher due to limitations in the quantity of the cord blood which may preclude further testing. Approximately 500 000 new volunteers are added annually to the current total of over 6 million worldwide.

Search strategies for donor identification

Ideally, HLA testing and a donor search are initiated for a patient with the diagnosis of one of over 60 diseases treatable through HSC transplantation.[159] The patient is typed and patient samples are stored for repeat and extended testing.[126] Initial testing of siblings and parents of the patient should be used to identify a HLA-matched sibling donor since the observed probability of a sibling match is 30%.[176] The family typing will also confirm the patient's HLA types and define the linkage of alleles at multiple loci; that is, define haplotypes. If the patient does not have a matched sibling, testing of the extended family, such as cousins, may identify an HLA-matched related donor.[177] The extended family search is most effective if there is consanguinity within the family and/or when the patient carries a haplotype which is common in the general population. Selection of an HLA mismatched relative may also be an alternative.[176]

Typing of HLA-A,-B and -DR (-DRB1) is routinely performed. Within a family, only minimal resolution typing using serology or DNA-based testing is required to establish the segregation of the inherited HLA complex and to identify HLA recombinants. The exceptions are families in which similar alleles are segregating within the family or in which parents are not available or when HLA mismatched relatives are being evaluated for donation. In these cases, higher resolution testing using DNA-based methods as well as testing of other MHC loci and polymorphisms (e.g. microsatellites) might also be performed.

Initial searches of the NMDP registry for an unrelated donor can be undertaken by any physician by contacting the NMDP headquarters; however, formal searches in which the patient has a reasonable likelihood of proceeding to transplantation and during which specific donors are contacted for additional evaluation may only be undertaken by an NMDP-accredited transplant center. Referrals to such centers can be obtained through the NMDP. Submission of patient HLA-typing information for HLA-A, -B, and -DR is preferred; the greater the resolution of the initial testing, the more likely it is that an accurate picture of the availability of HLA-matched donors will be obtained. In families, HLA alleles are inherited so that siblings who have inherited identical chromosomes have identical HLA alleles. In comparison, unrelated individuals carry a diverse collection of alleles found embedded within a large number of haplotypes. Thus, the identification of unrelated individuals who carry identical HLA alleles requires higher resolution typing approaches of both patient and selected donors.[126]

An additional tool in the search process is a database listing HLA phenotypes available on most registries worldwide provided through Bone Marrow Donors Worldwide (BMDW).[178,179] This listing is frequently useful for rapidly estimating the likelihood of finding an HLA-matched donor for a specific patient. BMDW should be used to provide supplementary information since not all registry updates are incorporated into the BMDW database and not all donors listed in BMDW will be suitable or available. This information can, however, assist the physician in identifying treatment options and can spare patients the expense and time of undertaking a futile donor search.

Many donors are typed for HLA-A and -B, but not for HLA-DR. Thus, for some patients who do not find an HLA-A,-B,-DR match in the initial search of a registy, HLA-DR typing may be required of HLA-A,-B matched potential donors. Likewise, transplant centers may wish to evaluate HLA-A,-B one antigen mismatched donors for a DR match. Software tools are available to determine the likelihood that a matched donor exists and to determine which donors should be tested for HLA-DR.[150,179] An informed search strategy is important since time and funding for additional typing is usually limited. The median time to identify a donor is approximately 4 months through the NMDP although search times will vary depending on the frequency of the HLA alleles and haplotypes of the patient.[180] This time can be significantly reduced where there is an urgent need for the graft. In the United States, the likehood of a successful search is higher for patients with common caucasoid haplotypes.[181] Since approximately half a million new donors are added to registries and banks each year, it is recommended that searches be continued if matches are not immediately found.

A list of HLA types from potentially matched volunteers is provided by a registry or bank to the patient's physician. From this list of potential matches, the physician selects donors for additional testing. Volunteer donors are contacted to determine whether they are interested in continuing participation. If required, a second sample is obtained from the volunteer or from the sample repository to determine the HLA-DR type. More than one potential donor should be evaluated since some donors may be unavailable due to, in some cases, poor health or inability to locate the donor. Donors who appear to be potential HLA-A, -B, -DR matches are requested for confirmatory typing (CT). At this stage, a fresh blood sample from the donor and the patient are tested to confirm HLA identity and additional histocompatibility testing may be performed. This may include a higher level of resolution for the three primary HLA loci or the testing of additional loci such as HLA-C, -DRB3, -DRB4, -DRB5 and -DQB1. These additional tests are used to identify the best matched donor if several HLA-A, -B, -DRB1 matched donors are available. Selection factors which HSC transplant centers use to identify the best donor for a patient are based on criteria that improve the likelihood of successful transplant outcome. In addition to HLA, these include donor age (outcomes from younger donors are better), CMV infection status, large donor size for large patients, and matching for ABO red blood cell type. Searches for the best HLA match for a patient must be balanced with the timing of the transplant in relationship to disease stage, since survival is reduced as the disease advances.[182]

Histocompatible matches for HSC transplantation

At a minimum, HSC transplant centers attempt to match HLA-A, -B and -DR assignments of patient and potential donor since these loci have been shown to be clinically important in outcome.[182,183] This level of match is sometimes referred to as a six antigen match, two serologic assignments at HLA-A, two at HLA-B, and two at HLA-DR. (A mismatch for a single antigen is termed a five of six antigen match and so forth.) As the typing technology improved, it was realized that many patients originally defined by serologic reagents as a six antigen match were actually mismatched with their donor at the allele level and that other HLA loci not routinely tested were also mismatched.[184] The impact of this mismatching is not yet clear. Determination of the relative importance of particular HLA loci has been difficult to evaluate because of the presence of mismatches at multiple loci. Furthermore, the impact of mismatching likely differs depending on a variety of recipient factors including disease, treatment and age,[182,185] as well as the source of the HSC. One source of stem cells which may offer a reduced risk of severe GVHD is umbilical cord blood. The relative immaturity of these cells may permit more HLA mismatching,[186–190] but ongoing studies of cord blood transplants have not yet clarified the extent of mismatch possible.

The impact of mismatching might also be determined by the direction (or vector) of the mismatch.[191] Donor or 'host vs graft' incompatibility is characterized by HLA antigens present in the donor but absent in the recipient (e.g donor is heterozygous expressing HLA-A1, -A2 and recipient is homozygous expressing only A2). Recipient or 'graft vs host' incompatibility is characterized by HLA antigens present in the recipient but absent in the donor (e.g. donor is A2 and recipient is A1, -A2). Donor incompatibility might result in graft failure if the remaining immune system of the recipient recognizes the foreign HLA molecules expressed by the graft. Recipient incompatibility might result in GVHD if the grafted immune system recognizes the foreign HLA molecules expressed by cells of the patient. These types of HLA disparity may also stimulate NK-cell recognition of missing self.

At present, most transplant centers attempt to match recipients and their donors for the split antigens of HLA-A and -B and for HLA-DRB1 alleles. There is a trend toward identification of HLA-A and -B alleles using DNA-based testing in order to select the best allele-matched donor and transplant centers may attempt to also select an HLA-C allele-matched donor.[143,192,193] The importance of matching at HLA-DRB3, -DRB4, -DRB5, -DQ and -DP is still unclear. The maximum level of mismatching considered acceptable by many transplant centers is a single difference at the serologic split antigen level (identified by either serology or DNA-based testing) for HLA-A and HLA-B or for a single allele of DRB1 (identified by DNA-based testing); however, the level of acceptable mismatch may depend on other factors such as patient age.

Today, most patients can find closely matched volunteer donors, although the likelihood of finding a matched donor varies depending on the frequency that various HLA haplotypes are found. Some individuals have thousands of identical volunteers listed on donor registries, while a few individuals have no matches. Since many mismatched donors have good outcome, it is hypothesized that the importance of matching each locus will vary and some mismatches at these loci may be tolerated. Therefore, a long-range solution to this problem may lie in advances in transplantation technology such as improved immunosuppressants, induction of tolerance to histocompatibility mismatches,[194] and advanced matching strategies which incorporate an intelligent mismatching approach.[195] These strategies may incorporate testing and matching for other histocompatibility molecules such as NK receptors and minor histocompatibility antigens once the importance of these other histocompatibility molecules has been established.

Summary

The classical human leukocyte antigens bind antigenic peptides, stimulating specific immune responses to microbial pathogens and malignant cells. These molecules also play a primary role in determining the outcome of the transplantation of tissues from one individual to another. Now it is known that the classical HLA molecules have additional roles in the immune system and are the ligand for many different receptors and that other molecules also participate in a variety of these functions. Transplantation outcome will only improve from the benefits of continued research efforts in these areas of study.

REFERENCES

1. Snell GD 1981 Studies in histocompatibility. Science 213: 172–178
2. Benacerraf B 1981 Role of MHC gene products in immune regulation. Science 212: 1229–1238
3. Dausset J 1981 The Nobel Lectures in Immunology. Lecture for the Nobel Prize for Physiology or Medicine: 1980: the major histocompatibility complex in man. Past, present, and future concepts. Science 213: 1459–1474
4. Groth CG, Brent LB, Calne RY et al 2000 Historic landmarks in clinical transplantation: conclusions from the consensus conference at the University of California, Los Angeles. World Journal of Surgery 24: 834–84
5. Payne R, Tripp M, Weigle J et al 1964 A new leukocyte isoantigen system in man. Cold Spring Harbor Symposia in Quantitative Biology 29: 285–295
6. Van Rood JJ 1993 HLA and I. Annual Review of Immunology 11: 1–28
7. Bach FH, Hirschhorn K 1964 Lymphocyte interaction: a potential histocompatibility test *in vitro*. Science 143: 813–814
8. Thorsby E, Piazza A 1975 Joint report from the sixth international histocompatibility workshop conference. II. Typing for HLA-D (LD-1 or MLC) determinants. In: Kissmeyer-Nielsen F (ed), Histocompatibility testing. Munksgaard Copenhagen 414–458
9. Forbes SA, Trowsdale J 1999 The MHC quarterly report. Immunogenetics 50: 152–159
10. The MHC sequencing consortium 1999 Complete sequence and gene map of a human major histocompatibility complex. Nature 401: 921–923
11. Beck S, Trowsdale J 1999 Sequence organization of the class II region of the human MHC. Immunological Reviews 167: 201–210
12. Shiina T, Tamiya G, Oka A et al 1999 Genome sequence analysis of the 1.8 Mb entire human MHC class I region. Immunological Reviews 167: 193–199
13. Auffray C, Strominger JL 1986 Molecular genetics of the human major histocompatibility complex. Advances in Human Genetics 15: 197–247
14. Kappes D, Strominger JL 1988 Human class II major histocompatibility complex genes and proteins. Annual Review of Biochemistry 57: 991–1028
15. Kwok WW, Kovats S, Thurtle P et al 1993 HLA-DQ allelic polymorphisms constrain patterns of class II heterodimer formation. Journal of Immunology 150: 2263–2272
16. Little A-M, Parham P 1999 Polymorphism and evolution of HLA class I and class II genes and molecules. Reviews in Immunogenetics 1: 105–123

17. Bodmer JG, Marsh SGE, Albert ED et al 1999 Nomenclature for factors of the HLA system, 1998. Tissue Antigens 53: 407–446
18. Anthony Nolan Bone Marrow Trust HLA Informatics Group; www.anthonynolan.org.uk/HIG/
19. Carrington M, Martin MP, Kissner T et al 1999 HLA and HIV-1: heterozygote advantage and B*35-Cw*04 disadvantage. Science 283: 1748–1752
20. Gilbert SC, Plebanski M, Gupta S et al 1998 Association of malaria parasite population structure, HLA, and immunological antagonism. Science 279: 1173–1177
21. Yeager M, Hughes AL 1999 Evolution of the mammalian MHC: natural selection, recombination, and convergent evolution. Immunological Reviews 167: 45–58
22. Carrington M 1999 Recombination within the human MHC. Immunological Review 167: 245–256
23. Begovich AB, McClure GR, Suraj VC et al 1992 Polymorphism, recombination, and linkage disequilibrium within the HLA class II region. Journal of Immunology 148: 249–258
24. Trachtenberg EA, Keyeux G, Bernal JE et al 1996 Results of Expediction Humana. I. Analysis of HLA class II (DRB1-DQA1-DPB1) alleles and DR-DQ haplotypes in nine Amerindian populations from Colombia. Tissue Antigens 48: 174–181
25. Bugawan TL, Mack SJ, Stoneking M et al 1999 HLA class I allele distributions in six Pacific/Asian populations: evidence of selection at the HLA-A locus. Tissue Antigens 53: 311–319
26. Mori M, Beatty PG, Graves M et al 1997 HLA gene and haplotype frequencies in the North American population – The National Marrow Donor Program Donor Registry. Transplantation 64: 1017–1027
27. Schipper RF, D'Amaro J, Bakker JT et al 1997 HLA gene and haplotype frequencies in bone marrow donors worldwide registries. Human Immunology 52: 54–71
28. Tang TF, Huang AY, Pappas A et al 2000 Relative frequencies of DRB1*11 alleles and their DRB3 associations in five major population groups in a U.S. bone marrow registry. Human Immunology 61: 820–827
29. American Society for Histocompatibility and Immunogenetics; www.ashihla.org.
30. Ellis JM, Henson V, Slack R et al 2000 Frequencies of HLA-A2 alleles in five U.S. population groups. Human Immunology 61: 334–340
31. Sintasath DM, Tang T, Slack R et al 1999 Relative HLA-DRB1*13 allele frequencies and DRB3 associations of unrelated individuals from five U.S. populations. Human Immunology 60: 1001–1010
32. Begovich AB, Klitz W, Steiner LL et al 2000 HLA-DQ haplotypes in 15 different populations. In: Kasahara M (ed), The major histocompatibility complex: evolution, structure and function. Springer, Tokyo 412–426
33. Imanishi T, Akaza T, Kimura A et al 1992 Allele and haplotype frequencies for HLA and complement loci in various ethnic groups. In: Tsuji K, Aizawa M, Sasazuki T (eds) HLA 1991, vol 1. Oxford University Press, New York 1065–1220
34. Prasad VK, Heller G, Kernan NA et al 1999 The probability of HLA-C matching between patient and unrelated donor at the molecular level: estimations based on the linkage disequilibrium between DNA typed HLA-B and HLA-C alleles. Transplantation 68: 1044–1050
35. Degli-Esposti MA, Leaver AL, Christiansen FT et al 1992 Ancestral haplotypes: conserved population MHC haplotypes. Human Immunology 34: 242–252
36. Van den Elsen PJ, Gobin SJP, Van Eggermond MC et al 1998 Regulation of MHC class I and II gene transcription: differences and similarities. Immunogenetics 48: 208–221
37. Mach B, Steimle V, Martinez-Soria E et al 1996 Regulation of MHC class II genes: Lessons from a disease. Annual Review of Immunology 14: 301–331
38. Khanna R 1998 Tumor surveillance: missing peptides and MHC molecules. Immunology and Cell Biology 76: 20–26
39. Brodsky FM, Lem L, Solache A et al 1999 Human pathogen subversion of antigen presentation. Immunological Reviews 168: 199–215
40. Parham P 1997 Filling in the blanks. Tissue Antigens 50: 318–321
41. Kimball ES, Coligan JE 1983 Structure of class I major histocompatibility antigens. Contemporary Topics in Molecular Immunology 9: 1–63
42. Maenaka K, Jones EY 1999 MHC superfamily structure and the immune system. Current Opinion in Structural Biology 9: 745–753
43. Madden DR 1995 The three-dimensional structure of peptide-MHC complexes. Annual Review of Immunology 13: 587–622
44. SYFPEITHI: Database for MHC ligands and peptide motifs; www.unituebingen.de/uni/kxi/
45. Ettinger RA, Kwok WW 1998 A peptide binding motif for HLA-DQA1*0102/DQB1*0602, the class II MHC molecule associated with dominant protection in insulin-dependent diabetes mellitus. Journal of Immunology 160: 2365–2373
46. Chicz RM, Graziano DF, Trucco M et al 1997 HLA-DP2 – Self peptide sequences and binding properties. Journal of Immunology 159: 4935–4942
47. Dong R-P, Kamikawaji N, Toida N 1995 Characterization of T cell epitopes restricted by HLA-DP9 in streptococcal M12 protein. Journal of Immunology 154: 4536–4545
48. Thorsby E 1997 Invited anniversary review: HLA associated diseases. Human Immunology 53: 1–11
49. Giles RC, Capra JD 1985 Biochemistry of MHC class II molecules. Tissue Antigens 25: 57–68
50. McDonald JC, Adamashvili I 1998 Soluble HLA: A review of the literature. Human Immunology 59: 387–403
51. Hammer J, Sturniolo T, Sinigaglia F 1997 HLA class II peptide binding specificity and autoimmunity. Advances in Immunology 66: 67–100
52. Reizis B, Eisenstein M, Mor F 1998 The peptide-binding strategy of the MHC class II I-A molecules. Immunology Today 19: 212–216
53. Maffei A, Papadopoulos K, Harris PE 1997 MHC class I antigen processing pathways. Human Immunology 54: 91–103
54. Rock KL, Goldberg AL 1999 Degradation of cell proteins and the generation of MHC class I- presented peptides. Annual Review of Immunology 17: 739–779
55. Watts C, Powis S 1999 Pathways of antigen processing and presentation. Reviews in Immunogenetics 1: 60–74
56. Pieters J 1997 MHC class II restricted antigen presentation. Current Opinion in Immunology 9: 89–96
57. Vogt AB, Kropshofer H 1999 HLA-DM – an endosomal and lysosomal chaperone for the immune system. Trends in Biochemical Sciences 24: 150–154
58. Arndt SO, Vogt AB, Hammerling GJ 1997 Selection of the MHC class II-associated peptide repertoire by HLA-DM. Immunologic Research 16: 261–272
59. Vogt AB, Kropshofer H, Hämmerling GJ 1997 How HLA-DM affects the peptide repertoire bound to HLA-DR molecules. Human Immunology 54: 170–179
60. Jensen PE 1998 Antigen processing: HLA-DO – a hitchhiking inhibitor of HLA-DM. Current Biology 8: R128–R131
61. Westerheide SD, Louis-Plence P, Ping D 1997 HLA-DMA and HLA-DMB gene expression functions through the conserved S-X-Y region. Journal of Immunology 158: 4812–4821
62. Fruh K, Gruhler A, Krishna RM 1999 A comparison of viral immune escape strategies targeting the MHC class I assembly pathway. Immunological Reviews 168: 157–166
63. Garcia KC 1999 Molecular interactions between extracellular components of the T-cell receptor signaling complex. Immunological Reviews 172: 73–85
64. Kaufmann SHE 1996 Gamma/delta and other unconventional T lymphocytes: what do they see and what do they do? Proceedings of the National Academy of Sciences USA 93: 2272–2279
65. Garcia KC, Teyton L, Wilson LA 1999 Structural basis of T cell recognition. Annual Review of Immunology 17: 369–397
66. Clements JL, Boerth NJ, Lee JR 1999 Integration of T cell receptor-dependent signaling pathways by adapter proteins. Annual Review of Immunology 17: 89–108
67. Germain RN, Stefanova I 1999 The dynamics of T cell receptor signaling: Complex orchestration and the key roles of tempo and cooperation. Annual Review of Immunology 17: 467–522
68. Viret C, Janeway CA, Jr 1999 MHC and T cell development. Reviews in Immunogenetics 1: 91–104
69. Devine L, Kavathas PB 1999 Molecular analysis of protein interactions mediating the function of the cell surface protein CD8. Immunologic Research 19: 201–210
70. Rowen L, Koop BF, Hood L 1996 The complete 685-kilobase DNA sequence of the human β T cell receptor locus. Science 272: 1755–1762
71. McVay LD, Carding SR 1999 Generation of human gamma/delta T-cell repertoires. Critical Reviews in Immunology 19: 431–460
72. Garboczi DN, Biddison WE 1999 Shapes of MHC restriction. Immunity 10: 1–7
73. Goldrath AW, Bevan MJ 1999 Selecting and maintaining a diverse T-cell repertoire. Nature 402: 255–262

74. Sebzda E, Mariathasan S, Ohteki T 1999 Selection of the T cell repertoire. Annual Review of Immunology 17: 829–874

75. Janeway CA 1999 members of the Janeway laboratory. The role of self-recognition in receptor repertoire development. Immunologic Research 19: 107–118

76. Hernadez-Fuentes MP, Baker RJ, Lechler RI 1999 The alloresponse. Reviews in Immunogenetics 1: 282–296

77. Benichou G, Tam RC, Soares LRB et al 1997 Indirect T-cell allorecognition: perspectives for peptide-based therapy in transplantation. Immunology Today 18: 67–71

78. Elliott TJ, Eisen HN 1990 Cytotoxic T lymphocytes recognize a reconstituted class I histocompatibility antigen (HLA-A2) as an allogeneic target molecule. Proceedings of the National Academy of Sciences USA 87: 5213–5217

79. Demotz S, Sette A, Sakaguchi K 1991 Self peptide requirement for class II major histocompatibility complex allorecognition. Proceedings of the National Academy of Sciences 88: 8730–8734

80. Heath WR, Kane KP, Mescher MF 1991 Alloreactive T cells discriminate among a diverse set of endogenous peptides. Proceedings of the National Academy of Sciences 88: 5101–5105

81. Harris PE, Cortesini R, Suciu-Foca N 1999 Indirect allorecognition in solid organ transplantation. Reviews in Immunogenetics 1: 297–308

82. Hansen JA, Yamamoto K, Petersdorf E 1999 The role of HLA matching in hematopoietic cell transplantation. Reviews in Immunogenetics 1: 359–373

83. Chicz RM, Urban RG, Lane WS 1992 Predominant naturally processed peptides bound to HLA-DR1 are derived from MHC-related molecules and are heterogeneous in size. Nature 358: 764–768

84. Posch PE, Borrego F, Brooks AG 1998 HLA-E is the ligand for the natural killer cell CD94/NKG2 receptors. Journal of Biomedical Science 5: 321–331

85. Leibson PJ 1998 Cytotoxic lymphocyte recognition of HLA-E: Utilizing a nonclassical window to peer into classical MHC. Immunity 9: 289–294

86. Braud VM, Allan DSJ, McMichael AJ 1999 Functions of nonclassical MHC and non-MHC-encoded class I molecules. Current Opinion in Immunology 11: 100–108

87. O'Callaghan CA, Bell JI 1998 Structure and function of the human class Ib molecules HLA-E, HLA-F and HLA-G. Immunological Reviews 163: 129–138

88. Wainwright SD, Biro PA, Holmes CH 2000 HLA-F is a predominantly empty, intracellular, TAP-associated MHC class Ib protein with a restricted expression pattern. Journal of Immunology 164: 319–328

89. Gobin SJP, Van den Elsen PJ 1999 The regulation of HLA class I expression: is HLA-G the odd one out? Seminars in Cancer Biology 9: 55–59

90. Kirszenbaum M, Djoulah S, Hors J 1999 Polymorphism of HLA-G gene and protein. Journal of Reproductive Immunology 43: 105–109

91. Ober C, Aldrich CL 1997 HLA-G polymorphisms: neutral evolution or novel function. Journal of Reproductive Immunology 36: 1–21

92. Le Bouteiller P, Blaschitz A 1999 The functionality of HLA-G is emerging. Immunological Reviews 167: 233–244

93. Munz C, Nickolaus P, Lammert E et al 1999 The role of peptide presentation in the physiological function of HLA-G. Cancer Biology 9: 47–54

94. Bahram S, Bresnahan M, Geraghty DE et al 1994 A second lineage of mammalian major histocompatibility complex class I genes. Proceedings of the National Academy of Sciences USA 91: 6259–6263

95. Visser CJT, Tilanus MGJ, Schaeffer V et al 1998 Sequencing based typing reveals six novel MHC class I chain related gene B (MICB) alleles. Tissue Antigens 51: 649–652

96. Petersdorf EW, Shuler KB, Longton GM et al 1999 Population study of allelic diversity in the human MHC class I-related MIC-A gene. Immunogenetics 49: 605–612

97. Groh V, Bahram S, Bauer S et al 1996 Cell stress-regulated human major histocompatibility complex class I gene expressed in gastrointestinal epithelium. Proceedings of the National Academy of Sciences USA 93: 12445–12450

98. Li P, Willie ST, Bauer S et al 1999 Crystal structure of the MHC class I homolog MIC-A, a gamma/delta T cell ligand. Immunity 10: 577–584

99. Groh V, Rhinehart R, Secrist H et al 1999 Broad tumor-associated expression and recognition by tumor-derived gamma-delta T cells of MICA and MICB. Proceedings of the National Academy of Sciences USA 96: 6879–6884

100. Groh V, Steinle A, Bauer S et al 1998 Recognition of stress-induced MHC molecules by intestinal epithelial gamma-delta T cells. Science 279: 1737–1740

101. Bauer S, Groh V, Wu J et al 1999 Activation of NK cells and T cells by NKG2D, a receptor for stress-inducible MICA. Science 285: 727–729

102. Kasahara M 1999 Genome dynamics of the major histocompatibility complex: insights from genome paralogy. Immunogenetics 50: 134–145

103. Porcelli SA, Modlin RL 1999 The CD1 system: Antigen-presenting molecules for T cell recognition of lipids and glycolipids. Annual Review of Immunology 17: 297–329

104. Fairhurst RM, Wang C-X, Sieling PA et al 1998 CD1-restricted T cells and resistance to polysaccharide-encapsulated bacteria. Immunology Today 19: 257–259

105. Warren EH, Gavin M, Greenberg PD et al 1998 Minor histocompatibility antigens as targets for T-cell therapy after bone marrow transplantation. Current Opinion in Hematology 5: 429–433

106. Den Haan JMM, Meadows LM, Wang W et al 1998 The minor histocompatibility antigen HA-1: A diallelic gene with a single amino acid polymorphism. Science 279: 1054–1057

107. Den Haan JMM, Sherman NE, Blockland E et al 1995 Identification of a graft versus host disease-associated human minor histocompatibility antigen. Science 268: 1476–1480

108. Wang W, Meadows LR, Den Haan JMM et al 1995 Human H-Y: a male-specific histocompatibility antigen derived from the SMCY protein. Science 269: 1588–1590

109. Meadows L, Wang W, Den Haan JMM et al 1997 The HLA-A*0201-restricted H-Y antigen contains a posttranslationally modified cysteine that significantly affects T cell recognition. Immunity 6: 273–281

110. Pierce RA, Field ED, Den Haan JMM et al 1999 The HLA-A*0101-restricted HY minor histocompatibility antigen originates from DFFRY and contains a cysteinylated cysteine residue as identified by a novel mass spectrometric technique. Journal of Immunology 163: 6360–6364

111. Dolstra H, Fredrix H, Preijers F et al 1997 Recognition of a B cell leukemia-associated minor histocompatibility antigen by CTL. Journal of Immunology 158: 560–565

112. Dolstra H, Fredrix H, Maas F et al 1999 A human minor histocompatibility antigen specific for B cell acute lymphoblastic leukemia. Journal of Experimental Medicine 189: 301–308

113. Goulmy E, Schipper R, Pool J et al 1996 Mismatches of minor histocompatibility antigens between HLA-identical donors and recipients and the development of graft-versus-host disease after bone marrow transplantation. New England Journal of Medicine 334: 281–285

114. Wilke M, Pool J, Den Haan JMM et al 1998 Genomic identification of the minor histocompatibility antigen HA-1 locus by allele-specific PCR. Tissue Antigens 52: 312–317

115. Long EO 1999 Regulation of immune responses through inhibitory receptors. Annual Review of Immunology 17: 875–904

116. Lopez-Botet M, Bellon T 1999 Natural killer cell activation and inhibition by receptors for MHC class I. Current Opinion in Immunology 11: 301–307

117. Boyington JC, Motyka SA, Schunk P et al 2000 Crystal structure of an NK cell immunoglobulin-like receptor in complex with its class I MHC ligand. Nature 405: 537–543

118. Urhberg M, Valiante NM, Shum BP et al 1997 Human diversity in killer cell inhibitory receptor genes. Immunity 7: 753–763

119. Witt CS, Dewing C, Sayer DC et al 1999 Population frequencies and putative haplotypes of the killer cell immunoglobulin-like receptor sequences and evidence for recombination. Transplantation 68: 1784–1789

120. Wilson MJ, Torkar M, Haude A et al 2000 Plasticity in the organization and sequences of human KIR/ILT gene families. Proceedings of the National Academy of Sciences USA 97: 4778–4783

121. Wu J, Song Y, Bakker ABH et al 1999 An activating immunoreceptor complex formed by NKG2D and DAP10. Science 285: 730–732

122. Brooks AG, Borrego F, Posch PE et al 1999 Specific recognition of HLA-E, but not classical, HLA class I molecules by soluble CD94/NKG2A and NK cells. Journal of Immunology 162: 305–313

123. Colonna M, Nakajima H, Navarro F et al 1999 A novel family of Ig-like receptors for HLA class I molecules that modulate function of lymphoid and myeloid cells. Journal of Leukocyte Biology 66: 375–381

124. Colonna M, Nakajima H, Cella M 1999 Inhibitory and activating receptors involved in immune surveillance by human NK and myeloid cells. Journal of Leukocyte Biology 66: 718–722

125. American Society for Histocompatibility and Immunogenetics Laboratory Manual 3rd edn. In: Phelan DL, Mickelson EM, Noreen HS et al 2000 (eds), Lenexa, Kansas: American Society for Histocompatibility and Immunogenetics;

126. Hurley CK, Wade JA, Oudshoorn M et al 1999 A special report: Histocompatibility testing guidelines for hematopoietic stem cell transplantation using volunteer donors. Human Immunology 60: 347–360

127. Lou CD, Cunniffe KJ, Garovoy MR 1997 Histocompatibility testing by immunologic methods: humoral assays. In: Rose NR, Conway de Macario E, Folds JD et al (eds), Manual of clinical laboratory immunology. ASM Press, Washington DC 1087–1097

128. Reinsmoen NL 1997 Histocompatibility testing by immunologic methods: cellular assays. In: Rose NR, Conway de Macario E, Folds JD et al (eds), Manual of clinical laboratory immunology. ASM Press, Washington DC 1080–1086

129. Mickelson EM, Longton G, Anasetti C et al 1996 Evaluation of the mixed lymphocyte culture (MLC) assay as a method for selecting unrelated donors for marrow transplantation. Tissue Antigens 47: 27–36

130. Spencer A, Szydlo RM, Brookes PA et al 1995 Bone marrow transplantation for chronic myeloid leukemia with volunteer unrelated donors using *ex vivo* or *in vivo* T-cell depletion: major prognostic impact of HLA class I identity between donor and recipient. Blood 86: 3590–3597

131. Pei J, Martin PJ, Longton G et al 1997 Evaluation of pretransplant donor antirecipient cytotoxic and helper T lymphocyte responses as correlates of acute graft- vs.- host disease and survival after unrelated marrow transplantation. Biology of Blood and Marrow Transplantation 3: 142–149

132. Middleton D. 1999 History of DNA typing for the human MHC. Reviews in Immunogenetics 1: 135–156

133. Hurley CK, Tang T, Ng J et al 1997 HLA typing by molecular methods. In: Rose NR, Conway de Macario E, Folds JD et al (eds), Manual of clinical laboratory immunology. ASM Press, Washington DC 1098–1111

134. Saiki RK, Gelfand DH, Stoffel S et al 1988 Primer-directed enzymatic amplification of DNA with a thermostable DNA polymerase. Science 239: 487–491

135. Olerup O, Zetterquist H 1992 HLA-DR typing by PCR amplification with sequence specific primers (PCR-SSP) in 2 hours: an alternative to serological DR typing in clinical practice including donor-recipient matching in cadaveric transplantations. Tissue Antigens 39: 225–235

136. Welsh K, Bunce M 1999 Molecular typing for the MHC with PCR-SSP. Reviews in Immunogenetics 1: 157–176

137. Cao K, Chopek M, Fernandez-Vina MA et al 1999 High and intermediate resolution DNA typing systems for Class I HLA-A, -B, -C genes by hybridization with sequence specific oligonucleotide probes (SSOP). Reviews in Immunogenetics 1: 177–208

138. Arguello JR, Madrigal JA 1999 HLA typing by reference strand mediated conformation analysis (RSCA). Reviews in Immunogenetics 1: 209–219

139. Kurz B, Steiert I, Heuchert G et al 1999 New high resolution typing strategy for HLA-A locus alleles based on dye terminator sequencing of haplotypic group- specific PCR-amplicons of exon 2 and exon 3. Tissue Antigens 53: 81–96

140. Scheltinga SA, Johnston-Dow LA, White CB et al 1997 A generic sequencing based typing approach for the identification of HLA-A diversity. Human Immunology 57: 120–128

141. Sanger F, Nicklen S, Coulson A et al 1977 DNA sequencing with chain terminating inhibitors. Proceedings of the National Academy of Sciences USA 74: 5463

142. Rozemuller EH, Eliaou JF, Baxter-Lowe LA et al 1995 An evaluation of a multicenter study on HLA-DPB 1 typing using solid-phase Taq-cycle sequencing chemistry. Tissue Antigens 46: 96–103

143. Mickelson EM, Petersdorf E, Anasetti C et al 2000 HLA matching in hematopoietic cell transplantation. Human Immunology 61: 92–100

144. Bodmer JG, Marsh SGE, Albert ED et al 1997 Nomenclature for factors of the HLA system, 1996. Tissue Antigens 49: 297–321

145. Parham P, Lawlor DA, Salter RD et al 1989 HLA-A,B,C: patterns of polymorphism in peptide-binding proteins. In: Dupont B (ed), Immunobiology of HLA. Springer, New York, 10–33

146. Rodey GE, Fuller TC 1987 Public epitopes and the antigenic structure of the HLA molecules. Critical Reviews in Immunology 7: 229–267

147. Rodey GE, Neylan JF, Whelchel JD et al 1994 Epitope specificity of HLA Class I alloantibodies. I. Frequency analysis of antibodies to private versus public specificities in potential transplant recipients. Human Immunology 39: 272–280

148. Thompson JS, Thacker LR 1996 CREG matching for first cadaveric kidney transplants (TNX) performed by SEOPF centers between October 1987 and September 1995. Southeastern Organ Procurement Foundation. Clinical Transplantation 10: 586–593

149. Takemoto SK, Cecka JM, Terasaki PI 1997 Benefits of HLA-CREG matching for sensitized recipients as illustrated in kidney regrafts. Transplantation Proceedings 29: 1417–1417

150. Mori M, Graves M, Milford EL et al 1996 Computer program to predict likelihood of finding and HLA-matched donor: methodology, validation, and application. Biology of Blood and Marrow Transplantation 2: 134–144

151. National Marrow Donor Program; www.marrow.org; www.nmdpresearch.org.

152. Hurley CK 1997 Acquisition and use of DNA-based HLA typing data in bone marrow registries. Tissue Antigens 49: 323–328

153. Schreuder GMTh, Hurley CK, Marsh SGE et al 1999 The HLA dictionary 1999: a summary of HLA-A, -B, -C, -DRB1/3/4/5, -DQB 1 alleles and their association with serologically defined HLA-A, -B, -C, -DR and -DQ antigens. Tissue Antigens 54: 409–437

154. World Marrow Donor Association; www.worldmarrow.org.

155. Ridgway WM, Fassò M, Fathman CG 1999 A new look at MHC and autoimmune disease. Science 284: 749–751

156. Allen RL, Bowness P, McMichael A 1999 The role of HLA-B27 in spondyloarthritis. Immunogenetics 50: 220–227

157. Smith AG, Martin PJ 1999 Analysis of amplified variable number tandem repeat loci for evaluation of engraftment after hematopoietic stem cell transplantation. Reviews in Immunogenetics 1: 255–264

158. United Network for Organ Sharing; www.unos.org.

159. International Bone Marrow Transplant Registry; www.ibmtr.org.

160. Collaborative Transplant Study; cts.med.uni-heidelberg.de.

161. Opelz G, Wujciak T, Dohler B et al 1999 HLA compatibility and organ transplant survival. Reviews in Immunogenetics 1: 334–342

162. Yankee RA, Grumet FC, Rogentine GN et al 1969 Platelet transfusion. The selection of compatible platelet donors for refractory patients by lymphocyte HLA typing. New England Journal of Medicine 281: 1208–1212

163. Juji T, Saji H, Satake M et al 1999 Typing for human platelet alloantigens. Reviews in Immunogenetics 1: 239–254

164. Anonymous 1997 Leukotye reduction and ultraviolet B irradiation of platelets to prevent alloimmunization and refractoriness to platelet transfusions. New England Journal of Medicine 337: 1861–1869

165. Claas FH, van Doorn R, Witvliet MD et al 1995 Occurrence of allogeneic HLA and non-HLA antibodies after transfusion of prestorage filtered platelets and red blood cells: a prospective study. Blood 85: 1736–1741

166. Moroff G, Garratty G, Heal JM et al 1992 Selection of platelets for refractory patients by HLA matching and prospective crossmatching. Transfusion 32: 633–640

167. Thomas ED 1999 A history of haemopoietic cell transplantation. British Journal of Haematology 105: 330–339

168. Beatty PG, Clift RA, Mickelson EM et al 1985 Marrow transplantation from related donors other than HLA- identical siblings. New England Journal of Medicine 313: 765–771

169. O'Reilly RJ, Dupont B, Pahwa S et al 1977 Reconstitution in severe combined immundeficiency by transplantation of marrow from an unrelated donor. New England Journal of Medicine 297: 1311–1318

170. Hansen JA, Clift RA, Thomas ED et al 1980 Transplantation of marrow from an unrelated donor to a patient with acute leukemia. New England Journal of Medicine 303: 565–567

171. McCullough J, Hansen J, Perkins H et al 1989 The National Marrow Donor Program: How it works, accomplishments to date. Oncology (Huntingt) 3: 63–72

172. Hansen JA 1996 Development of registries of HLA-typed volunteer marrow donors. Tissue Antigens 47: 460–463

173. Howe CW, Radde-Stepaniak T 1999 Hematopoietic cell donor registries. In: Thomas ED, Blume KG, Forman SJ (eds), Hematopoietic cell transplantation Blackwell Science, Malden MA, 503–512

174. Goldman JM 1994 A special report: bone marrow transplants using volunteer donors – recommendations and requirements for a standardized practice throughout the world – 1994 update. Blood 84: 2833–2839

175. Cleaver SA, Warren P, Kern M et al 1997 A special report: Donor work-up and transport of bone marrow – recommendations and

requirements for a standardized practice throughout the world. Bone Marrow Transplant 20: 621–629

176. Beatty PG 1997 Histocompatibility assessment in bone marrow transplantation. In: Rose NR, de Macario EC, Foplds JD et al (eds) Manual of clinical laboratory immunology. ASM Press, Washington DC 1123–1131

177. Schipper RF, D'Amaro J, Oudshoorn M 1996 The probability of finding a suitable related donor for bone marrow transplantation in extended families. Blood 87: 800–804

178. Oudshoorn M, van Leeuwen A, v.d.Zanden HG et al 1994 Bone marrow donors worldwide: a successful exercise in international cooperation. Bone Marrow Transplant 14: 3–8

179. Bone Marrow Donors Worldwide; www.bmdw.leidenuniv.nl.

180. Oudshoorn M, Cornelissen JJ, Fibbe WE et al 1997 Problems and possible solutions in finding an unrelated bone marrow donor. Results of consecutive searches for 240 Dutch patients. Bone Marrow Transplant 20: 1011–1017

181. Beatty PG, Mori M, Milford E 1995 Impact of racial genetic polymorphism on the probability of finding an HLA-matched donor. Transplantation 60: 778–783

182. Madrigal JA, Scott I, Arguello R et al 1997 Factors influencing the outcome of bone marrow transplants using unrelated donors. Immunological Reviews 157: 153–166

183. Hansen JA, Petersdorf E, Martin PJ et al 1997 Hematopoietic stem ell transplants from unrelated donors. Immunological Reviews 157: 141–151

184. Hurley CK, Baxter-Lowe LA, Begovich AB et al 2000 The extent of HLA class II allele level disparity in unrelated bone marrow transplantation: analysis of 1259 National Marrow Donor Program donor–recipient pairs. Bone Marrow Transplant 25: 385–393

185. Hansen JA, Gooley TA, Martin PJ et al 1998 Bone marrow transplants from unrelated donors for patients with chronic myeloid leukemia. New England Journal of Medicine 338: 962–968

186. Kurtzberg J, Laughlin M, Graham ML et al 1996 Placental blood as a source of hematopoietic stem cells for transplantation into unrelated recipients. New England Journal of Medicine 335: 157–166

187. Madrigal JA, Cohen SBA, Gluckman E et al 1997 Does cord blood transplantation result in lower graft-versus- host disease? It takes more than two to tango. Human Immunology 56: 1–5

188. Gluckman E, Rocha V, Boyer-Chammard A et al 1997 Outcome of cord-blood transplantation from related and unrelated donors. Eurocord Transplant Group and the European Blood and Marrow Transplantation Group. New England Journal of Medicine 337: 373–381

189. Rubinstein P, Carrier C, Scaradavou A et al 1998 Outcomes among 562 recipients of placental-blood transplants from unrelated donors. New England Journal of Medicine 339: 1565–1577

190. Rocha V, Wagner JE, Sobocinski KA et al 2000 Graft-versus-host disease in children who have received a cord-blood or bone marrow transplant from an HLA-identical sibling. New England Journal of Medicine 342: 1846–1854

191. Anasetti C, Beatty PG, Storb R et al 1990 Effect of HLA incompatibility on graft-versus-host disease, relapse, and survival after marrow transplantation for patients with leukemia or lymphoma. Human Immunology 29: 79–91

192. Sasazuki T, Juji T, Morishima Y et al 1998 Effect of matching of class I HLA alleles on clinical outcome after transplantion of hematopoietic stem cells from an unrelated donor. New England Journal of Medicine 339: 1177–1185

193. Petersdorf EW, Gooley TA, Anasetti C et al 1998 Optimizing outcome after unrelated marrow transplantation by comprehensive matching of HLA class I and II alleles in the donor and recipient. Blood 92: 3515–3520

194. Witzke O, Barbara JAJ, Wood KJ 1999 Induction of tolerance to alloantigen. Reviews in Immunogenetics 1: 374–386

195. Class FH, deMeester J, Witvliet MD et al 1999 Acceptable HLA mismatches for highly immunized patients. Reviews in Immunogenetics 1: 351–358

Index

A

ABC7 mutations, 208, 269
Abetalipoproteinemia, 600
ABL1, 618
ABO blood group system, 617–619
  A allele, 617
  ABH non-secretors, 617
  ABO antigens, 617
    expression in leukemia, 618
    malignant tissue, 618, 619
  B allele, 617
  blood typing
    autologous blood, 643
    donated blood, 646, 647
    urgent blood transfusion, 653
  H antigens, 617
  hemolytic disease of newborn, 193,
    618
  O allele, 617
  transfusion reactions, 192, 655
AC133, 72
Acanthocytes, 133–134, 245, 335
Aceruloplasminemia, 223
Acid phosphatase, 9, 12, 14, 19, 33, 34,
    47, 506
Aclarubicin, 348
Acquired amegakaryocytic
    thrombocytopenia, 531
Acquired coagulation inhibitors, 584,
    593–594
  management, 594
Acquired heparin-like anticoagulants,
    593
Acquired hyperfibrinolysis, 592
Acquired immune deficiency syndrome
    see AIDS/HIV infection
Actin, 6, 11, 57
  cytoskeleton organisation defects, 326
Activated partial thromboplastin time
    (APTT), 480, 483–484, 486, 488
  correction tests, 484
  misleading prolongation, 485

neonate, 579
Activated protein C inhibitor, 602
Activated protein C resistance, 604–605
Actomyosin, 18
Acute phase reaction, thrombosis risk,
    608
Acyclovir, 243
Adenosylcobalamin deficiency, 240
Adenosylcobalamin/methylcobalamin
    combined deficiency, 240
Adenylate kinase deficiency, 155
Adhesion molecules, 63, 76–78
  hematopoiesis, 76–77
  multiple myeloma, 443–444
  platelet plug formation, 474
  red cell surface proteins, 623–624
Adriamycin, 451, 452
Adult T-cell leukemia/lymphoma,
    392–393
  immunophenotype, 393
Afibrinogenemia, 479, 570, 572
Agnogenic myeloid metaplasia *see*
    Idiopathic myelofibrosis
Agranulocytosis, 310
  drug-induced, 306–307
  infantile genetic (Kostmann's
    syndrome), 309, 323–324
AIDS/HIV infection, 104–109
  aplastic anemia, 533
  blood banking/transfusion impact,
    640–641
    donation regulations, 641
    nucleic acid amplification testing
      (NAT), 658
  blood transfusion-related
    transmission, 640–641, 657–658
    clotting factor concentrates, 559, 560
  bone marrow changes, 105–106
    gelatinous transformation, 105–106,
      109, 120
    lymphoid aggregates, 105, 432
    reticulin fibrosis, 105, 109
    trilineage myelodysplasia, 106
Burkitt's lymphoma, 421

clinical AIDS, 105
clinically latent phase, 105
complement receptor-1 (CR1; CD35)
    deficiency, 625
granuloma formation impairment, 111
hemophagocytic syndrome, 100
hemopoietic cell abnormalities, 93, 94
lymphocyte counts, 105
  lymphocytopenia (lymphopenia),
    105, 310
  lymphocytosis, 315
mechanisms underlying hematologic
    changes, 108–109
myelodysplasia, 343
neutrophil precursor abnormalities,
    94, 95
opportunistic infections, 106–108, 109
peripheral blood changes, 105
primary infection, 105
thrombocytopenia, 537–538
thrombotic thrombocytopenic
    purpura–hemolytic uremic
    syndrome, 196
transfusion-induced graft-versus-host
    disease, 652
vitamin B_{12} deficiency, 239
ALAS2 mutations, 268, 271
Albumin preparations, 640, 650
Alcohol abuse, 97, 310
  erythropoietic cell abnormalities, 92, 93
  macrocytosis, 242
    megaloblastic erythropoiesis, 244
    normoblastic erythropoiesis,
      244–245
  megakaryocyte increase, 96
  neutrophil precursor abnormalities, 94
  sideroblastic anemia, 269, 271
  thrombocytopenia, 537
Alder–Reilly anomaly, 302
Aldolase deficiency, 155
Aleukia, congenital (reticular
    dysgenesis), 309
ALK rearrangements, 423
Alkaline phosphatase, 9, 34

Alkylating-agent-related acute myeloid leukemia, 365, 366
All-*trans*-retinoic acid (ATRA), 362
Allele-specific oligonucleotides (ASO), 358
Allergic disorders
  eosinophil leukocytosis, 95, 311
  see also Immediate-type hypersensitivity reactions
Alloantibody-mediated thrombocytopenia, 539–540
Alloimmune hemolytic anemia, 192–194
  hemolytic disease of newborn, 193–194
  transfusion reactions, 192–193
Allorecognition, 682, 683, 684
  direct, 682
  indirect, 682
α_1 antitrypsin, 21, 33, 603
α_2-antiplasmin, 583
  cardiopulmonary bypass response, 588
α_2-antiplasmin deficiency, 592
  clinical features, 479
  diagnosis, 489
α granules, 18, 19, 20, 494, 495–496, 501–503, 529
  contents, 501, 529
  inherited disorders
    combined dense granule deficiency, 505
    enlarged granules, 505–506
    gray platelet syndrome, 503–505, 514
  platelet release response, 501
  storage pool disorder diagnosis, 482
  structure, 501
α_2 macroglobulin, 603
α-arabinosidase, 506
α-globin genes, 160, 170
  acquired mutations, 172
  α thalassemias
    deletions, 169, 170
    point mutations, 169, 170
    unstable α-globin variants, 170
  deletions in α thalassemia with mental retardation (ATR) syndromes, 171
  HS-40 regulatory element, 161
    deletions, 170
α-globins, 160
  α thalassemia, 169
  β thalassemia
    aggregates (ragged inclusions), 163
    excess production, 163, 166
  high-oxygen affinity hemoglobin variants, 180
  synthesis during development, 161
α-heavy-chain disease, 463–464
  treatment, 464
α-mannosidase, 9
α-methyldopa, 194, 547
Alport's syndrome, 512, 514
Aluminum, deposition in bone/bone marrow, 112
Amidopyrine-induced agranulocytosis, 306, 307

Aminolevulinic acid (ALA) synthase, 268
Aminosalicylic acid, 195, 239
AML1 fusion genes, 357, 375
AML1/ETO, 375
AML1/TEL, 357
Amyloidosis, 461
  bleeding disorder, 549
  bone marrow, 121
  classification, 461
  factor X deficiency, 571, 593
Anabolic steroids
  acquired aplastic anemia, 257
  complications, 260
  Fanconi anemia, 260
Anagrelide, 292, 531
Aniline hair dyes, 252
Anaphylactic blood transfusion reactions, 656
Anaplastic large cell lymphoma (systemic subtype), 423–424
chromosomal translocations, 423
Anaplastic lymphoma-associated kinase (ALK), 423, 424
Androgens, 30, 31
Anemia, 135–137
  blood loss-related, 137
  blood transfusion therapy, 647
    transfusion-related hemosiderosis, 101–102
  compensatory mechanisms, 136–137
  Cooley's, 162
  hemolytic, 137–140
  mechanisms, 137
  morphological classification, 137
  symptoms/signs, 135–136
Anemia of chronic disorders, 101, 211, 213, 218–220
  bone marrow sideroblasts, 102
  diagnosis, 219
  HIV infection/AIDS, 109
  iron metabolism, 218–219
  pathogenesis, 218
  treatment, 219–220
Angiocentric T-cell lymphoma *see* Extranodal NK/T 'nasal type' lymphoma
Angiogenesis, 476
Angioimmunoblastic lymphadenopathy associated pure red cell aplasia, 267
  bone marrow lesions, 111–112
Angioimmunoblastic T-cell lymphoma, 424–425
Anion exchanger 1 (AE1), 142, 143
Anisocytosis, 132, 235, 269, 276
Anisopoikilocytosis, 163, 334
ANK1 mutations, 143
Ankyrin, 142, 143, 625
Annexin II, 592
Anorexia nervosa, 120, 310
Anti-D immunoglobulin prophylaxis, 620
Antibiotics, antiplatelet activity, 478, 582
  Antibody-dependent cell-mediated cytotoxicity, warm autoimmune hemolytic anemia, 187
  Antibody-detection test, 647

Anticoagulant factors, 600–603
  deficiency, 603–604
Anticoagulant therapy
  clinical examination, 479
  international normalized ratio (INR) monitoring, 483
  'third space' bleeds, 478
Anticonvulsants, 241, 242
  macrocytosis, 245
  megaloblastic erythropoiesis, 244
Antidepressives, anti-platelet effects, 478
Antigen processing, 15, 668
  disruption by pathogens, 680
  MHC class I molecules, 679
  MHC class II molecules, 679–680
  invariant chain (Ii) function, 680
Antilymphocyte globulin (ALG)
  acquired aplastic anemia, 253, 256, 257
  paroxysmal nocturnal hemoglobinuria, 198
Antinuclear antibodies, 391
Antiphospholipid syndrome, 267, 606–607
Antiplasmin deficiency, 606
Antiplatelet drugs, 481, 581
  complications, 581
  laboratory monitoring, 582
Antiretroviral drugs, 109
Antithrombin, 476, 583, 601
  anticoagulant activity, 601
  cardiopulmonary bypass response, 588
  heparin binding, 601
  pregnant women, 21
  structure, 601
Antithrombin concentrates, 591
Antithrombin deficiency, 603–604, 648
  management, 609
  type I, 604
  type II, 604
Antithymocyte globulin (ATG), 253, 348
Antithyroid drugs, 251, 306
AnWj, 625
Aortic aneurysm, 591, 592
Aorto-gonads-mesonephros (AGM) region, 72, 73, 75
AP12-MLT fusion gene, 415
Apheresis, 645
Apheresis donors, 646
Aplastic anemias, 18, 91, 96, 97, 250–258, 310, 354
  acquired, 91, 250–258
  bone marrow examination, 533
    scoring system, 533
  bone marrow hemosiderin, 101
  clinical features, 255, 533
  clonal evolution, 255–256
  definition, 250
  differential diagnosis, 250
  drug-induced, 250–251, 532
  erythropoietic cell abnormalities, 92, 93
  hematology, 254–255
    neutropenia, 533
  industrial chemicals exposure-related, 251–252

inherited, 258–261
laboratory findings, 533
leukemia association, 255, 256
management, 533
megakaryocyte decrease, 97
myelodysplastic syndromes association, 255, 256
paroxysmal nocturnal hemoglobinuria, 254, 255–256
pathophysiology, 252–254, 532
bone marrow microenvironment, 253
immune processes, 253–254
stem cells, 253
radiation-induced, 532–533
severity classification, 252, 253
thrombocytopenia, 532–533
transfusion-induced graft-versus-host disease, 652
treatment
anabolic steroids, 257
growth factors, 256–257
immunosuppressive therapy, 253, 254, 256, 257, 258
stem cell transplantation, 257
viral etiological agents, 252, 533
Aplastic crises
hemolytic anemia, 139
sickle cell disease, 175
Apoptosis, 39, 57, 342, 346, 440–442
Apparent erythrocytosis, 284, 294
management, 294
Aprotinin, 589
Aquaporin 1, Colton antigen activity, 622–623
Arabinosylcytosine (Ara-C; cytarabine), 178, 243, 348, 531
Arachidonic acid metabolism, 545
platelets, 19–20
Arsenic poisoning, 243
Arteriosclerotic bone marrow lesions, 122
Arteritis/arteriolitis, 121
Aryl sulfatase, 506
Ascorbate, 209
L-Aspariginase, 592
Aspirin, 197, 536, 548
anti-platelet activity, 478, 549, 550
mode of action, 544, 545, 581, 582
Ataxia-telangiectasia, 317
Atheromatous bone marrow embolism, 122
ATP-binding cassette 7 (ABC7) mutations, 208, 269
ATR-X syndrome, 171–172
ATR-16 syndrome, 171
Atransferrinemia, congenital, 210, 223
Atypical mycobacterial infection, 107
bone marrow granulomas, 110, 111
Atypical pneumonia, 266
Audit, hemostatic testing, 490
Auer rods, 270
acute myeloid leukemia, 360, 361, 362, 363, 364, 367
Autoantibody-mediated thrombocytopenia, 540–544
Autoimmune disease

anemia of chronic disorders, 218
bone marrow lymphoid aggregates, 97
complement receptor-1 (CR1; CD35)
acquired deficiency, 625
hemophagocytic syndrome, 100
HLA allele associations, 699
pathogenesis, 681
Autoimmune hemolytic anemia, 187–192
autoimmune neutropenia, 307
blood transfusion, 653–654
cold antibodies, 190–192
marrow macrophage erythrophagocytosis, 100
warm antibodies, 187–190
Autoimmune neutropenia, 306, 307–308, 631
Autoimmune thrombocytopenia, 654
Autoimmune thrombocytopenic purpura, 96
treatment, 650
Autoimmune vasculitis, 196
Autologous blood donation, 642
intraoperative blood salvage, 643
perioperative hemodilution (acute normovolemic hemodilution), 643
postoperative blood salvage, 643–644
preoperative, 642–643
Automated blood-counting machines, 4, 9
Autoplex, 565
Autosomal recessive sideroblastic anemias, 269
5-Azacytidine, 173, 178, 348
Azathioprine, 190, 243, 267, 544

B

B_1-cells, 64
B-cell lymphomas, 412–422
AIDS/HIV patients, 109
B-cells, 17
antigen-dependent maturation, 39
antigen-independent maturation, 39
bone marrow, 63
cytokines influencing maturation, 39
differentiation, 39
motile activity, 63
phenotypic characterization, 72
plasma cell differentiation, 64
surface markers, 63
progenitor cell lineage-specific, 39
B-lineage acute lymphoblastic leukemias, 353
Babesiosis, 135
transmission by blood transfusion, 641, 658
Bacterial endocarditis, 100
Bacterial infections
bone marrow smears, 103
HIV-related opportunistic infection, 107
neutropenia, 306
Bacterial permeability inducer, 9, 12
bak-b antibodies, 540

Band 3 (Diego system blood group antigen), 189, 622
structural function, 625
Band 4.1 protein, 6, 142
Band 4.1 protein Madrid, 145
Band 4.1R protein Aravis, 145
Band 4.2 protein, 6, 142, 143
Band 4.2 protein Nippon, 143
Barr bodies, 9
Bartonella, 107
Bartonellosis (Oroya fever), 135
Basement membrane migration, 9
Basic-fibroblast growth factor (b-FGF), 78
multiple myeloma, 443
Basopenia, 310
Basophil colony-forming unit (CFU-Baso), 35
Basophil count, 10, 11
Basophil leukocytosis, 314
Basophilic stippling, 134, 152, 163, 180, 269, 270, 276, 278, 335
Basophils, 13–14, 21
granules, 13, 36
granulocytopoiesis, 35–36, 60
disease-related changes, 95
piecemeal degranulation, 13–14
BCL1, 387, 388, 418
BCL2, 79, 419, 420
BCL6, 386, 419, 420
BCNU chemotherapy, 451
BCR-ABL fusion gene/fusion protein
acute lymphoblastic leukemia, 357
chronic granulocytic leukemia, 393, 396
chronic myeloid leukemia, 357
Beige-nude-severe combined immunodeficiency mice (BNX mice), 73
Bence Jones protein, 447
Benefix, 561
Benzene
aplastic anemia induction, 532
bone marrow damage, 251, 252
myelodysplastic syndrome induction, 332
neutropenia induction, 306
pure red cell aplasia induction, 267
Bernard–Soulier syndrome, 516–518, 627
diagnosis, 482
platelet glycoprotein defects, 516
β locus control region (β-LCR), 161
$β_2$ microblobulin, 9, 675
multiple myeloma, 448
β-adrenergic agents, antiplatelet activity, 582
β-globin gene mutations
β thalassemia, 163–164
compound heterozygotes, 166
deletions, 164, 165
'dominantly inherited', 164, 181
point mutations, 164, 165
'silent', 164
δβ thalassemia, 167
γδβ thalassemia, 167
hemoglobin E, 162, 179
hemoglobin S (sickle hemoglobin), 174

hereditary persistence of fetal hemoglobin (HPFH), 167
thalassemia intermedia, 168, 169
β-globin genes, 160–161
  β locus control region (β-LCR), 161
β-globins, 160
  β thalassemia defect, 163
  δβ thalassemia defect, 167
  hemoglobin H (β₄ tetramers), 169, 170
  synthesis during development, 160, 161
β-glucuronidase, 9, 12
β-N-acetylgalactoseaminidase, 506
Bilirubin metabolism, hemolytic anemia, 138, 157
Bisphosphonates, 452
Bite cells, 195
Blastomycosis, 103
Bleeding time (skin bleeding time), 20, 482, 582
  cardiopulmonary bypass, 588
  neonate, 579
  renal disease/uremia, 586
Blister cells, 195
Blood cells, 4–21
Blood component therapy, 639
  administration techniques, 655
  apheresis collection method, 645–646
  component separation/storage procedures, 644–645
  plasma derivatives, 640
  red blood cells, 647–648
  see also Coagulation factor replacement therapy
Blood donation
  adverse reactions, 642, 646
  AIDS epidemic impact, 641, 657–658
    nucleic acid amplification testing (NAT), 658
  apheresis, 646
  autologous, 642
    intraoperative blood salvage, 643
    perioperative hemodilution (acute normovolemic hemodilution), 643
    postoperative blood salvage, 643–644
    preoperative, 642–643
  blood collection procedure, 641–642
    anticoagulation, 642
  directed (patient-specific), 644
  laboratory tests, 646–647
  medical history, 641
  physical examination, 641
  plasmapheresis, 640
  recruitment, 639–640
  therapeutic bleeding, 644
  venepuncture
    procedure, 642
    site, 641–642
  volunteerism, 639
  whole blood, 641–642
Blood groups, 616–631
  red cell transporters, 622–623
  systems, 616
Blood loss see Hemorrhage
Blood salvage
  intraoperative, 643

postoperative, 643–644
Blood substitutes, 659–660
Blood transfusion, 639–660
  AIDS epidemic impact, 640–641
  anemia, 647
    of chronic disorders, 219
  antenatal, 274
  autoimmune hemolytic anemia, 653–654
  β thalassemia, 162–163, 172–173
    indications, 173
  cardiovascular surgery, 652
  coagulation factor-containing products, 648–649
  compatibility testing (cross-matching), 647
    emergencies, 653
  complications see Blood transfusion reactions
  congenital dyserythropoietic anemia type I, 274
  cytomegalovirus-negative blood, 650–651, 654
  Diamond–Blackfan anemia, 266
  disease transmission, 639, 646, 650, 657–659
    antibody-detection test, 647
  hemopoietic growth factor uses, 659
  intrauterine, 194, 274
  iron overload, 220, 223
  irradiated blood compounds, 651–652
  massive, 652
    coagulation factor replacement, 649
    coagulopathy, 584, 587
    thrombocytopenia, 537
  myelodysplastic syndromes, 347
  national blood supply systems, 639–640
  neonates, 652, 653
    exchange transfusion, 653
  paroxysmal cold hemoglobinuria, 192
  pregnant patients, 654
  rare blood types, 654–655
  regulations/standards, 639, 641
  sickle cell anemia, 177, 178
  stem cell transplantation, 652–653
  techniques, 655
  urgent situations, 653
  warm autoimmune hemolytic anemia, 190
  see also Blood component therapy; Exchange transfusion
Blood transfusion reactions, 192–193, 655–657
  allergic, 656
  anaphylactic, 656
  delayed, 192
  febrile, 656
  graft-versus-host disease, 656–657
  hemolytic, 192, 616, 655
  platelet transfusions, 656
  pulmonary, 656
Blood transfusion-related hemosiderosis, 101, 140
Blood-borne virus infections, 559, 560
Bohr effect, 7
Bombay phenotype, 617

Bone lesions, multiple myeloma, 445–447
  bisphosphonates treatment, 452
Bone marrow, 54–68, 91–122
  aluminum deposition, 112
  amyloidosis, 121
  arteritis/arteriolitis, 121
  blood vessels, 58–59
  erythropoiesis, 26–31, 59
  examination, 90–91
    aspirated marrow smears, 90
    post mortem, 90–91
    trephine biopsy, 90
  fat cells (adipose tissue), 54, 55, 56, 57
  fetal hemopoiesis, 24
  fibroblasts, 57
  fibrosis (myelofibrosis), 113–116
    causes, 114
    generalized, 113
  gelatinous transformation, 120–121
  granulocytopoiesis, 31
  granuloma-like lesions, 111–112
  granulomas, 109–112
    lipid, 111
  hemopoietic cells, 24–43
    disease-related alterations, 92–100
  infections, 103–109
  iron stores, 62
    assessment methods, 101
    disease-related changes, 101–102
  lymphocytes, 55, 63–64
  lymphoid aggregates, 97
  lymphoid nodules, 63
  lymphopoiesis, 39
  macrophages (phagocytic reticular cells), 43–44, 55, 57
    ultrastructure, 44–45
  mast cells, 46, 47, 55
  megakaryopoiesis, 36–38
  metastatic tumors, 112–113, 114
  monocytopoiesis, 34–35
  necrosis, 119–120
    associated conditions, 119
  nerves, 58
  non-phagocytic reticular cells, 45–46
  osteoblasts, 46–47, 57, 59, 75
  osteoclasts, 46, 47
  plasma cells, 39, 40, 41–43, 44, 64
  postnatal changes, 24–25
  progenitor cells, 25, 54, 59
  sinusoids, 43, 44, 56, 74
    endothelial cells, 74–75
  stem cells, 25, 54, 59
  storage cells in lysosomal storage disease
    mucopolysaccharidoses, 119
    sphingolipidoses, 117–118
  structural organization, 54–55
    histomorphometry, 54
    parenchyme, 54, 59
    topography/architecture, 56
    myelodysplastic syndromes, 340–342
  vascular/embolic lesions, 121–122
Bone marrow aspirate, 48
  lymphoma, 409
  marrow smears, 90

hemosiderin assessment, 101
myelodysplastic syndromes, 336–339
Bone marrow cellularity, 55–56
assessment, 48
differential counts, 48–49
changes with aging, 56, 91
changes in infants/children, 48–50
disease-related alterations, 91
hypercellularity, 56, 91
acute lymphoblastic leukemia, 354
atypical chronic myeloid leukemia, 397
chronic granulocytic leukemia, 394–395
chronic lymphocytic leukemia, 384
chronic myelomonocytic leukemia, 398
eosinophilic leukemia, 400
juvenile chronic myelomonocytic leukemia, 399
myelodysplastic syndromes, 332, 337, 339
pernicious anemia, 235
polycythemia vera, 288, 289, 291
hypocellularity, 55–56, 91
acquired aplastic anemia, 252, 255
acute myeloid leukemia, 371
immunohistology, 55
normocellularity, 55
Bone marrow sections
artifacts, 65
diagnostic evaluation, 65
hemosiderin assessment, 101
processing methods, 65–68
paraffin embedding, 67
plastic embedding, 65–67
rapid processing, 67
Bone marrow stroma, 54–55, 56, 57–59
cells, 39, 43–45, 54–55, 72, 73–74
cell lines, 73–74
HIV infection-related damage, 108–109
sialomucin receptors, 77–78
extracellular matrix, 57, 72
fibers, 58
microenvironment
acquired aplastic anemia, 253
hemopoiesis, 56–57, 79, 80
sinusoids, 57
Bone marrow transplantation
β thalassemia, 173
Diamond–Blackfan anemia, 266
dyserythropoiesis following, 93
HLA allele matching, 699–700
multiple myeloma, 452–453
myelodysplastic syndromes, 348
paroxysmal nocturnal hemoglobinuria, 198
sickle cell anemia, 178
Bone marrow trephine biopsy, 48
histologic sections, 90
iron status assessment, 213
lymphoid infiltrates assessment, 429–430
hematogones, 429
reactive lymphoid aggregates, 429–430

lymphoma, 409–410
lymphoproliferative disease, 407–408
metastatic tumors detection, 113
myelodysplastic syndromes, 339
paraffin embedded specimens, 90
plastic-mebedded specimens, 90
touch preparations, 90
Bone metastases, 100
Bone plasmacytoma, solitary, 456–458
Borrelia burgdorferi, transmission by blood transfusion, 659
brca-1, 258
Breast carcinoma, bone marrow metastasis, 112
Brucella, 111
Brucellosis, 111, 314
Bruising, hemostatic disorders, 478, 479
Budd–Chiari syndrome, 607
Buffy coat method, platelet concentrate preparation, 645
Burkitt's lymphoma, 353, 421–422
AIDS/HIV patients, 109
bone marrow aspirate, 421
bone marrow trephine biopsy, 421–422
chromosomal translocations, 421
endemic, 421
Epstein–Barr virus, 317, 421
demonstration, 422
immunodeficiency-related, 421
immunohistochemistry, 421
peripheral blood, 421
sporadic, 421
Burn injury, 197
Bursa of Fabricius, 39
Busulfan, 292
Butyrate/butyrate analogs, 173, 178

C

C1 esterase inhibitor, 603
C3 receptors, 9, 11, 12, 14, 34
C3d receptor (CD21), 315, 424
C4 receptors, 12
C5a, 13
c-kit, 75
c-*KIT* mutations, 403
C/EBP transcription factors, 324
C/EBPE mutations, 302, 324
CA 19-9 (sialated LeSas), 619
Caisson disease, 119
Calcium, platelet function, 19, 20
Calnexin, 679
Calreticulin, 679
CAMPATH 1H, 544
Campbell de Morgan spots, 479
Candida, 107
Candidiosis, 103
Carbamazepine, 547
Carbaminohemoglobin, 7
Carbimazole, 251, 307
Carbon dioxide, red cell transport, 7
Carbonic anhydrase, 7
Carboxyhemoglobinemia, 162
Carcinomatous infiltration, bone marrow necrosis, 119

Cardiac hemolysis, 197
Cardiopulmonary bypass, 652
coagulopathy, 584, 587–589
laboratory monitoring, 589
treatment, 589
Cardiovascular surgery, 652
Cartilage-hair hypoplasia, 309
Cathepsins, 9, 12, 46
CBFβ–MYH11 fusion gene, 364, 375
CC chemokines (β chemokines), 76
CC receptors, 13, 14
CCNU chemotherapy, 451
CCR2, 14
CCR3, 12, 13
CCR5, 14, 108
CD1, 681, 686
CD1a, 355, 356
CD2, 356, 391, 392, 393
CD3, 63, 290, 355, 356, 376, 389, 391, 392, 393, 423, 680
CD4, 63, 108, 355, 356, 389, 392, 393
CD4 T-cells, 17, 680
helper phenotype (Th), 681
MHC class II restriction, 680–681
CD5, 356, 386, 391, 392, 393, 419
CD7, 39, 72, 355, 356, 372, 389, 391, 392
CD8, 63, 355, 356, 389, 391
CD8 T-cells, 17, 680
cytotoxic phenotype (Tcyt), 681
MHC class I restriction, 680–681
CD9, 373
CD10, 39, 72, 290, 353, 355, 356, 418, 420, 421, 429, 621
CD11a, 629, 630
CD11a/CD18 (LFA-1), 325, 444, 630
CD11b, 629, 630
CD11b/CD18 (CR3; Mac-1), 325, 444, 630
CD11c, 388
CD11c/CD18 (p150,95), 325, 444
CD11d/CD18, 325
CD13, 60, 355, 356, 371, 372
CD14, 371, 373
CD15, 30, 344, 356, 371, 372, 373, 426
CD16 (FcγRIIIb), 391, 629–630
CD19, 39, 72, 355, 372, 386, 387, 388, 458
CD20, 63, 290, 355, 386, 387, 388, 413, 414, 415, 416, 418, 419, 420, 421, 426, 429, 431, 458
CD21 (C3d receptor), 315, 424
CD22, 355, 386, 387, 388, 458
CD23, 386, 413, 424
CD25, 393
CD29, 443
CD30, 423, 424, 426
CD31, 423, 450
CD33, 60, 72, 355, 371, 372, 373
CD34, 59, 60, 72, 75, 76, 77, 78, 79, 80, 290, 355, 356, 371, 372, 373, 395, 423, 450, 646
immunohistochemistry, 344
CD35 (complement receptor-1; CR1; Knopps antigen), 624–625
CD38, 39, 72, 355, 356, 393, 449, 450, 454, 456, 458
CD40, 439, 444
CD41, 369, 373

713

CD41/CD61 *see* GPIIb/IIIa
CD42, 369
CD42a *see* GPIX
CD42b (GPIbα), 373, 627
CD42c (GPIbβ), 627
CD42d *see* GPV
CD43, 77, 78, 371
CD44, 443, 444, 624, 625
CD45, 355, 371, 372, 423, 426
CD45RA, 413, 414
CD45RO, 450
CD47, 623
CD49/CD20 *see* GPIa/IIa
CD49d (VLA-4), 443, 444
CD54, 443
CD55 (decay-accelerating factor; DAF), 198, 624, 625
CD56 (NCAM), 372, 391, 423, 443, 444, 450
CD57, 391
CD58 (LFA-3), 443, 623
CD59 (membrane inhibitor of reactive lysis), 198, 624
CD61, 290, 369, 371, 373
immunohistochemistry, 344
CD64, 373
CD65, 355
CD68, 62, 371, 414, 416
CD68-DAKO PG-M1, 290
CD70a, 420, 421
CD71, 373
CD79, 376
CD79a, 290, 355, 386, 387, 388, 413, 414, 415, 416, 418, 419, 426, 429
CD79b, 386, 387, 388
CD94/NKG2, 689–690
CD99, 624
CD103, 392
CD109, human platelet antigens (HPA) expression, 538, 626, 628
CD117, 371, 372
CD138 (syndecan-1), 64, 444, 446, 449, 450, 454, 456
CD147 (Ok glycoprotein), 623, 624
CD164, 77–78
CDAN1, 275
CDAN2, 276
CDAN3, 277
Cdc42, 326
CDP-choline phosphotransferase deficiency, 152
Cephalosporins, 194
antiplatelet activity, 582
Cerebellar hemangioblastoma, 292, 293
Cerebrovascular accident, sickle cell disease, 175, 176, 177
Ceruloplasmin, 210
gene mutations, 223
Chagas' disease, transmission by blood transfusion, 641, 658
Charcot–Leyden crystals, 12, 13
Chédiak–Higashi syndrome, 94, 300–301
infection susceptibility, 300
neutropenia, 310
platelet defects, 500–501
lysosomes, 506–507
Chelation therapy, 205, 224, 347

β thalassemia, 172
post-bone marrow transplantation, 173
thalassemia intermedia, 173
Chemical-induced myelodysplastic syndromes, 332–333
Chemical-induced sideroblastic anemia, 269
Chemokines
eosinophil responses, 13
hematopoiesis regulation, 76
Chemotaxis
basophils, 14
eosinophils, 13
monocytes, 14
neutrophils, 11
phagocyte responses, 322
Chemotherapy
complications
acute myeloid leukemia induction, 365–366
thrombocytopenia, 545
multiple myeloma, 450, 451–452
myelodysplastic syndromes, 348
Chest syndrome, acute, sickle cell disease, 175, 176, 177
Chickenpox *see* Varicella
Chloramphenicol, 93, 94, 267
aplastic anemia, 251, 532
Chloroma (granulocytic sarcoma; extramedullary acute myeloid leukemia), 371
Chlorpromazine-induced neutropenia/agranulocytosis, 306, 307
Cholestyramine, 239
Chondroitin sulfate, 13, 46, 78
Chromogenic coagulation factor assays, 488–489
Chromosomal abnormalities
acute lymphoblastic leukemia, 356–357
acute myeloid leukemia, 374
aggressive NK-cell leukemia, 391
chronic granulocytic leukemia, 393, 396
chronic lymphocytic leukemia, 386
chronic myelomonocytic leukemia, 399
juvenile chronic myelomonocytic leukemia, 400
MALT-type extranodal marginal zone lymphoma, 415
multiple myeloma, 444–445
myelodysplastic syndromes, 286–287, 345
polycythemia vera, 286, 287
prolymphocytic leukemia, 387
Sézary syndrome/mycosis fungoides, 392
splenic lymphoma with villous lymphocytes, 388
T-cell granular lymphocytic leukemia, 391
T-lineage prolymphocytic leukemia, 389
therapy-related acute myeloid

leukemia, 365
see also Chromosomal translocations
Chromosomal translocations
acute lymphoblastic leukemia, 353, 356, 357–358
acute myeloid leukemia, 333, 361–364, 374
anaplastic large cell lymphoma (systemic subtype), 423
Burkitt's lymphoma, 421
diffuse large B-cell lymphoma, 419
eosinophilic leukemia, 401
lymphoplasmacytic lymphoma, 412
mantle cell lymphoma, 418
multiple myeloma, 445
non-Hodgkin's lymphoma, 409
Chymase, 13, 46
Class II transactivator (CIITA), 674–675
Clinical governance, hemostatic testing, 490
Clinical scoring systems, hemostatic tests results, 490–491
CLIP, 680
Clonality demonstration
methods, 287
polycythemia vera, 286–287
Clopidogrel, 582
Clostridium infection, 196
Clostridium perfringens, 195
cMYC rearrangements, 421
Coagulation factor concentrates, 640, 649, 650
blood-borne virus transmission, 559, 560
HIV in hemophiliacs, 640
inhibitors development, 564–565
virucidal treatment, 559–560
Coagulation factor replacement therapy
blood products, 648–649
disseminated intravascular coagulation (DIC), 591
hemophilia A, 559–560
prophylaxis, 563–564
therapeutic strategies, 562
treatment on demand, 562–563
recombinant clotting factors, 560–562
von Willebrand's disease, 568
see also Blood component therapy
Coagulation factors
deficiency diagnosis, 487
functional bioassays, 488
chromogenic, 488–489
one-stage, 488
two-stage, 488
immunoassays, 489
liver synthesis, 583
monocytes, 14
platelet α granules, 501, 529
specific assays, 487–488
Coagulation pathway, 475, 476, 600
initiation, 475
intrinsic tenase complex, 475
platelet function, 20
prothrombinase complex, 475
Coagulation tests, 480, 483–489
diagnostic, 487–489
screening tests, 483–487

logical use, 486–487
Coccidioidomycosis, 103
Colchicine, 239
Cold agglutin test, 191
Cold autoimmune hemolytic anemia, 190–191
  autoantibody specificities, 191
Cold hemagglutinin disease *see* Cold autoimmune hemolytic anemia
Collagen
  bone marrow
    grading, 114
    myelofibrosis, 113
  platelet adhesion, 19
Collagen vascular disease, 95
Collagenase, 9, 12, 14
Colloid solutions, 648
Colony-forming unit in spleen (CFU-S), 25, 46
Colony-forming unit-Mix assays, 72
Colton antigen, 622–623
Common variable immunodeficiency, 327
Compatibility testing (cross-matching), blood donations, 647
Complement activation
  cold autoimmune hemolytic anemia, 191
  neutrophil phagocytosis, 11
  paroxysmal cold hemoglobinuria, 191
  warm autoimmune hemolytic anemia, 188
Complement receptor-1 (CR1; CD35), 624–625
Complement regulatory glycoproteins, red cell membrane, 624–625
Constitutional erythroid hyperplasia *see* Diamond–Blackfan anemia
Cooley's anemia, 162
Coombs' negative autoimmune hemolytic anemia, 189
Coombs' test *see* Direct antiglobulin test
Corticosteroids
  acute neutrophilia response, 311
  Diamond–Blackfan anemia, 266
  erythropoiesis influence, 31
  granulocytopenia, 310
  idiopathic thrombocytopenic purpura, 543
  neonatal alloimmune thrombocytopenia, 539
  paroxysmal nocturnal hemoglobinuria, 198
  post-transfusion purpura, 540
  thrombotic thrombocytopenic purpura–hemolytic uremic syndrome, 197
  warm autoimmune hemolytic anemia, 190
CR1 (CD35; Knopps antigen), 624–625
CR3 (CD11b/CD18; Mac-1), 325, 444, 630
Crohn's disease, 238, 242
Cromer blood group antigens, 624
Cross-reactive epitope groups (CREGs), 695
Cryoglobulinemia, 465

Cryoprecipitate
  indications, 649
  irradiation, 652
  preparation procedure, 644–645
Cryptococcosis, 103
Cryptococcus neoformans, 107, 108, 111
Crystalloid solutions, 648
Cushing's syndrome, 310
CXC chemokine receptors, 9
CXC chemokines (α chemokines), 76
CXCR4, 76, 108
Cyclical neutropenia, 308–309, 323
  genetic aspects, 323
Cyclodeaminase deficiency, 243
Cyclophosphamide, 190, 243, 257, 260, 451, 465
Cyclosporin, 198, 256, 257, 348, 544
Cytapheresis, 646
Cytarabine *see* Arabinosylcytosine
Cytochrome b5 reductase, 150
  deficiency, 181
Cytokines
  extracellular matrix interactions, 76
  helper T_H1 T-cells, 17
  helper T_H2 T-cells, 17
  hemopoiesis regulation, 25, 72, 75–76, 79, 80
    anemia of chronic disorders, 218–219
    lymphopoiesis, 39–40
  MHC class I gene expression regulation, 673
  multiple myeloma pathogenesis, 439–442, 443
    bone lesions, 446
  osteoblasts, 75
  receptors, 75
Cytomegalovirus, 107, 111, 647, 675, 680
  bone marrow examination, 103
  lymphocytosis, 314
  post-transfusion hepatitis, 657
  transmission by blood transfusion, 658
Cytomegalovirus-negative blood products, 650–651, 654
Cytoskeletal network, erythrocytes, 6
Cytotoxic T-cells (T_C cells), 17

D

D-dimer, 476, 608
D-dimer assay, 485–486
  fibrinolytic system testing, 489
Danazol, 190, 544
Dapsone, 109, 195, 544
DDT, hematologic toxicity, 251, 252, 532
Decay-accelerating factor (DAF; CD55), 198, 624, 625
Decitabine, 348
Defensins, 9, 12, 14
Deferipone (L1), 172, 224
Dehydrated hereditary stomatocytosis, 146
Dehydration, bone marrow specimen preparation, 65
del(16)(q22), 360, 364

δ granules *see* Dense bodies
Delta-1, 79
Delta-4, 79
δ-aminolevulinic acid synthase (ALAS), 207, 218
  mutations, 208
δ-globins, 160
  δβ thalassemia defect, 167
Delta-like (dlk), 74, 79, 80
Dense bodies (δ granules), 18, 20, 494, 495, 496, 529
  contents, 496–497, 529
  inherited defects
    Chediak–Higashi syndrome, 500, 501
    combined α granule deficiency, 505
    giant dense body disorder, 507
    Hermansky–Pudlak syndrome, 498
    storage pool deficiency, 499, 500
    serotonin (5-hydroxytryptamine; 5-HT) demonstration, 497
Dental-extraction-related bleeding, 477
Dermatan sulfate, 78
Dermatopathic lymphadenopathy, 391, 392
Desferrioxamine, 172, 173, 224, 347
Desmopressin (DDAVP), 547, 586
  hemophilia A, 564, 565
  von Willebrand's disease, 567–568, 570
Dextrans, antiplatelet activity, 582
Dialysis patients
  bone/bone marrow aluminum deposition, 112
  folate deficiency, 242
  neutropenia, 308
Diamond–Blackfan anemia, 266
DiSbs antigen, 189
Diclofenac, 194, 547
Diego system blood group antigen (band 3), 189, 622, 625
Diffuse large B-cell lymphoma, 419–421
  AIDS/HIV patients, 109
  bone marrow aspirate, 420
  bone marrow trephine biopsy, 420–421
  chromosomal translocations, 419
  clinical features, 419
  extranodal presentation, 419
  immunohistochemistry, 420
  peripheral blood, 419–420
Dihydrofolate reductase deficiency, 243
Dihydrofolate reductase inhibitors, 242
2,3-Diphosphoglycerate, 136, 644
  congenital deficiency, 292
  oxygen dissociation effect, 7
  red cell enzyme disorders, 155, 156
Diphyllobothrium latum (fish tapeworm), 238
Dipyridamole, 197
  mode of action, 582
Direct antiglobulin (Coombs') test
  cold autoimmune hemolytic anemia, 191
  drug-induced hemolytic anemia, 194
  warm autoimmune hemolytic anemia, 189

Directed (patient-specific) blood donation, 644
Disseminated intravascular coagulation (DIC), 481, 487, 533–534, 584, 589–592
  associated disorders, 590
    bone marrow necrosis, 119
    liver disease, 585
    malignant disease, 592
    pre-eclampsia/HELLP syndrome, 537
  cardiopulmonary bypass, 589
  chronic, 591–592
  clinical evaluation, 591
  end-organ damage, 590
  laboratory diagnosis, 534, 591
  management, 534, 591
  microvascular thrombosis, 589, 590
  pathogenesis/triggers, 534
  schistocytic hemolytic anemia, 196
  trigger mechanisms, 590
DMT1, 206, 207, 209, 211
DNA strand gel mobility assays, 693
DNA-based HLA allele identification, 692–693
  DNA strand gel mobility assays, 693
  sequence-based typing, 693
  sequence-sepcific priming, 692–693
  sequence-specific oligonucleotide probe hybridization (SSOPH), 693
Docetaxel, 304
Döhle bodies, 21, 103, 302, 304, 311, 509, 510, 514
Donath–Landsteiner biphasic antibody, 191–192
Donath–Landsteiner test, 192
Down's syndrome, 368, 369
  transient leukemia of infancy, 514
DPA1, 669
DPA2, 669
DPB1, 669
DPB2, 669
DQA1, 669
DQB1, 669
DRA, 669
DrSas antigen, 625
DRB, 669
DRB1, 669
Drug reactions
  agranulocytosis, 100, 306–307
  AIDS/HIV patients, 109
  aplastic anemia, 250–252, 532
  bleeding disorders, 579–582
  hemolysis, 154
    G6PD deficiency-related hemolytic crisis, 153
  hemolytic anemia, 194–195
    autoantibody induction, 194
    bystander effects, 195
    drug (hapten)-dependent antibodies, 194
    red cell oxidative injury, 195
  hemostatic disorders, 478
  hypersensitivity
    bone marrow granulomas, 111
    bone marrow granulomatous vasculitis, 121

megakaryocyte hypoplasia, 531
megaloblastic anemia, 243
myelodysplastic syndromes, 332–333
neutropenia, 306–307
platelet dysfunction, 549–550
pure red cell aplasia, 267
sideroblastic anemia, 269
thrombocytopenia, 544–547
  clinical features, 544
  immune-mediated, 545
  laboratory investigations, 544
  management, 544
  predictable (non-immune) reactions, 544–545
Duffy antigen receptor for chemokines (DARC), 623
Duffy blood group system, 189
  antigens, 623
  null phenotype, Plasmodium vivax malaria resistance, 623
  transfusion reactions, 192
Duke test, 20
Duncan's syndrome (X-linked lymphoproliferative disease), 317
Duodenal cytochrome b (Dcytb), 209, 211
Duodenal mucosal iron uptake, 209–210
Dutcher bodies, 412, 433, 448, 458
Dutcher–Fahey bodies, 97
Dyserythropoietic anemias, congenital, 91, 92, 274–282
  bone marrow hemosiderin, 101
  characteristics, 274
  diagnosis, 282
  groups IV-VII, 278–282
    classification, 279
  iron overload from excess iron absorption, 224
  pseudo-Gaucher cells, 117
  single family cases, 281
  type I, 274–276
  type II (hereditary erythroblastic multinuclearity with positive acidified serum lysis test), 276–277
  type III, 277–278, 279, 280
Dysfibrinogenemia, 605
Dysgranulopoietic neutropenia, congenital, 310

E

Echinocytes, 133
Ehlers–Danlos syndrome, 479
ELA2, 323
Elastase, 9, 14, 32, 33
Elliptocytes, 143, 144, 625
myelodysplastic syndromes, 335
Elliptocytosis, hereditary, 143–144, 625
  EPB41 mutations, 145
  SPTA1 mutations, 144–145
  SPTB mutations, 145
Embden–Meyerhof pathway, 6, 8, 11, 150
  enzyme defects, 150

biochemical investigations, 155, 156
clinical features, 151
molecular basis, 157
Rapoport–Luerbering shunt, 7
Embolism, bone marrow, 122
Embryonic hemoglobins, 24, 160
Emperipolesis, 38, 61
Endothelial cell damage
  disseminated intravascular coagulation (DIC), 590
  thrombotic thrombocytopenic purpura/hemolytic uremic syndrome, 535
Endothelial cells
  adhesion molecules, 325
  bone marrow sinusoids, 43, 58, 74–75
  neutrophil adhesion, 9, 11
  platelet adhesion, 19, 530
  primary hemostasis, 474
  stem cell interactions, 75
Endothelial protein C receptor, 601–602
Endothelin-3, 621
Endotoxins, 311
Energy metabolism
  erythrocytes, 6, 150–151
  neutrophils, 11
  platelets, 19
Enolase 1 deficiency, 154
Enyeart anomaly, 518
Enzyme-linked direct antiglobulin test, 189
Eosinopenia, 310
Eosinophil cationic protein (Rnase 3), 12, 13
Eosinophil chemotactic factor of anaphylaxis (ECF-A), 13
Eosinophil colony-forming unit (CFU-Eo), 35
Eosinophil count, 10, 11, 13
Eosinophil leukocytosis, 311–312
  causes, 312
  idiopathic hypereosinophilic syndrome, 312–314
Eosinophil peroxidase, 12, 13
Eosinophil-derived neurotoxin (Rnase 2), 12, 13
Eosinophilia, chronic myelomonocytic leukemia, 398, 399
Eosinophils, 12–13, 17
  functions, 13
  granules, 12
    development, 35
  granulocytopoiesis, 35, 60
    cytochemistry, 35
    cytology, 35
    disease-related abnormalities, 95
    ultrastructure, 35, 36
  lifespan, 13
  morphology, 12–13
  pregnant women, 21
  surface receptors, 12
Eotaxin, 13, 14
EPB3 (SLC4A1) mutations, 143, 145
EPB41 mutations, 145
EPB42 mutations, 143
Epipodophyllotoxin-related acute myeloid leukemia, 365, 366

Epistaxis, hemostatic disorders, 477
Epithelioid cell granulomas, 109, 110
Epithelioid histiocytes, 62
Epstein–Barr virus, 100, 107
  X-linked lymphoproliferative disease
      (Duncan's syndrome), 317
  aggressive NK-cell leukemia, 389,
      391
  angio-immunoblastic T-cell
      lymphoma, 424
  aplastic anemia, 252, 533
  atypical manifestations of infection,
      316–317
  Burkitt's lymphoma, 421, 422
  chronic active infection, 317
  lymphoproliferative disorders in
      immunocompromised subjects,
      317
  post-transfusion hepatitis, 657
  thrombocytopenia, 537
  see also Infectious mononucleosis
Epstein's syndrome, 512–513
Erythemic myelosis, 101
Erythroblastic islands, 26, 44, 56, 59
Erythroblastic multinuclearity with
      positive acidified serum lysis test,
      hereditary (HEMPAS; congenital
      dyserythropoietic anemia type II),
      276–277
Erythroblastopenia, congenital *see*
      Diamond–Blackfan anemia
Erythroblastosis fetalis *see* Hemolytic
      disease of newborn
Erythroblasts, 26, 59
  cytochemistry, 27, 28
  cytology, 26–27
  disease-related changes
    infections, 103
    morphologic abnormalities, 92–94
    myeloid/erythroid (M/E) ratio, 92,
        103
    stainable non-hemoglobin iron
        alterations, 102
    ultrastructural abnormalities, 94, 95,
        96
  iron uptake, 208
  post mortem changes, 91
  ultrastructure, 28–29, 30, 31
    minor abnormalities, 93
Erythrocytes *see* Red cells
Erythrocytosis, 284
  absolute, 284, 292
    classification, 284, 285
    laboratory investigations, 286
    polycythemia vera, 285, 286
  apparent, 284, 294
  classification, 284
  idiopathic, 293–294
  packed cell volume (PCV) estimation,
      284
  red cell mass (RCM) estimation, 284
  secondary, 286, 292–293
    causes, 286
    management, 293
  see also Polycythemia vera
Erythroenzyme disorders *see* Red cell
      enzyme disorders

Erythrogenesis imperfecta *see*
      Diamond–Blackfan anemia
Erythroid burst-forming units (BFU-E),
      26, 208, 288
  assays, 72
  parvovirus B19 infection, 252
Erythroid colony-forming units (CFU-
      E), 26, 208
Erythroid hyperplasia
  congenital dyserythropoietic anemias,
      275, 277
  hemolytic anemia, 138, 139
  iron overload from excess absorption,
      224
  sideroblastic anemias, 270
Erythroid Krüppel-like factor (EKLF),
      161
Erythroid-specific transcription factors,
      161
Erythroleukemia *see* Leukemia, acute
      erythroid (FAB M6)
Erythropoiesis, 26–31, 54, 59
  assessment indices, 135, 136
  erythroblast iron uptake, 208
  globin gene expression regulation, 161
  hormonal influences, 30–31
  ineffective *see* Ineffective
      erythropoiesis
  myelodysplastic syndromes, 337
  progenitor cells, 26
  red cell surface glycoprotein
      expression, 624
  regulation, 29–31
Erythropoietin, 15, 24
  erythropoiesis regulation, 29–30, 31,
      208, 252, 253
  familial autonomous high production,
      292
  polycythemia vera, 287, 288
  postnatal/infantile production, 49
  renal production, 30, 31
    impairment in anemia of chronic
        disorders, 218
  secondary erythrocytosis, 286
Erythropoietin receptors, 208
Erythropoietin therapy, 173, 178, 210,
      659
  anemia of chronic disorders, 219–220
  autologous blood donation, 643
  functional iron deficiency, 213, 217
  myelodysplastic syndromes, 347
Escherichia coli, 625
  enterotoxin-producing, 196
Escherichia coli 0157.H7 verotoxin, 536
Essential cryoglobulinemia, 465
Essential thrombocythemia, 314
  megakaryocyte increase, 96
  platelet abnormalities, 548, 592
  thrombosis risk, 548, 607
Estrogens, 31, 531, 586–587
Ethanol-induced megakaryocyte
      hypoplasia, 531
Ethnic differences
  HLA alleles/haplotypes, 671–672
  neutrophil counts, 10, 309
  platelet counts, 19
Ethylenediamene tetracetic acid

(EDTA)-induced
      pseudothrombocytopenia, 531
Etiocholanolone, 311
Euglobulin clot lysis time, 489
EVI-1, 345
Ewing's sarcoma, bone marrow
      metastasis, 112, 113
Exchange transfusion, 653
  neonatal alloimmune neutropenia, 654
  neonatal alloimmune
      thrombocytopenia, 539, 654
Exfoliative dermatitis, 242
Extracellular matrix, 74
  bone marrow stroma, 57, 72
  cytokine interactions, 76
  hemopoiesis, 76–78
Extramedullary hemopoiesis
  bone marrow necrosis, 120
  hemolytic anemia, 139, 140
  idiopathic myelofibrosis, 115
  polycythemia vera, 291, 292
Extramedullary plasmacytoma, 458
Extranodal marginal zone lymphoma,
      mucosa-associated lymphoid
      tissue (MALT)-type, 415
  bone marrow involvement, 415
  chromosomal abnormalities, 415
  cryoglobulinemia, 465
  progression to large cell lymphoma,
      415
Extranodal NK/T 'nasal type'
      lymphoma, 422
Extrinsic factor pathway inhibitor *see*
      Tissue factor pathway inhibitor

F

F cells, 160
Fabry's disease, 118
Factor II *see* Prothrombin
Factor V, 19, 20
  acquired inhibitors, 589, 593
  coagulation pathway, 475, 600
  coagulation screen, 483, 484
  hepatic function assessment, 584
  inactivation, 476
  platelet α granules, 501, 529
  pregnant women, 21
  protein C–protein S system inhibition,
      601, 602
Factor V deficiency, 571, 572
  combined factor VIII deficiency, 487
  fresh frozen plasma (FFP)
      replacement therapy, 648
Factor V Leiden, 604–605, 609
Factor Va assay, 609
Factor VII, 20
  acquired inhibitors, 593
  activation, 600
  coagulation initiation, 475, 600
  coagulation screen, 483
  hepatic function assessment, 584
  pregnant women, 21
Factor VII deficiency, 571, 572
Factor VIIa–tissue factor complex, 475
Factor VIII, 20

acquired inhibitors, 593, 594
coagulation pathway, 475, 600
coagulation screen, 484, 486
elevation, thrombosis association, 605, 609
gene, 558
gene mutations, 558
inactivation, 476
pregnant women, 21
protein C–protein S system inhibition, 601, 602
replacement therapy
  cryoprecipitate, 644, 645
  fresh frozen plasma (FFP), 648
  see also Coagulation factor replacement therapy; Factor VIII concentrates
Factor VIII concentrates, 559–560, 649
  antibodies development, 564
  blood-borne virus transmission, 559, 560
  virucidal treatment, 559–560
  see also Recombinant Factor VIII
Factor VIII deficiency see Hemophilia A
Factor VIIIR:Ag, 61
Factor IX, 20
  activation, 600
  antithrombin inhibition, 601
  coagulation pathway, 475
  coagulation screen, 484, 486
  elevation, thrombosis association, 605
  gene, 558
  gene mutations, 558
  pregnant women, 21
  replacement therapy
    fresh frozen plasma (FFP), 648
    see also Coagulation factor replacement therapy; Factor IX concentrates
Factor IX concentrates, 649
  virucidal treatment, 560
  see also Recombinant Factor IX
Factor IX deficiency see Hemophilia B
Factor X, 20
  activation, 600
  antithrombin inhibition, 601
  coagulation pathway, 475
  coagulation screen, 483, 484
  fresh frozen plasma (FFP) replacement therapy, 648
  pregnant women, 21
  protein Z–ZPI interaction, 603
Factor X deficiency, 571, 572
  amyloidosis, 593
Factor XI
  antithrombin inhibition, 601
  coagulation screen, 484, 486
  elevation, thrombosis association, 605
  fresh frozen plasma (FFP) replacement therapy, 648
Factor XI deficiency, 571–573
Factor XII
  C1 esterase inhibitor activity, 603
  coagulation screen, 484
Factor XII deficiency, 606
Factor XIII, 606
  acquired inhibitors, 593

Factor XIII concentrate, 573
Factor XIII deficiency, 572, 573
  diagnosis, 487
Familial benign chronic neutropenia, 309
Familial high-density lipoprotein deficiency (Tangier disease), 119
Familial Mediterranean fever, 121
Familial pseudohyperkalemia, 146
Familial vacuolization of leukocytes (Jordan's anomaly), 94, 302
Fanconi anemia, 91, 258–261
  clinical course, 259
  genetic aspects, 258–259
  hematologic features, 259
    megakaryocyte hypoplasia/thrombocytopenia, 97, 496
  skin/skeletal abnormalities, 258, 259
  treatment, 260
Farnesyl transferase inhibitors, 348
Fava bean-related hemolytic crises, 153
Fc receptors, warm autoimmune hemolytic anemia, 187–188
FcγRIIIb (CD16), 391, 629–630
Febrile blood transfusion reactions, 656
Fecal occult blood test, 214
Fecal urobilinogen, 138
FEIBA, 565, 594
Felty's syndrome, 267, 307, 389
Ferritin, 101, 102, 206, 209, 210
  anemia of chronic disorders, 219
  iron status assessment, 211–212, 219, 220, 222
  regulation of synthesis, 207, 208
Ferrochelatase, 205, 268
Ferroportin, 210, 211
  iron overload-related mutations, 223
Ferrous gluconate, 217
Ferrous sulfate, 216–217
Fetal hemoglobin see Hemoglobin F
Fetal hemopoiesis
  bone marrow, 24
  liver, 24, 72, 73
Fetal liver tyrosine kinase receptor-3 (FLT3-R), 75
Fibrin clot
  formation, 20, 475, 476, 530
  removal, 476
Fibrin degradation products, 476, 608
Fibrin glue, 652
Fibrin–fibrinogen degradation products assay, 485–486, 487
Fibrinogen
  coagulation screen, 483, 484
  cryoprecipitate content, 644, 645
  platelet aggregation/binding, 19, 475
  integrin interactions, 530
  platelet α granules, 501, 529
  pregnant women, 21
  replacement therapy, 649
  thrombosis-related abnormalities (dysfibrinogenemia), 605
Fibrinogen assays, 485, 487
  fibrinolytic system testing, 489
Fibrinogen concentrate replacement therapy, 570

Fibrinolysis
  cardiopulmonary bypass, 588
  diagnostic tests, 489
  disseminated intravascular coagulation (DIC), 590
  liver disease, 585
  neonate, 579
  pathway, 475, 476
  renal disease, 586
  thrombosis, 605–606
Fibrinopeptide A assay, 608
Fibroblast growth factor, 15
Fibroblasts, 59
  bone marrow, 57
  cell lines, 74
  HIV infection, 108
Fibronectin, 76, 77, 80
  platelet α granules, 529
  platelet integrin interactions, 530
Fibronectin receptor (GPIc/IIa), 528
Filariasis
  cardiac damage (Löffler's endocarditis), 314
  tropical eosinophilia, 312
Fish tapeworm (Diphyllobothrium latum), 238
Fixation of bone marrow specimens, 65
Flavocytochrome b_{558}, 327
Flow cytometry
  acute lymphoblastic leukemia
    immunophenotypic diagnosis, 355
    residual disease detection, 356
  acute myeloid leukemia diagnosis, 372–373
  lymphoma investigation, 409
  multiple myeloma, 444, 450
Fluorescent in situ hybridization
  multiple myeloma, 444, 445
  myelodysplastic syndromes, 345
FMC7, 386, 387, 388, 458
Foam cells, 62
Foamy macrophages, 118, 119
Focal adhesion kinase, 77
Folate deficiency, 234, 241
  causes, 234, 241
    acquired abnormalities of metabolism, 242
    congenital metabolic disorders, 243
    dietary inadequacy, 241–242
    increased loss, 242
    increased requirement, 242
    malabsorption, 242
  dyserythropoiesis, 92
  hemolytic anemia, 139
  hemopoietic cell abnormalities, 94
  macropolycytes, 304
  neutrophil right shift, 302
  preterm infants, 242
  thrombocytopenia, 538
Folate malabsorption, hereditary, 243
Folate supplements
  β thalassemia intermedia, 173
  neural tube defect prevention, 241
  sickle cell disease in pregnancy, 177, 178
Folates, 241
  dietary sources, 241

metabolism, 241
requirement in pregnancy, 21, 242
Follicular lymphoma, 416–418, 432, 433
bone marrow aspirate, 416
bone marrow trephine biopsy,
416–418
clinical features, 416
cryoglobulinemia, 465
immunohistochemistry, 418
lymph node pathology, 416
peripheral blood, 416
Frataxin gene mutations, 208
Fresh frozen plasma (FFP), 534
cardiopulmonary bypass-related
coagulopathy, 589
coagulation factor replacement
therapy, 648–649
disseminated intravascular
coagulation (DIC), 591
factor V deficiency, 571
factor XI deficiency, 571
indications, 648–649
irradiation, 652
preparation procedure, 644
thawing procedure, 644
thrombotic thrombocytopenic
purpura, 535
vitamin K deficiency, 583
Friederich's ataxia, 208
Frizzled receptors, 79
Frozen deglycerolized red cell
preparations, 648
Fungal infection, 110
bone marrow changes, 103
HIV-related, 107
FUT1, 617
FUT2, 617
FUT3, 618
FySas, 623
FySbs, 623

G

Gallstones, 139, 157, 175
γ-globins, 160
δβ thalassemia/γδβ thalassemia
increased production, 167
hemoglobin Bart (γS4s tetramers), 170
γ-glutamylcysteine synthetase
deficiency, 156
red cell oxidative damage, 153
γ-heavy-chain disease, 464
Ganciclovir, 109
Gastrectomy, 214, 234, 237–238, 242
Gastrointestinal bleeding, hemostatic
disorders, 477
Gaucher cells, 62, 117
Gaucher's disease, 117
Geisböck's syndrome *see* Apparent
erythrocytosis
Gelatinase, 9
Gene therapy
β thalassemia, 173
Fanconi anemia, 260
Gerbich blood-group antigens, 625
Giant cells, 34, 62

granulomas, 109, 110
Giant dense body disorder, 507
Giant metamyelocytes, 94, 231, 232
Giardiasis, 239
Giemsa stain, 66, 67
Gilbert syndrome, 157
Glanzmann's thrombasthenia, 627
diagnosis, 482
Globin genes, 160–161
developmental stage-specific
expression, 160, 161
erythroid-specific transcription
factors, 161
tissue-dependent expression, 160, 161
upstream regulatory elements, 161
Globins, 7, 160
β thalassemia, 163
hyperunstable variants, 162
unstable hemoglobins, 179–180
see also α-globins; β-globins; δ-globins;
γ-globins
Glucose-6-phosphate dehydrogenase
(G6PD), 150
mosaicism, 25
variants
class I, 150, 151
geographical distribution, 151
Glucose-6-phosphate dehydrogenase
(G6PD) deficiency
biochemical investigations, 155, 156
bone marrow hemosiderin, 101
drug-induced hemolytic anemia, 195
drug/fava bean-induced hemolytic
crises, 153
Heinz bodies, 154
molecular pathology, 157
neonatal hyperbilirubinemia, 151
prenatal diagnosis, 156
red cell oxidative damage, 152–153
erythrocyte 'hemighosts', 153
Glucose-phosphate isomerase
deficiency, 150, 151
biochemical investigations, 155
prenatal diagnosis, 156
Glue sniffing, 93
Glutamate formiminotransferase
deficiency, 243
Glutathione pathway, 150
enzyme defects, 150–151
biochemical investigations, 155
clinical features, 151
drug-induced hemolytic anemia,
195
molecular basis, 157
Glutathione peroxidase deficiency, 155
Glutathione reductase deficiency, 153
Glutathione synthetase deficiency,
150–151, 156
red cell oxidative damage, 153
Gluten-sensitive enteropathy, 239, 242
Glycophorin A, 189, 290, 344, 371, 625
Glycophorin C, 344, 625
Glycophorin D, 625
Glycophorins, *Plasmodium falciparum*
ligands, 625
Glycosaminoglycans, 78, 80
Glycosylation disorders, congenital, 325

type I, 325
type II, 325
type IIc (leukocyte adhesion
deficiency type 2 (LAD 2),
325–326
Gold salts, 251, 544, 545, 547
Gov^a, 628
Gov^b, 628
gp91^{phox}, 327
gp130, 75, 76
GPIa, human platelet antigens (HPA)
expression, 626
GPIa/IIa (CD49/CD20; VLA-2), 528
human platelet antigens (HPA)
expression, 538, 627–628
GPIb
defects in Bernard–Soulier syndrome,
516, 517
human platelet antigens (HPA)
expression, 538, 626
GPIbα (CD42b), 373, 627
GPIbβ (CD42c), 627
GPIb/IX
autoantibodies, idiopathic
thrombocytopenic purpura (ITP),
540, 541, 542
GPV complex, human platelet
antigens (HPA) expression, 627
uremia-related abnormality, 547
GPIc/IIa (fibronectin receptor), 528
GPIc'/IIa (laminin receptor), 528
GPIIb, human platelet antigens (HPA)
expression, 626
GPIIb/IIIa (CD41/CD61), 19, 474, 528
autoantibodies, idiopathic
thrombocytopenic purpura (ITP),
540, 542
autoantigenic epitopes, 543
deficiency, 627
human platelet antigens (HPA)
expression, 538, 627
platelet adhesion, 530
polymorphisms, platelet function,
629
structure, 543, 627
GPIIIa, human platelet antigens (HPA)
expression, 626
GPIV, 19
human platelet antigens (HPA)
expression, 538
GPV (CD42d), 627
defects in Bernard–Soulier syndrome,
516, 517
human platelet antigens (HPA)
expression, 538
GPIX (CD42a), 19, 627
defects in Bernard–Soulier syndrome,
516, 517
human platelet antigens (HPA)
expression, 538
immunohistochemistry, 344
Graft-versus-host disease, 239, 310, 667,
682, 684, 686
transfusion-related, 651, 652, 656–657
Granulocyte antigens, 629–631
FcγRIIIb (CD16), 629–630
function, 629–630

polymorphisms, clinical relevance, 631
structure, 629–630
Granulocyte counts, 10, 11
Granulocyte transfusion, 650
Granulocyte-colony stimulating factor (G-CSF), 15, 25, 75, 256–257, 646
  acquired aplastic anemia, 252, 253
  myelodysplastic syndromes, 347
  neutropenia, 308, 309, 323
Granulocyte–macrophage colony stimulating factor (GM-CSF), 15, 25, 75, 78, 659
Granulocyte–macrophage colony-forming units (CFU-GM), 31
  assays, 72
Granulocytes (polymorphonuclear leukocytes), 9–15, 59
  blood component preparation procedure
    leukapheresis, 646
    whole blood, 645
  circulating pool (CGP), 10
  marginated pool (MGP), 10
  megaloblastic erythropoiesis-related abnormalities, 231
  morphological abnormalities
    acquired, 302–305
    inherited, 300–302
  post mortem changes, 90
  stem cells, 25
  toxic granulation of neutropenia, 254
Granulocytic sarcoma (chloroma; extramedullary acute myeloid leukemia), 371
Granulocytopoiesis (myelopoiesis), 54, 56, 322
  basophils, 35–36
  eosinophils, 35, 36
  myelodysplastic syndromes, 338
  myeloid/erythroid (M/E) ratio, 92
  neutrophils, 31–34, 60
  response to infection, 322
Granuloma-like bone marrow lesions, 111–112
Granulomas, bone marrow, 90, 103, 109–112
  AIDS/HIV infected patients, 107, 108
  cellular composition, 109
  lipid, 111
Granulomatous disease, chronic, 118, 326, 327
  genetic aspects, 327
Granulomatous vasculitis, 121
Gray platelet syndrome, 115, 503–505, 514–515
Growth factors, aplastic anemia treatment, 256–257
GYPC, 625

H

H antigens, 617
  Lewis antigens synthesis, 618
HA-1, 687
Haemophilus influenzae, 625

splenectomy patient vaccination, 173, 190
Hairy cell leukemia/hairy cell leukemia variant, 413–415
  bone marrow aspirate, 413
  bone marrow trephine biopsy, 413–415
  granuloma formation impairment, 111
  immunohistochemistry, 414–415
  peripheral blood, 413
  reticulin fibrosis, 113
  spleen involvement, 413
Ham's test, 198
Haplotype, 671
  extended, 673
  inheritance, 671
Haptoglobins, 138
Heat stroke, 304
Heavy chain disorders, 463–465
  α-heavy-chain disease, 463–464
  γ-heavy-chain disease, 464
  μ-heavy-chain disease, 464–465
Heinz bodies, 153–154, 179, 180, 195
Heinz body hemolytic anemia, congenital, 179, 180, 181
Helicobacter pylori, 625
HELLP syndrome, 536–537
Helper T-cells (T$_H$ cells), 17, 681
  hemopoiesis regulation, 17–18
  T$_H$0 subtype, 17
  T$_H$1 subtype, 17
  T$_H$2 subtype, 17
Hematin, 138
Hematocrit (packed cell volume; PCV), 4–5
  erythrocytosis, 284
Hematogones, 429
Heme, 160
  breakdown, 206
  dietary iron absorption, 209–210, 214
  intravascular hemolysis-related blood levels, 138
  synthesis, 205–206
Heme oxygenase, 206, 210
Hemochromatosis, hereditary, 101, 205, 220
  abnormal sideroblasts, 102
  hepatic iron index, 213
  HFE mutations, 208, 211
  HFE-related, 220–223
    clinical features, 222
    diagnosis, 222
    genetics, 220–221
    screening, 222–223
    treatment, 222
  iron metabolism, 208, 211
  non-HFE-related, 223
  transferrin receptor 2 (TfR2) gene mutations, 209
  type 2 (juvenile hemochromatosis), 223
  type 3, 223
Hemochromatosis, neonatal, 223
Hemochromatosis, secondary, 102
Hemoglobin
  abnormalities, 160–181
  acquired disorders, 162

concentration, 4, 5, 284
  pregnant women, 20
  red cell transfusion indications, 647
δβ fusion variants, 162
developmental switches, 160–161
embryonic, 24, 160
  switch to fetal hemoglobin (Hb F) production, 160
globin chains, 160
haptoglobin complexes clearance, 138
heme group, 160
inherited disorders, 161–181
oxygen affinity, 7
oxygen transport, 7, 160
solutions as blood substitutes, 660
structural variants *see* Hemoglobin variants
structure, 160
synthesis, 8
Hemoglobin A (Hba), 7, 160
  β thalassemia, 163
  fetal hemopoiesis, 24
  oxygen dissociation curve, 7
Hemoglobin A$_2$, β thalassemia, 163
Hemoglobin Bart's, 170
  α thalassemia, 169
Hemoglobin Bart's hydrops syndrome, 169, 170
Hemoglobin C, 173, 179
  dyserythropoiesis in homozygotes, 92
Hemoglobin C/hemoglobin S double heterozygotes *see* Hemoglobin SC disease
Hemoglobin Chesapeake, 180
Hemoglobin Constant Spring, 170, 171
Hemoglobin D-Punjab/hemoglobin S double heterozygotes, 134, 178
Hemoglobin E, 162, 173, 179, 181
  genetic aspects, 162, 167
  homozygous disease, 167
    bone marrow necrosis, 119
    dyserythropoiesis, 92
Hemoglobin E/hemoglobin H disease, 179
Hemoglobin E/β thalassemia, 166–167, 179
Hemoglobin E/hemoglobin S double heterozygotes, 134
Hemoglobin electrophoresis
  α thalassemias, 169
  β thalassemia, 163
  hemoglobin E/β thalassemia, 167
  sickle cell disease, 176
Hemoglobin F (fetal hemoglobin), 160
  β thalassemia, 163
    therapeutic gene activation, 173
  fetal hepatic hemopoiesis, 24
  hereditary persistence (HPFH), 162, 167–168
  levels in sickle cell disease, 177
    therapeutic augmentation, 178
  oxygen affinity, 160
  pregnant women, 21
  switch to adult hemoglobin production, 160
Hemoglobin G-Philadelphia, 181
Hemoglobin Geneva, 162

Hemoglobin Gower I, 24, 160
Hemoglobin Gower II, 24, 160
Hemoglobin H, 170
  α thalassemias, 169
Hemoglobin H disease, 169, 171, 335
  acquired, 162
  hemoglobin E interactions, 179
  iron overload from excess iron
      absorption, 224
  red blood cell inclusions, 171, 172
Hemoglobin H hydrops fetalis, 169, 171
Hemoglobin Hasharon, 180
Hemoglobin Icaria, 170
Hemoglobin Knossos, 181
Hemoglobin Koln, 180
Hemoglobin Koya Dora, 170
Hemoglobin Lepore, 162, 181
Hemoglobin Lepore/hemoglobin S
      double heterozygotes, 134
Hemoglobin M variants, 181
Hemoglobin O-Arab/hemoglobin S
      double heterozygotes, 134, 178
Hemoglobin Portland, 24, 160
Hemoglobin Quong Sze, 170
Hemoglobin S, 173, 174
  α thalassemia co-inheritance, 176, 177
  compound heterozygous states,
      sickling disorders, 134, 178–179
  deoxygenation-related
      polymerization, 176–177
  homozygotes (sickle cell anemia)
      bone marrow necrosis, 119
      sickle-shaped red cells, 134, 135
  molecular features, 174
  sickle cell disease diagnosis, 176
Hemoglobin S/β thalassemia, 174, 175,
      178–179
  bone marrow necrosis, 119
  diagnostic features, 176
  sickle-shaped red cells, 134
Hemoglobin SC disease, 174, 175, 178,
      179
  bone marrow necrosis, 119
  diagnostic features, 176
  red cell sickling, 134
Hemoglobin SD disease, 174
Hemoglobin Seal Rock, 170
Hemoglobin Tarrent, 180
Hemoglobin variants, 161
  abnormal oxygen binding, 180–181
  high-oxygen affinity, 180–181
  low-oxygen affinity, 181
  secondary erythrocytosis, 292
  unstable
      dyserythropoiesis, 92
      hemolytic anemia, 179, 180
Hemoglobinemia, 138
Hemoglobinuria, 138, 139
Hemolytic anemia, 91, 137–140
  abnormal sideroblasts, 102
  acquired, 186–198
      clinical features, 186
      pathogenesis, 187
  aplastic crises, 139
  bilirubin metabolism, 138
      gallstones formation, 139, 157
  biochemical features, 138, 186

bone marrow hemosiderin, 101
cardiac hemolysis, 197
classification, 140
erythroid hyperplasia-related bone
    deformities, 139
extramedullary hemopoiesis, 139, 140
extravascular hemolysis, 137–138, 186
hematologic features, 138–139
hepatic failure patients, 198
hereditary/acquired causes, 140
immune *see* Immune hemolytic
    anemia
infection-induced, 195
intravascular hemolysis, 138, 186
leg ulcers, 140
non-immune, 195–198
osmotic damage, 197
paroxysmal nocturnal
    hemoglobinuria, 197–198
red cell damage
    external impact, 195–196
    thermal, 197
    traumatic, 197
red cell enzyme disorders, 150,
    151–152
    clinical features, 151
red cell membrane defects, 142–146
renal failure patients, 198
Rhesus-deficiency syndrome, 620
schistocytic, 196
sickle cell disease, 174, 175, 177
splenomegaly, 139–140
thrombotic thrombocytopenic
    purpura–hemolytic uremic
    syndrome, 196–197
toxin-induced, 198
transfusion-related hemosiderosis, 140
unstable hemoglobins, 179, 180
venom-induced, 198
Hemolytic disease of newborn
    (erythroblastosis fetalis), 193–194,
    616
  ABO blood group system, 618
  Kell blood group system, 621
  prevention, 193, 620
  Rhesus blood-group system, 620
  therapeutic interventions, 193–194
Hemolytic states, 137
  bone marrow lymphoid aggregates,
    97
  compensation, 137, 138
  marrow macrophage
    erythrophagocytosis, 100
Hemolytic transfusion reactions, 616,
    655
Hemolytic uremic syndrome, 196–197,
    534
  children, 536
  classification, 534
  clinical features, 536
  diagnosis, 535
  etiology, 536
  laboratory investigations, 536
  management, 536
  pathogenesis, 535, 536
  see also Thrombotic thrombocytopenic
    purpura

Hemopexin, 138
Hemophagocytic syndromes, 98–100
  associated conditions, 100
    AIDS/HIV infection, 109
Hemophilia
  clinical features, 479
  coagulation factor therapy-related
    HIV infection, 640
  family history, 478
  'third space' bleeds, 478
Hemophilia A (factor VIII deficiency),
    558
  acquired inhibitors, 593
    development, 564–565
    treatment, 564–565
  carrier detection, 558
  clinical features, 559
  combined factor V deficiency, 487
  diagnosis, 484, 558
  inheritance, 558
  molecular basis, 558
  therapeutic strategies, 562
    prophylaxis, 563–564
    treatment on demand, 562–563
    vascular access, 564
  therapy
    cryoprecipitate, 645
    desmopressin (DDAVP), 564, 565
    factor VIII concentrates, 559–560
    recombinant Factor VIII, 560–561
    recombinant Factor VIIa, 561–562
Hemophilia B (factor IX deficiency),
    558–559
  acquired inhibitors, 593
  carrier detection, 559
  clinical features, 559
  diagnosis, 484, 558
  inheritance, 558
  therapeutic strategies, 562
    prophylaxis, 563–564
    vascular access, 564
  therapy
    factor IX concentrates, 560
    recombinant Factor IX, 561
    recombinant Factor VIIa, 561–562
Hemopoiesis, 54, 59–64, 72
  bone marrow microenvironment,
    56–57, 72, 79, 80
    proteoglycans, 78, 80
    stem cell/progenitor niches, 73, 74,
      80
  cell lineages, 527
  cell proliferation assessment, 54
  cell proliferation processes, 25
  cytodifferentiation processes, 25
  development, 24, 72
  myeloid/erythroid (M/E) ratio, 92
  progenitor cells, 25, 72, 79
  regulation, 73–81
    adhesion receptors, 76–77, 80
    chemokines, 76
    cytokines, 25, 72, 75–76, 79, 80
    extracellular matrix components,
      76–78
    Notch, 78–79
    proteoglycans, 78, 80
    Wnt/Frizzled, 79

sites in childhood/adults, 25, 54
stem cells, 25, 72–73, 79
see also Erythropoiesis;
    Granulocytopoiesis;
    Lymphopoiesis;
    Megakaryocytopoiesis;
    Monocytopoiesis
Hemopoietic cells, 24–43
    functional characteristics, 72–73
    HIV infection, 108
    phenotypic characterization, 72
Hemorrhage
    anemia following, 137
    blood transfusion, 647, 648
    chronic blood loss, 137
    iron deficiency, 214
    megakaryocyte increase, 96
    rapid, cardiovascular impact, 137
Hemorrhagic disease of newborn, 583
Hemosiderin, 101
Hemosiderinuria, 138, 139
Hemosiderosis, 101–102
Hemostasis
    coagulation pathway (fibrin clot
        generation), 20, 475, 476
    fibrinolytic pathway, 475
    physiology, 474–476
    platelet function, 19
    platelet plug formation, 19–20,
        474–475, 494
    primary, 474–475
    protein C pathway, 475
    secondary, 475
Hemostatic disorders
    acquired, 579–594
        acquired coagulation inhibitors, 584,
            593–594
        cardiopulmonary bypass, 584,
            587–589
        causes, 579
        disseminated intravascular
            coagulation *see* Disseminated
            intravascular coagulation (DIC)
        drug-induced, 579–582
        liver disease, 583–585
        malignant disease, 584, 592–593
        massive blood transfusion, 584, 587
        neonatal physiologic clotting factor
            deficiencies, 579
        renal disease/uremia, 584, 585–587
        snake venom, 584, 594
        toxic coagulopathies, 594
        vitamin K deficiency, 582–583, 585
    clinical approaches, 476–480
        clinical examination, 479–480
        history-taking, 477–479
        pretest probability of bleeding
            disorder, 480
        'mucosal' versus 'third space' pattern
            of bleeding, 478
        postoperative/traumatic blood loss,
            479–480
        screening tests, 480–481
        venepuncture precautions, 480
    see also Platelet disorders
Hemostatic tests, 480–491
    coagulation tests, 483–489

screening, 483–487
    fibrinolytic system, 489
    maximizing clinical utility, 490–491
        audit, 490
        clinical governance, 490
        clinical scoring systems, 490–491
    minimizing error, 489–490
        calibration/standards, 490
        confounding effects, 490
        pre-analytical phase, 489
        quality control, 490
        test methodology, 489–490
    molecular diagnosis, 489
    primary hemostasis, 480–483
        diagnostic tests, 482–483
        platelet function testing, 481–482
        screening tests, 480–481
        skin bleeding time (SBT), 482
Heparan sulfate, 76, 78
Heparin, 46
    anticoagulant activity, 579–580
        complications, 580
        laboratory monitoring, 484, 580
        protamine reversal, 589
    antithrombin binding, 601
    cardiopulmonary bypass, 588–589
    interference with coagulation
        screening tests, 485, 487
Heparin cofactor II, 583, 603
Heparin-induced thrombocytopenia,
    545–547
    clinical features, 546
    laboratory investigations, 546
    management, 547
    mechanism, 546
    thrombotic events, 546
    type I, 545
    type II, 545–546
Hepatic iron index, 213
Hepatitis A
    aplastic anemia association, 533
    transmission by blood transfusion,
        657
        clotting factor concentrates, 559
Hepatitis B
    aplastic anemia association, 533
    transmission by blood transfusion,
        657
        clotting factor concentrates, 559, 560
Hepatitis C
    transmission by blood transfusion,
        657
        clotting factor concentrates, 559, 560
        nucleic acid amplification testing
            (NAT), 658
Hepatitis, viral
    aplastic anemia association, 252, 533
    lymphocytosis, 315
    pure red cell aplasia association, 267
    transmission by blood transfusion,
        641, 657
Hepatocellular carcinoma, 222
Hepatocyte iron metabolism, 206, 209,
    211
Hepatosplenic γ-δ T-cell lymphoma,
    422–423
Hepcidin, 211, 219

Hephaestin, 210
Hereditary persistence of fetal
    hemoglobin (HPFH), 162, 167–168
Hermansky–Pudlak syndrome, 118,
    497–499
    ceroid storage, 497, 498
Herpes virus infection, 103, 109
Hess test, 20
Hexokinase deficiency, 150, 155
HFE, 163, 168, 208, 220
    hereditary hemochromatosis, 220–221
        diagnostic testing, 222
        screening, 222–223
HFE protein, 208
    knockout mouse studies, 211
High proliferative potential colony-
    forming cell (HPP-CFC) assay, 72
High-molecular weight kininogen, 484,
    501
Hirudin, 580
Histaminase, 12, 13
Histamine, 13, 14, 46
Histamine receptors, 13
Histidine-rich glycoprotein, 603
Histiocytes, 62
    see also Macrophages
Histiocytic medullary reticulosis, 98
Histocompatibility, 667–703
    HLA *see* HLA (human leukocyte
        antigens)
    measurement of sensitization to
        differences, 693–694
    minor antigens, 686–687
Histoplasma capsulatum, 107
Histoplasmosis, 100, 103, 111
HLA (human leukocyte antigens),
    668–685
    allele assignments, 694–699
        cellular, 694, 696
        DNA-based, 694, 696–697
        limitations, 697–698
        National Marrow Donor Program
            (NMDP) DNA nomenclature, 697,
            698
        serologic, 694–696
        serologic–DNA-based system
            correlations, 698–699
    alleles
        DNA-based identification, 692–693
        linkage disequilibrium, 672–673
    antigen binding site, 670
    clinical aspects, 699–703
        autoimmune disorders, 699
        identity establishment, 699
        platelet transfusion immune
            sensitization, 700
        stem cell transplantation *see* Stem
            cell transplantation
        transplantation biology, 699–701
    diversity, 670–673
    function, 679–684
        peptide processing/binding,
            679–680
    gene organization, 669–670
    haplotypes, 671
        ethnic differences, 671–672
        extended, 673

inheritance, 671, 672
population distribution, 671–672
specific allelic associations, 672
polymorphisms/allelic differences, 667, 670
evolutionary aspects, 670–671
identification techniques, 690–693
typing
lymphocyte microcytotoxicity testing, 690–691
mixed leukocyte culture (MLC)/mixed lymphocyte reaction (NLR), 690
HLA class I molecules *see* MHC class I molecules
HLA class II molecules *see* MHC class II molecules
HLA-A, 667, 668
alleles, 670
common, 671
assignments
cross-reactive epitope groups (CREGs), 695
DNA-based, 696–697
serologic, 694, 695
CD8 T-cell recognition, 680
expression, 673, 675
killer cell inhibitory receptor (KIR) interactions, 689
matching for stem cell transplantation, 700, 701, 702, 703
natural peptide binding, 678
polymorphism detection tests, 690
HLA-A1,B8,DR3 extended haplotype, 673
HLA-B, 667, 668
alleles, 670, 671
assignments
cross-reactive epitope groups (CREGs), 695
DNA-based, 697
serologic, 694, 695
CD8 T-cell recognition, 680
expression, 673, 675
killer cell inhibitory receptor (KIR) interactions, 689
matching for stem cell transplantation, 700, 701, 702, 703
polymorphism detection tests, 690
HLA-B27, 698, 699
HLA-C, 667, 668
alleles, 670
CD8 T-cell recognition, 680
expression, 673, 675
killer cell inhibitory receptor (KIR) interactions, 689
polymorphism detection tests, 690
serologic assignments, 694, 695
HLA-D, 667
cellular specificities, 695
HLA-DM, 667, 680
HLA-DO, 667, 680
HLA-DP, 667, 668
alleles, 671
CD4 T-cell recognition, 680
expression, 674, 675
gene organization, 669

polymorphism detection tests, 691
HLA-DQ, 667, 668
alleles, 671
CD4 T-cell recognition, 680
DQA1–DQB1 specific allelic associations, 672
expression, 674, 675
gene organization, 669
polymorphism detection tests, 690, 691
serologic assignments, 694, 695
HLA-DR, 72, 667, 668
alleles, 671
CD4 T-cell recognition, 680
expression, 674, 675
gene organization, 669–670
haplotypes, 673
matching for stem cell transplantation, 700, 701, 702, 703
natural peptide binding, 678
polymorphism detection tests, 690, 691
serologic assignments, 694, 695
structure, 678
HLA-DRA alleles, 671
HLA-DRB1 alleles, 670, 671
common, 671
ethnic differences, 671
HLA-DRB3 alleles, 671
HLA-E, 668, 684
CD94/NKG2 interaction, 689–690
expression, 684
HLA-F, 668, 684–685
polymorphism, 685
HLA-G, 668, 685
expression, 685
polymorphism, 685
HM1.24, 454
HNA-1a, 629, 631
HNA-1b, 630
HNA-1c, 630
HNA-2a (NB1), 630
HNA-3a, 630
HNA-4a, 630
HNA-5a, 630
Hodgkin's lymphoma, 117, 118, 310, 425–427
AIDS/HIV patients, 109
associated pure red cell aplasia, 267
autoimmune neutropenia, 307
bone marrow granulomas, 111
classical, 426–427
bone marrow aspirate, 426
bone marrow trephine biopsy, 427
peripheral blood, 426
eosinophil/eosinophil precursor number increase, 95
lymphocyte-depleted, 426, 427
lymphocyte-rich classical subtype, 426, 427
megakaryocyte increase, 96
mixed-cellularity subtype, 426, 427
nodular lymphocyte predominant, 425–426
nodular sclerosing subtype, 426, 427
staging, 407
Homocystinuria, 608

Hookworm infection, 214
Howell–Jolly bodies, 92, 133, 134, 176, 180, 335, 462
Hox transcription factors, 80
HPA-1, 529, 626
neonatal alloimmune thrombocytopenia, 654
polymorphisms, clinical relevance, 629
HPA-1a, 538, 539, 540, 627, 628, 629
HPA-1b, 539, 540, 627, 629
HPA-2, 529, 626
polymorphisms, clinical relevance, 629
HPA-2a, 539, 627
HPA-2b, 627, 629
HPA-3, 529, 626
polymorphisms, clinical relevance, 629
HPA-3a, 539, 540, 627
HPA-3b, 539, 627
HPA-4, 529, 626
polymorphisms, clinical relevance, 629
HPA-4a, 539, 540, 628
HPA-4b, 539, 627, 628
HPA-5, 529, 626
HPA-5a, 538, 539, 627
HPA-5b, 539, 540, 627
HPA-6bw-13bw (low frequency alloantigens), 626
HPA-6w, 627
HPA-7w, 627
HPA-8w, 627
HPA-9w, 627
HPA-10w, 627
HPA-11w, 627
HPA-12w, 627
HPA-13w, 627
HPA-PeSas, 627
HS-40, 161
Human immunodeficiency virus (HIV) *see* AIDS/HIV infection
Human platelet antigens (HPA), 529, 626–627
alloantibody-mediated thrombocytopenia, 539–540
alloimmunization disorders, 539
antibody response to non-self antigens, 538–539
CD109 expression, 628
GPIa/IIa (CD49/CD20; VLA-2) expression, 627–628
GPIb/IX/V complex expression, 627
GPIIb/IIIa expression, 627
molecular basis, 538
polymorphisms, platelet function impact, 629
post-transfusion purpura, 540
Human T lymphotropic virus (HTLV-1)
adult T-cell leukemia/lymphoma, 392
transmission by blood transfusion, 658
HUMARA probe, 287
Hunter-Hurler syndrome, 302
Hurler's disease
bone marrow storage cells, 119
sea-blue histiocytes, 118

HUT11, Kidd antigen activity, 622
Hyaluronic acid, 78
Hydrops fetalis
  α thalassemias, 169, 171
  Rhesus hemolytic disease of newborn, 193
Hydroxycobalamin, 236
Hydroxyurea, 173, 178, 243, 292
Hyperbilirubinemia
  hemolytic anemia, 138
  neonatal, red cell enzyme defects, 151
Hypercalcemia, 447
Hypercholesterolemia, 119
Hyperchylomicronemia, 119
Hyperfibrinolysis, acquired, 592
Hyperhomocystinemia, 608
Hyperlipidemias, 118, 119
Hyperosmolar diabetic coma, 93
Hypersegmentation of neutrophil nuceli, hereditary (myelokathexis), 300, 324–325
Hypersplenism, 531
  neutropenia, 306
Hyperthyroidism, 310
Hyperviscosity
  multiple myeloma, 447
  Waldenström's macroglobulinemia, 459, 460
Hypochromic erythrocytes, 132
Hypofibrinogenemia, 649
Hypogammaglobulinemia, 309
Hypoplastic anemias, 91
Hypothyroidism, 120, 245, 314
Hypoxemia, secondary erythrocytosis, 292–293

I

I antigen antibodies, 191, 195
[125]I-radioimmune direct antiglobulin test, 189
[125]I-staphylococcal protein A two-stage immunoradiometric assay, 189
Identity testing, 699
Idiopathic aplastic anemia, 532
Idiopathic chronic neutropenia, 308
Idiopathic erythrocytosis, 284, 293–294
Idiopathic hypereosinophilic syndrome, 95, 312–314
  cardiac damage, 314
Idiopathic myelodysplastic syndromes, 333
Idiopathic myelofibrosis, 113–114, 115–116, 548
Idiopathic thrombocytopenic purpura (ITP), 96, 118, 307, 511, 528, 540–544
  acute, 540–541
    management, 541
    adults, 541
    children, 540
  chronic, 541–544
    clinical features, 541, 542
    diagnosis, 542–543
    pathophysiology/anti-platelet antibodies, 542

treatment, 543–544
Idiopathic/primary acquired sideroblastic anemia see Refractory anemia with ringed sideroblasts
IgA autoantibodies, 188
IgE receptors
  basophils, 13
  eosinophils, 12
  mast cells, 46
  monocytes, 34
IgG autoantibodies, 187, 188
IgG-Fc receptors, 9, 11, 12
  basophils, 13
  monocytes, 14, 34
IgM autoantibodies, 188, 191
IgM paraprotein
  lymphoplasmacytic lymphoma, 412, 413
  lymphoproliferative disorders, 458–461
Ileal resection, 234, 238
Imerslund–Gräsbeck syndrome, 234, 238–239
Immediate-type hypersensitivity reactions
  basophils, 13, 14, 314
  blood transfusion reactions, 656
  eosinophils, 13
  mast cells, 13, 46
Immune deficiency syndromes, 310
Immune globulin preparations, 640, 650
Immune hemolytic anemia, 187–195
  acute transient in children, 191
  alloimmune, 192–194
  autoimmune see Autoimmune hemolytic anemia
  blood smear, 187
  drug-induced, 194–195
Immune thrombocytopenia, 481
  secondary, 544
Immunoassays
  coagulation factors, 489
  fibrinolytic system testing, 489
Immunocompromised patient
  Epstein–Barr virus-related lymphoproliferative disorders, 317
  fungal infection, 103
  granuloma formation impairment, 109–110, 111
  transfusion-induced graft-versus-host disease, 651, 652
Immunocytoma, 465
Immunoglobulin superfamily molecules, 623–624, 678, 681
Immunoglobulin-like transcripts (ILT), 690
Immunoglobulin-synthesizing cell abnormalities, 439–465
Immunoglobulins
  adhesion molecules, 63
  fresh frozen plasma (FFP) replacement therapy, 648–649
Immunohistology
  bone marrow cells, 55

bone marrow specimens processing, 67, 68
  lymphoma, 410
  myelodysplastic syndromes, 344–345
Immunophenotype
  acute lymphoblastic leukemia, 354–355
    precursor B-cell, 355–356
    precursor T-cell, 356
    residual disease monitoring, 358
  acute megakaryocytic leukemia, 369
  acute myeloid leukemia, 360
    diagnosis, 372–373
  adult T-cell leukemia/lymphoma, 393
  aggressive NK-cell leukemia, 391
  Burkitt's lymphoma, 421
  chronic lymphocytic leukemia, 385–386
  diffuse large B-cell lymphoma, 420
  extramedullary acute myeloid leukemia (chloroma; granulocytic sarcoma), 371
  follicular lymphoma, 418
  hairy cell leukemia/hairy cell leukemia variant, 414
  hematogones, 429
  hepatosplenic γ–δ T-cell lymphoma, 423
  lymphomas, 429
  lymphoplasmacytic lymphoma, 413
  mantle cell lymphoma, 419
  multiple myeloma plasma cells, 449
  non-Hodgkin's lymphoma, 409
  prolymphocytic leukemia, 387
  Sézary syndrome/mycosis fungoides, 392
  splenic lymphoma with villous lymphocytes, 388
  T-cell granular lymphocytic leukemia, 391
  T-lineage prolymphocytic leukemia, 389
Immunosuppressive therapy
  acquired aplastic anemia, 253, 254, 256, 257, 258
  myelodysplastic syndromes, 348
  paroxysmal nocturnal hemoglobinuria, 198
  pure red cell aplasia, 267
  warm autoimmune hemolytic anemia, 190
Indian (In^a/In^b) blood group polymorphism, 624
Indirect antiglobulin test, 189
Indomethacin, 251
Industrial solvents, 251
Ineffective erythropoiesis, 26
  β thalassemia, 166
  bone marrow hemosiderin, 101
  congenital dyserythropoietic anemias, 274, 276, 277, 278
  iron absorption effect, 210
  iron overload, 205
  malaria, 103
  megaloblastic erythropoiesis, 230–231

Infantile genetic agranulocytosis (Kostmann's syndrome; severe congenital neutropenia), 309, 323–324
Infection susceptibility
  Chediak–Higashi syndrome, 300
  infantile genetic agranulocytosis (Kostmann's syndrome), 309
  lactoferrin deficiency ('specific granule' deficiency), 302
  leukocyte adhesion deficiency type 1 (LAD 1), 325
  multiple myeloma, 447
  phagocyte functional disorders, 322
  red cell surface antigen associations, 625–626
  sickle cell disease, 175, 176
  see also Opportunistic infections
Infections
  anemia of chronic disorders, 218
  bone marrow, 103–109
  bone marrow changes
    hemopoietic cell abnormalities, 94
    hypercellularity, 91
    mast cells, 96
    neutrophil precursor abnormalities, 94
  hemolytic anemia, 195
  lymphocytosis, 314
  megakaryocyte increase, 96
  neutrophil responses
    left shift, 302, 303
    leukocytosis, 311
    morphologic abnormalities, 302, 303, 304, 311
  thrombocytopenia, 537–538
Infectious mononucleosis, 97, 111, 191, 315–316
  bone marrow appearance, 316
  clinical features, 315
  peripheral blood, 314, 315–316
  serology, 316
  pure red cell aplasia following, 266
Influenza, 191
Insecticides, 251–252
Integrins, 57, 63, 325, 528
  hemopoiesis, 76–77, 80
  leukocyte adhesion molecules, 325
  platelets, 528, 529
    functional aspects, 530
    ligands, 530
  RGD sequence recognition, 528
  signal pathways, 77
  structure, 528
Intercellular adhesion molecule-1 (ICAM-1), 325, 443, 623, 624
Intercellular adhesion molecule-2 (ICAM-2), 325
Intercellular adhesion molecule-3 (ICAM-3), 325
Interferon α
  congenital dyserythropoietic anemia type I, 276
  HIV infection-related thrombocytopenia, 538
  idiopathic thrombocytopenic purpura (ITP), 544

multiple myeloma, 452
polycythemia vera, 292
Interferon γ, 17
  acquired aplastic anemia pathogenesis, 254
  anemia of chronic disorders, 218, 219
  MHC class I gene expression enhancement, 673
  MHC class II gene expression enhancement, 674
Interferons, 76
Interleukin-1 (IL-1), 15, 218, 219, 592
Interleukin-1α (IL-1α), 75, 443
Interleukin-1β (IL-1β), 443
Interleukin-2 (IL-2), 17, 39, 594
Interleukin-3 (IL-3), 75, 78, 528
Interleukin-4 (IL-4), 17, 39, 46
Interleukin-5 (IL-5), 17, 39
Interleukin-6 (IL-6), 15, 39, 75
  myeloma
    apoptosis resistance, 440–442
    bone lesions pathogenesis, 446
    plasma cell growth stimulation, 439–440, 443
    signaling pathway, 440, 441
Interleukin-6 (IL-6) receptor, 75, 76
Interleukin-7 (IL-7), 78
Interleukin-8 (IL-8), 15
Interleukin-10 (IL-10), 39
Interleukin-11 (IL-11), 39, 75, 528
Interleukin-11 (IL-11) receptor, 75
International normalized ratio (INR), 483, 486
Intestinal lymphangiectasia (Waldman's disease), 120
Intraoperative blood salvage, 643
Intrauterine blood transfusion, 194
  congenital dyserythropoietic anemia type I, 274
Intrauterine death, 591
Intravenous immunoglobulin
  hemolytic disease of newborn, 193, 194
  neonatal alloimmune thrombocytopenia, 539
  post-transfusion purpura, 540
  warm autoimmune hemolytic anemia, 190
Intrinsic factor
  congenital abnormality, 238
  vitamin BU12u binding, 232
Intrinsic factor deficiency
  congenital, 238
  pernicious anemia, 236
inv14(q11q32), 389
inv(16) abnormalities, 333–334, 360, 364, 374, 375
Invariant chain (Ii), 680
Iron
  bone marrow stores, 62
    assessment methods, 101
    disease-related changes, 101–102
  dietary intake, 214
  pregnant women, 20–21
Iron deficiency, 205, 213–215
  causes, 214
  functional, 217

hemopoietic cell abnormalities, 94
stages of development, 215–216
  iron store exhaustion, 215
  iron-deficient erythropoiesis, 215
Iron deficiency anemia, 205, 213, 215–216
  bone marrow sideroblasts, 102
  chronic blood loss, 137
  clinical features, 215
  diagnosis, 216
  dyserythropoiesis, 92
  hematologic features, 215–216
  mechanism, 216
  non-hematologic effects, 216
  treatment, 216–217
Iron mal-distribution, 205
Iron metabolism
  absorption regulation, 210–211
  anemia of chronic disorders, 218–219
  dietary uptake, 209
  disorders, 205–224
    spectrum of pathology, 205
  exchange pathways, 205–206
  molecular mechanisms, 206–210
    cellular heomeostasis regulation, 206–207
    cellular release, 210
    cellular uptake from transferrin, 206
    duodenal mucosal cell uptake, 209–210
    erythroid progenitor iron uptake, 208
    hepatocyte iron uptake, 209
    HRE protein, 208
    macrophage iron uptake, 209
Iron overload, 97, 205, 220–224
  β thalassemia-treated children, 163
    chelation therapy, 163
  cardiac complications, 224
  clinical disorders, 220, 221
  congenital dyserythropoietic anemias, 274, 276, 277, 282
  definition, 220
  iron metabolism-regulating genes, 163
  liver damage, 206, 209, 224
  primary, 220–223
  secondary, 223–224
    increased absorption, 224
    parenteral iron loading, 223
    treatment, 224
  thalassemia intermedia, 168
Iron status assessment, 211–213
  serum ferritin, 211
  serum transferrin receptors, 211
  tissue biopsy, 213
Iron therapy
  oral, 216–217
  parenteral, 217
Iron-regulatory proteins (IRPs), 207, 211, 218, 219
Iron-responsive elements (IREs), 207, 218, 219
Irradiated blood compounds, 651–652
ITB2 mutations, 325
Ivy test, 20

J

Jacobsen–Paris–Trousseau syndrome, 505–506
Jagged-1, 74, 79, 80
Jaundice, 138
Jejunal resection, 242
Jordan's anomaly (familial vacuolization of leukocytes), 94, 302
Juvenile hemochromatosis (hereditary hemochromatosis type 2), 223
Juvenile pernicious anemia, 237

K

K (killer) cells, 17
Kala azar, 104, 105
    dyserythropoiesis, 93
    reticulin fibrosis, 113
Kaposi's sarcoma, patients, 109
Kasabach Merrit syndrome, 591
Kell blood group system, 189, 620–622
    hemolytic disease of newborn, 621
    null pehotype KU0u, 620, 621
    transfusion reactions, 192
Kell glycoprotein, 620–621
    Kx complex, 621–622
Keloid scars, 479
Kelp ingestion, 93
Keratocyte erythrocytes, 134
Ki67, 54, 59, 421, 422
Kidd antigen (HUT11), 622
Kidd system, 189
    transfusion reactions, 192
Killer cell inhibitory receptors (KIR), 682, 688–689
Kleihauer–Betke test, 193
Knopps antigen (CD35; complement receptor-1; CR1), 624–625
Kogenate, 560–561
    inhibitors development, 564
    treatment on demand, 563
Kostmann's syndrome (infantile genetic agranulocytosis; severe congenital neutropenia), 309, 323
    genetic aspects, 323–324
KP1 immunohistochemistry, 344
Kreb cycle, 11
Kx, 621
    Kell glycoprotein complex, 621–622

L

Lactoferrin, 9, 12, 32, 33, 209
Lactoferrin deficiency (neutrophil 'specific granule' deficiency), 302
Laminin receptor (GPIc'/IIa), 528
LAN, 630
Langerhans cell histiocytosis, 118
Langerhans'-type giant cells, 109, 110, 111
Large granular lymphocyte syndrome, 307

Large granular lymphocytes, 16, 17
Late-onset cholesterol ester storage disease, 119
Lazy leukocyte syndrome, 310
LCA, 63
LeSas, 618
    sialated (CA 19-9), 619
LeSbs, 618, 625
LeSxs, 618
LeSys, 618
Leach phenotype, 625
Lecithin-cholesterol acyltransferase deficiency, 118
Leg ulceration
    hemolytic anemia, 140
    sickle cell disease, 175–176, 177
Leishmania donovani, 104, 108, 111
Leishmaniasis, 107, 110
    bone marrow examination, 103, 104
    bone marrow gelatinous transformation, 120
    dyserythropoiesis, 103
Leprosy, 111
Lesch–Nyhan syndrome, 244
Leukapheresis, 646
Leukemia, acute, 352–376
    ABO antigen expression alteration, 618
    acquired aplastic anemia association, 255, 256
    bleeding disorders, 548–549, 592
    bone marrow cellularity, 91
    bone marrow necrosis, 119
    FAB classification, 352, 353
    megakaryocyte decrease, 97
    myelodysplastic syndrome transformation, 332, 333
    neutrophil myelocyte/metamyelocyte abnormalities, 94
    pseudo-Gaucher cells, 117
    WHO classification, 352, 353
Leukemia, acute basophilic, 369–370
Leukemia, acute biphenotypic, 375–376
Leukemia, acute erythroid (FAB M6), 368
    immunophenotypic diagnosis, 373
    megaloblastic erythropoiesis, 244
    pure erythroid leukemia, 368, 369
Leukemia, acute lymphoblastic (ALL), 352–358
    bone marrow trephine biopsy, 354
    clinical features, 352–353
    CNS infiltration, 354
    cytogenetic abnormalities, 356, 357
        chromosomal translocations, 353, 356, 357
        MLL gene rearrangement, 356, 357
        prognostic significance, 356
    cytology, 353–355
    disease monitoring, 357–358
    disseminated intravascular coagulation (DIC), 592
    FAB classification, 353
    immunophenotype diagnosis, 354–355
        prognostic significance, 355–356
    mature B-cell type (ALL-L3), 421

molecular pathology, 357–358
    Philadelphia chromosome positive, 357
    precursor B-cell, 353, 355–356, 357
    precursor T-cell, 353, 356
    relapse, 354
    residual disease detection, 356
    residual disease monitoring, 358
    reticulin fibrosis, 113
    testicular infiltration, 354
    WHO classification, 353
Leukemia, acute megakaryoblastic, 360
    myelofibrosis, 115
Leukemia, acute megakaryocytic (FAB M7), 369
    immunophenotypic diagnosis, 373
Leukemia, acute monocytic (FAB M5A/M5B), 367–368
    immunophenotypic diagnosis, 373
Leukemia, acute myeloid, 352, 358–375, 481
    ABO antigen expression alteration, 618
    acquired aplastic anemia association, 256
    blast cell morphology, 360
    chromosomal abnormalities, 333, 374
        inv(16) and t(16;16), 364, 374, 375
        molecular diagnosis, 375
        prognostic significance, 374
        recurrent chromosomal translocations, 361–364, 374
        residual disease monitoring, 375
        t(8;21), 361–362, 374
        t(15;17), 362–363, 374
        t(v;11)(v;q23), 364
    CNS involvement, 371–372
    cytochemistry, 361
    diagnostic criteria, 333
    disseminated intravascular coagulation (DIC), 592
    erythropoietic cell abnormalities, 92, 93
    extramedullary (chloromas; granulocytic sarcomas), 371
    FAB classification, 358, 359, 360, 366–371
    Fanconi anemia presentation, 258
    hypocellular forms, 371
    immunophenotypic diagnosis, 372–373
    Kostmann's syndrome association, 323
    multilineage dysplasia, 364–365
    myelodysplastic syndrome transformation, 333–334
    neutrophil precursor abnormalities, 94
    neutrophil 'specific granule' deficiency, 304
    'not otherwise categorized', 366
    platelet abnormalities, 548
    polycythemia vera acute transformation, 290
    residual disease detection, 373–374
    reticulin fibrosis, 113
    therapy-related, 365–366
    trilineage myelodysplasia, 364, 365

WHO classification, 360, 366
Leukemia, acute myeloid with maturation (FAB M2), 366–367
immunophenotypic diagnosis, 372
Leukemia, acute myeloid minimally differentiated (FAB MO), 360, 366
immunophenotypic diagnosis, 372
Leukemia, acute myeloid without maturation (FAB M1), 366
immunophenotypic diagnosis, 372
Leukemia, acute myelomonocytic with eosinophil precursor abnormalities, 360
chromosomal translocations, 364
Leukemia, acute myelomonocytic (FAB M4), 367
immunophenotypic diagnosis, 373
Leukemia, acute promyelocytic (AML-M3)
all-*trans*-retinoic acid (ATRA) responsiveness, 362
chromosomal translocations, 362, 375
disseminated intravascular coagulation (DIC), 592
hypergranular, 362–363
hypogranular, 363
immunophenotypic diagnosis, 372–373
molecular diagnosis, 375
Leukemia, aggressive NK-cell, 389
bone marrow, 390
chromosomal abnormalities, 391
peripheral blood, 390
Leukemia, atypical chronic myeloid, 396–397
Leukemia, basophilic, 314
Leukemia, chronic granulocytic, 25, 117, 118, 304, 314, 393–396
acquired platelet defects, 592
BCR-ABL fusion gene/fusion protein, 357, 393, 396
bone marrow, 95, 394–395
myelofibrosis, 115
chromosomal abnormalities
Philadelphia chromosome, 396
t(9;22)(q34;q11), 393, 396
clinical features, 394
megakaryocyte increase, 96
neutrophil precursor abnormalities, 94
peripheral blood, 314, 394
eosinophilia, 95
platelet functional abnormalities (bleeding/thrombotic complications), 548
polycythemia vera transformation, 290
progression to acute leukemia (blast crisis/blast transformation), 368, 393–394
pathological features, 395, 396
reticulin fibrosis, 113
splenic involvement, 396
Leukemia, chronic lymphocytic, 383–386
acquired factor VII inhibitors, 593
associated pure red cell aplasia, 267
bone marrow pathology, 96, 97, 384, 407

patterns of infiltration, 384, 385
chromosomal abnormalities, 386
clinical features, 383
FAB classification, 384
immunophenotype, 385–386
lymph node involvement, 385
μ-heavy-chain disease association, 464
peripheral blood pathology, 383–384
polycythemia vera transformation, 290
prolymphocytoid/large cell transformation (Richter's syndrome), 383, 385
pure red cell aplasia, 18
reticulin fibrosis, 113
tissue infiltration, 385
VUHu gene mutations, 383
WHO classification, 383
Leukemia, chronic myelogenous *see* Leukemia, chronic granulocytic
Leukemia, chronic myeloid *see* Leukemia, chronic granulocytic
Leukemia, chronic myelomonocytic, 333, 397–399
bone marrow, 398
chromosomal abnormalities, 399
clinical features, 397
eosinophilia, 398, 399
neutrophil 'specific granule' deficiency, 304
peripheral blood, 398
spleen involvement, 398–399
transformation to acute myeloid leukemia, 397
white cell characterisitcs, 335, 336
bone marrow, 338, 340
Leukemia, chronic neutrophilic, 94, 290
Leukemia, eosinophilic, 314, 400–401
bone marrow, 400–401
cardiac involvement, 401
chromosomal translocations, 401
clinical features, 400
peripheral blood, 400
eosinophilia, 95
Leukemia, hairy cell/hairy cell leukemia variant, 111, 113, 413–415
Leukemia inhibitory factor (LIF), 75
Leukemia, juvenile myelomonocytic, 333, 399–400
chromosomal abnormalities, 400
clinical features, 399
neurofibromatosis association, 346, 400
Leukemia of large granular lymphocytes, 267, 389–391
bone marrow, 390
clinical features, 389
immunophenotype, 391
peripheral blood, 389–390
Leukemia, plasma cell, 456
Leukemia, prolymphocytic, 386–387
chromosomal abnormalities, 387
immunophenotype, 387
Leukocyte abnormalities, 300–317
Leukocyte adhesion deficiency type 1 (LAD 1), 325

Leukocyte adhesion deficiency type 2 (LAD 2), 325–326
Leukocyte adhesion molecule deficiencies, 325–326
Leukocyte immunoglobulin-like receptors (LIR), 690
Leukocytosis, 310–317
basophil, 314
eosinophil, 311–312
lymphocytosis, 314
monocytosis, 314
neutrophil, 310–311
Leukoerythroblastic anemia, 112, 113
Leukopenia, 305–310
Leukoreduced red cell preparations, 648
Leukotriene B$_4$, 13
Leukotriene C$_4$, 13, 46
Levodopa, 194
Lewis antigens, 618
tumor cell expression, 618–619
LFA-1 (CD11a/CD18), 325, 444, 630
LFA-3 (CD58), 443, 623
Light-chain-associated amyloidosis, 461–463
clinical features, 461–462
disease progression, 463
pathology, 462–463
treatment, 463
Lindane, 251
Linkage disequilibrium, 672–673
Lipid granulomas, 111
Lipo-macrophages, 62
Littoral cells, 62
Livedo reticularis, 479
Liver biopsy, iron status assessment, 213
Liver disease
acquired hyperfibrinolysis, 592
chronic lymphocytic leukemia, 385
coagulopathy, 585–585
management, 585, 649
disseminated intravascular coagulation, 585
dyserythropoiesis, 93
laboratory findings, 585
systemic fibrinolysis, 585
thrombocytopenia, 531, 537, 585
Liver failure
hemolytic anemia, 198
thrombocytopenia, 537
LMP2, 667, 679
LMP7, 667, 679
Löffler's endocarditis, 314
Long-term-culture initiating cell (LTC-IC), 73, 78
Lonoma achelous toxic coagulopathy, 594
Low-molecular weight heparin, 547, 579
Lung carcinoma, bone marrow metastasis, 112
Lupus anticoagulant, 606–607
Lupus-like (phospholipid-dependent) inhibitors, 484
Lutheran glycoproteins, 623, 624
LW glycoprotein (ICAM-4), 623, 624
Lymph node involvement
adult T-cell leukemia/lymphoma, 393
chronic lymphocytic leukemia, 385
follicular lymphoma, 416

Lymph nodes, 39
Lymphoblasts, 39
Lymphocyte counts, 10, 11, 16
  HIV infection, 105
Lymphocyte microcytotoxicity test, 690
Lymphocytes, 15–18, 59, 63–64
  bone marrow, 55
    infants/children, 50
  life span, 17
  morphology, 15–16
  pregnant women, 21
  progenitors cells, 39
  recirculation, 16–17
  stem cells, 25
  see also B-cells; T-cells
Lymphocytopenia (lymphopenia), 310
Lymphocytosis, 314
  causes, 314
Lymphoid aggregates
  AIDS/HIV infection, 105, 432
  autoimmune disease, 97
  myelodysplastic syndromes, 432
  myeloproliferative disorders, 97, 432
  reactive, 429–430
Lymphoid cells, 63
Lymphoid nodules, 63
Lymphoid progenitor cells, 39
  functional characteristics, 72–73
  in vitro assays, 73
  lineage-specific markers, 39
  long-term-culture assays, 73
  phenotypic characterization, 72
Lymphoid stem cells, 25, 39, 59
Lymphoid tissue, B-cell maturation, 39
Lymphoma, 407–433
  anaplastic large cell (systemic
    subtype), 423–424
  angio-immunoblastic T-cell, 424–425
  autoimmune blood cell destruction,
    407
  B-cell, 412–422
  bone marrow involvement
    aspirate assessment, 429
    hematologic consequences, 407
  bone marrow trephine biopsy,
    429–433
    bone marrow hyperplastic/stromal
      reactions, 432
    discordance with lymph node
      findings, 431
    histologic diagnosis, 432–433
    infiltrates following chemotherapy,
      431–432
    lymphoid infiltrates, 429–430, 432
    lymphoma grade assessment,
      430–431
    necrotic deposits, 431
  Burkitt's, 109, 353, 421–422
  diagnosis, 408
  diffuse large B-cell, 109, 419–421
  extranodal marginal zone of mucosa-
    associated lymphoid tissue
    (MALT)-type, 415
  extranodal NK/T 'nasal type', 422
  follicular, 416–418, 432, 433, 465
  follow-up, 408
  hepatosplenic γ-δ T-cell, 422–423

Hodgkin's *see* Hodgkin's lymphoma
  laboratory investigations, 408–410
    blood specimens, 409
    bone marrow aspirate, 409
    bone marrow trephine biopsy,
      409–410
    immunohistochemistry, 410
  lymphoplasmacytic, 412–413, 432, 433
  mantle cell, 407, 418–419, 432
  megakaryocyte increase, 96
  nodal marginal zone (+/- monocytoid
    B-cells), 415–416
  paraprotein, 407
  peripheral blood involvement
    assessment, 428–429
  peripheral T-cell not otherwise
    characterized, 425
  REAL classification, 411
  speen involvement, 407
  splenic
    marginal zone, 458
    with villous lymphocytes, 458
  T-cell, 422–425
  treatment complications, 408
  WHO classification, 411–412
  see also Lymphoproliferative disease
Lymphoplasmacytic lymphoma,
  412–413, 432, 433
  bone marrow, 412–413
  chromosomal translocation, 412
  immunohistochemistry, 413
Lymphopoiesis, 39–40, 54
  disease-related changes, 97
Lymphoproliferative disease
  acquired inhibitors of coagulation, 593
  bone marrow biopsy, 407–408
  with IgM paraprotein, 458–461
  see also Lymphoma
Lysosomal storage disease, 100, 116–117
  mucopolysaccharidoses, 119
  sphingolipidoses, 117–118
Lysosomes, platelets (λ granules), 18, 19,
  495, 506
Lysozyme (muramidase), 9, 12, 14, 32,
  33, 34, 344, 371

M

Mac-1 (CD11b/CD18; CR3), 325, 444,
  630
McLeod syndrome, 622
Macrocytes, 132, 230, 231
Macrocytic anemia, 230–245
  megaloblastic erythropoiesis, 230–244
  normoblastic erytropoiesis, 244–245
Macrocytosis
  hemolytic anemia, 138, 139
  pernicious anemia, 235
Macrophage inflammatory protein 1α
  (MIP-1α), 14, 15, 76, 78, 446
Macrophage inflammatory protein 1β
  (MIP-1β), 14, 15, 78
Macrophage-colony-stimulating factor
  (M-CSF), 15
Macrophages, 14, 59, 62
  aged red cell destruction, 5, 62, 206

antigen processing/presentation, 15
bone marrow, 30, 43–44, 55, 62
  disease-related changes, 97–100, 103
  erythroblast interactions, 26
  infection-related changes, 103
  ultrastructure, 44–45
cytokines production, 15
epithelioid cell transformation, 34
erythroblast islands, 44, 57, 59
foamy, 118, 119
functions, 15
giant cell transformation, 34
granulomas, 109, 110, 111
hemophagocytosis/hemophagocytic
  syndromes, 98–100, 103
  anemia of chronic disorders, 218
  warm autoimmune hemolytic
    anemia, 187, 188
iron retention, 205, 211, 218
iron storage, 62
  assessment, 213
iron uptake, 209
monocyte transformation, 34
post mortem changes, 91
surface receptors, 26
Macropolycytes, 94, 302, 304
Majocchi's purpura, 479
Major basic protein, 13
Major histocompatibility complex
  (MHC), 667–668
genetic recombination, 671
genomic organization, 667–668,
  669–670
  class I region, 667, 668, 669
  class II region, 667, 669
  class III region, 667–668
historical aspects, 667
see also MHC class I molecules; MHC
  class II molecules
Malaria, 135, 195
  bone marrow aspirate, 103
  cerebral, 122
  dyserythropoiesis, 93, 103
  hemopoietic cell abnormalities, 94
  lymphocytosis, 315
  marrow macrophage
    hemophagocytosis, 100
  protective genetic alterations, 145, 157,
    162, 623
    hemoglobin E, 179
    hemoglobin S, 174
    red cell surface antigens, 625
  transmission by blood transfusion,
    641, 658
Malignant disease
  acquired inhibitors of coagulation, 593
  anemia of chronic disorders, 218
  bleeding disorders, 584, 592–593
  bone marrow hypercellularity, 91
  complement receptor-1 (CR1; CD35)
    acquired deficiency, 625
  disseminated intravascular
    coagulation (DIC), 590, 591, 592
  eosinophilia, 312
  hemophagocytic syndrome, 100
  hemopoietic cell abnormalities, 94
  hyperfibrinolysis, 592

megakaryocyte increase, 96
neutrophil leukocytosis, 311
pure red cell aplasia, 267
thrombotic thrombocytopenic
purpura–hemolytic uremic
syndrome, 196
transfusion-induced graft-versus-host
disease, 652
Malignant histiocytosis, 98, 99
Malignant hypertension, 196
Malignant mastocytosis, 113
MALT lymphomas (MALT-type
extranodal marginal zone
lymphoma), 415, 465
Mannose-binding lectin, 327
deficiency, 328
Mantle cell lymphoma, 418–419, 432
bone marrow aspirate, 418
bone marrow trephine biopsy,
418–419
chromosomal translocations, 418
clinical features, 418
immunohistochemistry, 419
peripheral blood, 418
March hemoglobinuria, 196, 197
Maroteaux–Lamy polydystrophic
dwarfism, 302
Massive blood transfusion, 652
coagulation factor replacement, 649
coagulopathy, 584, 587
thrombocytopenia, 537
Mast cells, 59
bone marrow, 46, 47, 55, 60–61
disease-related changes, 96
cell responses to secreted factors, 60
eosinophil chemotaxis, 13
granules, 46
piecemeal degranulation, 13–14, 46
progenitor cells, 46
stem cells, 25
Matrix metalloproteinases, 446, 476
May–Hegglin anomaly, 300, 509–512,
514
Mean cell hemoglobin concentration
(MCHC), 5
Mean cell hemoglobin (MCH), 5
Mean cell volume (MCV), 5
myelodysplastic syndromes, 334
pregnant women, 20
Mean platelet volume (MPV), 508
Measles, 191, 537
Medich giant inclusion disorder,
518–520
Mediterranean macrothrombocytopenia,
509
Medulloblastoma, bone marrow
metastasis, 112, 113
Mefenamic acid, 194
Megakaryoblasts, 36, 61
cytology, 37
ultrastructure, 37
Megakaryocyte burst-forming units
(BFU-Meg), 527, 528
Megakaryocyte colony-forming units
(CFU-Meg), 36, 528
Megakaryocyte disorders, 494–520
acquired, 527–550

inherited, 496
Megakaryocyte hypoplasia, congenital,
496
Megakaryocytes, 18, 36, 56, 59, 61–62,
527
bone marrow differential counts, 48
bone marrow topography, 61–62
cytology, 37
development, 527–528
emperipolesis, 38
granules, 37
platelets generation (thrombopoiesis),
527, 528
progenitor cells, 527
pulmonary, 37
structure, 494
dense bodies, 494, 497
ultrastructure, 37–38
Megakaryocytopoiesis
(thrombopoiesis), 36–38, 54,
61–62, 527
cytology, 37
disease-related changes, 96–97
myelodysplastic syndromes,
338–339
emperipolesis, 38, 61
megakaryocyte maturation, 494,
507–508
ultrastructure, 37–38
Megaloblastic anemia, 91, 97, 230–244
abnormal sideroblasts, 102
bone marrow hemosiderin, 101
characteristic features, 230
folate deficiency, 231, 234, 241–243
ineffective erythropoiesis, 230–231
infection-related bone marrow
necrosis, 119
nucleic acid synthesis abnormalities,
243–244
vitamin BU12u deficiency, 231,
234–241
Megaloblastic erythropoiesis, 93
Megaloblasts, 230
Melanoma, bone marrow metastasis,
112
Melphalan, 348, 451, 463
Membrane inhibitor of reactive lysis
(CD59), 198, 624
Memphis I polymorphism, 145
Meningococcus vaccination, 173, 190
Menorrhagia, 478
von Willebrand's disease, 569–570
Menstruation, hemostatic disorders, 478
Mercaptopurine, 243
Mesenchymal stem cells, 75
Metastatic bone marrow tumors,
112–113
histologic sections, 113
Metformin, 239
Methemalbuminemia, 138
Methemoglobin, 7
drug-induced oxidative hemolysis,
195
Methemoglobinemia, 162, 181
Methimazole, 251
Methionine synthase deficiency, 243
Methotrexate, 242, 306, 531

Methyl methacrylate embedding, 66
Methylcobalamin deficiency, 240–241
adenosylcobalamin combined
deficiency, 240
Methylene tetrahydrofolate reductase
(MTHFR) deficiency, 243
Methylmalonic acidurias, 240
Metiamide, 307
MHC class I chain-related (MIC) genes,
668
MHC class I chain-related (MIC)
molecules, 685–686
MHC class I genes, 668, 669
expression, 673–675
inheritance, 671, 672
polymorphism, 670
recombination frequency, 671
specific MHC class II gene
associations, 673
structure, 674
MHC class I molecules, 667, 668
cellular assays, 691
classical, 668
DNA-based allele identification,
692–693
function, 668
CD8 T-cell recognition, 680–682
peptide processing/binding, 679
killer cell inhibitory receptor (KIR)
interactions, 689
non-classical, 668–669, 684–685
serological detection, 690–691
structure, 675, 676
anchor residues, 677
antigen-binding groove/pockets,
675, 677
peptide-binding motifs, 677, 678
MHC class II genes, 667, 669
expression, 674–675
inheritance, 671, 672
polymorphism, 671
recombination frequency, 671
specific MHC class I gene
associations, 673
structure, 674
MHC class II molecules, 667, 668
cellular assays, 690–691
DNA-based allele identification,
692–693
function, 668
CD4 T-cell recognition, 680–682
invariant chain (Ii), 680
peptide processing/binding,
679–680
serological detection, 690–691
structure, 676, 678
antigen-binding groove/pockets,
678
peptide-binding motifs, 677, 678
MHC class III genes, 667–668
MICA, 668, 685, 686
MICB, 668, 685, 686
Microangiopathic hemolysis, 195
Microbial killing, 322
eosinophils, 13
monocytes, 15
neutrophils, 9, 11–12

mechanisms, 12
  oxygen-dependent, 11, 12
  oxygen-independent, 12
Microcytes, 132
Microfilaments, 18
Microspherocytes, 132
Minor histocompatibility antigens,
    686–687
Mithramycin, 196
Mitochondrial DNA mutations, 269, 270
Mitochondrial iron accumulation
    ringed sideroblasts, 337
    sideroblastic anemias, 271
      (iron laden) siderotic granules, 268,
      270
Mitochondrial iron metabolism
    abnormalities, 207–208
Mixed leukocyte culture, 690, 695
Mixed lymphocyte reaction (NLR), 690
MLL gene rearrangement, 356, 357, 364,
    375
MNS system, 189
Monoblasts, 31, 34
  cytochemistry, 34
  cytology, 34
Monoclonal gammopathy of
    undetermined significance
    (MGUS), 439, 455
  clinical features, 455
  IgM paraprotein, 458, 459
  pathology, 455
  platelet dyfunction, 549
  treatment, 455
Monocyte chemoattractant protein
    (MCP), 13, 14
Monocyte chemoattractant protein-1
    (MCP-1), 14, 15
Monocyte chemoattractant protein-2
    (MCP-2), 14
Monocyte chemoattractant protein-3
    (MCP-3), 14
Monocytes, 14–15, 34, 62, 590
  granules, 14
  phagocytosis/microbial killing, 15
  stem cells, 25
  surface receptors, 34
  transformation into macrophages, 14,
    34
  ultrastructure, 34–35
Monocytopenia, 310
Monocytopoiesis, 34–35
Monocytosis, 314
  causes, 315
Mononuclear cell concentrates, 646
Mononuclear phagocyte system, 62
  extravascular hemolysis, 137
  infection-related changes, 103
  monocytopoiesis, 34–35
Montreal platelet syndrome, 515–516
Mott cells, 97
μ-heavy-chain disease, 464–465
  clinical features, 464
  pathology, 464–465
  treatment, 465
MUC1, 454
Mucopolysaccharidoses, 119
  Alder–Reilly anomaly, 302

Mucormycosis, 119
Multiple myeloma, 117, 118, 439–455
  acquired factor VII inhibitors, 593
  adhesion molecule expression,
    443–444
    disease progression, 444
  AIDS/HIV patients, 109
  amyloid deposition, 462
  bone disease, 445–447
    bisphosphonate therapy, 452
  bone marrow plasma cell
    characteristics, 97, 98
  cell cycle regulatory protein
    abnormalities, 442
  chromosomal abnormalities, 444–445
    immunoglobulin gene
      rearrangements, 445
    translocations, 445
  coagulation disorders/platelet
    dysfunction, 549, 593
  cryoglobulinemia, 465
  diagnostic criteria, 446
  epidemiology, 439
  etiology, 439
  hypercalcemia, 447
  hyperviscosity, 447
  infection susceptibility, 447
  molecular pathology, 444–445
  μ-heavy-chain disease association, 464
  myeloma plasma cells, 439
    IL-6-mediated growth/survival,
      439–442
  neurological features, 447
  p53 mutations, 445
  paraprotein, 447
  pathogenesis, 439, 440
    cytokines, 443, 446
  pathology, 448–450
  plasma cell immunophenotype, 449
  prognostic features, 447–448
    β2 microglobulin levels, 448
  progression to plasma cell leukemia,
    442, 456
  Rb mutations, 442, 445
  renal failure, 447
  reticulin fibrosis, 113
  staging, 447–448
  treatment, 450–455
    chemotherapy, 450, 451–452
    immune-based, 454–455
    interferon α, 452
    monoclonal antibodies, 454
    radiotherapy, 452
    stem cell transplantation, 450, 452–453
    thalidomide, 453–454
MUM1/IRF4, 445
Mumps, 266, 537
Myasthenia gravis, 267, 464, 631
Mycobacterial infection, 109, 110, 117
  bone marrow changes, 100, 103
Mycobacterium avium intracellulare, 107,
    108, 110, 117
Mycobacterium leprae, 111, 625
Mycobacterium tuberculosis, 107, 110, 111
Mycoplasma pneumoniae, 191, 195
Mycosis fungoides, 391–392
  chromosomal abnormalities, 392

immunophenotype, 392
Myeloblasts, 31, 60
  cytochemistry, 32
  cytology, 31–32
  ultrastructure, 33
Myelocytes, 60
  eosinophil, 35
  neutrophil, 31
    cytochemistry, 32
    cytology, 31–32
    disease-related abnormalities, 94
    granules, 33–34
    post mortem changes, 90–91
    ultrastructure, 33–34
Myelodysplasia, 481
  congenital, 92
Myelodysplastic syndromes, 310,
    332–348
  acquired α thalassemia, 172
  acquired aplastic anemia, 255, 256
  apoptotic activity, 342, 346
  blood cell abnormalities, 332
  blood film examination, 334–336
    platelets, 336
    red cells, 334–335
    white cells, 335–336
  bone marrow aspirate, 336–339
    erythropoiesis, 337
    granulopoiesis, 338
    thrombopoiesis, 338–339
  bone marrow changes, 91, 96, 332, 343
    lymphoid aggregates, 432
  bone marrow progenitor cell culture,
    346
  bone marrow trephine biopsy, 339,
    340–342
    cytology, 342
    fluorescent *in situ* hybridization, 345
    hemopoietic cell topography,
      340–342
    immunohistochemistry, 344–345
  classification, 333–334
  clinical features, 334
  definition, 332
  diagnosis, 334–339
  epidemiology, 332–333
  FAB classification, 332, 333, 336,
    339–340
  familial forms, 333
  genetic abnormalities, 345–346
    karyotype analysis, 286, 345
  histologic features, 339–345
    abnormal localization of immature
      precursors (ALIP), 340, 342
    dysplastic erythropoiesis, 340–341,
      342
    hypoplastic bone marrow, 343
    megakaryocytes, 341–342
    secondary myelodysplasia, 343–344
  idiopathic, 333
  immune function impairment, 346
    lymphoid involvement, 347
  International Prognostic Scoring
    System (IPSS), 333
  laboratory abnormalities, 346, 347
  management, 347–348
  megaloblastic erythropoiesis, 244

natural history, 347
neutropenia, 335
neutrophil leukocytosis, 311
neutrophil myelocyte/metamyelocyte abnormalities, 94
neutrophil 'specific granule' deficiency, 304
pathogenesis, 346
platelet functional abnormalities (bleeding complications), 548–549
pure red cell aplasia, 267
secondary (drug/chemical-induced), 332–333
WHO classification, 333–334, 339–340
Myelofibrosis, 481
acquired platelet defects, 592
basophil changes, 95, 314
causes, 114
megakaryocyte increase, 96
polycythemia vera, 288, 289
Myeloid cell markers, 60
Myeloid progenitors cells
functional characteristics, 72–73
long-term-culture assyas, 73
phenotypic characterization, 72
Myeloid stem cells, 25, 31, 56, 59
Myeloid/erythroid (M/E) ratio, 92, 103, 135
causes of alteration, 92
chronic granulocytic leukemia, 394
hemolytic anemia, 139
pernicious anemia, 235
Myelokathexis (hereditary hypersegmentation of neutrophil nuceli), 300, 324–325
Myeloperoxidase, 9, 12, 14, 60, 290, 355, 361, 371, 376
Myeloperoxidase deficiency
acquired, 304
inherited, 301
Myelopoiesis *see* Granulocytopoiesis
Myeloproliferative disorders, chronic, 284
acquired platelet defects, 592–593
storage pool deficiency, 593
acquired von Willebrand disease, 593
bone marrow hypercellularity, 91
bone marrow lymphoid aggregates, 97, 432
myelofibrosis, 115
peripheral blood eosinophilia, 95
platelet functional abnormalities (bleeding/thrombotic complications), 548
polycythemia vera transformation, 290
thrombosis risk, 607
Myelosclerosis *see* Idiopathic myelofibrosis
Myoglobin, 7

N

N-ras mutations, 346
NADPH-oxidase, 326, 327
National blood programs, 639

National Marrow Donor Program (NMDP), 701
DNA-based HLA allele nomenclature, 697, 698
donor searches, 701–702
Natural anticoagulants, 600–603
Natural killer (NK) cells, 16, 17, 63
phenotypic characterization, 72
progenitor cell lineage-specific markers, 39
NB1 (HNA-2a), 630
NCAM (CD56), 372, 391, 423, 443, 444, 450
Neocyte transfusion, 652
Neomycin, 239
Neonatal alloimmune neutropenia, 306, 307, 308, 630–631, 654
clinical features, 630–631
granulocyte antigens, 630
Neonatal alloimmune thrombocytopenia, 539, 626, 628–629
clinical features, 539, 628–629
diagnosis, 539
future pregnacies, 539–540
human platelet antigens (HPA), 538, 539, 627, 628
HPA-1a, 627, 628, 654
management, 539, 654
pathophysiology, 628
platelet antibodies, 654
Neonatal hemochromatosis, 223
Neonatal hemolysis, glutathione biosynthesis impairment, 153
Neonatal hyperbilirubinemia
hemolytic disease of newborn (erythroblastosis fetalis), 193, 194
red cell enzyme defects, 151
Neonates
blood transfusion, 653
exchange transfusion, 653
transfusion-graft-versus-host disease, 652
physiological clotting factor deficiencies, 579
vitamin K deficiency, 582–583
Neural tube defects, 241
Neuroblastoma, bone marrow metastasis, 112, 113
Neurofibromatosis, 346, 400
Neuronal ceroid lipofuscinosis, 119
Neutropenia, 305–310
autoimmune of infancy, 631
causes, 305–306
chronic
familial benign, 309
idiopathic, 18, 308
congenital, 94
X-linked, 324
aleukia (reticular dysgenesis), 309
dysgranulopoietic, 310
neonatal alloimmune, 306, 307, 308, 630–631, 654
severe (Kostmann's syndrome), 309, 323–324
cyclical, 308–309, 323
dialysis-related, 308

drug-induced, 306–307
ethnic variations in neutrophil count, 309
immune, 307–308
myelodysplastic syndromes, 335
syndromic associations, 309–310
Neutrophil counts, 10, 11
ethnic variations, 10, 309
reference limits, 10
Neutrophil elastase, 324
endogenous inhibitors, 324
neutropenia-related defects, 323, 324
Neutrophil esterase, 290
Neutrophil leukocytosis, 310–311
causes, 311
Neutrophil 'specific granule' deficiency, 302, 304, 324
Neutrophil-specific antigens (NA1/NA2), 308
Neutrophils, 9–12
acquired abnormalities, 302, 303
botryoid nuclei, 304
left shift, 302, 303, 311
right shift, 302
'specific granule' deficiency, 304–305
toxic granulation, 302, 303, 311
basement membrane migration, 9
cell membrane receptors, 9, 11
chemotaxis, 11
disease-related bone marrow changes
infections, 103
myeloid/erythroid (M/E) ratio, 92
endothelial adhesion, 9, 11
energy metabolism, 11
FcγRIIIb (CD16), 629
functions, 11–12
granules, 9, 11
myelocytes, 33–34
granulocytopoiesis, 31–34, 60
cytochemistry, 32
disease-related abnormalities, 94–95
precursor cytology, 31–32
ultrastructure, 33–34
hereditary hypersegmentation of nuceli, 300
inherited defects, 300–302
life span, 10–11, 31
morphology, 9–10
numbers, 10–11
phagocytosis/microbial killing, 9, 11–12, 305
pregnant women, 21
NF1, 346, 400
Niemann–Pick disease, 118
Nitrofurantoin, 195
Nitrous oxide exposure, vitamin BU12u inactivation, 239–240
Nocturnal hypoxemia, 293
Nodal marginal zone lymphoma (+/- monocytoid B-cells), 415–416
Non-Hodgkin's lymphoma
acquired factor VII inhibitors, 593
autoimmune neutropenia, 307
bone marrow changes
lymphocytosis, 97
mast cells, 96
bone marrow granulomas, 111

chromosomal translocations, 409
immunophenotype, 409
molecular genetics, 409
polycythemia vera transformation, 290
pseudo-Gaucher cells, 117
pure red cell aplasia association, 267
staging, 407
Non-obese diabetic (NOD)-severe combined immunodeficiency (SCID) mice, 73
Non-steroidal anti-inflammatory drugs (NSAIDs)
anti-platelet activity, 478, 549, 582
aplastic anemia, 251
drug-induced hemolytic anemia, 194, 195
mode of action, 544
Normoblasts, 26–27
Normochromic erythrocytes, 132
Normocytes, 132
Normovolemic hemodilution, acute (perioperative hemodilution), 643
Notch, 78–79, 80
Notch-1, 79
Notch-2, 79
Nucleic acid amplification testing (NAT), 658

O

Obstructive airway disease, chronic, 293
Ok glycoprotein (CD147), 623, 624
Oncostatin-M, 75
Opportunistic infections
adult T-cell leukemia/lymphoma, 392
AIDS/HIV infection, 106–108, 109
see also Infection susceptibility
Oral contraceptive drugs, 243
Orotic aciduria, 243
Oroya fever (bartonellosis), 135
Osmotic red cell damage, 197
Osteoblasts
bone marrow, 46–47, 57, 59, 75
disease-related changes, 100
cytokines, 75
Osteoclasts, 59
bone marrow, 46, 47
disease-related changes, 100
multiple myeloma, 445, 446
stem cells, 25
Osteoprotegerin, 446
Ovalo-stomatocytes, 144, 145
Overhydrated hereditary stomatocytosis, 146
Oxygen affinity, 7
Oxygen dissociation curve, 7
Oxygen transport, 6–7
Oxygen-dependent microbial killing, 11, 12
Oxyphenbutazone, 251

P

p16, 442
p21rac, 327
p40Sphoxs, 327
p47Sphoxs, 327
p53, 346, 387, 445
p67Sphoxs, 326, 327
p150,95 (CD11c/CD18), 325, 444
P antigen, 625
autoantibodies, 191
parvovirus B19 cellular receptor, 626
P-selectin, 78
P-selectin glycoprotein ligand (PSGL-1), 78
Packed cell volume (PCV) see Hematocrit
Packed red cells, 644
Paclitaxel, 304
Pancreatitis
chronic, 239
disseminated intravascular coagulation (DIC), 590
Panmyelosis, acute with marrow fibrosis, 370–371
Pappenheimer bodies, 134, 208, 269, 270
Paraffin embedded specimens, 90
lymphoma investigation, 410
Paraffin embedding procedure, 67
Paraprotein/paraproteinemia
coagulation disorders, 593
cryoglobulinemia, 465
lymphoplasmacytic lymphoma, 412, 413
multiple myeloma, 447
platelet dyfunction, 549
see also IgM paraprotein
Parasite infections
basophil defences, 14
eosinophil leukocytosis, 311
eosinophil phagocytosis/killing, 13
eosinophil/eosinophil precursor number increase, 95
HIV-related opportunistic infection, 107
mast cell defences, 46
Parietal cell antibodies, 235–236
Paris–Trousseau syndrome, 505–506
Paroxysmal cold hemoglobinuria, 191–192
management, 192
Paroxysmal nocturnal hemoglobinuria, 91, 96, 114, 197–198, 205
associated acquired aplastic anemia, 254, 255–256
diagnosis, 198
dyserythropoiesis, 92–93
molecular pathology, 197–198, 624
thrombosis risk, 607
treatment, 198
Parvovirus B19, 107, 139, 142, 625
aplastic crises with sickle cell disease, 175
blood transfusion transmission, 659
bone marrow examination, 104
clotting factor concentrate transmission, 559
P antigen cellular receptor, 626
transient red cell aplasia, 104, 252, 266
AIDS patients, 109
Paternity testing, 699
Paul Bunnell test, 316
PAX5 rearrangements, 412, 458
Pearson's syndrome, 93, 269
Pelger–Huët anomaly, 94
acquired, 270, 300, 304, 394
inherited, 300
Penicillin prophylaxis
β thalassemia, 173
sickle cell disease, 177
Penicillin-induced hemolytic anemia, 194
Penicillium marneffei, 107
Pentachlorophenols, 251
Pentose phosphate pathway, 6, 8, 150
enzyme defects, 150
biochemical investigations, 156
clinical features, 151
molecular basis, 157
Perfluorocarbons, 660
Perioperative hemodilution (acute normovolemic hemodilution), 643
Peripheral blood stem cells, collection/preparation procedure, 646
Peripheral neuropathy
post-gastrectomy, 238
vitamin BU12u deficiency, 233, 234
pernicious anemia, 235, 237
Peripheral T-cell 'not otherwise characterized' lymphoma, 425
Pernicious anemia, 97, 231, 232, 234–237
associated autoimmune disorders, 234
associated hypogammaglobulinemia, 237
epidemiology, 234
histopathology, 236–237
gastric mucosal atrophy, 236
iron deficiency, 214, 216
juvenile form, 237
laboratory investigations, 235
parietal cell antibodies, 235–236
Schilling test, 236
peripheral neuropathy, 235, 237
subacute combined degeneration of spinal cord, 236–237
symptoms/signs, 235
treatment, 236
Peroxidase, 13, 14, 33, 35, 38
Peyer's patches, 39
PFA-100 analysis, 482
Phagocyte functional disorders, 322–328
extrinsic, 327–328
leukocyte adhesion molecule deficiencies, 325–326
maturation disorders, 323–325
primary (phagocyte immunodeficiency diseases), 322, 323
respiratory burst deficiencies, 326–327
signalling abnormalities, 326
Phagocytosis, 322
eosinophils, 13
macrophage hemophagocytosis, 98–100, 103, 187, 188, 218
monocytes, 15
neutrophils, 9, 11–12

Phenacetin, 195
Phenformin, 239
Phenylalanine deficiency, 93
Phenylbutazone, 251
Phenytoin, 267
Philadelphia chromosome, 25, 396, 618
Phlebotomy, 205
  apparent erythrocytosis, 294
  blood donations, 644
  hereditary hemochromatosis, 222
  idiopathic erythrocytosis, 294
  polycythemia vera, 292
  secondary erythrocytosis, 293
Phosphatidyl serine, 475
Phosphofructokinase deficiency, 150
  biochemical investigations, 155
Phosphogluconate dehydrogenase
    deficiency, 153
6-Phosphogluconolactonase deficiency,
    153
Phosphoglycerate kinase deficiency, 150
Phosphosomes, 9, 34
Piecemeal degranulation, 13–14, 46
pig-a mutations, 197, 624
Plasma cell leukemia, 456
Plasma cells, 39, 40, 41, 44, 54, 55
  bone marrow, 64
    age-related changes, 50
    disease-related changes, 97
    lymphoplasmacytoid, 64
    reticular ('Marschalko'), 64
  hemosiderin-containing granules, 97
  light chain restriction, 64
  reactive plasmacytosis, 97
  ultrastructure, 41–43
Plasma collection, 644
  plasmapheresis, 644, 646
Plasma derivatives, 640, 650, 651
  viral disease transmission, 640
    HIV, 640–641
Plasma exchange, thrombotic
    thrombocytopenic
    purpura–hemolytic uremic
    syndrome, 196–197, 535, 536
Plasma volume expansion, 137
Plasmacytoma
  extramedullary, 458
  solitary bone, 456–458
Plasmapheresis
  donors, 640
  plasma collection, 644, 646
Plasmin, 476
  cardiopulmonary bypass response, 588
Plasmin–antiplasmin complexes assay,
    608
Plasminogen, 583
  activators, 592
  cardiopulmonary bypass response,
    588
  deficiency, 606
Plasminogen activator inhibitor (PAI-1)
    deficiency, 606
Plasmodium falciparum
  glycophorin ligands, 625
  malaria, 93, 94, 100, 103, 174
Plasmodium malariae, 658
Plasmodium vivax, 625

Duffy antigen receptor for
    chemokines (DARC) interaction,
    623
  malaria, 93
Plastic embedding methods
  bone marrow specimens, 65–67, 68
  rapid processing, 67
Plastic-embedded specimens, 90
  lymphoma investigation, 410
Platelet aggregometry, 482
Platelet antigens, 626–629
  function, 626–627
  structure, 626–627
  see also Human platelet antigens
    (HPA)
Platelet clot
  generation, 530
  retraction, 18
    platelet function assessment, 20
Platelet concentrates, 645
  see also Platelet transfusion
Platelet count, 19, 480
  ethnic variations, 528
  normal reference range, 481
  pregnant women, 21
  primary hemostasis investigation,
    480–481, 486
  procedure, 480–481
  transient elevation, 528
Platelet disorders
  acquired, 527–550
    function abnormalities, 547–550
    myeloproliferative disorders,
      592–593
  inherited, 494–520
    giant granule anomaly, 501, 507
    giant platelet disorders, 509–518
    membrane inclusion disorders,
      518–520
    membrane/membrane organization
      defects, 507–518
    organelle defects, 496–507
    small platelets, 508–509
Platelet factor 3, 20, 475
Platelet factor 3 availability test, 20
Platelet factor 4, 19, 78, 115
  heparin-induced thrombocytopenia,
    545, 546
  platelet α granules, 501, 529
Platelet function testing, 20, 481–482
  whole blood platelet analysis, 481–482
Platelet growth factors, therapeutic
    applications, 659
Platelet plug formation, 19–20, 474–475,
    494
Platelet transfusion, 481, 659
  autoimmune thrombocytopenia, 654
  cardiopulmonary bypass-related
    coagulopathy, 589
  clinical response, 650
  complications, 656
  disseminated intravascular
    coagulation (DIC), 534, 591
  HLA antigen allosensitization, 700
  indications, 649–650
  inherited megakaryocyte disorders,
    496

massive blood transfusion,
    thrombocytopenia prevention, 537
neonatal alloimmune
    thrombocytopenia, 539, 654
  platelet concentrates, 645
  platelet functional abnormalities in
    leukemia/myelodysplastic
    syndromes, 548
Platelet-activating factor (PAF), 13
Platelet-derived growth factor (PGDF),
    15, 115
  platelet α granules, 501, 529
Platelet-rich plasma, platelet
    concentrate preparation
    procedure, 645
Plateletpheresis, 645
Platelets, 18–20, 59, 494
  activation, 18, 19, 530
    cardiopulmonary bypass, 588
    coagulation cascade, 600
    disseminated intravascular
      coagulation (DIC), 590
  adhesion, 19, 20, 530, 627
    primary hemostasis, 474
    shape change, 530
    uremia-related abnormalities, 547,
      586
  aggregation, 18, 19, 20, 530, 627
    myeloproliferative disorders-related
      abnormalities, 548
    primary hemostasis, 474–475
  alloantigens, 529
  α granules, 18, 19, 20, 494, 495–496,
    501–503, 529
    secretion response, 501–503
  dense bodies (δ granules), 18, 20, 494,
    495, 496, 529
  dense tubular system, 18, 495
  energy metabolism, 19
  function, 19–20, 494, 529–530
    drug interference, 549–550
    in vivo/in vitro assessment, 20,
      481–482
  giant, pseudothrombocytopenia, 531
  granules, 18–19
    structure/function investigations,
      482–483
  integrins, 528, 529
    functional aspects, 530
    ligands, 530
  life span, 19, 528
  lysosomal (lambda) granules, 18, 19,
    495, 506
  megakaryocyte production, 494,
    507–508
  membranes/membrane complexes,
    19, 495, 507, 510, 528, 529
    glycoproteins, 474, 528, 529
  morphology, 18
  open canalicular system, 18, 495, 502,
    503
  peroxisomes, 18, 19
  pooling in spleen, 531
  quantitative abnormalities *see*
    Thrombocytopenia
  release reaction, 19, 501–503
  satellitism, 531

stem cells, 25
structure, 494–496, 528–529
surface HPA antigens *see* Human
	Platelet Antigens
thrombosis mechanisms, 494
Plumbism, 152
PML/RARA fusion gene/gene product,
	362, 363, 373, 375
Pneumococcal vaccination, 173, 177, 190
POEMS syndrome, 458
Poikilocytes, 144
Poikilocytosis, 132
	congenital dyserythropoietic anemia
		type II, 276
	hereditary, 143–144
		EPB41 mutations, 145
		pyruvate kinase deficiency, 155
		SPTA1 mutations, 144–145
		SPTB mutations, 145
	iron deficiency anemia, 215
	myelodysplastic syndromes, 335
	pernicious anemia, 235
	polycythemia vera, 288
	sideroblastic anemia
		X-linked, 269
		refractory anemia with ringed
			sideroblasts, 270
Polyarteritis nodosa, 121
Polycythemia *see* Erythrocytosis
Polycythemia rubra vera, 91, 118
	basophil leukocytosis, 314
	megakaryocyte increase, 96
	myelofibrosis, 115
	platelet abnormalities, 548, 592
Polycythemia vera, 284–292
	BFU-E (burst-forming units-erythroid)
		culture in vitro, 288
	blood donations, 644
	bone marrow appearances, 288–290
		differential diagnosis, 291
		proliferative phase, 288
		spent phase, 288–289
		transformation, 290
	clinical features, 285
	clonal nature, 284, 285
		demonstration, 286–287
	diagnosis, 285–286
	erythropoietin levels, 287
	karyotype analysis, 286–287
	progression to acute myeloid
		leukemia/malignant disease, 290
	spleen histology, 291, 292
	splenomegaly, 285, 287, 288
	treatment, 292
Polymorphonuclear leukocytes *see*
	Granulocytes
Polymyalgia rheumatica, 307
Polymyositis, 307
Pompe's disease (type II glycogen
	storage disease), 100
Porphyria cutanea tarda, 97, 220
Post-transfusion hepatitis, 657
Post-transfusion purpura, 540
Post-transplant lymphoproliferative
	disease, 428
Postoperative blood salvage, 643–644
Prednisolone, 451, 463

Pre-eclampsia, 536–537
Pregnancy
	blood alterations, 20–21
	blood transfusion, 654
	fetal red cells/lymphocytes in
		maternal circulation, 21
	folate requirement, 242
	mean cell volume changes, 245
Prekallikrein, 484
Prenatal diagnosis
	α thalassemia, 172
	sickle cell disease, 178
Priapism, sickle cell disease, 175, 177
Procainamide, 194
Procarbazine, 243
Proerythroblasts, 26
Progenitor cells, 25, 54, 59, 79
	acquired aplastic anemia, 253
	assays, 72
	basophils, 35
	bone marrow microenvironment
		('niches'), 73, 74, 80
	eosinophils, 35
	erythropoiesis, 26
	extracellular matrix component
		interactions, 76–77
	granulocytopoiesis, 31
	HIV infection, 108
	long-term-culture initiating cell (LTC-
		IC) assay, 73
	lymphocytes, 39
	mast cells, 46
	megakaryocytes, 36, 527
	monocytopoiesis, 31
	phenotypic characterization, 72
	sialomucin receptors
		CD34, 77
		CD43, 77, 78
		CD164, 77–78
Proliferating cell nuclear antigen
	(PCNA), 54
Proliferative retinopathy, sickle cell
	disease, 176, 177
Propylthiouracil, 251
Prostaglandin D$_2$, 46
Prostaglandin E$_2$, 13
Prostaglandin metabolism, 544, 545
	anti-platelet drug actions, 549
Prostate carcinoma, bone marrow
	metastasis, 112
Prosthetic heart valves, 196
Protein C, 583, 602
	activated form anticoagulant activity,
		602
	activation, 476, 601, 602
		disseminated intravascular
			coagulation (DIC), 590
	clot regulation, 475, 476
	structure, 602
Protein C deficiency, 603–604
	management, 609
	type I, 604
	type II, 604
Protein C supplements, 591
Protein C–protein S system, 601
	endothelial protein C receptor,
		601–602

thrombomodulin, 601
Protein S, 476, 583, 602
	activated protein C cofactor function,
		602
	anticoagulant activity, 602
	structure, 602
Protein S deficiency, 603–604
	classification, 604
	management, 609
	type I, 604
	type II, 604
	type III, 604
Protein Z-ZPI, 603
Protein-energy malnutrition, 93, 94, 267
Proteinase 3, 9
Proteoglycans, 78, 80
Proteosome, 679
Prothrombin complex concentrates, 571
Prothrombin consumption test, 20
Prothrombin deficiency, congenital,
	570–571, 572
Prothrombin (factor II), 19, 20
	coagulation pathway, 475, 600
	coagulation screen, 483, 484, 486
	elevation, thrombosis association, 605,
		609
	pregnant women, 21
Prothrombin frament F1+2 assay, 608
Prothrombin time (PT), 480, 483, 486,
	488
	neonate, 579
Prothrombinase complex, 475
Protozoal infection, 111
Pseudo Pelger–Huët cells, 335, 342, 365
Pseudo-Chediak granules, 362
Pseudo-Gaucher cells, 62, 117, 277, 278
Pseudo-Pelger neutrophils, 362
Pseudopolycythemia *see* Apparent
	erythrocytosis
Pseudothrombocytopenia, 531
Psoriasis, 242
Pulmonary blood transfusion reactions,
	656
Pulmonary disease, chronic, 245, 293
Pure red cell aplasia, 266–267
	chronic lymphocytic leukemia, 18
	Diamond–Blackfan anemia, 266
	drug/chemical-induced, 267
	immunologic disorders, 267
	myelodysplastic syndromes, 267
	viral causes, 266–267
Pyk-2, 77
Pyrexia of unknown origin, 110
Pyridium (phenazopyridine), 195
Pyridoxine therapy, 268
Pyrimidine 5'-nucleotidase, 150
Pyrimidine 5'-nucleotidase deficiency,
	150, 152
	biochemical investigations, 155
Pyruvate kinase deficiency, 150
	biochemical investigations, 155, 156
	bone marrow hemosiderin, 101
	dyserythropoiesis, 92
	molecular basis, 157
	neonatal hyperbilirubinemia, 151
	parvovirus B19 infection, 104
	poikilocytes, 155

prenatal diagnosis, 156
spheroechinocytes, 154–155

Q

5q- syndrome, 334, 336, 339, 340, 342
Quality control, hemostatic testing, 490
Quinidine, 194, 195, 196
  drug-induced thrombocytopenia, 545, 547
Quinine, 194, 195, 196
  drug-induced thrombocytopenia, 544, 545, 547

R

Rac, 326
Rac2 mutation, 326
Radiotherapy
  aplastic anemia induction, 532–533
  multiple myeloma, 452
RANTES, 13, 14, 15
Rapid processing methods, 67
Rapoport–Luebering shunt, 7, 150
RARA rearrangements, 362, 375
ras mutations, 399, 400
  multiple myeloma, 445
  myelodysplastic syndromes, 346
Raynaud's phenomenon, 191
Rb mutations
  chronic lymphocytic leukemia, 386
  multiple myeloma, 442, 445
Reactive B lymphocytosis, 429
Reactive lymphoid aggregates, 429–430
Reactive macrophage hyperplasia, 98
Reactive plasmacytosis, 64
  bone marrow plasma cell characteristics, 97, 98
Reactive thrombocytosis, 96
Recombinant clotting factors, 560–562
  assay, 561
  inhibitors development, 564
  prophylaxis, 563–564
  therapeutic strategies, 562
  treatment on demand, 562–563
Recombinant Factor VIIa, 561–562, 565, 571
Recombinant Factor VIII, 560–561, 650
  Kogenate, 560–561
  Recombinate, 560, 561
  Refacto, 561
Recombinant Factor IX, 561, 650
Recombinate, 560, 561
  inhibitors development, 564
  treatment on demand, 563
Red cell count, 4, 5
Red cell damage, hemolytic anemia, 138, 195–196
  cardiac surgery/valvular lesions, 197
  drug-induced oxidative injury, 195
  external impact trauma, 197
  osmotic damage, 197
  thermal damage, 197
Red cell enzyme disorders, 150–157
  biochemical investigations, 155–156

blood cell morphology, 151–155
  clinical features, 151, 152
  molecular basis, 156–157
Red cell mass (RCM), 284
  erythrocytosis, 284
    absolute, 284, 292
  polycythemia vera, 285, 286
Red cell membrane, 6
  adhesion molecules, 623–624
  complement regulatory glycoproteins, 624–625
  hereditary defects, 142–146
    leakiness (stomatocytosis), 145–146
  immunoglobulin superfamily glycoproteins, 623–624
  membrane skeleton glycoprotein anchors, 625
  structural aspects, 142
  surface antigens, 616, 622–626
    infectious disease associations, 625–626
    null phenotypes, 616
    polymorphisms, 616
  surface receptors, 623–624
  transporters, 622–623
Red cell parameters, 4–5, 6
  children, 5
Red cell preparations, 647–648
  concentrate preparation procedure, 644
  effects of transfusion, 648
  frozen deglycerolized, 648
  leukoreduced, 648
  neocytes, 652
  washed, 648
Red cell transfusion therapy, 647–648
  indications, 647
  urgent situations, 653
Red cells (erythrocytes), 4–7, 59
  biconcave shape, 6, 7
  carbon dioxide transport, 7
  cytoskeletal network, 6
  energy metabolism, 6, 150–151
  life span, 5, 26
  maturation changes, 8
  membrane *see* Red cell membrane
  morphological abnormalities, 132–135
    causes, 136
  morphology, 4
  oxygen transport, 6–7
  stem cells, 25
Reduced glutathione (GSH), 155, 156
Reed–Sternberg cells, 426, 427
Refacto, 561
  treatment on demand, 563
Refractory anemia, 332, 333, 336, 337, 340
  see also Myelodysplastic syndromes
Refractory anemia with excess of blasts (RAEB), 334, 340
Refractory anemia with excess of blasts in transformation (RAEBt), 333, 334, 340, 360
Refractory anemia with ringed sideroblasts (RARS), 269, 270, 271, 333, 334, 335, 337, 340

Refractory cytopenias with multilineage dysplasia, 333
Refractory normoblastic anemia, 97
Relative polycythemia *see* Apparent erythrocytosis
Renal carcinoma, bone marrow metastasis, 112
Renal disease, 96
  anemia, 585
  chronic localised disseminated intravascular coagulation (DIC), 591
  coagulopathy, 547–548, 584, 585–587
    laboratory investigations, 586
    treatment, 586–587
  dialysis, 586
  erythropoietin therapy, 659
    functional iron deficiency, 213, 217
  hemolytic anemia, 198
  multiple myeloma, 447
  pure red cell aplasia, 267
  secondary erythrocytosis, 292
  sickle cell disease, 175
  thrombocytopenia, 585
Renal erythropoietin production, 30, 31
Renal transplantation, 100
Reopro, 582
Reptilase time, 485
Respiratory burst, 322
  inherited defects, 326–327
  neutrophil phagocytosis, 11
Respiratory burst oxidase, 12
Reticular cells *see* Macrophages
Reticular dysgenesis (congenital aleukia), 309
Reticulin, 113
  grading, 114
Reticulin fibrosis, 113
  AIDS/HIV infection, 105, 109
Reticulo-endothelial system (RES) *see* Mononuclear phagocyte system
Reticulocyte count, 8–9, 135
Reticulocytes, 7–9, 59
  basophilic stipling, 134
  cytology, 27
  maturation, 26
  pregnant women, 20
Reticulocytosis
  hemolytic anemia, 138
  unstable hemoglobins, 179, 180
Retinoblastoma, 112, 113
RGD sequences, 528
Rh-associated glycoprotein (RhAG), 620
Rh$_{mod}$, 620
Rh$_{null}$, 620
Rhabdomyosarcoma, bone marrow metastasis, 112, 113
RHAG, 620
RHCE, 619, 620
RHD, 619, 620
Rhesus antigens, 619, 622
  blood typing
    autologous blood, 643
    donated blood, 646, 647
    urgent blood trnasfusion, 653
  warm autoimmune hemolytic anemia, 188, 189

Rhesus blood-group system, 619–620
  hemolytic disease of newborn,
    193–194, 620
    prevention, 193, 620
  prenatal management of
    incompatibility, 193
  Rh-deficiency syndrome, 620
  Rh$_{mod}$, 620
  Rh$_{null}$, 620
Rhesus C/c polymorphism, 619, 620
Rhesus D, 619–620
Rhesus E/e polymorphism, 619, 620
Rhesus immune globulin, 193
Rhesus-deficiency syndrome, 620
Rheumatoid arthritis, 118, 218, 242, 267,
    307, 389, 464
  acquired inhibitors of coagulation, 593
  bone marrow amyloid deposits, 121
  bone marrow lymphoid aggregates,
    97
Rheumatoid factor, 391
Rho, 326
Riboflavin deficiency, 93
Richter's syndrome, 383, 461
  bone marrow pathology, 385
Rifampicin, 547
Ringed sideroblasts, 267, 271, 333, 337,
    361, 365
Ristocetin, 566
Ristocetin-induced platelet
    agglutination (RIPA), 566
Rubella, 104, 537
Russell bodies, 41, 43, 97, 412, 448
Russell's Viper venom clotting time, 488

S

Salazopyrine, 242
SAR, 630
Sarcoidosis, 110, 111
Schilling test, 236
Schistocytes, 132
Schistocytic hemolytic anemia, 196
Schwachmann's syndrome, 309
SCL gene disruption, 358
Scleroderma, 96, 307
Sea-blue histiocyte syndrome, 118
Sea-blue histiocytes, 62, 118
Selectins, 63, 325
Sequence-specific priming, 692–693
Sequence-specific oligonucleotide probe
    hybridization (SSOPH), 693
Serine proteinases, 46
Serum amyloid A, 461
Serum amyloid P, 461
Severe combine immunodeficiency
    (SCID) mice, 73
Severe congenital neutropenia, see
    infantile genetic agranulocytosis
Sézary cells, 391
Sézary syndrome, 391–392
  chromosomal abnormalities, 392
  immunophenotype, 392
Shiga toxin, 536
Shigella dysenteriae, 196
Sialomucin receptors, 77

CD34, 77
CD43, 77, 78
CD164, 77–78
signal pathways, 78
Sialyl-Lewis X, 325
Sickle cell disease, 174–178
  α thalassemia co-inheritance, 176, 177
  bone marrow appearances
    hemosiderin, 101
    macrophage erythrophagocytosis,
      100
    sea-blue histiocytes, 118
  bone marrow necrosis, 119
  clinical features, 174–175
    hemoglobin F level relationship,
      177
  compound heterozygous states, 174
    hemoglobin electrophoresis, 176
  genetic basis, 176–177
  geographic distribution, 174
  hand–foot syndrome, 175
  historical aspects, 174
  infection susceptibility, 175, 176
  management, 177–178
    anti-sickling therapy, 178
    bone marrow transplantation, 178
    hemoglobin F induction, 178
    pregnancy, 177, 178
  molecular pathophysiology, 176–177
  neonatal screening programs, 177
  parvovirus B19 infection, 104
  prenatal diagnosis, 176, 178
  sickle cell anemia, 174–175, 481
    diagnostic features, 176
  sickle cell trait (carrier status), 174, 176
  sickling crises, 175
    hospital care, 177
  skull X-ray ('hair on end' appearance),
    139
Sideroblastic anemia with
    spinocerebellar ataxia (Xq13-
    linked), 208
Sideroblastic anemias, 91, 102, 267–271,
    333
  bone marrow appearances, 101,
    267–268, 270–271
  classification, 269
  drug/chemical-induced, 269
  hereditary, 92, 268–269
    X-linked, 268–269
    autosomal recessive, 269
    iron overload, 224
    mitochondrial DNA mutations, 269
    thiamine-responsive, 269
  idiopathic (primary acquired) see
    Refractory anemia with ringed
    sideroblasts
Sideroblasts, 27, 62, 102, 208
  abnormal, 102
Siderocytes, 134
Siderosomes (ferritin bodies), 102
Siderotic granules, 102, 267, 268
Sjögren's syndrome, 307
Skin bleeding time see Bleeding time
Skin disease
  adult T-cell leukemia/lymphoma, 393
  chronic lymphocytic leukemia, 385

chronic myelomonocytic leukemia,
    399
eosinophil/eosinophil precursor
    number increase, 95
hemostatic disorders, 479
juvenile chronic myelomonocytic
    leukemia, 399
Sézary syndrome/mycosis fungoides,
    391, 392
systemic mastocytosis, 403
T-cell granular lymphocytic leukemia,
    390
T-lineage prolymphocytic leukemia,
    388
SLC4A1 (EPB3) mutations, 143
  Southeast Asian ovalocytosis, 145
SLC19A2 mutations, 269
Sleep apnea syndrome, 293
Small intestinal bacterial flora
    abnormalities, 234, 238
Smallpox, 314
Snake venom
  coagulopathies, 584, 594
    disseminated intravascular
      coagulation (DIC), 590
  hemolytic anemia, 198
Snake venom clotting time, 488
Sodium valproate, 267, 304, 582
Solid organ transplantation, HLA allele
    matching, 700
Solitary bone plasmacytoma, 456–458
Source plasma, 644
Southeast Asian ovalocytosis, 145, 625
SP1, 673
Spectrin, 6, 142, 143
  α-chain mutations, 143, 144
  β-chain mutations, 143, 145
Spectrin α^{LELY}, 144, 145
Spectrin α^{LEPRA}, 143
Spherocytes, 132, 134, 142, 144
Spherocytosis
  drug-induced oxidative hemolysis, 195
  hemolytic anemia, 138
  hereditary, 104, 142–143
    enolase 1 deficiency, 154
    molecular genetics, 143
Spheroechinocytes, 154
Sphingolipidoses, 117–118
Spider venom-induced hemolytic
    anemia, 198
Spleen, 39
  chronic granulocytic leukemia, 396
  chronic lymphocytic leukemia, 385
  chronic myelomonocytic leukemia,
    398–399
  hairy cell leukemia/hairy cell
    leukemia variant, 413
  juvenile chronic myelomonocytic
    leukemia, 399
  lymphoma, 407
  platelet pooling, 531
  prolymphocytic leukemia, 386
  systemic mastocytosis, 403
  T-cell granular lymphocytic leukemia,
    390
  T-lineage prolymphocytic leukemia,
    388

Splenectomy
  β thalassemia, 173
  congenital dyserythropoietic anemias, 276, 277, 279
  Haemophilus influenzae type B vaccination, 173
  pneumococcal vaccination, 173
  prophylactic penicillin, 173
  warm autoimmune hemolytic anemia, 190
Splenic lymphoma with villous lymphocytes, 387–388, 458
  chromosomal abnormalities, 388
  immunophenoytpe, 388
Splenic marginal zone lymphoma, 458
Splenic sequestration crisis, sickle cell disease, 175, 177
Splenomegaly
  hemolytic anemia, 139–140
  polycythemia vera, 285, 287, 288
  sickle cell disease, 175
SPTA1 mutations
  hereditary elliptocytosis/poikilocytosis, 144–145
  hereditary spherocytosis, 143
SPTB mutations
  hereditary elliptocytosis/poikilocytosis, 145
  hereditary spherocytosis, 143
Spurious polycythemia *see* Apparent erythrocytosis
Steel factor receptor *see* c-kit
Stem cell factor (SCF), 46, 75
  acquired aplastic anemia, 252, 253
Stem cell factor receptor *see* c-kit
Stem cell transplantation
  acquired aplastic anemia, 257
  blood transfusion strategies, 652–653
  chronic granulomatous disease, 327
  Fanconi anemia treatment, 260
  HLA allele matching, 667, 700–701
    donor search strategies, 701–702
    level of match, 702–703
    umbilical cord blood banks, 701
    unrelated donor registries, 701
  HLA mismatch consequences, 681–682
    allorecognition, 684
  lymphoma, 407
  multiple myeloma, 450, 452–453
  stem cell collection/preparation from peripheral blood, 646
  unrelated volunteer transplants, 257, 260
Stem cells, 25, 54, 59, 72–73, 79
  acquired aplastic anemia, 253
  bone marrow microenvironment ('niches'), 73, 74, 80
  endothelial cell interactions, 75
  extracellular matrix component interactions, 76–77
  functional characteristics, 72–73
  HIV infection, 108
  lymphopotent, 39
  phenotypic characterization, 72
  see also Mesenchymal stem cells

Stoddard's solvent, 251
Stomatocytes, 134, 144
Stomatocytosis, hereditary, 145–146
  dehydrated, 146
  overhydrated, 146
Storage pool deficiency, 499–500
  acquired with leukemia/myelodysplastic syndromes, 548
  diagnosis, 482
  myeloproliferative disorders, 593
Streptomycin, 195
Stress polycythemia *see* Apparent erythrocytosis
Stroma-derived factor-1 (SDF-1), 76
Structural hemoglobin variants, 173–181
  clinical disorders, 173
Sub-Saharah iron overload, 220
Subacute combined degeneration of spinal cord, 233, 234
  histopathology, 236–237
  pernicious anemia, 236
Sulfhemoglobin, 195
Sulfhemoglobinemia, 181
Sulfonamides, 195, 547
  drug-induced thrombocytopenia, 544
Sulfonylureas, 195
Sulindac, 251
Suppressor/cytotoxic T-cells (T_C cells), 17
Surface immunoglobulins
  chronic lymphocytic leukemia, 385
  prolymphocytic leukemia, 387
  splenic lymphoma with villous lymphocytes, 388
Syndecan-1 (CD138), 64, 444, 446, 449, 450, 454, 456
Syphilis, transmission by blood transfusion, 658
Systemic lupus erythematosus, 267, 306, 307, 310, 464
  acquired inhibitors of coagulation, 593
  bone marrow gelatinous transformation, 120
  complement receptor-1 (CR1; CD35) acquired deficiency, 625
  secondary immune thrombocytopenia, 544
Systemic mastocytosis, 401–403
  bone marrow, 96, 111, 401–402
  clinical features, 401
  genetic abnormalities, 403
  liver/skin involvement, 403
  peripheral blood, 401
  splenic involvement, 403

T

t(1;14)(p32;q11), 358
t(1;19), 353, 355, 356, 357, 358
t(1;19)(q23;p13), 353
t(1;22)(p13;q13), 369
t(2;8)(p12;q24), 353, 421
t(3;14)(q27;q32), 419
t(3;21), 375
t(4;11), 355, 356, 358

t(5;12), 346
t(5;12)(q31;p12), 399
t(5;12)(q33;p13), 398, 401
t(5;14)(q31.1;q32.3), 353
t(5;17)(q23;q12), 362
t(6;8)(q27;p11), 401
t(6;9)(p23;q34), 370, 374
t(6;14), 445
t(8;13)(p11;q12), 401
t(8;14)(q24;q32), 353, 421
t(8;16)(p11;p13), 368, 374
t(8;21), 333
  acute myeloid leukemia, 361–362, 372, 374, 375
t(8;22)(q24;q11), 353, 421
t(9;14)(p13;q32), 412, 458
t(9;22), 353, 357, 374, 376
  acute lymphoblastic leukemia, 353, 356, 357, 358
  chronic granulocytic leukemia, 393, 396
t(10;14), 356
t(11;14)(q13;q32), 387, 388, 418
t(11;17)(q3;q21), 362, 363
t(11;18)(q21;q21), 415
t(11;19), 355
t(11;22)(q11;q13), 418
t(12;21), 355, 356, 357, 358, 375
t(12;21)(p12;q22), 353
t(14;14)(q11;q32), 389
t(14;18)(q32;q21), 419
t(15;17), 333, 360, 373, 375
  acute myeloid leukemia, 362–363, 374
t(16;16)(p13;q22), 360, 364, 374, 375
t(16;21), 375
t(v;11)(v;q23), 353, 364
T-cell chronic lymphocytic leukemia, 267
T-cell granular lymphocytic leukemia, 389–391
  bone marrow, 390
  chromosomal abnormalities, 391
  clinical features, 389
  immunophenotype, 391
  peripheral blood, 389–390
  splenic involvement, 390
T-cell lymphomas, 422–425
T-cell receptor (TCR), 17
  αβ (TcR-2), 17
  γδ (TcR-1), 17
  HLA molecule/bound peptide recognition, 668, 680–682
  allorecognition, 682, 683, 684
  structure, 681
T-cells, 17
  αβ, 17
  bone marrow, 63
  class II molecules expression, 674
  cytokines influencing maturation, 39–40
  double negative (DN), 681
  γδ, 17
  motile activity, 63
  phenotypic characterization, 72
  surface markers, 63
    progenitor cell lineage-specific, 39
  thymic differentiation/education, 39, 40, 681

see also CD4 T-cells; CD8 T-cells; Cytotoxic T-cells (T_C cells); Helper T-cells (T_H cells)

T-lineage acute lymphoblastic leukemia, 353
  chromosomal abnormalities, 356
    molecular genetics, 357–358
  classification, 353
  clinical features, 352–353
  precursor T-cell acute lymphoblastic leukemia, 356

T-lineage prolymphocytic leukemia (T-PLL), 388–389
  bone marrow, 388, 389
  chromosomal abnormalities, 389
  clinical features, 388
  immunophenotype, 389
  peripheral blood, 388, 389
  tisse infiltration, 388

Taipan venom clotting time, 488
TAL-1 abnormalities, 357
Tangier disease (familial high-density lipoprotein deficiency), 119
TAP (transporter associated with antigen processing), 679
TAP1, 667, 679
TAP2, 667, 679
Tapasin, 679
Target cells, 132, 133, 163, 176, 215, 269
Tay-Sachs disease, 118
TCL1 rearrangements, 389
TEL/AML1 fusion gene, 357
TEL/PDGFRβ fusion gene, 399
Tenase complex, 475
Terminal deoxynucleotidyl transferase (TdT), 355, 356, 372, 375, 429
Thalassemia, 102, 118, 161, 162–173
  α, 162, 169–173
    acquired, 172
    antenatal screening, 172
    associated mental retardation (ATR) syndromes, 171–172
    carrier state, 169
    clinical features, 169
    diagnosis, 169
    genetic aspects, 170–171
    hemoglobin S co-inheritance, 176, 177
    pathophysiology, 171
    prevention programs, 172
  β, 162
    βS+s, 163
    bone changes, 162
    clinical features, 162–163, 166
    diagnosis, 163
    genetic aspects, 163–166
    globin-chain imbalance, 163, 166
    hemoglobin E/β thalassemia, 166–167, 179
    hemoglobin electrophoresis, 163
    hemoglobin S/β thalassemia, 179
    heterozygous state, 163, 169
    homozygous βS0s, 163
    ineffective erythropoiesis, 166
    intermediate forms (thalassemia intermedia), 104, 168–169, 172, 173, 224

iron overload, 223, 224
major, 117, 162–163
management, 172–173
minor, 163
pathophysiology, 166
classification, 162
δ, 162
δβ, 162, 167–168
εγδβ, 162
γ, 162
γδβ, 162, 167–168
geographic distribution, 162, 169
Thalassemia syndromes, 162
  bone marrow hemosiderin, 101
  dyserythropoiesis, 92
Thalassemic hemoglobinopathies, 162, 179, 181
Thalidomide, 348, 453–454
Thermal red cell damage, 197
Thiamine-responsive anemia, 92, 244, 269
Thiazides, 195, 531
Thioguanine, 243
Third world national blood programs, 639
Thrombin
  antithrombin inhibition, 601
  coagulation pathway, 475, 600
  thrombomodulin binding, 476, 601
    protein C activation, 601, 602
Thrombin time (TT), 480, 485, 486
Thrombin-activated fibrinolysis inhibitor (TAFI), 606
Thrombocytopenia, 481, 530–547
  AIDS/HIV patients, 109
  alloantibody-mediated, 539–540
  autoantibody-mediated, 540–544
  bone marrow failure syndromes, 532–533
  cardiopulmonary bypass, 588
  drug-induced, 544–547
  hematinics deficiencies, 538
  increased platelet destruction, 96, 533–547
    immune causes, 538–547
    non-immune causes, 533–538
  infection-related, 537–538
  liver disease, 531, 537
  massive blood transfusion, 537
  mechanisms, 530
  myelodysplastic syndromes, 336
  platelet production failure, 531–533
  renal disease, 585
Thrombocytopenia and absent radii (TAR) syndrome, 97, 496, 500
Thromboembolic bone marrow lesions, 122
Thrombolytic agents, 581, 592
  laboratory monitoring, 581
Thrombomodulin, 601
  disseminated intravascular coagulation (DIC), 590
  structure, 601
  thrombin binding, 476, 601
Thrombophilia, 603–609
  acquired, 606–608
  activation peptide assays, 608–609

management aspects, 609
multifactorial interactions, 608
Thromboplastin generation test, 20
Thrombopoiesis *see* Megakaryocytopoiesis
Thrombopoietin, 75, 528
  acquired aplastic anemia, 252, 253
  idiopathic thrombocytopenic purpura (ITP), 541
  therapeutic applications, 659
Thrombosis
  acquired predisposing causes, 607
  antiphospholipid syndrome, 607
  antithrombin deficiency, 604
  dysfibrinogenemia, 605
  factor V Leiden, 604–605
  GPIIb/IIIa polymorphism influence, 629
  heparin-induced thrombocytopenia, 546
  human platelet antigen (HPA) polymorphisms, 629
  lupus anticoagulant, 607
  platelet function, 494
  procoagulant factor elevation, 605
  protein C deficiency, 604
  protein S deficiency, 604
  reduced fibrinolysis, 606
  thrombophilic trait-related risk, 606
Thrombospondin, 19, 76
  platelet α granules, 501, 529
Thrombotic thrombocytopenic purpura, 96, 122, 196–197, 534–536
  classification, 534
  clinical features, 534–535
  diagnosis, 535
  laboratory investigations, 535
  management, 196–197, 535–536, 648
  pathogenesis, 535
    triggering factors, 196
    von Willebrand factor (vWF), 535
  see also Hemolytic uremic syndrome
Thromboxane AU2u, 18, 19
  antiplatelet drug mode of action, 582
ThyU1uSlows, 72
Thymic T-cell differentiation/education, 39, 40, 681
Thymic tumors, 267
Thymosin, 15
Thyroid carcinoma, bone marrow metastasis, 112
Thyroxine, 30, 31
Ticlopidine, 196, 197, 581
Tissue factor, 20, 600
  coagulation pathway, 475
  Factor VIIa complex, 475
Tissue factor pathway inhibitor (TFPI), 475, 600
Tissue plasminogen activator (tPA), 476, 606
  cardiopulmonary bypass response, 588
Toluidine blue stain, 67
Topoisomerase II-related acute myeloid leukemia, 365, 366
Toxic coagulopathies, 594
Toxic neutrophil granulation, 302, 303
  pregnant women, 21

Toxin-induced hemolytic anemia, 198
Toxocariasis, 314
Toxoplasma gondii, 108, 111
Toxoplasmosis, 107, 315
TRANCE (TNF-related activation-induced cytokine), 446
Tranexamic acid, 568, 570
Transcobalamin I, 9, 233
Transcobalamin II, 233
  congenital abnormality, 240
  deficiency, 94
    congenital, 234, 240
Transferrin, 205, 206, 208, 209
  anemia of chronic disorders, 218
  cellular iron uptake, 206, 207
  genetic polymorphism, 214–215
  pregnant women, 20
Transferrin receptor 1 (TfR1)
  duodenal mucosal cells, 209
  HRE protein binding, 208
Transferrin receptor 2 (TfR2), 209
Transferrin receptor 2 (TfR2) gene mutations, 209
  hereditary hemochromatosis type 3, 223
Transferrin receptors, 206, 218
  cellular iron uptake, 206, 207
  duodenal mucosal cells, 209
  iron deficiency-related upregulation, 215
  regulation of synthesis, 207, 208
  serum levels, iron status assessment, 211, 219, 220
Transforming growth factor β (TGF-β), 76, 115, 443
Transfusion reactions *see* Blood transfusion reactions
Transient erythroblastopenia of childhood, 267
Triamterene, 242
Trimethoprim, 242, 544, 545
Triose phosphate isomerase deficiency, 150, 151
  molecular basis, 157
  prenatal diagnosis, 156
Tropheryma whippelii, 103
Tropical eosinophilia, 312
Tropical sprue, 238, 242
Trypanosoma cruzi, 658
Trypanosomiasis, 107, 315
Tryptase, 46
Tuberculosis, 100, 242
  bone marrow granulomas, 110
  lymphocytosis/monocytosis, 314
Tubulin, 18
Tumor emboli, bone marrow, 122
Tumor necrosis factor (TNF), 15, 46, 76, 592, 673
  anemia of chronic disorders, 218, 219
Typhoid fever, 111

U

Ulcerative colitis, 314
Umbilical cord blood banks, 701

Unfractionated heparin, 579
Unstable hemoglobin variants, 179–180
  basophilic stippling, 152
  Heinz bodies, 154
Uremia
  hemostatic disorders, 547–548, 584, 585–587
  thrombocytopenia, 585
Uridine diphosphate glucuronosyltransferase (UGT1A1) gene promoter, 157
Urinary hemosiderin granules, 138
Urogenital bleeding, hemostatic disorders, 477
Urokinase, 476

V

Varicella, 191, 314, 604
  thrombocytopenia, 537
Varicella-zoster, 111
Vascular adhesion molecule-1 (VCAM), 76, 77, 80, 443, 444
Vascular endothelial growth factor (VEGF), 443
Vascular malformations, 591, 592
Vaso-occlusive crises, sickle cell disease, 175, 176, 177
Vegan diet, 234
Vegetarian diets, 205, 214
Venepuncture
  blood donation, 642
    site, 641–642
  precautions with bleeding disorders, 480
Venesection *see* Phlebotomy
Venom-induced hemolytic anemia, 198
V_H gene mutations, 383
Vimentin, 57
Vinca alkaloids, 190, 544
Vincristine, 197, 451, 452
Viral infections
  bone marrow changes, 100, 103
  eosinophil ribonucleases, 13
  HIV-related opportunistic infection, 107
  lymphocytosis, 314
Vitamin B_{12}, 232–234
  binding protein (R-binder), 232
  biochemical pathways, 233
  dietary sources, 232
  hepatic metabolism/storage, 233
  ileal absorption, 232–233
  intrinsic factor complex, 232
  pregnant women, 21
  structure, 232
Vitamin B_{12} deficiency, 231, 234
  AIDS/HIV patients, 109
  causes, 234–241
    chronic pancreatitis, 239
    dietary cobalamin malabsorption, 239
    dietary inadequacy, 234
    drug interactions, 239
    gastric lesions, 234–238
    HIV infection, 239

    intestinal lesions, 238–239
    Zollinger–Ellison syndrome, 239
  clinical features, 233
    biochemical mechanisms, 233–234
    neurologic abnormalities, 233, 234
  cobalamin metabolism
    acquired abnormalities, 239–240
    inherited disorders, 240–241
  dyserythropoiesis, 92
  hemopoietic cell abnormalities, 94, 304
  neutrophil right shift, 302
  thrombocytopenia, 538
Vitamin K deficiency, 583
  adults, 583
  neonates/infants, 582–583
Vitamin K_1, 582
Vitamin K_2, 582
Vitamin K_3, 582
Vitamin K-dependent clotting factors, 582
Vitronectin, 19
Vitronectin receptor, 528
VLA-2 (GPIa/IIa; CD49/CD20), 528, 538, 627–628
VLA-4 (CD49d), 443, 444
VLA-5, 444
von Willebrand factor (vWF), 19, 450, 474
  multimers, 535
  platelet α granules, 496, 501, 529
  platelet integrin interactions, 530
  structure, 568–569
  thrombotic thrombocytopenic purpura pathogenesis, 535
  uremia-related abnormality, 547
von Willebrand factor (vWF) concentrates, 568
von Willebrand factor (vWF) gene, 568, 569
  mutations, 569
von Willebrand's disease, 565–570
  acquired, 567
    myeloproliferative disorders, 593
  clinical features, 479
  diagnosis, 482, 487, 490
    immunoassays, 489
  molecular basis, 568–569
  platelet type (pseudo von Willebrand's disease), 567
  screening tests, 565–566
  skin bleeding time (SBT), 482
  treatment, 567–568
  type 1, 565, 566–567, 569
  type 2, 565, 567, 569
  type 3, 565, 567, 569
  women patients, 569–570
    pregnancy, 570

W

Waldenström's macroglobulinemia, 96, 97, 191, 458
  amyloid deposition, 462
  clinical features, 458
  coagulation disorders, 593

cryoglobulinemia, 465
disease progression, 460–461
μ-heavy-chain disease association, 464
pathology, 458–459
platelet dyfunction, 549
reticulin fibrosis, 113
treatment, 460
Waldeyer's ring, 39
Waldman's disease (intestinal
lymphangiectasia), 120
Warfarin
anticoagulant activity, 580
laboratory monitoring, 581
drug interactions, 580–581
reversal, 648
Warm autoimmune hemolytic anemia,
187–190
diagnostic evaluation, 189
hemolysis mechanisms
complement-mediated hemolysis,
188
Fc receptor-mediated immune
adherence, 187–188
immune specificity, 188–189
management, 189–190
WAS, 326
Washed red cell preparations, 648

WASp, 326
X-linked congenital
neutropenia/monocytopenia,
324
actin cytosekelton organisation, 326
WHIM syndrome, 325
Whipple's disease, 103
White blood cell counts, 10, 11
pregnant women, 21
Whole blood platelet analysis, 481–482
Whole blood transfusion, 647
Whooping cough, 314
Wilson's disease, 198
Wiskott–Aldrich syndrome, 326, 500
Epstein–Barr virus-related
lymphoproliferative disorders,
317
platelet disorders, 508–509
Wnt glycoproteins, 79, 80
Wnt-1, 79
Wnt-2b, 79
Wnt-5a, 79
Wnt-10b, 79
Wolman's disease, 118, 119
World Marrow Donor Association
(WMDA), 701
Wr^b antigen, 189

X

X-linked agammaglobulinemia, 327
X-linked congenital
neutropenia/monocytopenia, 324
X-linked hyper IgM syndrome, 327
X-linked lymphoproliferative disease
(Duncan's syndrome), 317
X-linked sideroblastic anemia, 208,
268–269
with ataxia, 269
X-linked thrombocytopenia, 326
Xenogeneic transplant models, 73
Xg, 624

Y

Yolk sac blood islands, 24
Yolk sac hemopoiesis, 24, 72, 73, 75

Z

Zidovudine, 109, 538
Zollinger–Ellison syndrome, 239